KEY TO ESSENTIAL TERMINOLOGY

PATIENT ASSESSMENT DATA BASE

Provides an overview of the more commonly occurring etiology and coexisting factors associated with a specific medical/surgical diagnosis as well as the signs/symptoms and corresponding abnormal diagnostic findings.

NURSING PRIORITIES

Establishes a general ranking of needs/concerns upon which the Nursing Diagnoses are ordered. In actual care plan construction, this ranking would be altered according to the individual patient situation.

DISCHARGE CRITERIA

Identifies generalized statements which could be developed into short-term and intermediate goals to be achieved by the patient before being "discharged" from nursing care. They may also provide guidance for creating long-term goals for the patient to work on after discharge.

NURSING DIAGNOSES

The general problem/concern (Diagnosis) is stated without the distinct cause and signs/symptoms, which would be added to create a *patient problem statement* when specific patient information is available. For example: when a patient displays increased tension, apprehension, quivering voice, and focus on self, the nursing diagnosis of Anxiety could be stated "Anxiety, Severe, related to unconscious conflict, threat to self-concept as evidenced by statements of increased tension, apprehension, observations of quivering voice, focus on self."

In addition, diagnoses identified within these care plan guides as actual or potential can be changed or deleted and new diagnoses added, depending entirely on the specific patient information.

MAY BE RELATED TO/POSSIBLY EVIDENCED BY

These lists provide the usual/common reasons (etiology) a particular problem may occur with probable signs/symptoms, which would be used to create the "related to" and "evidenced by" portions of the *patient problem statement* when the specific patient situation is known.

When a potential diagnosis has been identified, signs/symptoms have not yet developed and therefore are not included in the nursing diagnosis statement. However, interventions are provided to prevent progression to an *actual* problem. The exception to this occurs in the nursing diagnosis *Violence, potential for*, which has possible indicators that suggest the patient may be at risk.

PATIENT OUTCOMES/EVALUATION CRITERIA

These give direction to patient care as they identify what the patient/nurse hope to achieve. They are stated in general terms in this book to permit the practitioner to modify/individualize them by adding time lines and individual patient criteria so they become "measurable," e.g., "Patient appears relaxed and reports anxiety is reduced to a manageable level within 24 hours."

ACTIONS/INTERVENTIONS

Interventions are divided into independent and collaborative and are ranked in this book from most to least common. When creating the individual care plan, interventions would normally be ranked to reflect the patient's specific needs/situation. In addition, the division of independent/collaborative is arbitrary and is actually dependent on the individual nurse's capabilities and hospital/community standards.

RATIONALE

Although not commonly appearing in patient care plans, rationale has been included here to provide a pathophysiological basis to assist the nurse in deciding about the relevance of a specific intervention for an individual patient situation.

BOOKS OF RELATED INTEREST

Be accurate, quick, and confident with these practical care planning guides.

NURSE'S POCKET GUIDE: NURSING DIAGNOSIS WITH INTERVENTIONS, 2nd ed.
Marilynn E. Doenges, BSN, MA, RN, CS
Mary Frances Moorhouse, RN, CCP, CCRN

Details nursing diagnoses approved by NANDA. Includes etiology, defining characteristics, prioritized interventions, and desired patient outcomes. Includes latest (1988) NANDA diagnoses. 413 pp, 1988.

PSYCHIATRIC CARE PLANS: GUIDELINES FOR CLIENT CARE
Marilynn E. Doenges, BSN, MA, RN, CS
Mary C. Townsend, RN, MN
Mary Frances Moorhouse, RN, CCP, CCRN

Includes 31 comprehensive care plans and identifies nursing diagnoses (organized according to psychiatric disorders) with appropriate interventions while caring for psychiatric clients in both institutional and community settings. Major divisions conform to DSM-III-R categories. 426 pp, 1989.

NURSING DIAGNOSES IN PSYCHIATRIC NURSING: A POCKET GUIDE FOR CARE PLAN CONSTRUCTION
Mary C. Townsend, RN, MN

A quick reference to help prepare psychiatric nursing care plans. Concise and practical, it identifies nursing diagnoses common to specific psychiatric diagnoses. Conforms to DSM-III-R categories. 270 pp, 1989.

MATERNAL/NEWBORN CARE PLANS: GUIDELINES FOR CLIENT CARE
Marilynn E. Doenges, BSN, MA, RN, CS
Janet R. Kenty, BSN, MSN
Mary Frances Moorhouse, RN, CCP, CCRN

Contains 49 comprehensive care plans organized according to prenatal, intraparatal, postpartal, and newborn concepts. 549 pp, 1988.

CRITICAL CARE PLANS: GUIDELINES FOR PATIENT CARE
Mary Frances Moorhouse, RN, CCP, CCRN
Alice C. Geissler, RN, CCRN
Marilynn E. Doenges, BSN, MA, RN, CS

Offers 36 complete care plans for patients in advanced med-surg and ICU/CCU settings. 470 pp, 1987.

OTHER BOOKS OF RELATED INTEREST

NURSE'S MED DECK
Judith Hopfer Deglin, Pharm.D.
April Hazard Vallerand, RN, MSN

Includes vital facts on 400 most commonly prescribed drugs. The nursing implications and pharmacologic data are more comprehensive than *any* other card deck available. Gives you precise drug facts for preparation, administration, and aftercare. 375 cards, 1988.

DAVIS'S DRUG GUIDE FOR NURSES
Judith Hopfer Deglin, Pharm.D.
April Hazard Vallerand, RN, MSN

A practical handbook which offers comprehensive coverage on the most commonly prescribed drugs. This pocket-sized volume fully integrates the nursing process with each of the drugs described. 739 pp, 1988.

POCKET GUIDE TO THE OPERATING ROOM
Maxine A. Goldman, BS, RN

This handy pocket guide offers easily accessible and accurate information on the technical aspects of patient care in the operating room for more than 250 surgical procedures. 559 pp, 1988.

AVAILABLE FROM YOUR LOCAL BOOK SELLER

F.A. Davis Company
1915 Arch Street
Philadelphia, PA 19103

(800) 523-4049   (215) 568-2270

NURSING CARE PLANS
Guidelines for Planning Patient Care
Edition 2

Marilynn E. Doenges, BSN, MA, RN, CS
Clinical Specialist
Adult Psychiatric/Mental Health Nursing
Private Practice
Colorado Springs, Colorado

Mary Frances Moorhouse, RN, CCP, CCRN
Consultant and Contract Practitioner
Critical Care
Colorado Springs, Colorado

Alice C. Geissler, RN, CCRN
Contract Practitioner
Critical Care
Colorado Springs, Colorado

Mary F. Jeffries, BSN, MS, RN, LtC ANC (Deceased)

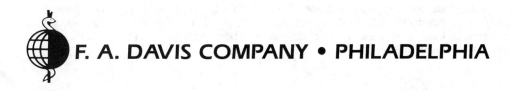

F. A. DAVIS COMPANY • PHILADELPHIA

Printed in the United States of America

Last digit indicates print number: 10 9 8 7 6 5 4 3 2 1

NOTE: As new scientific information becomes available through basic and clinical research, recommended treatments and drug therapies undergo changes. The author(s) and publisher have done everything possible to make this book accurate, up-to-date, and in accord with accepted standards at the time of publication. However, the reader is advised always to check product information (package inserts) for changes and new information regarding dose and contraindications before administering any drug. Caution is especially urged when using new or infrequently ordered drugs.

Library of Congress Cataloging-in-Publication Data

Nursing care plans.

   Rev. ed. of: Nursing care plans / Marilynn E. Doenges, Mary F. Jeffries, Mary Frances Moorhouse, c1984.
   Includes bibliographies.
   1. Diagnosis. 2. Nursing care plans.
I. Doenges, Marilynn E., 1922–   . II. Doenges, Marilynn E., 1922–   . Nursing care plans.
[DNLM: 1. Nursing Process—handbooks. 2. Patient Care Planning—handbooks. WY 39 N9745]
RT48.N877 1989   610.73   88-20282
ISBN 0–8036–2661–4

To our spouses, children, parents, and friends, who much of the time have had to manage without us as well as cope with us.

The Doenges families: Dean, Jim, and Barbara; David, Monita, Matthew, and Tyler; John, Theresa, and Nicole; and the Daigle family, Nancy, Jim, Jennifer, and Jonathan.

The Moorhouse family: Jan, Paul, and Jason.

The Geissler family: Bill and children.

To our FAD family, especially Bob Martone, Ruth De George, and Herb Powell, whose support has been so vital to the completion of a project of this magnitude.

To the nurses we are writing for, who daily face the challenge of caring for the acutely ill patient and are looking for a practical way to organize and document this care. We believe that Nursing Diagnosis and these guides will help.

Finally, to the memory of Mary Frances Lisk Jeffries, who initiated the original project and, though gravely ill, continued to work on this revision, with the support of her husband, Ken, until her death. We miss her.

PREFACE

One of the most significant achievements in the health care field during the last 20 years has been the emergence of the nurse as an active coordinator and initiator of patient care. Although the transition from helpmate to health care professional has been painfully slow and is not yet complete, the importance of the nurse within the system can no longer be denied or ignored. Today's nurse designs nursing care interventions that will move the total patient toward the goal of improved health.

The current state of the theory of nursing process, diagnosis, and intervention has been brought to the clinical setting to be implemented by the nurse. This book gives definition and direction to the development and use of individualized nursing care. Therefore, the book is not an end in itself, but a beginning for the future growth and development of the profession.

Professional care standards, physicians, and patients will continue to increase the expectations of nurses' performance. Each day brings advances in the struggle to understand the mysteries of normal body function and human response to actual and potential health problems. With this increased knowledge comes greater responsibility for the nurse. To meet this challenge competently, the nurse must have detailed, up-to-date physical assessment skills and knowledge of pathophysiologic concepts concerning the more common diseases/conditions presented on a general medical/surgical unit. This book is a tool, a means of attaining that competency.

In the past, care plans were viewed principally as a learning tool for students and seemed to have little relevance after graduation. However, as nursing has moved toward defining its professional status and accountability, the need for a written format to communicate and document individualized patient care has been recognized. In addition, governmental regulations and requirements of third-party payors have created the need to validate the appropriateness of care given and justify patient care charges and staffing patterns.

The practicing nurse, as well as the nursing student, will welcome this text as a ready reference in clinical practice. The book has been designed for use in the acute medical/surgical setting and is organized according to systems for easy reference. Rationales are given for the nurses' actions/interventions, each including brief related pathophysiology, when applicable, enhancing the reader's understanding. Each rationale serves as a catalyst for thought in planning and evaluating the care being rendered.

Chapter 1 discusses current issues and trends affecting the nursing profession. An overview of cultural, community, sociologic and ethical concepts with an impact on the nurse is included. The need for cooperation and coordination with other health care professionals is an important concept of the care plans.

Chapter 2 reviews the historic use of the nursing process in formulating plans of care and the nurse's role in the delivery of that care. Use of nursing diagnoses is discussed to provide the nurse with an understanding of their role in the nursing process.

Chapter 3 discusses care plan construction and the use and adaptation of the care-palnning guides that are presented in this book. A nursing-based history tool and sample patient situation, with data base and corresponding care plan, are presented.

Chapters 4 through 17 present nursing-oriented care plan guides and include information shared with other disciplines. Each care plan is developed by identifying nursing diagnoses with "related to" and "evidenced by" factors that provide an explanation of patient problems. Each plan includes a history and physical examination (presented in a nursing assessment format) and diagnostic studies, termed the *patient assessment data base.* After the data base is collected, *nursing priorities* are sifted from the information to delineate the overall goals of care. *Discharge criteria* are also listed, to identify which general goals should be accomplished by the time of discharge from care. *Outcomes/evaluation criteria* are stated in behavioral terms that can be measured in specific ways. The *actions/interventions* are designed to assist with problem resolution. *Rationales* for the actions are designed to enable the nurse to decide whether the intervention applies to a particular patient. Information is provided to assist the nurse in identifying and planning for rehabilitation as the patient progresses toward discharge.

This book is not intended to be a procedure manual, and efforts have been made to avoid detailed descriptions of techniques/protocols that might be viewed as individual/regional in nature. Instead, the reader is referred to a procedure manual/standards of care book for in-depth direction for these concerns.

M.E.D.

CONTRIBUTORS

Ida Marlene Beam, RN
Major, ANC Retired
Colorado Springs, Colorado

Pat Budd, RN, MS
Assistant Professor
Beth-El College of Nursing
Colorado Springs, Colorado

Nancy Lee Carter, RN, BSN, MA
Hospital Nursing and Management
Counseling of Children
Child Care Provider
Albuquerque, New Mexico

Mary Davignon, RN, BSN, CCRN
Medical Intensive Care Unit
St. Mary's Hospital and Health Center
Tucson, Arizona

Betty Hagge, RN, BS
Administrative Supervisor
Penrose Hospital
Colorado Springs, Colorado

Beth Hamstra, RN, MS
Nursing Supervisor
Memorial Hospital
Instructor
Beth-El College of Nursing
Colorado Springs, Colorado

Cindy Hindsley, RN, MSN
Clinical Nurse Specialist
Medical-Surgical
Private Practice
Monterey, California

Christie Hinds, RN, BSN, CSNP, PNP
Certified School Nurse Practitioner
HIV Program Coordinator
Fort Carson, Colorado

Laura Teigen Johnson, BSN, CNOR
Clinical Educator, Surgery
Penrose Community Hospital
Colorado Springs, Colorado

L. Michael Koenig, BSN, MS
Oncology Certified Nurse (OCN)
Veterans Administration Medical Center
Tucson, Arizona

Patricia Trinosky Lind, RN, MS
Assistant Professor
Beth-El College of Nursing
Colorado Springs, Colorado

Gwenyth Loughmiller Lynn, RN, BA
Oncology Staff Nurse (Retired)
Kettering Medical Center
Dayton, Ohio

Rebecca F. Murray, RN, MOT
Charge Nurse
Long Term Care Facility
Colorado Springs, Colorado

Linda Pfeffer, RN, MS
Assistant Professor
Beth-EL College of Nursing
Colorado Springs, Colorado

Betsy Philips, RN
Nurse Entrepreneur
Owner: American Beauty Salon
Clinical Director Center for Aging and Sun-Damaged
   Skin
Colorado Springs, Colorado

Leann Scroggins, RN, MS
Assistant Director
Quality Assurance/Research
Formerly Clinical Nurse Specialist
Cardiovascular Nursing
Saint Mary's Hospital
Rochester, Minnesota

Diana Kenney Woodhouse, RN, MS
Program Director
Oncology
Orthopedics and Surgery
Lutheran Medical Center
Wheat Ridge, Colorado

REVIEWERS/CONSULTANTS

Carolyn Ferree, RN, BSN, PHN
Tuberculosis Control Nurse
El Paso County Health Department
Colorado Springs, Colorado

Dorothy Gusa, RN, BSN
Assistant Clinical Manager, Cardiac Telemetry
Penrose Hospital
Colorado Springs, Colorado

Linda Langlais, RN, BSN, CTRS
International Rehabilitation Associates
Colorado Springs, Colorado

Cynthia Porter, RN

Roberta Smith, RN, BSN, ET
Enterostomal/Dermatology Nurse
St. Mary-Corwin Hospital
Pueblo, Colorado

Larry L. Maton, RPh
Executive Park Pharmacy
Colorado Springs, Colorado

Anne Zobek, RN, BS, MS
Oncology Nurse Specialist
Penrose Hospital
Colorado Springs, Colorado

Special Thanks to:
Anne Maria Nolan, RN, BS, MS
Dingoney, Victoria, Australia

ACKNOWLEDGEMENTS OF CONTRIBUTIONS FROM OTHER WORKS

(Psychiatric Care Plans)
Marti Davis Buffum, RN, MS
Nursing Faculty/Lecturer
San Francisco State University
Staff Nurse III
Inpatient Psychiatry
Marin General Hospital
Greenbrae, California

Wm. G. Cantin, BSN
Lieutenant US Navy Nurse Corps
Alcohol Rehabilitation Facility
Tripler Army Medical Center, Hawaii
Nurse/Administration Coordinator
Transformation Life Center
West Park, New York

MaryAnnie Lewis Hughes, MSN, BSN, RN, CS
Captain, US Army Nurse Corps
Clinical Head Nurse
Clinical Specialist at Tri-Service Alcoholism Recovery
   Facility (TRI-SARF)
Tripler Army Medical Center
Hawaii

(Critical Care Plans)
Karen Bell, RN, MSN, CEN
Major Army Nurse Corps
Director
Practical Nurse Course
Fitzsimmons Army Medical Center
Aurora, Colorado

Kathleen Crocker, RN, MSN, CNSN
Clinical Specialist
Nutrition Support Nursing
Director of Nursing
New England Critical Care, Inc.
Marlborough, Massachusetts

Pamela DeLoach, RN, BSN
Primary Nurse III
Neurotrauma Center
M.I.E.M.S.S.
Baltimore, Maryland

Kerry Fater, RN, PhD
Assistant Professor of Nursing
Salve Regina College
Newport, Rhode Island

Terry Mathew Foster, RN, CEN, CCRN
Critical Care and Emergency Nursing Instructor
Our Lady of Mercy Hospitals
Anderson/Mariemont
Cincinnati, Ohio
Staff Nurse, Emergency Department
Saint Elizabeth Medical Center
North Unit
Covington, Kentucky

Ruth Froyd, RN, BSN, CCRN
Critical Care Staff Nurse
Austin, Texas

M. Ann Jansen, MS, RN, CCRN
Critical Care Clinician
Memorial Hospital
Colorado Springs, Colorado

Merrily A. Mathewson, RN, PhD, CCRN
President/Director of Education
Educational Services
Hamburg, New York

Cynthia McCall May, RN, BSN, CCRN
Head Nurse
Memorial Hospital
Adult Critical Care Unit
Colorado Springs, Colorado

Linda S. Mayer, RN, MN
Pulmonary Clinical Nurse Specialist
Division of Pulmonary Medicine
University of Kansas Medical Center
Kansas City, Kansas

Linda J. Nielson, RN, CCRN
Charge Nurse
Intensive Care Unit
St. Peter Hospital
Olympia, Washington

Karen J. Replogle, RN, MS, CCRN
Critical Care Nursing Consultant
Healthcare Education and Computing
Dayton, Ohio

Sherry Smith, RN, BSN, MSN, EdD
Professor of Nursing
Director
School of Nursing
DePauw University
Greencastle/Indianapolis, Indiana

Brenda Lebowitz Stoller, BA, RN, CNA
Private Consultant for AIDS Projects and Programs
AMPC Fellow at New York University
Director of the Nurses Network on AIDS
New York, New York

Rita Bolek Trofino, RN, MNEd
Assistant Professor
Department of Nursing
Saint Francis College
Loretto, Pennsylvania

Connie Walleck, MS, RN, CNRN
Clinical Nurse Supervisor/Specialist
Neurotrauma Center
M.I.E.M.S.S.
Baltimore, Maryland

CONTENTS IN BRIEF

INDEX OF NURSING DIAGNOSES
appears on pages 951–956

INDEX OF NURSING DIAGNOSES appears on pages 951–956

INDEX OF NURSING DIAGNOSES appears on pages 951–956

APPENDIX 957

A table of contents including Nursing Diagnoses follows.

DETAILED CONTENTS

INDEX OF NURSING DIAGNOSES
appears on pages 951–956

INDEX OF NURSING DIAGNOSES appears on pages 951–956

INDEX OF NURSING DIAGNOSES appears on pages 951–956

INDEX OF NURSING DIAGNOSES appears on pages 951–956

INDEX OF NURSING DIAGNOSES appears on pages 951–956

INDEX OF NURSING DIAGNOSES appears on pages 951–956

INDEX OF NURSING DIAGNOSES appears on pages 951–956

INDEX OF NURSING DIAGNOSES appears on pages 951–956

INDEX OF NURSING DIAGNOSES appears on pages 951–956

INDEX OF NURSING DIAGNOSES appears on pages 951–956

CHAPTER 1

ISSUES AND TRENDS IN MEDICAL/SURGICAL NURSING

While the entire field of health care is changing, nowhere are these changes occurring at a more rapid rate than in the acute care arena. Here, nurses offer direct assistance to both patients and families who are facing illness or injury. This provides a tremendously exacting and exciting challenge for the nurse. The responsibility for coordinating this care requires planning and documentation that clearly identifies problems and interventions, as well as short- and long-range health care planning for individuals and families.

In this changing arena, what lies ahead? In this chapter we will examine some major trends that will have a lasting impact on nursing and patient care:

Decreasing health care dollars
Quantification of nursing care costs
Reduced length of stay
Increasing reliance on high technology
Requirement for advanced nursing knowledge
Need for collaboration and communication
Innovations in care planning through computerization

DECREASING HEALTH CARE DOLLARS

Major changes in payment mechanisms for hospital Medicare patients were introduced in 1983 in response to escalating costs for provision of health care within the United States. Implementation of prospective reimbursement has had an impact on nursing care and has implications for patient care planning.

The focus of health care under prospective reimbursement is cost containment, requiring that nursing redefine the minimum standards of care while still maintaining and providing effective nursing care. Implementation of prospective reimbursement has resulted in decreased lengths of stay and increased levels of patient acuity. Hospitals, no longer compensated on a cost basis but reimbursed by patient episode, benefit financially when less technology per patient is used. Hospitals have and will continue to respond to decreased dollars by reducing beds and staff. As never before, the patient care plan must reflect preparation for meeting patient needs within the restrictions of time limitations and fewer resources. As a result of these changes, the nurse must function more efficiently.

In addition, hospitals are merging or sharing services in order to spread the risks of operating in a tight economic environment. As a result, some services may be deleted or offered in only one, instead of every, facility. Furthermore, the use of alternative health care providers, such as freestanding emergency facilities, outpatient services, and long-term care/rehabilitation facilities, may delay or eliminate the need for hospital admission. Reduction in the number of low-priority admissions ultimately results in higher acuity of patients and loss of the "bell curve" of the usual patient load.

Rationing of health care dollars has occurred as a result of prospective reimbursement; and as the health care dollar shrinks, many questions arise. How shall allocation of a fixed number of resources to many possible users be determined? Beyond that, who will decide who receives the benefits purchased with these scarce dollars? Whether decision is by "ethics committees" or some other less formal mechanism, the patient care plan contributes to the decision-making process.

QUANTIFICATION OF NURSING CARE

Attention is thus focused on the cost of providing nursing care to patients within the acute care setting in the wake of prospective reimbursement, fewer dollars, limited time, and reduced beds and staff. Quantifying nursing time requires that the intensity of nursing care necessary for each patient be identified. Clinically, intensity may be measured by a patient classification system or directly by the patient care plan.

Quantification of nursing's contribution to patient care can be used to "cost" and "bill" for nursing care. Although only a few of the nation's hospitals currently cost and bill for nursing, a growing number of hospitals will adopt this practice as they are forced to monitor costs more closely. In those hospitals already billing for nursing services, the patient care plan is an integral part of the justification of nursing care costs. In addition, the care plan may be used for comparison from hospital to hospital to establish or evaluate competitive charges for nursing.

REDUCED LENGTH OF STAY

The provision of personalized care must be planned and provided with continuity as the quantity of care time decreases. Many patients who leave the hospital earlier are still in need of health care. Hospitals are responding to this need by creating transitional care floors/beds, creating their own health care agencies, or hiring hospital-based coordinators to work with private home health care agencies. Nurses are assuming a larger portion of responsibility for ensuring that patients are discharged on time according to their DRG classification. Aggressive discharge planning must begin on admission to the medical/surgical unit and incorporate knowledge of hospital and community resources available for the patient.

To facilitate early but safe discharge and to ensure continuity of care, nurses find many traditional unit boundaries loosening. Some may follow patients from admission to the general care units, through discharge into the community in an effort to achieve optimal outcomes. This "following" may be the active participation in discharge planning as the patient convalesces, the formation of a care plan early in the patient's stay that is passed on to other care givers, or telephone contacts, home visits, or consultation with postdischarge care givers. An effectively coordinated care plan can follow the patient, ensuring continuity of care between the health care system and the home or agency.

INCREASING RELIANCE ON HIGH TECHNOLOGY

Long before John Naisbett's *Megatrends* (New York, Warner Books, 1982) became a bestseller and "high tech/high touch" became a trendy phrase, nurses expressed concern that the patient was in danger of being lost among the tubes, monitors, and machines as complex technology became an increasingly larger part of health care. This has led nurses to advocate recognition of patient individuality and the holistic concept of "mind–soul–body" interaction by various means, such as adoption of the primary nurse concept and heightened awareness of ethical issues like the "quality of life/right to die" dilemma. Inclusion of these concepts and consideration of the individual's cultural/socioeconomic background can facilitate achieving balance between technologic advances and human needs.

REQUIREMENT FOR ADVANCED NURSING KNOWLEDGE

Increased patient acuity combined with shorter lengths of stay within the medical/surgical environment requires more intensive nursing interventions. The nurse needs greater clinical expertise, maturity, critical thinking ability, assertiveness, and patient management skills in order to handle these increased responsibilities.

Nursing specialty certification programs sponsored by various agencies such as American Nurses Association (ANA), the Nurses Association of the American College of Obstetricians and Gynecologists (NAACOG), and the Association of Operating Room Nurses (AORN) share common goals: to provide consumer protection, to enhance nursing knowledge and competency, to increase nursing autonomy, and to strengthen collaboration. Certification recognizes the attainment of predetermined standards established by the certifying group and takes on more importance in this cost-conscious era as managers seek to hire competent professionals. In addition, this type of credentialing can provide a framework for reimbursement by third-party payors.

Care planning serves as a means of enhancing nursing knowledge and improving nursing practice. Standardized care plans aid in establishing priorities of care and defining minimum standards of safe practice. Standardized care plans also serve as "memory joggers" to nurses caring for patients not usually seen in their area of clinical practice, thus providing information to promote effective practice.

NEED FOR COLLABORATION AND COMMUNICATION

As health care delivery becomes more complex and more economically centered, the need for communication and collaboration among health care professionals is intensified. Only through collaboration between departments/services/facilities can medical professionals deliver the most efficient and comprehensive care. The nurse, as the primary coordinator of overall patient care, strives to ensure that the patient receives quality but cost-efficient care.

Interdepartmental communication and collaboration may take form as a patient care conference. Information obtained from patient care conferences is incorporated into the overall plan of care by the nurse, who works as a liaison between health care providers. Thus, the care plan serves as the vehicle for and documentation of ongoing communication among nurses and other disciplines.

Patients and families, assuming responsibility for themselves (internal locus-of-control), are participating in more decisions determining the level and amount of health care they desire. The care plan should include moral/ethical concerns, such as "no code/living will" decisions, with date, time, and names of those participating. This provides legal and ethical documentation of the decision-making/communication process.

INNOVATIONS IN CARE PLANNING THROUGH COMPUTERIZATION

Many nurses believe that their limited time can be better spent at the bedside, giving patient care, rather than filling out paperwork. Institutions using computerized care planning report increased numbers of care plans being generated and maintained than occurred previous to computerization (Lombard and Light, 1983). In fact, computerized systems have had a favorable impact on the process, as nurses may quickly enter, display, update, evaluate, and print a care plan, thus improving the quality of record keeping.

Most computerized systems use standardized patient care plans, which are designed to meet specific needs, and which reflect standards of care for particular patient problems. Many use the nursing diagnoses accepted for testing by the North American Nursing Diagnosis Association (NANDA). Since computerized plans reflect a wealth of varied nursing knowledge and experience, they allow even novice practitioners to formulate effective care strategies. In addition, they provide all nurses with an efficient means of developing comprehensive, continuously updated, individualized, and legible care plans for each patient.

CONCLUSION

Rapid changes in the health care environment, with continuous technologic advances, increasing severity of illness, budget constraints, and expanding nursing knowledge, have greatly increased the responsibilities facing today's nurse.

In order to fulfill these responsibilities, planning and documentation of care are essential to satisfy patient needs and meet legal obligations. The use of care plans reflecting only functional divisions of tasks/duties perpetuates the notion that care plans are "busy work," unrelated to care-giving. Restructuring care plans to use "nursing models" could increase usage and provide succinct documentation, demonstrating the relationship between planning and documentation.

Efficient and effective use of the patient care plan can ensure that acutely ill patients receive individualized quality care in the midst of cost containment. Documentation of the impact of nursing on patient care also provides information for continuing care needs, legal concerns, and payment.

What lies ahead for nursing and care planning? Definitely, a tremendously exciting and exacting challenge!

CHAPTER 2

NURSING PROCESS, NURSING DIAGNOSIS, AND CARE PLAN CONSTRUCTION

There is a growing awareness that nursing care is a key factor in patient survival and in the maintenance, rehabilitative, and preventive aspects of health care. In 1980, the American Nurses Association Social Policy Statement defined nursing as the diagnosis and treatment of human responses to actual and potential health problems. The ANA Standards of Practice have provided impetus and support for the use of nursing diagnosis in the practice setting. With the development of prospective payment plans, movement away from acute care to other settings (i.e., long-term/convalescent, rehabilitation, home health services), and other changes in the health care system, the need for a common framework of communication and documentation has become a necessity to ensure continuity of care.

With the "knowledge explosion" that began in the late 1950s, many disciplines have expanded their horizons. Nursing is no exception, having accepted the concept of total, individualized care of patients as a basis for effective, therapeutic nursing actions. Philosophically, this is termed a holistic approach to health care. In implementing the concept, the nursing profession has identified a process that contributes to the prevention of illness as well as the restoration and maintenance of health. It is adapted from the scientific approach to problem solving and requires the skills of (1) assessment (systematic collection of data relating to patients and their problems/needs), (2) problem identification (interpretation of data), (3) planning (choice of solutions), (4) implementation (putting the plan into action), and (5) evaluation (assessing the effectiveness of the plan and changing the plan as indicated by the current needs). While nurses use these terms separately, in reality they are interrelated and form a continuous circle of thought and action, providing an efficient method of organization for clinical decision making. This "nursing process" is now included in the conceptual framework of most nursing curricula and accepted in the legal definition of nursing in most nurse practice acts.

Within the nursing process framework, the critical element for effective, therapeutic nursing care is the relevance of care based upon appropriately performed assessments. Understanding the individuality of patient care requires integration of a personal, sociologic, psychologic, and medical history with a thorough physical examination and the results of diagnostic studies. Looking at the data as a whole provides the nurse with a comprehensive picture of the patient in relation to the patient's past, present, and future health status.

Nursing diagnosis provides a format for expressing the nursing process. While there are differing definitions of nursing diagnosis, we have chosen to use Shoemaker's, taken from the Classification of Nursing Diagnosis, Proceedings of the Fifth National Conference (Kim et al., 1984): "Nursing diagnosis is a clinical judgment about an individual, family, or community which is derived through a deliberate, systematic process of data collection and analysis. It provides the basis for prescriptions for definitive therapy for which the nurse is accountable. It is expressed concisely and it includes the etiology of the condition when known."

The responsibility for establishing the nursing diagnosis varies according to the theoretic framework of nursing practice used by the particular service organization, e.g., functional method, team method, primary care, and case method. Although nursing practice is more than nursing diagnosis, it provides a common language for identifying patient problems, nursing interventions, and evaluation tools.

CARE PLAN CONSTRUCTION

PATIENT ASSESSMENT DATA BASE

The patient assessment data base is the foundation upon which identification of individual needs, responses, and problems is based and includes the history-taking interview, the physical examination, and diagnostic studies. The philosophy and policies of the health care agency may affect this process, and the data base may be read and used by numerous/all members of the health care team.

INTERVIEWING

Interviewing provides a specific set of data (history) that the nurse obtains from the patient and significant others through both conversation and observation. The information may be collected during one or more contact periods and should include all data (positive and negative) that is relevant to the situation. Organization of this data assists in identifying patient problems and desired patient outcomes. All participants in the conversation need to know that the information will be used in formulating the plan of patient care.

PHYSICAL EXAMINATION

During this aspect of information gathering, the nurse exercises perceptual and observational skills, using the senses of sight, hearing, touch, and smell. Physical examination skills vary from basic to advanced; however, the nurse needs to know the normal physical and emotional characteristics well enough to be able to recognize deviations from normal. The duration and depth of any physical examination depends on the condition of the patient and the urgency of the situation. Several different formats are available. Findings may be recorded according to (1) body systems being examined (medical model); (2) subjective data (e.g., may report) and objective data (e.g., may exhibit); (3) activity involved (inspection, palpation, and so forth); or (4) by a nursing model (e.g., Diagnostic Divisions, Functional Health Patterns). In this book we have chosen to use a nursing model, Diagnostic Divisions, as presented in Chapter 3.

DIAGNOSTIC STUDIES

Laboratory studies are included as part of the information-gathering process. Some tests are used to diagnose disease, while others are useful in following the course of a disease or in adjusting therapies. In many cases the relationship of the test to the pathologic physiology is clear, while in other cases it is not. This is the result of the interrelationships between the various organs and systems of the body. Interpretation of test results should be integrated with the history and physical findings. The nurse needs to be aware of significant test results that require reporting to the physician and/or initiation of specific nursing actions.

NURSING DIAGNOSIS (PROBLEM IDENTIFICATION)

Nursing diagnosis is now becoming a uniform way of identifying, focusing on, and dealing with specific problems or responses. Accurate diagnosis of a patient problem can provide a standard for nursing action, understood by all who are using the plan of care, thereby resulting in improved coordination and/or delivery of care.

 The nursing diagnosis may be a physical, sociologic, or psychologic finding. Physical nursing diagnoses include those that pertain to circulation, ventilation, elimination, and so forth. Psychosocial nursing diagnoses include anything that pertains to or deals with the mind, emotion, or lifestyle/relationships.

 There are several steps involved in the process of problem identification (nursing diagnosis):
1. Collecting a data base (nursing interview, physical examination) combined with information collected by other members of the health team (including diagnostic studies).
2. Analyzing and reviewing the data for relevant information (positive and negative findings) and for conflicts in findings that normally reinforce each other/information expected to exist that does not (e.g., complains of pain in RUQ, but does not flinch on abdominal examination).
3. Synthesizing (combining/organizing) the data into nursing diagnostic problems/concerns.
4. Comparing and contrasting the relationships among the diagnoses (according to established criteria of etiology, risk factors, defining characteristics) and determining interrelationships within or between diagnoses. This step is crucial to the creation of individual patient problem statements as the nurse identifies the meaning within and between each diagnosis listed.
5. Combining the nursing diagnosis with the etiology and signs/symptoms to create the patient problem statement (e.g., Comfort, altered, acute pain related to abdominal tissue trauma (incision) as evidenced by muscle guarding, restlessness, self-focus, grimacing).

Integrating these steps provides for a systematic approach to problem identification and writing of the patient problem statement.

After nursing diagnoses are identified, they are listed according to priority and classified according to status, e.g., active, inactive/potential, or resolved. Active diagnoses are those that require some form of action or intervention. Inactive/potential diagnoses are those that may occur/recur. Resolved diagnoses are those that no longer need action.

NURSING PRIORITIES

In this book, nursing priorities are listed in a certain order to facilitate prioritizing the nursing diagnoses that appear in these care plan guides. In the individual situation, nursing priorities may differ on the basis of specific patient needs, and nursing diagnoses would be reranked accordingly.

PATIENT OUTCOMES/EVALUATION CRITERIA

A patient outcome can be defined as a response that (1) may be achievable, (2) is desired by the patient, and (3) can be attained within a defined time period, given the present situation and resources. Useful *patient outcome statements* need to
1. be specific;
2. be realistic;
3. consider the patient's circumstances and desires;
4. indicate a time frame;
5. provide measurable evaluation criteria for determination of success or failure in achieving the desired outcome.

Desired outcomes are written by listing items/behavior to observe that can determine that a positive/acceptable outcome has been achieved (e.g., Verbalizes understanding of disease process and potential complications). This serves as the evaluation tool. Action verbs are used when the patient or nurse is asked to perform an action (e.g., verbalizes/demonstrates), with modifiers to add specificity (e.g., ambulates with use of cane). Time elements also provide measurable criteria (e.g., ambulates with cane without assistance within 3 days).

Outcomes involve different time frames, i.e., long-term, intermediate, or short-term. Long-term outcomes indicate the overall direction for actions as a result of the interventions of the health care team and/or patient. These outcomes may not be achieved prior to discharge. Intermediate outcomes are shorter-range activities directed toward accomplishing the long-range goal(s). Short-term outcomes require immediate action and usually must be achieved prior to discharge or movement to a less acute level of care, supervision or support.

When outcomes are properly written, they provide direction for planning and validating the choice of interventions. In the outcome "Identifies individual nutritional needs and formulates dietary plan based on these needs," the nurse knows that the patient's level of knowledge needs to be assessed, individual needs identified, and nutritional information presented to provide the patient with the tools necessary to formulate a dietary plan.

The nurse/patient outcomes are only part of the overall health care outcome(s). Each discipline involved in assisting the patient will have individual outcomes that contribute to the overall goal(s). The challenge is to write meaningful outcomes that avoid multidisciplinary conflicts and can be understood and used by all colleagues providing health care.

Some agencies separate patient goals from nursing goals. Nursing goals may replace outcomes in the patient who has little individual responsibility in achieving them (e.g., airway clearance in a comatose patient, control of gastric bleeding, or improved cardiac output). These goals are achieved by intervention of health team members. However, since the well-being of the patient may depend on the achievement of both patient and nurse goals, they are combined here for simplicity.

NURSING INTERVENTIONS

After information is gathered, problems identified, and outcomes formulated, actions are selected that can be expected to achieve the desired outcomes. In the patient care plan this basic unit is known as an intervention.

Nursing interventions are prescriptions for specific behaviors expected from the nurses and/or other members of the health team and the patient. The expectation is that the prescribed behavior/action benefits the patient in a predictable way related to the identified diagnosis and desired outcome. These interventions have the intent of individualizing and guiding nursing care.

Interventions begin with an action verb, communicating a specific behavior (e.g., "Instruct . . ."). Content area deals with the "what, where, and how" of the intervention, especially when continuity or repetition are described (e.g., time elements may be included indicating when, how often, or how long an intervention is to be implemented, depending on patient need and/or institutional policy, such as "every 2 hours × 4, then q.i.d.").

Independent nursing actions are an integral part of this process. Interdependent or collaborative actions are based on the medical regimen along with suggestions or orders from other disciplines involved with the care of the patient. The educational background and expertise of the nurse, established protocols or standards of care, and areas of practice (rural/urban, acute/community care settings) influence whether an intervention is an independent nursing function or requires collaboration.

Incorporation of the medical plan of care reveals the nursing interventions required to implement the orders (e.g., administer medications) and show nursing actions that need to be performed to achieve nursing goals related to the medical plan (e.g., monitoring effects of drugs or other therapeutic interventions).

RATIONALE

Although not commonly appearing on a care plan, rationales for interventions are included that reflect pathophysiologic and/or psychologic principles. This provides a sound basis for deciding the relevance of a specific intervention for an individual patient situation.

DISCHARGE CRITERIA

Discharge criteria represent goals that are to be achieved by the patient prior to discharge from the acute care setting. Unmet criteria reflect a need for further care/supervision in the acute care or an alternate care setting. Discharge planning, which is crucial to continuity of care, begins upon admission to the health care facility and should include the expected discharge destination (e.g., home, skilled nursing facility, and so forth). The nurse is committed to planning continuity of care in all its aspects: between nursing personnel, between services within the hospital, and between the hospital and the community. The nurse may also be responsible for initiating/cooperating in referrals to community services. The question needing an answer here is, Does the patient need continuation of care after leaving this health care agency? If the answer is Yes, the next question is, What is involved in the patient's care needs, and how and where can these needs be best met? Planning for an alternative to hospital care is dependent on answers to the above questions and provides the nurse with needed direction for patient/family learning to facilitate recovery and promote wellness.

One of the concerns associated with the identification of patient problems and the implementation of the care plan is what the nurse's responsibility is once a diagnosis is made and the patient is discharged before all short-term goals are met and/or problems are resolved. Whose responsibility is it for follow-through for provision and evaluation of care once discharge has occurred? Who is responsible for monitoring patient progress toward long-term goals? Should this information be shared with the patient's physician or office nurse? Is the nurse who has made a nursing diagnosis responsible for follow-through to its resolution? Nationally, this issue is unresolved, and patient goals often remain unmet. Ethically, it is up to the health care industry and the nursing community to formulate policies that will promote optimum patient recovery and health maintenance.

DOCUMENTATION

Once constructed, the care plan provides documentation of the planning process and serves as a framework for documentation of administered care. Nurses feel at risk in committing themselves to documenting a nursing diagnosis. However, many references are currently available to aid in identifying and formulating the problem statement. Unlike medical diagnoses, nursing diagnoses change as the patient progresses through various stages of illness/maladaption, to problem resolution. Documentation of these changes and actions taken are important for continuity of care. Finally, the care plan is used when the question of liability arises and information is required for determining whether actions were planned appropriately and care provided accordingly.

SUMMARY

This book is intended to facilitate the application of the nursing process to the medical/surgical patient and significant other(s). Each care plan is intended to be an informational guide so that the individual practitioner will be able to modify or extract that information which is pertinent to the specific patient situation. As noted, with few exceptions, we have presented NANDA's recommendations as formulated by the Conferences. Brackets indicate additions or changes the authors have made to clarify or enhance the accepted nursing diagnoses, e.g., "[learning need]." Some diagnoses have been combined for convenience, indicating that two factors may be involved, i.e., "fluid volume, altered [fluctuation]." It is anticipated that the nurse will choose "what fits." Nurses can be creative as they work with the standardized format redefining and sharing interventions as they are used with individual patients. We appreciate that not all diagnoses presented in these care plans may be appropriate for your patient or locale, and alternates should be chosen to meet individual patient needs.

CHAPTER 3

ADAPTATION OF THEORY TO PRACTICE

Given the formative stage of nursing diagnosis, the nurse is encouraged to investigate and learn in order to tailor the care plan to the individual patient. The care plans presented here are a guide for the nurse in the use of this process, rather than standard plans that "fit all." They are designed to give the nurse a sampling of information about general patient situations, identifying many factors that may or may not need to be given consideration in caring for any particular patient.

Patient assessment is the foundation upon which identification of individual needs, responses, and problems is based. In order to facilitate this step of the nursing process, an Assessment Tool has been constructed, combining history, physical examination, and several common diagnostic studies, using a nursing focus instead of the more familiar medical approach ("review of systems"). To achieve this nursing focus, the NANDA nursing diagnoses (Table 3–1) are grouped in related categories entitled Diagnostic Divisions (Table 3–2), which reflect a blending of Maslow's Hierarchy of Needs and a self-care philosophy. As data are collected, these divisions serve to direct the nurse to the appropriate corresponding nursing diagnosis labels. Since these divisions are based on human responses/needs and not specific "systems," information may be recorded in more than one area. For this reason, the nurse is encouraged to collect as much data as possible before choosing the nursing diagnosis that best reflects the patient's situation. The results (synthesis) of the collected data are written in concise diagnostic statements (patient problem statements).

Nursing priorities and diagnoses are arranged in a general order that can be altered to fit the individual patient. Each nursing diagnosis has been provided with a list of etiologic factors ("may be related to") and defining characteristics ("possibly evidenced by") which the nurse may select from or add to, in order to accurately represent the patient's situation.

Patient outcomes/goals are then identified to facilitate choosing appropriate interventions and to serve as evaluators of both nursing care and patient response. These goals are also a framework for documentation.

The interventions are designed to specify the action of the nurse, the patient, and/or significant other(s). They are not all inclusive, because such nursing actions as "bathe the patient" or "notify the physician of changes" have been left out. It is expected that these are included in patient care. Sometimes controversial issues or treatments are presented for the sake of information and/or because alternate therapies may be used in different care settings or geographic locations.

In addition to achieving physiologic stability, interventions need to promote movement toward independence. An important aspect of the self-care philosophy is the involvement of patients in their own care. Information is given at the level of the individual's understanding and ability to encourage participation in decisions about care and outcomes whenever possible. This promotes patient responsibility, negating the idea that health care providers control patient lives.

For visualizing the tailoring of a care plan guide, a specific Patient Situation (p. 21) is provided as an example of data collection and care plan construction. As the Patient Assessment Data Base is reviewed, the nurse can identify the etiologic factors and defining characteristics that were used to formulate the patient problem statements. The addition of time lines to specific patient outcomes/goals reflects anticipated length of stay and individual patient/nurse expectations. Interventions are based upon concerns/needs identified by the patient and nurse during data collection, as well as physician orders. Although not normally written in a care plan, rationales are included in this sample for the purpose of explaining or clarifying the choice of interventions and enhancing the nurse's learning.

TABLE 3-1. Nursing Diagnoses (Through the 8th NANDA Conference of 1988)

Activity intolerance
Activity intolerance, potential
Adjustment, impaired
Airway clearance, ineffective
*Anxiety [specify]
Aspiration, potential for
Body temperature, potential altered
Bowel elimination, altered: constipation
     Constipation, colonic
     Constipation, perceived
Bowel elimination, altered: diarrhea
Bowel elimination, altered: incontinence
Breastfeeding, ineffective
Breathing pattern, ineffective
Cardiac output, altered: decreased
Comfort, altered: pain, acute
Comfort, altered: pain, chronic
Communication, impaired: verbal
Coping, defensive
Coping, family: potential for growth
Coping, ineffective family: compromised
Coping, ineffective family: disabling
Coping, ineffective individual
Decisional conflict (specify)
Denial, ineffective
Disuse syndrome, potential for
Diversional activity deficit
Dysreflexia
Family process, altered
Fatigue
Fear
Fluid volume, altered: excess
†Fluid volume deficit, actual 1 [regulatory failure]
†Fluid volume deficit, actual 2 [active loss]
Fluid volume deficit, potential
Gas exchange, impaired
Grieving, anticipatory
Grieving, dysfunctional
Growth and development, altered
Health maintenance, altered
Health seeking behaviors (specify)
Home maintenance management, impaired
Hopelessness
Hyperthermia
†Hypothermia
Incontinence, functional
Incontinence, reflex
Incontinence, stress
Incontinence, total
Incontinence, urge
Infection, potential for
Injury, potential for: poisoning; suffocation; trauma
*Knowledge deficit [learning need] (specify)
Mobility, impaired physical
Neglect, unilateral
*Noncompliance [compliance, altered] (specify)
Nutrition, altered: less than body requirements
Nutrition, altered: more than body requirements

Nutrition, altered: potential for more than body requirements
Oral mucous membranes, altered
Parental role conflict
Parenting, altered: actual or potential
Post-trauma response
Powerlessness
Rape trauma syndrome
Self-care deficit: feeding; bathing/hygiene; dressing/grooming; toileting
Self-concept, disturbance in: body image; personal identity; role performance; self-esteem
 Self-esteem, chronic low
 †Self-esteem, disturbance in
 Self-esteem, situational low
Sensory-perceptual alteration: visual; auditory; kinesthetic; gustatory; tactile; olfactory
Sexual dysfunction
Sexuality patterns, altered
Skin integrity, impaired: actual
Skin integrity, impaired: potential
Sleep pattern disturbance
Social interaction, impaired
Social isolation
Spiritual distress (distress of the human spirit)
Swallowing, impaired
Thermoregulation, ineffective
Thought processes, altered
Tissue integrity, impaired
Tissue perfusion, altered: cerebral; cardiopulmonary; renal; gastrointestinal; peripheral
Urinary elimination: altered patterns
*Urinary retention [acute/chronic]
Violence, potential for: directed at self/others

---

*Information that appears in brackets has been added by the authors to clarify and enhance the use of
 nursing diagnoses.
†Revised.

TABLE 3-2. Diagnostic Divisions

After data have been collected and areas of concern/need have been identified, the nurse is directed to the Diagnostic Divisions to review the list of nursing diagnoses that fall within the individual categories. This will assist the nurse in choosing the specific diagnostic label to describe the data accurately. Then, with the addition of etiology (when known) and signs and symptoms, the patient problem statement emerges.

ACTIVITY/REST
Activity intolerance
Activity intolerance, potential
Disuse syndrome, potential for
Diversional activity deficit
Fatigue
Sleep pattern disturbance

CIRCULATION
Cardiac output, altered: decreased
Dysreflexia
Tissue perfusion, altered: (specify)

EGO INTEGRITY
Adjustment, impaired
*Anxiety [specify]
Coping, defensive
Coping, ineffective individual
Decisional conflict (specify)
Denial, ineffective
Fear
Grieving, anticipatory
Grieving, dysfunctional
Hopelessness
Post-trauma response
Powerlessness
Rape trauma syndrome
Self-concept, disturbance in: body image; personal identity; role performance; self-esteem
 Self-esteem, chronic low
 †Self-esteem, disturbance in
 Self-esteem, situational low
Spiritual distress (distress of the human spirit)

ELIMINATION
Bowel elimination, altered: constipation
 Constipation, colonic
 Constipation, perceived
Bowel elimination, altered: diarrhea
Bowel elimination, altered: incontinence
Incontinence, functional
Incontinence, reflex
Incontinence, stress
Incontinence, total
Incontinence, urge
Urinary elimination: altered patterns
*Urinary retention [acute/chronic]

FOOD/FLUID
Breastfeeding, ineffective
Fluid volume, altered: excess

*Fluid volume deficit, actual 1 [regulatory failure]
*Fluid volume deficit, actual 2 [active loss]
Fluid volume deficit, potential
Nutrition, altered: less than body requirements
Nutrition, altered: more than body requirements
Nutrition, altered: potential for more than body requirements
Oral mucous membranes, altered
Swallowing, impaired

HYGIENE

Self-care deficit: feeding; bathing/hygiene; dressing/grooming; toileting

NEUROSENSORY

Neglect, unilateral
Sensory-perceptual alteration: visual; auditory; kinesthetic; gustatory; tactile; olfactory
Thought processes, altered

PAIN/COMFORT

Comfort, altered: pain, acute
Comfort, altered: pain, chronic

RESPIRATION

Airway clearance, ineffective
Aspiration, potential for
Breathing pattern, ineffective
Gas exchange, impaired

SAFETY

Body temperature, potential altered
Health maintenance, altered
Home maintenance management, impaired
Hyperthermia
†Hypothermia
Infection, potential for
Injury, potential for: poisoning; suffocation; trauma
Mobility, impaired physical
Skin integrity, impaired: actual
Skin integrity, impaired: potential
Thermoregulation, ineffective
Tissue integrity, impaired
Violence, potential for: directed at self/others

SEXUALITY (Component of Social Interaction)

Sexual dysfunction
Sexuality patterns, altered

SOCIAL INTERACTION

Communication, impaired: verbal
Coping, family: potential for growth
Coping, ineffective family: compromised
Coping, ineffective family: disabling
Family process, altered
Parental role conflict
Parenting, altered: actual or potential
Self-concept, disturbance in: role performance
Social interaction, impaired
Social isolation

TEACHING/LEARNING
Growth and development, altered
Health seeking behaviors (specify)
*Knowledge deficit [learning need] (specify)
*Noncompliance [compliance, altered] (specify)

*Information that appears in brackets has been added by the authors to clarify and enhance the use of
nursing diagnoses.
†Revised.

MEDICAL/SURGICAL ASSESSMENT TOOL

This is a suggested guide/tool for development by an individual/institution to create a data base reflecting Diagnostic Divisions of Nursing Diagnoses. Although the divisions are alphabetized for ease of presentation, they can be prioritized or rearranged to meet individual needs.

Name: _____

Age: _____ DOB: _____ Sex: _____ Race: _____

Admission date: _____ Time: _____ From: _____

Source of information: _____ Reliability (1–4): _____

Family member/Significant other: _____

ACTIVITY/REST

Reports (Subjective)

Occupation: _____ Usual activities/Hobbies: _____

Leisure time activities: _____

Complaints of boredom: _____

Limitations imposed by condition: _____

Sleep: Hours: _____ Naps: _____ Aids: _____

    Insomnia: _____ Related to: _____

    Rested upon awakening: _____

Exhibits (Objective)

Observed response to activity: Cardiovascular: _____

                   Respiratory: _____

Mental status (i.e., withdrawn/lethargic): _____

Neuromuscular assessment:

    Muscle mass/tone: _____

    Posture: _____ Tremors: _____

    ROM: _____ Strength: _____

    Deformity: _____ Other: _____

CIRCULATION

Reports (Subjective)

History of: Hypertension: _____ Heart trouble: _____

       Rheumatic fever: _____ Ankle/leg edema: _____

       Phlebitis: _____ Slow healing: _____

       Claudication: _____ Other: _____

Extremities: Numbness: _____ Tingling: _____

Cough/hemoptysis: _____

Change in frequency/amount of urine: _____

Exhibits (Objective)

BP: R: Lying: _____ Sitting: _____ Standing: _____

    L: Lying: _____ Sitting: _____ Standing: _____

    Pulse pressure: _____ Auscultatory gap: _____

Pulse (palpation): Carotid: _____ Temporal: _____

            Jugular: _____ Radial: _____

            Femoral: _____ Popliteal: _____

            Post Tibial: _____ Dorsalis pedis: _____

Cardiac (palpation): PMI: _____

    Thrill: _____ Heaves: _____

Heart sounds: Rate: _____ Rhythm: _____ Quality: _____

Friction rub: _____ Murmur: _____
Breath sounds: _____
Vascular bruit: (specify): _____
Jugular vein distention: _____
Extremities: Temperature: _____ Color: _____
    Capillary refill: _____
    Homan's sign: _____ Varicosities: _____
    Nails (describe abnormalities): _____
    Distribution/quality of hair: _____
Color/cyanosis: Overall: _____ Mucous membranes: _____ Lips: _____
    Nail beds: _____ Conjunctiva: _____ Sclera: _____

EGO INTEGRITY

Reports (Subjective)

Report of stress factors: _____
Ways of handling stress: _____
Financial concerns: _____
Relationship status: _____
Cultural factors: _____
Religion: _____ Practicing: _____
Lifestyle: _____ Recent changes: _____
Feelings of: Helplessness: _____ Hopelessness: _____
    Powerlessness: _____

Exhibits (Objective)

Emotional status (check those that apply):
    Calm: _____ Anxious: _____ Angry: _____
    Withdrawn: _____ Fearful: _____ Irritable: _____
    Restive: _____ Euphoric: _____ Other (specify): _____
Observed physiologic response(s): _____

ELIMINATION

Reports (Subjective)

Usual bowel pattern: _____ Laxative use: _____
Character of stool: _____ Last BM: _____
History of bleeding: _____ Hemorrhoids: _____
Constipation: _____ Diarrhea: _____
Usual voiding pattern: _____ Incontinence: _____ When: _____
    Urgency: _____ Frequency: _____ Retention: _____
Character of urine: _____
Pain/burning/difficulty voiding: _____
History of kidney/bladder disease: _____

Exhibits (Objective)

Abdomen: Tender: _____ Soft/Firm: _____
    Palpable mass: _____ Size/girth: _____
    Bowel sounds: _____
Hemorrhoids (per rectal exam): Internal: _____ External: _____
Bladder palpable: _____ Overflow voiding: _____

FOOD/FLUID

Reports (Subjective)

Usual diet (type): _____ No. meals daily: _____
Last meal/intake: _____ Dietary pattern: _____

Loss of appetite: _____ Nausea/vomiting: _____

Heartburn/indigestion: _____ Related to: _____ Relieved by: _____

Allergy/Food intolerance: _____

Mastication/swallowing problems: _____

    Dentures: Upper: _____ Lower: _____

Usual weight: _____ Changes in weight: _____

Use of diuretics: _____

Exhibits (Objective)

Current weight: _____ Height: _____ Body build: _____

Skin turgor: _____ Mucous membranes moist/dry: _____

Hernia/masses: _____

Edema: General: _____ Dependent: _____

      Periorbital: _____ Ascites: _____

Jugular vein distention: _____

Thyroid enlarged: _____ Halitosis: _____

Condition of teeth/gums: _____

Appearance of tongue: _____

    Mucous membranes: _____

Bowel sounds (previously assessed): _____

Breath sounds (previously assessed): _____

Urine S/A or Chemstix: _____

HYGIENE

Reports (Subjective)

Activities of daily living: Independent: _____

    Dependent (specify): Mobility: _____ Feeding: _____

              Hygiene: _____ Dressing: _____

              Toileting: _____ Other: _____

    Equipment/prosthetic devices required: _____

    Assistance provided by: _____

    Preferred time of bath: _____ AM _____ PM

Exhibits (Objective)

General appearance: _____

Manner of dress: _____ Personal habits: _____

Body odor: _____ Condition of scalp: _____

Presence of vermin: _____

NEUROSENSORY

Reports (Subjective)

Fainting spells/dizziness: _____

Headaches: Location: _____ Frequency: _____

Tingling/Numbness/Weakness (location): _____

Stroke (residual effects): _____

Seizures: _____ Aura: _____ How controlled: _____

Eyes: Vision loss: R: _____ L: _____

    Glaucoma: _____ Cataract: _____

Ears: Hearing loss: R: _____ L: _____

Nose: Epistaxis: _____ Sense of smell: _____

Exhibits (Objective)

Mental status:

    Oriented/disoriented: Time: _____

Place: _____

Person: _____

Alert: _____ Drowsy: _____ Lethargic: _____

Stuporous: _____ Comatose: _____ Other: _____

Cooperative: _____ Combative: _____ Delusions: _____

Hallucinations: _____ Affect (describe): _____

Memory: Recent: _____ Remote: _____

Speech pattern: _____ Content: _____

Word choice: _____ Congruence: _____

Glasses: _____ Contacts: _____ Hearing Aids: _____

Pupil size/reaction: R: _____ L: _____

Facial droop: _____ Swallowing: _____

Handgrip/release: R: _____ L: _____ Posturing: _____

Deep tendon reflexes: _____ Paralysis: _____

PAIN/COMFORT

Reports (Subjective)

Location: _____ Intensity (1–10): _____ Frequency: _____

Quality: _____ Duration: _____ Radiation: _____

Precipitating factors: _____

How relieved: _____

Exhibits (Objective)

Facial grimacing: _____ Guarding affected area: _____

Emotional response: _____ Narrowed focus: _____

RESPIRATION

Reports (Subjective)

Dyspnea (related to): _____

Cough/sputum: _____

History of Bronchitis: _____ Asthma: _____

Tuberculosis: _____ Emphysema: _____

Recurrent pneumonia: _____ Other: _____

Exposure to noxious fumes: _____

Smoker: _____ Packs/day: _____ Number of years: _____

Use of respiratory aids: _____ Oxygen: _____

Exhibits (Objective)

Respiratory: Rate: _____ Depth: _____ Symmetry: _____

Use of accessory muscles: _____ Nasal flaring: _____

Fremitis: _____

Breath sounds: _____

Egophony: _____

Cyanosis: _____ Clubbing of fingers: _____

Sputum characteristics: _____

Mentation/restlessness: _____

Other: _____

SAFETY

Reports (Subjective)

Allergies/Sensitivity: _____ Reaction: _____

Previous alteration of immune system: _____ Cause: _____

History of sexually transmitted disease (date/type): _____

Blood transfusion: _____ When: _____
      Reaction (describe): _____
History of accidental injuries: _____
Fractures/dislocations: _____
Arthritis/Unstable joints: _____
Back problems: _____
Changes in moles: _____ Enlarged nodes: _____
Impaired: Vision: _____ Hearing: _____
Prosthesis: _____ Ambulatory devices: _____
Expressions of ideation of violence (self/others): _____

Exhibits (Objective)

Temperature: _____ Diaphoresis: _____
Skin integrity: _____
    Scars: _____ Rashes: _____
    Lacerations: _____ Ulcerations: _____
    Ecchymosis: _____ Blisters: _____
    Burns (degree/percent): _____
Mark location of above on diagram:

General strength: _____ Muscle tone: _____
    Gait: _____ ROM: _____
    Paresthesia/Paralysis: _____

SEXUALITY

Sexual concerns: _____

Female

Reports (Subjective)

Age at menarche: _____ Length of cycle: _____ Duration: _____
Last menstrual period: _____ Menopause: _____
Vaginal discharge: _____ Bleeding between periods: _____
Practices breast self-exam: _____ Last PAP smear: _____
Method of birth control: _____

Exhibits (Objective)

Breast exam: _____
Vaginal warts/lesions: _____

Male

Reports (Subjective)

Penile discharge: _____ Prostate disorder: _____

Vasectomy: _____ Use of condoms: _____
Practices self-exam: Breast: _____ Testicles: _____
Last proctoscopic exam: _____ Last prostate exam: _____

Exhibits (Objective)

Exam: Breast: _____ Testicles: _____

SOCIAL INTERACTION

Reports (Subjective)

Marital status: _____ Years in relationship: _____
   Living with: _____
   Concerns/Stresses: _____
Extended family: _____
Other support person(s): _____
Role within family structure: _____
Report of problems related to illness/condition: _____
Coping behaviors: _____
Do others depend on you for assistance? _____
   How are they managing? _____
Frequency of social contacts (other than work): _____

Exhibits (Objective)

Speech: Clear: _____ Slurred: _____
   Unintelligible: _____ Aphasic: _____
   Unusual speech pattern/impairment: _____
   Laryngectomy: _____ Speech aids: _____
Verbal/nonverbal communication with family/SO(s): _____
_____
Family interaction (behavioral) pattern: _____

TEACHING/LEARNING

Reports (Subjective)

Dominant language (specify): _____
Education level: _____
Learning disabilities (specify): _____
Cognitive limitations (specify): _____
Health beliefs/practices: _____
Special health care practices: _____
Familial risk factors (indicate relationship):
   Diabetes: _____ Tuberculosis: _____
   Heart disease: _____ Strokes: _____
   High BP: _____ Epilepsy: _____
   Kidney disease: _____ Cancer: _____
   Mental illness: _____ Other (specify): _____
Prescribed medications (circle last dose):

Drug	Dose	Times	Takes regularly	Purpose

Nonprescription drugs: OTC: _____
   Street drugs: _____ Smokeless tobacco: _____
Use of alcohol (amount/frequency): _____
Admitting diagnosis (physician): _____
Reason for hospitalization (patient): _____
History of current complaint: _____

Patient expectations of this hospitalization: _____

Previous illnesses and/or hospitalizations/surgeries: _____
_____

Evidence of failure to improve: _____

Last complete physical exam: _____ By: _____

Discharge Plan Considerations

Date data obtained: _____

1. Anticipated date of discharge: _____
2. Resources available: Persons: _____
   Financial: _____
3. Do you anticipate changes in your living situation after discharge? _____
4. If Yes: Areas that may require alteration/assistance:

   Food preparation: _____ Shopping: _____

   Transportation: _____ Ambulation: _____

   Medication/IV therapy: _____ Treatments: _____

   Wound care: _____ Supplies: _____

   Self-care assistance (specify): _____

   Physical layout of home (specify): _____

   Homemaker assistance (specify): _____

   Living facility other than home (specify): _____

PATIENT SITUATION: Diabetes Mellitus

Mr. R.S., non-insulin-dependent diabetic (NIDDM) for 5 years, presented to his physician's office with a nonhealing ulcer of 3 weeks' duration on his left foot. Laboratory studies at the doctor's office revealed blood sugar level per Chemstix >250 and urine Clinitest of 1%/small.

ADMITTING PHYSICIAN'S ORDERS

Culture/sensitivity and Gram stain of foot ulcer.
Random blood sugar on admission and fasting blood sugar every AM.
CBC, electrolytes, glycosylated Hb in AM.
Chest x-ray and ECG in AM.
NPH insulin 15 U q AM; begin insulin instruction for self-care after discharge.
Dicloxacillin 500 mg PO, q 6 hr, start after culture obtained.
Darvon 65 mg q 4 hr p.r.n., pain.
Diet—1800 cal ADA/3 meals with 2 snacks.
Up in chair ad lib with feet elevated.
Foot cradle for bed.
Betadine soak L foot t.i.d. × 15 min, then cover with dry sterile dressing.
Urine sugar/acetone a.c. and h.s.
Vital signs q.i.d.

PATIENT ASSESSMENT DATA BASE

Name: R.S.   Informant: Patient.   Reliability (1–4): 3+.
Age: 64.   DOB: 5/3/23.   Race: Caucasian.   Sex: M.
Admission date: 6/28/87.   Time: 7 PM.   From: Home.

ACTIVITY/REST

Reports:
Occupation: Farmer.
Usual activities/hobbies: Reading, playing cards. "Don't have time to do much. Anyway, I'm too tired most of the time to do anything after the chores."
Limitations imposed by illness: "Have to watch what I order in restaurants."
Sleep: Hours: 6–8 hr/night.   Naps: No.   Aids: No.   Insomnia: "Not unless I drink coffee after supper."   Feels rested when awakens at 4:30 AM.

Exhibits:
Observed response to activity: Favors L foot when walking.
Cardiovascular: 0.   Respiratory: 0.
Mental status: Alert/active.
Neuromuscular assessment: Muscle mass/tone: bilaterally equal/firm.
Posture: erect.   Tremors: 0.   ROM: Full.   Deformity: 0.
Strength: Equal 3 extremities/favors L leg currently.

CIRCULATION

Reports:
History of elevated BP: 0.   Heart trouble: 0.
Ankle edema: 0.   Claudication: 0.   Phlebitis: 0.
Slow healing: Lesion L foot, 3 weeks.
Extremities: Numbness/tingling: "My feet feel cold and tingling when I walk a lot."
Cough/character of sputum: Occasional/white.
Change in frequency/amount of urine: Yes, voiding more lately.

| **Exhibits:** | Peripheral pulses: Radials 3+, popliteal, dorsalis, posttibial-pedal, all 1+. |

Exhibits: Peripheral pulses: Radials 3+, popliteal, dorsalis, posttibial-pedal, all 1+.

BP: R: Lying: 146/90.   Sit: 140/86.   Stand: 138/90.
      L: Lying: 142/88.   Sit: 138/88.   Stand: 138/84.

Pulse: Apical: 86.   Radial: 86.   Quality: Strong.   Rhythm: Regular.

Chest auscultation: Few rhonchi clear with cough, no murmurs/rubs.

Jugular vein distention: 0.

Extremities: Temperature: Feet cool bilat/remainder warm.   Color: Skin: Legs pale.   Capillary refill: Slow both feet.   Homans' sign: 0.   Varicosities: Few enlarged superficial veins both calves.   Nails: Toenails thickened, yellow, brittle.   Distribution and quality of hair: Coarse hair to ankles, none on toes.

Color: General: Ruddy. Mucous membranes/lips: Pink.

Nail beds: Blanch well. Conjunctiva and sclera: White.

EGO INTEGRITY

Reports: Report of stress factors: "Normal farmer's problems, weather, pests, bankers, etc."

Ways of handling stress: "I get busy with the chores and talk things over with my livestock; they listen real good."

Financial concerns: No insurance/needs to hire someone while here.

Relationship status: Married.

Cultural factors: Rural/agrarian.

Religion: Protestant/practicing.

Lifestyle: Middle-class/self-sufficient farmer.   Recent changes: 0.

Feelings: "I'm in control of most things, except the weather and this diabetes."

Exhibits: Emotional status: Calm.

Other: Concerned re possible therapy change "from pills to shots."

Observed physiologic response(s): Occasionally sighs deeply/frowns, shrugs shoulders.

ELIMINATION

Reports: Usual bowel pattern: Most every PM.

Last BM: Last night.   Character of stool: Firm/brown.

Bleeding: 0.   Hemorrhoids: 0.   Diarrhea: 0.   Constipation: Occasional.

Laxative used: Hot prune juice.

Pain/burning/difficulty with urination: 0.

Incontinence: 0.   Character of urine: Pale yellow.

Kidney/bladder disease: 0.

Exhibits: Abdomen tender: No.   Soft/Firm: Soft.   Palpable mass: None. Size/girth: Deferred.   Bowel sounds: Active all 4 quadrants.

Hemorrhoids: Deferred.   Palpate bladder: Not palpable.

FOOD/FLUID

Reports: Usual diet (type): 1800 ADA (occasionally "cheats" with dessert, "but my wife watches it pretty closely"). Number of meals daily: 3.

Dietary pattern: B: Fruit juice/toast/ham/coffee.   L: Meat/potatoes/veg/fruit/milk.   D: Meat sandwich/soup/fruit/coffee.   Snack: Milk/crackers at HS. Usual beverage: skim milk, 2–3 cups decaffeinated coffee, and drinks a *lot* of water.

Last meal/intake: Dinner: Roast beef sandwich, vegetable soup, pear, decaf.

Loss of appetite: "Never, but lately I don't feel as hungry as usual."

Nausea/vomiting: 0.   Food allergies: None.

Heartburn/food intolerance: Cabbage causes gas.

Mastication/swallowing probs: No.   Dentures: Upper, partial.

Usual weight: 175 lb.

Recent changes: Has lost about 3 lb this month.

Diuretic therapy: No.

Exhibits: Weight: 171 lb.   Ht: 5 ft 10 in.   Build: Stocky.   Skin turgor: Good/leathery.

Edema: 0.   Jugular distention: 0.

Appearance of tongue: Midline, pink.   Mucous membranes: Pink, intact.

Halitosis: 0.   Condition of teeth/gums: Good, "no problem with bleeding."

Breath sounds: Few rhonchi cleared with cough.

Bowel sounds: Active all 4 quadrants.

Urine Chemstix: 1%/small.

HYGIENE

Reports: Activities of daily living: Independent in all areas.

Preferred time of bath: PM.

Exhibits: General appearance: Clean, shaven, short cut hair.

Hands rough and dry.   Scalp and eyebrows: Scaly white patches.

NEUROSENSORY

Reports: Fainting spells/dizziness: 0.

Headache: "Occasionally behind my eyes when I worry too much."

Weakness: 0.   Stroke: 0.   Seizures: 0.

Tingling/numbness: Feet, occasionally.

Eyes: Vision loss, far-sighted; exam 2 years ago.   Glaucoma: 0.   Cataract: 0.

Ears: Hearing loss: R: "Some."   L: No (has not been tested).

Nose: Epistaxis: 0.   Sense of smell: States no problem.

Exhibits: Mental status: Alert, oriented to time, place, person.   Affect: Concerned.

Memory: Remote and recent: Clear and intact.

Speech: Clear/coherent.

Pupil reaction: PERLA.   Glasses: Reading.   Hearing aid: No.

Handgrip/release: Strong/equal.

PAIN/DISCOMFORT

Reports: Location: L foot.   Intensity: 6½.   Quality: Dull ache.

Frequency/duration: "Seems like all the time."   Radiation: No.

Precipitating factors: Shoes, walking.   How relieved: ASA, not helping.

Other complaints: Sometimes has back pain following chores/heavy lifting relieved by ASA/liniment.

Exhibits: Facial grimacing: When lesion border palpated.

Guarding affected area: Pulls foot away.   Narrowed focus: No.

Emotional response: Tense, irritated.

RESPIRATION

Reports: Dyspnea: 0.   Cough: Occasional morning cough, white sputum.

Emphysema: 0.   Bronchitis: 0.   Asthma: 0.   Tuberculosis: 0.

Smoker: Filters.   Pack/day: ½.   Number of years: 40 + .

Use of respiratory aids: 0.

Exhibits: Respiratory rate: 22.   Depth: Good.   Symmetry: Equal, bilateral.

Use of accessory muscles: 0.   Nasal flaring: 0.

Auscultation: Few rhonchi, clear with cough.

Cyanosis: 0.   Clubbing of fingers: 0.

Sputum characteristics: None at present.

Mentation/restlessness: Alert/oriented/relaxed.

SAFETY

Reports: Allergies: 0.   Blood transfusions: 0.

Previous alteration of immune system: 0.

Sexually Transmitted Disease: None.

Fractures/dislocations: L clavicle, 1962, fell getting off tractor.

Arthritis/unstable joints: "Think I've got some in my knees."

Back problems: Occasional lower back pain.

Enlarged nodes: 0.   Changes in moles: 0.

Vision impaired: Requires glasses for reading.

Hearing impaired: Slightly, compensates by turning "good ear" toward speaker.

Prostheses: 0.   Ambulatory devices: 0.

Exhibits: Temperature: 99.4 oral.

Skin integrity: Impaired L foot.   Scars: R Ing, surgical.

Rashes: 0.   Bruises: 0.   Lacerations: 0.   Blisters: 0.

Ulcerations: Medial aspect L foot, 2.5 cm diameter, approximately 0.5 cm deep, draining small amount cream color/pink-tinged matter, no odor noted.

Strength (general): Equal all extremities.   Muscle tone: firm.

ROM: Good.   Gait: Favors L foot.   Paresthesia/Paralysis: 0.

SEXUALITY (Male)

Reports: Penile discharge: 0.   Prostate disorder: 0.   Vasectomy: 0.

Last proctoscopic exam: 2 years ago.   Prostate exam: 1 year ago.

Practice self-exam: Breast/testicles: No.

Problems/complaints: "I don't have any problems, but you'd have to ask my wife if there are any complaints."

Exhibits: Exam: Breast: No masses.   Testicles: Deferred.   Prostate: Deferred.

SOCIAL INTERACTION

Reports: Marital status: Married 40 years.   Living with: Wife.

Report of problems: None.

Extended family: 1 daughter lives in town (30 miles away); 1 daughter, married/grandson, living out of state.

Other: Several couples, he and wife play cards/socialize with 2 or 3 times a month.

Role: Works farm alone, husband/father/grandfather.

Report of problems related to illness/condition: None until now.

Coping behaviors: "My wife and I have always talked things out. You know the Eleventh Commandment is Thou shalt not go to bed angry."

Exhibits: Speech: Clear, intelligible.

Verbal/nonverbal communication with family/SO(s): Speaks quietly with wife, looking her in the eye with a slight smile.

Family interaction patterns: Wife sitting at bedside, relaxed, both reading paper, making occasional comments to each other.

TEACHING/LEARNING

Reports:

Dominant language: English.   Education level: 2 years college.

Health beliefs/practices: "I take care of the minor problems and only see the doctor when something's broken."

Familial risk factors/relationship:

Diabetes: Maternal uncle.   Tuberculosis: Brother, died age 27.
Heart disease: Father, died, age 78, heart attack.
Stroke: Mother died, age 81.   High BP: Mother.   Epilepsy: 0.
Kidney disease: 0.   Cancer: 0.   Mental illness: 0.

Prescribed medications:

Drug	Dose	Schedule (time/last dose)	Purpose
Orinase	250 mg	8 AM/6 PM; last dose 6 PM today	diabetes

Home glucose monitoring: "Stopped several months ago when I ran out of TesTape. It was always negative anyway."

Does patient take medications regularly? Yes.

Nonprescription (OTC) drugs: Occasionally ASA.

Use of alcohol (amount/frequency): Socially, occasionally beer.

Admitting diagnosis (physician): Hyperglycemia and L foot ulcer.

Reason for hospitalization (patient): Sore on foot and "My sugar is up."

History of current complaint: "Three weeks ago I got a blister on my foot from breaking in my new boots. It got sore so I lanced it, but it isn't getting any better."

Patient's expectations of this hospitalization? "Clear up this infection and control my diabetes."

Other relevant illness and/or previous hospitalizations/surgeries: 1965 R inguinal hernia repair.

Evidence of failure to improve: lesion L foot, 3 weeks.

Last physical exam: complete 1 year ago, office follow-up 3 months ago.

Discharge Plan Considerations (as of 6/28):

Anticipated discharge: 7/1/88 (3 days).

Resources: Person: Wife.   Financial: "If this doesn't take too long to heal, we got some savings to cover things."

Anticipated lifestyle changes: None.

Assistance needed: May require farm help for several days.

SAMPLE NURSING CARE PLAN: Diabetes Mellitus

PATIENT PROBLEM STATEMENT:	SKIN INTEGRITY, IMPAIRED: ACTUAL, related to pressure, altered metabolic state, circulatory impairment and decreased sensation evidenced by draining wound left foot.
PATIENT OUTCOMES/ GOALS:	Correction of metabolic state as evidenced by blood sugar within normal limits within 36 hours. Wound free of purulent drainage and wound edges clean/pink within 60 hours.

ACTIONS/INTERVENTIONS	RATIONALE
Obtain culture of wound drainage.	To identify pathogens and therapy of choice.
Administer dicloxacillin 500 mg PO starting 10 PM. Observe for signs of hypersensitivity, i.e., pruritis, urticaria, rash.	Treatment of infection/prevention of complications. Food interferes with drug absorption, which requires scheduling around meals. Although no prior history of penicillin reaction, it may occur at any time.
Soak foot in room temperature sterile water with betadine solution t.i.d. for 15 minutes. Dress wound with dry sterile dressing; use paper tape.	Local germicidal effective for surface wounds. Keeps wound clean/minimize cross-contamination. Adhesive tape may be abrasive to fragile tissues.
Administer 15 units NPH insulin SC q AM after daily laboratory sample drawn.	Treats underlying disease state, reducing hyperglycemia and promoting healing.

PATIENT PROBLEM STATEMENT:	COMFORT, ALTERED: PAIN, ACUTE, related to physical agent (wound left foot), evidenced by verbal complaint of discomfort, guarding behavior, and facial grimace.
PATIENT OUTCOMES/ GOALS:	Reports pain is minimized/relieved within 48 hours. Ambulating normally, full weight bearing by discharge.

ACTIONS/INTERVENTIONS	RATIONALE
Determine pain characteristics through patient's description.	Establishes baseline for assessing improvement/ changes.
Place foot cradle on bed/encourage use of loose-fitting slipper when up.	Avoids direct pressure to area of injury which could result in vasoconstriction/increased pain.
Administer Darvon 65 mg PO every 4 hours as needed. Document effectiveness.	Provides relief of discomfort when unrelieved by other measures.

PATIENT PROBLEM STATEMENT:	TISSUE PERFUSION, ALTERED: lower extremities related to decreased arterial flow evidenced by decreased pulses and hair growth, pale/cool feet, thick brittle nails, numbness/tingling of feet when walks "a lot."
PATIENT OUTCOMES/ GOALS:	Verbalizes understanding of relationship between chronic disease (diabetes mellitus) and circulatory

ACTIONS/INTERVENTIONS

Elevate feet when up in chair. Avoid long periods with feet dependent.

Assess for signs of dehydration. Monitor intake/output. Encourage oral fluids.

Instruct client to avoid constricting clothing/socks and ill fitting shoes.

Reinforce safety precautions re use of heating pads, hot water bottles/soaks.

Discuss complications of disease that result in vascular changes, i.e., ulceration, gangrene, muscle or bony structure changes.

Review proper foot care as outlined in ND: Knowledge Deficit.

RATIONALE

Maximizes blood flow, reduces venous pooling.

Glycosuria may result in dehydration, reducing circulating volume, and further alteration of peripheral perfusion.

Compromised circulation and decreased pain sensation may precipitate or aggravate tissue breakdown.

Heat increases metabolic demands on compromised tissues. Vascular insufficiency alters pain sensation, increasing risk of tissue injury.

Proper control of diabetes mellitus may not prevent complications but may minimize severity of effect.

Altered perfusion of lower extremities may lead to serious/persistent complications at the cellular level.

PATIENT PROBLEM STATEMENT:

KNOWLEDGE DEFICIT, related to misinterpretation of information and/or lack of recall evidenced by inaccurate follow-through of instructions regarding home glucose monitoring and foot care, and failure to recognize signs/symptoms of hyperglycemia.

PATIENT OUTCOMES/ GOALS:

Verbalizes basic understanding of disease process and treatment within 48 hours. Correctly performs procedure of home glucose monitoring and insulin administration, and explains reasons for actions within 72 hours.

ACTIONS/INTERVENTIONS

Determine patient's level of knowledge, priorities of learning needs, desire/need for including wife in instruction.

Provide teaching guide, "Understanding your Diabetes" 6/29 AM. Show film "Diabetes and You" 6/29 4 PM when wife is visiting. Include in group teaching session 6/30 AM. Review information and obtain feedback from patient and wife.

Discuss factors related to/altering diabetes control, e.g., stress, illness, exercise.

Review signs/symptoms of hyperglycemia, e.g., fatigue, nausea/vomiting, polyuria/polydipsia; discuss prevention and evaluation of situation and when to seek medical care. Have patient identify appropriate interventions.

RATIONALE

Establishes baseline and direction for teaching/planning. Involvement of wife, if desires, will provide additional resource for recall/understanding and may enhance follow-through.

Provides different methods for accessing/reinforcing information and enhances opportunity for learning/understanding.

Drug therapy/diet may require alteration in response to short- and long-term stressors.

Recognition/understanding of these signs/symptoms and timely intervention will aid patient in avoiding recurrences and preventing complications.

ACTIONS/INTERVENTIONS	RATIONALE
Review and provide information about routine examination of feet and proper foot care, e.g.: daily inspection for injuries, pressure areas, corns, calluses; proper nail cutting; daily washing; avoiding going barefoot; wearing loose-fitting socks, properly fitting shoes (breaking in new shoes gradually); if foot injury/skin break occurs, washing with soap/water and covering with sterile dressing, inspecting wound and change dressing daily, and reporting redness, swelling, or presence of drainage.	Reduces risk of tissue injury, promotes understanding and prevention of stasis ulcer formations and wound healing difficulties.
Instruct regarding prescribed insulin therapy:	May be a temporary treatment of hyperglycemia with infection, or may be permanent replacement of Orinase.
NPH insulin, SC	Intermediate-acting insulin generally lasts 18–24 hours, with peak effect 6–12 hours.
Keep vial in current use at room temperature; store extra in refrigerator.	Refrigeration prevents wide fluctuations in temperature, prolonging the drug shelf life but possibly impeding absorption.
Roll bottle and invert to mix (solution is milky). Do not shake vigorously.	Vigorous shaking may create foam, which can interfere with accurate dose withdrawal and may damage the insulin molecule.
Rotate injection sites/provide diagram.	Minimizes tissue damage and improves absorption of medication.
Demonstrate, then observe patient in drawing insulin into syringe, reading syringe markings, and administering dose. Assess for accuracy.	May require numerous instruction sessions and practice before patient and wife feel comfortable drawing up and injecting medication.
Instruct in signs/symptoms of insulin reaction/hypoglycemia, i.e., fatigue, nausea, headache, hunger, sweating, irritability, shakiness, anxiety, difficulty concentrating.	Knowing what to watch for and appropriate treatment, such as grape juice for immediate response or cheese for a sustained effect, may prevent/minimize complications and enhance diabetic control.
Review "Sick Day Rules," e.g., call the doctor if too sick to eat normally/stay active; take insulin as ordered; keep record as noted on Sick Day Guide.	Reminder of necessary actions in the event of mild/severe illness to reduce risk of hyper/hypoglycemia.
Encourage patient to maintain record of urine testing, insulin dosage/site, unusual physiologic response, dietary intake.	Provides accurate record for review by care givers for assessment of therapy effectiveness.
Refer to dietitian for revision of diet.	Calories are unchanged but have been redistributed to 3 meals and 2 snacks.
Discuss other health care issues, e.g., smoking habits, self-monitoring for cancer (breasts/testicles), and reporting changes in general well-being.	Encourages patient involvement, awareness, and responsibility for own health; promotes wellness.

CHAPTER 4
CARDIOVASCULAR

Hypertension: Severe _____

Hypertension is defined by the World Health Organization as blood pressure greater than 160/95 mmHg and is classified according to the degree of severity, ranging from high normal blood pressure to malignant hypertension. It is categorized as primary/essential (constituting approximately 90% of all cases) or secondary, occurring as a result of an identifiable, often correctable pathologic condition.

PATIENT ASSESSMENT DATA BASE

ACTIVITY/REST

May report: Weakness, fatigue, shortness of breath.

May exhibit: Elevated heart rate.

Change in heart rhythm.

Tachypnea.

CIRCULATION

May report: History of hypertension, atherosclerosis, valvular/coronary artery heart disease and cerebrovascular disease.

Episodes of palpitations, perspiration.

May exhibit: Blood pressure elevated (serial elevated measurements are necessary to confirm diagnosis).

Postural hypotension (may be related to drug regimen).

Pulse: bounding carotid, jugular, radial pulsations; pulse disparities, e.g., femoral delay as compared with radial or brachial pulsation; absence of/diminished popliteal, posterior tibial, pedal pulses.

Apical pulse: PMI possibly displaced and/or forceful.

Rate/rhythm: tachycardia, various dysrhythmias.

Heart sounds: accentuated S_2 at base, S_3 (early CHF), S_4 (rigid left ventricle/left ventricular hypertrophy).

Murmurs of valvular stenosis.

Vascular bruits audible over carotid, femoral, or epigastrium (artery stenosis).

Jugular vein distention (venous congestion).

Extremities: discoloration of skin, cool temperature (peripheral vasoconstriction); capillary refill possibly slow/delayed (vasoconstriction).

Skin: pallor, cyanosis, and diaphoresis (congestion, hypoxemia); flushing (pheochromocytoma).

EGO INTEGRITY

May report:
History of personality changes, anxiety, depression, euphoria, or chronic anger (may indicate cerebral impairment).

Multiple stress factors (relationship, financial, job-related).

May exhibit:
Mood swings, restlessness, narrowed attention span, outbursts of crying.

Emphatic hand gestures, tense facial muscles, particularly around the eyes, quick physical movement, expiratory sighs, accelerated speech pattern.

ELIMINATION

May report:
Past or present renal insult (e.g., infection/obstruction or past history of kidney disease).

FOOD/FLUID

May report:
Food preferences which may include high-salt, high-fat, high-cholesterol foods (e.g., fried foods, cheese, eggs); licorice; high caloric content.

Nausea, vomiting.

Recent weight changes (gain/loss).

History of diuretic use.

May exhibit:
Normal weight or obesity.

Presence of edema (may be generalized or dependent).

Venous congestion, jugular venous distention.

Glycosuria (almost 10% of hypertensive clients are diabetic).

NEUROSENSORY

May report:
Fainting spells/dizziness.

Throbbing, suboccipital headaches (present on awakening and disappearing spontaneously after several hours).

Episodes of numbness and/or weakness on one side of the body.

Visual disturbances (diplopia, blurred vision).

Episodes of epistaxis.

May exhibit:
Mental status changes: alertness, orientation, speech pattern/content, inappropriate affect, thought process, or memory.

Motor responses: hand grip, decreased deep tendon reflexes.

Optic fundi: examination of retinal changes: from mild sclerosis/arterial narrowing to marked retinal and sclerotic changes with edema or papilledema exudates, hemorrhages dependent on degree/duration of hypertension.

PAIN/DISCOMFORT

May report:
Angina (coronary artery disease/cardiac involvement).

Intermittent pain in legs/claudication (indicative of arteriosclerosis of lower extremity arteries).

Severe occipital headaches as previously noted.

Abdominal pain/masses (pheochromocytoma).

RESPIRATION

(Generally associated with advanced cardiopulmonary effects of sustained/severe hypertension.)

May report: Dyspnea related to activity/exertion.

         Tachypnea, orthopnea, paroxysmal nocturnal dyspnea.

         Cough with/without sputum production.

         Smoking history.

May exhibit: Respiratory distress/use of accessory muscles.

         Adventitious breath sounds (crackles/wheezes).

         Cyanosis.

SAFETY

May report: Impaired coordination/gait.

         Transient episodes of unilateral paresthesia.

         Postural hypotension.

         Use of oral contraceptives.

TEACHING/LEARNING

May report: Familial risk factors: hypertension, atherosclerosis, heart disease, diabetes mellitus, cerebrovascular/kidney disease.

         Ethnic/racial risk factors, e.g., Afro-American, Southeast Asian.

         Factors that may contribute to progression of hypertension and end/organ complications, e.g., excess salt intake, use of birth control pills or other hormones, smoking, obesity, drug/alcohol use, sedentary lifestyle.

Discharge Plan Considerations: Self-care assistance.

         Self-monitoring of blood pressure.

         Alterations in medication therapy.

DIAGNOSTIC STUDIES

Hemoglobin/hematocrit: not diagnostic but assesses relationship of cells to fluid volume (viscosity), and may indicate risk factors such as hypercoagulability, anemia.

BUN/creatinine: provides information about renal perfusion/function.

Glucose: hyperglycemia (diabetes mellitus is a precipitator of hypertension) may result from elevated catecholamine levels (increases hypertension).

Serum potassium: hypokalemia may indicate the presence of primary aldosteronism (cause) or be a side effect of diuretic therapy.

Serum calcium: elevation may contribute to hypertension.

Serum cholesterol and triglycerides: elevated level may indicate predisposition for/presence of atheromatous plaquing (cardiovascular effect).

Thyroid studies: hyperthyroidism may lead/contribute to vasoconstriction and hypertension.

Serum/urine aldosterone level: to assess for primary aldosteronism (cause).

Urinalysis: blood, protein, glucose suggests renal dysfunction and/or presence of diabetes.

Urine VMA (catecholamine metabolite): elevation may indicate presence of pheochromocytoma (cause); 24-hour urine VMA may be done for assessment of pheochromocytoma if hypertension is intermittent.

Uric acid: hyperuricemia has been implicated as a risk factor for the development of hypertension.

Urine steroids: elevation may indicate hyperadrenalism, pheochromocytoma or pituitary dysfunction, Cushing's syndrome; renin levels may also be elevated.

IVP: may identify cause of hypertension, e.g., renal parenchymal disease, renal/ureteral calculi.

Chest x-ray: may demonstrate obstructing calcification in valve areas; deposits in and/or notching of aorta; cardiac enlargement.

CT scan: assesses for cerebral tumor, CVA; encephalopathy; or to rule out pheochromocytoma.

ECG: may demonstrate enlarged heart, strain patterns, conduction disturbances. Note: Broad, notched P wave is one of the earliest signs of hypertensive heart disease.

NURSING PRIORITIES

1. Maintain/enhance cardiovascular functioning.
2. Prevent complications.
3. Provide information about disease process/prognosis and treatment regimen.
4. Support active patient control of condition.

DISCHARGE CRITERIA

1. Blood pressure within acceptable limits for individual.
2. Cardiovascular and systemic complications prevented/minimized.
3. Disease process/prognosis and therapeutic regimen understood.
4. Necessary lifestyle/behavioral changes initiated.

NURSING DIAGNOSIS:	**CARDIAC OUTPUT, ALTERED: DECREASED [POTENTIAL]**
May be related to:	**Increased afterload, vasoconstriction/SVR**
	Myocardial ischemia
	Ventricular hypertrophy/rigidity
Possibly evidenced by:	**[Not applicable; presence of signs and symptoms establishes an *actual* diagnosis.]**
PATIENT OUTCOMES/ EVALUATION CRITERIA:	**Participates in activities that reduce blood pressure/ cardiac workload. Maintains blood pressure within individually acceptable range. Demonstrates stable cardiac rhythm and rate within patient's normal range.**

ACTIONS/INTERVENTIONS	RATIONALE
Independent	
Monitor blood pressure. Measure in both arms/thighs for initial evaluation. Use correct cuff size and accurate technique.	Comparison of pressures provides a more complete picture of vascular involvement/scope of problem. Severe hypertension is classified (in the adult) as a diastolic pressure elevation to 130; progressive diastolic readings above 130 are considered first accelerated, then malignant. Systolic hypertension also is an established risk factor for cerebrovascular disease and ischemic heart disease when diastolic pressure is 90–115.
Note presence, quality of central and peripheral pulses.	Bounding carotid, jugular, radial and femoral pulses may be observed/palpated. Pulses in the legs may be diminished reflecting effects of vasoconstriction (increased SVR) and venous congestion.

ACTIONS/INTERVENTIONS	RATIONALE

Independent

Auscultate heart tones and breath sounds.

S_4 is likely to be present in severely hypertensive patient as it reflects atrial hypertrophy (increased atrial volume/pressure). Development of S_3 indicates ventricular hypertrophy and impaired functioning. Presence of crackles, wheezes may indicate pulmonary congestion secondary to developing/chronic heart failure.

Observe skin color, moisture, temperature, and capillary refill time.

Presence of pallor, cool, moist skin, and delayed capillary refill time may be due to peripheral vasoconstriction or reflect cardiac decompensation/decreased output.

Note dependent/general edema.

May indicate heart failure, impaired renal function, vascular damage.

Provide calm, restful surroundings, minimize environmental activity/noise. Limit the number of visitors and length of stay.

Helps to reduce sympathetic stimulation; promotes relaxation.

Maintain activity restrictions, e.g., bed/chair rest; schedule periods of uninterrupted rest; assist patient with self-care activities as needed.

Reduces stress and tension that affects blood pressure and the course of hypertension.

Provide routine comfort measures, e.g., back and neck massage, elevation of head.

Decreases discomfort and may reduce sympathetic stimulation.

Instruct in relaxation techniques, guided imagery, distractions.

Can reduce stressful stimuli, produce a calming effect, and thereby reduce blood pressure.

Monitor response to medications to control blood pressure.

Stepped drug therapy (consisting of diuretics, sympathetic inhibitors and vasodilators) is dependent on both the individual and synergistic effects of the drugs given at the lowest possible dosage to achieve desired effect(s), thereby minimizing side effects. Because of side effects, it is important to use the fewest number and lowest dosage of medications.

Collaborative

Administer medications as indicated, e.g.:

Thiazide diuretics, e.g., chlorothiazide (Diuril), hydrochlorothiazide (Esidrix/HydroDIURIL), bendroflumethiazide (Naturetin);

Most commonly used diuretics to decrease systemic vascular resistance/blood pressure by reducing intravascular fluid volume and producing slight vasodilation. Potentiates other antihypertensive agents by limiting fluid retention.

Loop diuretics, e.g., furosemide (Lasix), ethacrynic acid (Edecrin), bumetanide (Bumex);

These drugs produce marked diuresis and are effective antihypertensives, especially in patients who are resistant to thiazides or have renal impairment.

Potassium-sparing diuretics, e.g., spironolactone (Aldactone), triamterene (Dyrenium), amiloride (Midamor);

May be given in combination with a thiazide diuretic to minimize potassium loss.

Sympathetic inhibitors, e.g., propranolol (Inderal), metoprolol (Lopressor), atenolol (Tenormin), nadolol (Corgard), methyldopa (Aldomet), reserpine (Serpasil), clonidine (Catapres);

Specific actions of these drugs vary but generally reduce blood pressure through the combined effect of decreased total peripheral resistance, reduced cardiac output, inhibited sympathetic activity and suppression of renin release.

Vasodilators, e.g., minoxidil (Loniten), hydralazine (Apresoline), prazosin (Minipress); or calcium

May be necessary to treat severe hypertension when a combination of a diuretic and a sympathetic inhibitor

33

ACTIONS/INTERVENTIONS

Collaborative

channel blockers, e.g., nifedipine (Procardia), verapamil (Calan);

Ganglion blockers, e.g., guanethidine (Ismelin), trimethaphan (Arfonad); or ACE inhibitor, e.g., captopril (Capoten).

Maintain fluid and dietary sodium restrictions as indicated.

Prepare for surgery, when indicated.

RATIONALE

have not sufficiently controlled BP. Vasodilation of healthy cardiac vasculature and increased coronary blood flow are secondary benefits of vasodilator therapy.

The use of an additional sympathetic inhibitor may be required for its cumulative effect when other measures have failed to control BP and patient cooperation with the therapeutic regimen has been verified.

These restrictions can reduce fluid retention with associated hypertensive response, thereby decreasing myocardial workload.

When hypertension is due to the presence of pheochromocytoma, removal of the tumor will correct condition.

NURSING DIAGNOSIS:	ACTIVITY INTOLERANCE
May be related to:	**Generalized weakness**
	Imbalance between oxygen supply and demand
Possibly evidenced by:	**Verbal report of fatigue or weakness**
	Abnormal heart rate or BP response to activity
	Exertional discomfort or dyspnea
	ECG changes reflecting ischemia; dysrhythmias
PATIENT OUTCOMES/ EVALUATION CRITERIA:	**Participates in necessary/desired activities. Reports a measurable increase in activity tolerance. Demonstrates a decrease in physiologic signs of intolerance.**

ACTIONS/INTERVENTIONS

Independent

Assess the patient's response to activity noting pulse rate over 20 bpm above resting rate; marked increase in BP during/after activity (systolic pressure increase of 40 mmHg or diastolic pressure increase of 20 mmHg); dyspnea or chest pain; excessive fatigue and weakness; diaphoresis; dizziness or syncope.

Instruct patient in energy-saving techniques, e.g., using chair when showering, sitting to brush teeth or comb hair, carrying out activities at a slower pace.

Encourage progressive activity/self-care when tolerated. Provide assistance as needed.

RATIONALE

The stated parameters are helpful in assessing the patient's physiologic response to the stress of activity and, if present, are indicators of overexertion associated with the activity level.

Energy-saving techniques reduce the energy expenditure, thereby assisting in equalization of oxygen supply and demand.

Gradual activity progression prevents a sudden increase in cardiac workload. Providing assistance only as needed encourages independence in performing activities.

NURSING DIAGNOSIS:	COMFORT, ALTERED: PAIN, ACUTE (HEADACHE)
May be related to:	**Increased cerebral vascular pressure**
Possibly evidenced by:	**Reports of throbbing pain located in suboccipital region, present on awakening and disappearing spontaneously after being up and about**
	Reluctance to move head, rubbing head, avoidance of bright lights and noise, wrinkled brow, clenched fists
	Reports of stiffness of neck, dizziness, blurred vision, nausea and vomiting
PATIENT OUTCOMES/ EVALUATION CRITERIA:	**Reports pain/discomfort is relieved/controlled. Verbalizes methods that provide relief. Follows prescribed pharmacologic regimen.**

ACTIONS/INTERVENTIONS	RATIONALE
Independent	
Maintain bedrest during acute phase.	Minimizes stimulation/promotes relaxation.
Provide nonpharmacologic measures for relief of headache, e.g., cool cloth to forehead, back and neck rubs; quiet, dimly lit room; relaxation techniques, guided imagery, distraction, and diversional activities.	Measures that reduce cerebral vascular pressure and which slow/block sympathetic response are effective in relieving headache and associated complications.
Eliminate/minimize vasoconstricting activities that may aggravate headache, e.g., straining at stool, prolonged coughing, bending over.	Activities that increase vasoconstriction accentuate the headache, in the presence of increased cerebral vascular pressure.
Assist patient with ambulation as needed.	Dizziness and blurred vision frequently are associated with headache. The patient may also experience episodes of postural hypotension.
Provide liquids, soft foods, frequent mouth care if nose bleeds occur or nasal packing has been done to stop bleeding.	Promotes general comfort. Nasal packing may interfere with swallowing or require mouth breathing, leading to stagnation of oral secretions and drying mucous membranes.
Collaborative	
Administer medications as indicated:	
Analgesics;	Reduces/controls pain, and stimulation of the sympathetic nervous system.
Tranquilizers, e.g., lorazepam (Ativan), diazepam (Valium).	May aid in the reduction of tension and discomfort that is intensified by stress.

NURSING DIAGNOSIS:	NUTRITION, ALTERED: MORE THAN BODY REQUIREMENTS
May be related to:	**Excessive intake in relation to metabolic need**
	Sedentary lifestyle
	Cultural preferences

Possibly evidenced by:	Weight 10–20% over ideal for height and frame
	Triceps skin fold greater than 15 mm in men (critical defining characteristic) and 25 mm in women
	Reported or observed dysfunctional eating patterns
PATIENT OUTCOMES/ EVALUATION CRITERIA:	Identifies correlation between hypertension and obesity. Demonstrates change in eating patterns, e.g., food choices, quantity, etc., in order to attain desirable body weight with optimal maintenance of health. Initiates/ maintains individually appropriate exercise program.

INTERVENTIONS

Independent

Assess patient understanding of direct relationship between hypertension and obesity. Discuss necessity for decreased caloric intake and limiting intake of salt, fats, and sugar as indicated.

Determine patient's desire to lose weight.

Review usual daily caloric intake and dietary choices.

Establish a realistic weight reduction plan with the patient, e.g., a 1–2-lb weight loss/week.

Encourage patient to maintain a diary of food intake including when and where eating takes place and the circumstances and feelings around which the food was eaten.

Instruct and assist in appropriate food selection, avoiding foods high in saturated fat (butter, cheese, eggs, ice cream, meat), and cholesterol (fatty meats, egg yolks, whole dairy products, shrimp, organ meats).

Collaborative

Refer to dietician as indicated.

RATIONALE

Obesity is an added risk with high blood pressure because of the disproportion between fixed aortic capacity and increased cardiac output associated with increased body mass. Faulty eating habits contribute to atherosclerosis and obesity, which predispose to hypertension and subsequent complications, e.g., stroke, kidney disease, heart failure. Excessive salt intake expands the intravascular fluid volume and may damage kidneys, which can further aggravate hypertension.

Motivation for weight reduction is internal. The individual must want to lose weight, or program may not succeed.

Identifies current strengths/weaknesses in dietary program. Aids in determining individual need for adjustment/teaching.

One pound of adipose tissue has the energy potential of 3500 calories. Reducing one's daily caloric intake by 500 calories for 1 week theoretically yields a weight loss of 1 lb.

Provides a data base for both the adequacy of nutrients eaten as well as the emotional conditions of eating. Helps to focus attention on factors which patient has control over/can change.

Avoiding foods high in saturated fat and cholesterol is important in preventing progressing atherogenesis.

Provides assistance with developing plan to meet individual dietary needs and additional teaching resource.

NURSING DIAGNOSIS:	COPING, INEFFECTIVE INDIVIDUAL
May be related to:	Situational/maturational crisis
	Multiple life changes
	Inadequate relaxation

Inadequate support systems

Little or no exercise

Poor nutrition

Unmet expectations

Work overload

Unrealistic perceptions

Inadequate coping methods

Possibly evidenced by: Verbalization of inability to cope or ask for help

Inability to meet role expectations/basic needs/problem-solve

Destructive behavior toward self; overeating, lack of appetite; excessive smoking/drinking and alcohol proneness

High blood pressure

Chronic fatigue/insomnia; muscular tension; frequent head/neck aches; chronic worry/irritability/anxiety/emotional tension, depression

PATIENT OUTCOMES/ EVALUATION CRITERIA: Identifies ineffective coping behaviors and consequences. Verbalizes awareness of own coping abilities/strengths. Identifies potential stressful situations and takes steps to avoid them. Demonstrates the use of effective coping skills/methods.

ACTIONS/INTERVENTIONS	RATIONALE
Independent	
Assess effectiveness of coping strategies by observing behaviors, ability to verbalize feelings and concerns, and willingness to participate in the treatment plan.	Adaptive mechanisms are necessary to appropriately alter one's lifestyle, deal with the chronicity of hypertension, and integrate prescribed therapies into activities of daily living.
Note complaints of sleep disturbances, increasing fatigue, impaired concentration, irritability, decreased tolerance of headache, verbalization of inability to cope/problem-solve.	Manifestations of maladaptive coping mechanisms such as keeping anger contained which have been found to be major determinants of diastolic blood pressure.
Assist patient to identify specific stressors and possible strategies for coping with them.	Recognition of stressors is the first step in altering one's response to the stressor.
Include patient in planning of care and encourage maximum participation in treatment plan.	Involvement provides the patient with an ongoing sense of control, improves coping skills and can enhance cooperation with therapeutic regimen.
Encourage patient to evaluate life priorities/goals. Ask questions such as, "Is what you are doing getting you what you want?"	Focuses patient attention on reality of present situation related to patient's view of what is wanted. Strong work ethic, need for "control," outward focus may have led to lack of attention to personal needs.
Assist patient to identify and begin planning for necessary lifestyle changes. Assist to adjust, rather than abandon personal/family goals.	Necessary changes should be realistically prioritized to avoid being overwhelmed and feeling powerless.

NURSING DIAGNOSIS:	KNOWLEDGE DEFICIT [LEARNING NEED] (SPECIFY)
May be related to:	Lack of knowledge about hypertension
	Lack of recall
	Information misinterpretation
	Cognitive limitation
	Denial of diagnosis
Possibly evidenced by:	Verbalization of the problem
	Request for information
	Statement of misconception
	Inaccurate follow-through of instruction
	Inadequate performance of procedures
	Inappropriate or exaggerated behaviors, e.g., hysterical, hostile, agitated, apathetic
PATIENT OUTCOMES/ EVALUATION CRITERIA:	Verbalizes understanding of disease process and treatment regimen. Identifies drug side effects and possible complications that necessitate attention. Maintains blood pressure within normal parameters.

ACTIONS/INTERVENTIONS	RATIONALE
Independent	
Assess readiness and blocks to learning. Include SO.	Misconceptions, denial of the diagnosis because of long-standing feelings of well-being may interfere with patient's/SO's willingness to learn about disease, progression, and prognosis. If the patient does not accept the reality of a life condition requiring continuing treatment, lifestyle/behavioral changes will not be initiated/ sustained.
Define and state the limits of normal blood pressure. Explain hypertension and its effects on the heart, blood vessels, kidneys, and brain.	Provides basis for understanding elevations of blood pressure and clarifies frequently used medical terminology. Understanding that high blood pressure can exist without symptoms is central to enabling patient to continue treatment even when feeling well.
Avoid saying "normal" blood pressure, and use the term "well-controlled" when describing patient's blood pressure within desired limits.	Because treatment for hypertension is life-long, conveying the idea of "control" helps the patient to understand the need for continued treatment/medication.
Assist the patient in identifying modifiable cardiovascular risk factors, e.g., obesity, diet high in saturated fats and cholesterol, sedentary lifestyle, smoking, alcohol intake (more than 2 oz/day on a regular basis), stressful lifestyle.	These risk factors have been shown to contribute to hypertension and cardiovascular and renal disease.
Problem-solve with patient to identify ways in which appropriate lifestyle changes can be made to reduce the above factors.	Risk factors may accelerate the disease process or exacerbate symptoms. Changing "comfortable/usual" behavior patterns can be very stressful. Support, guidance, and empathy can enhance the patient's success in accomplishing these tasks.

ACTIONS/INTERVENTIONS	RATIONALE

Independent

Discuss importance of eliminating smoking and assist patient in formulating a plan to quit smoking.

Nicotine increases catecholamine discharge, resulting in increased heart rate, BP, and vasoconstriction, reducing tissue oxygenation, and increasing the myocardial workload.

Reinforce the importance of cooperation with treatment regimen and keeping follow-up appointments.

Lack of cooperation is a common reason for failure of antihypertensive therapy; therefore, ongoing evaluation of patient compliance is critical to successful treatment. Effective therapy reduces the incidence of stroke, heart failure, renal impairment, and possibly MI.

Instruct and demonstrate technique of self-monitoring of blood pressure (assess the patient for hearing, visual acuity, manual dexterity, and coordination).

Teaching the patient or SO to monitor the blood pressure is reassuring to the patient, provides visual/positive reinforcement for patient efforts and helps in guiding therapy.

Help in developing a simple, convenient schedule for taking medications.

Individualizing medication schedule to fit the patient's personal habits/needs may facilitate compliance with long-term regimen.

Explain the rationale, dosage, side effects, and importance of taking prescribed medications, e.g.:

Adequate information enhances cooperation with treatment plan.

Diuretics: take daily dose (or larger dose) in the early morning;

Scheduling minimizes nighttime urination.

weigh self daily and record;

Primary indicator of effectiveness of diuretic therapy.

avoid/limit alcohol intake;

The combined vasodilating effect of alcohol and volume-depleting effect of a diuretic greatly increase the risk of orthostatic hypotension.

increase intake of foods/fluids high in potassium (e.g., oranges, bananas, figs, dates, tomatoes, potatoes, raisins, apricots, Gatorade, fruit juices) as indicated;

Diuretic use can deplete potassium levels. Dietary replacement is more palatable than drug supplements and may be all that is needed to correct deficit.

notify physician if unable to tolerate food or fluid;

Dehydration can develop rapidly if intake is poor and patient continues to take a diuretic.

identify signs/symptoms requiring notification of health care provider: e.g., weight gain of 2 lb in a day or 5 lb in a week, swelling of ankles/feet or abdomen, excessive thirst, severe dizziness or episodes of fainting, muscle weakness/cramping, nausea/vomiting, irregular pulse or increased pulse rate;

Early detection of developing complications, decreased effectiveness, or adverse reactions to drug regimen allows for timely intervention and may prevent progression of the disease process.
May indicate a need to evaluate electrolyte status (specifically potassium) and alter medication regimen.

Antihypertensives: take prescribed dose on a regular schedule, avoid skipping, altering, or making up doses, and do not discontinue without the health care provider;

Abruptly discontinuing drug causes rebound hypertension that may lead to severe complications.

be alert to expected and adverse side effects. Report those that interfere with lifestyle;

Side effects such as mood changes, weight gain, and dry mouth are common and often subside with time. A change in drug or dosage may also be needed for more serious side effects, e.g., impotence.

rise slowly from a lying to standing position, sitting for a few minutes before standing. Sleep with the head slightly elevated.

Measures reduce severity of orthostatic hypotension associated with the use of vasodilators and diuretics.

Avoid prolonged standing. Do leg exercises when lying down.

Decreases peripheral venous pooling that may be potentiated by vasodilators.

ACTIONS/INTERVENTIONS

Independent

Avoid hot baths, steam rooms, and saunas and concomitant use of alcoholic beverages.

Instruct the patient to consult health care provider before taking other prescription or nonprescription medication.

Explain rationale for prescribed dietary regimen (usually a diet low in sodium, saturated fat, and cholesterol is recommended).

Help patient to identify sources of and reduce sodium intake, e.g., table salt, salty snacks, processed meats and cheeses, sauerkraut, sauces, canned soups and vegetables, baking soda, baking powder, monosodium glutamate. Stress importance of reading ingredient labels of foods and OTC drugs;

Decrease intake of foods high in saturated (animal) fat (e.g., butter, cheese, eggs, ice cream, meat) and cholesterol (e.g., fatty meats, egg yolks, whole dairy products, shrimp, organ meats).

Encourage patient to decrease or eliminate caffeine, e.g., coffee, tea, cola, chocolate.

Stress importance of planning/accomplishing daily rest periods.

Recommend patient monitor own physiologic response to activity (e.g., pulse rate, shortness of breath); report a decreased tolerance to activity; and stop activity that causes chest pain, shortness of breath, dizziness, extreme fatigue, or weakness.

Establish an individual exercise program incorporating aerobic exercise (walking, swimming) within the patient's capabilities. Stress the importance of avoiding isometric activity.

Instruct the patient to report the following: headache present on awakening; sudden and continued increase of BP; chest pain/shortness of breath; significant weight gain or peripheral edema; visual disturbance; frequent uncontrollable nose bleeds; depression/emotional lability; side effects of medications.

Demonstrate application of ice pack to the back of the neck and pressure over the distal third of nose, and recommend the patient lean the head forward if nose bleed occurs.

Provide information regarding community resources and support the patient in making lifestyle changes. Initiate a referral if indicated.

RATIONALE

Prevents unnecessary vasodilation with dangerous side effect of syncope and hypotension.

Precaution is important in preventing potentially dangerous drug interaction. Any drug that contains a sympathetic nervous stimulant may increase BP or may counteract antihypertensive effects.

Excess saturated fats, cholesterol, sodium, alcohol, and caloric consumption have been defined as nutritional risks with hypertension.

Two years on a moderately low-salt diet may be sufficient to control mild hypertension or reduce the amount of medication required.

Food high in saturated fats and cholesterol contribute to the atherosclerotic process. A low-fat and high-polyunsaturated-fat diet reduces BP, possibly through prostaglandin balance, in both normotensive and hypertensive people.

Caffeine is a cardiac stimulant and may adversely affect cardiac function/reserves.

Alternating rest and activity increases tolerance to activity progression.

The patient's involvement in monitoring his or her own activity tolerance is vital to safely resuming and/or modifying activities of daily living.

Besides helping to lower BP, aerobic activity aids in toning the cardiovascular system. Isometric exercise can increase serum catecholamine levels further elevating BP.

These may be indicators of inadequate management, disease complications, or side effects of therapy.

Nasal capillaries may rupture as a result of excessive vascular pressure. Cold and pressure constricts capillaries, which slows or halts bleeding. Leaning forward reduces the amount of blood that is swallowed.

Community resources such as the American Heart Association, "coronary clubs," stop smoking, alcohol rehabilitation, weight loss programs, stress management classes, and counseling services may be helpful to the patient's efforts to make lifestyle changes.

Congestive Heart Failure: Chronic _____

CARDIOVASCULAR: Congestive Heart Failure

PATIENT ASSESSMENT DATA BASE

ACTIVITY/REST

May report: Fatigue/exhaustion progressing throughout the day.
Insomnia.
Chest pain with activity.
Dyspnea at rest or with exertion.

May exhibit: Restlessness, mental status changes, e.g., lethargy.
Vital sign changes with activity.

CIRCULATION

If CHF, then ↓ Cardiac Output

May report: History of hypertension, recent/acute MI, episodes of CHF, valvular heart disease, cardiac surgery, endocarditis, SLE, anemia, septic shock.
Use of cardiosuppressive drugs, e.g., beta-blockers, calcium channel blockers.

May exhibit: Blood pressure: may be low (pump failure); normal (mild or chronic CHF); or high (fluid overload/increased SVR).
Pulse pressure: may be narrow, reflecting reduced stroke volume.
Heart rate: tachycardia.
Heart rhythm: dysrhythmias, e.g., atrial fibrillation, premature ventricular contractions/tachycardia, heart blocks.
Apical pulse: PMI may be diffuse and displaced inferiorly to the left.
Heart sounds: S_3 is diagnostic, S_4 may occur, and S_1 and S_2 may be softened. Systolic and diastolic murmurs may indicate the presence of valvular stenosis or insufficiency.
Pulses: peripheral pulses diminished; alteration in strength of beat may be noted; central pulses may be bounding, e.g., visible jugular, carotid, abdominal pulsations.
Color: ashen, pale, dusky, cyanotic.
Nailbeds: pale or cyanotic with slow capillary refill.
Liver: enlarged/palpable, positive hepatojugular reflex.
Breath sounds: crackles, rhonchi.
Edema: ankle, dependent or generalized; jugular venous distention.

EGO INTEGRITY

May report: Fear, anxiety, apprehension.
Stress related to illness/financial concerns (job/cost of medical care).

May exhibit: Various behavioral manifestations, e.g., anxiety, anger, fearful, irritable.

ELIMINATION

May report: Decreased voiding, dark urine.
Night voiding (nocturia).
Constipation.

FOOD/FLUID

If CHF then fluid retention

May report: Loss of appetite.
Nausea/vomiting; diarrhea/constipation.
Significant weight gain.
Lower extremity swelling.

Tight clothing/shoes.
Diet high in salt/processed foods, fat, sugar, caffeine.
Use of diuretics.

May exhibit: Rapid weight gain.
Abdominal distention, ascites, edema (general, dependent, brawn, pitting).

HYGIENE

May report: Fatigue/weakness, exhaustion during self-care activities.
May exhibit: Appearance indicative of neglect of personal care.

NEUROSENSORY

May report: Weakness, dizziness, fainting episodes.
May exhibit: Lethargy, confusion, disorientation.
Behavior changes.

PAIN/COMFORT

May report: Chest pain, chronic or acute angina.
Right upper abdominal pain.
Muscle aches.

May exhibit: Nervousness, restlessness.
Narrowed focus (withdrawal).
Guarding behavior.

RESPIRATION

of CHF, then respiratory change.

May report: Dyspnea on exertion, sleeping sitting up, or with several pillows.
Cough with/without sputum production.
History of chronic lung disease.
Use of respiratory aids, e.g., oxygen or medications.

May exhibit: Respirations: tachypnea; shallow, labored breathing; use of accessory muscles, nasal flaring.
Cough: dry/hacking/nonproductive or may be gurgling with/without sputum production.
Sputum: may be blood-tinged, pink/frothy (pulmonary edema).
Breath sounds: may be diminished, with bibasilar crackles and wheezes.
Mentation: restlessness, lethargy.
Color: pallor or cyanosis.

SAFETY

May exhibit: Changes in mentation.
Loss of strength/muscle tone.
Skin excoriations.

SOCIAL INTERACTION

May report: Decreased participation in usual social activities.

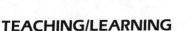

TEACHING/LEARNING

May report: Use/misuse of cardiac medications.
Evidence of failure to improve.

Discharge Plan Considerations: Assistance with shopping, transportation, self-care needs, homemaker tasks.
Alteration in medication use/therapy, physical layout of home.

DIAGNOSTIC STUDIES

ECG: Ventricular or atrial hypertrophy, axis deviation, ischemia, and damage patterns may be present. Persistent ST/T segment elevation 6 weeks or more after MI suggests presence of ventricular aneurysm (may cause cardiac dysfunction/failure). Dysrhythmias, e.g., tachycardia, atrial fibrillation, frequent PVCs may be present.

Echocardiography: May reveal enlarged chamber dimensions, alterations in valvular function/structure, or areas of decreased ventricular contractility.

Nuclear imaging scan: measures ejection fraction and estimates wall motion.

Cardiac catheterization: may be indicated to differentiate right versus left heart failure and/or assess patency of coronary arteries.

Chest x-ray: may show enlarged cardiac shadow reflecting chamber dilatation/hypertrophy, or changes in blood vessels reflecting increased pulmonary pressure. Abnormal contour, e.g., bulging of left cardiac border, may suggest ventricular aneurysm.

Liver enzymes (SGOT, SGPT): elevated in liver congestion/failure.

Electrolytes: may be altered due to fluid shifts/decreased renal function, diuretic therapy.

Ear/pulse oximetry: oxygen saturation may be low, especially when acute CHF is imposed upon COPD or chronic CHF.

ABGs: left ventricular failure is characterized by mild respiratory alkalosis (early); hypoxemia with an increased PCO_2 (late).

BUN, creatinine: elevated BUN suggests decreased renal perfusion. Elevation of both BUN and creatinine is indicative of renal failure.

Serum albumin/transferrin: may be decreased as a result of reduced protein intake or reduced protein synthesis in congested liver.

CBC: may reveal anemia, polycythemia, or dilutional changes indicating water retention. WBCs may be elevated, reflecting recent/acute MI, pericarditis, or other inflammatory or infectious states.

Sedimentation rate (ESR): may be elevated, indicating acute inflammatory reaction.

Thyroid studies: increased thyroid activity suggests thyroid hyperactivity as precipitator of CHF.

NURSING PRIORITIES

1. Improve myocardial contractility/systemic perfusion.
2. Reduce fluid volume overload.
3. Prevent complications.
4. Provide information about disease/prognosis, therapy needs and prevention of recurrences.

DISCHARGE CRITERIA

1. Cardiac output adequate for individual needs.
2. Complications prevented.
3. Optimum level of activity/functioning attained.
4. Disease process/prognosis and therapeutic regimen understood.

NURSING DIAGNOSIS:	CARDIAC OUTPUT, ALTERED: DECREASED
May be related to:	**Altered myocardial contractility/inotropic changes**
	Alterations in rate, rhythm, electrical conduction

	Structural changes (e.g., valvular defects, ventricular aneurysm)
Possibly evidenced by:	**Increased heart rate (tachycardia)**
	Changes in blood pressure (hypo/hypertension)
	Extra heart sounds (S_3, S_4), dysrhythmias, ECG changes
	Decreased urine output
	Diminished peripheral pulses
	Cool, ashen skin; diaphoresis
	Orthopnea, crackles
	JVD, liver engorgement, edema
	Chest pain
PATIENT OUTCOMES/ EVALUATION CRITERIA:	**Displays vital signs within acceptable limits, dysrhythmias absent/controlled, and free of individual symptoms of failure. Reports decreased episodes of dyspnea, angina. Participates in activities that reduce cardiac workload.**

ACTIONS/INTERVENTIONS	RATIONALE
Independent	
Auscultate apical pulse. Assess heart rate, rhythm. (Document dysrhythmia if telemetry available.)	Tachycardia is usually present (even at rest) to compensate for decreased LV contractility. PACs, PAT, MAT, PVCs, and AF are common dysrhythmias associated with CHF, although others may also occur. Note: Intractable ventricular dysrhythmias unresponsive to medication suggests ventricular aneurysm.
Note heart sounds.	S_1 and S_2 may be weak because of diminished pumping action. Gallop rhythms are common (S_3 and S_4), produced as blood flows into noncompliant/distended chambers. Murmurs may reflect valvular incompetence/stenosis.
Palpate peripheral pulses.	Decreased cardiac output may be reflected in diminished radial, popliteal, dorsalis pedis, and posttibial pulses. Pulses may be fleeting or irregular to palpation, and pulsus alternans (strong beat alternating with weak beat) may be present.
Monitor blood pressure.	In early, moderate, or chronic CHF, BP may be elevated due to increased SVR. In advanced CHF, the body may no longer be able to compensate and profound/irreversible hypotension may occur.
Inspect skin for pallor, cyanosis, diaphoresis.	Indicative of diminished peripheral perfusion secondary to decreased/inadequate cardiac output vasoconstriction and anemia. Cyanosis may develop in refractory CHF. Dependent areas are often blue or mottled as venous congestion increases.
Monitor urine output, noting fluctuations of/decreasing output and dark/concentrated urine.	Kidneys respond to reduced cardiac output by retaining water and sodium. Urine output is usually de-

ACTIONS/INTERVENTIONS

Independent

Assess changes in sensorium, e.g., lethargy, confusion, disorientation, anxiety, and depression.

Provide rest semirecumbent in bed or chair. Assist with physical care as indicated.

Provide for psychological rest by quiet environment; explaining medical/nursing management; helping patient avoid stressful situations, listening/responding to expressions of feelings/fears. (Refer to CP: Psychosocial Aspects of Acute Care, ND: Anxiety, p. 774.)

Provide bedside commode. Avoid activities eliciting a Valsalva response, e.g., straining at stool, holding breath during position changes.

Elevate legs, avoid pressure under knee. Encourage active/passive exercises. Increase ambulation/activity as tolerated.

Check for calf tenderness, diminished pedal pulse, swelling, local redness, or pallor of extremity.

Withhold digitalis preparation and notify physician if marked changes occur in cardiac rate or rhythm, or signs of digitalis toxicity occur. (Refer to CP: Digitalis Toxocity, p. 53.)

Collaborative

Administer supplemental oxygen by nasal cannula/mask as indicated.

Administer medications as indicated:

Diuretics, e.g., furosemide (Lasix), bumetanide (Bumex); spironolactone (Aldactone);

Vasodilators, e.g., nitrates (Nitro-Dur, Isordil); arteriodilators, e.g., hydralazine (Apresoline); combination drugs, e.g., prazosin (Minipress);

Digoxin (Lanoxin);

Captopril (Capoten);

RATIONALE

creased during the day because of fluid shifts into tissues but may be increased at night as fluid returns to circulation when patient is recumbent.

May indicate inadequate cerebral perfusion secondary to decreased cardiac output.

Physical rest should be maintained during acute or refractory CHF to improve efficiency of cardiac contraction and to decrease myocardial oxygen demand/consumption and workload.

Emotional stress produces vasoconstriction, elevating BP and increasing heart rate/work.

Commode decreases work of getting to bathroom or struggling to use bedpan. Valsalva maneuver causes vagal stimulation followed by rebound tachycardia which further compromises cardiac output function/output.

Decreases venous stasis and may reduce incidence of thrombus/embolus formation.

Reduced cardiac output, venous pooling/stasis, enforced bedrest increases risk of thrombophlebitis.

Incidence of toxicity is high because of narrow margin between therapeutic and toxic ranges. Digoxin may have to be discontinued in the presence of toxic drug levels, a slow heart rate, or low potassium level.

Increases available oxygen for myocardial uptake to combat effects of hypoxia/ischemia.

A variety of medications may be used to increase stroke volume, improve contractility and reduce congestion.

Preload reduction is most useful in treating patients with a relatively normal cardiac output accompanied by congestive symptoms.

Vasodilators are used to increase output, reducing ventricular volume (venodilators) and decreasing systemic vascular resistance (arteriodilators), thereby reducing ventricular stretch/workload.

Increases force of myocardial contraction and slows heart rate by decreasing conduction velocity and prolonging refractory period of the AV junction to increase cardiac efficiency/output.

May be used to control heart failure by inhibiting angiotensin conversion in the lungs, reduce vasoconstriction, SVR, and blood pressure.

ACTIONS/INTERVENTIONS	RATIONALE
Collaborative	
Morphine sulfate;	Decreases vascular resistance and venous return reducing myocardial workload. Allays anxiety and breaks the feedback cycle of anxiety/catecholamine release/anxiety.
Tranquilizers/sedatives;	Promotes rest/relaxation reducing oxygen demand and myocardial workload.
Anticoagulants, e.g., low-dose heparin, warfarin (Coumadin).	Occasionally used prophylactically to prevent thrombus/emboli formation in presence of risk factors such as venous stasis, enforced bedrest, cardiac dysrhythmias, history of previous thrombolic episodes.
Administer IV solutions, restricting total amount as indicated. Avoid saline solutions.	Because of existing elevated left ventricular pressure, patient may not tolerate increased fluid volume (preload). CHF patients also excrete less sodium, which causes fluid retention and increases myocardial workload.
Monitor/replace electrolytes.	Fluid shifts and use of diuretics can alter electrolytes (especially potassium and chloride), which affect cardiac rhythm and contractility.
Monitor serial ECG and chest x-ray changes.	ST segment depression and T wave flattening can develop because of increased myocardial oxygen demand, even if no coronary artery disease is present. Chest x-ray may show enlarged heart and changes of pulmonary congestion.
Monitor laboratory studies, e.g.,	
BUN, creatinine;	Elevation of BUN/creatinine reflects kidney hypoperfusion/failure.
Liver function studies (SGOT, LDH);	SGOT/LDH may be elevated due to liver congestion and indicate need for smaller dosages of medications that are detoxified by the liver.
PT/APTT/coagulation studies.	Measures changes in coagulation processes or effectiveness of anticoagulant therapy.
Prepare for insertion/maintain pacemaker, if indicated.	May be necessary to correct bradydysrhythmias unresponsive to drug intervention, which can aggravate congestive failure/produce pulmonary edema.
Prepare for surgery as indicated.	Congestive failure due to ventricular aneurysm or valvular dysfunction may require aneurysmectomy or valve replacement to improve myocardial contractility/function. (Refer to CP: Cardiac Surgery, p. 98.)

NURSING DIAGNOSIS: **ACTIVITY INTOLERANCE**

May be related to: Imbalance between oxygen supply/demand

            Generalized weakness

            Prolonged bedrest/immobility

Possibly evidenced by: Weakness, fatigue

            Changes in vital signs, presence of dysrhythmias

            Dyspnea

Pallor

Diaphoresis

PATIENT OUTCOMES/ EVALUATION CRITERIA: **Participates in desired activities, meeting own self-care needs. Achieves measurable increase in activity tolerance, evidenced by reduced fatigue and weakness, and vital signs within acceptable limits during activity.**

ACTIONS/INTERVENTIONS

Independent

Check vital signs before and immediately after activity, especially if patient is on vasodilators, diuretics, beta-blockers.

Document cardiopulmonary response to activity. Note: tachycardia, dysrhythmias, dyspnea, diaphoresis, pallor.

Assess for other precipitators/causes of fatigue, e.g., treatments, pain, medications.

Evaluate accelerating activity intolerance.

Encourage verbalization of feelings regarding limitations.

Provide assistance with self-care activities as indicated. Intersperse activity periods with rest periods.

Collaborative

Follow graded cardiac rehabilitation/activity program.

RATIONALE

Orthostatic hypotension can occur with activity because of medication effect (vasodilation), fluid shifts (diuresis), compromised cardiac function.

Compromised myocardium/inability to increase stroke volume during activity, may cause an immediate increase in heart rate and oxygen demands thereby aggravating weakness and fatigue.

Fatigue is a side effect of some medications (beta blockers, tranquilizers and sedatives). Pain and stressful regimens also extract energy and produce fatigue.

May denote increasing cardiac decompensation rather than overactivity.

Expression of feelings/concerns may decrease stress/anxiety which is an energy drain and can contribute to feelings of fatigue.

Meets patient's personal care needs without undue myocardial stress/excessive oxygen demand.

Gradual increase in activity avoids excessive myocardial workload/oxygen consumption. Strengthens and improves cardiac function under stress.

NURSING DIAGNOSIS: **FLUID VOLUME, ALTERED: EXCESS**

May be related to: **Reduced glomerular filtration rate (decreased cardiac output)/increased ADH production, and sodium/water retention**

Possibly evidenced by: **Orthopnea**

S₃ heart sound

Oliguria

Edema, jugular vein distention, positive hepatojugular reflex

Weight gain

Hypertension

Respiratory distress, abnormal breath sounds

ACTIONS/INTERVENTIONS	RATIONALE
Independent	
Monitor urine output, noting amount and color in addition to time of day when diuresis occurs.	Urine output may be scanty and concentrated especially during the day because of reduced renal perfusion. Recumbency favors diuresis therefore urine output may be increased at night/during bedrest.
Monitor/calculate 24-hour intake and output balance.	Diuretic therapy may result in sudden/excessive fluid loss (hypovolemia) even though edema/ascites remains.
Maintain chair or bedrest in semi-Fowler's position.	Recumbency increases glomerular filtration and decreases production of ADH, thereby enhancing diuresis.
Establish fluid intake schedule, incorporating beverage preferences when possible. Give frequent mouth care, ice chips as part of fluid allotment.	Involving patient in therapy regimen may enhance sense of control and cooperation with restrictions.
Weigh daily.	Documents changes in edema in response to therapy. Gain of 5 lb represents approximately two liters of fluid. Conversely, diuretics can result in excessive fluid and weight loss.
Assess for distended neck and peripheral vessels. Inspect dependent body areas for edema with/without pitting; note presence of generalized body edema (anasarca).	Excessive fluid retention may be manifested by venous engorgement and edema formation. Peripheral edema begins in feet/ankles (or dependent areas), and ascends as failure worsens. Pitting edema is generally obvious only after retention of at least 10 lb of fluid. Increased vascular congestion (associated with right heart failure) eventually results in systemic tissue edema.
Change position frequently. Elevate feet when sitting. Inspect skin surface, keep dry and provide padding as indicated. (Refer to ND: Skin Integrity, Impaired [Potential], p. 50.)	Edema formation, slowed circulation, altered nutritional intake and prolonged immobility/bedrest are cumulative stressors affecting skin integrity which require close supervision and preventive interventions.
Auscultate breath sounds, noting decreased and/or adventitious sounds, e.g., crackles, wheezes. Note presence of increased dyspnea, tachypnea, orthopnea, paroxysmal nocturnal dyspnea, persistent cough.	Fluid volume excess often leads to pulmonary congestion. Symptoms of pulmonary edema may reflect left acute heart failure. Right heart failure's respiratory symptoms (dyspnea, cough, orthopnea) may have slower onset, but are more difficult to reverse.
Investigate sudden extreme dyspnea/air hunger, sitting straight up, sensation of suffocation, feelings of panic.	May indicate development of complications (pulmonary edema/embolus) and differs from orthopnea and paroxysmal nocturnal dyspnea in that it develops much more rapidly and requires immediate intervention.
Monitor blood pressure and CVP (if available).	Hypertension and elevated CVP suggests fluid volume excess and may reflect developing/increasing pulmonary congestion, heart failure.
Assess bowel sounds. Note complaints of anorexia, nausea, abdominal distention, constipation.	Visceral congestion (occurring in progressive CHF), can alter gastric/intestinal function.

ACTIONS/INTERVENTIONS	RATIONALE
Independent	
Provide small, frequent easily digestible meals.	Reduced gastric motility can adversely affect digestion and absorption. Small frequent meals may enhance digestion/prevent abdominal discomfort.
Measure abdominal girth, if indicated.	In progressive right heart failure, fluid pressure can exceed oncotic pressure, resulting in fluid shifting into the peritoneal space evidenced by increasing abdominal girth (ascites).
Palpate for hepatomegaly; note complaints of right upper quadrant pain/tenderness.	Advancing heart failure leads to venous congestion resulting in abdominal distention, liver engorgement, and pain. This can alter liver function, e.g., impair/prolong drug metabolism.
Note increased lethargy, hypotension, muscle cramping.	Signs of potassium and sodium deficits that may occur due to fluid shifts and diuretic therapy.
Collaborative	
Administer medications as indicated:	
Diuretics, e.g., furosemide (Lasix), bumetanide (Bumex);	Increases rate of urine flow and may inhibit reabsorption of sodium/chloride in the renal tubules.
Thiazides with potassium-sparing agents, e.g., spironolactone (Aldactone);	Promotes diuresis without excessive potassium losses.
Potassium supplements.	Potassium wasting is a common side effect of diuretic therapy which can adversely affect cardiac function.
Maintain fluid/sodium restrictions as indicated.	Reduces total body water/prevents fluid reaccumulation.
Consult with dietician.	May be necessary in order to provide diet acceptable to patient that meets caloric needs within sodium restriction.
Monitor chest x-ray.	Reveals changes indicative of increase/resolution of pulmonary congestion.
Assist with rotating tourniquets/phlebotomy as indicated.	Although not frequently needed/used, may be carried out to reduce circulating volume, especially in pulmonary edema refractory to other therapies.

NURSING DIAGNOSIS:	**GAS EXCHANGE, IMPAIRED [POTENTIAL]**
May be related to:	**Alveolar-capillary membrane changes, e.g., fluid collection/shifts into interstitial space/alveoli**
Possibly evidenced by:	**[Not applicable; presence of signs and symptoms establishes an *actual* diagnosis.]**
PATIENT OUTCOMES/ EVALUATION CRITERIA:	**Demonstrates adequate ventilation and oxygenation of tissues by ABGs within patient's normal ranges and free of symptoms of respiratory distress. Participates in treatment regimen within level of ability/situation.**

ACTIONS/INTERVENTIONS

Independent

Auscultate breath sounds noting crackles, wheezes.

Instruct patient in effective coughing, deep breathing. Encourage frequent position changes.

Maintain chair/bedrest in semi-Fowler's position.

Collaborative

Monitor/graph serial ABGs.

Administer supplemental oxygen as indicated.

Administer medications as indicated:

    Diuretics, e.g., furosemide (Lasix);

    Bronchodilators, e.g., aminophylline.

RATIONALE

Reveals presence of pulmonary congestion/collection of secretions indicating need for further intervention.

Clears airways and facilitates oxygen delivery.

Reduces oxygen consumption/demands and promotes maximal lung inflation.

May show severe hypoxemia during acute pulmonary edema or reveal compensatory changes in chronic CHF.

Increases alveolar oxygen concentration and may enhance arterial oxygenation to correct/reduce tissue hypoxemia.

Reduces alveolar congestion, enhancing gas exchange.

Increases oxygen delivery by dilating small airways and exerts mild diuretic effect to aid in reducing pulmonary congestion.

NURSING DIAGNOSIS:	SKIN INTEGRITY, IMPAIRED: POTENTIAL
May be related to:	Prolonged bedrest
	Edema, decreased tissue perfusion
Possibly evidenced by:	[Not applicable; presence of signs and symptoms establishes an *actual* diagnosis.]
PATIENT OUTCOMES/ EVALUATION CRITERIA:	Maintains skin integrity. Demonstrates behaviors/techniques to prevent skin breakdown.

ACTIONS/INTERVENTIONS

Independent

Inspect skin noting skeletal prominences, presence of edema, areas of altered circulation/pigmentation, obesity/emaciation.

Massage reddened or blanched areas.

Reposition frequently in bed/chair. Assist with active/passive range of motion exercises.

Provide frequent skin care. Minimize contact with moisture/excretions.

Check fit of shoes/slippers.

RATIONALE

Skin is at risk because of impaired peripheral circulation, physical immobility, and alterations in nutritional status.

Improves blood flow, minimizing tissue hypoxia.

Improves circulation/reduces time any one area is deprived of blood flow.

Excessive dryness or moisture damages skin and hastens breakdown.

Presence of dependent edema may result in poor fit which can cause pressure and skin breakdown.

ACTIONS/INTERVENTIONS

Independent

Avoid intramuscular medication.

Collaborative

Provide alternating pressure/egg crate mattress, sheep skin, elbow/heel protectors.

RATIONALE

Interstitial edema and slowed circulation impair drug absorption predisposing to tissue breakdown/development of infection.

Reduces pressure to skin, may improve circulation.

NURSING DIAGNOSIS:	KNOWLEDGE DEFICIT [LEARNING NEED] (SPECIFY)
May be related to:	Lack of understanding/misconceptions about interrelatedness of cardiac function/disease/failure
Possibly evidenced by:	Questions
	Statements of concern/misconceptions
	Recurrent, preventable episodes of congestive heart failure
PATIENT OUTCOMES/ EVALUATION CRITERIA:	Verbalizes signs/symptoms that require immediate intervention. Identifies own stress/risk factors and some techniques for handling. Initiates necessary lifestyle changes and participates in treatment. Identifies relationship of treatment program in reducing recurrent episodes and complications.

ACTIONS/INTERVENTIONS

Independent

Discuss normal heart function. Include information regarding patient's variance from normal function.

Reinforce treatment rationale.

Discuss importance of being active if possible, but not becoming exhausted; to rest between activities.

Discuss importance of sodium limitation, signs/symptoms of imbalance. Provide list of foods high in sodium that are to be avoided/limited. Encourage reading of labels on food and drug packages.

Discuss medications, purpose and side effects. Give instructions both verbally and in writing.

RATIONALE

Knowledge of disease process and expectations can facilitate adherence to prescribed treatment regimen.

Patient may alter postdischarge regimen when "feeling well and symptom-free" or when feeling "below par." Understanding of regimen, medications, restrictions, may augment cooperation.

Excessive physical activity can further weaken the heart, exacerbating failure.

Dietary intake of sodium above 3 g daily will offset diuretic effect. Most common source of sodium is table salt and obviously salty foods although canned soups/vegetables, luncheon meats, and dairy products also may contain high levels of sodium.

Understanding therapeutic needs and importance of prompt reporting of side effects can prevent occurrence of drug-related complications. Anxiety may block comprehension of input or details and patient/SO may refer to written material at later date to refresh memory.

ACTIONS/INTERVENTIONS	RATIONALE

Independent

Recommend taking diuretic early in morning.

Provides adequate time for drug effect before bedtime to prevent/limit interruption of sleep.

Instruct and receive return demonstration of ability to take and record daily pulse and when to notify health care provider, e.g., pulse above/below preset rate, changes in rhythm/regularity.

Promotes self-monitoring of condition/drug effect. Early detection of changes allows for timely intervention and may prevent complications, such as digitalis toxicity.

Explain and discuss patient's role in control of risk factors, e.g., smoking, etc., and precipitating or aggravating factors, e.g., high salt diet, inactivity/overexertion, exposure to extremes in temperature.

Adds to body of knowledge and permits patient to make informed decisions regarding control of condition and prevention of recurrence/complications. Smoking potentiates vasoconstriction; sodium intake promotes water retention/edema formation; improper balance between activity/rest and exposure to extremes in temperature may result in exhaustion/increased myocardial workload and increased risk of respiratory infections.

Review signs/symptoms that require immediate medical attention, e.g., rapid weight gain, edema, shortness of breath, increased fatigue, cough, hemoptysis, fever.

Participation in health monitoring increases patient responsibility in health maintenance and aids in prevention of complications, e.g., pulmonary edema, pneumonia.

Provide opportunities for patient/SO to ask questions discuss concerns and ability to make necessary lifestyle changes.

Chronicity and recurrent/debilitating nature of condition may exhaust coping abilities and supportive capacity of both patient and SO leading to depression. (Refer to CP: Psychosocial Aspects of Acute Care, p. 773.)

Stress importance of reporting signs/symptoms of digitalis toxicity, e.g., development of GI and visual disturbances, changes in pulse rate/rhythm, worsening of congestive failure.

Recognition of developing complication and involvement of health care provider may prevent toxicity/hospitalization.

Collaborative

Refer to community resources/support groups and VNA as indicated.

May need additional assistance with self-monitoring/home management.

Digitalis Toxicity

PATIENT ASSESSMENT DATA BASE

ACTIVITY/REST

May report: Insomnia, fatigue.

May exhibit: Exertional dyspnea, fatigue, weakness.
Abnormal pulse/blood pressure response to activity.

CIRCULATION

May report: History of recent/acute myocardial infarction, congestive heart failure.
Changes in usual heart rate/rhythm.

May exhibit: Excessive slowing of pulse (increasing AV block).
Characteristic ECG changes (see diagnostic studies).
Dysrhythmias: frequent premature beats, ventricular bigeminy, PAT.

EGO INTEGRITY

May report: Feelings of helplessness/hopelessness or powerlessness.

May exhibit: Irritability, restlessness, agitation.
Confusion, depression, delirium, psychosis (with high serum levels).

ELIMINATION

May report: Use of diuretics.
Presence of diarrhea.

May exhibit: Decreased urine output.
Dependent edema.

FOOD/FLUID

May report: Loss of appetite.
Nausea, vomiting.
Changes in weight.
Use of diuretics.

May exhibit: Changes in weight/decrease in muscle mass, subcutaneous fat.
Signs of altered fluid balance (excess or deficit).

NEUROSENSORY

May report: Visual disturbances, e.g., double, blurry, flickering lights, yellow/green tint to vision, colored dots.
Vertigo, faintness.
Seizure activity.
Headache.

May exhibit: Disorientation.
Restlessness.
Irritability, confusion, agitation/combative behavior.
Slurred speech.
Hallucinations, psychoses.
Seizures.

PAIN/COMFORT

May report: Chest/abdominal pain.

May exhibit: Guarding/distraction behaviors.

Self-focusing.

Autonomic responses (changes in vital signs).

SAFETY

May report: Concurrent use of drugs/substances that may lead to increased digitalis effect/toxicity, interactions, e.g., thiazide or loop diuretics, steroids, Quinidine, nifedipine, verapamil, beta-blockers, thyroid hormones, caffeine.

May exhibit: Muscle weakness.

Vision impairment.

TEACHING/LEARNING

May report: Improper use of digitalis, use of medications that produce interactions (see above).

Evidence of failure to improve.

Discharge Plan Considerations: Alteration in medication use/therapy.

DIAGNOSTIC STUDIES

Serum digoxin/digitoxin level: usually elevated above therapeutic range of particular preparation.

ECG: prolonged P–R interval, dysrhythmias, and heart blocks are associated with digitalis toxicity. Other changes (T wave and ST segment depression) characteristically produced by the therapeutic digitalis effect on the heart can mimic ischemic changes.

Electrolytes: imbalance in potassium, magnesium, calcium are known to aggravate digitalis toxicity.

NURSING PRIORITIES

1. Document current digitalis therapy and usage.
2. Prevent/control dysrhythmias.
3. Correct/maintain fluid balance.
4. Educate patient/SO regarding proper drug usage/signs/symptoms of developing toxicity.

DISCHARGE CRITERIA

1. Cardiac rate/rhythm within patient's expected range.
2. Free of signs and symptoms of digitalis toxicity.
3. Adequate fluid balance maintained.
4. Cognitive/perceptual abilities improved.
5. Digitalis regimen, and what/when to report to health care provider understood.

NURSING DIAGNOSIS:	CARDIAC OUTPUT, ALTERED: DECREASED
May be related to:	**Altered myocardial contractility**
	Alterations in rate, rhythm, electrical conduction
	Long drug half-life and narrow therapeutic dose range of digitalis preparation used; patient's age, organ function, amount of muscle mass, nutrition status, electrolyte/acid–base balance, and concurrent use of other medications

Possibly evidenced by:	Dysrhythmias
	Changes in mentation
	Variations in hemodynamic readings
	Worsening of congestive heart failure
	Elevated serum digitalis levels
PATIENT OUTCOMES/ EVALUATION CRITERIA:	Demonstrates heart rate and rhythm within patient's expected range with absence/control of dysrhythmias. Maintains usual mentation.

ACTIONS/INTERVENTIONS	RATIONALE

Independent

ACTIONS/INTERVENTIONS	RATIONALE
Assess/monitor blood pressure.	Dysrhythmias may diminish cardiac output, decreasing tissue perfusion, promoting hypoxemia, and worsening digitalis toxicity.
Palpate radial pulse, noting rate and regularity. Auscultate apical pulse, noting rate/rhythm and presence of extra heart sounds.	Rapid irregular pulse/heart rate or excessively slow pulse/heart rate may indicate digitalis toxicity. Extra heart sounds (e.g., S_3) are common in the presence of congestive heart failure.
Monitor/document cardiac rhythm.	Numerous dysrhythmias can occur, including several which are life-threatening. Premature ventricular contractions (PVCs) are common with possible bigeminal and trigeminal rhythms. Digitalis-induced tachydysrhythmias can lead to potentially lethal ventricular dysrhythmias.
Evaluate for presence of dependent/generalized edema, increased jugular venous distention/hepatojugular reflux. Auscultate breath sounds noting development of crackles.	Digitalis toxicity has been found to be responsible for deterioration of preexisting CHF, and/or development of heart failure during digitalization. In severe/refractory CHF, altered cardiac binding of digitalis may result in toxicity even with previously appropriate drug doses. (Refer to CP: Congestive Heart Failure, p. 41.)
Investigate changes in sensorium and behavior, e.g., confusion, restlessness, agitation, delirium.	Although psychic disturbances may be the result of decreased cardiac output, drug effect, or electrolyte imbalance, they could indicate developing pathology unrelated to drug toxicity/electrolyte imbalance.
Note presence of gastrointestinal symptoms, e.g., vomiting, diarrhea, abdominal discomfort.	May be direct effect of drug toxicity or reflect altered electrolytes or cardiac output/organ perfusion.
Assess factors that may alter drug absorption/excretion (e.g., small bowel disease, cirrhosis, hyperthyroidism; use of certain drugs, e.g., barbiturates, Dilantin).	Digitalis absorption, effectiveness, or half-life may be reduced by these factors thereby necessitating higher dosage of digitalis to achieve desired effect. When any of these factors change without alteration in digitalis dosage, toxicity can occur. Diminished renal/liver function and loss of body fat/muscle mass may slow drug metabolism necessitating reduction in drug dosage.
Note concomitant use of drugs which increase potential for digitalis toxicity or dysrhythmias.	Quinidine can double serum digitalis level, Verapamil can increase digitalis level by 60%; some antibiotics can increase digitalis level by 10–40%. Thiazide and loop diuretics potentiate potassium, calcium, and magnesium loss. Steroids and laxatives enhance potassium loss. Propanolol (Inderal), other beta-blockers, and thyroid preparations also fall in this category.

55

ACTIONS/INTERVENTIONS

RATIONALE

Collaborative

Monitor serum digoxin (Lanoxin) or digitoxin (Crystodigin) level.

Useful when evaluated in conjunction with clinical manifestations and ECG to determine individual therapeutic levels/resolution of toxicity.

Monitor laboratory studies which may be impacted by digitalis preparations, e.g., electrolytes, BUN, creatinine, liver function studies.

Abnormal levels of potassium, calcium, or magnesium increase heart's sensitivity to digitalis. Impaired kidney function can cause Lanoxin (mainly excreted by the kidney) to accumulate to toxic levels. Crystodigin levels (mainly excreted by the bowel) are affected by impaired liver function.

Administer potassium, calcium, magnesium as indicated.

Returning these electrolytes to normal may correct many dysrhythmias.

Administer appropriate antidysrhythmia medications. (Refer to CP: Dysrhythmias, p. 81.)

May be necessary to maintain/improve cardiac output.

Prepare patient for transfer to critical care unit, as indicated.

Patients with digitalis toxicity frequently require intensive monitoring until therapeutic levels have been restored. Because all digitalis preparations have long serum half-lives, stabilization can take several days.

Prepare patient for insertion of temporary pacemaker if indicated.

May be required to maintain adequate heart rate until digitalis levels are within therapeutic range.

NURSING DIAGNOSIS:	FLUID VOLUME DEFICIT/EXCESS, POTENTIAL
May be related to:	Gastrointestinal side effects of digitalis toxicity, e.g., nausea/vomiting, diarrhea
	Continued use of diuretics in face of reduced intake
	Excess sodium/fluid retention
	Decreased plasma proteins/malnutrition
Possibly evidenced by:	[Not applicable; presence of signs and symptoms establishes an *actual* diagnosis.]
PATIENT OUTCOMES/ EVALUATION CRITERIA:	Demonstrates stabilized fluid volume with balanced intake/output, stable weight, vital signs within patient's norms, and absence of edema. Verbalizes relief from nausea and absence of vomiting/diarrhea.

ACTIONS/INTERVENTIONS

RATIONALE

Independent

Monitor intake/output. Calculate fluid balance, noting insensible losses. Weigh as indicated.

Direct evaluator of fluid status. Sudden changes in weight suggest fluid loss/retention.

Evaluate skin turgor, mucous membrane moisture; presence of dependent/generalized edema.

Indirect indicators of fluid status/resolution of imbalance.

Monitor vital signs, e.g., blood pressure, pulse and respiratory rate. Auscultate breath sounds, noting presence of crackles.

Fluid deficits may be manifested by hypotension, tachycardia, as heart tries to maintain cardiac output. Fluid excess/developing failure may be manifested by

ACTIONS/INTERVENTIONS

Independent

Review fluid requirements. Establish 24-hour schedule and routes to be used. Ascertain patient beverage/food preferences.

Eliminate noxious sights and smells from the environment. Provide frequent oral hygiene.

Instruct patient to take fluids and food slowly as indicated.

Collaborative

Provide IV fluids via control device.

Administer antiemetics, e.g., prochlorperazine maleate (Compazine), trimethobenzamide (Tigan), as indicated.

Monitor laboratory studies as indicated, e.g., Hb/Hct, BUN/Cr, plasma proteins, electrolytes.

RATIONALE

hypertension, tachycardia, tachypnea, crackles, respiratory distress.

Dependent upon situation, fluids may be restricted or forced. Providing information involves patient in formulating schedule with individual preferences, enhances a sense of control and cooperation with regimen.

May reduce stimulation of the vomiting center.

May reduce occurrence of vomiting in nausea.

Fluids may be needed to prevent dehydration, although fluid restrictions may be required if the patient is in CHF.

May be helpful in reducing nausea/vomiting (considered to be central, rather than gastric in origin) enhancing fluid/food intake.

Evaluates hydration status, renal function and causes/effects of imbalance.

NURSING DIAGNOSIS:	**THOUGHT PROCESSES, ALTERED [POTENTIAL]**
May be related to:	**Physiologic effects of toxicity/reduced cerebral perfusion**
Possibly evidenced by:	**[Not applicable; presence of signs and symptoms establishes an *actual* diagnosis.]**
PATIENT OUTCOMES/ EVALUATION CRITERIA:	**Usual mentation is maintained.**

ACTIONS/INTERVENTIONS

Independent

Assess/investigate changes in mentation/sensorium. Talk to family members about patient's usual mentation.

Stay with/arrange for companion when patient is severely agitated.

Explain procedures, repeatedly if indicated. Reorient to surroundings as needed.

RATIONALE

The elderly patient may already have problems in mentation associated with age, cerebral vascular impairment, and/or multiple system failure in addition to digitalis toxicity. Information from the family concerning usual mentation is helpful in understanding the patient's progress in resolution of the toxic state. Exaggerated symptoms usually resolve as digitalis level returns to therapeutic range.

Protects patient from bodily harm until normal functioning is regained.

May reduce agitation/anxiety, promoting sense of security as toxicity clears.

ACTIONS/INTERVENTIONS

Independent

Provide emotional support to the patient/SO. Stress temporary nature of recent changes in mentation. (Refer to CP: Psychosocial Aspects of Care, p. 773.)

Collaborative

Administer supplemental oxygen if indicated.

RATIONALE

Provides reassurance and reduces level of fear in stressful situation.

May be helpful in improving level of mentation/thought processes, especially in the presence of severe heart disease, CHF, or acid–base imbalance.

NURSING DIAGNOSIS:	KNOWLEDGE DEFICIT [LEARNING NEED] (SPECIFY)
May be related to:	Lack of information concerning specific digitalis therapy or ways to monitor safety/effectiveness of therapy
Possibly evidenced by:	Failure to follow prescribed regimen. Failure to recognize toxic side effects.
PATIENT OUTCOMES/ EVALUATION CRITERIA:	Verbalizes understanding of why drug is needed, when it is toxic, how it interacts with other drugs. Demonstrates how to count pulse rate. Recognizes signs of digitalis overdose, developing CHF, and what to report to physician.

ACTIONS/INTERVENTIONS

Independent

Provide information about why digitalis preparation is needed, e.g., to strengthen heart muscle contraction, and to correct irregular heartbeat.

Explain patient's specific type of digitalis.

Instruct patient not to change dose for any reason, not to omit dose, not to increase dose or take extra doses, and to contact doctor if more than one dose is omitted.

Show patient how to count pulse for 1 full minute, and have patient demonstrate this skill. Instruct patient to contact doctor before taking dose if pulse is below or above predetermined levels or is more irregular.

Advise patient that digitalis may react with any other drug(s) (e.g., barbiturates, neomycin, quinidine) presently taken, and to provide physician with information that digitalis is taken whenever new medications are prescribed. Advise patient not to take OTC drugs (e.g., laxatives, antidiarrheals, antacids, cold remedies, diuretics) without first checking with the pharmacist or physician.

Provide information and have the patient/SO verbalize understanding of toxic signs/symptoms to report to the physician.

RATIONALE

Understanding need for using potentially dangerous drug may enhance compliance with therapeutic regimen.

Reduces confusion due to digitalis preparations varying in name (although they may be similar), dosage strength, and onset and duration of action.

Alterations in drug regimen can reduce therapeutic effects/result in toxicity, and development of complications.

Digitalis may potentiate/cause dangerous dysrhythmias, impairing cardiac output/patient safety.

Knowledge may help prevent dangerous drug interactions.

Nausea, vomiting, diarrhea; unusual drowsiness, confusion; very slow or very fast irregular pulse, thumping in chest; double/blurred vision, yellow/green tint or ha-

ACTIONS/INTERVENTIONS	RATIONALE

Independent

los around objects, flickering color forms or dots, altered color perception are warning signs that patient should be aware of and report to physician immediately.

Provide written instructions to take home. Involve SO in education.

Patient teaching card listing important facts in large, readable print and simple terms can minimize misinterpretation.

Collaborative

Arrange for visiting nurse, home assistance if responsible SO is not readily available.

If elderly patient lives alone and/or is visually or cognitively impaired, home follow-up is essential to reduce risk of overdose.

Angina Pectoris _____

PATIENT ASSESSMENT DATA BASE

ACTIVITY/REST

May report: Fatigue, weakness, sedentary lifestyle.
Chest pain with exertion.

May exhibit: Exertional dyspnea.

CIRCULATION

May report: History of heart disease, hypertension, obesity.
High stress levels.
Diabetes.

May exhibit: Tachycardia, dysrhythmias.
Blood pressure normal, elevated, or decreased.
Heart sounds: may be normal; late S_4 or transient late systolic murmur (papillary muscle dysfunction) may be evident during pain.
Moist, cool, pale skin/mucous membranes in presence of vasoconstriction.

FOOD/FLUID

May report: Nausea.
Diet high in cholesterol/fats, salt, caffeine, liquor.

May exhibit: Belching, gastric distention.

EGO INTEGRITY

May report: Stressors of work, family, others.

May exhibit: Apprehension, uneasiness.

PAIN/COMFORT

May report: Substernal, anterior chest pain that may radiate to jaw, neck, shoulders, upper extremities (to left side more than right).
Quality: varies, mild to moderate, heavy pressure, tightness, squeezing, burning.
Duration: usually less than 15 minutes, not more than 30 minutes (average 3 minutes).
Precipitating factors: pain may be related to physical exertion or great emotion, such as anger or sexual arousal; exercise in weather extremes; or may be unpredictable and/or occur during rest.
Relieving factors: pain may be responsive to particular relief mechanisms (e.g., rest, antianginal medications).
New or ongoing chest pain which has changed in frequency, duration, character or predictability (i.e., unstable, variant, Prinzmetal's).

May exhibit: Facial grimacing, muscle tension, restlessness.
Autonomic responses.

RESPIRATION

May report: Dyspnea with exertion.
History of smoking.

May exhibit: Respirations: increased rate/rhythm, and alteration in depth.

TEACHING/LEARNING

May report: Familial history of heart disease, hypertension, stroke, diabetes.

Use/misuse of cardiac, hypertensive, or OTC drugs.

Regular alcohol use.

Discharge Plan Considerations: Alteration in medication use/therapy.

Assistance with homemaker tasks.

Physical layout of home.

DIAGNOSTIC STUDIES

Cardiac enzymes/isoenzymes: usually within normal limits (WNL); elevation indicates myocardial damage.

ECG: usually normal when patient at rest; but flattening or depression of the ST segment of T wave signifies ischemia; transient ST elevation or decrease greater than 1mm during pain with no abnormalities when pain-free demonstrates transient myocardial ischemia. Dysrhythmias, heart block may also be present.

24-hour ECG monitoring (Holter): done to see whether pain periods correlate with ST segment changes. ST depression without pain is highly indicative of ischemia.

Chest x-ray: usually normal; however, infiltrates may be present (cardiac decompensation or pulmonary complications).

PCO_2, potassium and myocardial lactate: may be elevated during anginal attack (all play a role in myocardial ischemia and may perpetuate it).

Serum cholesterol/triglycerides: may be elevated (CAD risk factor).

Echocardiogram: may reveal abnormal valvular action as cause of angina.

Paced stress-atrial tachycardia: may show ST segment change. LV end diastolic pressure (LVEDP) may rise or remain static with ischemia. Rise with chest pain or ST change is diagnostic of ischemia.

Nuclear imaging studies: (thallium 201) ischemic myocardial regions appear as areas of decreased thallium uptake.

Gated imaging (MUGA): evaluates specific and general ventrical performance, regional wall motion and ejection fraction.

Coronary angiography: used to demonstrate levels of blockage in main coronary vessels, as well as collateral vessels. Note: Ten percent of patients with unstable angina have normal-appearing coronary arteries.

Ergonovine (Ergotrate): injected in patients who have angina at rest to demonstrate hyperspastic coronary vessels. Patients with resting angina usually experience chest pain, ST elevation, or depression and/or pronounced rise in LVEDP, fall in systemic systolic pressure, and/or high-grade coronary artery narrowing. Some patients may also have severe ventricular dysrhythmias.

NURSING PRIORITIES

1. Relieve/control pain.
2. Prevent/minimize development of myocardial complications.
3. Provide information about disease process/prognosis and treatment.
4. Support patient/SO in initiating necessary lifestyle/behavioral changes.

DISCHARGE CRITERIA

1. Achieves desired activity level; meets self-care needs with minimal or no pain.
2. Complications prevented.
3. Disease process/prognosis and therapeutic regimen understood.
4. Participating in treatment program, behavioral changes.

Refer to CPs: Acute Myocardial Infarction, p. 69; Congestive Heart Failure, p. 41; Dysrhythmias, p. 81.

NURSING DIAGNOSIS:	COMFORT, ALTERED: PAIN, ACUTE
May be related to:	Decreased myocardial blood flow
	Increased cardiac workload/oxygen consumption
Possibly evidenced by:	Reports of pain varying in frequency, duration and intensity (as condition worsens)
	Narrowed focus
	Distraction behaviors (moaning, crying, pacing, restlessness)
	Autonomic responses, e.g., diaphoresis, blood pressure and pulse rate changes, pupillary dilation, increased/decreased respiratory rate
PATIENT OUTCOMES/ EVALUATION CRITERIA:	Verbalizes relief of pain. Reports anginal episodes decreased in frequency, duration and severity.

ACTIONS/INTERVENTIONS	RATIONALE
Independent	
Instruct patient to notify nurse immediately when chest pain occurs.	Pain and decreased cardiac output may stimulate the sympathetic nervous system to release excessive amounts of norepinephrine, increasing platelet aggregation and release of thromboxane A_2. This potent vasoconstrictor causes coronary artery spasm which can precipitate, complicate and/or prolong an anginal attack. Unbearable pain may cause vasovagal response, decreasing BP and heart rate.
Assess and document patient response/effects of medication.	Provides information about disease progression. Aids in evaluating effectiveness of interventions and may indicate need for change in therapeutic regimen.
Identify precipitating event, if any, frequency, duration, intensity and location of pain.	Helps differentiate this chest pain and aids in evaluating possible progression to unstable angina. (Stable angina usually lasts 3–5 minutes while unstable angina is more intense and may last up to 45 minutes.)
Observe for associated symptoms, e.g., dyspnea, nausea/vomiting, dizziness, palpitations, desire to micturate.	Decreased cardiac output (which may occur during ischemic myocardial episode) stimulates sympathetic/parasympathetic nervous system, causing a variety of vague aches/sensations that patient may not identify as related to anginal episode.
Evaluate complaints of pain in jaw, neck, shoulder, arm or hand (typically on left side).	Cardiac pain may radiate, e.g., pain is often referred to more superficial sites served by the same spinal cord level.
Place patient at complete rest during anginal episodes.	Reduces myocardial oxygen demand to minimize risk of tissue injury/necrosis.
Elevate head of bed if short of breath.	Facilitates diaphragmatic expansion, increasing area for gas exchange to decrease hypoxia and resultant shortness of breath.
Monitor heart rate/rhythm.	Unstable angina patients have an increased risk of acute life-threatening dysrhythmias, which occur in response to ischemic changes and/or stress.

ACTIONS/INTERVENTIONS	RATIONALE

Independent

Monitor vital signs every 5 minutes during anginal attack.

Blood pressure may rise initially due to sympathetic stimulation, then fall if cardiac output is compromised. Tachycardia also develops in response to sympathetic stimulation and may be sustained as a compensatory response if cardiac output falls.

Stay with patient experiencing pain or appearing anxious.

Anxiety increases catecholamines which increases myocardial workload and increases or prolongs ischemic pain. Presence of nurse can reduce feelings of fear and helplessness.

Maintain quiet, comfortable environment; restrict visitors as necessary.

Mental/emotional stress increases myocardial workload.

Provide light meals. Have patient rest for 1 hour after meals.

Decreases myocardial workload associated with work of digestion, reducing risk of anginal attack.

Collaborative

Provide supplemental oxygen as indicated.

May increase oxygen available for myocardial uptake/reversal of ischemia. Unstable angina is thought to be a preinfarction syndrome, and that MI can occur at any time due to the narrow margin separating reversible ischemia and tissue damage.

Administer antianginal medication(s) promptly as indicated:

Nitroglycerine sublingual (Nitrostat) or

Rapid vasodilator whose effect lasts 10–30 minutes. Can be used prophylactically to prevent, as well as abort, anginal attacks. May, however, enhance vasospastic angina.

Long-acting, e.g., Nitro-Dur, Transderm-Nitro, isosorbide (Isordil, Sorbitrate);

Reduces frequency and severity of attack by producing prolonged/continuous vasodilation. May cause headache, dizziness, lightheadedness, but these symptoms usually pass quickly. If headache is intolerable, alteration of dosage or discontinuation may be necessary.

Beta-blockers, e.g., atenolol (Tenormin), metroprolol (Lopressor), propranolol (Inderal);

Reduces angina by decreasing heart rate and systolic blood pressure. (Refer to ND: Cardiac Output, Altered: Decreased, p. 64.)

Analgesics, i.e., acetaminophen (Tylenol);

Usually sufficient analgesia for relief of headache caused by dilatation of cerebral vessels in response to nitrates.

Morphine (IV).

Potent narcotic analgesic that has several beneficial effects, e.g., causes peripheral vasodilation, reducing myocardial workload; has a sedative effect to produce relaxation; interrupts the flow of vasoconstricting catecholamines, and thereby effectively relieves severe chest pain. It is given IV for rapid action as decreased cardiac output may compromise peripheral tissue absorption.

Monitor serial ECG changes.

Ischemia during anginal attack may cause transient ST segment depression or elevation and T wave inversion. Verifies ischemic changes which may not be evident when patient is not experiencing pain. Also helpful as baseline with which to compare later pattern changes.

NURSING DIAGNOSIS:	CARDIAC OUTPUT, ALTERED: DECREASED
May be related to:	Inotropic changes (transient/prolonged myocardial ischemia, effects of medications)
	Alterations in rate/rhythm and electrical conduction
Possibly evidenced by:	Changes in hemodynamic readings
	Dyspnea
	Restlessness
	Decreased tolerance for activity, fatigue
	Diminished peripheral pulses
	Cool/pale skin
	Change in mental status
	Continued chest pain
PATIENT OUTCOMES/ EVALUATION CRITERIA:	Reports/displays decreased episodes of dyspnea, angina, and dysrhythmias. Demonstrates an increase in activity tolerance. Participates in activities that reduce workload of the heart.

ACTIONS/INTERVENTIONS	RATIONALE
Independent	
Monitor vital signs, e.g., heart rate, blood pressure.	Tachycardia may be present because of pain, anxiety, hypoxemia, drop in cardiac output. Changes may also occur in blood pressure (hypertension or hypotension) because of cardiac response.
Evaluate mental status, noting development of confusion, disorientation.	Reduced perfusion to vital organs can produce observable and documentable changes in sensorium.
Note skin color, and presence/quality of pulses.	Peripheral circulation is reduced as cardiac output falls giving the skin a pale or grey color (depending on level of hypoxia) and diminishing the strength of peripheral pulses.
Auscultate heart/breath sounds and for presence of murmurs.	S_3, S_4 or crackles may indicate cardiac decompensation or effects of medication especially beta-blockers. Development of murmurs may reveal a valvular cause for chest pain, e.g., AS, MS, MVP. (Refer to CP: Valvular Heart Disease, p. 88.)
Maintain bedrest in position of comfort during acute episodes.	Decreases oxygen consumption/demand reducing myocardial workload and risk of decompensation.
Provide for adequate rest periods. Assist with/perform self-care activities, as indicated.	Conserves energy, reduces cardiac workload.
Stress importance of avoiding straining/bearing down for stool.	Valsalva maneuver causes vagal stimulation, reducing heart rate (bradycardia), which may be followed by rebound tachycardia, both of which may impair cardiac output.
Encourage immediate reporting of pain for prompt administration of medications as indicated.	Timely interventions can reduce oxygen consumption and myocardial workload and may prevent/minimize cardiac complications.

ACTIONS/INTERVENTIONS	RATIONALE

Independent

Monitor for and document effects/adverse response of pharmacotherapeutics, noting blood pressure, heart rate and AV conduction especially when giving combination of calcium antagonists, propranolol, and nitrates.

Overall effect is to decrease myocardial oxygen demand by decreasing wall stress. Beta-blockers are given for negative inotropic effect, which may decrease perfusion to already ischemic myocardium. Combination of nitrates, beta-blockers may have cumulative effect on cardiac output.

Assess for signs and symptoms of congestive heart failure.

Angina is only a symptom of underlying pathology causing myocardial ischemia. Disease may compromise cardiac function to point of decompensation. (Refer to CP: Congestive Heart Failure, p. 41.)

Collaborative

Administer supplemental oxygen as needed.

Given to increase oxygen available for myocardial uptake to improve contractility by reducing ischemia and lactic acid levels.

Administer medications, as indicated, e.g.:

Calcium channel blockers: diltiazem (Cardizem), nifedipine (Procardia), verapamil (Calan);

Although differing in mode of action, calcium channel blockers play a major role in preventing and terminating myocardial ischemia induced by coronary artery spasm and in reducing vascular resistance, thereby decreasing BP and cardiac workload.

Beta-blockers, e.g., atenolol (Tenormin), nadolol (Corgard), propranolol (Inderal).

Decreases cardiac workload by reducing heart rate, workload and systolic BP. Note: Overdosage produces decompensation.

Discuss purpose for cardiac catheterization.

Identifies areas of obstruction/damage that may require surgical intervention.

Prepare for surgical intervention (CABG, valve replacement, PTCA) if indicated. (Refer to CP: Cardiac Surgery [Postoperative Care], p. 98.)

CABG is recommended when testing confirms myocardial ischemia as a result of left main coronary artery disease or symptomatic three-vessel disease. Note: PTCA may be performed in specific situations to increase coronary blood flow by compression of atheromatous lesions and dilatation of vessel lumen in an occluded coronary artery.

Prepare for transfer to critical care unit if condition warrants.

Profound/prolonged decrease in cardiac output reflects progression of disease process/development of complications requiring more intense/emergent interventions.

NURSING DIAGNOSIS: **ANXIETY [SPECIFY LEVEL]**

May be related to: **Situational crises**

Threat to self-concept (altered image/abilities)

Underlying pathophysiologic response

Threat to or change in health status (disease course which can lead to further compromise, debility, even death)

Negative self-talk

Possibly evidenced by:	Expressed concern regarding changes in life events
	Increased tension/helplessness
	Apprehension, uncertainty, restlessness
	Association of diagnosis with loss of healthy body image, loss of place/influence as family member
	View of self as noncontributing member of family/society
	Fear of death as an imminent reality
PATIENT OUTCOMES/ EVALUATION CRITERIA:	Verbalizes awareness of feelings of anxiety and healthy ways to deal with them. Reports anxiety is reduced to a manageable level. Expresses concerns about effect of disease on lifestyle, position within family and society. Demonstrates effective coping strategies/problem-solving skills.

ACTIONS/INTERVENTIONS

Independent

Explain purpose of tests and procedures, e.g., stress testing.

Promote expression of feelings and fears, e.g., denial, depression and anger; let patient/SO know these are normal reactions. Note statements of concern, e.g., "Heart attack is inevitable."

Encourage family and friends to treat patient as before.

Tell patient the medical regimen has been designed to reduce/limit future attacks and increase cardiac stability.

(Refer to CP: Psychosocial Aspects of Acute Care, p. 773.)

Collaborative

Administer sedatives, tranquilizers, as indicated.

RATIONALE

Reduces anxiety attributable to fear of prognosis which may disrupt beliefs about body image.

Unexpressed feelings may create internal turmoil and may affect self-image. Verbalization of concerns reduces tension, verifies level of coping, and facilitates dealing with feelings. Presence of negative self-talk can increase level of anxiety and may contribute to exacerbation of anginal attacks. This is part of the grieving process, which is necessary before patient can adapt to altered self-image.

Reassures patient that role in the family and business has not been altered.

Encourages patient to test symptom control (e.g., no angina with certain levels of activity) to increase confidence in medical program and integrate abilities into perceptions of self.

May be desired to help patient to relax until physically able to reestablish adequate coping strategies.

NURSING DIAGNOSIS:	KNOWLEDGE DEFICIT [LEARNING NEED] (SPECIFY)
May be related to:	Lack of exposure
	Inaccurate/misinterpretation of information
	Unfamiliarity with information resources

Possibly evidenced by:	Questions
	Request for information
	Statement of concerns
	Inaccurate follow-through of instructions
PATIENT OUTCOMES/ EVALUATION CRITERIA:	Participates in learning process. Assumes responsibility for own learning, looking for information and asking questions. Verbalizes understanding of condition/ disease process and treatment. Participates in treatment regimen and initiates necessary lifestyle changes.

ACTIONS/INTERVENTIONS

Independent

Review pathophysiology of condition. Stress need for preventing anginal attacks and progression of atherosclerotic process.

Encourage avoidance of factors/situations that may precipitate anginal episode, e.g., emotional stress, physical exertion, ingestion of large/heavy meal, exposure to extremes in environmental temperature.

Assist patient/SO to identify sources of physical and emotional stress and discuss ways that they can be avoided.

Review importance of weight control, cessation of smoking, dietary changes, exercise.

Encourage patient to follow prescribed reconditioning program; caution to avoid exhaustion.

Discuss impact of illness on desired lifestyle and activities, including work, driving, sexual activity, and hobbies. Provide information, privacy, or consultation, as indicated.

Demonstrate/encourage patient to monitor own pulse during activities, schedule/simplify activities, avoid strain.

Discuss steps to take when anginal attacks occur, e.g., cessation of activity, administration of p.r.n. medication, use of relaxation techniques.

Discuss proper times, doses, and medications for control/prevention of anginal attacks. Stress importance of checking with physician prior to taking OTC drugs.

Review use of aspirin (ASA) as a regularly prescribed drug.

RATIONALE

This is the focus of therapeutic management in order to reduce likelihood of myocardial infarction.

May reduce incidence/severity of ischemic episodes.

This is a crucial step in limiting/preventing anginal attacks.

Knowledge of the significance of risk factors provides patient with opportunity to make needed changes.

Fear of triggering attacks may cause patient to avoid participation in activity which has been prescribed to enhance recovery (increase myocardial strength and form collateral circulation).

Patient may be reluctant to resume/continue usual activities because of fear of anginal attack/death.

Allows patient to identify how activities can be modified to avoid increased cardiac stress. Helps to limit increases in oxygen demand/consumption and cardiac workload in order to keep cardiac stress below anginal threshold.

Being prepared for an event takes away the fear that patient will not know what to do if attack occurs.

Angina is a complicated illness which often requires the use of many drugs given to decrease myocardial workload and control the occurrence of attacks. OTC drugs may potentiate or negate prescribed medications.

May be given prophylactically on a daily basis to prevent platelet aggregation.

ACTIONS/INTERVENTIONS

Independent

Review symptoms to be reported to physician, e.g., increase in frequency/duration of attacks, changes in response to medications.

Discuss importance of follow-up appointments.

RATIONALE

Knowledge of expectations can avoid undue concern for insignificant reasons or delay in treatment of important symptoms.

Angina is a progressive disease and may require adjustment of treatment regimen to prevent myocardial damage.

Myocardial Infarction

PATIENT ASSESSMENT DATA BASE

ACTIVITY/REST

May report: Weakness, fatigue, loss of sleep.

May exhibit: Tachycardia, dyspnea with rest/activity.

CIRCULATION

May report: History of previous MI, coronary artery disease, CHF, BP problems, diabetes mellitus.

May exhibit: Blood pressure: may be normal or increased/decreased; postural changes may be noted from lying to sitting/standing.

Pulse: may be normal; full/bounding, or weak/thready quality with delayed capillary refill; irregularities (dysrhythmias) may be present.

Heart sounds: extra heart sounds, S_3/S_4 may reflect cardiac failure/loss of ventricular contractility (resistance).

Murmurs: if present, may reflect valvular insufficiency or papillary muscle dysfunction.

Friction rub: suggests pericarditis.

Heart rate: may be abnormal (tachycardia, bradycardia).

Heart rhythm: can be regular or irregular.

Edema: jugular vein distention, peripheral/dependent edema, generalized edema, crackles may be present with cardiac failure.

Color: pallor or cyanosis/mottling of skin, nailbeds, mucous membranes, lips may be noted.

EGO INTEGRITY

May report: Fear of dying, feelings of impending doom.
Anger at inconvenience of illness/"unnecessary" hospitalization.
Worry about family, job, finances.

May exhibit: Denial, withdrawal, anxiety, lack of eye contact, irritability, anger.
Combative behavior.
Focus on self/pain.

ELIMINATION

May exhibit: Normal or decreased bowel sounds.

FOOD/FLUID

May report: Nausea, loss of appetite.

May exhibit: Decreased skin turgor; dry/diaphoretic skin.
Vomiting.
Weight change.

HYGIENE

May exhibit: Exertional dyspnea/chest pain or tachycardia during care tasks.

NEUROSENSORY

May report: Dizziness, fainting spells.

May exhibit: Changes in mentation.

PAIN/COMFORT

May report:
Sudden onset chest pain (may/may not be associated with activity), unrelieved by rest or nitroglycerin.

Location: typically anterior chest, substernal, precordium; may radiate to arms, jaws, face.

May have atypical location such as epigastrium, elbow, jaw.

Quality: crushing, constricting viselike, steady.

Intensity: usually 10 on a scale of 1–10; may be "worst pain ever experienced."

May exhibit:
Facial grimacing, changes in body posture.

Crying, groaning.

Withdrawal, loss of eye contact.

Changes in heart rate/rhythm, ECG; blood pressure, respirations, skin color/moisture, level of consciousness.

RESPIRATION

May report:
Dyspnea, with/without exertion, nocturnal dyspnea.

Cough, with/without sputum production.

History of smoking, chronic respiratory disease.

May exhibit:
Increased respiratory rate, shallow/labored breathing.

Pallor or cyanosis.

Breath sounds: clear, or crackles/wheezes.

Sputum: clear, pink-tinged.

SOCIAL INTERACTION

May report:
Recent stress, e.g., work, family.

Difficulty coping with current stressors, e.g., illness, hospitalization.

May exhibit:
Difficulty resting quietly, overemotional responses (intense anger, fear).

TEACHING/LEARNING

May report:
Family history of heart disease, diabetes, stroke, hypertension, peripheral vascular disease.

Use of tobacco.

Discharge Plan Considerations:
Assistance with food preparation, shoppinng, transportation, homemaking tasks; physical layout of home.

DIAGNOSTIC STUDIES

ECG: shows S-T wave elevation, signifying ischemia; depressed or inverted T wave, indicating injury; and presence of Q waves, signifying necrosis.

Cardiac enzymes and isoenzymes: CPK-MB elevates within 4–12 hours and peaks in 24 hours. LDH elevates within 24–48 hours, peaks within 3–6 days, and may take as long as 2 weeks to return to normal. SGOT elevations (less reliable/specific) occur in 6–12 hours and peak in 36 hours.

Electrolytes: imbalances may occur that alter conduction and can compromise contractility, e.g., hypo/hyperkalemia.

WBC: Leukocytosis (10,000–20,000) usually appears on the second day after MI due to inflammation.

Sedimentation rate: rises on second to third day after MI, indicating inflammation.

Chemistry profiles: may be abnormal depending on acute/chronic abnormal organ function/perfusion.

ABGs: indicate hypoxia or acute/chronic lung disease processes.

Serum cholesterol/triglycerides: elevation may reflect arteriosclerosis.

Chest x-ray: may be normal or show an enlarged cardiac shadow suggestive of congestive heart failure or ventricular aneurysm.

Echocardiogram: may be done to determine dimensions of chambers, septal/ventricular wall motion, and valve configuration/function.

Nuclear imaging studies:

Thallium: evaluates myocardial blood flow and status of myocardial cells, e.g., location/extent of acute/previous MI.

Technetium: detects acute MI.

Cardiac blood imaging/MUGA: evaluates specific and general ventricular performance, regional wall motion and ejection fraction.

Coronary arteriography: visualizes narrowing/occlusion of coronary arteries and is usually done in conjunction with measurements of chamber pressures and assessment of left ventricular function (ejection fraction). Procedure not usually done in acute phase of MI unless angioplasty/emergency heart surgery is imminent.

Digital subtraction angiography (DSA): technique being used to visualize arterial bypass grafts and to detect peripheral artery disease.

Nuclear magnetic resonance (NMR): allows visualization of blood flow, cardiac chambers/intraventricular septum, and valves and detection of vascular lesions, plaque formations, infarction, and blood clots.

Exercise stress test: determines cardiovascular response to activity (often done in conjunction with thallium imaging in the recovery phase).

NURSING PRIORITIES

1. Relieve pain, anxiety.
2. Reduce myocardial workload.
3. Prevent/detect and assist in treatment of life-threatening dysrhythmias or complications.
4. Promote cardiac health, self-care.

DISCHARGE CRITERIA

1. Chest pain absent/controlled.
2. Heart rate/rhythm sufficient to sustain adequate cardiac output/tissue perfusion.
3. Achievement of activity level sufficient for basic self-care.
4. Anxiety reduced/managed.
5. Disease process, treatment plan, and prognosis understood.

NURSING DIAGNOSIS:	COMFORT, ALTERED: PAIN, ACUTE
May be related to:	Tissue ischemia secondary to coronary artery occlusion
Possibly evidenced by:	Complaints of chest pain with/without radiation to arms, jaws, back, epigastrium
	Facial grimacing
	Restlessness, changes in level of consciousness
	Changes in pulse, blood pressure
PATIENT OUTCOMES/ EVALUATION CRITERIA:	Verbalizes relief/control of chest pain. Demonstrates reduced tension, relaxed manner.

ACTIONS/INTERVENTIONS	RATIONALE

Independent

Monitor/document characteristics of pain, noting verbal complaints, nonverbal cues and hemodynamic response (e.g., moaning, crying, restlessness, diaphoresis, clutching chest, rapid breathing, blood pressure/heart rate changes).

Variation of appearance and behavior of patients in pain may present a challenge in assessment. Most patients with an acute MI appear acutely ill, distracted, and focused on pain. Verbal history and deeper investigation of precipitating factors should be postponed until pain is relieved. Respirations may be increased as a result of pain and associated anxiety, while release of stress induced catecholamines will increase heart rate and blood pressure.

Obtain full description of pain from patient; including location, intensity (1–10), duration, quality (dull/crushing), and radiation.

Pain is a subjective experience, and must be described by the patient. Assist patient to quantify pain by comparing it to other experiences.

Review history of previous angina, anginal equivalent, or myocardial infarction pain.

May differentiate current pain from preexisting patterns, as well as identify complications such as extension of infarction, pulmonary embolus, or pericarditis.

Instruct patient to report pain immediately.

Delay in reporting pain hinders pain relief/may require increased dosage of medication to achieve relief. In addition, severe pain may induce shock by stimulating the sympathetic nervous system.

Provide quiet environment, and calm activities, and comfort measures (e.g., dry/wrinkle-free linens, backrub). Approach the patient calmly and with confidence.

Decreases external stimuli which may aggravate anxiety and cardiac strain, and limit coping abilities.

Assist/instruct in relaxation techniques, e.g., deep/slow breathing, distraction behaviors, visualization, guided imagery.

Helpful in decreasing perception of/response to pain. Provides a sense of having some control over the situation.

Check vital signs before and after narcotic medication.

Hypotension/respiratory depression can occur as a result of narcotic administration.

Collaborative

Administer supplemental oxygen, by means of nasal cannula, face mask as indicated.

Increases amount of oxygen available for myocardial uptake, and may relieve discomfort associated with tissue ischemia or dyspnea, in addition to reducing cardiac work.

Administer medications as indicated, e.g.:

    Antianginals, e.g., nitroglycerin (Nitro-Bid, Nitro-stat, Nitro-Dur);

Nitrates are useful for pain control by coronary vasodilating effects which increases coronary blood flow and myocardial perfusion. Peripheral vasodilation effects reduce the volume of blood returning to the heart (preload), thereby decreasing myocardial work and oxygen demand.

    Beta-blockers, e.g., atenolol (Tenormin), pindolol (Visken), propranolol (Inderal);

Important secondline agents for pain control through effect of blocking sympathetic stimulation, thereby reducing heart rate, systolic BP, and myocardial oxygen demand. May be given alone or with nitrates. Note: Beta-blockers may be contraindicated if myocardial contractility is severely impaired, because negative inotropic properties can further reduce contractility.

    Analgesics, e.g., morphine/meperidine (Demerol);

Although IV morphine is the usual drug of choice, other injectable narcotics may be used in acute phase/

ACTIONS/INTERVENTIONS

Collaborative

Calcium channel blockers, e.g., verapamil (Calan), diltiazem hydrochloride (Cardizem), nifedipine (Procardia).

RATIONALE

recurrent chest pain unrelieved by nitroglycerin to reduce severe pain, provide sedation, and decrease myocardial workload. Intramuscular injections should be avoided, if possible, because they can alter the CPK diagnostic indicator and are not well absorbed in underperfused tissue.

Vasodilation effects can increase coronary blood flow, encourage collateral circulation, and reduce preload and myocardial oxygen demands. Some of these agents also have antidysrhythmic properties.

NURSING DIAGNOSIS:	ACTIVITY INTOLERANCE
May be related to:	Imbalance between myocardial oxygen supply and demand
	Presence of ischemia/necrotic myocardial tissues
	Cardiac depressant effects of certain drugs (beta-blockers, antidysrhythmics)
Possibly evidenced by:	Alterations in heart rate and blood pressure with activity
	Development of dysrhythmias
	Changes in skin color/moisture
	Exertional angina
	Generalized weakness
PATIENT OUTCOMES/ EVALUATION CRITERIA:	Demonstrates measurable/progressive increase in tolerance for activity with heart rate/rhythm and blood pressure within patient's normal limits and skin warm, pink, dry. Reports angina absent/controlled.

ACTIONS/INTERVENTIONS

Independent

Record/document heart rate, rhythm and blood pressure changes before, during, after activity, as indicated. Correlate with complaints of chest pain/shortness of breath. (Refer to ND: Cardiac Output, Altered: Decreased [Potential], p. 75.)

Promote rest (bed/chair) initially. Limit activity on basis of pain/hemodynamic response. Provide nonstress diversional activities.

Instruct patient to avoid straining at stool.

RATIONALE

Trends determine patient's response to activity and may indicate myocardial oxygen deprivation that may require decrease in activity level/return to bedrest, changes in medication regimen, use of supplemental oxygen.

Reduces myocardial workload/oxygen consumption, reducing risk of complications (e.g., extension of MI).

Activities that require holding the breath and bearing down (Valsalva maneuver) can result in bradycardia, temporarily reduced cardiac output, and rebound tachycardia with elevated BP.

ACTIONS/INTERVENTIONS

Independent

Explain pattern of graded increase of activity level, e.g., getting up in chair when there is no pain, progressive ambulation, and resting for 1 hour after meals. Take vital signs before and after activity.

Review signs/symptoms reflecting intolerance of present activity level, requiring notification of nurse/physician.

Collaborative

Refer to hospital/community cardiac rehabilitation program.

RATIONALE

Progressive activity provides a controlled increase of demand on the heart, increasing strength and preventing overexertion.

Palpitations/pulse irregularities, development of chest pain/dyspnea may indicate need for changes in exercise regimen or medication.

Provides continued support/supervision after discharge.

NURSING DIAGNOSIS:	ANXIETY/FEAR [SPECIFY LEVEL]
May be related to:	Threat to or change in health and socioeconomic status
	Threat of loss/death
	Unconscious conflict about essential values, beliefs, and goals of life
Possibly evidenced by:	Fearful attitude
	Apprehension, increased tension, restlessness, facial tension
	Uncertainty
	Feelings of inadequacy
	Somatic complaints/sympathetic stimulation
	Focus on self, expressions of concern about current events
	Fight or flight behavior
PATIENT OUTCOMES/EVALUATION CRITERIA:	Recognizes feelings and identifies causes, contributing factors. Verbalizes reduction of anxiety/fear. Demonstrates positive problem-solving skills. Identifies/uses resources appropriately.

ACTIONS/INTERVENTIONS

Independent

Identify and acknowledge patient's perception of threat/situation. Encourage expressions of and do not deny feelings, e.g., anger, grief, sadness, fear. Note complaints of insomnia; presence of hostility, withdrawal, and/or denial (inappropriate affect or refusal to comply with medical regimen).

RATIONALE

Coping with pain and emotional trauma of an MI is difficult. Patient may fear death and/or be anxious about immediate environment. Ongoing anxiety (related to concerns about impact of heart attack on future lifestyle, matters left unattended/unresolved, and effects of illness on family) may be present in varying degrees for some time and be manifested by symptoms of depression. Note: Research into survival rates between Type A/Type B individuals and the impact of

ACTIONS/INTERVENTIONS	RATIONALE
Independent	
	denial has been ambiguous; and although there seems to be some connection between personality and heart disease, the need for further research is indicated.
Maintain confident manner without false reassurance.	Patient and SO can be affected by the anxiety/uneasiness displayed by health team members.
Observe for verbal/nonverbal signs of anxiety and stay with patient. Intervene if patient displays destructive behavior.	Patient may not express concern overtly, but words/actions may convey sense of agitation. Actions may take the form of aggression and hostility and intervention can help patient to control own behavior.
Accept but do not reinforce use of denial. Avoid confrontations.	Denial can be beneficial in decreasing anxiety but can postpone dealing with the reality of the current situation. Confrontation can increase use of denial reducing cooperation and impeding recovery.
Orient patient/SO to routine procedures, and expected activities.	Predictability and information can decrease anxiety for patient who has been transferred to a new setting and is still recovering from acute episode.
Answer all questions factually. Provide consistent information, and repeat as indicated.	Accurate information about the situation reduces fear, strengthens patient–nurse relationship, assists patient/SO to deal realistically with situation. Attention span may be short, and repetition of information helps with retention.
Encourage patient/SO to communicate with one another, sharing questions and concerns.	Sharing information elicits support/comfort and can relieve tension of unexpressed worries.
Provide rest periods/uninterrupted sleep time.	Conserves energy, enhances coping abilities as well as reducing myocardial workload and oxygen consumption.
Support normality of grieving behavior.	Can provide reassurance that feelings are normal response to situation/perceived changes.
Provide privacy for patient and SO.	Allows needed time for expression of feelings, relief of anxiety, and the establishing of more adaptive behaviors.
Encourage independence, self-care, and decision-making during recuperation.	Increased independence from staff promotes self-confidence and prevents feelings of abandonment that can accompany transfer from coronary unit/discharge from hospital.
Encourage discussion about postdischarge expectations.	Helps patient/SO identify realistic goals, reducing risk of discouragement in face of the reality of limitations of condition/pace of recuperation.
Collaborative	
Administer sedatives/hypnotics as indicated, e.g., diazepam (Valium), flurazepam hydrochloride (Dalmane), lorazepam (Ativan).	Promotes relaxation/rest, and reduces feelings of anxiety.

NURSING DIAGNOSIS:	CARDIAC OUTPUT, ALTERED: DECREASED [POTENTIAL]
May be related to:	Changes in rate, rhythm, electrical conduction
	Reduced preload/increased SVR

Infarcted/dyskinetic muscle, structural defects, e.g., ventricular aneurysm, septal defects

Possibly evidenced by: [Not applicable; presence of signs and symptoms establishes *actual* diagnosis.]

**PATIENT OUTCOMES/
EVALUATION CRITERIA:**   Reports decreased episodes of dyspnea, angina. Demonstrates an increase in activity tolerance, decrease in dysrhythmias.

ACTIONS/INTERVENTIONS	RATIONALE
Independent	
Auscultate blood pressure. Compare both arms and obtain lying, sitting, standing pressures when able.	Hypotension may occur related to ventricular dysfunction, hypoperfusion of the myocardium, and vagal stimulation. However, hypertension is also a common phenomenon, possibly related to pain, anxiety, catecholamine release, or preexisting vascular problems. Orthostatic (postural) hypotension may be associated with complications of infarct, e.g., CHF.
Evaluate quality and equality of pulses, as indicated.	Decreased cardiac output results in diminished weak/thready pulses. Irregularities suggest dysrhythmias, which may require further evaluation/monitoring.
Note development of S_3, S_4;	S_3 is usually associated with CHF, but it may also be noted with mitral insufficiency (regurgitation) and LV overload that can accompany severe infarction. S_4 may be associated with myocardial ischemia, ventricular stiffening, and pulmonary or systemic hypertension.
Presence of murmurs/rubs.	Indicates disturbances of normal blood flow within the heart, e.g., incompetent valve, septal defect, or vibration of papillary muscle/chordae tendinae (complication of MI). Presence of rub with an infarction is also associated with inflammation, e.g., pericardial effusion and pericarditis.
Auscultate breath sounds.	Crackles reflecting pulmonary congestion may develop because of depressed myocardial function.
Monitor heart rate and rhythm. Document dysrhythmias via telemetry. (Refer to CP: Dysrhythmias, p. 81.)	Reveals response to medication and activity, as well as developing complications/dysrhythmias (especially premature ventricular contractions or progressive heart blocks), which could compromise cardiac function or increase ischemic damage. Acute or chronic atrial flutter/fibrillation may be seen with coronary artery or valvular disease and may or may not be pathologic.
Note response to activity, and promote rest appropriately. (Refer to ND: Activity Intolerance, p. 73.)	Overexertion increases oxygen consumption/demand and can compromise myocardial function.
Provide bedside commode if unable to use bathroom facilities.	Attempts at using bedpan can be exhausting and psychologically stressful, thereby increasing oxygen demand and cardiac workload.
Provide small/easily digested meals. Restrict caffeine intake, e.g., coffee, chocolate, cola.	Large meals may increase myocardial workload and cause vagal stimulation resulting in bradycardia/ectopic beats. Caffeine is a direct cardiac stimulant which can increase heart rate.

ACTIONS/INTERVENTIONS	RATIONALE

Independent

Have emergency equipment/medications available.

Sudden coronary occlusion, lethal dysrhythmias, extension of infarct, or unrelenting pain are situations that may precipitate cardiac arrest requiring immediate life-saving therapies/transfer to critical care unit.

Collaborative

Administer supplemental oxygen, as indicated.

Increases amount of oxygen available for myocardial uptake reducing ischemia and resultant dysrhythmias.

Maintain IV access as indicated.

Patent line is important for administration of emergency drugs in presence of persistent dysrhythmias or chest pain.

Review serial ECGs.

Provides information regarding progression/resolution of infarction, status of ventricular function, electrolyte balance, and effects of drug therapies.

Review chest x-ray.

May reflect pulmonary edema related to ventricular dysfunction.

Monitor laboratory data: e.g., cardiac enzymes, ABGs, electrolytes.

Enzymes monitor resolution/extension of infarction. Presence of hypoxia indicates need for supplemental oxygen. Electrolyte imbalance, e.g., hypo/hyperkalemia adversely affects cardiac rhythm/contractility.

Administer antidysrhythmic drugs as indicated. (Refer to CP: Dysrhythmias, p. 81.)

Dysrhythmias are usually treated symptomatically.

Assist with insertion/maintain pacemaker, when used.

Pacing may be a temporary support measure during acute/healing phase, or may be needed permanently if infarction severely damages conduction system.

NURSING DIAGNOSIS: TISSUE PERFUSION, ALTERED: DECREASED (SPECIFY) [POTENTIAL]

May be related to: Reduction/interruption of blood flow, e.g., vasoconstriction, hypovolemia/shunting, and thromboembolic formation

Possibly evidenced by: [Not applicable; presence of signs and symptoms establishes an *actual* diagnosis.]

PATIENT OUTCOMES/ EVALUATION CRITERIA: Demonstrates adequate perfusion as individually appropriate, e.g., skin warm and dry, peripheral pulses present/strong, vital signs within patient's normal range, alert/oriented, balanced intake/output, absence of edema, free of pain/discomfort.

ACTIONS/INTERVENTIONS	RATIONALE

Independent

Investigate sudden changes or continued alterations in mentation, e.g., anxiety, confusion, lethargy, stupor.

Cerebral perfusion is directly related to cardiac output and is also influenced by electrolyte/acid–base variations, hypoxia, or systemic emboli.

ACTIONS/INTERVENTIONS	RATIONALE
Independent	
Inspect for pallor, cyanosis, mottling, cool/clammy skin. Note strength of peripheral pulse.	Systemic vasoconstriction resulting from diminished cardiac output may be evidenced by decreased skin perfusion, diminished pulses. (Refer to ND: Cardiac Output, Altered: Decreased [Potential], p. 75.)
Assess for Homans' sign (pain in calf on dorsiflexion), erythema, edema.	Indicators of deep vein thrombosis.
Encourage active/passive leg exercises, avoidance of isometric exercises.	Reduces venous stasis enhancing venous return and decreasing risk of thrombophlebitis. However, isometric exercises can adversely affect cardiac output by increasing myocardial work and oxygen consumption.
Instruct patient in application/periodic removal of anti-embolic hose, when used.	Limits venous stasis, improves venous return and reduces risk of thrombophlebitis in patient who is limited in activity.
Monitor respirations, note work of breathing.	Cardiac pump failure may precipitate respiratory distress. However, sudden/continued dyspnea may indicate thromboembolic pulmonary complications.
Assess gastrointestinal function, noting anorexia, decreased/absent bowel sounds, nausea/vomiting, abdominal distention, constipation.	Reduced blood flow to mesentery can produce gastrointestinal dysfunction, e.g., abdominal pain, nausea and loss of peristalsis. Problems may be potentiated/aggravated by use of analgesics, decreased activity and dietary changes.
Monitor intake, note changes in urine output. Record specific gravity as indicated.	Decreased intake/persistent nausea may result in reduced circulating volume negatively impacting perfusion and organ function. Specific gravity measurements reflect hydration status and renal function.
Collaborative	
Monitor laboratory data, e.g., ABGs, BUN, creatinine, electrolytes when done.	Indicators of organ perfusion/function.
Administer medications as indicated, e.g.:	
Heparin/warfarin sodium (Coumadin)	Low-dose heparin may be given prophylactically in high-risk patients (e.g., atrial fibrillation, obesity, ventricular aneurysm, or history of thrombophlebitis) to reduce risk of thrombophlebitis or mural thrombus formation. Coumadin is drug of choice for long-term/postdischarge anticoagulant therapy.
Cimetidine (Tagamet), ranitidine (Zantac); antacids.	Reduces or neutralizes gastric acid, preventing discomfort and gastric irritation especially in presence of reduced mucosal circulation.

NURSING DIAGNOSIS:	**FLUID VOLUME, ALTERED: EXCESS [POTENTIAL]**
May be related to:	**Decreased organ perfusion (renal)**
	Increased sodium/water retention
	Increased hydrostatic pressure or decreased plasma proteins (sequestering of fluid in interstitial space/tissues)

Possibly evidenced by:	[Not applicable; presence of signs and symptoms establishes an *actual* diagnosis.]
PATIENT OUTCOMES/ EVALUATION CRITERIA:	Maintains fluid balance as evidenced by blood pressure within patient's normal limits; absence of peripheral/ venous distention and dependent edema; lungs clear and weight stable.

ACTIONS/INTERVENTIONS	RATIONALE
Independent	
Auscultate breath sounds for presence of crackles.	May indicate pulmonary edema secondary to cardiac decompensation.
Note jugular venous distention (JVD); development of dependent edema.	Suggests developing congestive failure/fluid volume excess.
Measure intake/output, noting decrease in output, concentrated appearance. Calculate fluid balance.	Decreased cardiac output results in impaired kidney perfusion, sodium/water retention, and reduced urine output. Recurrent positive fluid balance in presence of other symptoms suggests volume excess/cardiac failure.
Weigh daily.	Sudden changes in weight reflect alterations in fluid.
Maintain total fluid intake at 2000 ml/24 hours within cardiovascular tolerance.	Meets normal adult body fluid requirements, but may require alteration/restriction in presence of cardiac decompensation.
Collaborative	
Provide low sodium diet/beverages.	Sodium enhances fluid retention and should therefore be restricted.
Administer diuretics, e.g., furosemide (Lasix), hydralazine (Apresoline), spirolactone with hydrochlorothiazide (Aldactazide). Monitor potassium as indicated.	May be necessary to correct fluid overload. Drug choice is usually dependent on acute/chronic nature of symptoms. Note: Hypokalemia can limit effectiveness of therapy and can occur with use of potassium-depleting diuretics.

NURSING DIAGNOSIS:	**KNOWLEDGE DEFICIT [LEARNING NEED] (SPECIFY)**
May be related to:	**Lack of factual information regarding cardiac functioning/implications of heart disease and future health status**
	Need for lifestyle changes
	Unfamiliarity with postdischarge therapy/self-care needs
Possibly evidenced by:	**Statements of concern/misconceptions, questions**
	Development of preventable complications
PATIENT OUTCOMES/ EVALUATION CRITERIA:	**Verbalizes understanding of own heart disease, symptoms that require immediate attention, dietary/exercise program, purpose of medications and side effects. Identifies/plans for necessary lifestyle changes.**

ACTIONS/INTERVENTIONS	RATIONALE

Independent

Assess patient/SO's level of knowledge and ability/desire to learn. Continue orientation to unit/procedures/equipment on an ongoing basis.

Necessary for creation of individual teaching plan. Reinforces expectation that this will be a "learning experience." Verbalization identifies misunderstandings and allows for clarification.

Be alert to signs of avoidance, e.g., changing subject away from information being presented, or extremes of behavior (withdrawal/euphoria).

Natural defense mechanisms such as anger, denial of significance of situation can block learning, affecting patient's response and ability to assimilate information. Changing to a less formal/structured style may be more effective until patient/SO is ready to accept/deal with current situation.

Present information in varied learning formats, e.g., programmed books, audio/visual tapes, question/answer sessions, group activities.

Using multiple learning methods enhances retention of material.

Reinforce explanations of risk factors, dietary/activity restrictions, medications, and symptoms requiring immediate medical attention.

Provides opportunity for patient to retain information and to assume control/participate in rehabilitation program.

Encourage identification/reduction of individual risk factors, e.g., smoking/alcohol consumption, obesity.

These behaviors/chemicals have direct adverse effect on cardiovascular function and may impede recovery.

Warn against isometric activity, Valsalva maneuver and activity requiring arms positioned above head.

These activities greatly increase cardiac work/myocardial oxygen consumption and may adversely affect myocardial contractility/output.

Review programmed increases in levels of activity. Educate patient regarding gradual resumption of activities, e.g., walking, work, recreational and sexual activity.

Gradual increase in activity increases strength and prevents overexertion, may enhance collateral circulation, and allow return to normal lifestyle.

Identify alternate activities for "bad weather" days, such as measured walking in house or shopping mall.

Provides for continuing daily activity program.

Review signs/symptoms requiring reduction in activity and notification of health care provider.

Pulse elevations beyond established limits, development of chest pain, dyspnea may require changes in exercise and medication regimen.

Stress importance of follow-up care and identify community resources/support groups, e.g., cardiac rehabilitation programs, "Coronary Clubs," smoking cessation clinics.

Emphasizes that this is an ongoing/continuing health problem for which support/assistance is available postdischarge.

Emphasize importance of contacting physician if chest pain, change in anginal pattern, or other symptoms recur.

Timely evaluation/intervention may prevent complications.

Stress importance of reporting development of fever in association with diffuse/atypical chest pain (pleural, pericardial) and joint pain.

Post-MI complication of pericardial inflammation of unknown etiology (Dressler's syndrome) requires further medical evaluation/intervention.

(Refer to ND: Knowledge Deficit [Learning Need] in CPs: Angina Pectoris, p. 60; Dysrhythmias, p. 81; Congestive Heart Failure, p. 41; Digitalis Toxicity, p. 51; and Inflammatory Cardiac Conditions, p. 109, for information regarding pharmacologic needs and complications.)

Dysrhythmias

PATIENT ASSESSMENT DATA BASE

ACTIVITY/REST

May report: Weakness, generalized, and exertional fatigue.

May exhibit: Changes in heart rate/blood pressure with activity/exercise.

CIRCULATION

May report: History of previous/acute myocardial infarction (90–95% experience dysrhythmias), cardiomyopathy, CHF, valvular heart disease, hypertension.

History of pacemaker insertion.

Pulse: fast, slow or irregular; palpitations, skipped beats.

May exhibit: Blood pressure changes, e.g., hypertension or hypotension during episodes of dysrhythmia.

Pulses: may be irregular, e.g., skipped beats, pulsus alternans (regular strong beat/weak beat), bigeminal pulse (irregular strong beat/weak beat).

Pulse deficit (difference between apical pulse and radial pulse).

Heart sounds: irregular rhythm, extra sounds, dropped beats.

Skin: color and moisture changes, e.g., pallor, cyanosis, diaphoresis (heart failure, shock).

Edema: dependent, generalized, jugular venous distention (in presence of heart failure).

Urine output: decreased if cardiac output is severely diminished.

EGO INTEGRITY

May report: Feeling nervous (certain tachydysrhythmias).

Stressors related to current medical problems.

May exhibit: Anxiety, fear, withdrawal, anger, irritability, crying.

FOOD/FLUID

May report: Loss of appetite.

Food intolerance (with certain medications).

Nausea/vomiting.

Changes in weight.

May exhibit: Anorexia.

Changes in weight.

Edema.

Changes in skin moisture/turgor.

Respiratory crackles.

NEUROSENSORY

May report: Dizzy spells, fainting, headaches.

May exhibit: Mental status/sensorium changes, e.g., disorientation, confusion, loss of memory, changes in usual speech pattern, consciousness, stupor, coma.

Behavioral changes, e.g., combativeness, lethargy, hallucinations.

Pupil changes (equality and reaction to light).

Loss of deep tendon reflexes with life-threatening dysrhythmias (ventricular tachycardia, severe bradycardia).

PAIN/COMFORT

May report: Chest pain (unstable angina), mild to severe, which may or may not be relieved by antianginal medication.

May exhibit: Distraction behaviors, e.g., restlessness.

RESPIRATION

May report: Chronic lung disease.

Tobacco use.

Shortness of breath.

Coughing (with/without sputum production).

May exhibit: Changes in respiratory rate/depth during dysrhythmia episode.

Breath sounds: crackles may be indicative of left heart failure (pulmonary edema) or pulmonary thromboembolic phenomena or accompany tachydysrhythmias.

SAFETY

May report: Reactions to medications.

May exhibit: Fever.

Skin rashes/gastrointestinal symptoms (medication reaction).

Thromboembolic phenomena (superficial/deep vein thrombosis, pulmonary, cerebral).

Loss of muscle tone/strength.

TEACHING/LEARNING

May report: Familial risk factors, e.g., heart disease, stroke.

Use/misuse of prescribed medications, e.g., heart medications (digitalis), anticoagulants (Coumadin), or OTC medications, e.g., cough syrup, and analgesics containing aspirin.

Lack of understanding about disease process/therapeutic regimen.

Evidence of failure to improve, e.g., recurrent/intractable dysrhythmias that are life-threatening.

Discharge Plan Considerations: Alteration of medication use/therapy.

Refer to CPs: Myocardial Infarction, p. 69; Congestive Heart Failure, p. 41; Pulmonary Embolism, p. 118; and Inflammatory Cardiac Conditions, p. 109, for additional information regarding underlying cause/complications.

DIAGNOSTIC STUDIES:

ECG: demonstrates patterns of ischemia/injury and conduction aberrance. Reveals type/source of dysrhythmia, effects of electrolyte imbalance and cardiac medications.

Holter monitor: extended ECG tracing (24 hours) may be desired to determine which dysrhythmias may be causing specific symptoms when patient is active (home/work). May also be used to evaluate pacemaker function/antidysrhythmia drug effect.

Chest x-ray: may show enlarged cardiac shadow due to ventricular or valve dysfunction.

Myocardial imaging scans: may demonstrate ischemic/damaged myocardial areas that could impede normal conduction.

Multiple-gated acquisition (MUGA): evaluates regional wall motion and determines ejection fraction; when performed after exercise, is used to evaluate changes in cardiac output.

Exercise stress test: may be done to demonstrate exercise-induced dysrhythmias.

Electrolytes: elevated or decreased levels of potassium, calcium can cause dysrhythmias.

Drug screen: may reveal toxicity of cardiac drugs or suggest interaction of drugs, e.g., digitalis, quinidine, etc. resulting in dysrhythmias.

Thyroid studies: elevated serum thyroid levels can cause/aggravate dysrhythmias.

Sedimentation rate: elevation may indicate acute/active inflammatory process, e.g., endocarditis.

NURSING PRIORITIES

1. Prevent/treat life-threatening dysrhythmias.
2. Support patient/SO in dealing with anxiety/fear of potentially life-threatening situation.
3. Assist in identification of cause/precipitating factors.
4. Review information regarding condition/prognosis/treatment regimen.

DISCHARGE CRITERIA

1. Free of life-threatening dysrhythmias, and complications of impaired cardiac output/tissue perfusion.
2. Anxiety reduced/managed.
3. Disease process, therapy needs, prevention of complications understood.

NURSING DIAGNOSIS:	CARDIAC OUTPUT, ALTERED: DECREASED [POTENTIAL]
May be related to:	Altered electrical conduction Reduced myocardial contractility
Possibly evidenced by:	[Not applicable; presence of signs and symptoms establishes an *actual* diagnosis.]
PATIENT OUTCOMES/ EVALUATION CRITERIA:	Maintains/achieves adequate cardiac output as evidenced by absence of signs/symptoms of decompensation. Observed decrease in frequency of dysrhythmia(s). Participates in activities that reduce myocardial workload.

ACTIONS/INTERVENTIONS

Independent

Palpate pulses (radial, carotid, femoral, dorsalis pedis) noting rate, regularity, amplitude (full/thready), and symmetry. Document presence of pulsus alternans, bigeminal pulse, or pulse deficit.

Auscultate heart sounds noting rate, rhythm. Note presence of extra heart beats, dropped beats.

Monitor vital signs and assess adequacy of cardiac output/tissue perfusion. Report significant variations in blood pressure; pulse rate/equality; respirations; changes in skin color/temperature; level of consciousness/sensorium; and urine output during episodes of dysrhythmias.

RATIONALE

Differences in equality, rate, and regularity of pulses are indicative of the effect of altered cardiac output on systemic/peripheral circulation.

Specific dysrhythmias are more clearly detected audibly than by palpation. Hearing extra heart beats or dropped beats helps identify dysrhythmias in the unmonitored patient.

Although not all dysrhythmias are considered life-threatening, immediate treatment to terminate dysrhythmia may be required in the presence of alterations in cardiac output and tissue perfusion.

ACTIONS/INTERVENTIONS	RATIONALE

Independent

Determine type of dysrhythmia and document with rhythm strip (if cardiac/telemetry monitoring is available):

Useful in determining need for/type of intervention required.

    Tachycardia;

Tachycardia can occur in response to stress, pain, fever, infection, coronary artery blockage, valvular dysfunction, hypovolemia, hypoxia; or as a result of decreased vagal tone or increased sympathetic nervous system activity with the release of catecholamines. Persistent tachycardia may worsen underlying pathology in patients with ischemic heart disease because of shortened diastolic filling time and increased oxygen demands.

    Bradycardia;

Bradycardia is common in patients with acute myocardial infarction (especially inferior) and is the result of excessive parasympathetic activity, blocks in conduction to the SA or AV nodes, or loss of automaticity of the heart muscle. Patients with severe heart disease may not be able to compensate for a slow rate by increasing stroke volume. Therefore, decreased cardiac output, CHF, and potentially lethal ventricular dysrhythmias may occur.

    Atrial dysrhythmias;

PACs can occur as a response to ischemia and are normally harmless, but can precede or precipitate AF. Acute and chronic atrial flutter and/or fibrillation can occur with coronary artery or valvular disease, and may or may not be pathologic. Rapid atrial flutter/fibrillation reduces cardiac output as a result of incomplete ventricular filling (shortened cardiac cycle) and increased oxygen demand.

    Ventricular dysrhythmias;

Premature ventricular contractions (PVCs) reflect cardiac irritability and are commonly associated with MI, digitalis toxicity, coronary vasospasm, misplaced temporary pacemaker leads. Frequent, multiple, or multifocal PVCs result in diminished cardiac output and may lead to potentially lethal dysrhythmias, e.g., ventricular tachycardia (VT), or sudden death/cardiac arrest from ventricular flutter/fibrillation. Note: Intractable ventricular dysrhythmias unresponsive to medication may reflect ventricular aneurysm.

    Heart blocks.

Reflect altered transmission through normal conduction channels (slowed, altered) and may be the result of MI; coronary artery disease with reduced blood supply to SA or AV nodes; drug toxicity; and sometimes cardiac surgery. Progressing heart block is associated with slow ventricular rates, decreased cardiac output, and potentially lethal ventricular dysrhythmias or cardiac standstill.

Provide calm/quiet environment. Review reasons for limitation of activities during acute phase.

Reduces stimulation and release of stress-related catecholamines, which cause/aggravate dysrhythmias and vasoconstriction and increase myocardial workload.

Demonstrate/encourage use of stress management behaviors, e.g., relaxation techniques, guided imagery, slow/deep breathing.

Promotes patient participation, in exerting some sense of control in a potentially very stressful situation.

ACTIONS/INTERVENTIONS	RATIONALE

Independent

Investigate complaints of chest pain documenting location, duration, intensity, relieving/aggravating factors. Note non-verbal pain cues, e.g., facial grimacing, crying, changes in BP/heart rate.

Reasons for chest pain are variable, dependent on underlying cause of dysrhythmias. However, chest pain may indicate ischemia due to decreased myocardial perfusion or increased oxygen need (impending/evolving MI). (Refer to CP: Myocardial Infarction, p. 69.)

Be prepared for/initiate cardiopulmonary resuscitation (CPR) as indicated.

Development of life-threatening dysrhythmias requires prompt intervention to prevent ischemic damage/death.

Collaborative

Monitor laboratory studies, e.g.:

Electrolytes;

Electrolyte imbalance (e.g., hypo/hyperkalemia or hypocalcemia) adversely affects cardiac rhythm and contractility.

Drug levels.

Reveals therapeutic/toxic level of medications which may affect/contribute to presence of dysrhythmias.

Administer supplemental oxygen as indicated.

Increases amount of oxygen available for myocardial uptake, which decreases irritability caused by hypoxia.

Administer medications as indicated:

Dysrhythmias are generally treated symptomatically except for ventricular prematures which may be treated prophylactically in acute MI.

Potassium:

Correction of hypokalemia may be sufficient to terminate some ventricular dysrhythmias.

Antidysrhythmics:

Type I, e.g.: disopyramide (Norpace), procainamide (Pronestyl), quinidine (Quinaglute);

Useful for treatment of atrial and ventricular premature beats, repetitive dysrhythmias (e.g., atrial tachycardias and atrial flutter/fibrillation). Note: Myocardial depressant effects may be potentiated when used in conjunction with any drugs possessing similar properties.

Type II, e.g.: lidocaine (Xylocaine), phenytoin (Dilantin), tocainide (Tonocard), mexiletine (Mexitil);

Drugs of choice for ventricular dysrhythmias. Effective for automatic and reentrant ventricular dysrhythmias and for digitalis-induced dysrhythmias. Action depends on the tissue affected and the level of extracellular potassium. Note: These drugs may aggravate myocardial depression.

Type III, e.g.: propranolol (Inderal), nadolol (Corgard);

Beta-adrenergic blockers are useful in the treatment of dysrhythmias occurring because of SA and AV node dysfunction (e.g., supraventricular tachycardias, atrial flutter or fibrillation). Note: These drugs may exacerbate bradycardia and cause myocardial depression (especially when combined with drugs with similar properties).

Type IV, e.g.: bretylium tosylate (Bretylol);

Occasionally used to terminate ventricular fibrillation if lidocaine/pronestyl not effective.

Type V, e.g.: verapamil (Calan), nifedipine (Procardia), diltiazem (Cardizem);

Calcium antagonists slow conduction time through the AV node to decrease ventricular response in supraventricular tachycardias, atrial flutter/fibrillation.

Others, e.g.: atropine sulfate, isoproterenol (Isuprel); and cardiac glycosides: digitalis (Lanoxin).

Useful in treating bradycardia by increasing SA and AV conduction and enhancing automaticity. Cardiac glycosides may be used alone or in combination with

ACTIONS/INTERVENTIONS	RATIONALE
Collaborative	
	other antidysrhythmic drugs to reduce ventricular rate in presence of uncontrolled/poorly tolerated atrial tachycardias or flutter/fibrillation.
Prepare for/assist with elective cardioversion.	May be used in atrial fibrillation or certain unstable dysrhythmias to restore normal heart rate/relieve symptoms of heart failure.
Assist with insertion/maintain pacemaker function.	Temporary pacing may be necessary to accelerate impulse formation or override tachydysrhythmias and ectopic activity in order to maintain cardiovascular function until spontaneous pacing is restored or permanent pacing is initiated by correcting conduction disturbance.
Insert/maintain IV access.	Patent access line may be required for administration of emergency drugs.
Prepare for invasive diagnostic procedures/surgery as indicated.	Differential diagnosis of underlying cause may be required in order to formulate appropriate treatment plan. Resection of ventricular aneurysm may be required to correct intractable ventricular dysrhythmias unresponsive to medical therapy, CABG may be indicated to enhance circulation to myocardium and conduction system.

NURSING DIAGNOSIS:	KNOWLEDGE DEFICIT [LEARNING NEED] (SPECIFY)
May be related to:	Lack of information/understanding of medical condition/therapy needs
	Unfamiliarity with information resources
	Lack of recall
Possibly evidenced by:	Questions
	Statement of misconception
	Failure to improve on previous regimen
	Development of preventable complications
PATIENT OUTCOMES/ EVALUATION CRITERIA:	Verbalizes knowledge of disease and treatment regimen, desired action and possible adverse side effects of medications. Correctly performs necessary procedures and explains reasons for actions. Demonstrates understanding of function of pacemaker (if used) and verbalizes signs of pacemaker failure.

ACTIONS/INTERVENTIONS	RATIONALE
Independent	
Review normal cardiac function/electrical conduction.	Provides a knowledge base to understand individual variations and reasons for therapeutic interventions.

ACTIONS/INTERVENTIONS	RATIONALE

Independent

Explain/reinforce specific dysrhythmia problem and therapeutic measures to patient/SO.

Ongoing/updated information (e.g., about whether the problem is resolving or may require long-term control measures) can decrease anxiety associated with the unknown, and prepare patient/SO to make necessary lifestyle adaptations. Educating the SO may be especially important if the patient is elderly, visually or hearing impaired, or unable to learn/follow instructions. Repeated explanations may be needed, because anxiety and/or bulk of new information can block/limit learning.

Identify adverse effects/complications of specific dysrhythmias, e.g., fatigue, dependent edema, progressing changes in mentation, vertigo.

Dysrhythmias may decrease cardiac output manifested by symptoms of developing cardiac failure/altered cerebral perfusion. Tachydysrhythmias may also be accompanied by debilitating anxiety/feelings of impending doom.

Instruct/document teaching regarding medications. Include why the drug is needed (desired action); how and when to take the drug; what to do if a dose is forgotten (dosage and usage information); expected side effects, or possible adverse reactions/interactions with other prescribed/OTC drugs or substances (alcohol, tobacco); as well as what and when to report to the physician.

Information necessary for patient to make informed choices and to manage medication regimen.

Encourage development of regular exercise routine, avoiding overexertion. Identify signs/symptoms requiring immediate cessation of activities, e.g., dizziness, lightheadedness, dyspnea, chest pain.

When dysrhythmias are properly managed, normal activity should not be affected. Exercise program is useful in improving overall cardiovascular well-being.

Review individual dietary needs/restrictions, e.g., potassium, caffeine.

Depending upon specific problem, patient may need to increase dietary potassium such as when potassium depleting diuretics are used. Caffeine may be limited to prevent cardiac excitation.

Provide information in written form for patient/SO to take home.

Follow-up reminders may enhance patient's understanding and cooperation with the desired regimen. Written instructions are a helpful resource when patient is not in direct contact with health care team.

Demonstrate how to take own pulse. Encourage daily recording before medication/during exercise, and identify situations requiring immediate medical intervention.

Continued self-observation/monitoring provides for timely intervention to avoid complications. Medication regimen may be altered, depending on pulse rate, or further evaluation may be required when heart rate varies from desired rate or pacemaker's preset rate.

Review safety precautions, techniques to evaluate/maintain pacemaker function, and symptoms requiring medical interventions.

Promotes self-care, provides for timely interventions to prevent serious complications. Instructions/concerns will be dependent upon type of pacemaker, batteries, and lead placement.

Collaborative

Review procedures to terminate PAT, e.g., carotid/sinus massage, Valsalva maneuver.

These procedures may be deemed necessary in some patients to restore regular rhythm/cardiac output in emergency situations.

Valvular Heart Disease _____

Aortic stenosis (AS), regurgitation (AR); mitral stenosis (MS), regurgitation (MR), prolapse (MVP).

PATIENT ASSESSMENT DATA BASE

ACTIVITY/REST

May report:
Weakness, fatigue.

Dizziness, fainting spells.

Dyspnea on exertion, palpitations.

Sleep disturbance (orthopnea, paroxysmal nocturnal dyspnea, nocturia, night sweats).

May exhibit:
Tachycardia, alterations in BP.

Effort syncope.

Tachypnea, dyspnea.

Cough.

CIRCULATION

May report:
History of predisposing conditions, e.g., rheumatic fever, subacute bacterial endocarditis, streptococcal infection or congenital conditions (e.g., atrial-septal defect, Marfan's syndrome).

History of heart murmur, palpitations.

Hoarseness, hemoptysis.

Cough, with/without sputum production.

May exhibit:
Decreased systolic blood pressure (late AS).

Pulse pressure: narrowed (AS); widened (AR).

Pulse: carotid pulse: slow with small pulse volume (AS); bounding, with visible arterial pulsations (AR).

Apical pulse: PMI forceful and displaced downward and to the left (MR); forceful and displaced laterally (AR).

Thrills: Diastolic thrill at apex (MS). Systolic thrill at base (AS). Diastolic thrill along left sternal border; systolic thrill in jugular notch and along carotid arteries (AR).

Heaves: apical heave during systole (AS).

Heart sounds: Loud S_1; opening snap (MS). Diminished or absent S_1, wide splitting of S_2; development of S_3, S_4 (severe MR). Systolic ejection click (AS). Systolic click: accentuated by standing/squatting (MVP).

Rate: tachycardia (MVP); resting tachycardia (MS).

Rhythm: irregular, atrial fibrillation (MS and MR). Dysrhythmias and first degree AV block (AS).

Murmurs: Low-pitched, rumbling diastolic murmur (MS). Systolic murmur heard best at apex (MR). Systolic murmur heard best at base with radiation to neck (AS). Diastolic murmurs (blowing), high-pitched and heard best at base (AR).

Jugular vein distention: may be present in the presence of right ventricular failure (AR, AS, MR, MS).

Extremities: capillary beds flush and pale with each pulse (AR).

Color/cyanosis: skin warm, damp and flushed (AR).

EGO INTEGRITY

May exhibit:
Signs of anxiety, e.g., restlessness, pallor, diaphoresis, trembling, narrowed focus.

FOOD/FLUID

May report: Dysphagia (chronic MR).
Changes in weight.
Use of diuretics.

May exhibit: Generalized or dependent edema.
Hepatomegaly and ascites (MS and MR).
Warm, flushed and damp skin (AR).
Labored, wet and noisy respirations with audible crackles and wheezes.

NEUROSENSORY

May report: Episodes of dizziness/fainting related to exertion.

PAIN/DISCOMFORT

May report: Chest pain angina (AS, AR).
Nonanginal/atypical chest pain (MVP).

RESPIRATION

May report: Dyspnea (exertion, orthopnea, paroxysmal nocturnal).
Persistent or nocturnal cough (may/may not be productive of sputum).

May exhibit: Tachypnea.
Adventitious breath sounds (crackles and wheezes).
Frothy, blood tinged sputum (pulmonary edema).
Restlessness/apprehension (in the presence of pulmonary edema).

SAFETY

May report: Recent infectious process/sepsis, radiation chemotherapy.
Recent dental care (cleaning, fillings, etc.)

May exhibit: Need for oral/dental care.

TEACHING/LEARNING

May report: Recent/chronic use of IV drugs (illicit).

Discharge Plan Considerations: Assistance with self-care needs, homemaker tasks.
Alteration in medication therapy.
Physical layout of home.

DIAGNOSTIC STUDIES

Radionuclide studies (MUGA): determines resting and exercise ventricular ejection fractions.

Cardiac catheterization: provides the following diagnostic information:
MS: pressure gradient in diastole between the left atrium and left ventricle across the mitral valve; decreased valve orifice (1.5 cm); elevated left atrial, pulmonary artery, and right ventricular pressures; low cardiac output.
MR: back flow of contrast media through the mitral valve during systole; elevated left atrial, pulmonary artery pressures.
AS: pressure gradient in systole across the aortic valve; increased LVEDP.
AR: back flow of contrast media through the aortic valve during diastole, increased LVEDP.

Left ventriculography: used to demonstrate mitral cusp prolapse (MVP).

ECG:
MVP: T-wave abnormalities.
MS: left atrial enlargement, right ventricular hypertrophy; chronic atrial fibrillation.

MR: left atrial enlargement; left ventricular hypertrophy; premature atrial contractions and atrial fibrillation.
AS: left ventricular hypertrophy, ST/T wave changes, conduction defects (first degree AV block, left bundle branch block) and atrial fibrillation.
AR: left ventricular hypertrophy, atrial fibrillation present if congestive failure is severe.

Chest x-ray:
MS: increased vasculature, enlarged right ventricle and left atrium, and signs of pulmonary congestion/ edema.
MR: increased vascularity in the upper lung lobe, calcification of the mitral annulus, dilation of cardiac chambers and signs of pulmonary edema.
AS: aortic and left ventricular dilation/hypertrophy; aortic valve calcification.
AR: left ventricular enlargement, dilated ascending aorta.

Echocardiograms:
MS: left atrial enlargement, altered movement of valve leaflets.
MR: left atrial enlargement, hyperdynamic left ventricle, prolapse of mitral valve leaflet.
AS: restricted movement of aortic valve.
AR: left ventricular dilation, calcification or vegetation on the aortic valve, enlargement of the aortic root of ascending aorta.
MVP: leaflets bulge posteriorly into left atrium during ventricular systole.

NURSING PRIORITIES

1. Maintain adequate cardiac output.
2. Maintain and/or increase activity tolerance.
3. Relieve/control pain.
4. Provide information about disease process, management, and prevention of complications.

DISCHARGE CRITERIA

1. Free of signs/symptoms of cardiac decompensation.
2. Meeting self-care needs with improved activity tolerance.
3. Pain/discomfort minimized/controlled.
4. Disease process, management, and prevention of complications understood.

Refer to CP: Congestive Heart Failure, p. 41, when this occurs with valvular disease.

NURSING DIAGNOSIS:	CARDIAC OUTPUT, ALTERED: DECREASED
May be related to:	**Alteration in preload/increased atrial pressure and venous congestion (MR, AR)**
	Alteration in afterload/increased LVEDP and SVR (AS)
	Alteration in electrical conduction (AS), rate/rhythm (MS, MR)
	Left ventricular inflow obstruction (MS)
Possibly evidenced by:	**Variations in hemodynamic parameters**
	Dysrhythmias/ECG changes
	Dyspnea
	Jugular vein distention
	Cold, clammy skin
	Cyanosis/pallor of skin and mucous membranes

Oliguria/anuria

Weak peripheral pulses

Fatigue

Exhaustion

Crackles

PATIENT OUTCOMES/ EVALUATION CRITERIA:	Reports/displays decreased episodes of dyspnea, angina, and dysrhythmias. Participates in activities that reduce cardiac workload. Demonstrates increased activity tolerance. Identifies signs of cardiac decompensation, alters activities, and seeks help appropriately.

ACTIONS/INTERVENTIONS	RATIONALE
Independent	
Monitor blood pressure, apical pulse, peripheral pulses.	Clinical indicators of the adequacy of cardiac output. Monitoring enables early detection/treatment of decompensation.
Monitor cardiac rhythm as indicated.	Dysrhythmias are common in patient with valve disease. Atrial dysrhythmias are most common, due to increased atrial pressures and volumes. Conduction abnormalities can also occur with aortic valve disease because of deceased coronary artery perfusion.
Promote/encourage bedrest with head of bed elevated to 45 degrees.	Reduces blood volume returning to the heart (preload), which increases oxygenation, deceases dyspnea, and may reduce cardiac strain.
Assist with activities as indicated (e.g., walking) when patient is able to be out of bed.	Gradual resumption of activities prevents overtaxing cardiac reserves.
Discuss/demonstrate techniques of stress management. (Refer to ND: Anxiety, p. 94.)	Reduction of anxiety can reduce sympathetic cardiac stimulation and workload.
Collaborative	
Administer supplemental oxygen as indicated. Monitor ABGs.	Provides optimal oxygen for myocardial uptake in an attempt to compensate for increasing oxygen demand. Alterations in myocardial circulation (in combination with pulmonary congestion) affect oxygenation and may result in increased cardiac workload.
Administer medications as indicated, e.g., antidysrhythmics; inotropic drugs; vasodilators; diuretics. (Refer to CP: Dysrhythmias, p. 81.)	Treatment of atrial and ventricular dysrhythmias, is specific to underlying condition and symptomatology, but is aimed at sustaining/enhancing cardiac efficiency/output. Vasodilators are used to decrease hypertension by reducing systemic vascular resistance (afterload). This reduces regurgitation and outflow resistance. Diuretics decrease circulating volume (preload), which reduces blood pressure across dysfunctional valve, thereby improving cardiac function and reducing venous congestion.
Prepare for surgical intervention as indicated. (Refer to CP: Cardiac Surgery, p. 98.)	Replacement of diseased/compromised valve(s) may be necessary to enhance cardiac output, or control/reverse cardiac decompensation.

NURSING DIAGNOSIS:	FLUID VOLUME, ALTERED: EXCESS [POTENTIAL]
May be related to:	Altered glomerular filtration Increased fluid and sodium retention
Possibly evidenced by:	[Not applicable; presence of signs and symptoms establishes an *actual* diagnosis.]
PATIENT OUTCOMES/ EVALUATION CRITERIA:	Demonstrates balanced intake and output, stable weight, vital signs within normal range, and absence of edema. Verbalizes understanding of individual dietary/fluid restrictions.

ACTIONS/INTERVENTIONS

Independent

Monitor intake and output, note fluid balance (positive or negative). Weigh daily.

Auscultate breath and heart sounds.

Asssess for jugular venous distension/elevation of CVP.

Monitor blood pressure.

Note complaints of dyspnea, orthopnea. Evaluate presence/degree of edema (dependent/generalized).

Explain purpose of fluid/sodium restriction to patient/SO. Involve in planning fluid intake schedule/choosing appropriate diet.

Collaborative

Administer diuretics, e.g., furosemide (Lasix), ethacrynic acid (Edecrin) as indicated.

Monitor serum electrolytes, particularly potassium. Provide potassium-rich diet, potassium supplement, if indicated.

Administer IV fluids via control device.

RATIONALE

Important in ongoing assessment of cardiac and kidney function, effectiveness of diuretic therapy. Continued positive fluid balance (intake greater than output) and weight gain reflect worsening cardiac failure.

Adventitious breath sounds (crackles) may indicate the onset of acute pulmonary edema or reflect chronic CHF. An audible S_3 is one of the first clinical findings associated with cardiac decompensation. It may be transient (acute pulmonary congestive failure); or permanent (chronic or advancing heart and end-organ failure associated with severe valvular disease).

Clinical indicator of right-sided heart failure and systemic congestion present in advanced valvular (2- or 3-valve) disease.

Hypertension is a common result of certain valvular disorders, e.g., aortic stenosis. However, increases in blood pressure above patient's usual range may indicate fluid volume excess, especially if it occurs suddenly, along with signs of pulmonary congestion.

Development/resolution of symptoms reflect status of fluid balance and effectiveness of therapy.

May enhance patient cooperation. Provides some sense of control in face of enforced limitations.

Inhibits reabsorption of sodium/chloride which enhances fluid excretion and reduces total body water excess and pulmonary edema.

Hypokalemia predisposes the patient to further cardiac rhythm disturbance. Electrolyte values change in response to diuresis and alterations in oxygenation and metabolism.

Intravenous pump prevents inadvertent excess administration of fluid.

ACTIONS/INTERVENTIONS

Collaborative

Restrict fluids as indicated (both oral and intravenous).

Provide sodium restricted diet as indicated.

RATIONALE

May be necessary to decrease extracellular fluid volume/edema.

Decreases fluid retention.

NURSING DIAGNOSIS:	TISSUE PERFUSION, ALTERED: DECREASED (SPECIFY) [POTENTIAL]
May be related to:	Interruption of arterial-venous flow, e.g., systemic emboli (mitral valve involvement); or venous thrombosis (venous stasis, decreased activity)
Possibly evidenced by:	[Not applicable; presence of signs and symptoms establishes an *actual* diagnosis.]
PATIENT OUTCOMES/ EVALUATION CRITERIA:	Maintains/demonstrates improved tissue perfusion as individually appropriate.

Refer to CP: Inflammatory Cardiac Conditions, ND: Tissue Perfusion, Altered: Decreased [Potential], p. 113.

NURSING DIAGNOSIS:	COMFORT, ALTERED: PAIN, ACUTE [POTENTIAL]
May be related to:	Ischemia of myocardial tissues (AS and AR)
	Stretching of left atrium (MVP)
Possibly evidenced by:	[Not applicable; presence of signs and symptoms establishes an *actual* diagnosis.]
PATIENT OUTCOMES/ EVALUATION CRITERIA:	Reports pain is relieved/controlled. Verbalizes methods that provide relief.

ACTIONS/INTERVENTIONS

Independent

Evaluate complaints of chest pain and compare with previous episodes. Use pain scale (1–10) for rating intensity. Note verbal/nonverbal expressions of pain, autonomic response to pain (diaphoresis, BP, and pulse changes, increased or decreased respiratory rate).

Investigate complaints of chest pain in response to medication administration.

Provide restful environment and limit activity as needed.

RATIONALE

Differentiation of symptoms is necessary to identify causes of pain. Behaviors and changes in vital signs help determine the degree of discomfort the patient is experiencing.

Useful in establishing drug therapy/dosage. Note: pain that is unrelieved or increased with nitrates may indicate MVP which is associated with atypical/ nonanginal chest pain.

Activities which increase myocardial oxygen demands (e.g., sudden exertion, stress, heavy meals, cold exposure) may precipitate chest pain.

ACTIONS/INTERVENTIONS

Independent

Instruct patient in appropriate response to angina (e.g., stopping angina-producing activity, resting, and taking appropriate antianginal medication).

Collaborative

Administer vasodilators, e.g., nitroglycerin, nifedipine, (Procardia) as indicated.

RATIONALE

Ceasing activity reduces oxygen demands and cardiac workload and often stops angina. (Refer to CP: Angina Pectoris, p. 60.)

Medications given to enhance myocardial circulation (vasodilation) reduces angina associated with ischemic myocardium.

NURSING DIAGNOSIS:	ACTIVITY INTOLERANCE
May be related to:	**Imbalance between oxygen supply and demand (decreased/fixed cardiac output)**
Possibly evidenced by:	**Verbal report of fatigue or weakness**
	Abnormal heart rate or blood pressure in response to activity
	Exertional discomfort or dyspnea
PATIENT OUTCOMES/ EVALUATION CRITERIA:	**Demonstrates a measurable increase in activity tolerance. Identifies factors which influence activity tolerance and reduces those with a negative effect.**

ACTIONS/INTERVENTIONS

Independent

Assess patient's tolerance to activity using the following parameters: pulse rate >20 bpm above resting rate, marked increase in BP, dyspnea or chest pain, excessive fatigue and weakness, diaphoresis, dizziness or syncope.

Assess readiness for increased activity, e.g., reduction in fatigue/weakness, stable BP/pulse rate, increased interest in activities and self-care.

Encourage progression in activity/self-care as tolerated.

Provide assistance as needed and suggest use of shower chair, sitting to brush teeth/hair.

Encourage patient to participate in alternating rest periods with activity.

RATIONALE

The stated parameters reflect the patient's physiologic response to the stress of activity, and are indicators of the degree of overexertion/cardiac compromise.

Physiologic stability at rest is essential prior to progressing the individual's activity level.

The required myocardial oxygen consumption during various activities may exceed the amount of oxygen available. Gradual activity progression prevents a sudden increase in cardiac workload.

Energy-saving techniques reduce the energy expenditure and thereby assist in equalizing oxygen supply and demand.

Such scheduling increases tolerance to activity progression and prevents fatigue.

NURSING DIAGNOSIS:	ANXIETY [SPECIFY LEVEL]
May be related to:	**Threat to or change in health status (chronicity of disease)**

	Physiologic effects
	Situational crisis (hospitalization/absence from family)
Possibly evidenced by:	Sympathetic stimulation: cardiovascular excitation, restlessness, insomnia
	Increased tension; apprehension
	Increased helplessness
	Uncertainty
	Fear of unspecified consequences
	Focus on self
	Expressed concerns regarding changes in life events
PATIENT OUTCOMES/ EVALUATION CRITERIA:	Verbalizes awareness of feelings of anxiety. Reports anxiety reduced/controlled. Appears relaxed. Demonstrates behaviors to manage stress.

ACTIONS/INTERVENTIONS

Independent

Identify/evaluate patient's perception of the threat represented by the situation.

Monitor physical responses, e.g., palpitations, tachycardia, repetitive movements, restlessness.

Provide routine comfort measures (e.g., shower/bath, back rub, position change).

Provide time for rest, diversional activities appropriate for condition.

Encourage ventilation of feelings about disease, its effect on lifestyle and future health status. Assess the effectiveness of coping with stressors.

Include patient/SO in planning care and encourage maximum participation in treatment plan.

Instruct patient in relaxation techniques, e.g., deep breathing, guided imagery, progressive relaxation. (Refer to CP: Psychosocial Aspects of Acute Care, p. 773.)

RATIONALE

Aids in defining the scope of the problem and choice of interventions.

Helpful in determining degree of anxiety as well as cardiac status. Useful in evaluating congruency of verbal and nonverbal responses.

Helps to redirect attention and promotes relaxation, enhancing coping abilities.

Provides patient a sense of control in managing some aspects of treatment (e.g., care activities, private time, etc.)

Adaptive mechanisms are necessary to cope with the chronicity of valvular heart disease and appropriately alter one's lifestyle, integrating prescribed therapies into daily living.

Involvement will help focus patient's attention in a positive manner and provide a sense of control.

Provides a means of altering response to anxiety, refocuses attention, promotes relaxation enhancing coping abilities.

NURSING DIAGNOSIS:	**KNOWLEDGE DEFICIT [LEARNING NEED] (SPECIFY)**
May be related to:	Lack of exposure to information about valvular heart disease
	Misconceptions/misinterpretation of information

Possibly evidenced by:	Request for information
	Statement of concerns
	Inappropriate or exaggerated behaviors, e.g., excessive anxiety, agitation (particularly in MVP)
	Inaccurate follow-through of instruction
PATIENT OUTCOMES/ EVALUATION CRITERIA:	Verbalizes understanding of disease process, treatment regimen, and potential complications. Identifies behaviors/lifestyle changes to prevent complications. Recognizes need for cooperation and follow-up care.

ACTIONS/INTERVENTIONS

Independent

Explain basic pathophysiology of valve abnormality.

Explain medication rationale, dosage, side effects, and importance of taking as prescribed, e.g., diuretics, antidysrhythmics, inotropic agents, vasodilators.

Instruct the patient taking a diuretic to take daily dose (or larger dose) in the morning.

Recommend monitoring own weight and maintaining a record. Encourage reporting weight gain of 2 lb in 1 day or 5 lb in 1 week; swelling of ankles, feet or abdomen; weight loss of > 5 pounds in 1 week.

Stress importance of reporting excessive thirst, severe dizziness or episodes of fainting.

Instruct and have patient demonstrate skill in self-monitoring of pulse if the patient is discharged on digitalis.

Discuss safety precautions which will minimize orthostatic hypotension if the patient is discharged on vasodilators, e.g., rise slowly from a lying to standing position, sit for a few minutes before standing; avoid prolonged standing; wear support stockings when up and around; avoid hot baths, steam rooms, and saunas.

Explain rationale for the prescribed dietary regimen (usually a diet low in sodium).

Discuss with patient need to balance activity and rest. Explain importance of consistency in activity/exercise.

Provide instructions on appropriate activity regimen: regular low intensity exercise, e.g., walking program (stable/asymptomatic patients); self-care activities, active or assisted range-of-motion, energy saving techniques (symptomatic patients).

RATIONALE

The patient should have a basic understanding of own valve abnormality, and the hemodynamic consequences of the defect, as a basis for explaining rationale for various aspects of treatment.

May enhance cooperation with drug therapy, prevent unauthorized discontinuation of medication; and/or adverse drug interactions.

Scheduling minimizes nighttime urination/interruption of sleep.

Weight is a primary indicator of the effectiveness of diuretic therapy and should be measured on a regular basis for monitoring trends.

May indicate a need to evaluate electrolyte status (specifically potassium) and/or alter medication regimen.

Any change in pulse rate (typically below 60 in adults) and rhythm (onset of irregularity) may be an indication of digitalis toxicity and should be reported to the physician for evaluation.

Measures help to minimize untoward side effects of vasodilation and enhance postural adjustments in blood pressure (may prevent syncope/falls).

Increased sodium results in water retention and increased cardiac workload.

A consistent, appropriately paced activity program is best to minimize deconditioning and fatigue, while preventing overexertion, which can increase cardiac workload/decompensation.

Activity regimen needs to be individualized, as some patients tolerate only range-of-motion exercises while others participate in more active programs.

ACTIONS/INTERVENTIONS	RATIONALE

Independent

Instruct patient to (1) monitor own physiologic response to activity, e.g., pulse rate, shortness of breath; (2) stop activity that causes chest pain, shortness of breath, dizziness, or extreme fatigue or weakness; (3) report decreased tolerance to activity.

The patient's involvement in monitoring own activity tolerance is vital to safely resuming and/or modifying activities of daily living.

Stress importance of informing health care provider of effort syncope or chest pain.

These are indicative of intolerance to activity which are related to inadequate cardiac output/worsening valve dysfunction.

Provide information concerning significance of endocarditis. (Refer to CP: Inflammatory Cardiac Conditions, p. 109.)

Patients with valvular heart disease are at risk for endocarditis (due to the adherence of infected vegetations on cardiac structures), which can lead to further valvular scarring, retraction of leaflets, and loss of function, requiring surgical intervention.

Instruct the patient requiring antithrombotic therapy in the purpose, dosage and side effects of the medication prescribed, e.g., warfarin (Coumadin), dipyridamole (Persantine), aspirin.

The patient with an enlarged left atrium, chronic atrial fibrillation and certain prosthetic valves are at increased risk for embolization, and therefore may be discharged on anticoagulant medications.

Reinforce the importance of taking the anticoagulant according to physician instructions, and reporting for prothrombin times.

Drugs need to be taken at the same time every day to maintain therapeutic level. The therapeutic range for Coumadin is based on patient prothrombin time.

Identify the most common signs of early bleeding, e.g., develops bruises without trauma. Stress importance of reporting bleeding to health care provider.

Prompt evaluation and intervention may prevent more serious complications.

Instruct patient to avoid OTC medications, use electric shaver, rather than blade razors, floss and brush teeth gently, cut nails carefully, avoid straining at stool.

Anticoagulant action is affected by many OTC products. Attention to safety measures will help minimize the risk of traumatic bleeding.

Stress importance of maintaining a minimum fluid intake of 2500 ml/day (unless contraindicated).

This will help to prevent increased blood viscosity which leads to hypercoagulability and potentiates thrombus formation.

Review necessary dietary modification.

Alcohol and foods high in vitamin K alter the prothrombin time and should be avoided.

Encourage patient to wear an identification bracelet/tag.

Alerts emergency personnel that patient is taking anticoagulants.

Collaborative

Identify/refer to community resources and support group.

Chronic nature of condition may affect ability to meet self-care needs/home maintenance management, increasing risk of social isolation/depression.

Cardiac Surgery: Coronary Artery Bypass Graft; Valve Replacement (Postoperative Care)

PATIENT ASSESSMENT DATA BASE

The preoperative data presented here are dependent on the specific disease process and underlying cardiac condition/reserve.

ACTIVITY/REST

May report:
History of exercise intolerance.
Generalized weakness, fatigue.
Concern about ability to perform expected/usual life activities.

May exhibit:
Abnormal heart rate, blood pressure response to activity.
Exertional discomfort or dyspnea.
ECG changes/dysrhythmias.

CIRCULATION

May report:
History of recent/acute MI, three vessel coronary artery disease, valvular heart disease, hypertension.

May exhibit:
Variations in blood pressure, heart rate/rhythm.
Dysrhythmias/ECG changes.
Abnormal heart sounds: S_3/S_4, murmurs.
Pallor/cyanosis of skin or mucous membranes.
Cool/cold, clammy skin.
Edema, jugular vein distention.
Diminished peripheral pulses.
Crackles.
Restlessness/other changes in mentation or sensorium (severe cardiac decompensation).

EGO INTEGRITY

May report:
Feeling scared/apprehensive, helpless.
Distress over current events (anger/fear).
Fear of death/eventual outcome of surgery (complications).
Fear about changes in lifestyle/role functioning.

May exhibit:
Apprehension.
Restlessness.
Insomnia/sleep disturbance.
Facial/general tension.
Withdrawal/lack of eye contact.
Crying.
Focus on self, hostility, anger.
Changes in heart rate, blood pressure, breathing patterns.

FOOD/FLUID (REFLECTING ADVANCED CARDIAC INVOLVEMENT)

May report:
Change in urine frequency/amount.
Change in weight.

Loss of appetite.
Abdominal pain, nausea/vomiting.

May exhibit: Changes in urine output.
Weight gain/loss.
Dry skin, poor skin turgor.
Postural hypotension.
Diminished/absent bowel sounds.
Edema (generalized, dependent, pitting).
Vomiting.

NEUROSENSORY

May report: Fainting spells, vertigo.

May exhibit: Changes in orientation or usual response to stimuli.
Restlessness.
Irritability.
Apathy.
Exaggerated emotional responses.

PAIN/COMFORT

May report: Chest pain, angina.

Postoperative:
Incisional discomfort.
Pain/paresthesia of shoulders, arms, hands, legs.

May exhibit: *Postoperative:*
Guarding.
Facial mask of pain.
Grimacing.
Distraction behaviors.
Moaning.
Restlessness.
Changes in blood pressure/pulse/respiratory rate.

RESPIRATION

May report: Shortness of breath.

Postoperative:
Inability to cough or take a deep breath.

May exhibit: *Postoperative:*
Decreased chest expansion.
Splinting/muscle guarding.
Dyspnea (normal response to thoracotomy).
Areas of diminished or absent breath sounds (atelectasis).
Anxiety.
Changes in ABGs.

SAFETY

May report: Infectious episode with valvular involvement.

Postoperative:
Oozing/bleeding from chest or leg incisions.

TEACHING/LEARNING

May report: Familial risk factors of diabetes, heart disease, hypertension, strokes.

Use of various cardiovascular drugs.

Failure to improve.

Discharge Plan Considerations: Assistance with food preparation, shopping, transportation, self-care needs and homemaker tasks.

DIAGNOSTIC STUDIES (POSTOPERATIVE)

Hemoglobin/hematocrit: decreased Hb reduces oxygen-carrying capacity and indicates need for red blood cell replacement. Elevation of Hct suggests dehydration/ need for fluid replacement.

Electrolytes: imbalances (hyper/hypokalemia, hyper/hyponatremia, and hypocalcemia) can affect cardiac function and fluid balance.

ABGs: identifies oxygenation status/effectiveness of respiratory function and acid/base balance.

Ear/pulse oximetry: noninvasive measure of oxygenation at tissue level.

BUN/creatinine: reflects adequacy of renal and liver perfusion function.

Amylase: elevation is occasionally seen in high-risk patients, e.g., those with heart failure undergoing valve replacement.

Glucose: fluctuations may occur due to rate of dextrose infusions, preoperative nutritional status, presence of diabetes/organ dysfunction.

Cardiac enzymes/isoenzymes: elevated in the presence of acute, recent or perioperative myocardial infarction.

Chest x-ray: reveals heart size and position, pulmonary vasculature, and changes indicative of pulmonary complications (e.g., atelectasis). Verifies condition of valve prosthesis and sternal wires, position of pacing leads, intravascular/cardiac lines.

ECG: identifies changes in electrical/mechanical function such as might occur in immediate postoperative phase, acute/perioperative myocardial infarction, valve dysfunction, and/or pericarditis.

NURSING PRIORITIES

1. Support hemodynamic stability/ventilatory function.
2. Promote relief of pain/discomfort.
3. Promote healing.
4. Provide information about postoperative expectations and treatment regimen.

DISCHARGE CRITERIA

1. Exercise tolerance adequate to meet self-care needs.
2. Pain is alleviated/managed.
3. Complications prevented/minimized.
4. Incisions healing.
5. Postdischarge medications, exercise, diet therapy understood.

NURSING DIAGNOSIS:	CARDIAC OUTPUT, ALTERED: DECREASED [POTENTIAL]
May be related to:	Decreased myocardial contractility secondary to temporary factors (e.g., ventricular wall surgery, recent myocardial infarction, response to certain medications/ drug interactions)
	Decreased preload (hypovolemia)
	Alterations in electrical conduction (dysrhythmias)

Possibly evidenced by:	[Not applicable; presence of signs and symptoms establishes an *actual* diagnosis.]
PATIENT OUTCOMES/ EVALUATION CRITERIA:	Reports/displays decreased episodes of angina and dysrhythmias. Demonstrates an increase in activity tolerance. Participates in activities that maximize/enhance cardiac function.

ACTIONS/INTERVENTIONS	RATIONALE
Independent	
Monitor/document trends in heart rate and blood pressure, especially noting hypertension. Be aware of specific systolic/diastolic limits defined for patient.	Tachycardia is a common response to discomfort and anxiety, inadequate blood/fluid replacement, and the stress of surgery. However, sustained tachycardia increases cardiac workload and can decrease effective cardiac output. Hypertension can occur (fluid excess or preexisting condition), placing stress on suture lines of new grafts and changing blood flow/pressure within heart chambers/across valves, with increased risk for thromboembolic phenomena. Hypotension may result from fluid deficit, dysrhythmias, heart failure/shock.
Monitor/document cardiac dysrhythmias. Observe patient response to dysrhythmias, e.g., drop in BP.	Life-threatening dysrhythmias can occur due to electrolyte imbalance, myocardial ischemia, or alterations in the heart's electrical conduction. Decreased cardiac output and hemodynamic compromise occurring with dysrhythmias require prompt intervention.
Observe for changes in usual mental status/orientation/body movement or reflexes, e.g., onset of confusion, disorientation, restlessness, reduced response to stimuli, stupor.	May indicate decreased cerebral blood flow or oxygenation as a result of diminished cardiac output (sustained or severe dysrhythmias, low BP, heart failure, or thromboembolic phenomena).
Record skin temperature/color, and quality/equality of peripheral pulses.	Warm, pink skin and strong, equal pulses are general indicators of adequate cardiac output.
Measure/document intake, output and fluid balance.	Useful in determining fluid needs or identifying fluid excesses which can compromise cardiac output.
Schedule uninterrupted rest/sleep periods. Assist with self-care activities.	Prevents fatigue/overexhaustion and excessive cardiovascular stress.
Monitor graded activity program. Note patient response, vital signs before/during/after activity; development of dysrhythmias.	Regular exercise stimulates circulation/cardiovascular tone and promotes feeling of well-being. Progression of activity is dependent on cardiac tolerance.
Evaluate presence/degree of anxiety/emotional duress. Encourage the use of relaxation techniques, e.g., deep breathing, diversional activities.	Excessive/escalating emotional reactions can affect vital signs and systemic vascular resistance eventually affecting cardiac function.
Inspect for jugular vein distention, peripheral or dependent edema, congestion in lungs, shortness of breath, change in mental status.	May be indicative of heart failure (acute or chronic). (Refer to CP: Congestive Heart Failure, p. 41.)
Investigate complaints of angina/severe chest pain, accompanied by restlessness, diaphoresis, ECG changes.	Although not a common complication of CABG, perioperative or postoperative myocardial infarction can occur. (Refer to CP: Myocardial Infarction, p. 69.)
Investigate/report profound hypotension (unresponsive to fluid challenge), tachycardia, distant heart sounds, stupor/coma.	Development of cardiac tamponade can rapidly progress to cardiac arrest due to inability of the heart to fill adequately for effective cardiac output. Note: this is a relatively rare life-threatening complication that usually occurs in the immediate postoperative period, but can occur later in the recovery phase.

ACTIONS/INTERVENTIONS	RATIONALE
Collaborative	
Review serial ECGs.	Most frequently done to follow the progress in normalization of electrical conduction patterns/ventricular function after surgery, or to identify complications, e.g., perioperative myocardial infarction.
Administer IV fluids/blood transfusions as indicated.	IV fluids may be discontinued prior to discharge from the intensive care unit, or one line (central/peripheral) may remain in place for fluid replacement and/or emergency cardiac medications. Red blood cell replacement may be indicated on occasion to restore/maintain adequate circulating volume and enhance oxygen-carrying capacity.
Administer supplemental oxygen as indicated.	Promotes maximal oxygenation, which may reduce cardiac workload, aid in resolving myocardal ischemia and dysrhythmias.
Administer electrolytes, and medications as indicated, e.g., electrolyte solutions/potassium; antidysrhythmics, beta-blockers, digitalis, diuretics, anticoagulants.	Patient needs are variable, depending on type of surgery (CABG or valve replacement), response to surgical intervention, and preexisting conditions (e.g., general health, age, type of heart disease). Electrolytes, antidysrhythmics, and other heart medications may be required on a short-term or long-term basis to maximize cardiac contractility/output.
Maintain surgically placed pacing wires (atrial/ventricular), and initiate pacing if indicated.	May be required to support cardiac output in presence of conduction disturbances (severe dysrhythmias) which compromise cardiac function.

NURSING DIAGNOSIS:	**COMFORT, ALTERED: PAIN, ACUTE [DISCOMFORT]**
May be related to:	**Sternotomy (mediastinal incision) and/or donor site (leg/arm incision)**
	Myocardial ischemia (acute MI, angina)
	Tissue inflammation/edema formation
	Intraoperative nerve trauma
Possibly evidenced by:	**Complaints of incisional discomfort/pain**
	Discomfort, paresthesia, pain in hand/arm/shoulder
	Anxiety, restlessness, irritability
	Distraction behaviors
	Increased heart rate
PATIENT OUTCOMES/ EVALUATION CRITERIA:	**Verbalizes relief/absence of pain. Demonstrates relaxed body posture, ability to rest/sleep appropriately. Differentiates surgical discomfort from angina/preoperative heart pain.**

ACTIONS/INTERVENTIONS	**RATIONALE**

Independent

Encourage patient to report type, location and intensity of pain, rating on a scale of 1–10. Ask the patient how this compares with preoperative chest pain.

Pain is perceived, manifested, and tolerated individually. It is important for the patient to differentiate incisional pain from other types of chest pain, e.g., angina. Many CABG patients do not experience severe discomfort in chest incision, and may complain more often of donor site incision discomfort. Severe pain in either area should be investigated further for possible complications.

Observe for anxiety, irritability, crying, restlessness, sleep disturbances.

These nonverbal cues may indicate the presence/degree of pain being experienced.

Monitor vital signs.

Heart rate usually increases with pain, although a bradycardiac response can occur in a severely diseased heart. Blood pressure may be elevated slightly with incisional discomfort but may be decreased or unstable if chest pain is severe and/or myocardial damage is occurring.

Identify/promote position of comfort using adjuncts as necessary.

Pillows/blanket rolls are useful in supporting extremities, maintaining body alignment, and splinting incisions to reduce muscle tension/promote comfort.

Provide routine comfort measures (e.g., back rubs, position changes), assist with self-care activities and encourage diversional activities as indicated.

May promote relaxation/redirect attention and reduce analgesic dosage needs/frequency.

Schedule care activities to balance with adequate periods of sleep/rest.

Rest and sleep are vital for cardiac healing (balance between oxygen demand and consumption), and can enhance coping with stress and discomfort.

Identify/encourage use of behaviors such as guided imagery, distractions, visualizations, deep breathing.

Relaxation techniques aid in management of stress, promote sense of well-being, may reduce analgesic needs, and promote healing.

Tell patient that it is acceptable, even preferable to request analgesics when discomfort becomes noticeable.

Presence of pain causes muscle tension which can impair circulation and slow healing process.

Medicate prior to procedures/activities as indicated.

Patient comfort and cooperation in respiratory treatments, ambulation and procedures (e.g., removal of chest tubes, pacemaker wires and suture removal) are facilitated by prior analgesic administration.

Investigate complaints of pain in unusual areas (e.g., calves of legs, abdomen) or vague complaints of discomfort, especially when accompanied by changes in mentation, vital signs, respiratory rate.

May be an early manifestation of developing complication, e.g., thrombophlebitis, infection, gastrointestinal dysfunction.

Note complaints of pain and/or numbness in ulnar area (fourth and fifth digits) of the hand often accompanied by pain/discomfort of the arms and shoulders. Tell the patient that the problem usually resolves with time.

Indicative of a stretch injury of the brachial plexus as a result of the position of the arms during surgery. No specific treatment is currently useful.

Collaborative

Administer medications as indicated, e.g., propoxyphene and acetaminophen (Darvocet-N), acetaminophen and oxycodone (Tylox).

Usually provides for adequate control of pain, reduces muscle tension to improve patient comfort and promote healing.

NURSING DIAGNOSIS:	SELF-CONCEPT, DISTURBANCE IN: ROLE PERFOR-MANCE
May be related to:	Situational crisis (dependent role)/recuperative process Uncertainty about future
Possibly evidenced by:	Delay/alteration in physical capacity to resume role Change in usual role or responsibility Change in self/others' perception of role
PATIENT OUTCOMES/ EVALUATION CRITERIA:	Reports anxiety is reduced to a manageable level. Verbalizes realistic perception and acceptance of self in changed role. Talking with SO about situation and changes that have occurred. Developing realistic plans for adapting to perceived role changes.

ACTIONS/INTERVENTIONS	RATIONALE
Independent	
Assess patient role in family constellation. Identify concerns about role dysfunction/interruption, e.g., recuperation, health–illness transitions.	Helps to know patient responsibilities and how illness affects this role. Dependent role of the patient provokes anxiety and concern about how the patient will be able to manage usual role responsibilities.
Assess level of anxiety, patient's perception of degree of threat to self/life.	Information provides baseline for identifying/individualizing plan of care.
Note cultural factors affecting role changes.	Cultural expectations regarding male/female illness role can determine how patient/SO react to and deal with current situation and may affect future adaptation to perceived changes.
Maintain positive attitude toward the patient, providing opportunities for the patient to exercise control as much as possible.	Helps patient to accept changes that are occurring and begin to realize that control over self is possible.
Assist patient/SO to develop strategies for dealing with changes, e.g., shifting of responsibilities to other family members/friends or neighbors, acquiring temporary assistance (homemaker/yardwork), investigate avenues for financial assistance.	Planning for changes which may occur/be required, promotes sense of control and accomplishment without loss of self-esteem.
Acknowledge reality of grieving process related to role change and help patient to deal realistically with feelings of anger and sadness.	Cardiac surgery constitutes a dramatic point in the patient's life and it will never be the same again. Patient needs to recognize these feelings in order to deal with them and move forward.

NURSING DIAGNOSIS:	BREATHING PATTERN, INEFFECTIVE [POTENTIAL]
May be related to:	Inadequate ventilation (pain/muscular weakness) Diminished oxygen-carrying capacity (blood loss) Decreased lung expansion (atelectasis or pneumo/hemothorax)

Possibly evidenced by:	[Not applicable; presence of signs and symptoms establishes an *actual* diagnosis.]
PATIENT OUTCOMES/ EVALUATION CRITERIA:	Maintains a normal/effective respiratory pattern free of cyanosis and other signs/symptoms of hypoxia with breath sounds equal bilaterally, lung fields clear(ing). Displays complete reexpansion of lungs with absence of pneumo/hemothorax.

ACTIONS/INTERVENTIONS

Independent

Evaluate respiratory rate and depth. Note respiratory effort, e.g., presence of dyspnea, use of accessory muscles, nasal flaring.

Auscultate breath sounds. Note areas of diminished/absent breath sounds, presence of adventitious sounds, e.g., crackles or rhonchi.

Observe chest excursion. Investigate decreased expansion or lack of symmetry in chest movement.

Observe character of cough and sputum production.

Inspect skin and mucous membranes for cyanosis.

Elevate head of bed, place in upright or semi-Fowler's position. Assist with early ambulation/increased time out of bed.

Encourage patient participation/responsibility for deep breathing exercises, use of adjuncts (blow bottles) and coughing as indicated.

Reinforce splinting of chest with pillows during deep breathing/coughing.

Explain that coughing/respiratory treatments will not loosen/damage grafts or reopen chest incision.

RATIONALE

Patient responses are variable. Rate and effort may be increased by pain, fear, fever, diminished circulating volume (blood or fluid loss), accumulation of secretions, hypoxia, or gastric distention. Respiratory suppression (decreased rate) can occur from excessive use of narcotic analgesics. Early recognition and treatment of abnormal ventilation may prevent complications.

Breath sounds are often diminished in lung bases for a period of time following surgery due to normally occurring atelectasis. Loss of active breath sounds in an area of previous ventilation may reflect collapse of lung, especially if chest tubes have recently been removed. Crackles or rhonchi may be indicative of fluid accumulation (interstitial edema, pulmonary edema, or infection) or partial airway obstruction (pooling of secretions).

Air or fluid in the pleural space prevents complete expansion (usually on one side) and is indicative of need for further assessment of ventilation status.

Frequent coughing may simply be throat irritation or can reflect pulmonary congestion. Purulent sputum suggests onset of pulmonary infection.

Cyanosis of lips, nailbeds, earlobes or general duskiness may indicate a hypoxic condition due to heart failure or pulmonary complications. General pallor (commonly present in immediate postoperative period) may indicate anemia from blood loss/insufficient blood replacement or red blood cell destruction from cardiopulmonary bypass pump.

Stimulates respiratory function/lung expansion. Effective in preventing and resolving pulmonary congestion.

Aids in reexpansion/maintaining patency of small airways especially after removal of chest tubes. Coughing is not necessary unless wheezes/rhonchi are present indicating retention of secretions.

Reduces incisional tension, promotes maximal lung expansion and may enhance effectiveness of cough effort.

Provides reassurance that injury will not occur, may enhance cooperation with therapeutic regimen.

105

ACTIONS/INTERVENTIONS	RATIONALE

Independent

Encourage maximal fluid intake within cardiac reserves.

Medicate with analgesic before respiratory treatments as indicated.

Record response to deep breathing exercises or other respiratory treatment noting breath sounds (before/after treatment), cough/sputum production.

Investigate/report respiratory distress, diminished/absent breath sounds, tachycardia, severe agitation, drop in blood pressure.

Adequate hydration helps liquefy secretions facilitating expectoration.

Allows for easier chest movement and reduces discomfort related to incisional pain, facilitating patient cooperation with/effectiveness of respiratory treatments.

Documents effectiveness of therapy or need for more aggressive interventions.

Although not a common complication, hemo/pneumothorax may occur following removal of the chest tubes and requires prompt intervention to maintain respiratory function. (Refer to CP: Hemothorax/Pneumothorax, p. 165.)

Collaborative

Review chest x-ray reports and laboratory studies (ABGs, hemoglobin) as indicated.

Monitors effectiveness of respiratory therapy and/or documents developing complications. A blood transfusion may be needed if blood loss is the reason for respiratory hypoxemia.

Assist with use of incentive spirometer/blow bottles.

Used to maximize lung inflation, reduce atelectasis, and prevent pulmonary complications.

Administer supplemental oxygen by cannula or mask as indicated.

Enhances oxygen delivery to the lungs for circulatory uptake, especially in presence of reduced/altered ventilation.

Assist with reinsertion of chest tubes or thoracentesis if indicated.

Reexpands lung by removal of accumulated blood/air and restoration of negative pleural pressure.

NURSING DIAGNOSIS:	SKIN INTEGRITY, IMPAIRED: ACTUAL
Related to:	Surgical incisions, puncture wounds
Evidenced by:	Disruption of skin surface
PATIENT OUTCOMES/ EVALUATION CRITERIA:	Demonstrates behaviors/techniques to promote healing, prevent complications. Displays timely wound healing.

ACTIONS/INTERVENTIONS	RATIONALE

Independent

Encourage patient to inspect all incisions. Evaluate healing progress. Review expectations for healing with patient.

Healing begins immediately but complete healing will take time. Chest incision heals first (minimal muscle tissue) but donor site incision (leg) will require more time (more muscle tissue, longer incision, slower circulation). As healing progresses, the incision lines may appear dry with crusty scabs. Underlying tissue may look bruised and feel tense, warm, and lumpy (resolving hematoma).

Suggest wearing soft cotton shirts, loose fitting clothing; cover/pad incisions as indicated; leave incisions open to air as much as possible.

Reduces suture line irritation and pressure from clothing. Leaving incisions open to air promotes healing process and may reduce risk of infection.

ACTIONS/INTERVENTIONS

Independent

Shower in warm water, washing incisions gently. Avoid tub baths until approved by physician.

Support incisions with Steristrips (as needed) when sutures are removed.

Encourage elevation of legs when sitting up in chair.

Watch for/report to physician: places in incision that do not heal; reopening of healed incision; any drainage (bloody or purulent); localized area of swelling with redness, increased pain, hot to touch.

Promote adequate nutritional and fluid intake.

Collaborative

Obtain specimen of wound drainage as indicated.

RATIONALE

Keeps incision clean, promotes circulation/healing. Note: "Climbing" out of tub requires use of arms and pectoral muscles, which can put undue stress on sternotomy.

Aids in maintaining approximation of wound edges to promote healing.

Promotes circulation, reduces edema to improve tissue healing.

Signs/symptoms indicating failure to heal, development of complications requiring further evaluation/intervention.

Helps to maintain good circulating volume for tissue perfusion and meets cellular energy requirements to facilitate tissue regeneration/healing process.

If infection occurs, local and systemic treatments may be required, e.g., peroxide/saline/Betadine soaks, antibiotic therapy.

NURSING DIAGNOSIS:	**KNOWLEDGE DEFICIT [LEARNING NEED] (SPECIFY)**
May be related to:	**Lack of exposure**
	Information misinterpretation
	Lack of recall
Possibly evidenced by:	**Questions/requests for information**
	Verbalization of problem
	Statement of misconception
	Inaccurate follow-through of instructions
PATIENT OUTCOMES/ EVALUATION CRITERIA:	**Participates in learning process. Assumes responsibility for own learning. Begins to look for information/ask questions. Verbalizes understanding of condition, prognosis, and therapeutic needs.**

ACTIONS/INTERVENTIONS

Independent

Reinforce surgeon's explanation of particular surgical procedure providing diagram as appropriate. Incorporate this information into discussion about short/long-term recovery expectations.

RATIONALE

Provides individually specific information creating knowledge base for subsequent learning regarding home management. Length of rehabilitation and prognosis is dependent on type of surgical procedure, preoperative physical condition, and duration of complications.

ACTIONS/INTERVENTIONS	RATIONALE

Independent

Review prescribed exercise program, and progress to date. Assist patient/SO to set realistic goals.

Individual capabilities and expectations are dependent on type of surgery, underlying cardiac function, and prior physical conditioning.

Encourage alternating rest periods with activity, and light tasks with heavy tasks. Avoid heavy lifting, isometric/strenuous upper body exercise.

Prevents excessive fatigue/overexhaustion. Note: Strenuous use of arms can place undue stress on sternotomy.

Problem-solve with patient/SO ways to continue progressive activity program, during temperature extremes, high wind/pollution days, e.g., walking predetermined distance within own house or local indoor shopping mall/exercise tract.

Having a plan will forestall giving up exercise because of interferences such as weather.

Schedule rest periods several times a day and take short naps.

Rest and sleep enhances coping abilities, reduces nervousness (common in this phase) and promotes healing.

Reinforce physician's time limitations about lifting, driving, returning to work, resumption of sexual activity.

These restrictions are present until after the first postoperative office visit for assessment of sternum healing.

Discuss issues concerning resumption of sexual activity, e.g., correlation of stress of sex to other activities;

Concerns about sexual activity often go unexpressed, but patients usually desire information about what to expect. In general, one can safely engage in sex when activity level has advanced to point where patient can climb two flights of stairs (which is about the same amount of energy expenditure).

Position recommendations;

Patient should avoid positions that restrict breathing (sex increases oxygen demand and consumption). Patient should not support self or partner with arms (chest bone healing, support muscles stretched).

Expectations of sexual performance;

Impotence appears to occur with some regularity in postoperative cardiac surgery patients. Although etiology is unknown, condition usually resolves in time without specific intervention. If situation persists, may require further evaluation.

Appropriate timing, e.g., avoid sex following heavy meal; during periods of emotional distress, when patient is fatigued/exhausted;

Timing of sexual activity may reduce occurrence of complications/angina.

Pharmacologic considerations.

Some patients may require antianginal medications (prophylactically) before sexual activity.

Inflammatory Cardiac Conditions: Pericarditis, Myocarditis, Endocarditis

Pericarditis: inflammation of the visceral and parietal pericardium.
Myocarditis: focal or diffuse inflammation of the myocardium.
Endocarditis: inflammation of the cardiac endothelial lining.

PATIENT ASSESSMENT DATA BASE

ACTIVITY/REST

May report: Fatigue, weakness.

May exhibit: Tachycardia.
Decreased blood pressure.
Dyspnea with activity.

CIRCULATION

May report: History of rheumatic fever, congenital heart disease, myocardial infarction, cardiac surgery (CABG/valve replacement/prolonged cardiopulmonary bypass).
Palpitations.
Fainting spells.

May exhibit: Tachycardia, dysrhythmias.
PMI displaced left and inferior (cardiac enlargement).
Pericardial friction rub.
Murmurs of aortic, mitral, tricuspid stenosis/insufficiency; change in preexisting murmurs; papillary muscle dysfunction.
Gallop rhythm (S_3/S_4 heart sounds).
Edema, jugular vein distention (congestive heart failure).
Petechia (conjunctiva, mucous membranes).
Splinter hemorrhages (nail beds).
Osler's nodes (fingers/toes).
Janeway lesions (palms, soles).

ELIMINATION

May report: History of kidney disease/renal failure.
Reduced urine frequency/amount.

May exhibit: Dark concentrated urine.

PAIN/COMFORT

May report: Pain in anterior chest (mild to severe/sharp) aggravated by breathing, movement, lying down; relieved by sitting up, leaning forward (pericarditis).
Chest/back/joint pain (endocarditis).

May exhibit: Distraction behaviors, e.g., restlessness.

RESPIRATION

May report: Shortness of breath; chronic shortness of breath worse at night (myocarditis).

May exhibit: Dyspnea, nocturnal dyspnea.
Cough.

SAFETY

May report: History of viral, bacterial, fungal or parasitic infections (myocarditis); chest trauma; malignant disease/thoracic irradiation; recent dental work; endoscopic examination of GI/GU system.

Compromised immune system, e.g., course of immunosuppressive therapy, SLE, other collagen diseases.

Long-term IV therapy or indwelling catheter use, or parenteral drug abuse.

May exhibit: Fever.

TEACHING/LEARNING

Discharge Plan Considerations: Assistance with food preparation, shopping, transportation, self-care needs, homemaker tasks.

DIAGNOSTIC STUDIES

ECG: may show ischemia, hypertrophy, conduction blocks, dysrhythmias.

Echocardiogram: may reveal pericardial effusion, cardiac hypertrophy, valvular dysfunction, dilatation of chambers.

Angiography: may show valvular stenosis and regurgitation, and/or decreased wall motion.

Chest x-ray: may show cardiac enlargement, pulmonary infiltrates.

CBC: may reveal acute/chronic infectious process; anemia.

Blood cultures: done to isolate causative bacteria, virus, fungus.

ASO titer: elevated with rheumatic fever (possible precipitator).

ANA titer: positive with autoimmune diseases, e.g., SLE (possible precipitator).

BUN: may be done to evaluate for uremia (possible precipitator).

Pericardiocentesis: pericardial fluid may be examined for etiology of infection.

NURSING PRIORITIES

1. Relieve pain.
2. Promote rest, provide self-care assistance.
3. Assist in treatment/alleviation of underlying cause.
4. Prevent complications.
5. Instruct in disease etiology, treatment, and prevention.

DISCHARGE CRITERIA

1. Pain alleviated/controlled.
2. Achieves activity level sufficient to meet basic self-care needs.
3. Infection resolved/controlled; fever absent.
4. Hemodynamic stability maintained; free of symptoms of heart failure.
5. Lifestyle changes initiated to prevent recurrence.

NURSING DIAGNOSIS:	**COMFORT, ALTERED: PAIN, ACUTE**
May be related to:	**Inflammation of myocardium or pericardium**
	Local or systemic infection
	Ischemia of myocardium
Possibly evidenced by:	**Chest pain, radiating to neck/back**
	Joint pain

Pain increased by deep inspiration, movement/activity, position

Fever, chills

| PATIENT OUTCOMES/ EVALUATION CRITERIA: | Reports pain is relieved/controlled. Verbalizes methods that provide relief. Demonstrates use of relaxation skills and diversional activities as indicated for individual situation. |

ACTIONS/INTERVENTIONS

Independent

Investigate complaints of chest pain, noting onset, aggravating and relieving factors. Note nonverbal clues of discomfort, e.g., lying very still/restlessness, muscle tension, crying.

Provide quiet environment and comfort measures, e.g., change of position, back rubs, use of heat/cold, emotional support.

Provide diversional activities.

Collaborative

Administer medications as indicated:

Nonsteroidal agents, e.g., indomethacin (Indocin); acetylsalicylic acid (aspirin);

Antipyretics, e.g., aspirin/acetaminophen (Tylenol).

Administer supplemental oxygen as indicated.

RATIONALE

Pain of pericarditis is typically located substernally and may radiate into neck and back. However, this differs from myocardial ischemia/infarction pain, in that it becomes worse with deep inspiration, movement or lying down and is relieved by sitting up/leaning forward. Note: chest pain may or may not accompany endocarditis and myocarditis, depending upon the presence of ischemia.

These measures can decrease patient's physical and emotional discomfort.

Redirects attention, provides distraction.

May provide relief of pain, reduces inflammatory response.

To reduce fever, promote comfort.

Maximizes oxygen available for uptake to reduce myocardial workload and decrease discomfort associated with ischemia.

NURSING DIAGNOSIS:	ACTIVITY INTOLERANCE
May be related to:	Inflammation and degeneration of myocardial muscle cells
	Restriction of cardiac filling/ventricular contraction, reduced cardiac output
	Toxins from infecting organism
Possibly evidenced by:	Complaints of weakness/fatigue/dyspnea with activity
	Changes in vital signs with activity
	Signs of congestive heart failure
PATIENT OUTCOMES/ EVALUATION CRITERIA:	Reports/displays measurable increase in activity tolerance. Demonstrates a decrease in physiologic signs of

intolerance. Verbalizes understanding of necessary therapeutic restrictions.

ACTIONS/INTERVENTIONS	RATIONALE
Independent	
Assess patient response to activity. Note presence of and changes in complaints of weakness, fatigue, and dyspnea associated with activity.	Myocarditis causes inflammation and possible damage to functioning myocardial cells with resultant congestive heart failure. Diminished cardiac filling and output may develop as fluid collects in the pericardial sac when pericarditis is present. Lastly, endocarditis may present with dysfunctional valves, negatively affecting cardiac output.
Assess/monitor heart rate/rhythm, blood pressure, respiratory rate before/after activity.	Helps determine the degree of cardiac and pulmonary decompensation/restoration. Decreased blood pressure, tachycardia, dysrhythmias, and tachypnea are indicative of impaired cardiac tolerance to activity.
Maintain bedrest during febrile periods and as indicated.	Promotes resolution of inflammation during acute phase of pericarditis/endocarditis. Note: Fever increases oxygen demand and consumption, thereby increasing cardiac workload and reducing activity tolerance.
Plan care with uninterrupted rest/sleep periods.	Provides for balance in demands that activity places on the heart, enhances healing process and emotional coping ability.
Assist patient with gradual progressive exercise program as soon as able to be out of bed, noting vital sign response and patient tolerance to increased activity.	As inflammation resolves/underlying condition is treated, patient may be able to resume most desired activities, unless permanent myocardial damage/complications have occurred.
Evaluate emotional response to situation/provide support.	Anxiety will be present because of inflammation/infection and cardiac response (physiologic), as well as the degree of patient's fear and demands upon emotional coping skills imposed by a potentially life-threatening illness (psychologic). Encouragement and support will be needed to cope with the frustration of prolonged hospital stay/recovery period.
Collaborative	
Administer supplemental oxygen.	Increases available oxygen for myocardial uptake to offset increased oxygen consumption that occurs with activity.

NURSING DIAGNOSIS:	CARDIAC OUTPUT, ALTERED: DECREASED [POTENTIAL]
May be related to:	Accumulation of fluid within the pericardial sac (pericarditis)
	Valvular stenosis/insufficiency
	Depressed/constricted ventricular function
	Degeneration of cardiac muscle (myocarditis)
Possibly evidenced by:	[Not applicable; presence of signs and symptoms establishes an *actual* diagnosis.]

PATIENT OUTCOMES/ EVALUATION CRITERIA:	Reports/displays decreased episodes of dyspnea, angina, and dysrhythmias. Identifies behaviors to reduce cardiac workload.

ACTIONS/INTERVENTIONS	RATIONALE
Independent	
Monitor heart rate/cardiac rhythm.	Tachycardia and numerous dysrhythmias can occur as the heart attempts to increase output in response to fever, hypoxia, acidosis because of ischemia.
Auscultate heart sounds. Note distant/muffled heart tones, murmurs, S_3 and S_4 gallops.	Provides for early detection of developing complications, e.g., CHF, cardiac tamponade.
Encourage bedrest in semi-Fowler's position.	Reduces cardiac workload, maximizes cardiac output.
Provide routine comfort measures, e.g., back rub and position change, and diversional activities within cardiac tolerance.	Promotes relaxation, and redirects attention.
Encourage use of stress management techniques, e.g., guided imagery, breathing exercises. (Refer to CP: Psychosocial Aspects of Acute Care, p. 773.)	Behaviors useful to control anxiety, promote relaxation and reduce cardiac workload.
Investigate rapid pulse, hypotension, narrow pulse pressure, elevated CVP/jugular venous distention, changes in heart tones, diminishing level of consciousness.	Clinical manifestations of cardiac tamponade which may occur in pericarditis when accumulation of fluid/exudate within the pericardial sac restricts cardiac filling and output.
Evaluate complaints of fatigue, dyspnea, palpitations, continuous chest pain. Note presence of adventitious breath sounds, fever.	Clinical manifestations of congestive heart failure that may accompany endocarditis (infection/valve dysfunction) or myocarditis (acute myocardial muscle dysfunction).
Collaborative	
Administer supplemental oxygen.	Enhances available oxygen for myocardial function, and reduces effects of anaerobic metabolism which occurs as a result of hypoxia and acidosis.
Administer medications as indicated, e.g., digitalis, diuretics;	May be given to increase myocardial contractility and reduce workload in presence of congestive heart failure (myocarditis).
Intravenous antibiotics/antimicrobials.	Given to treat identified pathogen(s) (endocarditis, pericarditis, myocarditis), preventing further cardiac involvement/damage.
Assist with emergency pericardiocentesis.	Procedure may be performed at the bedside to reduce fluid pressure around the heart which can rapidly restore cardiac output (pericarditis).
Prepare patient for surgery, if indicated.	Valve replacement may be necessary to improve cardiac output (endocarditis). Pericardectomy may be required because of recurrent pericardial fluid accumulation or scar tissue and constriction of cardiac function (pericarditis).

NURSING DIAGNOSIS:	**TISSUE PERFUSION, ALTERED: DECREASED [POTENTIAL]**
May be related to:	**Embolization of thrombi/valvular vegetations secondary to endocarditis**

113

<table>
<tr><td>Possibly evidenced by:</td><td>[Not applicable; presence of signs and symptoms establishes an *actual* diagnosis.]</td></tr>
<tr><td>PATIENT OUTCOMES/ EVALUATION CRITERIA:</td><td>Maintains/demonstrates increase in tissue perfusion as individually appropriate, e.g., usual mentation, stable vital signs, skin warm and dry, peripheral pulses present/ strong, balanced intake/output.</td></tr>
</table>

ACTIONS/INTERVENTIONS	RATIONALE
Independent	
Evaluate mental status. Note development of hemiparalysis, aphasia, seizures, vomiting, elevated blood pressure.	Indicators suggesting systemic embolization to brain.
Investigate chest pain, sudden dyspnea accompanied by tachypnea, pleuritic pain, pallor/cyanosis.	Arterial emboli, affecting the heart and/or other vital organs, may occur as a result of valvular disease, and/ or chronic dysrhythmias. Venous congestion/stasis may lead to thrombus formation in deep veins and embolization to lungs.
Observe extremities for swelling, erythema. Note tenderness/pain, positive Homans' sign.	Prolonged inactivity/bedrest predisposes to venous stasis increasing risk of developing venous thrombosis.
Observe for hematuria, accompanied by back/flank pain, oliguria.	Indicative of emboli to kidney(s).
Note complaints of pain in upper left abdomen radiating to left shoulder, local tenderness, abdominal rigidity.	May indicate splenic emboli.
Promote bedrest as appropriate.	May help prevent the formation or migration of emboli in the patient with endocarditis. Prolonged bedrest (often required for patients with endocarditis and myocarditis), however, carries its own risk of development of thromboembolic phenomena.
Encourage active exercises/assist with range-of-motion as tolerated.	Enhances peripheral circulation and venous return, thereby decreasing risk of thrombus formation.
Collaborative	
Apply/remove antiembolism stockings as indicated.	Use is controversial, but may promote venous circulation and decrease risk of superficial/deep vein thrombus formation.
Administer anticoagulants, e.g., heparin, warfarin (Coumadin).	Heparin may be used prophylactically when the patient requires prolonged bedrest; has sepsis, congestive heart failure; and/or before and after valve replacement surgery. Note: Heparin is contraindicated in pericarditis and cardiac tamponade. Coumadin is drug of choice for long-term/discharge therapy after valve replacement, or in presence of peripheral thrombi.

<table>
<tr><td>NURSING DIAGNOSIS:</td><td>KNOWLEDGE DEFICIT [LEARNING NEED] (SPECIFY)</td></tr>
<tr><td>May be related to:</td><td>Lack of information about disease process, ways to prevent recurrence or complications

Need for long-term therapy and follow-up</td></tr>
</table>

Possibly evidenced by:	Requests for information
	Failure to improve
	Preventable recurrences/complications
PATIENT OUTCOMES/ EVALUATION CRITERIA:	**Verbalizes understanding of inflammatory process, treatment needs, and possible complications. Identifies/ initiates necessary lifestyle or behavior changes to prevent recurrence/development of complications.**

ACTIONS/INTERVENTIONS

Independent

Explain effects of inflammation upon the heart, individualizing for particular patient. Educate concerning symptoms associated with complications/relapse, and symptoms to report immediately to health care provider, e.g., fever, increased/unusual chest pain, weight gain, increasing intolerance to activity, etc.

Instruct patient/SO in dose, purpose, side effects of medications; dietary needs/special considerations; activity allowances/limitations. Review necessity of prolonged antibiotic/antimicrobial therapy.

Discuss prophylactic use of antibiotics.

Identify actions to prevent endocarditis:

Good oral hygiene and dental care;

Avoidance of people with current infectious process (especially respiratory);

Appropriate choice of birth control method for female patient;

Avoidance of illicit IV drug use;

Promote practices of general well-being such as good nutritional intake, balance between activity/ rest, monitoring of own health status and reporting signs of infection;

Obtain immunizations, e.g., influenza vaccines as indicated.

Identify support person(s)/resources available post discharge to meet self-care/home maintenance needs.

RATIONALE

In order to take responsibility for own health, the patient needs to understand the specific cause, treatment, and expected long-term effects of the particular inflammatory condition, as well as signs/symptoms indicating recurrence/complications.

Information necessary to promote self-care, enhance compliance with therapeutic regimen, prevent complications. Lengthy hospital/home IV administration of antibiotics/antimicrobials may be necessary until blood cultures are negative/other blood work indicates absence of infection.

Patients with a history of rheumatic fever are at high risk for recurrences and usually require long-term antibiotic prophylaxis. Patients with a valvular deformity (who do not have a history of rheumatic fever) require short-term antibiotic protection for procedures that may cause transient bacteremia. Such procedures include dental procedures; tonsillectomy and/or adenoidectomy; surgical procedures/biopsy of respiratory mucosa; bronchoscopy; incision/drainage of infected tissue; and GU/GI procedures, childbirth.

Bacteria commonly found in mouth can enter easily into systemic circulation through the gums.

Development of infections, particularly respiratory streptococcal/pneumococcal or influenza, increases risk of cardiac involvement.

Use of IUDs has been linked to increased risk of pelvic inflammatory processes/infection.

Reduces risk of direct access of pathogens to systemic circulation.

Strengthens immune system and resistance to infection.

Reduces risk of acquiring severe infections that can lead to cardiac infections.

Activity intolerance/limitations may impair patient's ability to perform desired/needed tasks.

ACTIONS/INTERVENTIONS	RATIONALE
Independent	
Stress importance of regular follow-up medical care. Assist patient in making initial appointments.	Understanding reasons for medical supervision and planning for/accepting responsibility for follow-up care reduces risk of recurrence/complications.
Identify predisposing risk factors over which patient may have control, e.g., IV drug use (endocarditis), and problem-solve solutions.	Patient may be motivated by present cardiac problems to seek support to stop drug abuse/detrimental activities.

Thrombophlebitis: Deep Vein Thrombosis _____

Thrombophlebitis is a condition in which a clot forms in a vein secondary to inflammation/trauma of the vein wall, or because of a partial obstruction of the vein. Clot formation is related to (1) stasis of blood flow, (2) abnormalities in the vessel walls, and (3) alterations in the clotting mechanism.

Thrombophlebitis can affect superficial or deep veins, and while both conditions can cause symptoms, deep vein thrombosis (DVT) is more serious in terms of potential complications, including pulmonary embolism and postphlebotic syndrome.

PATIENT ASSESSMENT DATA BASE

ACTIVITY/REST

May report: History of occupation which requires sitting or standing for long periods of time.

History of lengthy immobility, e.g., orthopedic trauma, long hospitalization/bedrest, complicated pregnancy.

Pain with activity/prolonged standing.

CIRCULATION

May report: History of previous venous thrombosis, preexisting varices.

History of other predisposing factors, e.g., hypertension (pregnancy-induced); diabetes mellitus, myocardial infarction/valvular heart disease; thrombotic cerebrovascular accident, malignancy.

History of direct or indirect injury to extremity or vein (e.g., major trauma, orthopedic/pelvic surgery, prolonged labor with fetal head pressure on pelvic veins, intravenous therapy).

May exhibit: Affected extremity (calf/thigh): Skin color/temperature: pale, cool, edematous (DVT); pinkish red along the course of the vein (superficial).

Varicosities and/or hardened, bumpy/knotty vein (thrombus).

Peripheral pulse diminished in the affected extremity (DVT).

Homans' sign (absence does not rule out DVT).

Heart rate and temperature elevations (superficial and DVT).

FOOD/FLUID

May exhibit: Poor skin turgor, dry mucous membranes (dehydration predisposes to hypercoagulability).

Obesity (predisposes to stasis and pelvic vein pressure).

Edema of affected extremity (dependent on location of thrombus).

PAIN/COMFORT

May report: Throbbing, tenderness, aching pain aggravated by standing or movement (affected extremity).

May exhibit: Guarding of affected extremity.

SAFETY

May report: History of fractures/orthopedic surgery.

TEACHING/LEARNING

May report: Use of oral contraceptives; previous anticoagulant therapy (predisposes to hypercoagulability).

History of previous thrombophlebitis.

DIAGNOSTIC STUDIES

Hematocrit: hemoconcentration (elevated Hct) potentiates risk of thrombus formation.

Coagulation studies: may reveal hypercoagulability.

Noninvasive vascular studies (Doppler, oscillometry, exercise tolerance, plethysmography): may help pinpoint partially or totally occluded vessels.

Trendelenburg test: may demonstrate vessel valve incompetence.

Venography: may help confirm diagnosis by examining blood flow and size of channels.

Magnetic resonance imaging (MRI): may be useful in assessing blood flow turbulence and movement, venous valvular competence.

NURSING PRIORITIES

1. Maintain/enhance tissue perfusion, facilitate resolution of thrombus.
2. Promote optimal comfort.
3. Provide information about disease process/prognosis and treatment regimen.

DISCHARGE CRITERIA

1. Tissue perfusion of affected limb improved.
2. Pain/discomfort relieved.
3. Complications prevented/resolved.
4. Disease process/prognosis and therapeutic needs are understood.

NURSING DIAGNOSIS:	TISSUE PERFUSION, ALTERED: DECREASED, PERIPHERAL
May be related:	Deceased blood flow (venous stasis due to partial or complete venous obstruction)
Possibly evidenced by:	Tissue edema Diminished peripheral pulses, slow/diminished capillary refill Skin color changes (pallor, erythema)
PATIENT OUTCOMES/ EVALUATION CRITERIA:	Demonstrates improved perfusion as evidenced by peripheral pulses present/equal, skin color and temperature normal, absence of edema. Engages in behaviors/ actions to enhance tissue perfusion. Displays increasing tolerance to activity.

ACTIONS/INTERVENTIONS	RATIONALE
Independent Inspect extremity for skin color changes, and for edema (from groin to foot). Note symmetry of calves; measure and record calf circumference. Report proximal progression of inflammatory process.	Symptoms help distinguish between superficial thrombophlebitis and DVT. Redness, heat, tenderness, and localized edema are characteristic of superficial involvement. Pallor and coolness of extremity are characteristic of DVT. Calf vein involvement of DVT is asso-

ACTIONS/INTERVENTIONS	RATIONALE
Independent	
	ciated with absence of edema; femoral vein involvement is associated with mild to moderate edema; ileofemoral vein thrombosis is characterized by severe edema.
Examine extremity for obviously prominent veins. Palpate (gently) for local tissue tension, stretched skin, knots/bumps along course of vein.	Distention of superficial veins can occur in DVT because of backflow through communicating veins. Evidence of thrombophlebitis in superficial veins may be visible or palpable.
Assess capillary refill, and check for Homans' sign.	Diminished capillary refill usually present in DVT. Positive Homans' sign (pain in affected area upon dorsiflexion of foot) is not a consistent clinical manifestation as once thought and may or may not be present.
Promote bedrest during acute phase.	Reduces oxygen and nutrient demands on affected extremity and minimizes the possibility of dislodging thrombus and creating emboli.
Elevate legs when in bed or chair. Periodically elevate feet and lower legs above heart level.	Reduces tissue swelling and rapidly empties superficial and tibial veins, preventing overdistention and thereby increasing venous return. Note: Some physicians believe that elevation may potentiate release of thrombus and increase risk of embolization.
Initiate active or passive exercises while in bed (e.g., flex/extend/rotate foot periodically). Assist with gradual resumption of ambulation (e.g., walking 10 minutes each hour) as soon as patient is permitted out of bed.	These measures are designed to increase venous return from lower extremities and reduce venous stasis, as well as improve general muscle tone/strength.
Caution patient to avoid crossing legs and hyperflexion at knee (seated position with legs dangling, or lying in jackknife position).	Physical restriction of circulation impairs blood flow and increases venous stasis in pelvic, popliteal, and leg vessels.
Instruct patient to avoid rubbing/massaging the affected extremity.	Activity potentiates risk of fragmenting/dislodging thrombus, and embolization.
Encourage deep breathing exercises.	Produces increased negative pressure in thorax, which assists in emptying large veins.
Increase fluid intake to at least 2000 ml/day within cardiac tolerance.	Dehydration leads to increased blood viscosity and stasis, predisposing to thrombus formation.
Collaborative	
Apply warm, moist compresses to affected extremity as indicated.	Increases circulation to area; promotes vasodilation, venous return and resolution of local edema. Note: May be contraindicated in presence of arterial insufficiency, in which heat can increase cellular oxygen consumption/nutritional needs, furthering imbalance between supply and demand.
Administer anticoagulants, e.g., heparin (via continuous IV drip, intermittent intravenous or subcutaneous administration) and/or coumarin derivatives (Coumadin).	Heparin is preferred initially because of its prompt, predictable antagonistic action on thrombin formation and its prevention of further clot formation. Coumadin, which blocks formation of prothrombin from vitamin K, may be used for long-term/postdischarge therapy.
Monitor laboratory studies as indicated; prothrombin time (PT), partial thromboplastin time (PTT), activated partial thromboplastin time (APTT), CBC.	Monitors effectiveness of anticoagulant therapy and risk factors, e.g., hemoconcentration and dehydration, which potentiate clot formation.
Apply/regulate graduated compression stockings, intermittent pneumatic compression if indicated.	Sequential compression devices may be used (when anticoagulants are contraindicated or ineffective) to improve blood flow velocity and emptying of vessels.

ACTIONS/INTERVENTIONS

Collaborative

Apply elastic support hose following acute phase. Note that care must be taken to avoid tourniquet effect.

Prepare for surgical intervention when indicated.

RATIONALE

Properly fitted support hose are useful (once ambulation has begun) to minimize or delay development of postphlebotic syndrome, because they exert a sustained, evenly distributed pressure over entire surface of calves and thighs that reduces caliber of superficial veins, thus increasing blood flow to deep veins.

Thrombectomy (excision of thrombus) is occasionally necessary if inflammation extends proximally/circulation is severely restricted. Multiple/recurrent thrombotic episodes unresponsive to medical treatment (or when anticoagulant therapy is contraindicated) may require insertion of a vena caval screen/umbrella.

NURSING DIAGNOSIS:	COMFORT, ALTERED: PAIN, ACUTE [DISCOMFORT]
May be related to:	Diminished arterial circulation and oxygenation of tissues with production/accumulation of lactic acid in tissues
	Inflammatory process
Possibly evidenced by:	Complaints of pain, tenderness, aching/burning
	Guarding of affected limb
	Restlessness, distraction behaviors
PATIENT OUTCOMES/ EVALUATION CRITERIA:	Reports pain/discomfort is relieved/controlled. Verbalizes methods that provide relief. Displays relaxed manner, able to sleep/rest and engage in desired activity.

ACTIONS/INTERVENTIONS

Independent

Assess degree of discomfort/pain. Note guarding of extremity. Palpate leg with caution.

Maintain bedrest during acute phase.

Elevate affected extremity.

Provide foot cradle.

Encourage patient to change position frequently, keeping extremity elevated.

Monitor vital signs, noting elevated temperature.

RATIONALE

Degree of pain is directly related to extent of circulatory deficit, inflammatory process, degree of hypoxia, and extent of edema associated with thrombus development.

Reduces discomfort associated with muscle contraction and movement.

Encourages venous return to facilitate circulation, reducing stasis/edema formation.

Cradle keeps pressure of bed clothes off the affected leg, thereby reducing pressure discomfort.

Decreases/prevents fatigue, helps minimize muscle spasm and increases venous return.

Elevations in heart rate may indicate increased pain/discomfort or occur in response to fever and inflammatory process. Fever can also increase patient's discomfort.

ACTIONS/INTERVENTIONS

Independent

Investigate complaints of sudden and/or sharp chest pain, accompanied by dyspnea, tachycardia, and apprehension.

Collaborative

Administer medications, as indicated:

Analgesics (narcotic/nonnarcotic);

Antipyretics, anti-inflammatory agents, e.g., aspirin, phenylbutazone (Butazolidin).

Apply moist heat to extremity.

RATIONALE

These signs/symptoms suggest presence of pulmonary emboli as a complication of DVT. (Refer to CP: Pulmonary Embolism, p. 148.)

Relieves pain and decreases muscle tension.

Reduces fever and inflammation.

Causes vasodilation which increases circulation, relaxes muscles and may stimulate release of natural endorphins.

NURSING DIAGNOSIS:	KNOWLEDGE DEFICIT [LEARNING NEED] (SPECIFY)
May be related to:	**Lack of exposure**
	Misinterpretation of information
	Unfamiliarity with information resources
	Lack of recall
Possibly evidenced by:	**Statement of misconception**
	Verbalization of the problem
	Request for information
	Inaccurate follow-through of instruction
	Development of preventable complications
PATIENT OUTCOMES/ EVALUATION CRITERIA:	**Verbalizes understanding of disease process, treatment regimen and limitations. Participates in learning process. Identifies signs/symptoms requiring medical evaluation. Correctly performs therapeutic procedure(s) and explains reasons for actions.**

ACTIONS/INTERVENTIONS

Independent

Review pathophysiology of condition and signs/ symptoms of possible complications, e.g., pulmonary emboli, chronic venous insufficiency, venous stasis ulcers (postphlebotic syndrome).

Explain purpose of activity restrictions and need for balance between activity/rest.

Establish appropriate exercise/activity program.

RATIONALE

Provides a knowledge base from which patient can make informed choices and understand/identify health care needs.

Rest reduces oxygen and nutrient needs of compromised tissues, and decreases risk of fragmentation of thrombosis. Balance of activity prevents exhaustion and further impairment of cellular perfusion.

Aids in developing collateral circulation and enhances venous return. Aids in prevention of recurrence.

ACTIONS/INTERVENTIONS	RATIONALE

Independent

Problem-solve solutions to predisposing factors that may be present, e.g., employment that requires prolonged standing/sitting, wearing of restrictive clothing (girdles/garters), use of oral contraceptives, obesity, prolonged bedrest/immobility, dehydration.

Actively involves patient in identifying and initiating lifestyle/behavior changes to promote health and prevent recurrence of condition/development of complications.

Discuss purpose, dosage of anticoagulant. Emphasize importance of taking drug as prescribed.

Promotes patient safety by reducing risk of inadequate therapeutic response/deleterious side effects.

Identify safety precautions, e.g., use of soft toothbrush, electric razor for shaving, gloves for gardening; avoiding sharp objects (including toothpicks), walking barefoot, engaging in rough sports/activities, or forceful blowing of nose.

Reduces the risk of traumatic injury/bleeding.

Review possible drug interactions and stress need to read ingredient labels of OTC drugs.

Salicylates and excess alcohol decrease prothrombin activity, whereas vitamin K (multivitamins, bananas, green leafy vegetables) increases prothrombin activity. Barbiturates increase metabolism of coumarin drugs; antibiotics alter intestinal flora and may interfere with vitamin K synthesis.

Identify untoward anticoagulant effects requiring medical attention, e.g., bleeding from mucous membranes (nose, gums), severe bruising after minimal trauma, development of petechiae, continued oozing from cuts/punctures.

Early detection of deleterious effects of therapy (prolongation of clotting time) allows for timely intervention and may prevent serious complications.

Stress importance of medical follow-up/laboratory testing.

Understanding that close supervision of anticoagulant therapy is necessary (therapeutic dosage range is narrow and complications may be deadly) encourages patient participation.

Encourage wearing of identification bracelet/tag as indicated.

Alerts emergency health care givers to use of anticoagulants.

Review purpose and demonstrate correct application/removal of antiembolic hose.

Understanding may enhance cooperation with prescribed therapy and prevent improper/ineffective use.

Instruct in meticulous skin care of lower extremities, e.g., prevent/promptly treat breaks in skin, report development of lesions/ulcers or changes in skin color.

Chronic venous congestion/postphlebotic syndrome may develop (especially in presence of severe vascular involvement and/or recurrent episodes) potentiating risk of stasis ulcers/infection.

Raynaud's Disease

PATIENT ASSESSMENT DATA BASE

CIRCULATION

May report: History of migraines, hypertension, or correlation with menses/menopause, (vasospasm/hormonal effects).

History of color changes of affected parts on exposure to cold (onset in early adulthood).

Paresthesia of affected part during attack.

May exhibit: Skin color on fingers/affected parts (dependent upon phase at time of observation): may appear dead white (blanching), then cyanotic, then hyperemic (red). Late/progressive signs: skin is white or discolored, shiny, taut, smooth.

Pulses: radial and ulnar may be normal (early) or absent (late).

Nail clubbing/deformities may occur (late).

Ulcerations and/or areas of gangrene (rare).

EGO INTEGRITY

May report: Stress and strong emotional reactions (precipitator).

NEUROSENSORY

May report: Paresthesia, numbness in fingers.

May exhibit: Awkwardness/loss of fine coordination.

PAIN/COMFORT

May report: Throbbing pain during rubor phase of color change (vasodilation).

Sensitivity to pressure on affected part.

May exhibit: Guarding, restlessness, self-focus.

RESPIRATION

May report: Use of tobacco.

SAFETY

May report: Occupation which involves use of vibratory tools or requires frequent squeezing/repetitive movements, e.g., mechanics, farmers, typists, pianists, jackhammer/chainsaw operators (precipitator).

May exhibit: Lesions/areas of gangrene on fingertips, from the size of a pin to those involving the entire fingertip (very advanced).

TEACHING/LEARNING

May report: Other member(s) of family affected with vascular disease, e.g., hypertension, migraine headaches, or Raynaud's disease.

Discharge Plan Considerations: Alteration in medications.

Change in occupation.

DIAGNOSTIC STUDIES

Allen test: may show occlusion of radial or ulnar pulse proximal to wrist during attack.

Peripheral pulses: Doppler evaluation usually normal but may be reduced or absent during an attack.

Digital plethysmography: abnormal perfusion pulse contour and pressure during attacks.
Peripheral arteriography: may be done to visualize small peripheral arteries/rule out arteriovascular disease.

NURSING PRIORITIES

1. Minimize/eliminate ischemic attacks.
2. Support patient responsibility in prevention of complications.
3. Provide information about disease process/prognosis and treatment.

DISCHARGE CRITERIA

1. Frequency/severity of attacks is decreasing.
2. Complications are prevented/minimized.
3. Stress reduction techniques used appropriately.
4. Disease progression and therapeutic regimen are understood.

NURSING DIAGNOSIS:	COMFORT, ALTERED: PAIN, ACUTE/CHRONIC
May be related to:	Vasospasm/altered perfusion of affected tissues
	Ischemia/destruction of tissues
Possibly evidenced by:	Verbal complaints
	Guarding of affected parts
	Self-focusing
	Restlessness
PATIENT OUTCOMES/ EVALUATION CRITERIA:	Verbalizes decreased frequency of painful episodes. Identifies interventions that provide relief/prevent recurrence.

ACTIONS/INTERVENTIONS	RATIONALE
Independent	
Note characteristics of pain and paresthesia.	Changes in severity/duration may indicate progression of disease process/development of complications.
Discuss with patient how and why pain is produced.	Knowledge of pain-producing mechanism allows patient to intervene more effectively to minimize occurrences.
Assist patient to identify precipitating factors or situations, e.g., smoking, exposure to cold, and problem-solve solutions.	Vasoconstriction is to be limited as it may lead to tissue damage and gangrene.
Encourage use of stress management techniques, diversional activities.	Promotes relaxation/focusing attention to help in breaking the stress/anxiety/stress cycle which can worsen vasoconstrictive response and increase pain.
Immerse affected part in warm water.	This method of rewarming encourages vasodilation, stopping vasospasm.
Provide warm room, free of drafts, e.g., block air conditioner vent, keep hallway door closed as indicated.	Eliminates environmental factors which may precipitate an attack.

ACTIONS/INTERVENTIONS

Independent

Monitor effects of medications and treatment.

Collaborative

Administer medications as indicated. (Refer to ND: Tissue Perfusion, Altered: Peripheral, p. 125.)

Prepare for surgical intervention if indicated.

RATIONALE

Individual responses to prescribed therapies may not be adequate to control disease or may produce untoward side effects, indicating need for change in regimen.

Use of vasodilators/antihypertensives may relieve vasospasm, and reduce pain.

Sympathetic ganglionectomy is sometimes performed when relief of severe symptoms is not obtained by other methods. However, surgical relief is often temporary with return of symptoms within 6 months.

NURSING DIAGNOSIS:	TISSUE PERFUSION, ALTERED: PERIPHERAL
May be related to:	Interruption of arterial blood flow
Possibly evidenced by:	Coolness of affected areas during attack
	Intermittent color changes of tissue, e.g., blanching, cyanosis, reactive hyperemia
	Decreased sensation
	Slow healing of lesions
	Development of ulcerations/gangrene (rare)
PATIENT OUTCOMES/ EVALUATION CRITERIA:	Reports/displays decreased frequency/severity of vasospastic attacks with healing/absence of lesions.

ACTIONS/INTERVENTIONS

Independent

Observe skin color of affected parts.

Note diminshed pulses, delayed capillary refill, trophic skin changes (discoloration, shiny/taut); clubbing of nails.

Evaluate sensation in affected parts, e.g., sharp/dull, hot/cold.

Protect from injury, e.g., refrain from activities using sharp implements, requiring fine motor function, or involving heat/cold (drinking coffee/testing water for bath).

Inspect and assess skin for ulcerations, lesions, gangrenous areas.

RATIONALE

Typcial skin color changes occur in phases with intermittent blanching (result of sudden vasospasm), cyanosis (ischemia); and rubor (vasodilation/reactive hyperemia). During color changes, affected parts are first cold and numb, then throbbing, with tingling sensations and swelling.

These changes indicate progressive/chronic process.

Sensation is often diminished during attack or chronically in advanced disease.

Lack of awareness when sensation is diminished can lead to situations where the affected parts are damaged.

Lesions can occur from pinpoint size to those involving an entire fingertip and may result in infection/serious tissue damage/loss.

125

ACTIONS/INTERVENTIONS

Independent

Encourage proper nutrition, vitamins.

Collaborative

Administer medications as indicated:

Vasodilators, e.g., cyclandelate (Cyclospamol), tolazoline (Priscoline); antihypertensives, e.g., methyldopa (Aldomet), reserpine (Serpasil), phenoxybenzamine (Dibenzyline).

Obtain specimen of lesion drainage for culture and sensitivity.

RATIONALE

A well-balanced diet, including adequate protein and hydration, is necessary for proper healing and tissue regeneration.

Individual drugs or combinations may be used but effectiveness varies and use may be outweighed by presence of undesired side-effects.

Although site/mechanism of action varies, intended results are reduction of vasoconstriction, relaxation of vasospasm, and a more even blood flow/narrowing of pulse pressure.

Lesions may become secondarily infected, further damaging tissues and preventing healing. C&S identifies organism and identifies the antibiotic most useful in treating the organism.

NURSING DIAGNOSIS:	KNOWLEDGE DEFICIT [LEARNING NEED] (SPECIFY)
May be related to:	Lack of knowledge about cause and treatment of disease
	Misconceptions/misunderstanding
Possibly evidenced by:	Request for information
	Recurrence of attacks
PATIENT OUTCOMES/ EVALUATION CRITERIA:	Verbalizes understanding of need for protection from cold. Demonstrates understanding of medical regimen and symptoms to report to physician. Displays lifestyle/ behavior changes to reduce occurrence of attacks.

ACTIONS/INTERVENTIONS

Independent

Encourage avoidance of exposure to cold. Educate about the use of extra protection for cold, e.g., warm environment, adequate clothing, mittens, warm boots, avoiding direct contact with cold objects, when possible.

Keep environmental temperature at/above 70 degrees, eliminate drafts.

Discuss possible move to warmer climate, change of occupation as indicated.

Stress importance of cessation of smoking, provide information on clinics/support groups.

RATIONALE

Cold exposure is major precipitator of vasoconstriction. Warm clothing and environment help prevent vasoconstriction of digits by keeping the entire body warm. Note: Mittens are preferred, because gloves allow cold to surround and absorb heat from each finger.

Reduces risk of precipitating attack.

May be necessary if severe vasospasm attacks continue or ischemic tissue changes occur that cannot be controlled by other means.

Causes vasoconstriction, which may precipitate/ potentiate attacks. Patient usually requires support to accomplish elimination of this activity.

ACTIONS/INTERVENTIONS	RATIONALE
Independent	
Assist patient in designing methods to avoid or modify stressful episodes; help patient learn biofeedback and other relaxation techniques.	Allows patient to deal successfully with stress, which acts to stimulate catecholamine release by the sympathetic nervous system and produces vasoconstriction.
Prevent trauma to distal parts (hands, feet). Carefully trim nails. Advise patient to stop activity/protect affected part when spasm occurs.	Reduces risks of injury from sharp objects such as knives/needles, and from burns when sensitivity is diminished.
Discuss and provide information about how to terminate attacks, e.g., immersion of affected part in warm water.	Attack may subside spontaneously or be terminated by slow rewarming (encourages vasodilation). Information can reduce anxiety when patient takes measures to reduce pain.
Discuss purpose, dosage, side effects of medications.	Information necessary for patient to follow through with therapeutic regimen and evaluate effectiveness.
Recommend avoiding use of beta-blockers, e.g., propanolol (Inderal).	Contraindicated because they worsen vasospasm.
Investigate water therapy for behavior modification, e.g., soaking hands in warm water three to six times every other day indoors, then progressing to exposing body to cold while hands are submerged in warm water.	An experimental technique used to "retrain" body response to cold that has met with success in some trials.
Stress importance of daily inspection and proper skin care practices.	Maintaining integrity/health of compromised tissues may prevent progression/development of complications, e.g., lesions, infection, necrosis.

CHAPTER 5

RESPIRATORY

Chronic Obstructive Pulmonary Disease (COPD) _____

Chronic bronchitis: widespread inflammation of airways, narrowing or blocking of airways, and increased production of mucoid sputum, leading to ventilation–perfusion mismatch and marked cyanosis.

Emphysema: recurrent inflammation damages/eventually destroys alveolar walls creating large blebs or bullae (air spaces) and collapse of bronchioles upon expiration (air-trapping). However, pulmonary capillary destruction also occurs, which prevents ventilation–perfusion mismatch and cyanosis.

PATIENT ASSESSMENT DATA BASE

ACTIVITY/REST

May report:	Fatigue.
	Inability to perform basic activities of daily living because of breathlessness.
	Inability to sleep, need to sleep sitting up.
	Exhaustion.
May exhibit:	Fatigue.
	Insomnia.
	General debilitation/loss of muscle mass.

CIRCULATION

May report:	Swelling of lower extremities.
May exhibit:	Elevated heart rate, severe tachycardia.
	Distended neck veins (advanced disease).
	Dependent edema, may not be related to heart disease.
	Faint heart sounds (due to increased AP chest diameter).
	Skin color: bluish/cyanotic (chronic bronchitis) or pink (emphysema).

FOOD/FLUID

May report:	Nausea/vomiting.
	Poor appetite.

Inability to eat because of respiratory distress.

Persistent weight loss (emphysema).

May exhibit: Poor skin turgor.

Dependent edema.

Weight loss, decreased muscle mass/subcutaneous fat.

RESPIRATION

May report: History of persistent cough with sputum production on most days for minimum of 3 consecutive months each year for at least 2 years (chronic bronchitis).

History of long-term exposure to chemical pollution/respiratory irritants (e.g., cigarette smoke) or occupational dust/fumes (e.g., cotton hemp, asbestos, coal dust, sawdust).

History of recurrent respiratory infections.

History of oxygen use at home.

Shortness of breath, especially on exertion.

Chronic "air hunger."

Recurrent, persistent cough; intermittent cough episodes, usually productive of mucoid sputum.

Increased sputum production, particularly upon arising.

Thick, copious sputum (advanced chronic bronchitis).

Anxiety, restlessness.

May exhibit: Dyspnea, obvious "air hunger"/respiratory distress.

Assumption of three-point ("tripod") position for breathing (elbows may be callused).

Color: pallor with cyanosis of lips, nailbeds; overall duskiness; ruddy color.

Respirations: usually rapid; may be shallow; prolonged expiratory phase (emphysema).

Breath sounds: may be faint with expiratory wheezes (emphysema); scattered, moist crackles (bronchitis).

Chest: may appear hyperinflated with increased AP diameter (barrel-shaped); minimal diaphragmatic movement. May observe evidence of use of accessory muscles of respiration, e.g., elevated shoulder girdle, retraction of supraclavicular fossae.

Percussion: Hyperresonant over lung fields (e.g., air-trapping with emphysema); dull over lung fields (e.g., consolidation, fluid, mucus).

SEXUALITY

May report: Decreased libido.

SOCIAL INTERACTION

May report: Dependent relationship(s).

Lack of support systems.

Insufficient support from and/or to SO.

Prolonged disease or disability progression.

May exhibit: Inability to converse/maintain voice because of respiratory distress.

Limited physical mobility.

Neglectful relationships with other family members.

TEACHING/LEARNING

May report: Use/misuse of respiratory drugs.

Difficulty stopping smoking.

Regular use of alcohol.
Failure to improve.

Discharge Plan Considerations: Assistance with shopping, transportation, self-care needs, homemaker tasks.
Changes in medication/therapeutic treatments.

DIAGNOSTIC STUDIES

Chest x-ray: may reveal hyperinflation of lungs, flattened diaphragm, increased retrosternal air space; decreased vascular markings/bullae (emphysema).

Pulmonary function tests: done to determine cause of dyspnea; determine whether functional abnormality is obstructive or restrictive, and estimate degree of dysfunction; evaluate effects of therapy, e.g., bronchodilators.

Total lung capacity (TLC): increased in bronchitis; decreased in emphysema.

Inspiratory capacity: reduced in emphysema.

Residual volume: elevated in emphysema (may be markedly elevated).

FEV_1/FVC: ratio of forced expiratory volume to forced vital capacity is decreased in bronchitis.

ABGs: most often PaO_2 is decreased, and $PaCO_2$ is increased, pH normal or acidotic. Estimates progression of chronic disease process, e.g., chronically high $PaCO_2$.

Bronchogram: cylindrical dilation of bronchi on inspiration, bronchial collapse on forced expiration, enlarged mucous ducts seen in bronchitis.

Blood chemistry—α_1-antitrypsin: done to verify deficiency and a diagnosis of primary emphysema.

Sputum: culture to determine presence of infection, identify pathogen; cytologic examination to rule out underlying malignancy or allergic disorder.

Exercise ECG, stress test: helps in assessing degree of pulmonary dysfunction; evaluating effectiveness of bronchodilator therapy; planning/evaluating exercise program.

NURSING PRIORITIES

1. Maintain airway patency.
2. Assist with measures to facilitate gas exchange.
3. Enhance nutritional intake.
4. Prevent complications.
5. Provide information about disease process/prognosis and treatment regimen.

DISCHARGE CRITERIA

1. Ventilation/oxygenation adequate to meet self-care needs.
2. Nutritional intake meeting caloric needs.
3. Free of infection.
4. Disease process/prognosis and therapeutic regimen understood.

NURSING DIAGNOSIS:	AIRWAY CLEARANCE, INEFFECTIVE
May be related to:	Increased production of secretions; retained secretions; thick, viscous secretions
	Decreased energy/fatigue
Possibly evidenced by:	Statement of difficulty breathing
	Changes in depth/rate of respirations, use of accessory muscles
	Abnormal breath sounds, e.g., wheezes, rhonchi, crackles

Cough (persistent, with sputum production)

PATIENT OUTCOMES/ EVALUATION CRITERIA:	Maintains patent airway with breath sounds clear/ clearing. Demonstrates behaviors to improve airway clearance, e.g., coughs effectively and expectorates secretions.

[handwritten: ineffective Airway Clear]

Inde[pendent]

Auscu[ltate breath]
soun[ds]

Asse[ss]
expir[ation]

Note
"air[...]
tress; use of accessory muscles.

[handwritten: ineffective Airway Clearn]

Assist the patient to assume position of comfort, e.g., elevate head of bed, sitting on edge of bed.

Keep environmental pollution to a minimum, e.g., dust, smoke, feather pillows according to individual situation.

Encourage/assist with abdominal or pursed-lip breathing exercises.

Observe characteristics of cough, e.g., persistent, hacking, moist. Assist with measures to improve effectiveness of cough.

Increase fluid intake to 2000 ml/day within level of cardiac reserve. Provide warm/tepid liquids instead of cold.

Collaborative

Administer medications as indicated:

Bronchodilators, e.g., methylxanthines: aminophylline, oxtriphylline (Choledyl), theophylline (Bronkodyl, Theo-Dur);

Inhaled sympathomimetics: albuterol (Proventil), terbutaline (Brethine), isoetharine (Bronkometer);

Antimicrobials; steroids: methylprednisolone (Medrol) or cromolyn (Intol);

RATIONALE

Some degree of bronchospasm is present with obstructions in airway and may/may not be manifested in adventitious breath sounds, e.g., scattered, moist crackles (bronchitis) or faint, with expiratory wheezes (emphysema).

Tachypnea is usually present in some degree, and may be pronounced on admission or during stress, concurrent acute process. Respirations may be shallow and rapid. Chronic emphysema patients usually have prolonged expiration in comparison to inspiration (greater than 2:1).

Respiratory dysfunction is variable dependent upon stage of chronic process in addition to acute process that precipitated hospitalization, e.g., infection, allergic reaction.

Elevation of the head of the bed facilitates respiratory function by use of gravity. However, the patient in severe distress will seek the position that most eases breathing.

Precipitators of allergic type of respiratory reactions that can trigger onset of acute episode.

Provides the patient with some means to cope with and control dyspnea and reduce air-trapping.

Cough can be persistent but ineffective, especially if the patient is elderly, acutely ill, or debilitated. Coughing is most effective in an upright or in a head-down position after chest percussion.

Hydration helps decrease the viscosity of secretions, facilitating expectoration. Using warm liquids may decrease bronchospasm.

Decreases mucosal edema and smooth muscle spasm (bronchospasm), reducing wheezing.

Promotes relaxation of smooth muscles reducing airway spasm and wheezing.

Various antimicrobials may be indicated for control of respiratory infection. Corticosteroids may be used orally and/or inhaled to prevent allergic reactions/

Collaborative

inhibit release of histamine, reducing severity and frequency of airway spasm, respiratory inflammation, and dyspnea.

Analgesics, cough suppressants/antitussives, e.g., codeine, dextromethorphan products (Benylin DM, Comtrex, Novahistine).

Persistent, exhausting cough may need to be suppressed to conserve energy and permit the patient to rest.

Administer supplemental humidification, e.g., ultrasonic nebulizer, room humidifier.

Humidity reduces viscosity of secretions facilitating expectoration and may reduce/prevent formation of thick mucous plug in bronchioles.

Assist with respiratory treatments, e.g., IPPB, chest physiotherapy.

Postural drainage and percussion are an important part of the treatment for removal of sticky secretions and improved ventilation of bottom lung segments.

Monitor/graph serial ABGs, ear/pulse oximetry, chest x-ray.

Establishes baseline for monitoring progression/regression of disease process.

NURSING DIAGNOSIS:	GAS EXCHANGE, IMPAIRED
May be related to:	Altered oxygen supply (obstruction of airways by secretions, bronchospasm; air-trapping)
	Alveoli destruction
Possibly evidenced by:	Dyspnea
	Confusion, restlessness
	Inability to move secretions
	Abnormal ABG values (hypoxia and hypercapnea)
	Changes in vital signs
	Reduced tolerance for activity
PATIENT OUTCOMES/ EVALUATION CRITERIA:	Demonstrates improved ventilation and adequate oxygenation of tissues by ABGs within patient's normal range and free of symptoms of respiratory distress. Participates in treatment regimen within level of ability/situation.

ACTIONS/INTERVENTIONS   RATIONALE

Independent

Assess respiratory rate, depth. Note use of accessory muscles, pursed-lip breathing.

Useful in evaluating the degree of respiratory distress, and/or chronicity of the disease process.

Elevate head of bed, assist patient to assume position to ease work of breathing. Encourage deep slow or pursed-lip breathing as individually needed/tolerated.

Oxygen delivery may be improved by upright position and breathing exercises to decrease airway collapse, dyspnea, and work of breathing.

Assess/continuously monitor skin and mucous membrane color.

Cyanosis may be peripheral (noted in nailbeds) or central (noted around lips/or earlobes). Duskiness and central cyanosis would indicate advanced hypoxemia.

ACTIONS/INTERVENTIONS	RATIONALE
Independent	
Encourage expectoration of sputum; suction when indicated.	Thick, tenacious, copious secretions are a major source of impaired gas exchange in small airways. Deep suctioning may be required when cough is ineffective for expectoration of secretions.
Auscultate breath sounds, noting areas of decreased airflow and/or adventitious sounds.	May be faint because of decreased airflow, areas of consolidation. Presence of wheezes may indicate bronchospasm/retained secretions. Scattered moist crackles may indicate interstitial fluid/cardiac decompensation.
Palpat...	Decrease of vibratory tremors suggests fluid collection or air-trapping.
Asse... gate...	Restlessness and anxiety are common manifestations of hypoxia. Worsening ABGs, accompanied by confusion/somnolence, are indicative of cerebral dysfunction due to respiratory failure.
As... en... re... a...	During severe/acute/refractory respiratory distress the patient may be totally unable to perform basic self-care activities because of hypoxemia and dyspnea. Rest remains an important part of treatment regimen interspersed with care activities. However, an exercise program is aimed at increasing endurance and strength without causing severe dyspnea, and can enhance sense of well-being.
Monitor vit...	Tachycardia, dysrhythmias, and changes in blood pressure can reflect effect of systemic hypoxemia on cardiac function.
Collaborative	
Monitor/graph serial ABGs and ear/pulse oximetry.	$PaCO_2$ usually elevated and PaO_2 is generally decreased, so that hypoxia is present in a lesser or greater degree.
Administer supplemental oxygen judiciously as indicated by ABG results and patient tolerance.	Chronic COPD patient's respiratory drive is determined by the CO_2 level and may be eliminated by excess elevation of PaO_2.
Assist with intubation, institution/maintenance of mechanical ventilation and transfer to critical care area as indicated. (Refer to CP: Ventilatory Assistance [Mechanical], p. 191.)	Development of respiratory failure requires prompt life-saving measures.

(handwritten note: Impaired Gas Exchange)

NURSING DIAGNOSIS:	NUTRITION, ALTERED: LESS THAN BODY REQUIREMENTS
May be related to:	**Dyspnea**
	Fatigue
	Medication side effects
	Sputum production
	Anorexia, nausea/vomiting

Possibly evidenced by:	Weight loss
	Loss of muscle mass, poor muscle tone
	Fatigue
	Reported altered taste sensation
	Aversion to eating, lack of interest in food
PATIENT OUTCOMES/ EVALUATION CRITERIA:	Displays progressive weight gain toward goal. Demonstrates behaviors/lifestyle changes to regain and/or maintain appropriate weight.

ACTIONS/INTERVENTIONS

Independent

Assess dietary habits, recent food intake. Note degree of difficulty with eating. Evaluate weight and body size (mass).

Auscultate bowel sounds

Give frequent oral care; remove expectorated secretions promptly; provide specific container for disposal of secretions and tissues.

Provide frequent small feedings.

Avoid gas-producing foods and carbonated beverages.

Avoid very hot or very cold foods.

Weigh as indicated.

Collaborative

Consult dietician/nutritional support team to provide easily digested, nutritionally balanced meals by appropriate means, e.g., oral/supplemental/tube feedings, parenteral nutrition. (Refer to CP: Total Nutritional Support, p. 894.)

Review laboratory studies, e.g., serum albumin, transferrin, amino acid profile, iron, nitrogen balance studies, glucose, liver function studies, electrolytes. Administer vitamins/minerals/electrolytes as indicated.

Administer supplemental oxygen during meals as indicated.

RATIONALE

The patient in acute respiratory distress is often anorexic because of dyspnea, sputum production, medications. In addition, many COPD patients habitually eat poorly, even though respiratory insufficiency creates a hypermetabolic state with increased caloric needs. As a result, patient often is admitted with some degree of malnutrition, evidenced by thin appearance and wasted muscles.

Diminished/hypoactive bowel sounds may reflect decreased gastric motility and constipation (common complication) related to limited fluid intake, poor food choices, decreased activity, and hypoxemia.

Noxious tastes, smells, and sights are prime deterrents to appetite.

Helps to reduce fatigue during mealtime, provides opportunity to increase total caloric intake.

Can produce abdominal distention which hampers abdominal breathing and diaphragmatic movement, and can increase dyspnea.

Extremes in temperature can precipitate/aggravate coughing spasms.

Useful in determining caloric needs, setting weight goal and evaluating adequacy of nutritional plan. Note: Weight loss may continue initially in spite of adequate intake as edema is resolving.

Method of feeding and caloric requirements is based on individual situation/needs to provide maximal nutrients with minimal patient effort/energy expenditure.

Evaluates/treats deficits and monitors effectiveness of nutritional therapy.

Decreases dyspnea and increases energy for eating enhancing intake.

NURSING DIAGNOSIS: INFECTION, POTENTIAL FOR

May be related to: Inadequate primary defenses (decreased ciliary action, stasis of secretions)

Inadequate acquired immunity (tissue destruction, increased environmental exposure)

Chronic disease process

nutrition

applicable; presence of signs and symptoms establ an *actual* diagnosis.]

lizes understanding of individual causative/risk . Identifies interventions to prevent/reduce risk tion. Demonstrates techniques, lifestyle changes ote safe environment.

Infection, potential for (handwritten note)

RATIONALE

Ind

Mor

Revie _____ reathing exercises, effective cough _____ position changes and adequate fluid intake.

Observe color, character, odor of sputum.

Demonstrate and assist the patient in disposal of tissues and sputum. Stress proper handwashing (nurse and patient) and use gloves when handling/disposing of tissues, sputum containers.

Monitor visitors; provide masks as indicated.

Encourage balance between activity and rest.

Discuss need for adequate nutritional intake.

Fever may be present because of infection and/or dehydration.

These activities promote mobilization and expectoration of secretions to reduce risk of developing pulmonary infection.

Odorous, yellow or greenish secretions probably indicate the presence of pulmonary infection.

Prevents spread of fluid-borne pathogens.

Reduces potential for exposure to illnesses, (e.g., URI).

Reduces oxygen consumption/demand imbalance and improves patient's resistance to infection, promoting healing.

Malnutrition can affect general well-being and lower resistance to infection.

Collaborative

Obtain sputum specimen by deep coughing or suctioning for gram stain, culture/sensitivity.

Administer antimicrobials as indicated.

Done to identify causative organism and susceptibility to various antimicrobials.

May be given for specific organisms identified by culture and sensitivity, or be given prophylactically because of high risk.

135

NURSING DIAGNOSIS:	KNOWLEDGE DEFICIT [LEARNING NEED] (SPECIFY)
May be related to:	Lack of information necessary to make informed choices regarding condition, therapies, treatment plan
	Information misinterpretation
	Lack of recall/cognitive limitation
Possibly evidenced by:	Request for information
	Statement of concerns/misconception
	Inaccurate follow-through of instructions
	Development of preventable complications
PATIENT OUTCOMES/ EVALUATION CRITERIA:	Verbalizes understanding of condition/disease process and treatment. Identifies relationship of current signs/ symptoms to the disease process and correlates with causative factors. Initiates necessary lifestyle changes and participates in treatment regimen.

ACTIONS/INTERVENTIONS

Independent

Explain/reinforce explanations of individual disease process. Encourage patient/SO to ask questions.

Instruct/reinforce rationale for breathing exercises, as well as general conditioning exercises.

Discuss respiratory medications, side effects, adverse reactions. *N.B Specific meds for this pt as f have been discussed in Med Section Provide information i walla as well as Needed Form.*

Devise system for recording prescribed intermittent drug/inhaler usage.

Stress importance of oral care/dental hygiene.

Discuss importance of avoiding people with active respiratory infections.

Discuss factors that may aggravate condition, e.g., excessively dry air; wind, environmental temperature extremes; pollen, tobacco smoke, aerosol sprays, air pollution. Encourage patient/SO to explore ways to control these factors in and around the home.

Provide information about the harmful effects of smoking on the lungs, and encourage cessation of smoking by patient and/or SO.

RATIONALE

Decreases anxiety and can lead to improved participation in treatment plan.

Pursed-lip and abdominal breathing exercises strengthen muscles of respiration, help minimize collapse of small airways, and provide the individual with means to control dyspnea. General conditioning exercises increase activity tolerance and muscle strength.

These patients are frequently on several respiratory drugs at once, which have similar side effects and potential drug interactions. It is important that the patient understands the difference between nuisance side effects (medication continued), and untoward side effects (medication possibly discontinued/changed).

Reduces risk of improper use/overdosage of p.r.n. medications, especially during acute exacerbations, when cognition may be impaired.

Decreases bacterial growth in the mouth, gums, which can lead to pulmonary infections.

Decreases exposure to and incidence of acquired upper respiratory infections.

These environmental factors can induce/aggravate bronchial irritation leading to increased secretion production and airway blockage.

Even when patient wants to stop smoking, support groups and medical monitoring may be needed. Recent studies indicate that "side-stream" or "second

ACTIONS/INTERVENTIONS	RATIONALE

Independent

Provide information about limitations of activity, alternating activities with rest periods to prevent fatigue; ways to conserve energy during activities (e.g., pulling instead of pushing; sitting instead of standing while performing tasks); use of pursed-lip breathing, side-lying position and possible need for supplemental oxygen during sexual activity.

Discuss importance of medical follow-up care, periodic chest x-rays, sputum cultures.

Instruct patient/SO in safe use of oxygen and refer to supplier as indicated.

Collaborative

Review oxygen requirements/dosa~~ge~~
is discharged on supplemental

Refer to/encourage partic~~ipation~~
e.g., American Lung
partment. Refer f~~o~~
cated.

---

hand'' smoke can be as detrimental as actually smoking.

Having this knowledge can enable patient to make informed choices/decisions to reduce dyspnea, perform most desired activity, and prevent complications.

Monitoring disease process allows for alterations in therapeutic regimen to meet changing needs and r~~may~~ help prevent complications.

~~Prom~~otes environmental/physical safety.

~~Redu~~ces risk of misuse (too little/too much) and resul~~ting c~~omplications.

~~Some~~ patients and their SOs may experience anxiety, ~~depres~~sion and other reactions as they deal with a ~~chronic~~ disease that has an impact on their desired ~~lifestyle.~~ Support groups and/or home visits may be ~~wanted~~ or needed to provide assistance, emotional ~~support~~ or respite care.

137

Bacterial Pneumonia

PATIENT ASSESSMENT DATA BASE

ACTIVITY/REST

May report: Fatigue.
Insomnia.

May exhibit: Lethargy.
Decreased tolerance to activity.

CIRCULATION

May report: History of recent/chronic CHF.

May exhibit: Tachycardia.
Flushed appearance.

FOOD/FLUID

May report: Loss of appetite, nausea/vomiting.

May exhibit: Distended abdomen.
Hyperactive bowel sounds.
Dry skin with poor turgor.

NEUROSENSORY

May exhibit: Changes in mentation (confusion, somnolence).

PAIN/COMFORT

May report: Headache.
Chest pain (pleuritic), aggravated by cough.

May exhibit: Splinting/guarding over affected area (patient commonly lies on affected side to restrict movement).

RESPIRATION

May report: History of recurrent/chronic upper respiratory infection (URI), COPD, AIDS, lung cancer, cigarette smoking.
Exposure to pollutants/chemical toxins.
Shortness of breath.
Cough: dry hacking (initially) progressing to productive cough.

May exhibit: Tachypnea, progressive dyspnea.
Use of accessory muscles, nasal flaring.
Sputum: pink, rusty, or purulent.
Percussion: dull over consolidated areas.
Fremitus: tactile and vocal gradually increases with consolidation.
Pleural friction rub.
Breath sounds: diminished or absent over involved area, or bronchial breath sounds over area(s) of consolidation. Coarse inspiratory crackles.
Color: pallor or cyanosis.

SAFETY

May report: History of altered immune system: steroid or chemotherapy use; SLE, AIDS; institutionalization; general debilitation.

Fever.

May exhibit: Diaphoresis.

Shaking chills.

TEACHING/LEARNING

Discharge Plan Considerations: Assistance with self-care, homemaker tasks.

DIAGNOSTIC STUDIES

Chest x-ray: usually shows scattered or localized infiltration and identifies structural distribution (e.g., lobar, bronchial).

ABGs: abnormalities may be present, depending on extent of lung involvement and underlying lung disease.

Gram stain/cultures of sputum (and blood): to recover causative organism. More than one type of organism may be present; common bacteria include Diplococcus pneumoniae, Staphylococcus aureus, A-hemolytic streptococcus, Hemophilus influenzae.

CBC: leukocytosis usually present, though a low WBC may be present in viral infection, immunosuppressed conditions such as AIDS, overwhelming bacterial pneumonia.

Serologic studies, e.g., viral or Legionella titers, cold agglutinins: assist in differential diagnosis of specific organism.

ESR: increased.

Electrolytes: sodium and chloride may be low.

Bilirubin: may be increased.

NURSING PRIORITIES

1. Maintain/improve respiratory function.
2. Prevent complications.
3. Support recuperative process.
4. Provide information about disease process/prognosis and treatment.

DISCHARGE CRITERIA

1. Ventilation and oxygenation adequate for individual needs.
2. Complications prevented/minimized.
3. Disease process/prognosis and therapeutic regimen understood.
4. Lifestyle changes identified/initiated to prevent recurrence.

NURSING DIAGNOSIS:	AIRWAY CLEARANCE, INEFFECTIVE
May be related to:	**Tracheal broncheal inflammation, edema formation, increased sputum production**
	Pleuritic pain
	Decreased energy, fatigue
Possibly evidenced by:	**Changes in rate, depth of respirations**
	Incessant, painful cough

139

Abnormal breath sounds, use of accessory muscles

Dyspnea, cyanosis

Cough, effective or ineffective; with/without sputum production

PATIENT OUTCOMES/ EVALUATION CRITERIA: Identifies/displays behaviors to achieve airway clearance. Demonstrates patent airway with breath sounds clearing, absence of dyspnea, cyanosis.

ACTIONS/INTERVENTIONS	RATIONALE

Independent

Assess rate and depth of respirations and chest movement.

Tachypnea, shallow respirations and unsymmetric chest movement are frequently present because of discomfort of moving chest wall and/or fluid in lung.

Auscultate lung fields, noting areas of decreased/absent airflow and adventitious breath sounds, e.g., crackles, wheezes.

Decreased airflow occurs in areas consolidated with fluid. Bronchial breath sounds (normal over bronchus) can also occur in consolidated areas. Crackles, rhonchi, and wheezes are heard on inspiration and/or expiration in response to fluid accumulation, thick secretions, and airway spasm/obstruction.

Elevate head of bed, change position frequently.

Lowers diaphragm, promoting chest expansion, aeration of lung segments, mobilization and expectoration of secretions.

Assist patient in deep breathing exercises on a frequent basis. Demonstrate/help patient learn to perform coughing, e.g., splinting chest and upright position.

Deep breathing facilitates maximum expansion of the lungs/smaller airways. Coughing is a natural self-cleaning mechanism and a major means of assisting the cilia in maintaining patent airways. Splinting chest reduces discomfort, and upright position favors deeper, more forceful cough effort.

Suction as indicated.

Stimulates cough or mechanically clears airway in patient who is unable to do so because of ineffective cough, decreased level of consciousness.

Force fluids to at least 2500 ml/day (unless contraindicated). Offer warm, rather than cold, fluids.

Fluids (especially warm liquids) aid in mobilization and expectoration of secretions.

Collaborative

Assist with/monitor effects of nebulizer treatments and other respiratory physiotherapy, e.g., incentive spirometer, IPPB, blow bottles, percussion, postural drainage.

Facilitates liquefication and removal of secretions. Postural drainage may not be effective in interstitial pneumonias or those causing alveolar exudate/destruction.

Administer medications as indicated: mucolytics, expectorants, bronchodilators, analgesics.

Aids in reduction of bronchospasm as well as mobilization of secretions. Analgesics are given to improve cough effort by reducing discomfort but may decrease cough effort or depress respirations and should be used cautiously.

Provide supplemental fluids, e.g., IV, humidified oxygen and room humidification.

Fluids are required to replace losses (including insensible) and aid in mobilization of secretions.

140

ACTIONS/INTERVENTIONS

Collaborative

Monitor serial chest x-rays, ABGs, ear/pulse oximetry readings. (Refer to ND: Gas Exchange, Impaired, p. 141.)

Assist with bronchoscopy/thoracentesis, if indicated.

RATIONALE

Follows progress and effects of disease process and facilitates necessary alterations in therapy.

Occasionally needed to remove mucous plugs and/or prevent atelectasis.

NURSING DIAGNOSIS:	GAS EXCHANGE, IMPAIRED
May be related to:	Alveolar-capillary membrane changes (inflammatory effects)
	Altered oxygen-carrying capacity of blood (fever, shifting oxyhemoglobin curve)
	Altered delivery of oxygen (hypoventilation)
Possibly evidenced by:	Dyspnea, cyanosis
	Tachycardia
	Restlessness/changes in mentation
	Hypoxia
PATIENT OUTCOMES/ EVALUATION CRITERIA:	Demonstrates improved ventilation and oxygenation of tissues by ABGs within patient's normal range and absence of symptoms of respiratory distress. Participates in actions to maximize oxygenation.

ACTIONS/INTERVENTIONS

Independent

Assess respiratory rate, depth, and ease; use of accessory muscles.

Observe color of skin, mucous membranes, nailbeds, noting presence of peripheral (nailbeds) cyanosis, or central (circumoral) cyanosis.

Assess mental status.

Monitor heart rate/rhythm.

Monitor body temperature, as indicated. Assist with comfort measures to reduce fever and chills, e.g.,

RATIONALE

Hypoventilation (pleuritic pain/abdominal distention), pleural effusion/alveolar edema, and incomplete airway clearance (general weakness/fatigue and pain) impair gas exchange, resulting in respiratory insufficiency/distress. Manifestations are dependent on degree of lung involvement and underlying pulmonary/general health status

Cyanosis of nailbeds may indicate vasoconstriction or body response to fever/chills. However, cyanosis of earlobes, mucous membranes, and around the mouth is indicative of systemic hypoxemia.

Restlessness, irritation, confusion, somnolence may reflect hypoxemia/decreased cerebral oxygenation.

Tachycardia usually present as a result of fever/dehydration, but may represent a response to hypoxemia.

High fever (common in bacterial pneumonia) greatly increases metabolic demands and oxygen consump-

Independent

addition/removal of bedcovers, comfortable room temperature, tepid or cool water sponges.

Maintain bedrest. Encourage use of relaxation techniques and diversional activities.

Elevate head and encourage frequent position changes, deep breathing, and effective cough.

Assess level of anxiety. Encourage verbalization of concerns/feelings. Answer questions honestly. Visit frequently, stay with patient, arrange for SO to stay with patient as indicated.

Observe for deterioration in condition, noting hypotension, copious amounts of pink/bloody sputum, pallor, cyanosis, change in level of consciousness, severe dyspnea, restlessness.

Collaborative

Administer oxygen therapy by appropriate means, e.g., nasal prongs, mask, Venturi mask.

Monitor ABGs, ear/pulse oximetry readings.

tion, and alters oxyhemoglobin curve reducing cellular oxygenation.

Prevents overexhaustion and reduces oxygen consumption/demands and energy needs to facilitate resolution of infection.

These measures promote maximal inspiration, enhance expectoration of secretions to improve ventilation. (Refer to ND: Airway Clearance, Ineffective, p. 139.)

Anxiety is a manifestation of psychologic concerns as well as physiologic response to hypoxia. Providing reassurance, enhancing sense of security can reduce the psychologic component, thereby decreasing oxygen demand and adverse physiologic response.

Shock and pulmonary edema are the most common causes of death in pneumonia and require immediate medical intervention.

Oxygen therapy is usually aimed at maintaining PaO_2 above 60 mmHg and is administered by the method that provides appropriate delivery of oxygen within the patient's tolerance. It is possible that intubation and mechanical ventilation will be required in the event of severe respiratory insufficiency.

Follows progress of disease process and facilitates alterations in pulmonary therapy.

NURSING DIAGNOSIS:	INFECTION, POTENTIAL FOR [SPREAD]
May be related to:	Inadequate primary defenses (decreased ciliary action, stasis of respiratory secretions)
	Inadequate secondary defenses (presence of existing infection)
Possibly evidenced by:	[Not applicable; presence of signs and symptoms establishes an *actual* diagnosis.]
PATIENT OUTCOMES/ EVALUATION CRITERIA:	Achieves timely resolution of current infection without complications. Identifies intervention to prevent/reduce risk of infection.

ACTIONS/INTERVENTIONS
RATIONALE

Independent

Monitor vital signs closely, especially during initiation of therapy.

During this period of time, potentially fatal complications (hypotension/shock) may develop.

ACTIONS/INTERVENTIONS

Independent

Instruct patient concerning the disposition of secretions (e.g., raising and expectoration versus swallowing) and reporting changes in color, amount, odor of secretions.

Demonstrate/encourage good handwashing technique.

Change position frequently and provide good pulmonary toilet.

Limit visitors as indicated, e.g., persons with upper respiratory infections.

Institute isolation precautions as individually appropriate.

Encourage adequate rest balanced with moderate exercise. Promote adequate nutritional intake.

Monitor effectiveness of antimicrobial therapy.

Investigate sudden changes/deterioration in condition. Note: Increasing chest pain, extra heart sounds, altered sensorium, recurring fever, changes in sputum characteristics.

Administer antimicrobials as indicated by results of sputum/blood cultures, antibiotics, e.g., penicillins, erythromycin, tetracycline, amikacin (Amikin), cephalosporins.

RATIONALE

Patient may find expectoration offensive and will attempt to limit or avoid it.

Effective means of reducing spread/acquisition of infection.

Promotes expectoration, clearing of infection.

Reduces likelihood of exposure to other infectious pathogens and recurrence of pneumonia.

Dependent on type of infection response to antibiotics, patient's general health and development of complications, isolation techniques may be desired to prevent spread/protect patient from other infectious processes.

Facilitates healing process and enhances natural resistance.

Signs of improvement in condition should occur within 24–48 hours. Delayed response or increase in severity of symptoms suggest resistance to antibiotics, or may reflect secondary infection.

Complications affecting any/all organ systems include: lung abscess/empyema, bacteremia, pericarditis/endocarditis, meningitis/encephalitis, and superinfections.

Used to combat most of the bacterial pneumonias. These medications may be combined with antiviral and antifungal agents when the pneumonia is a result of mixed organisms.

NURSING DIAGNOSIS:	ACTIVITY INTOLERANCE
May be related to:	**Imbalance between oxygen supply and demand**
	General weakness
	Exhaustion associated with interruption in usual sleep pattern due to discomfort, excessive coughing, and dyspnea
Possibly evidenced by:	**Verbal reports of weakness, fatigue, exhaustion**
	Exertional dyspnea, tachypnea
	Tachycardia in response to activity
	Development/worsening of pallor/cyanosis
PATIENT OUTCOMES/ EVALUATION CRITERIA:	**Reports/demonstrates a measurable increase in tolerance to activity with absence of dyspnea, excessive fatigue; and vital signs within patient's normal range.**

ACTIONS/INTERVENTIONS

Independent

Evaluate patient's response to activity. Note complaints of dyspnea, increased weakness/fatigue; and changes in vital signs during and after activities.

Provide a quiet environment, and limit visitors as indicated. Encourage use of stress management and diversional activities as appropriate.

Explain importance of rest in treatment plan, and necessity for balancing activities with rest.

Assist the patient to assume comfortable position for rest and/or sleep.

Assist with self-care activities as necessary. Provide for progressive increase in activities during recovery phase.

RATIONALE

Establishes patient's capabilities/needs and facilitates choice of interventions.

Reduces stress and excess stimulation, promoting rest.

Bedrest is maintained during acute phase to decrease metabolic demands, conserving energy for healing. Activity restrictions thereafter are determined by individual patient response to activity and resolution of respiratory insufficiency.

Patient may be comfortable with head of bed elevated, or need to sleep in a chair, or resting forward on overbed table with pillow support.

Minimizes exhaustion and helps to balance oxygen supply and demand.

NURSING DIAGNOSIS:	COMFORT, ALTERED: PAIN, ACUTE
May be related to:	**Inflammation of lung parenchyma**
	Cellular reactions to circulating toxins
	Persistent coughing
Possibly evidenced by:	**Pleuritic chest pain**
	Headache, muscle/joint pain
	Guarding of affected area
	Distraction behaviors, restlessness
PATIENT OUTCOMES/ EVALUATION CRITERIA:	**Verbalizes relief/control of pain. Demonstrates relaxed manner, resting/sleeping and engaging in activity appropriately.**

ACTIONS/INTERVENTIONS

Independent

Determine pain characteristics, e.g., sharp, constant, stabbing. Investigate changes in character/location of pain.

Monitor vital signs.

Provide routine comfort measures, e.g., backrubs, change of position, quiet music/conversation, relaxation breathing exercises.

RATIONALE

Chest pain, usually present to some degree with pneumonia, may also herald the onset of complications of pneumonia such as pericarditis and endocarditis. (Refer to CP: Inflammatory Cardiac Conditions: Pericarditis, Myocarditis, Endocarditis, p. 109.)

Changes in heart rate or BP may indicate that the patient is experiencing pain, especially when other reasons for changes in vital signs have been ruled out.

Nonanalgesic measures administered with a gentle touch can alleviate discomfort and augment therapeutic effects of analgesics.

ACTIONS/INTERVENTIONS	RATIONALE
Independent	
Offer frequent oral hygiene.	Mouth breathing and oxygen therapy can irritate and dry out mucous membranes, potentiating general discomfort.
Instruct and assist patient in chest splinting techniques during coughing episodes. (Refer to ND: Airway Clearance, Ineffective, p. 139.)	Aids in control of chest discomfort while enhancing effectiveness of cough effort.
Collaborative	
Administer analgesics and antitussives as indicated.	Codeine may be used to suppress nonproductive/ paroxysmal cough, enhancing general comfort/rest.

NURSING DIAGNOSIS:	**NUTRITION, ALTERED: LESS THAN BODY REQUIRE-MENTS [POTENTIAL]**
May be related to:	**Increased metabolic needs secondary to fever and infectious process**
	Anorexia associated with bacterial toxins, the odor and taste of sputum, and certain aerosol treatments
	Abdominal distention/gas associated with swallowing air during dyspneic episodes
Possibly evidenced by:	**[Not applicable; presence of signs and symptoms establishes an *actual* diagnosis.]**
PATIENT OUTCOMES/ EVALUATION CRITERIA:	**Maintains/regains desired body weight.**

ACTIONS/INTERVENTIONS	RATIONALE
Independent	
Identify factors that are contributing to nausea/ vomiting, e.g., copious sputum, aerosol treatments, severe dyspnea, pain.	Choice of interventions is dependent on the underlying cause of the problem.
Provide covered container for sputum and remove at frequent intervals. Provide/assist with oral hygiene after emesis, after aerosol and postural drainage treatments, and before meals.	Eliminates noxious sights, taste, smell from the patient environment and can reduce nausea.
Schedule respiratory treatments at least one hour before meals.	Reduces effects of nausea associated with these treatments.
Auscultate for bowel sounds. Observe/palpate for abdominal distention.	Bowel sounds may be diminished/absent if the infectious process is severe/prolonged. Abdominal distention may occur as a result of air swallowing, or reflect the influence of bacterial toxins on the GI tract.
Provide small, frequent meals, including dry foods (toast, crackers) and/or foods that are appealing to patient.	These measures may enhance intake even though appetite may be slow to return.

NURSING DIAGNOSIS:	FLUID VOLUME DEFICIT, POTENTIAL
May be related to:	Excessive fluid loss (fever, profuse diaphoresis, mouth breathing/hyperventilation, vomiting)
	Decreased oral intake
Possibly evidenced by:	[Not applicable; presence of signs and symptoms establishes an *actual* diagnosis.]
PATIENT OUTCOMES/ EVALUATION CRITERIA:	Demonstrates fluid balance evidenced by individually appropriate parameters, e.g., moist mucous membrane, good skin turgor, prompt capillary refill; stable vital

ACTIONS/INTERVEN[...]NALE

Independent

Assess vital sign changes, e.g., i[...]ture/prolonged fever, tachycardia, [...]sion.

[...] olonged fever increases [...]s through evaporation. Or- [...] changes and increasing [...] systemic fluid deficit.

Assess skin turgor, moisture of m[...] (lips, tongue).

[...] quacy of fluid volume, al- [...] branes may be dry because [...] upplemental oxygen.

Note complaints of nausea/vomiti[...]

[...] ms reduces oral intake.

Monitor intake, output, noting colo[...] Calculate fluid balance. Be aware [...] Weigh as indicated.

[...] t adequacy of fluid volume [...]

Force fluids to at least 2500 ml/day or as individually appropriate.

Meets basic fluid needs reducing risk of dehydration.

Collaborative

Administer medications as indicated, e.g., antipyretics, antiemetics.

Useful in reducing fluid losses.

Provide supplemental IV fluids as necessary.

In presence of reduced intake/excessive loss, use of parenteral route may correct/prevent deficiency.

NURSING DIAGNOSIS:	KNOWLEDGE DEFICIT [LEARNING NEED] (SPECIFY)
May be related to:	Lack of exposure
	Misinterpretation of information
	Altered recall
Possibly evidenced by:	Requests for information
	Statement of misconception
	Failure to improve/recurrence

PATIENT OUTCOMES/ EVALUATION CRITERIA:	Verbalizes understanding of condition, disease process and treatment. Initiates necessary lifestyle changes and participates in treatment program.

ACTIONS/INTERVENTIONS	RATIONALE
Independent	
Review normal lung function, pathology of condition.	Promotes understanding of current situation and importance of cooperating with treatment regimen.
Discuss debilitating aspects of disease, length of convalescence and recovery expectations. Identify self-care and homemaker needs.	Fatigue and weakness can persist for an extended period of time and may be associated with depression. Respiratory symptoms may also be slow to resolve. Information can help reduce anxiety, excessive concern.
Provide information in written as well as verbal form.	Fatigue and depression can affect ability to assimilate information/follow medical regimen.
Stress importance of continuing effective coughing/ deep breathing exercises.	During initial 6–8 weeks after discharge, patient is at greatest risk for recurrence.
Emphasize necessity for continuing antibiotic therapy for prescribed period of time.	Early discontinuation of antibiotics may result in failure to completely resolve infectious process.
Review importance of cessation of smoking.	Smoking destroys tracheobronchial cilial action, irritates bronchial mucosa, and inhibits alveolar macrophages, compromising body's natural defense against infection.
	Increases natural defenses/immunity to pathogens.
Outline steps to enhance general health and well-being, e.g., balanced rest and activity, well-rounded diet, avoidance of crowds during cold/flu season or persons with upper respiratory infections.	
Stress importance of continuing medical follow-up, obtaining vaccinations/immunizations as appropriate.	May prevent recurrence of pneumonia/associated complications.
Identify signs/symptoms requiring notification of health care provider, e.g., increasing dyspnea, chest pain, prolonged fatigue, weight loss, fever/chills, persistence of productive cough, changes in alertness.	Prompt evaluation and timely intervention may prevent/minimize complications.

Pulmonary Embolism

PATIENT ASSESSMENT DATA BASE

ACTIVITY/REST

May report: Fatigue and/or weakness.

May exhibit: Exertional dyspnea or discomfort.
Abnormal heart rate or BP response to activity.
Sleep disturbances.

CIRCULATION

May report: History of conditions predisposing to thrombus formation, e.g., (1) hypercoagulable blood (pregnancy, rebound after discontinuation of anticoagulants, use of oral contraceptives); (2) vessel wall damage (following trauma to iliac and pelvic veins, previous venous disease, sepsis, burns); (3) venous stasis (prolonged immobility, polycythemia).
History of transmural/subendocardial/RV myocardial infarction.
History of dysrhythmias, e.g., chronic atrial fibrillation.

May exhibit: Tachycardia.
Dysrhythmias.
Extra heart sounds, e.g., S_3 or S_4.
Murmur of valvular insufficiency.
Hypotension.
Pulses may be normal, weak/thready (shock) or full/bounding (polycythemia vera).
Extremities: signs of thrombophlebitis, e.g., phlebotic veins, tense muscle tissue; shiny, edematous skin; increased skin temperature.

EGO INTEGRITY

May report: Apprehension.
Fear of death, feelings of impending doom.

May exhibit: Restlessness, trembling.
Facial tension.
Increased perspiration.
Panic behavior.

NEUROSENSORY

May report: Difficulty in concentrating, altered memory/thinking ability.

May exhibit: Altered attention span.
Disorientation.
Changes in remote/recent/immediate memory.
Lethargy/stupor.

PAIN/COMFORT

May report: Chest pain.
Nausea.
Discomfort in extremities (if thrombophlebitis is present).

May exhibit: Self-focusing/narrowed focus.
Distraction behaviors, facial grimacing, moaning, restlessness.

RESPIRATION

May report:	"Air hunger"/dyspnea. Cough, pink/bloody/brown sputum.
May exhibit:	Tachypnea. Dyspnea, gasping/shallow respirations. Decreased breath sounds; crackles, wheezes; pleural rub (if pulmonary infarction has occurred). Cough (hacking/dry or productive of bloody sputum).

SAFETY

May report:	History of cancer, systemic infection, fractures/trauma to lower extremities, burns.
May exhibit:	Fever.

TEACHING/LEARNING

Discharge Plan Considerations:	Alteration of medication regimen. Assistance with self-care, homemaker tasks.

DIAGNOSTIC STUDIES

ABGs: may show decreased PaO_2, $PaCO_2$ (hypoxemia/hypocarbia) and elevated pH (respiratory alkalosis) especially if pulmonary obstruction is severe.

Chest x-ray: frequently normal (especially in subacute PE), but may demonstrate shadow of a clot, abrupt vessel cutoff, diaphragmatic elevation on affected side, pleural effusion, infiltrates/consolidation.

ECG: may be normal or demonstrate changes indicative of right ventricular strain, e.g., changes in T waves/S-T segment, axis deviation/right bundle branch block. Tachycardia and dysrhythmias (new onset of atrial fibrillation) frequently present.

Pulmonary angiography: most specific study for pulmonary embolus. Presence of a filling defect or artery "cutoff" with no distal blood flow confirms diagnosis.

Lung scan (ventilation/perfusion scan): may reveal pattern of abnormal perfusion in areas of ventilation (ventilation/perfusion mismatch), or absence of both ventilation and perfusion (confirms diagnosis of PE).

NURSING PRIORITIES

1. Restore/maintain adequate oxygenation/ventilation.
2. Minimize/prevent complications.
3. Relieve anxiety and pain.
4. Provide information about disease process and treatment.

DISCHARGE CRITERIA

1. Respiratory function adequate for individual needs.
2. Complications minimized/prevented.
3. Anxiety reduced, pain controlled.
4. Disease process, therapy needs, prevention of complications/recurrence understood.

NURSING DIAGNOSIS:	**BREATHING PATTERN, INEFFECTIVE**
May be related to:	**Tracheobronchial obstruction by blood clot, copious secretions or active bleeding**
	Deceased lung expansion
	Inflammatory process

Possibly evidenced by:	**Changes in depth and/or rate of respiration**
	Dyspnea/use of accessory muscles of respiration
	Altered chest excursion
	Abnormal breath sounds, e.g., crackles, wheezes
	Cough, with or without sputum production
PATIENT OUTCOMES/ EVALUATION CRITERIA:	**Demonstrates effective respiratory pattern with rate and depth within patient's normal range and lungs clear/clearing.**

ACTIONS/INTERVENTIONS

Independent

Assess respiratory rate, depth, and chest expansion. Note respiratory effort, including use of accessory muscles/nasal flaring.

Auscultate breath sounds, and note presence of adventitious sounds such as crackles, wheezes, pleural rub.

Elevate head of bed and assist with frequent changes of position. Get patient out of bed and ambulate as soon as able.

Observe cough pattern, and character of secretions.

Encourage/assist patient in deep breathing and coughing exercises. Suction orally or nasotracheally if indicated.

Assist client to deal with fear/anxiety that may be present. (Refer to ND: Fear/Anxiety [Specify Level], p. 153.)

Collaborative

Administer supplemental oxygen.

Provide supplemental humidification, e.g., ultrasonic nebulizers, room humidifier.

Assist with chest physiotherapy (e.g., postural drainage and percussion of nonaffected area), blow bottles/ incentive spirometer.

Prepare for/assist with bronchoscopy.

RATIONALE

Rate is usually increased. Dyspnea ("air hunger") and increased work of breathing is present (may be first or only sign in subacute PE). Depth of respirations varies depending on degree of respiratory failure. Chest expansion may be limited due to atelectasis and/or pleuritic chest pain.

Breath sounds may be decreased/absent if airway obstruction is secondary to bleeding, clotting, or small airway collapse (atelectasis). Rhonchi and wheezing also accompanies airway obstruction/respiratory failure.

Upright position favors lung expansion and facilitates respiratory effort. Turning and ambulation enhances aeration of different lung segments, thereby improving gas diffusion.

Alveolar congestion may produce a dry/irritated cough. Bloody sputum may be the result of tissue destruction (pulmonary infarction) or overanticoagulation.

May have increased/copious secretions which impair ventilation and add to the discomfort of breathing effort.

Feelings of fear and severe anxiety are associated with inability to breathe/development of hypoxemia and may actually increase oxygen consumption/demand.

Maximizes respiratory effort and may reduce work of breathing.

Delivers moisture to mucous membranes, and helps liquefy secretions to facilitate airway clearance.

Facilitates deeper respiratory effort and promotes drainage of secretions from lung segments into bronchi, where they may more readily be removed by coughing/suctioning.

Occasionally useful to remove blood clots and clear airways.

NURSING DIAGNOSIS:	GAS EXCHANGE, IMPAIRED
May be related to:	Altered blood flow to alveoli or to major portions of the lung
	Atelectasis, airway/alveolar collapse
	Pulmonary edema/effusion
	Excessive secretions/active bleeding
Possibly evidenced by:	Profound dyspnea, restlessness, apprehension, somnolence, cyanosis
	Changes in ABGs, e.g., hypoxemia and hypercapnea
PATIENT OUTCOMES/ EVALUATION CRITERIA:	Demonstrates adequate ventilation/oxygenation by ABGs within patient's normal range. Reports/displays resolution/absence of symptoms of respiratory distress.

ACTIONS/INTERVENTIONS

Independent

Note respiratory rate and depth, use of accessory muscles, pursed-lip breathing. (Refer to ND: Breathing Pattern, Ineffective, p. 149.)

Auscultate lungs for areas of decreased/absent breath sounds, and the presence of adventitious sounds, e.g., crackles.

Observe for generalized duskiness and cyanosis in "warm tissues" such as earlobes, lips, tongue, and buccal membranes.

Institute measures to restore/maintain patent airways, e.g., coughing, suctioning, etc. (Refer to ND: Breathing Pattern, Ineffective, p. 149.)

Elevate head of the bed as patient requires/tolerates.

Monitor vital signs.

Assess level of consciousness/mentation changes.

Assess activity tolerance, e.g., complaints of weakness/fatigue during any exertion, vital signs changes. Encourage rest periods and limit activities to within patient tolerance.

Collaborative

Monitor serial ABGs.

RATIONALE

Tachypnea and dyspnea accompany pulmonary obstruction. More severe respiratory failure accompanies moderate to severe loss of functional lung units.

Nonventilated areas may be identified by absence of breath sounds. Crackles occur in fluid-filled tissues/airways or may reflect cardiac decompensation.

Indicative of systemic hypoxemia.

Plugged/collapsed airways reduce number of functional alveoli, negatively affecting gas exchange.

Promotes maximal chest expansion, making it easier to breathe which enhances physiologic/psychologic comfort.

Tachycardia, tachypnea, and changes in blood pressure occur with advancing hypoxemia and acidosis.

Systemic hypoxemia may be reflected first by restlessness and irritability, then by progressively decreased mentation.

Hypoxemia reduces ability to participate in activity without profound dyspnea, tachycardia, dysrhythmias, and possible hypotension. These parameters assist in determining patient response to resumed activities and ability to participate in self-care.

Hypoxemia is present in varying degrees, depending on the amount of airway obstruction, prior cardiopulmonary function, and presence/absence of shock.

151

ACTIONS/INTERVENTIONS

Collaborative

Administer oxygen by appropriate method.

RATIONALE

Respiratory alkalosis and metabolic acidosis can also occur.

Maximizes available oxygen for gas exchange. Oxygen is usually administered by nasal cannula in partial pulmonary obstruction. Note: If the obstruction is large, or hypoxemia does not respond to supplemental oxygenation, it may be necessary to move patient to critical care area for intubation and mechanical ventilation.

NURSING DIAGNOSIS:	TISSUE PERFUSION, ALTERED: DECREASED CARDIO-PULMONARY [ACTUAL] AND SPECIFY [POTENTIAL]
May be related to:	Interruption of blood flow: arterial/venous
	Exchange problems at alveolar level, or at tissue level (acidotic shifting of the oxyhemoglobin curve)
Possibly evidenced by: Actual (pulmonary)	Radiology/laboratory evidence of ventilation/perfusion mismatch
	Dyspnea
	Central cyanosis
Potential (specify)	[Not applicable; presence of signs and symptoms establishes an *actual* diagnosis.]
PATIENT OUTCOMES/ EVALUATION CRITERIA:	Demonstrates increased perfusion as individually appropriate, e.g., usual/normal mental status, cardiac rhythm/rate and peripheral pulses within normal limits, absence of central/peripheral cyanosis, warm/dry skin, urine output and specific gravity within normal limits.

ACTIONS/INTERVENTIONS

Independent

Observe for changes in mental status.

Auscultate heart rate and rhythm. Note development of extra heart sounds.

Observe skin/mucous membrane color and temperature.

RATIONALE

Restlessness, confusion, disorientation, and/or sensory/motor changes may indicate hypoxia; or impaired blood flow, or cerebral vascular accident (CVA) as a result of hypoxia or systemic emboli.

Tachycardia is present as a result of hypoxemia and a compensatory effort to increase blood flow and tissue perfusion. Rhythm alterations are related to hypoxemia, electrolyte imbalance, and/or increased right heart strain. Extra heart sounds, e.g., S_3, S_4, may be noted as cardiac workload increases/decompensation occurs.

Pallor or cyanosis of the skin, nailbeds, lips/buccal membranes or cool mottled skin are indicative of peripheral vasoconstriction (shock) and/or impaired systemic blood flow.

ACTIONS/INTERVENTIONS	RATIONALE

Independent

Measure urine output and note specific gravity.

Progressing shock/reduced cardiac output leads to decreased kidney perfusion, manifested by decreased urine output with normal or increased specific gravity.

Evaluate extremities for presence/absence/quality of pulses. Note calf tenderness/swelling.

Pulmonary embolus is frequently precipitated by thrombus arising from deep veins (pelvis or legs). Signs/symptoms may or may not be readily apparent.

Elevate legs/feet when in bed/chair. Encourage patient to exercise legs by flexing/extending feet at the ankles. Avoid use of knee gatch and sitting or standing for long periods of time. Apply/demonstrate how to apply and remove elastic stockings if used.

These measures are intended to promote peripheral blood flow, reduce venous stasis in the legs and pooling of blood in the pelvic veins to reduce risk of thrombus formation.

Collaborative

Administer fluids (IV/PO) as indicated.

Increased fluids may be required to reduce hyperviscosity of blood (potentiates thrombus formation), or to support circulating volume/tissue perfusion.

Monitor diagnostic/laboratory studies, e.g., ECG, electrolytes, BUN/Cr, ABGs, PTT, and PT.

Evaluates changes in organ function and monitors effects of heparin and Coumadin, which may require alterations in therapy.

Administer medications as indicated:

Heparin (intermittent or continuous IV infusion);

Heparin prevents further thrombus formation by preventing clot propagation. Continuous infusion is preferred to prevent peak and ebb levels from increasing coagulation imbalances. Heparin dosage is gradually reduced during addition of oral anticoagulant for long-term therapy.

Warfarin sodium (Coumadin);

Oral agent used for long-term therapy after initial anticoagulation is achieved.

Thrombolytic agents, e.g., streptokinase (Streptase), urokinase (Breakinase).

Usually indicated in massive pulmonary obstruction when the patient is seriously hemodynamically threatened. Note: These patients will probably be initially cared for in the critical care setting.

Prepare for surgical intervention if indicated.

Vena caval ligation or insertion of an intracaval umbrella may be useful for patients who experience recurrent emboli despite adequate anticoagulation, when anticoagulation is contraindicated, or when septic emboli arising from below the renal veins do not respond to treatment.

NURSING DIAGNOSIS:	FEAR/ANXIETY [SPECIFY LEVEL]
May be related to:	Severe dyspnea/inability to breathe normally
	Perceived threat of death
	Threat to/change in health status
	Physiologic response to hypoxemia/acidosis
	Concern regarding unknown outcome of situation

Possibly evidenced by:	Restlessness, irritability
	Withdrawal or attack behavior
	Sympathetic stimulation, e.g., cardiovascular excitation, pupil dilation, sweating, vomiting, diarrhea
	Crying, voice quivering
PATIENT OUTCOMES/ EVALUATION CRITERIA:	Reports fear/anxiety relieved or reduced to manageable level. Appears relaxed and resting/sleeping appropriately.

ACTIONS/INTERVENTIONS

Independent

Note degree of anxiety and fear. Inform the patient/SO that the feelings are normal and encourage expression of feelings.

Explain disease process and procedures within level of patient's ability to understand and handle the information. Review current situation and measures being taken to remedy the problems.

Stay with the patient or make arrangements for someone else to be there during acute attack.

Provide routine comfort measures, e.g., backrub, position changes. Assist the patient to identify helpful behaviors, e.g., assuming position of comfort, focused breathing, relaxation techniques.

Support patient/SO in dealing with the realities of the situation, especially in planning for long recovery period. Involve patient in planning and participating in care.

Develop activity program within limits of physical ability.

Be alert for out-of-control behavior or escalating cardiopulmonary dysfunction, e.g., worsening dyspnea and tachycardia.

(Refer to CP: Psychosocial Aspects of Acute Care, p. 773.)

RATIONALE

Understanding that feelings, which are based on stressful situation plus an oxygen imbalance that is being treated, are normal may help the patient regain some feeling of control over emotions.

Allays anxiety related to the unknown and reduces fears concerning personal safety. In the early phases of the illness, explanations need to be short and repeated frequently because the patient will have a reduced attention span.

Helpful in reducing anxiety associated with perceived abandonment in presence of severe dyspnea/feelings of impending doom.

Aids in reducing stress and redirecting attention to enhance relaxation and coping abilities.

Coping mechanisms and participation in treatment regimen may be enhanced as patient learns to deal with the outcomes of the illness and regains some sense of control.

Provides a healthy outlet for energy generated by feelings.

Development of incapacitating anxiety requires further evaluation and possible intervention with supervised sedatives.

NURSING DIAGNOSIS:	**KNOWLEDGE DEFICIT [LEARNING NEED] (SPECIFY)**
May be related to:	**Lack of information regarding disease process, complications, and long-term therapy**
Possibly evidenced by:	**Statements of concern**
	Requests for information

| PATIENT OUTCOMES/ EVALUATION CRITERIA: | Verbalizes understanding of disease process, possible complications, and measures to prevent recurrence. Identifies potential risk factors of therapy and signs/ symptoms requiring intervention. |

ACTIONS/INTERVENTIONS

Independent

Provide information about importance of:

Adhering to prescribed medication schedule;

Being alert for bleeding from mucous membranes (nose and gums), severe bruising after minimal trauma, development of petechiae, continued oozing from cuts or mild punctures;

Appropriate safety factors, e.g., use of electric instead of regular razor; gentle brushing of teeth and gums; avoiding forceful blowing of nose and scratching/rubbing of skin;

Need to report for scheduled follow-up laboratory monitoring and physicians visits;

Avoiding inactivity, e.g., sitting or standing for periods longer than an hour, avoiding constricting clothing, wearing/removing elastic stockings as prescribed;

Informing dentists and other care givers of anticoagulation, avoiding use of new medications (including OTC) without prior clearance by heatlh care provider.

Encourage patient to wear an identification bracelet/ tag.

Discuss and provide a written list of signs/symptoms to report to the physician, e.g., severe dyspnea, tachypnea and chest pain, excessive fatigue, unexplained weight gain, dependent edema, chest tightness;

Palpitations;

Calf pain/swelling.

RATIONALE

Anticoagulation may be required for 6 weeks to 6 months following initial episode. Taking the medication at the same time each day in the prescribed amount will help maintain serum anticoagulation levels within the narrow therapeutic range.

Signs of excessive prolongation of clotting time, which may indicate need for reduction or cessation of anticoagulant therapy.

Enables the patient to avoid trauma-induced bleeding.

Drug therapy may be altered/discontinued, depending on information obtained.

Reduces venous pooling and risk of thrombus formation.

May need to postponse procedures or alter therapy to reduce risk of hemorrhage. Drugs such as antacids, antihistamines, and vitamin C can decrease the effect of Coumadin. Alcohol, antibiotics, and ibuprofen (e.g., Motrin) can increase the effect of Coumadin.

Alerts emergency personnel that patient is taking anticoagulants.

Precautions are particularly relevant to those patients who have forced immobility, have recurrent thrombophlebitis, or a history of recurrent pulmonary emboli. Note: Patients surviving severe/multiple pulmonary embolus have increased risk of development of right-sided cardiac failure.

Pulmonary embolus can precipitate dysrhythmias such as atrial fibrillation/flutter.

Thrombophlebitis can occur or recur and precipitate pulmonary embolism.

Lung Cancer: Surgical Intervention (Postoperative Care)

Surgical procedures for operable tumors of the lung include (1) pneumonectomy (removal of an entire lung), performed for lesions originating in the mainstem bronchus or lobar bronchus; (2) lobectomy (removal of one lobe), preferred for peripheral carcinoma localized in a lobe; and (3) segmental resection, performed when lesion is small and well contained within one segment.

PATIENT ASSESSMENT DATA BASE (PREOPERATIVE)

ACTIVITY/REST

May report: Fatigue.

May exhibit: Lassitude (usually in advanced stage).

EGO INTEGRITY

May report: Scared feelings, fear of outcome of surgery.
Denial of severity of condition/potential for malignancy.

May exhibit: Restlessness, insomnia, repetitive questioning.

FOOD/FLUID

May report: Weight loss, poor appetite, decreased food intake.

May exhibit: Thin, emaciated or wasted appearance (late stages).

PAIN/COMFORT

May report: Chest pain (not usually present in early stages, and not always in advanced stages).

RESPIRATION

May report: History of smoking.
Occupational exposure to pollutants, industrial dusts, radioactive material.
Shortness of breath.
Hoarseness.
Mild cough or change in usual cough pattern and/or sputum production.

May exhibit: Dyspnea, aggravated by exertion.
Increased tactile fremitus (indicating consolidation).
Brief crackles/wheezes on inspiration or expiration (impaired airflow).
Persistent crackles/wheezes, tracheal shift (space-occupying lesion).

TEACHING/LEARNING

May report: Familial risk factors: cancer (especially lung), tuberculosis.
Failure to improve.

Discharge Plan Considerations: Assistance with transportation, medications, treatments, self-care, homemaker tasks.

DIAGNOSTIC STUDIES

Chest x-ray (PA and lateral), chest tomography: outlines shape, size and location of lesion; may reveal mass of air in hilar region, pleural effusion, atelectasis, erosion of ribs or vertebrae.

Cytologic examinations (sputum, pleural, or lymph node): performed to assess presence/stage of carcinoma.

Fiberoptic bronchoscopy: allows for visualization, regional washings and cytologic brushing of lesions (large percent of bronchogenic carcinomas may be visualized).

Biopsy: may be performed on scalene nodes, hilar lymph nodes, pleura to establish diagnosis.

Mediastinoscopy: used for staging of carcinoma.

Radioisotope scans: may be done on lungs, liver, brain, bones, distant organs for evidence of metastasis.

Pulmonary function studies and ABGs: may be done to assess lung capacity to meet postoperative ventilatory needs.

Skin tests, absolute lymphocyte counts: may be done to evaluate for immunocompetence (common in lung cancers).

NURSING PRIORITIES

1. Maintain/improve respiratory function.
2. Control/alleviate pain.
3. Support efforts to cope with diagnosis/situation.
4. Provide information about disease process/prognosis and therapeutic regimen.

DISCHARGE CRITERIA

1. Oxygenation/ventilation adequate to meet individual activity needs.
2. Pain controlled.
3. Anxiety/fear decreased to manageable level.
4. Free of preventable complications.
5. Disease process/prognosis and planned therapies understood.

Refer to CPs: Surgical Intervention, p. 789; Cancer, p. 872; Radical Neck Surgery, p. 171, Hemothorax/Pneumothorax, p. 165.

NURSING DIAGNOSIS:	GAS EXCHANGE, IMPAIRED
May be related to:	**Removal of lung tissue** **Altered oxygen supply (hypoventilation)** **Decreased oxygen-carrying capacity of blood (blood loss)**
Possibly evidenced by:	**Dyspnea** **Restlessness/changes in mentation** **Hypoxemia and hypercapnea** **Cyanosis**
PATIENT OUTCOMES/ EVALUATION CRITERIA:	**Demonstrates improved ventilation and adequate oxygenation of tissues by ABGs within patient's normal range, free of symptoms of respiratory distress.**

ACTIONS/INTERVENTIONS	RATIONALE
Independent Note respiratory rate, depth, and ease of respirations. Observe for use of accessory muscles, pursed-lip breathing, changes in skin/mucous membrane color, e.g., pallor, cyanosis.	Respirations may be increased as a result of pain or as an initial compensatory mechanism to accommodate for loss of lung tissue. However, increased work of breathing and cyanosis may indicate increasing oxy-

ACTIONS/INTERVENTIONS	RATIONALE

Independent

Auscultate lungs for air movement and abnormal breath sounds.

gen consumption and energy expenditures and/or reduced respiratory reserve, e.g., elderly patient or extensive chronic obstructive lung disease.

Consolidation and lack of air movement on operation side is normal in the pneumonectomy patient. However, the lobectomy patient should demonstrate normal airflow.

Assess for restlessness and changes in mentation/level of consciousness.

May indicate increased hypoxia or complications such as mediastinal shift in pneumonectomy patient when accompanied by tachypnea, tachycardia, and tracheal deviation.

Maintain patent airway by positioning, suctioning, use of adjuncts.

Airway obstruction impedes ventilation impairing gas exchange. (Refer to ND: Airway Clearance, Ineffective, p. 159.)

Reposition frequently, placing patient in sitting positions as well as supine to side position.

Maximizes lung expansion and drainage of secretions.

Avoid positioning the patient with a pneumonectomy with the remaining lung dependent.

This position reduces lung expansion and could foster the development of a tension pneumothorax secondary to a mediastinal shift and accumulation of fluid in the remaining lung.

Encourage/assist with deep breathing exercises.

Promotes maximal ventilation and oxygenation and reduces/prevents atelectasis.

Maintain patency of chest drainage system for lobectomy patient. (Refer to CP: Hemothorax/Pneumothorax, p. 165.)

Drains fluid from mediastinal cavity to promote reexpansion of remaining lung segments.

Note changes in amount/type of chest tube drainage.

Bloody drainage should decrease in amount and change to a more serous composition as recovery progresses. A sudden increase in amount of bloody drainage or return to frank bleeding suggests thoracic bleeding/hemothorax; sudden cessation suggests blockage of tube, requiring further evaluation and intervention.

Assess patient response to activity. Encourage rest periods/limit activities to patient tolerance.

Increased oxygen consumption/demand and stress of surgery can result in increased dyspnea and changes in vital signs with activity. However, early mobilization is desired to help prevent pulmonary complications and to obtain and maintain respiratory and circulatory efficiency. Adequate rest/balance with activity can prevent respiratory compromise.

Note development of fever.

Fever within the first 24 hours after operation is almost always due to atelectasis. Temperature elevation within the fifth to 10th postoperative day usually indicates an infection, e.g., wound or elsewhere in body.

Collaborative

Administer supplemental oxygen, via nasal cannula, partial rebreathing mask, or high humidity face mask, as indicated.

Maximizes available oxygen, while ventilation may be reduced from anesthetic depression, pain, as well as operative reduction of alveolar capillary surface.

Assist with/encourage use of incentive spirometer or blow bottles.

Prevents/reduces atelectasis, and promotes reexpansion of small airways.

ACTIONS/INTERVENTIONS	RATIONALE

Collaborative

Monitor/graph ABGs, ear/pulse oximetry readings. Note Hb levels.

Decreasing PaO_2 or increasing $PaCO_2$ may indicate need for ventilatory support. Significant blood loss can result in decreased oxygen-carrying capacity, reducing PaO_2.

NURSING DIAGNOSIS:	AIRWAY CLEARANCE, INEFFECTIVE
May be related to:	**Increased amount/viscosity of secretions**
	Restricted chest movement/pain
	Fatigue/weakness
Possibly evidenced by:	**Changes in rate/depth of respiration**
	Abnormal breath sounds
	Ineffective cough
	Dyspnea
PATIENT OUTCOMES/ EVALUATION CRITERIA:	**Demonstrates patent airway, fluid secretions that are easily expectorated, clear breath sounds, and noiseless respirations.**

ACTIONS/INTERVENTIONS	RATIONALE

Independent

Auscultate chest for character of breath sounds and presence of secretions.

Noisy respirations, rhonchi, and wheezes are indicative of retained secretions and/or airway obstruction.

Assist patient with/instruct in effective deep breathing and coughing with upright position (sitting) and splinting of incision.

Upright position favors maximal lung expansion, and splinting improves force of cough effort to mobilize and remove secretions. Splinting may be done by nurse (placing hands anteriorly and posteriorly over chest wall) and by patient (with pillows) as strength improves.

Observe amount and character of sputum/aspirated secretions. Investigate changes as indicated.

Increased amounts of colorless (or blood-streaked)/ watery secretions are normal initially and should decrease as recovery progresses. Presence of thick/ tenacious, bloody or purulent sputum suggests development of secondary problems (e.g., dehydration, pulmonary edema, local hemorrhage, or infection) requiring correction/treatment.

Avoid deep endotracheal/nasotracheal suctioning in pneumonectomy patient if possible.

Deep tracheal suctioning is generally contraindicated following pneumonectomy to reduce the risk of rupture of the bronchial stump suture line. If suctioning is unavoidable, it should be done gently only to induce effective coughing.

Encourage oral fluid intake (at least 2500 ml/day) within cardiac tolerance.

Adequate hydration aids in keeping secretions loose/ and enhances expectoration.

Assess for pain/discomfort and medicate on a routine basis and prior to breathing exercises.

Encourages the patient to move, cough more effectively and breathe more deeply to prevent respiratory insufficiency.

159

ACTIONS/INTERVENTIONS

Collaborative

Provide/assist with IPPB, incentive spirometer, blow bottles, postural drainage/percussion as indicated.

Use room humidifier/ultrasonic nebulizer. Provide additional fluids IV as indicated.

Administer bronchodilators, expectorants and/or analgesics as indicated.

RATIONALE

Improves pulmonary expansion/ventilation and facilitates removal of secretions. Note: Postural drainage may be contraindicated in some patients and in every event must be performed cautiously to prevent respiratory embarrassment and incisional discomfort.

Providing maximal hydration helps loosen, liquefy secretions to promote expectoration.

Relieves bronchospasm to improve airflow. Expectorants increase mucous production to liquefy and reduce viscosity of secretions, facilitating removal. Alleviation of chest discomfort promotes cooperation with breathing exercises and enhances effectiveness of respiratory therapies.

NURSING DIAGNOSIS:	**COMFORT, ALTERED: PAIN, ACUTE**
May be related to:	**Surgical incision, tissue trauma and disruption of intercostal nerves**
	Presence of chest tube(s)
	Cancer invasion of pleura, chest wall
Possibly evidenced by:	**Verbal reports of discomfort**
	Guarding of affected area
	Distraction behaviors, e.g., restlessness
	Narrowed focus (withdrawal)
	Changes in blood pressure, heart/respiratory rate
PATIENT OUTCOMES/ EVALUATION CRITERIA:	**Reports pain relieved/controlled. Appears relaxed and sleeps/rests appropriately. Participates in desired/needed activities.**

ACTIONS/INTERVENTIONS

Independent

Assess patient's verbal and nonverbal pain cues. Have patient rate intensity on a 1–10 scale. Be aware of possible pathophysiologic and psychologic causes of pain.

Evaluate effectiveness of drug regimen. Encourage sufficient medication to control pain; change medication or time span as appropriate.

RATIONALE

Use of rating scale aids patient in assessing level of pain, provides tool for evaluating effectiveness of analgesics, enhancing patient control of pain. A posterolateral incision is more uncomfortable for the patient than an anterolateral incision. The presence of chest tubes can greatly increase discomfort. In addition, fear, distress, anxiety, and grief over confirmed diagnosis of cancer can impair ability to cope.

Pain perception and pain relief is subjective and thus pain management is best left to the patient's discretion. If the patient is unable to provide input, the nurse should observe physiologic and nonverbal signs of pain and administer medications on a regular basis.

ACTIONS/INTERVENTIONS	RATIONALE
Independent	
Encourage verbalization of feelings about the pain.	Fears/concerns can increase muscle tension and lowers threshold of pain perception. (Refer to ND: Fear/Anxiety, p. 161.)
Provide routine comfort measures, e.g., frequent changes of position, backrubs, support with pillows. Encourage use of relaxation techniques, e.g., visualization, guided imagery, and appropriate diversional activities.	Promotes relaxation and redirects attention. Relieves discomfort and augments therapeutic effects of analgesia.
Schedule rest periods, provide quiet environment.	Decreases fatigue and conserves energy, enhancing coping abilities.
Assist with self-care activities, breathing/arm exercises and ambulation.	Prevents undue fatigue and incisional strain. Encouragement and physical assistance/support may be needed for some time before the patient is able or confident enough to perform these activities because of pain, or fear of pain.
Collaborative	
Administer analgesics routinely as indicated. Assist with patient controlled administration (PCA).	Maintaining a more constant drug level avoids "peak" periods of pain to aid in muscle healing, improved respiratory function, and emotional comfort/coping.

NURSING DIAGNOSIS:	**FEAR/ANXIETY [SPECIFY LEVEL]**
May be related to:	**Situational crises**
	Threat to/change in health status
	Perceived threat of death
Possibly evidenced by:	**Withdrawal**
	Apprehension
	Anger
	Increased pain, sympathetic stimulation
	Expressions of denial, shock, guilt
	Insomnia
PATIENT OUTCOMES/ EVALUATION CRITERIA:	**Acknowledges and discusses fears. Demonstrates appropriate range of feelings and lessened fear. Verbalizes accurate knowledge of situation and is beginning to cope with diagnosis, treatment and prognosis.**

ACTIONS/INTERVENTIONS	RATIONALE
Independent	
Evaluate patient/SO level of understanding of diagnosis.	Patient and SO are hearing and assimilating new information that includes changes in self-image and lifestyle. Understanding perceptions of those involved sets the tone for individualizing care and provides in-

ACTIONS/INTERVENTIONS

Independent

Acknowledge reality of patient's fears/concerns and encourage expression of feelings.

Provide opportunity for questions and answer them honestly. Be sure that patient and care providers have the same understanding of terms used.

Accept, but do not reinforce patient's denial of the situation.

Involve patient/SO in care planning. Provide time to prepare for events/treatments.

Provide for patient's physical comfort.

RATIONALE

formation necessary for choosing appropriate interventions.

Support may enable the patient to begin exploring/dealing with the reality of cancer and its treatment. Patient may need time to identify feelings, and even more time to begin to express them.

Establishes trust and reduces misperceptions/misinterpretation of information.

If extreme denial or anxiety is interfering with progress of recovery, the issues facing the patient need to be explained and resolutions explored.

May help restore some feeling of control/independence to patient who feels powerless in dealing with diagnosis and treatment.

It is difficult to deal with emotional issues when experiencing extreme/persistent physical discomfort.

NURSING DIAGNOSIS:	KNOWLEDGE DEFICIT [LEARNING NEED] (SPECIFY)
May be related to:	**Lack of exposure**
	Information misinterpretation
	Lack of recall
	Unfamiliarity with information/resources
Possibly evidenced by:	**Statements of concern**
	Request for information
	Inadequate follow-through of instruction
	Inappropriate or exaggerated behaviors, e.g., hysterical, hostile, agitated, apathetic
PATIENT OUTCOMES/ EVALUATION CRITERIA:	**Verbalizes understanding of ramifications of diagnosis, treatment regimen. Correctly performs necessary procedures and explains reasons for the actions. Participates in learning process. Initiates necessary lifestyle changes and participates in treatment regimen.**

ACTIONS/INTERVENTIONS

Independent

Discuss diagnosis, current/planned therapies and expected outcomes.

RATIONALE

Provides individually specific information creating knowledge base for subsequent learning regarding home management. Radiation or chemotherapy may follow surgical intervention and information is essential to enable the patient/SO to make informed decisions.

ACTIONS/INTERVENTIONS

Independent

Reinforce surgeon's explanation of particular surgical procedure providing diagram as appropriate. Incorporate this information into discussion about short/long-term recovery expectations.

Discuss necessity of follow-up care and help to make initial appointments prior to discharge.

Identify signs/symptoms requiring medical evaluations, e.g., changes in appearance of incision, development of respiratory difficulty, fever, increased chest pain, changes in appearance of sputum.

Help patient determine activity tolerance and set goals.

Evaluate availability/adequacy of supports and necessity for assistance in self-care/home management.

Recommend alternating rest periods with activity, and light tasks with heavy tasks. Avoid heavy lifting, isometric/strenuous upper body exercise. Reinforce physician's time limitations about lifting.

Recommend stopping any activity that causes undue fatigue, increased shortness of breath.

Encourage inspection of incisions. Review expectations for healing with patient.

Instruct to watch for/report places in incision that do not heal, reopening of healed incision; any drainage (bloody or purulent); localized area of swelling with redness, increased pain, hot to touch.

Suggest wearing soft cotton shirts, loose fitting clothing; cover/pad incision as indicated; leave incision open to air as much as possible.

Shower in warm water, washing incision gently. Avoid tub baths until approved by physician.

Support incision with Steristrips as needed when sutures are removed.

Instruct in/provide rationale for arm/shoulder exercises. Have patient/SO demonstrate exercises. En-

RATIONALE

Length of rehabilitation and prognosis is dependent on type of surgical procedure, preoperative physical condition, and duration of complications.

Follow-up assessment of respiratory status and general health is imperative to assure optimal recovery. Also provides opportunity to readdress concerns/questions at a less stressful time.

Early detection and timely intervention may prevent/minimize complications.

Weakness and fatigue should lessen as lung(s) heal and respiratory function improves during recovery period, especially if cancer was completely removed. If cancer is advanced, it is emotionally helpful for the patient to be able to set realistic activity goals in order to achieve positive results.

General weakness and activity limitations may reduce individuals ability to meet own needs.

Generalized weakness and fatigue are usual in the early recovery period, but should diminish as respiratory function improves and healing progresses. Rest and sleep enhances coping abilities, reduces nervousness (common in this phase), and promotes healing. Note: Strenuous use of arms can place undue stress on incision because chest muscles may be weaker than normal for 3–6 months following surgery.

Exhaustion aggravates respiratory insufficiency.

Healing begins immediately, but complete healing will take time. As healing progresses, incision lines may appear dry, with crusty scabs. Underlying tissue may look bruised and feel tense, warm, and lumpy (resolving hematoma).

Signs/symptoms indicating failure to heal, development of complications requiring further medical evaluation/intervention.

Reduces suture line irritation and pressure from clothing. Leaving incisions open to air promotes healing process and may reduce risk of infection.

Keep incision clean, promotes circulation/healing. Note: "Climbing" out of tub requires use of arms and pectoral muscles, which can put undue stress on incision.

Aids in maintaining approximation of wound edges to promote healing.

Simple arm circles and lifting arms over the head or out to the affected side are initiated on the first or sec-

ACTIONS/INTERVENTIONS

Independent

courage following graded increase in number/intensity of routine repetitions.

Stress importance of avoiding exposure to smoke, air pollution, and contact with individuals with upper respiratory infections.

Promote adequate fluid intake and nutrition.

Refer to appropriate community resources, e.g., American Cancer Society, Visiting Nurse Association, social services.

RATIONALE

ond postoperative day to restore normal range of motion of shoulder and to prevent ankylosis of the affected shoulder.

Protects lung(s) from irritation and reduces risk of infection.

Helps to maintain good circulating volume for tissue perfusion and meets cellular energy requirements to facilitate tissue regeneration/healing process.

Agencies such as these offer a broad range of services that can be tailored to provide support and meet individual needs.

Hemothorax/Pneumothorax _____

The lung may collapse partially/completely due to collection of air (pneumothorax), blood (hemothorax), or other fluid (pleural effusion) in the pleural/potential space. The intrathoracic pressure changes induced by increased pleural space volumes reduce lung capacity, causing respiratory distress and gas exchange problems, and producing tension on mediastinal structures that can impede cardiac and systemic circulation.

PATIENT ASSESSMENT DATA BASE

Findings vary, depending on the amount of air and/or fluid accumulation, rate of accumulation, and underlying lung function. Pain is dependent on the size/area involved.

CIRCULATION

May exhibit:
Tachycardia

Irregular rate/dysrhythmias.

S_3 or S_4/gallop heart rhythm (heart failure secondary to effusion).

Apical pulse (PMI) displaced in presence of mediastinal shift (with tension pneumothorax).

Hamman's sign (crunching sound correlating with heart beat, reflecting air in mediastinum).

Blood pressure: hypertension/hypotension.

PAIN/COMFORT

May report:
Unilateral chest pain.

Sudden onset of symptoms while coughing or straining (spontaneous pneumothorax).

Sharp stabbing pain aggravated by deep breathing, possibly radiating to neck, shoulders, abdomen (pleural effusion).

May exhibit:
Guarding affected area.

Distraction behaviors.

Facial grimacing.

RESPIRATION

May report:
History of recent chest surgery/trauma.

History of chronic lung disease, lung inflammation/infection (empyema/effusion), diffuse interstitial disease (sarcoidosis).

History of malignancies, e.g., obstructive tumor, malignant cells in pleural space; lung biopsy.

Previous spontaneous pneumothorax; spontaneous rupture of emphysematous bulla, subpleural bleb (COPD).

Current positive pressure mechanical ventilation/PEEP therapy.

Difficulty breathing, "air hunger."

Coughing (may be presenting symptom).

May exhibit:
Respirations: increased rate/tachypnea.

Increased work of breathing, use of accessory muscles in chest, neck; intercostal retractions, forced abdominal expiration.

Breath sounds decreased (involved site).

Fremitus decreased (involved site).

Chest percussion: hyperresonance over air-filled area (pneumothorax); dullness over fluid-filled area (hemothorax).

Chest observation and palpation: unequal (paradoxical) chest movement (if trauma, flail); reduced thoracic excursion (affected side).

Skin: pallor, cyanosis, diaphoresis, subcutaneous crepitation (air in tissues).

Mentation: anxiety, restlessness, confusion, stupor.

SAFETY

May report: Recent chest fractures.

Lung cancer, history of radiation/chemotherapy.

TEACHING/LEARNING

May report: History of familial risk factors: tuberculosis, cancer.

Evidence of failure to improve.

Discharge Plan Considerations: Assistance with self-care, homemaker tasks.

DIAGNOSTIC STUDIES

Chest x-ray: reveals air and/or fluid accumulation: may show shift of mediastinal structures (heart).

ABGs: variable dependent on degree of compromised lung function, altered breathing mechanics and ability to compensate. $PaCO_2$ occasionally elevated, PaO_2 may be normal or decreased, oxygen saturation usually decreased.

NURSING PRIORITIES

1. Promote/maintain lung reexpansion for adequate oxygenation/ventilation.
2. Minimize/prevent complications.
3. Reduce discomfort/pain.
4. Provide information about disease process, treatment regimen, and prognosis.

DISCHARGE CRITERIA

1. Adequate ventilation/oxygenation maintained.
2. Complications prevented.
3. Pain absent/controlled.
4. Disease process/prognosis and therapy needs understood.

NURSING DIAGNOSIS: **BREATHING PATTERN, INEFFECTIVE**

May be related to: Decreased lung expansion (air/fluid accumulation)

Musculoskeletal impairment

Pain/anxiety

Inflammatory process

Possibly evidenced by: Dyspnea, tachypnea

Changes in depth/equality of respirations

Use of accessory muscles, nasal flaring

Altered chest excursion

Cyanosis; abnormal ABGs

PATIENT OUTCOMES/ EVALUATION CRITERIA:	**Establishes a normal/effective respiratory pattern with absence of cyanosis/other signs/symptoms of hypoxia and ABGs within patient's normal range.**

ACTIONS/INTERVENTIONS

Independent

Identify etiology/precipitating factors, e.g. spontaneous collapse, trauma, malignancy, infection, complication of mechanical ventilation.

Evaluate respiratory function, noting rapid/shallow respirations, dyspnea, complaints of "air hunger," development of cyanosis, changes in vital signs.

Auscultate breath sounds.

Note chest excursion and position of trachea.

Assess fremitus.

Assist patient with splinting painful area when coughing, deep breathing.

Maintain position of comfort, usually with head of bed elevated. Turn to affected side. Encourage to sit up as much as possible.

Assist patient in dealing with anxiety/fear by maintaining a calm attitude, assisting patient to "take control" by the use of slower/deeper respirations.

Once chest tube inserted:

Check suction control chamber for correct amount of suction (by water level, wall/table regulator at correct setting).

Check fluid level in water-seal chamber/bottle; maintain at prescribed level.

Observe water-seal chamber bubbling.

Evaluate for abnormal/continuous water-seal chamber bubbling.

RATIONALE

Understanding the cause of lung collapse is necessary for proper chest tube placement (hemo/pneumothorax) and choice of other therapeutic measures.

Signs of respiratory distress and changes in vital signs may indicate increasing shock due to hypoxia, stress, pain.

May be diminished or absent in a lobe, lung segment, entire lung field (unilateral). Atelectatic area will have no breath sounds and partially collapsed areas have decreased sounds. Evaluation establishes areas of exchange and documents baseline to evaluate increasing atelectasis.

Chest excursion is unequal until lung reexpands. Trachea deviates away from affected side with tension pneumothorax.

Voice and tactile fremitus (vibration) is reduced in fluid-filled/consolidated tissue.

Supporting chest and abdominal muscles makes coughing more effective/less traumatic.

Promotes maximal inspiration; enhances lung expansion and ventilation in unaffected side.

Anxiety is present because of severe difficulty breathing and the physiologic effects of hypoxia.

Maintains prescribed intrapleural negativity which promotes optimum lung expansion and/or fluid drainage.

Water in a sealed chamber serves as a barrier that prevents atmospheric air from entering the pleural space should the suction source be disconnected, and aids in evaluating whether the chest drainage system is functioning appropriately.

Bubbling during expiration reflects venting of pneumothorax (desired action). Bubbling usually decreases as the lung expands or may occur only during expiration or coughing as the pleural space diminishes. Absence of bubbling may indicate complete lung reexpansion (normal) or represent complications, e.g., obstruction in the tube.

With suction applied, this indicates a persistent air leak that may be from a large pneumothorax, at the chest insertion site (patient-centered) or chest drainage unit (system-centered).

ACTIONS/INTERVENTIONS	RATIONALE

Independent

Determine location of air leak (patient- or system-centered) by clamping thoracic catheter just distal to exit from chest.

If bubbling stops when catheter is clamped at insertion site, leak is patient-centered (at insertion site or within the patient).

    Place Vaseline gauze and/or other appropriate material around the insertion as indicated.

Usually corrects insertion site air leak.

    Clamp tubing in stepwise fashion downward toward drainage unit if air leak continues.

Isolates location of a system-centered air leak.

    Seal drainage tubing connection sites securely with lengthwise tape or bands according to established policy.

Prevents/corrects air leaks at connector sites.

Note water-seal chamber "tidaling."

The water-seal chamber serves as an intrapleural manometer (gauges intrapleural pressure); therefore, fluctuation (tidaling) reflects pressure differences between inspiration and expiration. Tidaling of 2–6 cm during inspiration is normal.

Monitor for abnormal "tidaling" and note whether change is transient or permanent.

Tidal fluctuation increases briefly during coughing episodes. If airway obstruction exists or large pneumothorax is present, excessive tidal fluctuations may continue.

Position drainage system tubing for optimal function, e.g., coil extra tubing on bed, making sure tubing is not kinked or hanging below entrance to drainage container. Drain accumulated fluid as necessary.

Improper position, kinking, or accumulation of clots/fluid in the tubing changes the desired negative pressure and impedes air/fluid evacuation.

Evaluate need for tube stripping ("milking").

Although it is unlikely that serous or serosanguinous drainage will obstruct tubes, stripping may be necessary to assure/maintain drainage in the presence of fresh/large blood clots or purulent exudate (empyema).

Strip tubes carefully per protocol, in a manner which minimizes excess negative pressure.

Stripping is usually uncomfortable for the patient because of the change in intrathoracic pressure which may induce coughing or chest discomfort. Vigorous stripping can create very high intrathoracic suction pressure, which can be injurious (e.g., invagination of tissue into catheter eyelets, collapse of tissues around the catheter, and/or bleeding from rupture of small blood vessels).

If thoracic catheter is disconnected/dislodged:

Observe for signs of respiratory distress. Reconnect thoracic catheter to tubing/suction, if possible, using clean technique. If the catheter is dislodged from the chest, cover insertion site immediately with dressing and apply firm pressure. Notify physician at once.

Pneumothorax may recur.

After thoracic catheter is removed:

Observe for signs/symptoms which may indicate recurrence of pneumothorax, e.g., shortness of breath, complaints of pain. Cover insertion site with sterile occlusive dressing. Observe for insertion site drainage.

Early detection of developing complication is essential, e.g., recurrence of pneumothorax or infections.

Collaborative

Review serial chest x-rays.

Monitors progress of resolving hemo/pneumothorax and reexpansion of lung.

ACTIONS/INTERVENTIONS

Collaborative

Monitor/graph serial ABGs and ear/pulse oximetry. Review vital capacity/tidal volume measurements.

Administer supplemental oxygen as indicated.

RATIONALE

Assesses status of gas exchange and ventilation and/or reveals need for alterations in therapy.

Aids in reducing work of breathing, promotes relief of respiratory distress and cyanosis associated with hypoxemia.

NURSING DIAGNOSIS:	INJURY, POTENTIAL FOR: TRAUMA/SUFFOCATION
May be related to:	Concurrent disease/injury process
	Dependence on external device (chest drainage system)
	Lack of safety education/precautions
Possibly evidenced by:	[Not applicable; presence of signs and symptoms establishes an *actual* diagnosis.]
PATIENT OUTCOMES/ EVALUATION CRITERIA:	Recognizes need for/seeks assistance to prevent complications. Corrects/avoids environmental/physical hazards (care-giver-directed).

ACTIONS/INTERVENTIONS

Independent

Review with patient purpose/function of chest drainage unit, taking note of safety features.

Anchor thoracic catheter to chest wall and provide extra length of tubing before turning or moving patient:

Secure tubing connection sites;

Pad banding sites with gauze/tape.

Secure drainage unit on patient's bed or stand/cart placed in low-traffic area.

Provide safe transportation if patient is sent off unit for diagnostic purposes. Before transporting: check water-seal chamber for correct fluid level, presence/absence of bubbling; presence/degree/timing of tidaling. Ascertain whether or not chest tube can be clamped or disconnected from suction source.

Monitor thoracic insertion site, noting condition of skin, presence/characteristics of drainage from around the catheter. Change/reapply sterile occlusive dressing as needed.

Instruct patient to refrain from lying/pulling on tubing.

Identify changes/situations that should be reported to care givers, e.g., change in sound of bubbling, sudden "air hunger" and chest pain, disconnection of equipment.

RATIONALE

Information on how system works provides reassurance, reducing patient anxiety.

Prevents thoracic catheter dislodgment or tubing disconnection, and reduces pain/discomfort associated with pulling or jarring of tubing.

Prevents tubing disconnection.

Protects skin from irritation/pressure.

Maintains upright position and reduces risk of accidental tipping/breaking of unit.

Promotes continuation of optimal evacuation of fluid/air during transport. If patient is draining large amounts of chest fluid or air, tube should not be clamped or suction interrupted because of risk of reaccumulation of fluid/air, compromising respiratory status.

Provides for early recognition and treatment of developing skin/tissue erosion or infection.

Reduces risk of obstructing drainage/inadvertently disconnecting tubing.

Timely intervention may prevent serious complications.

ACTIONS/INTERVENTIONS

Independent

Observe for signs of respiratory distress if thoracic catheter is disconnected/dislodged. (Refer to ND: Breathing Pattern, Ineffective, p. 166.)

RATIONALE

Pneumothorax may recur/worsen, compromising respiratory function and requiring emergency intervention.

NURSING DIAGNOSIS:	KNOWLEDGE DEFICIT [LEARNING NEED] (SPECIFY)
May be related to:	Lack of exposure
Possibly evidenced by:	Expressions of concern, request for information Recurrence of problem
PATIENT OUTCOMES/ EVALUATION CRITERIA:	Verbalizes understanding of cause of problem. Identifies signs/symptoms requiring medical follow-up. Follows treatment regimen and demonstrates lifestyle changes necessary to prevent recurrence.

ACTIONS/INTERVENTIONS

Independent

Review pathology of individual problem.

Identify likelihood for recurrence/long-term complications.

Review signs/symptoms requiring immediate medical evaluation, e.g., sudden chest pain, dyspnea/air hunger, progressive respiratory distress.

Review significance of good health practices, e.g., adequate nutrition, rest, exercise.

RATIONALE

Information reduces fear of unknown. Provides knowledge base for understanding underlying dynamics of condition and significance of therapeutic interventions.

Certain underlying lung disease such as severe COPD and malignancies may increase incidence of recurrence. In otherwise healthy patients who suffered a spontaneous pneumothorax, incidence of recurrence is 10–50%. Those who have a second spontaneous episode are at high risk for a third incident (60%).

Recurrence of pneumo/hemothorax requires medical intervention to prevent/reduce potential complications.

Maintenance of general well-being promotes healing and can prevent/limit recurrences.

Radical Neck Surgery: Laryngectomy (Postoperative Care)

Partial laryngectomy: Tumors that are limited to only one vocal cord are removed and a tracheotomy performed to maintain the airway. After surgery, the patient's voice will be hoarse.

Hemilaryngectomy: When there is a chance the cancer has spread to a false cord. One true vocal cord, a false cord, an arytenoid cartilage, and half of the thyroid cartilage are removed and tracheotomy performed. The patient's voice will be hoarse.

Supraglottic laryngectomy: When the tumor is located in the epiglottis or false vocal cords, radical neck dissection is done and tracheotomy performed. The patient's voice remains intact; however, swallowing is more difficult because the epiglottis has been removed.

Total laryngectomy: Advanced cancers that involve a large portion of the larynx require removal of the entire larynx, the hyoid bone, the cricoid cartilage, two or three tracheal rings, and the strap muscles connected to the larynx. A permanent opening is created in the neck for the trachea, and a laryngectomy tube may be inserted to keep the stoma open. The lower portion of the posterior pharynx is removed when the tumor extends beyond the epiglottis with the remaining portion sutured to the esophagus after a nasogastric tube is inserted. The patient must breathe through a permanent tracheostomy with normal speech no longer possible, although swallowing is not a problem, because there is no connection between the upper and lower respiratory tracts.

PATIENT ASSESSMENT DATA BASE

Preoperative data presented here is dependent on specific type/location of cancer process and underlying complications.

EGO INTEGRITY

May report: Feelings of fear about loss of voice, dying, occurrence/recurrence of cancer.
Concern about how surgery will affect family relationships, ability to work, and finances.

May exhibit: Anxiety, depression, anger and withdrawal.
Denial.

FOOD/FLUID

May report: Difficulty/pain on swallowing.

May exhibit: Difficulty swallowing, chokes easily.
Swelling, ulcerations, masses may be noted dependent on location of cancer.
Inflammation/drainage/poor dental hygiene.
Leukoplakia, erythroplasia of oral cavity.
Halitosis.
Swelling of tongue.
Altered gag reflex and facial paralysis.

HYGIENE

May exhibit: Neglect of dental hygiene.
Need for assistance in basic care.

NEUROSENSORY

May report: Diplopia (double vision).
Deafness.
Tingling, paresthesia of facial muscles.

May exhibit:	Hemiparalysis of face (parotid and submandibular involvement).
	Persistent hoarseness.
	Difficulty swallowing.
	Conduction deafness.
	Disruption of mucous membranes.

PAIN/COMFORT

May report: Chronic sore throat, "lump in throat."

Referred pain to ear, facial pain.

Pain with swallowing, local pain in oropharynx.

Postoperative:

Sore throat or mouth (pain is not usually reported as severe following head and neck surgery, as compared with pain noted prior to surgery).

May exhibit: Guarding behaviors.

Restlessness.

Facial mask of pain.

Alteration in muscle tone.

RESPIRATION

May report: History of smoking/chewing tobacco.

Occupation working with hardwood sawdust, toxic chemicals/fumes, heavy metals.

History of voice overuse, e.g., professional singer or auctioneer.

History of chronic lung disease.

Cough with/without sputum.

Bloody nasal drainage.

May exhibit: Blood-tinged sputum, hemoptysis.

Dyspnea (late).

SAFETY

May report: Visual/hearing changes.

May exhibit: Masses/enlarged nodes.

SOCIAL INTERACTION

May report: Lack of family/support system (may be result of age group or behaviors, e.g., alcoholism).

May exhibit: Persistent hoarseness, change in voice pitch.

Muffled/garbled speech, reluctance to speak.

Hesitancy/reluctance of SO to provide care/be involved in rehabilitation.

TEACHING/LEARNING

May report: Nonhealing of oral lesions.

Concurrent use of alcohol.

Discharge Plan Considerations: Assistance with wound care, treatments, supplies; transportation, shopping; food preparation; self-care, homemaker tasks.

DIAGNOSTIC STUDIES

CBC: may reveal anemia which is a common problem.

Immunologic surveys: may be done for patients receiving chemo/immunotherapy.

Biochemical profile: changes may occur in organ function as a result of cancer, metastasis, and therapies.

ABGs: may be done to monitor status of lungs (ventilation).

Pulmonary function studies, bone scans, or other organ scans: may be indicated if distant metastasis is suspected.

Chest x-ray: done to establish baseline lung status.

NURSING PRIORITIES

1. Maintain patent airway, adequate ventilation.
2. Assist patient in developing alternate communication methods.
3. Restore/maintain skin integrity.
4. Reestablish/maintain adequate nutrition.
5. Provide emotional support for acceptance of altered body image.
6. Provide information about disease process/prognosis and treatment.

DISCHARGE CRITERIA

1. Ventilation/oxygenation adequate for individual needs.
2. Communicating effectively.
3. Complications prevented/minimized.
4. Beginning to cope with change in body image.
5. Disease process/prognosis and therapeutic regimen understood.

NURSING DIAGNOSIS:	AIRWAY CLEARANCE, INEFFECTIVE
May be related to:	**Partial/total removal of the glottis altering ability to breathe, cough, and swallow.**
	Procedure which results in temporary or permanent neck breathing (dependent on patent stoma)
	Edema formation (surgical manipulation and lymphatic accumulation)
	Copious and thick secretions
Possibly evidenced by:	**Dyspnea/difficulty breathing**
	Changes in rate/depth of respiration
	Use of accessory respiratory muscles
	Abnormal breath sounds
	Cyanosis
PATIENT OUTCOMES/ EVALUATION CRITERIA:	**Maintains patent airway with breath sounds clear/ clearing. Expectorates/clears secretions, and aspiration is prevented. Demonstrates behaviors to improve/ maintain airway clearance within level of ability/ situation.**

ACTIONS/INTERVENTIONS	RATIONALE

Independent

Monitor respiratory rate/depth; note ease of breathing. Auscultate breath sounds. Investigate restlessness, dyspnea, development of cyanosis.

Changes in respirations, use of accessory muscles and/or presence of rhonchi/wheezes suggests retention of secretions. Airway obstruction (even partial) can lead to ineffective breathing patterns and impaired gas exchange resulting in complications, e.g., pneumonia or respiratory arrest.

Elevate head of bed 30–45 degrees.

Facilitates drainage of secretions, work of breathing, and lung expansion.

Encourage swallowing, if patient is able.

Prevents pooling of oral secretions reducing risk of aspiration. Note: Swallowing is impaired when the epiglottis is removed and/or significant postoperative edema and pain are present.

Encourage effective coughing and deep breathing.

Mobilizes secretions to clear airway and helps prevent respiratory complications.

Suction laryngectomy/tracheostomy tube, oral and nasal cavities. Note amount, color, consistency of secretions.

Prevents secretions from obstructing airway especially when swallowing ability is impaired and patient cannot blow nose. Changes in character of secretions may indicate developing problems (e.g., dehydration, infection, and need for further evaluation/treatment).

Demonstrate and encourage patient to begin self-suction procedures as soon as possible. Educate patient in "clean" techniques.

Assists patient to exercise some control in postoperative care and prevention of complications. Reduces anxiety associated with difficulty in breathing or inability to handle secretions when alone.

Maintain proper position of laryngectomy/tracheostomy tube. Check/adjust ties as indicated.

As edema develops/subsides, tube can be displaced compromising airway. Ties should be snug but not constrictive to surrounding tissue or major blood vessels.

Observe tissue surrounding tube for bleeding. Change patient's position to check for pooling of blood behind neck or on posterior dressings.

Small amount of oozing may be present. However, continued bleeding or sudden eruption of uncontrolled hemorrhage presents a sudden and very real possibility of airway obstruction/suffocation.

Cleanse tube/inner cannula as indicated. Instruct patient in cleaning procedures.

Prevents accumulation of secretions and thick mucous plugs from obstructing airway. Note: This is a common cause of respiratory distress/arrest in later postoperative period.

Collaborative

Provide supplemental humidification: e.g., compressed air/oxygen mist collar, room humidifier, increased fluid intake.

Normal physiologic (nose/nasal passages) means of filtering/humidifying air is bypassed. Supplemental humidity decreases mucous crusting and facilitates coughing/suctioning of secretions through stoma.

Monitor serial ABGs; chest x-ray.

Pooling of secretions/presence of atelectasis may lead to pneumonia requiring more aggressive therapeutic measures.

NURSING DIAGNOSIS:	COMMUNICATION, IMPAIRED: VERBAL
May be related to:	Anatomic deficit (removal of vocal cords)
	Physical barrier (tracheostomy tube)

	Required voice rest
Possibly evidenced by:	**Inability to speak**
	Change in vocal characteristics
PATIENT OUTCOMES/ EVALUATION CRITERIA:	**Communicating needs in an effective manner. Identifies/ plans for appropriate alternate speech methods post healing.**

ACTIONS/INTERVENTIONS	RATIONALE
Independent	
Review preoperative instructions/discussion of why speech and breathing are altered, using anatomic drawings or models to assist in explanations.	Reinforces teaching at a time when "fear of surviving surgery" is past.
Determine whether patient has other communication impairment, e.g., hearing, vision, literacy.	Presence of other problems will influence plan for alternate communication.
Provide immediate and continual means to summon nurse, e.g., call light/bell. Let the patient know the summons will be answered immediately. Stop by to check on patient periodically without being summoned. Make note at central answering system/ nursing station that patient is unable to speak.	Patient needs assurance that nurse is vigilant and will respond to summons. Trust and self-esteem are fostered when the nurse cares enough to come at times other than when called by the patient.
Prearrange signals for obtaining immediate help.	May decease anxiety about inability to speak.
Provide alternate means of communication appropriate to patient need, e.g., pad and pencil, magic slate, alphabet/picture board. Consider placement of IV.	Permits patient to "express" needs/concerns. Note: IV positioned in hand/wrist may limit ability to use written form of communication.
Allow sufficient time for communication.	Loss of speech and stress of alternate communication can cause frustration and block expression, especially when care givers seem "too busy" or preoccupied.
Provide nonverbal communication, e.g., touching and physical presence. Anticipate needs.	Communicates concern and meets need for contact with others. Touch is believed to generate complex biochemical events with possible release of endorphins contributing to reduction of anxiety.
Encourage ongoing communication with "outside world," e.g., newspapers, television, radio, calendar, clock.	Maintains contact with "normal lifestyle" and continued communication through other avenues.
Refer to loss of speech as temporary depending on type of laryngectomy performed and/or availability of voice prosthetics.	Provides encouragement and hope for future with the thought that alternate means of communication and speech are available and possible.
Arrange for meeting with other persons who have experienced this procedure if appropriate.	Provides role model, enhancing motivation for problem solving and learning new ways to communicate.
Collaborative	
Consult with appropriate health team members/ therapists/rehabilitation agency (e.g., speech pathologist, social services, laryngectomee clubs) for hospital based rehabilitation as well as community resources, such as Lost Chord/New Voice Club, International Association of Laryngectomees, American Cancer Society.	Ability to use alternate voice and speech methods varies greatly, dependent on extent of surgical procedures, patient's age, emotional state and motivation to return to an active life. Rehabilitation time may be lengthy and require a number of agencies/resources to facilitate/support learning process.

```
┌─────────────────────────────────────────────────────────────────────────┐
│  NURSING DIAGNOSIS:          SKIN/TISSUE INTEGRITY, IMPAIRED              │
│                                                                           │
│      May be related to:      Surgical removal of tissues/grafting        │
│                                                                           │
│                              Radiation or chemotherapeutic agents         │
│                                                                           │
│                              Altered circulation/reduced blood supply     │
│                                                                           │
│                              Compromised nutritional status               │
│                                                                           │
│                              Edema formation                              │
│                                                                           │
│                              Pooling/continuous drainage of secretions    │
│                              (oral, lymph or chyle)                        │
│                                                                           │
│   Possibly evidenced by:     Disruption of skin surface                   │
│                                                                           │
│                              Destruction of skin layers                   │
│                                                                           │
│  PATIENT OUTCOMES/           Displays timely wound healing without        │
│  EVALUATION CRITERIA:        complications. Demonstrates techniques to    │
│                              promote healing/prevent complications.       │
└─────────────────────────────────────────────────────────────────────────┘
```

ACTIONS/INTERVENTIONS	RATIONALE
Independent	
Assess skin color/temperature and capillary refill in operative and skin graft areas.	Skin should be pink or similar to color of surrounding skin. Skin graft flaps should be pink and warm and should blanch (when gentle finger pressure is applied), with return of color within seconds. Cyanosis and slow refill may indicate venous congestion, which can lead to tissue ischemia/necrosis.
Keep head of bed elevated 30–45 degrees. Monitor facial edema (usually peaks by 3rd to 5th postoperative day).	Minimizes post operative tissue congestion and edema related to excision of lymph channels.
Protect skin flaps and suture lines from tension or pressure. Provide pillows/rolls and instruct patient to support head/neck during activity.	Pressure from tubings, tracheostomy tapes; or tension on suture lines can alter circulation/cause tissue injury.
Monitor bloody drainage from surgical sites, suture lines, drains. Measure hemovac drainage (if used).	Bloody drainage usually declines steadily after first 24 hours. Steady oozing or frank bleeding indicates problem requiring medical attention.
Note/report any milky appearing drainage.	Milky drainage may indicate thoracic lymph duct leakage (can result in depletion of body fluids and electrolytes). Such a leak may heal spontaneously or require surgical closure.
Change dressings as indicated when used.	Damp dressings increase risk of tissue damage/infection. Note: Pressure dressings are not used over skin flaps, because blood supply is easily compromised.
Cleanse incisions with sterile saline and peroxide (mixed 1:1) after dressings have been removed.	Prevents crust formation, which can trap purulent drainage, destroy skin edges, and increase size of wound. Peroxide is not used full strength, because it may cauterize wound edges and impair healing.
Monitor donor site if graft performed: check dressings as indicated.	Donor site may be adjacent to operative site or a distant site (e.g., thigh). Pressure dressings are usually

ACTIONS/INTERVENTIONS

Independent

Cleanse thoroughly around stoma and neck tubes (if in place), avoiding soap or alcohol. Show patient how to do self stoma/tube care with clean water and peroxide, and using cloth, not tissue or cotton.

Monitor all sites for signs of wound infection, e.g., unusual redness, increasing edema, pain, exudates, and temperature elevation.

Collaborative

Administer oral, IV, and topical antibiotics as indicated.

Cover donor sites with vaseline gauze or moisture-impermeable dressing.

RATIONALE

removed within 24–48 hours and wound left open to air to promote healing.

Keeping area cleansed promotes healing and comfort. Soap and other mucous drying agents can lead to stomal irritation and possible inflammation. Materials other than cloth may leave fibers in stoma that can irritate or be inhaled into lungs.

Impedes healing, which may already be slow because of changes induced by cancer or cancer therapies and/or malnutrition.

Prevents/controls infection.

Nonadherent dressing covers exposed sensory nerve endings and protects site from contamination.

NURSING DIAGNOSIS:	ORAL MUCOUS MEMBRANES, ALTERED
May be related to:	Dehydration/absence of oral intake
	Poor/inadequate oral hygiene
	Pathologic condition (oral cancer)
	Mechanical trauma (oral surgery)
	Decreased saliva production secondary to radiation (common) or surgical procedure (rare)
	Difficulty swallowing and pooling/drooling
	Nutritional deficits
Possibly evidenced by:	Xerostomia (dry mouth), oral discomfort
	Thick/mucoid saliva, decreased saliva production
	Dry, crusted, coated tongue; inflamed lips
	Absent teeth/gums; poor dental health; halitosis
PATIENT OUTCOMES/ EVALUATION CRITERIA:	Reports/demonstrates a decrease in symptoms/complaints. Identifies specific interventions to promote healthy oral mucosa. Demonstrates techniques to restore/maintain mucosal integrity.

ACTIONS/INTERVENTIONS

Independent

Inspect oral cavity and note changes in:

Saliva;

RATIONALE

Damage to salivary glands may decrease production of saliva, resulting in dry mouth. Pooling and drooling

ACTIONS/INTERVENTIONS	RATIONALE
Independent	
	of saliva may occur because of compromised swallowing capability or pain in throat and mouth.
Tongue;	Surgery may have included partial resection of tongue, soft palate and pharynx. This patient will have decreased sensation and movement of tongue, with difficulty swallowing and increased risk of aspiration of secretions, as well as potential for hemorrhage.
Lips;	Surgery may have removed part of lip resulting in uncontrollable drooling.
Teeth and gums;	Teeth may not be intact (surgical) or may be in poor condition because of malnutrition, chemical therapies, neglect. Gums may also be surgically altered or inflamed because of poor hygiene, long history of smoking/chewing, or chemical therapies.
Mucous membranes.	May be excessively dry, ulcerated, erythematous, edematous.
Suction oral cavity gently/frequently. Have patient perform self-suctioning when possible, or use gauze wick to drain secretions.	Saliva contains digestive enzymes which may be erosive to exposed tissues. Since drooling may be constant, patient can promote own comfort and enhance oral hygiene.
Show patient how to brush inside of mouth, palate, tongue, and teeth frequently.	Reduces bacteria and risk of infection, promotes tissue healing and comfort.
Apply lubrication to lips; provide oral irrigations as indicated.	Counteracts drying effects of therapeutic measures, negates erosive nature of secretions.

NURSING DIAGNOSIS:	**COMFORT, ALTERED: PAIN, ACUTE**
May be related to:	**Surgical incisions**
	Tissue swelling
	Presence of nasogastric/orogastric feeding tube
Possibly evidenced by:	**Discomfort in surgical areas/pain with swallowing**
	Facial mask of pain
	Distraction behaviors, restlessness
	Guarding behavior
PATIENT OUTCOMES/ EVALUATION CRITERIA:	**Reports/indicates pain is relieved/controlled. Demonstrates relief of pain/discomfort by reduced tension and relaxed manner, sleeping/resting appropriately.**

ACTIONS/INTERVENTIONS	RATIONALE
Independent	
Support head and neck with pillows. Show patient how to support neck during activity.	Muscle weakness results from muscle and nerve resection of the structures in the neck and/or shoulders.

ACTIONS/INTERVENTIONS	RATIONALE
Independent	
	Lack of support aggravates discomfort and may result in injury to suture areas.
Provide routine comfort measures (e.g., backrub, position change) and diversional activities (e.g., television, visiting, reading).	Promotes relaxation and helps the patient refocus attention on something besides self/discomfort. May reduce analgesic dosage needs/frequency.
Encourage patient to expectorate saliva or to suction mouth gently if unable to swallow.	Swallowing causes muscle activity that may be painful because of edema/strain on suture lines.
Investigate changes in complaints/characteristics of pain. Check mouth, throat suture lines for fresh trauma.	May reflect developing complications requiring further evaluation/intervention. Tissues are inflamed and congested and may be easily traumatized by suction catheter, feeding tube, etc.
Note nonverbal indicators and autonomic responses to pain. Evaluate effects of analgesics.	Aids in determining presence of pain, need for/effectiveness of medication.
Medicate before activity/treatments as indicated.	May enhance cooperation and participation in therapeutic regimen.
Schedule care activities to balance with adequate periods of sleep/rest.	Prevents fatigue/exhaustion and may enhance coping with stress/discomfort.
Recommend use of stress management behaviors, e.g., relaxation techniques, guided imagery.	Promotes sense of well-being, may reduce analgesic needs and enhance healing.
Collaborative	
Provide oral irrigations, anesthetic sprays and gargles. Instruct patient in self-irrigations.	Improves comfort and reduces halitosis. Commercial mouthwashes containing alcohol or phenol are to be avoided because of their drying effect.
Administer analgesics, e.g., codeine, ASA, Darvon as indicated.	Degree of pain is related to extent and psychologic impact of surgery as well as general body condition. Studies appear to support the idea that many patients experience less pain after head and neck surgery than prior to surgery.

NURSING DIAGNOSIS:	**NUTRITION, ALTERED: LESS THAN BODY REQUIREMENTS**
May be related to:	**Temporary or permanent alteration in mode of food intake**
	Altered feedback mechanisms of desire to eat, taste, and smell because of surgical/structural changes, radiation or chemotherapy.
Possibly evidenced by:	**Inadequate food intake, perceived inability to ingest food**
	Aversion to eating, lack of interest in food
	Reported altered taste sensation
	Weight loss
	Weakness of muscles required for swallowing or mastication

ACTIONS/INTERVENTIONS	RATIONALE
Independent	
Auscultate bowel sounds.	Feedings are begun only after bowel sounds are restored postoperatively.
Maintain feeding tube, e.g., check for tube placement; flush with water (or carbonated beverages, cranberry juice) as indicated.	Tube is inserted in surgery and usually sutured in place. Initially the tube may be attached to suction to reduce nausea and/or vomiting. Flushing aids in maintaining patency of tube.
Monitor intake and weigh as indicated. Show patient how to monitor and record weight on a scheduled basis.	Provides information regarding nutritional needs and effectiveness of therapy.
Instruct patient/SO in self-feeding techniques, e.g., bulb syringe, bag and funnel method, blending soft foods if the patient is to go home with a feeding tube. Make sure patient and SO are able to perform this procedure prior to discharge, and that appropriate food and equipment are available at home.	Helps promote nutritional success and preserves dignity in the adult who is now forced to be dependent on others for very basic needs in the social setting of meals.
Begin with small feedings and advance as tolerated. Note signs of gastric fullness, regurgitation, diarrhea.	Content of feeding may result in GI intolerance, requiring change in rate or type of formula.
Provide supplemental water by feeding tube or orally if patient can swallow.	Keeps patient hydrated to offset insensible losses and drainage from surgical areas. Meets free water needs associated with enteral feeding.
Resume oral feedings when feasible. Stay with patient during meals the first few days.	Oral feedings can usually resume after suture lines are healed (8–10 days) unless further reconstruction is required, or patient will be going home with feeding tube. The patient may experience pain or difficulty with chewing and swallowing initially and may require suctioning during meals in addition to support and encouragement.
Encourage the development of a pleasant environment for meals.	Promotes socialization and maximizes patient comfort when eating difficulties cause embarrassment.
Help patient/SO develop nutritionally balanced home meal plans.	Promotes understanding of individual needs and significance of nutrition in healing and recovery process.
Collaborative	
Consult with dietician/nutritional support team as indicated. Incorporate and reinforce dietitican's teaching.	Useful in establishing individual nutritional needs to promote healing and tissue regeneration. Discharge teaching and follow-up by the dietician may be needed to evaluate patient needs for diet/equipment modifications and meal planning in the home setting.
Provide nutritionally balanced diet (e.g., semisolid/soft foods) or tube feedings (e.g., blended soft food or commercial preparations) as indicated.	Variations can be made to add or limit certain factors such as fat, sugar; or to provide a food that the patient prefers. (Refer to CP: Total Nutritional Support, p. 894.)
Monitor laboratory studies, e.g., BUN, glucose, liver function, protein, electrolytes.	Indicators of utilization of nutrients as well as organ function.

NURSING DIAGNOSIS:	SELF-CONCEPT, DISTURBANCE IN: (SPECIFY)
May be related to:	Loss of voice
	Changes in anatomic contour of face and neck (disfigurement and/or severe functional impairment)
	Presence of chronic illness
Possibly evidenced by:	"Verbalization" of fear of rejection by/reaction of others
	Negative feelings about body change
	Refusal to verify actual change or preoccupation with change/loss, not looking at self in mirror
	Change in social involvement
	Discomfort in social situations
	Change in self/others' perception of role
	Anxiety, depression, lack of eye contact
	Failure of family members to adapt to change or deal with experience constructively
PATIENT OUTCOMES/ EVALUATION CRITERIA:	Identifies feelings and methods for coping with negative perception of self. Demonstrates initial adaptation to body changes. "Communicates" with SO about changes in role that have occurred. Begins to develop plans for altered lifestyle. Participates in team efforts toward rehabilitation.

ACTIONS/INTERVENTIONS	RATIONALE
Independent	
Discuss meaning of loss/change with patient, identifying perceptions of current situation/future expectations.	Aids in identifying/defining the problem(s) to focus attention and interventions constructively.
Note nonverbal body language, negative attitudes/self-talk. Assess for self-destructive/suicidal behavior.	May indicate depression/despair, need for further assessment/more intense intervention.
Note emotional reactions, e.g., grieving, depression, anger. Allow patient to progress at own rate.	May experience immediate depression after surgery or react with shock and denial. Acceptance of changes cannot be forced. Grieving process needs time for resolution.
Maintain calm, reassuring manner. Acknowledge and accept expression of feelings of grief, hostility.	May help allay patient's fears of dying, suffocation, inability to communicate or mutilation. Patient and SO need to feel supported and know that all feelings are appropriate for the type of experience they are going through.
Allow/but do not participate in patient's use of denial, e.g., when patient is reluctant to participate in self-care (suctioning stoma), provide care without comment in a nonjudgmental manner.	May be most helpful defense for the patient in the beginning, permitting the individual to begin to deal with difficult adjustment slowly.

181

ACTIONS/INTERVENTIONS	RATIONALE

Independent

Set limits on maladaptive behaviors, assisting patient to identify positive behaviors that will aid recovery.	Acting-out can result in lowered self-esteem, impede adjustment to new self image.
Encourage SO to treat patient normally and not as an invalid.	Distortions of body image may be unconsciously reinforced by SO.
Alert staff that facial expressions and other nonverbal behaviors need to convey acceptance and not revulsion.	This patient is very sensitive to nonverbal communication and may make negative assumptions about others' body language.
Encourage identification of anticipated personal/work conflicts that may arise.	Expressions of concern brings problems into the open where they can be examined/dealt with.
Recognize behavior indicative of overconcern with future lifestyle/relationship functioning.	Ruminating about anticipated losses/reactions of others is nonproductive and is a block to problem solving.
Encourage patient to deal with situation in small steps.	May feel overwhelmed/have difficulty coping with larger picture, but can manage one piece at a time.
Provide positive reinforcement for efforts/progress made.	Encourages patient to feel a sense of movement toward recovery.
Encourage patient/SO to communicate feelings to each other.	All those involved may have difficulty in this area (because of the loss of voice function and/or disfigurement) but need to understand that they may gain courage and help from one another.

Collaborative

Refer patient/SO to supportive resources, e.g., psychotherapy, social workers, family counseling, pastoral care.	A multifaceted approach is required to assist patient toward rehabilitation and wellness. Families need assistance in understanding the processes that the patient is going through and to help them with their own emotions. The goal is to enable them to guard against the tendency to withdraw from/isolate the patient from social contact.

NURSING DIAGNOSIS:	**KNOWLEDGE DEFICIT [LEARNING NEED] (SPECIFY)**
May be related to:	**Lack of information**
	Misinterpretation of information
	Lack of recall
	Poor assimilation of material presented
	Lack of interest in learning
Possibly evidenced by:	**Indications of concern/request for information**
	Inaccurate follow-through of instruction
	Inappropriate or exaggerated behaviors, e.g., hysterical, hostile, agitated, apathetic
PATIENT OUTCOMES/ EVALUATION CRITERIA:	**Indicates basic understanding of disease process, surgical intervention. Demonstrates ability to provide safe care. Uses resources (rehabilitation team members) ap-**

propriately. **Identifies symptoms requiring medical intervention and makes follow-up appointments.**

ACTIONS/INTERVENTIONS	RATIONALE

Independent

Ascertain amount of preoperative preparation and retention of information. Assess level of anxiety related to diagnosis and surgery.

Information can provide clues to patient's postoperative reactions. Anxiety may have interfered with understanding of information given before surgery.

Provide/repeat explanations at patient's level of acceptance. Discuss inaccuracies in perception of disease process and therapies with patient and SO.

Overwhelming stressors are present, and may be coupled with limited knowledge. Misconceptions are inevitable, but failure to explore and correct them can result in the patient's failing to progress toward health.

Provide written directions for the patient/SO to read/have available for future reference.

Reinforces proper information and may be used as a home reference.

Educate the patient and SO about basic information regarding stoma:

Tub baths instead of showers (initially); shampoo by leaning forward; no swimming or water sports;

Prevents water from entering airway/stoma.

Cover stoma with bib/natural fiber scarf (e.g., cotton or silk);

Prevents dust and particles from being inhaled.

Cover stoma when coughing or sneezing;

Normal airways are bypassed, and mucus will exit from stoma.

Smoking is prohibited.

Necessary to preserve lung function. Note: Patient may need extra support and encouragement to understand that quality of life can be improved by cessation of smoking.

Discuss importance of reporting to care giver/physician immediately such symptoms as stoma narrowing, presence of "lump" in throat, dysphagia, or bleeding.

May be signs of tracheal stenosis, recurrent cancer, or carotid erosion.

Develop a means of emergency communication at home.

Permits patient to summon assistance when needed.

Recommend wearing identification tag/bracelet. Encourage family members to become CPR-certified if they are interested/able to do so.

Provides for appropriate care if the patient becomes unconscious, or suffers a cardiopulmonary arrest.

Collaborative

Give careful attention to the provision of needed rehabilitative measures, e.g., temporary/permanent prosthesis, dental care, speech therapy, surgical reconstruction, vocational/sexual/marital counseling, financial assistance.

These services can contribute to patient's well-being and have a positive effect on patient's quality of life.

Adult Respiratory Distress Syndrome (ARDS) (Pre/post-acute Care)

ARDS is the result of pulmonary insult/injury in previously healthy lungs. Acute care is generally managed in the critical care setting.

PATIENT ASSESSMENT DATA BASE

An initial insult is usually followed by a latent period when pulmonary function appears normal, but gradually deteriorates by stages into respiratory failure. Physical findings vary, depending on the stage at which the diagnosis is made. Early signs are often missed, because abnormal findings are not evident until later stages.

CIRCULATION

May report:
History of recent cardiac surgery/cardiopulmonary bypass, current embolic phenomena (blood, air, fat), anaphylactic episode.

May exhibit:
Blood pressure: may be normal or elevated initially (progressing hypoxemia), hypotension occurs in later stages (shock).

Heart rate: tachycardia usually present.

Heart sounds: normal in early stages; S_2 (pulmonic component) may develop. Dysrhythmias can occur.

Skin and mucous membranes: may be pale, cool. Cyanosis usually develops (late stages).

EGO INTEGRITY

May report:
Feelings of impending doom.

May exhibit:
Restlessness, trembling, irritability, changes in mentation, or obtundation.

Insomnia.

Cardiovascular excitation.

FOOD/FLUID

May report:
Loss of appetite, nausea.

May exhibit:
Edema formation/changes in weight.

Loss of/diminished bowel sounds.

NEUROSENSORY

May report/ exhibit:
Current head trauma.

RESPIRATION

May report:
Current aspiration/near drowning, smoke/gas inhalation, diffuse pulmonary infections.

Sudden or gradual onset of breathing difficulty, "air hunger."

May exhibit:
Increased respirations.

Increased work of breathing; use of accessory muscles of respiration, e.g., intercostal or substernal retractions, nasal flaring.

Breath sounds: may be normal initially. Crackles, rhonchi, and bronchial breath sounds may develop.

Chest percussion: dull over consolidated areas.

Decreased or unequal chest expansion.

Increased fremitus (vibratory tremors in chest wall noted with palpation).

Pallor or cyanosis.

SAFETY

May report: Current history of orthopedic trauma/fractures, sepsis.

TEACHING/LEARNING

May report: Current drug ingestion/overdose.

Discharge Plan Considerations: Assistance with self-care, homemaker tasks.

DIAGNOSTIC STUDIES

Chest x-ray: unremarkable in initial stages or may reveal minimal scattered infiltrates. In later stages, diffuse bilateral interstitial and alveolar infiltrates become evident and may involve all lung lobes.

ABGs: serial comparisons show progressing hypoxemia (decreasing PaO_2 which does not respond to therapy), poorly responsive to increased concentrations of inspired oxygen. Hypocapnea (decreased level of carbon dioxide) may be present in initial stages due to compensatory hyperventilation. Hypercapnea ($PaCO_2$ greater than 50) reflects ventilatory failure. Respiratory alkalosis (pH greater than 7.45) may occur in early stages, but respiratory acidosis occurs in later stages due to increased deadspace and decreased alveolar ventilation. Metabolic acidosis may also occur in later stages due to rising blood lactate levels, resulting from anaerobic metabolism.

Pulmonary function tests: lung compliance and lung volumes are decreased, especially functional residual capacity (FRC). Increased deadspace (V_D/V_T) is produced by areas where vasoconstriction and microemboli have occurred.

Shunt measurement (Qs/Qt): measures pulmonary blood flow versus systemic blood flow, which provides a clinical measurement of intrapulmonary shunting.

Alveolar–arterial gradient (A–a gradient): provides a comparison of the oxygen tension within alveoli and arterial blood.

NURSING PRIORITIES

1. Promote/maintain optimal respiratory function and oxygenation.
2. Minimize/prevent complications.
3. Maintain adequate nutrition for healing/respiratory function.
4. Provide for emotional support of patient and family.
5. Provide information about disease process, prognosis, and treatment needs.

DISCHARGE CRITERIA

1. Breathing spontaneously with appropriate lung tidal volumes.
2. Breath sounds clear/clearing.
3. Free of preventable complications.
4. Dealing realistically with current situation.
5. Disease process, prognosis, and individual therapeutic regimen understood.

NURSING DIAGNOSIS:	**AIRWAY CLEARANCE, INEFFECTIVE**
May be related to:	**Loss of airway cilia function (hypoperfusion)**
	Increased amount/viscosity of pulmonary secretions
	Increased airway resistance (interstitial edema)
Possibly evidenced by:	**Complaints of dyspnea**
	Changes in depth/rate of respiration, use of accessory muscles for breathing

185

Cough (effective or ineffective) with/without sputum production

Anxiety/restlessness

PATIENT OUTCOMES/ EVALUATION CRITERIA: Verbalizes relief from dyspnea. Maintains patent airway with breath sounds clear/absence of rhonchi. Expectorates secretions without difficulty. Demonstrates behaviors to improve/maintain airway clearance.

ACTIONS/INTERVENTIONS	RATIONALE

Independent

Note changes in respiratory effort and patterns of breathing.

Use of intercostal/abdominal/neck muscles and flaring of nares reflects increased respiratory effort.

Observe for decreased chest wall expansion and presence of/increase in fremitus.

Chest expansion may be limited or unequal due to accumulation of fluid, edema, and secretions in sections/lobes. Lung consolidation and fluid-filled areas may increase fremitus.

Note characteristics of breath sounds. (Refer to ND: Gas Exchange, Impaired, p. 187.)

Breath sounds reflect air flow through the tracheobronchial tree and are affected by the presence of fluid, mucus, or other obstruction to air flow. Wheezes may be evidence of bronchoconstriction or airway narrowing due to edema. Rhonchi clear with cough and reflect collection of mucus in the airway.

Note characteristics of cough (e.g., persistent, effective/ineffective) as well as production and characteristics of sputum.

Cough characteristics may change depending on the cause/etiology of the respiratory failure. Sputum, if present, may be thick/viscous, bloody, copious, and/or purulent.

Facilitate maintenance of patent upper airways by proper positioning, and the use of airway adjuncts as needed.

Altered levels of consciousness, sedation, and maxillofacial trauma are some conditions that alter patient's ability to protect airway and require intervention.

Assist with coughing/deep breathing exercises, position changes, and suctioning as indicated.

Pooled secretions impair ventilation and predispose to the development of atelectasis and pulmonary infections.

Increase oral intake if possible.

In the absence of heart failure or pulmonary edema and if the patient is not intubated, an increased oral fluid intake may liquefy secretions/enhance expectoration.

Collaborative

Administer humidified oxygen, IV fluids, and/or room humidity.

Humidity loosens and mobilizes secretions, and promotes the transport of oxygen.

Provide aerosol therapy, ultrasonic nebulization.

Treatments may be initiated to forcefully deliver oxygen/bronchodilation/humidity to alveoli and to mobilize secretions.

Assist with/administer chest physiotherapy, e.g., postural drainage, chest percussion/vibration, as indicated.

Enhances drainage/elimination of lung secretions into central bronchi, where they may more readily be coughed or suctioned out. Promotes efficient use of respiratory muscles and helps reexpand alveoli.

Administer bronchodilators, e.g., aminophylline, albuterol (Proventil), isoetharine (Bronkosol); mucolytic agents, e.g., acetylcysteine (Mucomyst), guaifenesin (Robitussin). Monitor for adverse side effects, e.g., tachycardia, hypertension, tremor, insomnia.

Medications are given to relieve bronchospasm, reduce viscosity of secretions, improve ventilation and facilitate removal of secretions.

186

NURSING DIAGNOSIS: GAS EXCHANGE, IMPAIRED

May be related to: Accumulation of protein and fluid in interstitial/alveolar spaces

Alveolar hypoventilation

Loss of surfactant causing alveolar collapse

Possibly evidenced by: Tachypnea, use of accessory muscles, cyanosis

Changes in ABGs, A–a gradient, and shunt measurement

Ventilation/perfusion mismatching with increased dead-space and intrapulmonary shunting

PATIENT OUTCOMES/ EVALUATION CRITERIA: Demonstrates improved ventilation and adequate oxygenation by ABGs within normal ranges and free of symptoms of respiratory distress. Participates in treatment regimen within ability/situation.

ACTIONS/INTERVENTIONS	RATIONALE
Independent	
Assess respiratory status frequently, noting increased respiratory rate/effort, or change in breathing pattern.	Tachypnea is a compensatory mechanism for hypoxemia, and increased respiratory effort may reflect the degree of hypoxemia.
Note presence/absence of breath sounds, and the presence of adventitious sounds, e.g., crackles, wheezes.	Breath sounds may be muffled, unequal, or absent in affected areas. Crackles are evidence of increased fluid in tissue spaces as a result of increased alveolar–capillary membrane permeability. Wheezes may be evidence of bronchoconstriction and/or airway narrowing due to mucus/edema.
Assess for presence of cyanosis.	Usually a significant drop in oxygenation (desaturation of 5 g of hemoglobin) occurs before cyanosis appears. Central cyanosis of "warm organs," e.g., tongue, lips, and earlobes, is most indicative of systemic hypoxemia. Peripheral cyanosis of nailbeds/extremities is associated with vasoconstriction.
Observe for drowsiness, apathy, inattentiveness, restlessness, confusion, somnolence.	May reflect progressing hypoxemia and/or acidosis.
Auscultate heart rate and rhythm.	Hypoxemia can cause irritability of the myocardium, producing a variety of dysrhythmias.
Provide for rest periods and a quiet environment.	Conserves patient's energy reducing oxygen requirements.
Demonstrate/encourage the use of pursed-lip breathing if indicated.	May be especially helpful for patients who are recovering from prolonged/severe illness, resulting in lung parenchymal destruction.
Collaborative	
Administer supplemental oxygen by cannula/mask as indicated.	Maximizes available oxygen for exchange, and reduces work of breathing.

187

ACTIONS/INTERVENTIONS	RATIONALE

Collaborative

Assist with/provide IPPB treatments.

Promotes full expansion of lungs to improve oxygenation and to administer nebulized medications into respiratory passages. Intubation and ventilatory support are suggested when the PaO_2 is less than 60 mmHg and does not respond to other methods of oxygenation.

Review serial chest x-rays.

Shows progression or resolution of pulmonary congestion.

Monitor/graph serial ABGs.

Reflects ventilation/oxygenation and acid/base status. Used as a basis for evaluating effectiveness of therapies or indicator of need for changes in therapy.

Administer medications as indicated, e.g., steroids, antibiotics, bronchodilators, expectorants.

Steroids may be of benefit in reducing inflammation, and promoting surfactant production. Bronchodilators/expectorants promote airway clearance. Antibiotics may be indicated in presence of pulmonary infections/sepsis to treat causative pathogen.

NURSING DIAGNOSIS:	FLUID VOLUME DEFICIT, POTENTIAL
May be related to:	**Use of diuretics**
	Compartmental fluid shifts
Possibly evidenced by:	**[Not applicable; presence of signs and symptoms establishes an *actual* diagnosis.]**
PATIENT OUTCOMES/ EVALUATION CRITERIA:	**Demonstrates normal fluid volume as evidenced by blood pressure, heart rate, weight, urine output within patient's normal limits and clearing breath sounds.**

ACTIONS/INTERVENTIONS	RATIONALE

Independent

Monitor vital signs, e.g., blood pressure, heart rate, pulses (equality and volume).

Volume depletion/fluid shifts may increase heart rate, lower BP, and diminish volume of pulses.

Note changes in mentation, skin turgor, hydration of mucous membranes, character of sputum.

Decreased cardiac output affects cerebral perfusion/function. Fluid deficit can also be identified by decreased skin turgor, dry mucous membranes, and thick viscous secretions.

Measure/calculate intake, output, and fluid balance. Note insensible losses.

Provides information about general fluid status. Sequential negative fluid balances may indicate developing deficit.

Weigh daily.

Rapid changes suggest alterations in total body water.

Collaborative

Administer fluids under close observation/with control devices as indicated.

Restores/maintains circulatory volume and osmotic pressure. Note: In spite of fluid deficits, fluid administration may result in increased pulmonary congestion, negatively affecting respiratory function.

ACTIONS/INTERVENTIONS

Collaborative

Monitor/replace electrolytes as indicated.

RATIONALE

Electrolytes, especially potassium, sodium may be depleted as a result of diuretic therapy.

NURSING DIAGNOSIS:	ANXIETY/FEAR [SPECIFY LEVEL]
May be related to:	Situational crisis
	Threat to/change in health status; fear of death
	Physiologic factors (hypoxemia)
Possibly evidenced by:	Expressed concern regarding changes in life events
	Increased tension and helplessness
	Apprehension, fear, restlessness
PATIENT OUTCOMES/ EVALUATION CRITERIA:	Verbalizes awareness of feelings of anxiety and healthy ways to deal with them. Acknowledges and discusses fears. Appears relaxed and reports anxiety is reduced to a manageable level. Demonstrates problem solving and uses resources effectively.

ACTIONS/INTERVENTIONS

Independent

Identify patient's perception of the threat represented by the situation.

Encourage patient to acknowledge and express feelings.

Acknowledge reality of stress without denial or reassurance that everything will be all right. Provide information about measures being taken to correct/ alleviate condition.

Identify techniques patient has used previously to cope with anxiety.

Assist SO to respond in a positive manner to patient/ situation.

RATIONALE

Helps with recognition of extent of anxiety/fear and identification of measures that may be helpful for the individual.

Initial step in managing feelings is identification and expression. Encourages acceptance of situation and own ability to handle.

Helps patient to accept what is happening and can reduce level of anxiety. False reassurance is not helpful, because neither nurse nor patient knows the final outcome. Information can provide reassurance/help reduce fear of the unknown.

Focuses attention on skills patient already possesses, promoting sense of control.

Promotes reduction of anxiety to see others remaining calm. Because anxiety is contagious, if SO/staff exhibit their anxiety, the patient's coping abilities can be adversely affected.

(Refer to CP: Psychosocial Aspects of Acute Care, p. 773.)

NURSING DIAGNOSIS:	KNOWLEDGE DEFICIT [LEARNING NEED] (SPECIFY)
May be related to:	Lack of information about disease process and related therapies

	Misinterpretation of information
	Lack of recall
Possibly evidenced by:	Request for information
	Statement of concerns
PATIENT OUTCOMES/ EVALUATION CRITERIA:	Explains relationship between disease process and therapy. Describes/verbalizes dietary, medication, and activity regimen. Correctly identifies signs and symptoms requiring medical attention, and plans for follow-up care.

ACTIONS/INTERVENTIONS

Independent

Provide information concerning the cause/onset of disease process to patient/SO.

Instruct in preventive measures, if needed. Discuss avoidance of overexertion and importance of maintaining regular rest periods; avoiding chilling/cold environment and persons with infections.

Pace learning sessions to meet patient's needs. Give information in clear/concise ways. Assess potential for cooperation with home treatment regimen. Include SO in sessions as indicated.

Provide verbal and written information concerning medications, e.g., purpose, side effects, route, dose, schedules.

Provide guidelines for activity program.

Discuss follow-up care plan, e.g., doctor visits, diagnostic pulmonary function tests, and signs/symptoms requiring emergent and/or nonemergent medical attention.

(Refer to CP: Chronic Obstructive Pulmonary Disease (COPD), p. 128.)

RATIONALE

ARDS is a complication, not a primary diagnosis. Patient/SO are often confused by its development in a previously "healthy" respiratory system.

Lowered resistance persists for a period of time following recovery. Control/avoidance of exposure to environmental factors such as smoke inhalation, allergic reactions to drugs, or infections may be required to avoid further complications.

Recovery from respiratory compromise/failure may severely hamper the patient's attention span, concentration and energy for accepting new information/tasks. SO especially needs to be involved when disease process is severe or recovery limited.

Providing instruction for safe medication use enables patient to appropriately follow through with medical regimen. Written guidelines are useful for later referral.

Patient should avoid overfatigue and intersperse rest periods with activity in order to increase strength/stamina and prevent excessive oxygen consumption/demand.

Understanding reason and need for follow-up care as well as what constitutes a need for medical attention promotes patient participation and may enhance cooperation with medical regimen.

Ventilatory Assistance (Mechanical) _____

More and more patients on ventilators are being transferred from ICU to medical–surgical units with problems such as (1) neuromuscular deficits, e.g., quadriplegia with phrenic nerve injury or high C-spine injuries, Guillain-Barré and ALS; (2) chronic obstructive pulmonary disease with respiratory atrophy and malnutrition (inability to wean); (3) restrictive conditions of chest or lungs, e.g., kyphoscoliosis, interstitial fibrosis.

Volume-cycled ventilators are usually used for long-term ventilation of those patients whose permanent changes in lung compliance and resistance require increased pressure to provide adequate ventilation (e.g., COPD).

Pressure-cycled ventilators are desirable for those patients with relatively normal lung compliance who cannot initiate or sustain respiration because of muscular/phrenic nerve involvement (e.g., quadriplegics).

PATIENT ASSESSMENT DATA BASE

Data gathered are dependent on the underlying pathophysiology and/or reason for ventilatory support. Refer to the appropriate care plan.

DIAGNOSTIC STUDIES

ABGs: assesses status of oxygenation and ventilation and acid–base balance.

Vital capacity (VC): is reduced in restrictive chest or lung conditions; is normal or increased in COPD; normal to decreased in neuromuscular diseases (Guillain-Barré); decreased in conditions limiting thoracic movement (kyphoscoliosis).

Forced vital capacity (FVC): reduced in restrictive conditions, reduced in asthma, normal to reduced in COPD.

Tidal volume (V_T): may be decreased in both restrictive and obstructive processes.

Minute ventilation (V_E): reflects muscle endurance and is a major determinant of work of breathing.

Inspiratory pressure (Pi_{max}): measures respiratory muscle strength (less than -20 cm H_2O is considered insufficient for weaning).

Forced expiratory volume (FEV): usually decreased.

NURSING PRIORITIES

1. Promote adequate ventilation and oxygenation.
2. Prevent complications.
3. Provide emotional support for patient/SO.
4. Provide information about disease process/prognosis and treatment needs.

DISCHARGE CRITERIA

1. Respiratory function adequate to meet individual needs.
2. Complications prevented/minimized.
3. Effective means of communication established.
4. Disease process/prognosis and therapeutic regimen (including home ventilatory support if indicated) understood.

NURSING DIAGNOSIS:	BREATHING PATTERN, INEFFECTIVE
May be related to:	**Respiratory center depression**
	Respiratory muscle weakness/paralysis
	Noncompliant lung tissue (decreased lung expansion)
	Alteration of patient's usual O_2/CO_2 ratio

Possibly evidenced by:	Tachypnea/bradypnea or cessation of respirations when off the ventilator
	Changes in depth of respirations
	Dyspnea/increased work of breathing, use of accessory muscles
	Reduced vital capacity/total lung volume
	Cyanosis
	Anxiety, restlessness
PATIENT OUTCOMES/ EVALUATION CRITERIA:	**Reestablishes/maintains effective respiratory pattern via ventilator (if unable to wean) with absence of retractions/use of accessory muscles, cyanosis, or other signs of hypoxia, and ABGs within acceptable range.** *Care giver* **demonstrates behaviors necessary to maintain respiratory function.**

ACTIONS/INTERVENTIONS	RATIONALE

Independent

Investigate etiology of problem requiring ventilation.	Understanding the underlying cause of the patient's particular ventilatory problem is essential to the care of the patient, decisions about future patient capabilities/ventilation needs and type of ventilatory support that is most appropriate for long-term care.
Evaluate overall breathing pattern.	Patients on ventilator can experience dyspnea/air hunger, and attempt to correct deficiency by over-breathing if able.
Auscultate chest periodically, noting presence/absence and equality of breath sounds, adventitious breath sounds, as well as symmetry of chest movement.	Provides information regarding airflow through the tracheobronchial tree, and the presence/absence of fluid, mucous obstruction. Note: Frequent crackles or rhonchi that do not clear with coughing/suctioning may indicate developing complications (atelectasis, pneumonia, acute bronchospasm, pulmonary edema). Changes in chest symmetry may indicate improper placement of ET tube, development of barotrauma.
Count patient's respirations for 1 full minute and compare to desired/ventilator set rate.	Respirations vary depending on problem requiring ventilatory assistance, e.g., patient may be totally ventilator dependent, or be able to take breath(s) on own between ventilator-delivered breaths. Rapid patient respirations can produce respiratory alkalosis and/or prevent desired volume from being delivered by ventilator. Slow patient respirations/hypoventilation increases $PaCO_2$ levels and may cause acidosis.
Verify that patient's respirations are in phase with the ventilator.	Adjustments may be required in tidal volume, respiratory rate, and/or deadspace of the ventilator; or the patient may need sedation in order to synchronize respirations and reduce work of breathing/energy expenditure.
Elevate head of bed or place in orthopedic chair if possible.	Elevation of the patient's head or getting out of bed while still on the ventilator is physically and psychologically beneficial.

ACTIONS/INTERVENTIONS	RATIONALE

Independent

Inflate tracheal/endotracheal tube cuff properly using minimal leak/occlusive technique. Check cuff inflation every 4–8 hours and whenever cuff is deflated/reinflated.

The cuff must be properly inflated to insure adequate ventilation/delivery of desired tidal volume. Note: In long-term patients the cuff may be deflated most of the time, or a noncuffed tracheostomy tube used.

Keep resuscitation bag at bedside and ventilate manually whenever indicated.

Provides/restores adequate ventilation when patient or equipment problems require that the patient be temporarily removed from the ventilator.

Assist patient in "taking control" of breathing if weaning is attempted/ventilatory support is interrupted during procedure/activity.

Coaching the patient to take slower, deeper breaths, practice abdominal/pursed-lip breathing, assume position of comfort, and use relaxation techniques can be helpful in maximizing respiratory function.

Collaborative

Assess ventilator settings routinely and readjust as indicated:

Controls/settings are adjusted according to patient's primary disease and results of diagnostic testing to maintain parameters within appropriate limits.

Observe oxygen concentration percentage (FIO_2). Verify that oxygen line is in proper outlet/tank; monitor in-line oxygen analyzer or perform periodic oxygen analysis.

FIO_2 is adjusted to maintain an acceptable oxygen percentage and saturation for patient's condition. Because machine dials are not always accurate, an oxygen analyzer may be used to ascertain that patient is receiving the desired concentration of oxygen.

Assess tidal volume (10–15 ml/kg). Verify proper function of spirometer, bellows or computer readout of delivered volume. Note alterations from desired volume delivery.

Monitors amount of air inspired and expired. Changes may indicate alteration in lung compliance or leakage through machine/around tube cuff (if used).

Note airway pressure.

Airway pressure should remain relatively constant. Increased pressure reading reflects (1) increased airway resistance as may occur with bronchospasm; (2) retained secretions; and/or (3) decreased lung compliance asmay occur with obstruction of the ET tube, development of atelectasis, ARDS, pulmonary edema, worsening COPD, or pneumothorax.

Monitor inspiratory and expiratory (I:E) ratio.

Expiratory phase is usually twice the length of the inspiratory rate, but may be longer to compensate for air-trapping to improve gas exchange in the COPD patient.

Check sigh rate intervals (usually 1½ to 2 times tidal volume).

Sighing promotes ventilation of alveoli to prevent/reduce atelectasis, and enhances movement of secretions.

Note inspired humidity and temperature.

Usual warming and humidifying function of nasopharynx is bypassed with intubation. Dehydration can dry up normal pulmonary fluids, cause secretions to thicken, and increase risk of infection. Temperature should be maintained at about body temperature to reduce risk of damage to cilia and hyperthermia reactions.

Check tubing for obstruction, e.g., kinking or accumulation of water. Drain tubing as indicated, avoiding draining toward the patient or back into the reservoir.

Kinks in tubing prevent adequate volume delivery. Water prevents proper gas distribution and predisposes to bacterial growth.

Check ventilator alarms for proper functioning. Do not turn off alarms, even for suctioning. Ascer-

Ventilators have a series of visual and audible alarms, e.g., oxygen, low/high pressure, I:E ratio, etc. Turning

ACTIONS/INTERVENTIONS

Collaborative

tain that alarms can be heard in the nurses' station.

RATIONALE

off/failure to reset alarms places patient at risk for unobserved ventilator failure or respiratory distress/arrest.

NURSING DIAGNOSIS:	AIRWAY CLEARANCE, INEFFECTIVE
May be related to:	Foreign body (artificial airway) in the trachea
	Inability to cough/ineffective cough
Possibly evidenced by:	Changes in rate or depth of respiration
	Cyanosis
	Abnormal breath sounds
	Anxiety/restlessness
PATIENT OUTCOMES/ EVALUATION CRITERIA:	Maintains patent airway with breath sounds clear and aspiration prevented. Patient/care giver identifies potential complications and initiates appropriate actions.

ACTIONS/INTERVENTIONS

Independent

Assess airway patency.

Evaluate chest movement and auscultate for bilateral breath sounds.

Monitor endotracheal tube placement when used. Note lip line marking, and compare with desired placement. Secure tube carefully with tape or tube holder.

Note excessive coughing, increased dyspnea, pressure alarm sounding on ventilator, visible secretions in ET/tracheostomy tube, increased rhonchi.

Suction as needed, limiting duration of suction to 15 seconds or less. Choose appropriate suction catheter. Instill sterile normal saline, if indicated. Hyperventilate with bag before suctioning, using 100% oxygen if appropriate.

Teach coughing techniques, e.g., splinting, timing of breathing, quad cough as indicated.

RATIONALE

Obstruction may be caused by accumulation of secretions, mucous plugs, hemorrhage, bronchospasm, and/or problems with the position of tracheostomy/endotracheal tubes.

Symmetrical chest movement with breath sounds throughout lung fields indicates proper tube placement/unobstructed airflow. Lower airway obstruction (e.g., pneumonia/atelectasis) produces changes in breath sounds such as rhonchi, wheezing.

The endotracheal tube may slip into the right mainstem bronchus, thereby obstructing airflow to the left lung and putting patient at risk for a tension pneumothorax.

The intubated patient has an ineffective cough reflex, or the patient may have neuromuscular or neurosensory problem which causes inability to cough. These patients are dependent on alternate means such as suctioning to remove secretions.

Suctioning should not be routine and duration should be limited to reduce hazard of hypoxia. Suction catheter diameter should be less than 50% of the internal diameter of the ET/tracheostomy tube for prevention of hypoxia. Hyperventilation with bag or ventilator sigh on 100% oxygen may be desired to reduce atelectasis and to reduce accidental hypoxia.

Enhances effectiveness of cough effort.

ACTIONS/INTERVENTIONS

Independent

Reposition/turn periodically.

Encourage increased fluid intake within individual capability.

Collaborative

Administer chest physiotherapy as indicated, e.g., postural drainage, percussion.

Administer IV and aerosol bronchodilators as indicated, e.g., aminophylline, metaproterenol sulfate (Alupent), idoetharine hydrochloride (Bronkosol).

Assist with fiberoptic bronchoscopy, if indicated.

RATIONALE

Promotes drainage of secretions and ventilation to all lung segments, reducing risk of atelectasis.

Helps liquefy secretions, enhancing expectoration.

Promotes ventilation of all lung segments and aids drainage of secretions.

Promotes ventilation and removal of secretions by relaxation of smooth muscle/bronchospasm.

May be performed to remove secretions/mucous plugs.

NURSING DIAGNOSIS:	COMMUNICATION, IMPAIRED: VERBAL
May be related to:	**Physical barrier, e.g., endotracheal/tracheostomy tube**
Possibly evidenced by:	**Inability to speak**
PATIENT OUTCOMES/ EVALUATION CRITERIA:	**Establishes method of communication in which needs can be expressed.**

ACTIONS/INTERVENTIONS

Independent

Assess patient's ability to communicate by alternate means.

Establish means of communication, e.g., maintain eye contact; ask "yes" and "no" questions; provide magic slate, paper/pencil, picture/alphabet board; validate meaning of attempted communications.

Place call light/bell within reach, making certain patient is alert and physically capable of using it. Answer call light/bell immediately. Anticipate needs. Tell patient that nurse is immediately available should assistance be required.

Place note at central call station letting staff know patient is unable to speak.

Encourage family/SO to talk with patient, providing information about family and daily happenings.

RATIONALE

Reasons for long-term ventilatory support are various; patient may be alert and be adept at writing (chronic COPD with inability to be weaned) or may be lethargic, comatose, or paralyzed. Method of communicating with patient is therefore highly individualized.

Eye contact assures patient of interest in communicating; if patient is able to move head, blink eyes, or is comfortable with simple gestures, a great deal can be done with yes/no questions. Pointing to boards or writing is often tiring to patients, who can then become frustrated with the effort needed to attempt conversations. Family members/other care givers may be able to assist/interpret needs.

Ventilator dependent patient may be better able to relax, feel safe (not abandoned) and breathe with the ventilator knowing that nurse is vigilant and needs will be met.

Alerts all staff members to respond to the patient at the bedside instead of over intercom.

SO may feel self-conscious in one-sided conversation, but knowledge that s/he is assisting patient to regain/maintain contact with reality as well as enabling patient

ACTIONS/INTERVENTIONS

Independent

Collaborative

Evaluate need for/appropriateness of talking tracheostomy tubes.

RATIONALE

to feel part of family unit can reduce feelings of awkwardness.

Patients with adequate cognitive/muscular skills may have the ability to manipulate talking tracheostomy tube.

NURSING DIAGNOSIS:	ANXIETY/FEAR
May be related to:	**Situational crises; threat to self-concept**
	Threat of death/dependency on mechanical support
	Change in health/socioeconomic/role functioning
	Interpersonal transmission/contagion
Possibly evidenced by:	**Increased muscle/facial tension**
	Feelings of inadequacy
	Fearfulness, uncertainty, apprehension
	Focus on self/negative self-talk
	Expressed concern regarding changes in life events
	Insomnia; restlessness
PATIENT OUTCOMES/ EVALUATION CRITERIA:	**Verbalizes/communicates awareness of feelings and healthy ways to deal with them. Demonstrates problem-solving skills/behaviors to cope with current situation. Reports anxiety/fear is reduced to manageable level. Appears relaxed and sleeping/resting appropriately.**

ACTIONS/INTERVENTIONS

Independent

Identify patient's perception of threat represented by situation.

Observe/monitor physical responses, e.g., restlessness, changes in vital signs, repetitive movements. Note congruency of verbal/nonverbal communication.

Encourage patient/SO to acknowledge and express fears.

Acknowledge the anxiety and fear of the situation. Avoid meaningless reassurance that everything will be all right.

RATIONALE

Defines scope of individual problem and influences choice of interventions.

Useful in evaluating extent/degree of concerns, especially when compared with "verbal" comments.

Provides opportunity for discussion of concerns, clarifies reality of fears, focuses attention on what needs to be dealt with, and reduces anxiety to a more manageable level.

Validates the reality of the situation without minimizing the emotional impact. Provides opportunity for the patient/SO to accept and begin to deal with what has happened, reducing anxiety.

ACTIONS/INTERVENTIONS	RATIONALE

Independent

Identify/review with patient/SO the safety precautions/measures being taken, e.g., backup power and oxygen supplies, emergency equipment at hand for suction. Discuss/review the meanings of alarm system.

Provides reassurance to help allay unnecessary anxiety, reduce concerns of the unknown; preplans for response in emergency situation.

Note reactions of SO.

Family members have individual responses to what is happening and their anxiety may be communicated to the patient intensifying these emotions.

Identify previous coping strengths, current areas of control/ability.

Focuses attention on own capabilities, increasing sense of control.

Demonstrate/encourage use of relaxation techniques, e.g., focused breathing, guided imagery, progressive relaxation.

Provides active management of situation to reduce feelings of helplessness.

Provide/encourage sedentary diversional activities, e.g., handicrafts, writing, television.

Although handicapped by dependence on ventilator, activities that are normal/desired by the individual should be encouraged to enhance quality of life.

Collaborative

Refer to support groups, therapy as needed. (Refer to CP: Psychosocial Aspects of Acute Care, p. 773.)

May be necessary to provide additional assistance if patient/SO is not managing anxiety or when patient is "identified with the machine."

NURSING DIAGNOSIS:	ORAL MUCOUS MEMBRANES, ALTERED [POTENTIAL]
May be related to:	Inability to swallow oral fluids
	Presence of tube in mouth
	Lack of or decreased salivation
	Ineffective oral hygiene
Possibly evidenced by:	[Not applicable; presence of signs and symptoms establishes an *actual* diagnosis.]
PATIENT OUTCOMES/EVALUATION CRITERIA:	Reports/demonstrates a decrease in symptoms/complaints. Patient/care giver identifies specific interventions to promote healthy oral mucosa as appropriate.

ACTIONS/INTERVENTIONS	RATIONALE

Independent

Routinely inspect oral cavity, teeth, gums for sores, lesions, bleeding.

Early identification of problems provides opportunity for appropriate intervention/preventive measures.

Administer mouth care routinely (and as needed) in the patient with an oral intubation tube, e.g., cleanse mouth with water, saline, or preferred mouthwash. Brush teeth with soft toothbrush, Waterpik, or moistened swab.

Prevents drying/ulceration of mucous membranes and reduces medium for bacterial growth. Promotes comfort.

Change position of endotracheal tube/airway on a regular/prn schedule.

Reduces risk of lip and mouth ulceration.

Apply lip balm, administer oral lubricant solution.

Maintains moisture, prevents drying.

197

NURSING DIAGNOSIS:	NUTRITION, ALTERED: LESS THAN BODY REQUIREMENTS
May be related to:	Altered ability to ingest and properly digest food
	Increased metabolic demands
Possibly evidenced by:	Weight loss
	Aversion to eating
	Reported altered taste sensation
	Poor muscle tone
	Sore, inflamed buccal cavity
	Absence of/hyperactive bowel sounds
PATIENT OUTCOMES/ EVALUATION CRITERIA:	Indicates understanding of individual dietary needs. Demonstrates progressive weight gain toward goal with normalization of laboratory values.

ACTIONS/INTERVENTIONS

Independent

Evaluate ability to eat.

Observe/monitor for generalized muscle wasting, loss of subcutaneous fat.

Weigh as indicated.

Document oral intake if/when resumed. Offer foods that patient enjoys.

Encourage/administer fluid intake of at least 2500 ml/ day within cardiac tolerance.

Assess GI function: presence/quality of bowel sounds; note changes in abdominal girth, nausea/vomiting. Observe/document changes in bowel movements, e.g., diarrhea/constipation; test all stools for occult blood.

Collaborative

Adjust diet to meet respiratory needs as indicated.

RATIONALE

Patient with a tracheostomy tube may be able to eat, but patients with endotracheal tubes must be tube fed or parenterally nourished. (Refer to CP: Total Nutritional Support, p. 894.)

These symptoms are indicative of depletion of muscle energy and reduced respiratory muscle function.

Significant and recent weight loss (7–10% body weight) and poor nutritional intake provide clues regarding catabolism, muscle glycogen stores, and ventilatory drive sensitivity.

Appetite is usually poor and intake of essential nutrients may be reduced. Offering favorite foods can enhance oral intake.

Prevents dehydration that can be exacerbated by increased insensible losses (e.g., ventilator) and reduces risk of constipation.

A functioning GI system is essential for the proper utilization of enteral feedings. Mechanically ventilated patients are at risk of developing abdominal distention (trapped air or ileus) and gastric bleeding (stress ulcers).

High carbohydrates, protein and calories may be desired/needed to improve respiratory muscle function. Carbohydrates may be reduced and fat somewhat increased just prior to weaning attempts to prevent excessive CO_2 production and reduced respiratory drive.

ACTIONS/INTERVENTIONS	RATIONALE
Collaborative	
Provide small frequent feedings of soft/easily digested foods if able to swallow.	Prevents excessive fatigue, enhances intake and reduces risk of gastric distress.
Monitor laboratory studies as indicated, e.g., serum, transferrin, BUN/Cr, glucose.	Provides information about adequacy of nutritional support/need for change.

NURSING DIAGNOSIS:	**INFECTION, POTENTIAL FOR**
May be related to:	**Inadequate primary defenses (traumatized lung tissue, decreased ciliary action, stasis of body fluids)**
	Inadequate secondary defenses (immunosuppression)
	Chronic disease; malnutrition
	Invasive procedure (intubation)
Possibly evidenced by:	**[Not applicable; presence of signs and symptoms establishes an *actual* diagnosis.]**
PATIENT OUTCOMES/ EVALUATION CRITERIA:	**Indicates understanding of individual risk factors. Identifies interventions to prevent/reduce risk of infection. Demonstrates techniques to promote safe environment.**

ACTIONS/INTERVENTIONS	RATIONALE
Independent	
Note risk factors for occurrence of infection.	Intubation, prolonged mechanical ventilation, general debilitation, malnutrition are factors which potentiate patient's risk of acquiring infection and prolonging recovery.
Observe color/odor/characteristics of sputum. Note drainage around tracheostomy tube.	Yellow/green, purulent odorous sputum is indicative of infection; while thick, tenacious sputum suggests dehydration.
Reduce nosocomial risk factors, e.g., proper handwashing by all care givers, maintaining sterile suction techniques.	These factors may be the simplest but are the most important keys to prevention of hospital-acquired infection.
Encourage deep breathing, coughing and frequent position changes.	Maximizes lung expansion and mobilization of secretions to prevent/reduce atelectasis and accumulation of sticky, thick secretions.
Auscultate breath sounds.	Presence of rhonchi/wheezes suggests retained secretions requiring expectoration/suctioning.
Monitor/screen visitors. Avoid contact with persons with upper respiratory infection.	Individual is already compromised and is at increased risk for development of infections.
Instruct patient in proper secretion disposal, e.g., tissues, soiled tracheostomy dressings.	Reduces transmission of fluid-borne organisms.
Provide respiratory isolation when indicated.	Dependent on specific diagnosis the patient may require protection from others or must prevent transmission of infection to others (e.g., tuberculosis).

Independent

Maintain adequate hydration and nutrition. Encourage fluids to 2500 ml/day or cardiac tolerance.

Helps improve general resistance to disease and reduces risk of infection from static secretions.

Encourage self-care/activities to limit of tolerance. Assist with graded exercise program.

Improves general well-being and muscle strength and may stimulate immune system recovery.

Collaborative

Obtain sputum cultures as indicated.

May be needed to identify pathogens and appropriate antimicrobials.

Administer antimicrobials as indicated

One or more agents may be used dependent on identified pathogen(s) if infection does occur.

NURSING DIAGNOSIS:	KNOWLEDGE DEFICIT [LEARNING NEED] (SPECIFY)
May be related to:	**Lack of exposure/recall**
	Misinterpretation of information
	Unfamiliarity with information resources
	Stress of situational crisis
Possibly evidenced by:	**Questions about care, request for information**
	Inaccurate follow-through of instruction
	Reluctance to learn new skills
	Development of preventable complications
PATIENT/SO OUTCOMES/ EVALUATION CRITERIA:	**Participates in learning process. Exhibits increased interest, shown by verbal/nonverbal cues. Assumes responsibility for own learning and begins to look for information and to ask questions. Indicates understanding of mechanical ventilation therapy. Demonstrates behaviors/new skills to meet individual needs/prevent complications.**

Independent

Determine patient/SO ability and willingness to learn.

Physical condition may preclude patient involvement in care before and after discharge. SO may feel inadequate and afraid of machinery and have reservations about ability to learn or deal with overall situation.

Discuss with patient/SO specific condition requiring ventilatory support, what measures are being tried for weaning; short- and long-term goals of treatment.

Provides knowledge base to aid patient/SO in making informed decisions. Weaning efforts may continue for several weeks (extended period of time). Dependence is evidenced by repeatedly increased Pco_2, and/or decline in Pao_2 during weaning attempts, plus dypsnea, anxiety, tachycardia, perspiration, cyanosis.

Encourage patient/SO to evaluate impact of ventilatory dependence on their lifestyle and what changes

Quality of life must be resolved by the ventilator-dependent patient and care givers who need to un-

ACTIONS/INTERVENTIONS	RATIONALE

Independent

they are willing or unwilling to make. Problem-solve solutions to issues raised.

Promote participation in self-care/diversional activities and socialization as appropriate.

Review issues of general well-being: role of nutrition; assistance with feeding/cooking, shopping, etc.; graded exercise/specific restrictions, rest periods, alternated with activity.

Recommend SO/care givers learn CPR.

derstand that home ventilatory support is a 24-hour job that will affect everyone.

Refocuses attention back toward more normal life activities, increases endurance, and helps to prevent depersonalization.

Enhances recuperation and assures that individual needs will be met.

Provides sense of security about ability to handle emergency situations that might arise until help can be obtained.

Collaborative

Schedule team conference. Establish in-hospital training for care givers if patient is to be discharged home on ventilator.

Instruct care giver and/or patient in handwashing techniques, use of sterile technique for suctioning, tracheostomy/stoma care, and chest physiotherapy.

Provide both demonstration and "hands on" sessions as well as written material about specific type of ventilator to be used, function and care of equipment.

Discuss what/when to report to the health care provider, e.g., signs of respiratory distress, infection.

Ascertain that all needed equipment is in place and that safety concerns have been addressed, e.g., alternate power source (generator, batteries), backup equipment, patient call/alarm system.

Contact community/hospital-based services.

Refer to vocational/occupational therapist.

Nurses (e.g., VNA, private), pulmonary services, rehabilitation team need to coordinate care and teaching program to meet individual needs.

Reduces risk of infection and promotes optimal respiratory function.

Enhances familiarity reducing anxiety and promoting confidence in implementation of new tasks/skills.

Helps to reduce general anxiety while promoting timely/appropriate evaluation and intervention to prevent complications.

Predischarge preparations can reduce anxiety associated with transfer. Planning for potential problems increases sense of security for patient/SO.

Suppliers of home equipment, physical therapy, emergency power providers, social services, financial assistance aid in procuring equipment and facilitating transition to home.

Some ventilator-dependent patients are able to resume vocations either while on the ventilator or during the day (while ventilator-dependent at night).

Pulmonary Tuberculosis

Although most frequently seen as a pulmonary disease, tuberculosis may be extrapulmonary and affect organs and tissues other than the lungs. Most patients are treated as outpatients, but may be hospitalized for diagnostic evaluation, adverse drug reactions, or severe illness/debilitation.

PATIENT ASSESSMENT DATA BASE

Data are dependent on stage of disease and degree of involvement.

ACTIVITY/REST

May report: Generalized weakness and fatigue.

Shortness of breath with exertion.

Difficulty sleeping.

Evening or night fever with chills and/or sweats.

Nightmares.

May exhibit: Tachycardia.

Tachypnea/dyspnea on exertion.

Inattention, marked irritability, change in consciousness (advanced stages).

Muscle wasting, pain and stiffness (advanced stages).

EGO INTEGRITY

May report: Recent/long standing stress factors.

Financial concerns.

Feelings of helplessness/hopelessness.

May exhibit: Denial (especially during early stages).

Anxiety, apprehension.

FOOD/FLUID

May report: Anorexia.

Indigestion.

History of weight loss.

May exhibit: Poor skin turgor, dry/flaky skin.

Muscle wasting/loss of subcutaneous fat.

PAIN/COMFORT

May report: Chest pain aggravated by recurrent cough.

May exhibit: Guarding of affected area.

Distraction behaviors, restlessness.

RESPIRATION

May report: Cough, productive or nonproductive.

Shortness of breath.

Chest pain.

May exhibit: Increased respiratory rate (extensive disease or fibrosis of the lung parenchyma and pleura).

Asymmetry in respiratory excursion (pleural effusion).

Dullness to percussion and decreased fremitus (pleural fluid or pleural thickening).

Breath sounds: diminished/absent bilaterally or unilaterally (pleural effusion/ pneumothorax). Tubular breath sounds and/or whispered pectoriloquies over large lesions. Crackles may be noted over apex of lungs during quick inspiration after a short cough (posttussic crackles).

Sputum characteristics: green/purulent, yellowish mucoid, or blood-tinged.

Tracheal deviation (bronchogenic spread).

SAFETY

May report:	Presence of immunosuppressed conditions, e.g., ARC, AIDS, cancer. Positive HIV test.
May exhibit:	Low-grade fever or acute febrile illness.

SOCIAL INTERACTION

May report:	Feelings of isolation/rejection because of communicable disease. Change in usual patterns of responsibility/change in physical capacity to resume role.

TEACHING/LEARNING

May report:	History of exposure to TB. General debilitation/poor health status. Failure to improve/reactivation of TB. Nonparticipation in therapy.
Discharge Plan Considerations:	May require assistance with/alteration in drug therapy; assistance in self-care/home-maker tasks.

DIAGNOSTIC STUDIES

Sputum culture: positive for *Mycobacterium tuberculosis* in the active stage of the disease.

Ziehl-Neelsen (Acid-fast stain applied to a smear of body fluid): positive for acid-fast bacilli.

Skin tests (PPD, Mantoux, tine, Vollmer patch): a positive reaction (area of induration 10 mm or greater, occurring 48–72 hours after interdermal injection of the antigen) indicates past infection and the presence of antibodies but is not indicative of active disease.

ELISA/Western Blot: may reveal presence of human immunodeficiency virus (HIV).

Chest x-ray: may show small infiltrations of early lesions in the upper lung field, calcium deposits of healed primary lesions, or fluid of an effusion. Changes indicating more advanced tuberculosis may include cavitation, fibrous areas.

Histologic or tissue culture: positive for *M. tuberculosis*.

Needle biopsy of lung tissue: presence of giant cells indicating necrosis.

Electrolytes: may be abnormal depending on the location and severity of infection; e.g., hyponatremia caused by abnormal water retention may be found in extensive chronic pulmonary tuberculosis.

ABGs: may be abnormal depending on location, severity and residual damage to the lungs.

Pulmonary function studies: decreased vital capacity, increased dead space, increased ratio of residual air to total lung capacity, and decreased oxygen saturation are secondary to parenchymal infiltration/fibrosis, loss of lung tissue, and pleural disease (extensive chronic pulmonary tuberculosis).

NURSING PRIORITIES

1. Achieve/maintain ventilation/oxygenation.
2. Prevent spread of infection.
3. Support behaviors/tasks to maintain health.
4. Promote effective coping strategies.
5. Provide information about disease process/prognosis and treatment needs.

DISCHARGE CRITERIA

1. Respiratory function adequate to meet individual need.
2. Complications prevented.
3. Lifestyle/behavior changes adopted to prevent spread of infection.
4. Disease process/prognosis and therapeutic regimen understood.

NURSING DIAGNOSIS:	**INFECTION, POTENTIAL FOR [SPREAD/REACTIVATION]**
May be related to:	**Inadequate primary defenses, decreased ciliary action/stasis of secretions**
	Tissue destruction/extension of infection
	Lowered resistance/suppressed inflammatory process
	Malnutrition
	Environmental exposure
	Insufficient knowledge to avoid exposure to pathogens
Possibly evidenced by:	**[Not applicable; presence of signs and symptoms establishes an *actual* diagnosis.]**
PATIENT OUTCOMES/ EVALUATION CRITERIA:	**Identifies interventions to prevent/reduce risk of spread of infection. Demonstrates techniques/initiates lifestyle changes to promote safe environment.**

ACTIONS/INTERVENTIONS	RATIONALE
Independent	
Review pathology of disease (active/inactive phases; dissemination of infection through bronchi to adjacent tissues or via bloodstream/lymphatic system) and potential spread of infection via airborne droplet during coughing, sneezing, talking, laughing, singing.	Helps patient realize/accept necessity of adhering to medication regimen to prevent reactivation/complication. Understanding of how the disease is passed and awareness of transmission possibilities help patient/SO to take steps to prevent infection of others.
Identify others at risk, e.g., household members, close associates/friends.	Those exposed may require a course of drug therapy to prevent spread/development of infection.
Instruct patient to cough and expectorate into tissue. Review proper disposal of tissue and good hand washing techniques. Encourage return demonstration.	Behaviors necessary to prevent spread of infection.
Review necessity of temporary infection control measures, e.g., mask or isolation.	May help to reduce the patient's sense of isolation and remove the social stigma associated with communicable diseases.
Monitor temperature as indicated.	Febrile reactions are an indicator of continuing presence of infection.
Identify individual risk factors for reactivation of tuberculosis, e.g., lowered resistance (alcoholism, malnutrition/intestinal bypass surgery); use of immunosuppression drugs/corticosteroids; presence of diabetes mellitus, cancer; post partum.	Knowledge about these factors helps patient to alter lifestyle and avoid/reduce incidence of exacerbation.

ACTIONS/INTERVENTIONS	RATIONALE

Independent

Stress importance of uninterrupted drug therapy.

Contagious period may last only 2–3 days after initiation of chemotherapy but in presence of cavitation or moderately advanced disease, risk of spread of infection may continue up to 3 months.

Review importance of follow-up and periodic re-culturing of sputum for the duration of therapy.

Aids in monitoring the effects and effectiveness of medications and the patient's response to therapy.

Collaborative

Administer medications as indicated, e.g.:

Isoniazid (INH), ethambutal (Myambutol), rifampin (RMP/Rifadin);

INH is usually drug of choice for patient and those at risk for developing TB. Usually used in combination with other "primary" drugs, especially in the presence of extensive disease. Short-course chemotherapy of INH and rifampin for 9 months with inclusion of ethambutal for first 2 months may be sufficient treatment of uncomplicated pulmonary TB. However, extended therapy (up to 24 months) is indicated for reactivation cases, extrapulmonary TB, or in the presence of other medical problems, e.g., diabetes mellitus or silicosis.

Pyrazinamide (PZA/Aldinamide), para-amino salicylic (PAS), cycloserine (Seromycin), streptomycin (Strycin).

These "secondary" drugs may be required when infection is resistant to primary drugs.

Monitor sputum smear results.

Patient who has three consecutive negative sputum smears, is adhering to drug regimen, and is asymptomatic, judged to be a nontransmitter.

NURSING DIAGNOSIS:	AIRWAY CLEARANCE, INEFFECTIVE
May be related to:	**Thick, viscous or bloody secretions**
	Fatigue, poor cough effort
	Tracheal/pharyngeal edema
Possibly evidenced by:	**Abnormal respiratory rate, rhythm, depth**
	Abnormal breath sounds (rhonchi, wheezes), stridor
	Dyspnea
PATIENT OUTCOMES/ EVALUATION CRITERIA:	**Maintains patent airway. Expectorates secretions without assistance. Demonstrates behaviors to improve/ maintain airway clearance. Participates in treatment regimen, within the level of ability/situation. Identifies potential complications and initiates appropriate actions.**

ACTIONS/INTERVENTIONS	RATIONALE

Independent

Assess respiratory function, e.g., breath sounds, rate, rhythm and depth; use of accessory muscles; ability to

Diminished breath sounds may reflect atelectasis. Rhonchi, wheezes indicate accumulation of

ACTIONS/INTERVENTIONS

Independent

expectorate mucous/cough effectively; character, amount of sputum, presence of hemoptysis.

RATIONALE

secretions/inability to clear airways that may lead to use of accessory muscles and increased work of breathing. Secretions may be very thick because of the infection. Blood-tinged or frankly bloody sputum results from tissue breakdown (cavitation) in the lungs or bronchial ulceration.

Place patient in semi or high Fowler's position. Assist patient with coughing and deep breathing exercises.

Positioning helps maximize lung expansion and decreases respiratory effort. Maximal ventilation may open atelectic areas, promote movement of secretions into larger airways for expectoration.

Clear secretions from mouth and trachea; suction as necessary.

Prevents obstruction/aspiration. Suctioning may be necessary if patient is unable to expectorate secretions.

Maintain fluid intake of at least 2500 ml/day unless contraindicated.

High fluid intake helps to thin secretions, making them easier to clear.

Collaborative

Humidify inspired air/oxygen.

Prevents drying of mucous membranes; helps to thin secretions.

Administer medications as indicated:

Mucolytic agents, e.g., acetylcysteine (Mucomyst);

Mucolytic agents reduce the thickness and stickiness of pulmonary secretions to facilitate clearance.

Bronchodilators, e.g., oxtriphylline (Choledyl), theophylline (Theo-Dur);

Bronchodilators increase lumen size of the tracheobronchial tree, thus decreasing resistance to airflow.

Corticosteroids (Prednisone).

May be useful in presence of extensive involvement with profound hypoxemia and when inflammatory response is life-threatening.

Be prepared for/assist with emergency intubation.

Intubation may be necessary in rare cases of bronchogenic tuberculosis accompanied by laryngeal edema or acute pulmonary bleeding.

NURSING DIAGNOSIS:	GAS EXCHANGE, IMPAIRED [POTENTIAL]
May be related to:	**Decrease in effective lung surface, atelectasis**
	Destruction of alveolar-capillary membrane
	Thick viscous secretions
	Bronchial edema
Possibly evidenced by:	**[Not applicable; presence of signs and symptoms establishes an *actual* diagnosis.]**
PATIENT OUTCOMES/ EVALUATION CRITERIA:	**Reports absence of/decreased dyspnea. Demonstrates improved ventilation and adequate oxygenation of tissues by ABGs within patient's normal ranges and free of symptoms of respiratory distress.**

ACTIONS/INTERVENTIONS	RATIONALE
Independent	
Assess for dyspnea, tachypnea; abnormal/diminished breath sounds; increased respiratory effort; limited chest wall expansion; and fatigue.	Pulmonary tuberculosis can cause a wide range of effects in the lungs ranging from a small patch of bronchopneumonia to diffuse intense inflammation, caseous necrosis, pleural effusion, and extensive fibrosis, resulting in profound symptoms of respiratory distress.
Evaluate change in level of consciousness. Note cyanosis and/or change in skin color, including mucous membranes and nail beds.	Accumulation of secretions/airway compromise can impair oxygenation of vital organs and tissues. (Refer to ND: Airway Clearance, Ineffective, p. 205.)
Demonstrate/encourage pursed-lip breathing during exhalation, especially for patients with fibrosis or parenchymal destruction.	Creates resistance against outflowing air, to prevent collapse/narrowing of the airways, thereby helping to distribute air throughout the lungs and relieving/reducing shortness of breath.
Promote bedrest/activity restriction and assist with self-care activities as necessary.	Reducing oxygen consumption/demand during periods of respiratory compromise may reduce severity of symptoms.
Collaborative	
Monitor serial ABGs.	Decreased oxygen content (PaO$_2$), and/or saturation, or increased PaCO$_2$ indicates need for/change in therapeutic regimen.
Provide supplemental oxygen.	Aids in correcting the hypoxemia that may occur secondary to decreased ventilation/diminished alveolar lung surface.

NURSING DIAGNOSIS:	**NUTRITION, ALTERED: LESS THAN BODY REQUIREMENTS**
May be related to:	**Fatigue**
	Frequent cough/sputum production; dyspnea
	Anorexia
	Insufficient financial resources
Possibly evidenced by:	**Weight 10–20% below ideal for frame and height**
	Reported lack of interest in food, altered taste sensation
	Poor muscle tone
PATIENT OUTCOMES/ EVALUATION CRITERIA:	**Demonstrates progressive weight gain toward goal with normalization of laboratory values and free of signs of malnutrition. Demonstrates behaviors, lifestyle changes to regain and/or to maintain appropriate weight.**

ACTIONS/INTERVENTIONS	RATIONALE
Independent	
Assess and document patient's nutritional status upon admission, noting skin turgor, current weight and de-	Useful in defining degree/extent of problem and appropriate interventions.

207

ACTIONS/INTERVENTIONS	RATIONALE

Independent

gree of weight loss, integrity of oral mucosa, ability/inability to swallow, presence of bowel tones, history of nausea/vomiting or diarrhea.

Ascertain patient's usual dietary patterns, likes/dislikes.	Helpful in identifying specific needs/strengths. Consideration of individual preferences may improve dietary intake.
Monitor intake/output and weight periodically.	Useful in measuring effectiveness of nutritional and fluid support.
Note reports of anorexia, nausea and vomiting and ascertain if related to medications. Monitor frequency, volume, consistency of stools.	May affect dietary choices and identify areas for problem solving to enhance intake/utilization of nutrients.
Encourage and provide for frequent rest periods.	Helps to conserve energy especially when metabolic requirements are increased with fever.
Provide oral care before and after respiratory treatments.	Reduces bad taste left from sputum or medications used for respiratory treatments that can stimulate the vomiting center.
Encourage small frequent meals with foods high in protein and carbohydrates.	Maximizes nutrient intake without undue fatigue/energy expenditure from eating large meals and reduces gastric irritation.
Encourage SO to bring foods from home and to share meals with patient unless contraindicated.	Creates a more normal social environment during meal time and helps meet personal, cultural preferences.

Collaborative

Refer for dietary consult.	Provides assistance in planning a diet with nutrients adequate to meet patient's metabolic requirements and dietary preferences.
Consult with respiratory therapy to schedule treatments 1–2 hours before/after meals.	May help to reduce the incidence of nausea and vomiting associated with medications, or the effects of respiratory treatments on a full stomach.
Monitor laboratory studies, e.g., BUN, serum protein and albumin.	Low values reflect malnutrition and indicate need for/change in therapeutic regimen.
Administer antipyretics as appropriate.	Fever increases metabolism and therefore calorie consumption.

NURSING DIAGNOSIS:	KNOWLEDGE DEFICIT [LEARNING NEED] (SPECIFY)
May be related to:	**Lack of exposure to/misinterpretation of information**
	Cognitive limitations
	Inaccurate/incomplete information presented
Possibly evidenced by:	**Request for information**
	Expressed misconceptions about health status
	Lack of or inaccurate follow-through of instructions/behaviors
	Expressing or exhibiting feelings of being overwhelmed

PATIENT OUTCOMES/ EVALUATION CRITERIA:	**Verbalizes understanding of disease process/prognosis and treatment needs. Initiates behaviors/lifestyle changes to improve general well-being and reduce risk of reactivation of TB. Identifies symptoms for which a physician should be notified. Describes a plan for receiving adequate follow-up care.**

ACTIONS/INTERVENTIONS	RATIONALE

Independent

ACTIONS/INTERVENTIONS	RATIONALE
Assess patient's ability to learn, e.g., level of fear, concern, fatigue, participation level, best environment in which patient can learn, how much content, best media, who should be included.	Learning is dependent on emotional and physical readiness and is achieved at an individual pace.
Identify symptoms that should be reported to physician, e.g., hemoptysis, chest pain, fever, difficulty breathing, hearing loss, vertigo.	May indicate progression or reactivation of disease or side effects of medications requiring further evaluation.
Emphasize the importance of maintaining high protein and carbohydrate diet and adequate fluid intake. (Refer to ND: Nutrition, Altered: Less than Body Requirements, p. 207.)	Meeting metabolic needs helps to minimize fatigue. Fluids aid in liquefying/expectorating of secretions.
Provide instruction and specific written information for the patient to refer to, e.g., schedule for medications.	Written information relieves the patient of the burden of having to remember large amounts of information. Repetition strengthens learning.
Explain medication dosage, frequency of administration, expected action, and the reason for prolonged treatment. Review potential interactions with other drugs/substances.	Enhances cooperation with therapeutic regimen and may prevent discontinuation of medication as patient's condition improves.
Review potential side effects of treatment (e.g., dryness of mouth, constipation, visual disturbances, headache, orthostatic hypertension) and problem-solve solutions.	May prevent/reduce discomfort associated with therapy and enhance cooperation with regimen.
Abstain from alcohol while on INH.	Daily use of alcohol has been linked with increased incidence of hepatitis.
Refer for eye examination after starting and then monthly while taking ethambutal.	Major side effect is reduced visual acuity; initial sign may be decreased ability to perceive green.
Encourage patient/SO to verbalize fears/concerns. Answer questions factually. Note prolonged use of denial.	Provides opportunity to correct misconceptions/alleviate anxiety. Inadequate finances/prolonged denial may affect coping with/managing the tasks necessary to regain/maintain health.
Evaluate job-related risk factors, e.g., working in foundry/rock quarry, sandblasting.	Excessive exposure to silicone dust enhances risk of silicosis, which may negatively affect respiratory function/bronchitis.
Encourage abstaining from smoking.	Although smoking does not stimulate recurrence of TB, it does increase the likelihood of respiratory dysfunction/bronchitis.
Review how TB is transmitted (e.g., primarily by inhalation of airborne organisms but may also spread through stools or urine if infection is present in these systems) and hazards of reactivation.	Knowledge may reduce risk of transmission/reactivation. Complications associated with reactivation include cavitation, abscess formation, destructive emphysema, spontaneous pneumothorax, diffuse interstitial fibrosis, serous effusion, empyema, bronchiectasis, hemoptysis, GI ulceration, bronchopleural fistula, tuberculous laryngitis, and miliary spread.

209

CHAPTER 6
NEUROLOGIC

Headache

Headaches may be the most common of all pains experienced by people, are usually a symptom of an underlying disorder, and may occur with or without the presence of organic disease.

Migraine:
Cause: Unknown, however thought to result from intracranial blood vessel spasms. Similar periodic episodes can occur over an extended period of time.

Population: More frequently seen in teenage and early adult women; may be associated history of asthma or allergies; may be familial.

Pain characteristics: May be generalized or unilateral, throbbing quality. May begin around one eye and/or spread to both. May be preceded by aura and/or accompanied by symptoms of gastric distress (anorexia, nausea, vomiting).

Associated with: Stress, overwork, fatigue, bright lights, loud noise, alcohol, other dietary sources (chocolate, cheese, wines, onions, avocados, MSG).

Cluster:
Cause: Thought to be vascular; however, histamine seems to play a role.

Population: More common in adolescents and adult males.

Pain characteristics: Paroxysmal, abrupt, nonthrobbing, unilateral, intense; involves eye, temple, neck, face. Nasal stuffiness, fluid accumulation under eyes, rhinorrhea, facial flushing. Usually lasts 30–90 minutes. Periods of remission occur.

Associated with: REM sleep, frequently awakening patient; may follow alcohol consumption; emotional upset.

Muscle Tension:
Cause: Sustained muscle contractions around scalp, face, neck, upper body, possible cranial artery vasodilation.

Population: Adults, increased incidence in females.

Pain characteristics: Gradual onset, bilateral, pressure, nonthrobbing, intermittent, moderate, fronto-occipital, feeling of tightness/stiffness, aching. May be unrelieved for extended periods of time.

Associated with: Fatigue, strain/stress, depression.

Other:
Meningeal headache: Result of meningeal irritation. Severe, generalized, constant pain. May radiate down the neck. Associated with malaise, fever, vomiting, confusion, irritability, excitability, and nuchal rigidity.

Brain tumor headache: Result of a space-occupying lesion creating increased intracranial pressure. Pain is intense, steady, generalized or intermittent, frequently awakens patient. May be localized, positional. Associated with visual changes, aphasia, seizures, mental changes, papilledema, progressive weakness on one side.

Temporal arteritis headache: Unilateral or bilateral pain over the temporal area, usually unremitting, throbbing, severe, aching, burning. Occurs in patients 50 and over. Anorexia and fever may accompany the headache.

Exertion headache: Transient. Frontal area with severe pain during exertion such as coughing, sneezing, stooping, straining.

Posttraumatic headache: Occurs after head injury trauma. May be severe, chronic, continuous or intermittent, localized or generalized, variable in intensity, worsened by emotional disturbances, position changes. Vertigo, irritability, insomnia, inability to concentrate may be present.

Sinus headache: Gradual onset. Morning headache is worse. Pain is dull, the pressure positionally aggravated, and may be severe, frontal, or occur on one side of face. Purulent nasal drainage may be present.

PATIENT ASSESSMENT DATA BASE

Data gathered are dependent on type/cause of headache.

ACTIVITY/REST

May report:	Limitations imposed by condition.
	Eye strain, difficulty reading, weakness.
	Insomnia, early morning awakening with pain.
	Aggravation of headache by changes in posture or exertion.

CIRCULATION

May report:	History of hypertension.
May exhibit:	Hypertension.
	Vascular pulsation, e.g., temporal area.
	Pallor, facial flushing.

EGO INTEGRITY

May report:	Specific emotional/environmental stress factors.
	Feelings of helplessness, hopelessness, powerlessness.
May exhibit:	Apprehension, anxiety, irritability (during headache).
	Repression/defense mechanisms (chronic headaches).

FOOD/FLUID

May report:	Intake of foods high in vasoactive substances: e.g., caffeine, chocolate, onions, cheese, alcohol, wine, avocados, MSG, sausages, hot dogs, lunch meats, tomatoes, fatty foods, oranges.
	Nausea/vomiting (during headache).
	Weight loss.

NEUROSENSORY

May report:	History of recent head injury, trauma, stroke, cranial infection, craniotomy.
	History of seizures.
	Aura: visual, olfactory, tinnitus.
	Dizziness, disorientation (during headache).
	Visual changes.
	Epistaxis.
	Paresthesias, temporary one-sided paralysis.
May exhibit:	Changes in speech pattern/thought processes.
	Decreased deep tendon reflexes.

PAIN/COMFORT

May report:	Characteristics of pain dependent on type of headache.
	Unsuccessful attempts at self medication with OTC or prescription drugs.

May exhibit:	Facial mask of pain, flushing, pallor.
	Narrowed focus.
	Self-focus.
	Emotional response, e.g., crying.
	Nuchal rigidity.
	Tense musculature in neck area.

SAFETY

| *May report:* | History of allergies/allergic reactions. |
| *May exhibit:* | Gait disturbances, paresthesia, paralysis. |

SOCIAL INTERACTION

| *May report:* | Changes in role responsibilities/social interaction related to illness. |

TEACHING/LEARNING

May report:	Family history of hypertension, migraines, stroke, mental illness.
	Use of oral contraceptives.
	Use of alcohol/other drugs.
Discharge Plan Considerations:	May require alteration of medication/treatments.

DIAGNOSTIC STUDIES

Lumbar puncture: to evaluate/document increased cerebrospinal pressure, presence of abnormal cells, blood, infection.

Electroencephalography: records brain activity during various activities.

Echoencephalography: documents displacement of brain structure due to trauma, cerebrovascular accident, or space-occupying lesion.

CT scans:

Brain: detects intracranial masses, ventricular shifts, or intracranial hemorrhage.

Sinus: detects presence of infection in sphenoidal and ethmoidal areas.

MRI: detects lesions/tissue abnormalities; provides information about biochemistry, physiology, anatomic structures.

Cerebral arteriography: identifies/substantiates vascular lesions (aneurysm, malformations, space-occupying lesions).

Skull x-rays: detects fractures, deviation of structures.

Sinus x-rays: confirms diagnosis of sinusitis and identifies structural problems, jaw malformations (TMJ).

Visual tests: acuity, visual fields, refraction, assists in making differential diagnosis.

CBC: leukocytosis is suggestive of infection; presence of anemia may stimulate migraine.

Sedimentation rate: may be normal, ruling out temporal arteritis.

Electrolytes: imbalance, hypercalcemia may stimulate migraine.

NURSING PRIORITIES

1. Develop strategies to decrease frequency and duration of headaches.
2. Enhance patient comfort.
3. Assist in the detection/elimination of underlying disease.
4. Provide information about cause/treatment/prevention and complications.

DISCHARGE CRITERIA

1. Pain alleviated/managed.
2. Lifestyle changes/behaviors initiated to control/prevent recurrence.
3. Disease condition/process, therapeutic needs understood.

NURSING DIAGNOSIS:	**COMFORT, ALTERED: PAIN, ACUTE/CHRONIC**
May be related to:	**Stress and tension**
	Nerve irritation/pressure
	Vasospasm
	Increased intracranial pressure
Possibly evidenced by:	**Verbal complaints of pain, possibly affected by other factors, e.g., position changes**
	Facial mask of pain, pallor
	Guarding/distraction behaviors, restlessness
	Self-focusing; narrowed focus
	Changes in sleep patterns, insomnia
	Preoccupation with pain
	Autonomic responses
PATIENT OUTCOMES/ EVALUATION CRITERIA:	**Reports pain relieved/controlled. Demonstrates/uses behaviors to reduce recurrence.**

ACTIONS/INTERVENTIONS	RATIONALE
Independent	
Ascertain duration of problem/episodes, who has been consulted, and what drugs and/or therapies have been used.	Expedites choice of appropriate interventions. Helps identify actions that may have been overlooked/not tried or have failed to help in past episodes.
Investigate complaints of pain; note intensity (1–10 scale), characteristics (e.g., dull, throbbing, constant), location, duration, aggravating and relieving factors.	Pain is a subjective experience and must be described by the patient. Identification of pain characteristics and associated factors is essential to choosing appropriate interventions and evaluating effectiveness of therapy.
Identify specific probable pathophysiology, e.g., brain/meningeal/sinus infection, cervical spine injury, hypertension, trauma.	Understanding of underlying condition aids in choosing appropriate interventions.
Observe nonverbal pain cues, e.g., facial expressions, body position, restlessness; crying, withdrawal; diaphoresis; changes in heart/respiratory rate, blood pressure.	Indirect indicators of the presence/degree of pain being experienced. Headaches may be both acute and chronic; so physiologic manifestations may or may not be present.
Assess/correlate emotional/physical components of individual situation.	Factors that affect presence/perception of pain.
Evaluate pain behavior.	May be exaggerated because patient's perception of pain is not believed, or because patient believes SO/care givers are discounting complaints of pain.

213

ACTIONS/INTERVENTIONS	RATIONALE
Independent	
Note effects of pain, e.g., loss of interest in life, decreased activity, weight loss.	Pain may be interfering with life to a serious extent and may lead to development of depression.
Assess degree of personal maladjustment of the patient, such as isolationism.	Patient may be withdrawing from involvement with others/activities because of pain.
Determine issues of secondary gain for the patient/SO, e.g., insurance, mate/family.	These issues need to be recognized/dealt with in order to help patient recover.
Discuss the physiologic dynamics of tension/anxiety with patient/SO.	Knowledge about how these factors influence headache can help with management.
Instruct patient to report pain as soon as it begins.	Prompt recognition promotes early intervention and may reduce severity of attack.
Place in darkened room as indicated.	May be sensitive to light (photosensitivity), which can intensify attack.
Encourage rest in quiet room.	Decreases excessive stimulation, which may aggravate headache.
Apply cold compresses to head.	Promotes comfort by decreasing vasodilation.
Massage head/neck/shoulder area if patient can tolerate touch.	Relieves tension and promotes relaxation of muscles.
Use therapeutic touch, visualization, biofeedback, self-hypnosis, other stress reduction and relaxation techniques.	Provides the patient with some control over pain and/or may alter the pain-sensing mechanism and pain perception.
Encourage patient to use positive affirmations: "I am healing; I am relaxed; I love this life." Ask patient to be aware of internal-external dialogue and say "Stop," "Cancel," when negative thoughts develop.	Negative thinking can increase tension, increasing pain and disability of headache, making situation more intolerable. Recognition of negative messages and use of positive self-talk can reduce tension, decreasing pain of headache.
Observe for nausea/vomiting. Provide ice chips, carbonated beverages, crackers as indicated.	Often accompanies severe headache. Measures may promote comfort.
Collaborative	
Apply moist/dry heat to head, neck, shoulders.	Increases circulation to muscles, promoting relaxation, easing tension.
Administer medications as indicated:	
Analgesics, e.g., acetylsalicylic acid (aspirin), acetaminophen (Tylenol);	Primary treatments of common tension headaches, are only occasionally useful for vascular headaches.
Mild muscle relaxants, e.g., diazepam (Valium);	Used for general relaxation, sedation and prevention of migraines.
Nonsteroidal antiinflammatory agents, e.g., ibuprofen (Motrin), meclofenamate (Meclomen);	Used for antiinflammatory, analgesic, and antipyretic effect.
Narcotics, e.g., Demerol/codeine;	May be required at times to abort severe headache. Regular use should be restricted/avoided.
Vasoactive agents, e.g., ergotamine tartrate (Gynergen) or methysergide maleate (Sansert);	Cranial vasoconstrictive agents are useful for reducing frequency and intensity of migraine/cluster headaches. Note: Ergot preparations must be given at onset of headache attack.
Beta-blockers, e.g., propanalol (Inderal);	Used to decrease frequency of recurrent vascular headaches.

ACTIONS/INTERVENTIONS	RATIONALE
Collaborative	
Antidepressants, e.g., amitriptyline (Elavil), MAO inhibitors, e.g., isocarboxazid (Marplan);	Alleviates depression, reduces vascular/muscular tension and helps patient cope with situation.
Antiemetics (Tigan);	Reduces discomfort of associated symptoms of nausea and vomiting.
Antibiotics.	Used when brain or sinus infection is present.
Investigate the use of acupressure/acupuncture.	Pressure over the unilateral common carotid decreases blood flow to the brain, resulting in lessening of the pain.
Administer supplemental oxygen as indicated.	Shortens the headache attack by 60–70% in some patients by decreasing hypoxia associated with vascular spasm/constriction.
Assist with/prepare for application of transcutaneous electrical nerve stimulator (TENS) unit.	This device offers a measure of auto-control by interfering with/blocking the transmission of painful stimuli.
Refer to outpatient headache/pain clinic as indicated.	Ongoing team approach to chronic pain control, which may include counseling, highly structured relaxation sessions, exercise, and medications. May be helpful when other relief measures have failed.

NURSING DIAGNOSIS:	**COPING, INEFFECTIVE INDIVIDUAL [POTENTIAL]**
May report:	**Situation crisis**
	Personal vulnerability
	Inadequate support systems
	Work overload/no vacations
	Inadequate relaxation
	Inadequate coping methods
	Severe pain, overwhelming threat to self
Possibly evidenced by:	**[Not applicable; presence of signs and symptoms establishes an *actual* diagnosis.]**
PATIENT OUTCOMES/ EVALUATION CRITERIA:	**Identifies ineffective coping behaviors and consequences. Verbalizes awareness of own coping abilities. Assesses the current situation accurately. Demonstrates lifestyle changes necessary/appropriate to situation.**

ACTIONS/INTERVENTIONS	RATIONALE
Independent	
Assess current functional capacity.	Pain of headache (acute or chronic process) can interfere with coping ability.
Discuss usual coping methods, e.g., alcohol intake, smoking habits, eating patterns, physical and mental relaxation strategies.	Maladaptive behaviors may be used to cope with constant pain or may be contributors to continued pain.

ACTIONS/INTERVENTIONS	RATIONALE

Independent

Treat the patient with courtesy and respect. Take advantage of teachable moments.

Meets psychologic needs, enhancing self-esteem and promoting opportunities for learning new ways to cope with situation.

Assist patient in dealing with change in concept of body image.

Patient may view self as a person "who has headaches" and beginning to see self as well entails seeing self as "one who does not have headaches."

Encourage expression of feelings and discussion of how headaches interfere with work and enjoyment of life.

Enables patient to recognize feelings in relation to pain. Patient may be frustrated with occurrence of headache/treatments and adjustments that need to be made in lifestyle.

Ascertain impact of illness on sexual needs.

Chronic headache interferes with many aspects of the individual's life, and patient may not broach subject unless asked.

Provide information about cause of headache, treatment and expected course.

Understanding this information can help the patient make informed choices, learn to cope with events, and gain a sense of control over situation enhancing self esteem.

Collaborative

Refer for counseling and/or family therapy, assertiveness training classes as indicated.

May need additional help to solve associated problems that are interfering with progress toward wellness.

NURSING DIAGNOSIS:	KNOWLEDGE DEFICIT [LEARNING NEED] (SPECIFY)
May be related to:	Lack of exposure/lack of recall
	Unfamiliarity with information
	Cognitive limitation
Possibly evidenced by:	Request for information
	Statement of misconception
	Inappropriate, exaggerated behavior, e.g., hysterical, hostile, agitated, apathetic
	Development of preventable complications
	Inaccurate follow-through of instructions
PATIENT OUTCOMES/ EVALUATION CRITERIA:	Verbalizes understanding of condition and treatment. Identifies relationship of signs/symptoms to condition. Initiates appropriate lifestyle/behavior changes. Identifies stress situations and specific methods to deal with them.

ACTIONS/INTERVENTIONS	RATIONALE
Independent	
Discuss individual etiology of headache when known.	Influences choice of treatment and progress for recovery.
Assist patient to identify possible precipitating factors, e.g., emotional stressors, temperature extremes, food/environmental allergies.	Avoiding/limiting these factors can often prevent recurrence or frequency of attacks.
Discuss medication regimen/side effects. Review need to reduce/alter medications as indicated.	These patients may become drug-dependent and ignore other forms of therapy.
Instruct patient/SO in activity/exercise program, dietary considerations, and physical comfort measures, e.g., massage.	Exercise when done correctly can alleviate pain by increasing endorphin levels in the brain and patient's pain threshold. Dietary restrictions of vasoactive substances will decrease the frequency of headaches. Massage therapy is important in improving circulation to relax muscle tension.
Discuss importance of good body mechanics/posture.	Decreases strain on the muscles of the neck and shoulder areas, and can provide overall relief of body tension.
Encourage patient/SO to take time for relaxation and fun.	Overzealous sense of duty can lead to neglect of own well-being, adding to stress and contributing to headache.
Encourage use of right brain activities, love and laughter.	Releases body's natural painkillers (endorphins) helping patient to reduce pain of headache.
Encourage use of subliminal music with positive affirmations.	Bypasses logical part of the brain, promoting relaxation.
Encourage patient to keep log of headaches and associated factors/precipitators.	Provides opportunity to identify/control factors that may precipitate a headache.
Provide written information/guidelines.	Resource for the patient to refer to when in doubt about a certain exercise, diet, drug effect/interaction, or side effect.
Identify and discuss potential hazards of unproven and/or nonmedical therapies/remedies.	Patients can become discouraged with lack of relief from standard treatments and seek other sources that not only may not provide relief but may even be harmful.

Seizure Disorders _____

The main causes for seizures can be divided into six categories:

Drugs: poisons, alcohol, overdoses of prescription/nonprescription drugs—the leading cause of seizures.
Chemical imbalances: hyperkalemia, hypoglycemia, and acidosis.
Fever: the most frequent cause in young children.
Cerebral pathology: resulting from head injury, trauma, infections, increased intracranial pressure.
Eclampsia (prenatal hypertension): toxemia of pregnancy.
Idiopathic: unknown origin.

The phases of seizure activity are prodromal (aura), ictal, and postictal. The prodromal phase involves mood or behavior changes that may precede seizure by hours/days. The aura is a premonition of impending seizure activity and may be visual, auditory, gustatory. The ictal stage is seizure activity, usually musculoskeletal. The postictal stage is a period of confusion/somnolence/irritability that occurs after the seizure.

PATIENT ASSESSMENT DATA BASE

ACTIVITY/REST

May report: Fatigue, general weakness.

Limitation of activities/occupation imposed by self/SO/health care provider or others.

May exhibit: Altered muscle tone/strength.

CIRCULATION

May exhibit: Ictal: hypertension, increased pulse, cyanosis.

Postictal: vital signs normal or may be depressed with decreased pulse and respiration.

EGO INTEGRITY

May report: Internal/external stressors related to condition.

Irritability; sense of helplessness/hopelessness.

Changes in relationships.

May exhibit: Wide range of emotional responses.

ELIMINATION

May report: Episodic incontinence.

May exhibit: Ictal: increased bladder pressure and sphincter tone.

Postictal: muscles relaxed resulting in incontinence (urinary/fecal).

FOOD/FLUID

May report: Food sensitivity correlating with seizure activity.

May exhibit: Dental/soft tissue damage (injury during seizure).

Gingival hyperplasia (side effect of Dilantin).

NEUROSENSORY

May report: History of headaches, recurring seizure activity (epilepsy), fainting, dizziness.

History of head trauma, anoxia, cerebral infections.

Presence of aura (stimulation of visual, auditory areas).

Postictal: weakness, muscle pain, areas of parathesia/paralysis.

May exhibit:	*Seizure characteristics:*

Prodromal phase: Vague changes in emotional reactivity or affective response preceding aura in some cases and lasting minutes to hours.

Generalized seizures:

Tonic-clonic (grand mal): Loss of consciousness, dilated pupils, stertorous respiration, excessive saliva (froth).

Postictal: Patient sleeps 30 minutes to several hours; then weak, confused, and amnesic for the episode; with nausea and stiff, sore muscles.

Absence (petit mal): Periods of altered consciousness lasting 5–30 seconds; minor motor seizures may be akinetic (loss of movement), myoclonic (repetitive motor contractions), or atonic (loss of muscle tone).

Partial seizures (complex):

Psychomotor (temporal lobe): Patient generally remains conscious, with psychologic reactions such as irritability, hallucinations, hostility, or fear; involuntary motor symptoms, and behaviors that appear purposeful but are inappropriate (automatism) and include impaired judgment, and on occasion, antisocial acts.

Postictal: Absence of memory for these events.

Partial seizures (simple):

Focal-motor: Often preceded by aura, lasts 2-15 minutes. May produce drowsiness postictally. No loss of consciousness (unilateral), or loss of consciousness (bilateral). Convulsive movements and temporary disturbance in part controlled by the brain region involved (e.g., frontal lobe [motor dysfunction]; parietal [numbness, tingling]; occipital [bright, flashing lights]; posterotemporal [difficulty speaking]). If restrained during seizure, patient may exhibit combative and uncooperative behavior.

Jacksonian: No loss of consciousness (unilateral), or loss of consciousness (bilateral). Seizure activity marches along limb or side of body in orderly progression.

Status epilepticus: Continuous seizure activity (related to abrupt withdrawal of anticonvulsants and other metabolic phenomena).

PAIN/COMFORT

May report:	Headache, muscle/back soreness postictally.
	Paroxysmal abdominal pain during ictal phase (may occur during some partial/focal seizures without loss of consciousness).
May exhibit:	Guarding behavior.
	Alteration in muscle tone.
	Distraction behavior/restlessness.

RESPIRATION

May exhibit:	Ictal: clenched teeth, cyanosis, decreased or rapid respirations; increased mucous secretions.
	Postictal: apnea.

SAFETY

May report:	History of accidental falls/injuries, fractures.
	Presence of allergies.
May exhibit:	Soft tissue injury/ecchymosis.
	Decreased general strength/muscle tone.

SOCIAL INTERACTION

May report:	Problems with interpersonal relationships within family/socially.

TEACHING/LEARNING

May report: Familial history of epilepsy; history of head trauma.

Drug (alcohol) use/misuse.

Increased frequency of episodes/failure to improve.

Discharge Plan Considerations: May require: changes in medications, assistance with self-care activities, and transportation.

DIAGNOSTIC STUDIES

Electrolytes: imbalances may affect/predispose to seizure activity.

Glucose: hypoglycemia may precipitate seizure.

BUN: elevation may potentiate seizure activity or may indicate nephrotoxicity related to medication regimen.

CBC: aplastic anemia may result from drug therapy.

Serum drug levels: to verify therapeutic range of antiepileptic drugs.

Lumbar puncture: detects abnormal pressure, signs of infections, bleeding (subarachnoid, subdural hemorrhage).

Skull x-rays: identifies presence of space-occupying lesions, fractures.

Electroencephalogram: locates area of cerebral dysfunction; measures brain activity.

Video-EEG monitoring, 24 hours (video picture obtained at same time as EEG): identifies exact focus of seizure activity (advantage of repeated viewing of event with EEG recording).

CT scan: identifies localized cerebral lesions, infarcts, hematomas, cerebral edema, trauma, abscesses, tumor; can be done with or without contrast medium.

PET: demonstrates metabolic alterations, e.g., decreased metabolism of glucose at site of lesion.

MRI: localizes focal lesions.

Magnetoencephalogram: maps the electrical impulses/potential of brain for abnormal discharge patterns.

Wada: to determine hemispheric dominance (done as a presurgical evaluation prior to temporal lobectomy).

NURSING PRIORITIES

1. Control seizure activity; protect patient from injury.
2. Maintain airway/respiratory function.
3. Promote positive self-esteem.
4. Provide information about disease process, prognosis, and treatment needs.

DISCHARGE CRITERIA

1. Seizure activity controlled.
2. Complications/injury prevented.
3. Capable/competent self-image displayed.
4. Disease process/prognosis, therapeutic regimen, and limitations understood.

NURSING DIAGNOSIS:	INJURY, POTENTIAL FOR: TRAUMA, SUFFOCATION AND/OR POISONING
May be related to:	**Weakness, balancing difficulties**
	Cognitive/altered consciousness
	Loss of large or small muscle coordination
	Emotional difficulties
	Narrow therapeutic range of medications

Possibly evidenced by:	[Not applicable; presence of signs and symptoms establishes an *actual* diagnosis.]
PATIENT OUTCOMES/ EVALUATION CRITERIA:	Verbalizes understanding of factors that contribute to possibility of trauma, suffocation, and drug toxicity and takes steps to correct situations. Demonstrates behaviors, lifestyle changes to reduce risk factors and protect self from injury. Modifies environment as indicated to enhance safety. Maintains treatment regimen to control/eliminate seizure activity. *Care givers* identify actions/measures to take when seizure occurs.

ACTIONS/INTERVENTIONS	RATIONALE

Independent

ACTIONS/INTERVENTIONS	RATIONALE
Explore with patient the various stimuli that may precipitate a seizure.	Alcohol and various drugs may decrease the seizure threshold. Other stimuli (e.g., loss of sleep, flashing lights, prolonged television viewing) may increase brain activity, thereby increasing the potential for seizure activity.
Keep side rails up and padded with bed in lowest position.	Minimizes injury should seizures (frequent/generalized) occur while patient is in bed.
Encourage patient to smoke only while supervised.	May cause burns if cigarette is accidentally dropped during aura/seizure activity.
Evaluate need for/provide protective headgear.	Use of helmet may provide added protection for individual who suffers recurrent/severe seizures.
Use metal thermometer or obtain temperature via axillary or rectal route if necessary.	Reduces risk of patient biting and breaking glass thermometer if sudden seizure activity should occur.
Keep on strict bedrest if prodromal signs/aura experienced. Explain necessity for these actions.	Patient may feel restless/need to ambulate or even defecate during aura phase, thereby inadvertently removing self from safe environment and easy observation. Understanding importance of providing for own safety needs may enhance patient cooperation.
Stay with patient during/after seizure.	Promotes patient safety.
Insert plastic airway/bite block between teeth (if jaw relaxed). Turn head to side/suction airway as indicated.	Reduces risk of oral trauma but should not be "forced" or inserted when teeth are clenched, because dental and soft tissue damage may result. Also helps maintain airway. Note: wooden tongue blades should not be used, because they may splinter and break in patient's mouth. (Refer to ND: Airway Clearance/Breathing Pattern, Ineffective, p. 222.)
Cradle head, place on soft area, or assist to floor if out of bed. Do not attempt to restrain.	Gentle guiding of extremities reduces risk of physical injury when patient lacks voluntary muscle control. Note: If attempt is made to restrain patient during seizure, erratic movements may increase, and patient may injure self or others.
Document type of seizure activity (e.g., location/ duration of motor activity, loss of consciousness, incontinence) and frequency/recurrence.	Helps to localize the cerebral area of involvement.
Perform neurologic/vital sign check after seizure, e.g., level of consciousness, orientation, BP, pulse/ respiratory rate.	Documents postictal state, and time/completeness of recovery to normal state.

221

ACTIONS/INTERVENTIONS	RATIONALE

Independent

Reorient patient following seizure activity.

Patient will be confused and disoriented after the seizure and need help to regain control, and alleviate anxiety.

Allow postictal "automatic" behavior, without interfering, while providing environmental protection.

May display behavior (of motor or psychic origin) that seems inappropriate/irrelevant for time and place. Attempts to control or prevent activity may result in patient becoming aggressive/combative.

Observe for status epilepticus, e.g., one tonic-clonic seizure after another in rapid succession.

This is a life-threatening emergency that may cause respiratory arrest, severe hypoxia and/or brain and nerve cell damage. Immediate intervention is required to control seizure activity.

Discuss seizure warning signs (if appropriate) and usual seizure pattern. Teach SO to recognize warning signs and how to care for patient during and after seizure.

Enables patient to protect self from injury, and recognize changes that require notification of physician/further intervention. Knowing what to do when seizure occurs can prevent injury/complications and decrease SO's feelings of helplessness.

Collaborative

Administer medications as indicated:

  Antiepileptic drugs (AEDs), e.g., phenytoin (Dilantin), primidone (Mysoline), carbamazepine (Tegretol), clonazepam (Clonopin), valproic acid (Depakene);

These drugs raise the seizure threshold by stabilizing nerve cell membranes, reducing the excitability of the neurons, or through direct action on the limbic system, thalamus, and hypothalamus. Goal is for optimal suppression of seizure activity with lowest possible dose of drug and with fewest side effects.

  Phenobarbital (Luminal);

Potentiates/enhances effects of AEDs and allows for lower dosage to reduce side effects.

  Diazepam (Valium);

May be used as a first-line drug to suppress status seizure activity.

  Glucose, thiamine.

May be given to restore metabolic balance if seizure is induced by hypoglycemia or alcohol.

Monitor/document AED drug levels, corresponding side effects and frequency of seizure activity.

Standard therapeutic level may not be optimal for individual patient if untoward side effects develop/seizures are not controlled.

Monitor CBC, electrolytes, glucose levels.

Identifies factors that aggravate/decrease seizure threshold.

Prepare for surgery/electrode implantation as indicated.

Lobectomy, hemispherectomy or other surgical intervention may be done for intractable seizures, well-localized epileptogenic lesions when patient is disabled and at high risk for serious injury.

NURSING DIAGNOSIS:	**AIRWAY CLEARANCE, INEFFECTIVE [POTENTIAL]/ BREATHING PATTERN, INEFFECTIVE [POTENTIAL]**
May be related to:	**Neuromuscular impairment**
	Tracheobronchial obstruction
	Perceptual/cognitive impairment

Possibly evidenced by:	[Not applicable; presence of signs and symptoms establishes an *actual* diagnosis.]
PATIENT OUTCOMES/ EVALUATION CRITERIA:	Maintains effective respiratory pattern with airway patent/aspiration prevented.

ACTIONS/INTERVENTIONS	RATIONALE
Independent	
Encourage patient to empty mouth of dentures/foreign objects if aura occurs, or to avoid chewing gum/ sucking lozenges if seizures occur without warning.	Reduces risk of aspiration/foreign bodies lodging in pharynx.
Place in lying position, flat surface; turn head to side during seizure activity.	Promotes drainage of secretions; prevents tongue from obstructing airway.
Loosen clothing from neck/chest and abdominal areas.	Facilitates breathing/chest expansion.
Insert bite stick/airway as indicated.	If inserted prior to tightening of the jaw, may prevent biting of tongue and facilitate suctioning/respiratory support if required. Airway adjunct may be indicated after cessation of activity if patient is unconscious and unable to maintain safe position of tongue.
Suction as needed.	Reduces risk of aspiration/asphyxiation.
Collaborative	
Administer supplemental oxygen/hand ventilate as needed.	May reduce cerebral hypoxia resulting from decreased circulation/oxygenation secondary to vascular spasm during seizure.
Prepare for/assist with intubation.	Presence of prolonged apnea postictally may require ventilatory support, which is best accomplished by securing an airway via endotracheal intubation.

NURSING DIAGNOSIS:	**SELF-CONCEPT, DISTURBANCE IN: SELF-ESTEEM; PERSONAL IDENTITY**
May be related to:	**Stigma of epilepsy**
	Perception of being out of control
Possibly evidenced by:	**Verbalization about changed lifestyle**
	Fear of rejection; negative feelings about body
	Change in self-perception of role
	Change in usual patterns of responsibility
	Lack of follow-through/nonparticipation in therapy
PATIENT OUTCOMES/ EVALUATION CRITERIA:	**Identifies feelings and methods for coping with negative perception of self. Verbalizes increased sense of self-esteem in relation to diagnosis. Verbalizes realistic perception and acceptance of self in changed role/lifestyle.**

223

ACTIONS/INTERVENTIONS	RATIONALE

Independent

Discuss feelings about diagnosis, perception of threat to self. Encourage expression of feelings.

Reactions vary among individuals and previous knowledge/experience with this condition will affect acceptance of therapeutic regimen. Verbalization of fears, anger, and concerns about future implications can help patient begin to accept situation.

Identify possible/anticipated public reaction to condition. Encourage patient to refrain from concealing problem.

Provides opportunity to problem-solve responses and provides measure of control over situation. Concealment is destructive to self-esteem (potentiates denial), blocking progress in dealing with problem, and may actually increase risk of injury/negative response when seizure does occur.

Explore with patient current/past successes and strengths.

Focusing on positive aspects can help to alleviate feelings of guilt/self-consciousness and help patient begin to accept manageability of condition.

Avoid overprotecting patient; encourage activities providing supervision when indicated.

Participation in as many experiences as possible can lessen depression about limitations. Supervision needs to be provided for such activities as gymnastics, climbing, water sports.

Determine attitudes/capabilities of SO.

Negative expectations from SO may affect patient's sense of competency/self-esteem and interfere with support received from SO, limiting potential for optimal management.

Stress importance of staff/SO remaining calm during seizure.

Anxiety of care givers is contagious and can be conveyed to the patient, increasing/multiplying individual's own negative perceptions of situation/self.

Collaborative

Refer to support group, Epilepsy Society.

Provides opportunity to gain information, support, and ideas for dealing with problems from others who share similar experiences.

Discuss referral for psychotherapy with patient/SO.

Epilepsy has a profound effect on personal self-esteem, and patient/SO may feel guilt over perceived limitations and public stigma. Counseling can help overcome feelings of inferiority/self-consciousness.

NURSING DIAGNOSIS: KNOWLEDGE DEFICIT [LEARNING NEED] (SPECIFY)

May be related to: Lack of exposure

Information misinterpretation; lack of recall

Cognitive limitation

Failure to improve

Possibly evidenced by: Questions

Increased/lack of control of seizure activity

Noncompliance with drug regimen

PATIENT OUTCOMES/ EVALUATION CRITERIA:	Verbalizes understanding of disorder and various stimuli that may increase/potentiate seizure activity. Initiates necessary lifestyle/behavior changes as indicated. Adheres to prescribed drug regimen.

ACTIONS/INTERVENTIONS

Independent

Review pathology/prognosis of condition, and lifelong need for treatment as indicated.

Review medication regimen, necessity of taking drugs as ordered and not discontinuing therapy without physician supervision. Include directions for missed dose.

Recommend taking drugs with meals if appropriate.

Discuss adverse side effects of particular drugs, e.g., gingival hypertrophy, visual disturbances, nausea/vomiting, rashes, syncope/ataxia, birth defects, aplastic anemia.

Provide information about potential drug interactions, and necessity of notifying other health care providers of drug regimen.

Stress need for routine follow-up care/laboratory testing as indicated; e.g., CBC should be monitored biannually and in presence of sore throat/fever.

Discuss significance of maintaining good general health, e.g., adequate diet, rest; avoidance of exhaustion, alcohol, caffeine, and stimulant drugs.

Review importance of good oral hygiene and regular dental care.

Identify necessity/promote acceptance of actual limitations; discuss safety measures concerned with driving, using mechanical equipment, climbing ladders, etc.

Encourage patient to wear identification tag/bracelet stating the presence of a seizure disorder.

Review possible effects of hormonal changes.

Discuss local laws/restrictions pertaining to persons with epilepsy. Encourage awareness but not necessarily acceptance of these policies.

RATIONALE

Provides opportunity to clarify/dispel misconceptions and present condition as something that is manageable within a normal lifestyle.

Noncompliance is a leading cause of seizure breakthrough. Patient needs to know risks of status epilepticus resulting from abrupt withdrawal of anticonvulsants. Dependent on drug and frequency, patient may be instructed to take missed dose if remembered within a predetermined time frame.

May reduce incidence of gastric irritation, nausea/vomiting.

Promotes involvement/participation in decision-making process, awareness of potential long-term effects of drug therapy and provides opportunity to minimize/prevent complications.

Knowledge of anticonvulsant use reduces risk of prescribing drugs that may interact, altering seizure threshold or therapeutic effect; e.g., Dilantin potentiates anticoagulant effect of Coumadin, whereas INH and chloromycetin increase the effect of Dilantin.

Therapeutic needs may change, and/or serious drug side effects (e.g., agranulocytosis or toxicity) may develop.

May aid in reducing/controlling precipitating factors; enhances sense of general well-being, strengthening coping ability and self-esteem.

Reduces risk of oral infections and gingival hyperplasia.

Reduces risk of injury to self or others, especially if seizures occur without warning.

Expedites treatment and diagnosis in emergency settings.

Alterations in hormonal levels occurring during menstruation and pregnancy may increase risk of seizures.

Although legal/civil rights of persons with epilepsy have improved during the past decade, restrictions still exist in some states pertaining to obtaining driver's license, sterilization, worker's compensation, and required reportability to state agencies.

Craniocerebral Trauma (Acute Rehabilitative Phase)

Craniocerebral trauma (open and closed) includes skull fractures, concussion, cerebral contusion/laceration and cerebral hemorrhage (subarachnoid, subdural, epidural, intracerebral, brainstem).

Primary injury may occur from direct blow to head or indirect (acceleration/deceleration of brain).

Secondary brain injury can result from intracranial hypertension, hypoxemia, hypercapnea, or systemic hypotension.

Consequences range from no neurologic disturbance to a persistent vegetative state or death. Therefore, every head injury must be considered potentially serious.

PATIENT ASSESSMENT DATA BASE

Data are dependent on type, location, and severity of injury and may be complicated by additional injury to other vital organs.

ACTIVITY/REST

May report: Weakness, fatigue.

May exhibit: Altered consciousness, lethargy.

Hemiparesis, quadriparesis.

Unsteady gait (ataxia).

Balance problems.

Orthopedic injuries (trauma).

Loss of muscle tone, muscle spasticity.

CIRCULATION

May exhibit: Normal or altered BP (hypertension).

Changes in heart rate (bradycardia, tachycardia alternating with bradycardia, other dysrhythmias).

EGO INTEGRITY

May report: Behavior changes (subtle or dramatic).

May exhibit: Anxiety, irritability, delirium, agitation, confusion.

ELIMINATION

May exhibit: Bowel/bladder incontinence.

FOOD/FLUID

May report: Nausea/vomiting.

May exhibit: Vomiting (may be projectile).

Swallowing problems (coughing, drooling, dysphagia).

NEUROSENSORY

May report: Transient loss of consciousness.

Vertigo, syncope.

Tingling, numbness in extremity.

Visual changes, e.g., acuity, diplopia, photophobia, loss of part of visual field.

May exhibit: Alteration in consciousness, coma.

Mental status changes (orientation, alertness/responsiveness, attention, concentration, problem solving, emotional affect/behavior, memory).

Pupillary changes (response to light, symmetry), deviation of eyes, inability to follow.

Loss of senses, e.g., taste, smell, hearing.

Facial asymmetry.

Unequal, weak handgrip.

Absent/weak deep tendon reflexes.

Apraxia, hemiparesis, quadriparesis.

Posturing (decorticate, decerebrate); seizure activity.

Heightened sensitivity to touch and movement.

Loss of sensation to parts of body.

Difficulty in understanding self/limbs in relation to environment (proprioception).

PAIN/COMFORT

May report: Headache of variable intensity and location.

May exhibit: Facial grimacing, withdrawal response to painful stimuli, restlessness, moaning.

RESPIRATION

May exhibit: Changes in breathing patterns (e.g., periods of apnea alternating with hyperventilation).

Noisy respirations, stridor, choking.

Rhonchi, wheezes (possible aspiration).

SAFETY

May report: Current trauma/accidental injuries.

May exhibit: Fractures/dislocations.

Impaired vision.

Skin: head/facial lacerations, abrasions, discoloration, e.g., raccoon eyes, Battles' sign around ears (trauma signs).

Drainage from ears/nose (CSF).

Impaired cognition.

Range of motion impairment, loss of muscle tone, general strength; paralysis.

Fever, altered body temperature regulation.

SOCIAL INTERACTION

May exhibit: Expressive or receptive aphasia, unintelligible speech, repetitive speech, dysarthria, anomia.

TEACHING/LEARNING

May report: Use of alcohol/other drugs.

Discharge Plan Considerations: May require assistance with self-care, ambulation, transportation, food preparation, shopping, treatments, medications, homemaker tasks; change in physical layout of home or placement in living facility other than home.

DIAGNOSTIC STUDIES

CT scan (with/without contrast): identifies space-occupying lesions, hemorrhage, determines ventricular size, brain tissue shift.

MRI: uses similar to those of CT scan without use of radioactive contrast.

Cerebral angiography: demonstrates cerebral circulatory anomalies, e.g., brain tissue shifts secondary to edema, hemorrhage, trauma.

227

Brain scan: may be done to locate/identify intracranial hematoma.

Skull x-rays: detect changes in bony structure (fractures), shifts of midline structures (bleeding/edema).

Evoked potentials (BAERs): determines levels of cortical and brainstem function.

PET: detects changes in metabolic activity in the brain.

Lumbar puncture: may be diagnostic for suspected subarachnoid hemorrhage.

ABGs: determines presence of ventilation or oxygenation problems that may exacerbate/increase intracranial pressure.

Serum chemistry/electrolytes: may reveal imbalances that contribute to increased intracranial pressure (IICP)/changes in mentation.

Toxicology screen: detects drugs which may be responsible for/potentiate loss of consciousness.

Serum anticonvulsant levels: may be done to ensure that therapeutic level is adequate to prevent seizure activity.

NURSING PRIORITIES

1. Maximize cerebral perfusion/function.
2. Prevent/minimize complications.
3. Promote optimal functioning/return to preinjury level.
4. Support coping process and family recovery.
5. Provide information about disease process/prognosis, treatment plan, and resources.

DISCHARGE CRITERIA

1. Cerebral function improved; neurologic deficits resolving/stabilized.
2. Complications prevented or minimized.
3. ADL needs met by self or with assistance of other(s).
4. Family acknowledging reality of situation and involved in recovery program.
5. Disease process/prognosis and treatment regimen understood and available resources identified.

NURSING DIAGNOSIS:	TISSUE PERFUSION, ALTERED: CEREBRAL
May be related to:	**Interruption of blood flow by space-occupying lesions (hemorrhage, hematoma); cerebral edema (localized or generalized response to injury, metabolic alterations, drug/alcohol overdose); decreased systemic BP/hypoxia (hypovolemia, cardiac dysrhythmias)**
Possibly evidenced by:	**Altered level of consciousness; memory loss**
	Changes in motor/sensory responses, restlessness
	Changes in vital signs
PATIENT OUTCOMES/ EVALUATION CRITERIA:	**Maintains usual/improved level of consciousness, cognition, and motor/sensory function. Demonstrates stable vital signs and absence of signs of increased intracranial pressure.**

ACTIONS/INTERVENTIONS	RATIONALE
Independent	
Determine factors related to individual situation/cause for coma/decreased cerebral perfusion, and potential for increased intracranial pressure.	Influences choice of interventions. Deterioration in neurologic signs/symptoms or failure to improve after initial insult may require that the patient be transferred

ACTIONS/INTERVENTIONS	RATIONALE

Independent

Monitor/document neurologic status frequently and compare with baseline, such as Glasgow Coma Scale;

to critical care for monitoring of intracranial pressure and/or surgical intervention.

Assesses trends in level of consciousness (LOC) and potential for IICP and is useful in determining location, extent, and progression/resolution of central nervous system (CNS) damage.

Evaluate eye opening, e.g., spontaneous (awake), opens only to painful stimuli, keeps eyes closed (coma);

Determines arousal ability/level of consciousness.

Assess verbal response; note whether patient is alert, oriented to person, place, time, or is confused; uses inappropriate words/phrases that make little sense;

Measures appropriateness of speech and content of consciousness. If minimal damage has occurred in the cerebral cortex, the patient may be aroused by verbal stimuli but may appear drowsy or uncooperative. More extensive damage to the cerebral cortex may be displayed by slow response to commands, lapsing into sleep when not stimulated, disorientation, and stupor. Damage to midbrain, pons, and medulla are manifested by lack of appropriate responses to stimuli.

Assess motor response to simple commands, noting purposeful (obeys command, attempts to push stimulus away) and nonpurposeful (posturing) movement. Note limb movement and document right and left sides separately.

Measures overall awareness and ability to respond to external stimuli and best indicates state of consciousness in the patient whose eyes are closed because of trauma or who is aphasic. Consciousness and involuntary movement are integrated if the patient can both grasp and release the tester's hand or hold up two fingers upon command. Purposeful movement can include grimacing or withdrawing from painful stimuli, or movements that the patient desires, e.g., sitting up. Other movements (posturing and abnormal flexion of extremities) usually indicate diffuse cortical damage. Absence of spontaneous movement on one side of the body indicates damage to the motor tracts in the opposite cerebral hemisphere.

Monitor vital signs, e.g.:

Blood pressure, noting onset of/continuing systolic hypertension and widening pulse pressure; observe for hypotension in multiple trauma patient;

Normally, autoregulation maintains constant cerebral blood flow despite fluctuations in systemic BP. Loss of autoregulation may follow local or diffuse cerebral vascular damage. Elevating systolic BP accompanied by decreasing diastolic BP (widening pulse pressure) is an ominous sign of IICP when accompanied by decreased level of consciousness. Hypovolemia/hypotension (associated with multiple trauma) may also result in cerebral ischemia/damage.

Heart rate/rhythm, noting bradycardia, alternating bradycardia/tachycardia, other dysrhythmias;

Changes in rate (most often bradycardia) and dysrhythmias may develop, reflecting brainstem pressure/injury in the absence of underlying cardiac disease.

Respirations, noting patterns and rhythm, e.g., periods of apnea after hyperventilation, Cheyne–Stokes breathing.

Irregularities can suggest location of cerebral insult/increasing ICP and need for further intervention including possible respiratory support. (Refer to ND: Breathing Pattern, Ineffective [Potential], p. 231.)

Evaluate pupils, noting size, shape, equality, light reactivity.

Pupil reactions are regulated by the oculomotor (III) cranial nerve and are useful in determining if the brainstem is intact. Pupil size/equality is determined by bal-

229

ACTIONS/INTERVENTIONS

Independent

Assess for changes in vision, e.g., blurred vision, alterations in visual field, depth perception.

Assess position/movement of eyes, noting whether in midposition or deviated to side or downward. Note loss of doll's eyes (oculocephalic reflex).

Note presence/absence of reflexes (e.g., blink, cough, gag, Babinski).

Monitor temperature and regulate environmental temperature as indicated. Limit use of blankets; administer tepid sponge bath in presence of fever. Wrap extremities in blankets when hypothermia blanket is used.

Monitor intake and output. Weigh as indicated. Note skin turgor, status of mucous membranes.

Maintain head/neck in midline or neutral position, support with small towel rolls/pillows. Avoid placing head on large pillows.

Provide rest periods between care activities and limit duration of procedures.

Decrease extraneous stimuli, and provide comfort measures, e.g., back massage, quiet environment, soft voice, gentle touch.

Help patient avoid/limit coughing, vomiting, straining at stool/bearing down when possible.

Avoid/limit use of restraints.

Encourage SO to talk to patient.

Investigate increasing restlessness, moaning, guarding behaviors.

Palpate for bladder distention, maintain patency of urinary drainage if used. Monitor for constipation.

RATIONALE

ance between parasympathetic and sympathetic enervation. Response to light reflects combined function of optic (II) and oculomotor (III) cranial nerves.

Visual alterations reflect area of brain involved, indicate safety concerns and influence choice of interventions.

Position and movement of eyes helps localize area of brain involvement. An early sign of increased ICP is impaired abduction of eyes, indicating pressure/injury to the fifth cranial nerve. Loss of doll's eyes indicates deterioration in brainstem function and poor prognosis.

Alterations in reflexes reflect injury at level of midbrain or brainstem and have direct implications for patient safety. Loss of blink reflex suggests damage to the pons and medulla. Absence of cough and gag reflexes reflect damage to medulla. Presence of Babinski reflex indicates injury along pyramidal pathways in the brain.

Fever may reflect damage to hypothalamus. Increased metabolic needs and oxygen consumption occur (especially with fever and shivering), which can further increase ICP.

Useful indicators of total body water which is an integral part of tissue perfusion. Cerebral trauma/ischemia can result in diabetes insipidus (DI) or syndrome of inappropriate ADH secretion (SIADH). Alterations may lead to hypovolemia or vascular engorgement, either of which can negatively affect cerebral pressure.

Turning head to one side compresses the jugular veins and inhibits cerebral venous drainage, thereby increasing ICP.

Continual activity can increase ICP by producing a cumulative stimulant effect.

Provides calming effect, reduces adverse physiologic response and promotes rest to maintain/lower ICP.

These activities increase intrathoracic and intraabdominal pressures, which can increase ICP.

Mechanical restraints may enhance "fight" response, increasing ICP. Note: Cautious use may be indicated to prevent injury to patient.

Familiar voices of family/SO appear to have a relaxing effect on many comatose patients, which can reduce ICP.

These nonverbal cues may indicate increasing ICP or reflect presence of pain when patient is unable to verbalize complaints. Unrelieved pain can in turn aggravate/potentiate IICP.

May trigger autonomic responses potentiating elevation of ICP.

ACTIONS/INTERVENTIONS	RATIONALE
Independent	
Observe for seizure activity and protect patient from injury. (Refer to CP: Seizure Disorders, p. 218.)	Seizures can occur as a result of cerebral irritation, hypoxia or IICP and seizures can further elevate ICP, compounding cerebral damage.
Assess for nuchal rigidity, twitching, increased restlessness, irritability, onset of seizure activity.	Indicative of meningeal irritation, which may occur due to interruption of dura, and/or development of infection during acute or recovery period of brain injury.
Collaborative	
Elevate head of bed 15–45 degrees as tolerated/indicated.	Promotes venous drainage from head, thereby reducing cerebral congestion and edema/risk of IICP.
Administer IV fluids with control device. Restrict fluid intake as indicated.	Fluid restriction may be needed to reduce cerebral edema, minimize fluctuations in vascular load, BP, and ICP.
Administer supplemental oxygen.	Reduces hypoxemia, which may increase cerebral vasodilation and blood volume, elevating ICP.
Monitor ABGs/pulse oximetry.	Determines respiratory sufficiency (presence of hypoxia/acidosis) and indicates therapy needs.
Administer medications as indicated:	
Diuretics, e.g., mannitol (Osmitrol), furosemide (Lasix);	Diuretics may be used in acute phase to draw water from brain cells, reducing cerebral edema and ICP.
Steroids, e.g., dexamethasone (Decadron), methylprednisolone (Medrol);	Decreases inflammation, reducing tissue edema.
Anticonvulsant, e.g., phenytoin (Dilantin);	Drug of choice for treatment and prevention of seizure activity.
Chlorpromazine (Thorazine);	Useful in treating posturing and shivering which can increase ICP. Note: This drug can lower the seizure threshold or precipitate Dilantin toxicity.
Mild analgesics, e.g., codeine;	May be indicated to relieve pain and its negative effect on ICP but should be used with caution to prevent respiratory embarrassment.
Sedatives, e.g., diphenhydramine (Benadryl);	May be used to control restlessness, agitation.
Antipyretics, e.g., acetaminophen (Tylenol).	Reduces/controls fever and its deleterious effect on cerebral metabolism/oxygen needs.
Prepare for surgical intervention if indicated.	Craniotomy or trephination ("burr" holes) may be done to remove bone fragments, elevate depressed fractures, evacuate hematoma, control hemorrhage, debride necrotic tissue.

NURSING DIAGNOSIS:	**BREATHING PATTERN, INEFFECTIVE [POTENTIAL]**
May be related to:	**Neuromuscular impairment (injury to respiratory center of brain)**
	Perception or cognitive impairment
	Tracheobronchial obstruction
Possibly evidenced by:	**[Not applicable; presence of signs and symptoms establishes an *actual* diagnosis.]**

ACTIONS/INTERVENTIONS	RATIONALE
Independent	
Monitor rate, rhythm, depth of respiration. Note breathing irregularities.	Changes may indicate onset of pulmonary complications (common following brain injury), or indicate location/extent of brain involvement. Slow respiration, periods of apnea may indicate need for mechanical ventilation.
Note competence of gag/swallow reflexes and patient's ability to protect own airway. Insert airway adjunct as indicated.	Ability to mobilize or clear secretions is important to airway maintenance. Loss of swallow or cough reflex may indicate need for artificial airway/intubation. Note: Soft nasopharyngeal airways may be preferred to prevent stimulation of the gag reflex by hard oropharyngeal airway, which can lead to excessive coughing and increased ICP.
Elevate head of bed as permitted, position on sides as indicated.	Facilitates lung expansion/ventilation and reduces risk of airway obstruction by tongue.
Encourage deep breathing if patient is conscious.	Prevents/reduces atelectasis.
Suction with extreme caution, no longer than 10–15 seconds. Note character, color, odor of secretions.	Suctioning is usually required if patient is comatose or is immobile and unable to clear own airway. Deep tracheal suctioning should be done with caution, because it can cause or aggravate hypoxia, which produces vasoconstriction, adversely affecting cerebral perfusion.
Auscultate breath sounds, noting areas of hypoventilation and presence of adventitious sounds (crackles, rhonchi, wheezes).	Identifies pulmonary problems such as atelectasis, congestion, airway obstruction which may jeopardize cerebral oxygenation and/or indicate onset of pulmonary infection (common complication of head injury).
Monitor use of respiratory depressant drugs, e.g., sedatives.	Can increase respiratory embarrassment/complications.
Collaborative	
Monitor/graph serial ABGs, pulse oximetry.	Determines respiratory sufficiency, acid–base balance, and therapy needs.
Review chest x-rays.	Reveals ventilatory state and signs of developing complications (e.g., atelectasis, pneumonia).
Administer supplemental oxygen.	Maximizes arterial oxygenation and aids in prevention of hypoxia. If respiratory center is depressed, mechanical ventilation may be required.
Assist with chest physiotherapy when indicated.	Although contraindicated in patient with acute IICP, these measures are often necessary in acute rehabilitation phase to mobilize and clear lung fields and reduce atelectasis/pulmonary complications.

NURSING DIAGNOSIS:	SENSORY-PERCEPTUAL ALTERATION: (SPECIFY)
May be related to:	Altered sensory reception, transmission and/or integration (neurologic trauma or deficit)

Possibly evidenced by:	Disorientation to time, place, persons
	Change in usual response to stimuli
	Motor incoordination, alterations in posture, inability to tell position of body parts (proprioception)
	Altered communication patterns
	Visual and auditory distortions
	Poor concentration, altered thought processes/bizarre thinking
	Exaggerated emotional responses, change in behavior pattern
PATIENT OUTCOMES/ EVALUATION CRITERIA:	Regains/maintains usual level of consciousness and perceptual functioning. Acknowledges changes in ability and presence of residual involvement. Demonstrates behaviors/lifestyle changes to compensate for/overcome deficits.

ACTIONS/INTERVENTIONS	RATIONALE

Independent

Evaluate/continually monitor changes in orientation, ability to speak, mood/affect, sensorium, thought process.

Upper cerebral functions are often the first to be affected by altered circulation, oxygenation. Damage may occur at time of initial injury or develop sometime afterward because of swelling or bleeding. Motor, perceptual, cognitive, and personality changes may develop and persist, with gradual normalization of responses, or remain permanently to some degree.

Assess sensory awareness, e.g., response to touch, hot/cold, dull/sharp, and awareness of motion and location of body parts. Note problems with vision, other senses. (Refer to CP: Cerebrovascular Accident/ Stroke, ND: Sensory-Perceptual Alteration, p. 251.)

Information is essential to patient safety. All sensory systems may be affected with changes involving an increase or decrease in sensitivity or loss of sensation/ ability to perceive and respond appropriately to stimuli.

Observe behavioral responses, e.g., hostility, crying, inappropriate affect, agitation, hallucinations. (Refer to ND: Thought Processes, Altered, p. 234.)

Individual responses may be variable but commonalities, such as emotional lability, lowered frustration level, apathy, impulsiveness exist during recovery from brain injury. Documentation of behavior provides information needed for development of structured rehabilitation.

Document specific changes in abilities, e.g., focusing/ tracking with both eyes, following simple verbal instructions, answering "yes" or "no" to questions, feeding self with dominant hand.

Helps localize areas of cerebral dysfunction and identifies signs of progress toward improved neurologic function.

Eliminate extraneous noise/stimuli as necessary.

Reduces anxiety, exaggerated emotional responses/ confusion associated with sensory overload.

Speak in calm, quiet voice. Use short, simple sentences. Maintain eye contact.

Patient may have limited attention span/understanding during acute and recovery stages, and these measures can help patient to attend to communication.

Ascertain/validate patient's perceptions, provide feedback. Reorient patient frequently to environment, staff, and procedures, especially if vision is impaired.

Assists patient to separate reality from altered perceptions. Cognitive dysfunction and/or visual deficits can potentiate disorientation and anxiety.

ACTIONS/INTERVENTIONS	RATIONALE
Independent	
Provide meaningful stimulation: verbal (talk to patient), olfactory (e.g., oil of clove, coffee), tactile (touch, hand holding), and auditory (tapes, television, radio, visitors). Avoid physical or emotional isolation of patient.	Carefully selected sensory input may be useful for coma stimulation as well as during cognitive retraining.
Provide structured environment, including therapies, activities. Write out schedule for patient (if appropriate) and refer to regularly.	Provides consistency and reassurance, reducing anxiety associated with the unknown. Promotes sense of control/cognitive retraining.
Schedule adequate rest/uninterrupted sleep periods.	Reduces fatigue, prevents exhaustion, provides for REM sleep (absence of which can aggravate sensory-perceptual deficits).
Use day/night lighting.	Provides for normal sense of passage of time and sleep/wake pattern.
Allow adequate time for communication and performance of activities.	Reduces frustration associated with altered abilities/delayed response pattern.
Provide patient safety, e.g., padded side rails, assistance with ambulation, protection from hot/sharp objects. Note perceptual deficit on chart and at bedside.	Agitation, impaired judgment, poor balance, and sensory deficits increase risk of patient injury.
Identify alternate ways of dealing with perceptual deficits, e.g., arrange bed, personal articles, food to take advantage of functional vision; describe where affected body parts are located.	Enables patient to progress toward independence, enhancing sense of control, while compensating for neurologic deficits.
Collaborative	
Refer to physical, occupational, speech, and cognitive therapists.	Interdisciplinary approach can create an integrated treatment plan based on the individual's unique combination of abilities/disabilities with focus on evaluation and functional improvement in physical, cognitive, and perceptual skills.

NURSING DIAGNOSIS:	**THOUGHT PROCESSES, ALTERED**
May be related to:	**Physiologic changes; psychologic conflicts**
Possibly evidenced by:	**Memory deficit/changes in remote, recent, immediate memory**
	Distractibility, altered attention span/concentration
	Disorientation to time, place, person, circumstances and events
	Impaired ability to make decisions, to problem-solve, reason, abstract, or conceptualize
	Personality changes; inappropriate social behavior
PATIENT OUTCOMES/ EVALUATION CRITERIA:	**Maintains/regains usual mentation and reality orientation. Recognizes changes in thinking/behavior. Participates in therapeutic regimen/cognitive retraining.**

ACTIONS/INTERVENTIONS	RATIONALE
Independent	
Assess attention span, distractibility. Note level of anxiety.	Attention span/ability to attend/concentrate may be severely shortened, which both causes and potentiates anxiety, affecting thought processes.
Confer with SO to compare past behaviors/preinjury personality with current responses.	Recovery from head injury includes a phase of agitation, angry responses, and disordered thought sequences/conversation. Presence of hallucinations or alteration in interpretation of stimuli may have been present independent of current condition or be part of developing sequelae of brain injury. Note: SOs often have difficulty accepting and dealing with patient's aberrant behavior and may require assistance in coping with situation.
Maintain consistency in staff assigned to patient as much as possible.	Provides patient with feelings of stability and control of situation.
Present reality concisely and briefly, avoid challenging illogical thinking.	Patient may be totally unaware of injury (amnesic) or of extent of injury, and therefore deny reality of injury. Structured reality orientation can reduce defensive reactions.
Explain procedures and reinforce explanations given by others. Provide information about disease process in relationship to symptoms.	Loss of internal structure (changes in memory, reasoning, and ability to conceptualize) as well as fear of the unknown affect processing and retention of information, compounding anxiety, confusion, and disorientation.
Review necessity of recurrent neurologic evaluations.	Understanding that assessments are done frequently to prevent/limit complications and do not necessarily reflect seriousness of patient's condition may help reduce anxiety.
Reduce provocative stimuli, negative criticism, arguments and confrontations.	Reduces risk of triggering fight/flight response. Severely brain-injured patient may become violent or physically/verbally abusive.
Listen with regard to patient's verbalizations in spite of speech pattern/content.	Conveys interest and worth to individual, enhancing self-esteem and encouraging continued efforts.
Promote socialization within individual limitations.	Reinforcement of positive behaviors (e.g., appropriate interaction with others) may be helpful in relearning internal structure.
Encourage SO to provide current news/family happenings, etc.	Promotes maintenance of contact with usual events, enhancing reality orientation and normalization of thinking.
Instruct in relaxation techniques. Encourage diversional activities.	Can help refocus attention and reduce anxiety to manageable levels.
Maintain realistic expectations of patient's ability to control own behavior, comprehend, remember information.	It is important to maintain an expectation of the ability to improve and progress to a higher level of functioning to maintain hope and promote continued work of rehabilitation.
Avoid leaving patient alone when agitated, frightened.	Anxiety can lead to loss of control and escalate to panic. Support may provide calming effect, reducing anxiety and risk of injury.
Implement measures to control emotional outbursts/aggressive behavior if needed; e.g., tell patient to "stop," speak in a calm voice, remove from the situa-	Patient may need help/external control to protect self or others from harm until internal control is regained. Restraints (physical holding, mechanical, pharmaco-

ACTIONS/INTERVENTIONS

Independent

tion, provide distraction. May need restraint for brief periods of time.

Inform patient/SO that intellectual function, behavior and emotional functioning will gradually improve, but that some effects may persist for months or even be permanent.

Collaborative

Coordinate/participate in cognitive retraining program as indicated.

Refer to support groups, e.g., Brain Injury Association, social services, VNA, and counseling/therapy as needed.

RATIONALE

logic) should be used judiciously to avoid escalating violent, irrational behavior.

Most brain-injured patients have problems with concentration and memory and may think more slowly, have difficulty problem solving. Recovery may be complete, or residual effects may remain.

Assists with learning methods to compensate for disruption of cognitive skills and addresses problems in concentration, memory, judgment, sequencing, and problem-solving.

Additional assistance may be helpful in supporting/sustaining recovery efforts.

NURSING DIAGNOSIS:	MOBILITY, IMPAIRED PHYSICAL
May be related to:	Perceptual or cognitive impairment
	Decreased strength/endurance
	Restrictive therapies/safety precautions, e.g., bedrest, immobilization
Possibly evidenced by:	Inability to purposefully move within the physical environment, including bed mobility, transfer, ambulation
	Impaired coordination; limited range of motion; decreased muscle strength/control
PATIENT OUTCOMES/ EVALUATION CRITERIA:	Regains/maintains optimal position of function, as evidenced by absence of contractures, footdrop. Maintains/increases strength and function of affected and/or compensatory body part(s). Demonstrates techniques/behaviors that enable resumption of activities. Maintains skin integrity, bladder and bowel function.

ACTIONS/INTERVENTIONS

Independent

Review functional ability and reasons for impairment.

Assess degree of immobility, using a scale to rate dependence (0–4).

RATIONALE

Identifies probable functional impairments and influences choice of interventions.

The patient may be completely independent (0) or require minimal assistance/equipment (1), moderate assistance/supervision/teaching (2), extensive assistance/equipment, and devices (3), or be completely dependent on care givers (4). Persons in all categories are at risk for injury, but those in categories 2–4 are at greatest risk for hazards associated with immobility.

ACTIONS/INTERVENTIONS	RATIONALE
Independent	
Position patient to avoid pressure damage. Turn at regular intervals, and make small position changes between turns.	Regular turning more normally distributes body weight and promotes circulation to all areas. If paralysis or limited cognition is present, patient should be repositioned frequently and positioned on affected side for only brief periods of time.
Maintain functional body alignment, e.g., hips, feet, hands. Monitor for proper placement of devices and/or signs of pressure from devices.	Use of high-top tennis shoes, "space boots," and T-bar sheepskin devices can help prevent footdrop. Handsplints are variable and designed to prevent hand deformities and promote optimal function. Use of pillows, bedrolls, and sandbags can help prevent abnormal hip rotation.
Support head and trunk, arms and shoulders, feet and legs when patient is in wheelchair/recliner. Pad chair seat with foam or water-filled cushion, and assist patient to shift weight at frequent intervals.	Maintains comfortable, safe, and functional posture and prevents/reduces risk of coccyx skin breakdown.
Provide/assist with range-of-motion exercises.	Maintains mobility and function of joints/functional alignment of extremities and reduces venous stasis.
Instruct/assist patient with exercise program and use of mobility aids. Increase activity and participation in self-care as tolerated.	Lengthy convalescence often follows brain injury, and physical reconditioning is an essential part of the program. Involving patient in planning and performing activities is important to promote patient cooperation/sustain program.
Provide meticulous skin care, massaging with emollients and removing wet linen/clothing, keeping bedding free of wrinkles.	Promotes circulation and skin elasticity and reduces risk of skin excoriation.
Provide eye care, artificial tears; patch eyes as indicated.	Protects delicate tissues from drying. Patient may require eye patches during sleep to protect eyes from trauma if unable to keep eyes closed.
Monitor urinary output. Note color and odor of urine. Assist with bladder retraining when appropriate.	Indwelling catheter used during the acute phase of injury may be needed for an extended period of time before bladder retraining is possible. Once the catheter is removed, several methods of continence control may be tried, e.g., intermittent catheterization (for residual and complete emptying), external catheter, planned intervals on commode, incontinence pads.
Provide fluids within individual tolerance (e.g., neurologic and cardiac), including cranberry juice as indicated.	Once past the acute phase of head injury and if patient has no other contraindicating factors, forcing fluids will decrease risk of urinary tract infections/stone formation as well as provide other positive effects such as normal stool consistency, optimal skin turgor.
Monitor bowel elimination and provide for/assist with a regular bowel routine. Check for impacted stool; use digital stimulation as indicated. Sit patient upright on commode or stool at regular intervals. Add fiber/bulk/fruit juice to diet as appropriate.	A regular bowel routine requires simple but diligent measures to prevent complications. Stimulation of the internal rectal sphincter will stimulate bowel to empty automatically if stool is soft enough to do so. Upright position aids evacuation.
Inspect for localized tenderness, redness, skin warmth, muscle tension, and/or ropy veins in calves of legs. Observe for sudden dyspnea, tachypnea, fever, respiratory distress, chest pain.	Patient is at risk for development of deep vein thrombosis and pulmonary embolus (especially after trauma), requiring prompt medical evaluation/intervention to prevent serious complications.

ACTIONS/INTERVENTIONS

Collaborative

Provide air/water mattress, kinetic therapy as appropriate.

RATIONALE

Equalizes tissue pressure, enhances circulation, and helps reduce venous stasis to decrease risk of tissue injury.

NURSING DIAGNOSIS:	INFECTION, POTENTIAL FOR
May be related to:	**Traumatized tissues, broken skin, invasive procedures**
	Decreased ciliary action, stasis of body fluids
	Nutritional deficits
	Suppressed inflammatory response (steroid use)
	Altered integrity of closed system (CSF leak)
Possibly evidenced by:	**[Not applicable; presence of signs and symptoms establishes an *actual* diagnosis.]**
PATIENT OUTCOMES/ EVALUATION CRITERIA:	**Maintains normothermia, free of signs of infection. Achieves timely wound healing when present.**

ACTIONS/INTERVENTIONS

Independent

Provide meticulous/aseptic care, maintain good handwashing techniques.

Observe areas of impaired skin integrity (e.g., wounds, suture lines, invasive line insertion sites), noting drainage characteristics and presence of inflammation.

Monitor temperature routinely. Note presence of chills, diaphoresis, changes in mentation.

Encourage deep breathing, aggressive pulmonary toilet. Observe sputum characteristics.

Provide perineal care. Maintain integrity of closed urinary drainage system if used. Encourage adequate fluid intake.

Observe color/clarity of urine. Note presence of foul odor.

Screen/restrict access of visitors or care givers with upper respiratory infections.

Collaborative

Administer antibiotics as indicated.

RATIONALE

First-line defense against nosocomial infections.

Early identification of developing infection permits prompt intervention and prevention of further complications.

May indicate developing sepsis requiring further evaluation/intervention.

Enhances mobilization and clearing of pulmonary secretions to reduce risk of pneumonia, atelectasis. Note: Postural drainage should be used with caution if risk of IICP exists.

Reduces potential for bacterial growth/ascending infection.

Indicators of developing urinary tract infection requiring prompt intervention.

Reduces exposure of "compromised host."

Prophylactic therapy may be used in the presence of CSF leak or after surgical procedures to reduce risk of nosocomial infections.

ACTIONS/INTERVENTIONS	RATIONALE
Collaborative	
Obtain specimens as indicated.	Culture/sensitivity, Gram stain may be done to verify presence of infection, identify causative organism and appropriate treatment choices.

NURSING DIAGNOSIS:	**NUTRITION, ALTERED: LESS THAN BODY REQUIREMENTS [POTENTIAL]**
May be related to:	**Altered ability to ingest nutrients (decreased level of consciousness)**
	Weakness of muscles required for chewing, swallowing
	Hypermetabolic state
Possibly evidenced by:	**[Not applicable; presence of signs and symptoms establishes an *actual* diagnosis.]**
PATIENT OUTCOMES/ EVALUATION CRITERIA:	**Demonstrates maintenance of/progressive weight gain toward goal, with normalization of laboratory values and free of signs of malnutrition.**

ACTIONS/INTERVENTIONS	RATIONALE
Independent	
Assess ability to chew, swallow, cough, handle secretions.	These factors determine choice of feeding as patient must be protected from aspiration.
Auscultate bowel sounds, noting decreased/absent or hyperactive sounds.	Gastrointestinal functioning is usually preserved in brain injured patients; so bowel sounds help in determining response to feeding or development of complications, e.g., ileus.
Weigh as indicated.	Evaluates effectiveness or need for changes in nutritional therapy.
Provide for feeding safety, e.g., elevate head of bed while eating or during tube feeding;	Reduces risk of regurgitation and/or aspiration.
Divide feedings into small amounts and give frequently.	Enhances digestion and patient's tolerance of nutrients and can improve patient cooperation in eating.
Promote pleasant, relaxing environment, including socialization during meals. Encourage SO to bring in food that patient enjoys.	Although the recovering patient may require assistance with feeding and/or use of assistive devices, meal time socialization with SO or friends can improve intake and normalize the life function of eating.
Check stools, gastric aspirant, vomitus for blood.	Acute/subacute bleeding may occur (Cushing's ulcer) requiring intervention and alternate method of feeding. (Refer to CP: Upper Gastrointestinal/Esophageal Bleeding, p. 397.)
Collaborative	
Consult with dietician/nutritional support team. (Refer to CP: Total Nutritional Support, p. 894.)	Effective resource for identifying caloric/nutrient needs dependent on age, body size, desired weight, concurrent conditions (trauma, cardiac/metabolic problems).

ACTIONS/INTERVENTIONS

Collaborative

Monitor laboratory studies, e.g., serum albumin, transferrin, amino acid profile, iron, BUN, nitrogen balance studies, glucose, SGOT/SGPT, electrolytes.

Administer feedings by appropriate means, e.g., tube feeding, oral feedings with soft foods, and thick liquids.

Involve speech/occupational/physical therapists when mechanical problem exists, e.g., impaired swallow reflexes, wired jaws, contractures of hands, paralysis.

RATIONALE

Identifies nutritional deficiencies, organ function, and response to nutritional therapy.

Choice of route is dependent on patient needs/capabilities. Tube feedings (orogastric, gastric) may be required initially. If the patient is able to swallow, soft foods or semiliquid foods may be more easily managed without aspiration.

Individual strategies/devices may be needed to improve ability to eat.

NURSING DIAGNOSIS:	FAMILY PROCESS, ALTERED
May be related to:	**Situational transition and crisis**
	Uncertainty about outcomes/expectations
Possibly evidenced by:	**Difficulty adapting to change or dealing with traumatic experience constructively**
	Family not meeting needs of its members
	Difficulty accepting or receiving help appropriately
	Inability to express or to accept feelings of members
FAMILY OUTCOMES/ EVALUATION CRITERIA:	**Beginning to express feelings freely and appropriately. Identifies internal and external resources to deal with the situation. Directs energies in a purposeful manner to plan for resolution of crisis. Encourages and allows injured member to progress toward independence.**

ACTIONS/INTERVENTIONS

Independent

Note components of family unit, availability/involvement of support systems.

Encourage expression of concerns about seriousness of condition, possibility of death, or incapacity.

Listen for expressions of helplessness/hopelessness.

Encourage expression of/acknowledge feelings. Do not deny or reassure patient/SO that everything will be all right.

Reinforce previous explanations about extent of injury, treatment plan, and prognosis. Provide accurate infor-

RATIONALE

Defines family resources and identifies areas of need.

Verbalization of fears gets concerns out in the open and can decrease anxiety and enhance coping with reality.

Joy of survival of victim is replaced by grief/anger at "loss" and necessity of dealing with "new" person that family does not know and may not even like. Prolongation of these feelings may result in depression.

Because it is not possible to predict the outcome, it is more helpful to assist the person to deal with feelings about what is happening instead of giving false reassurance.

Patient/SO are unable to absorb/recall all information and blocking can occur because of emotional trauma.

ACTIONS/INTERVENTIONS	RATIONALE
Independent	
mation at current level of understanding/ability to accept.	As time goes by, reinforcement of information can help reduce misconceptions, fear about the unknown/future expectations.
Stress importance of continuous open dialog between family members.	Provides opportunity to get feelings out in the open. Recognition and awareness promotes resolution of guilt, anger.
Evaluate/discuss family goals and expectations.	May initially believe patient is going to live, so with rehabilitation will be cured. In spite of accurate information, expectations may be unrealistic. Also, patient's early recovery may be rapid, then plateau, resulting in disappointment/frustration.
Identify individual roles and anticipated/perceived changes.	Responsibilities/roles may have to be partially or completely assumed by others, which can further complicate family coping.
Assess energy direction, e.g., efforts at resolution/problem solving are purposeful or scattered.	May need assistance to focus energies in an effective way/enhance coping.
Identify and encourage use of previously successful coping behaviors.	Focuses on strengths and reaffirms individuals' ability to deal with current crisis.
Demonstrate and encourage use of stress management skills, e.g., relaxation techniques, breathing exercises, visualization.	Helps redirect attention toward revitalizing self to enhance coping ability.
Help family recognize needs of all members.	Attention may be so focused on injured member that other members feel isolated/abandoned, which can compromise family growth and unity.
Support family grieving for "loss" of member. Acknowledge normality of wide range of feelings and ongoing nature of process.	Although grief may never be fully resolved, and family may vacillate among various stages, understanding that this is typical may help members accept/cope with the situation.
Collaborative	
Include family in rehabilitation team meetings and care planning/placement decisions.	Facilitates communication, enables family to be an integral part of the rehabilitation and provides sense of control.
Identify community resources, e.g., VNA, homemaker service, day care facility, legal/financial counselor.	Provides assistance with problems that may arise because of altered role function.
Refer to family therapy, support groups.	Cognitive/personality changes are usually very difficult for family to deal with. Decreased impulse control, emotional lability, inappropriate sexual or aggressive/violent behavior can disrupt family and result in abandonment/divorce, etc. Trained therapists and peer role models may assist family to deal with feelings/reality of situation and provide support for decisions that are made.

NURSING DIAGNOSIS:	**KNOWLEDGE DEFICIT [LEARNING NEED] (SPECIFY)**
May be related to:	**Lack of exposure, unfamiliarity with information/resources**
	Lack of recall/cognitive limitation

Possibly evidenced by:	Request for information, statement of misconception
	Inaccurate follow-through of instruction
PATIENT/SO OUTCOMES/ EVALUATION CRITERIA:	Participates in learning process. Verbalizes understanding of condition, treatment regimen, potential complications. Initiates necessary lifestyle changes and/or involved in rehabilitation program. Correctly performs necessary procedures.

ACTIONS/INTERVENTIONS	RATIONALE
Independent	
Evaluate capabilities and readiness to learn of both patient and SO.	Permits presentation of material based on individual needs. Note: Patient may not be emotionally/mentally capable of assimilating information.
Review information regarding injury process and after-effects.	Aids in establishing realistic expectations and promotes understanding of current situation and needs.
Review/reinforce current therapeutic regimen. Identify ways of continuing program after discharge.	Recommended activities, limitations, medication/ therapy needs have been established on the basis of a coordinated interdisciplinary approach, and follow-through is essential to progression of recovery/prevention of complications.
Discuss plans for meeting self-care needs.	Varying levels of assistance may be required/need to be planned for based on individual situation.
Provide written instructions, and schedules for activity, medication, important facts.	Provides visual reinforcement and reference source after discharge.
Identify signs/symptoms of individual risks, e.g., delayed CSF leak, posttraumatic seizures.	Recognizing developing problems provides opportunity for prompt evaluation and interventions to prevent serious complications.
Discuss with patient/SO development of symptoms, such as reexperiencing traumatic event (flashbacks, intrusive thoughts, repetitive dreams/nightmares), psychic/emotional numbness, changes in lifestyle, including adoption of self-destructive behaviors.	May indicate occurrence/exacerbation of posttrauma response, which can occur months to years after injury, requiring further evaluation and supportive interventions.
Collaborative	
Identify community resources, e.g., head injury support groups, social services, rehabilitation facilities, outpatient programs, VNA.	May be needed to provide assistance with physical care, home management, adjustment to lifestyle changes, as well as emotional and financial concerns.
Refer/reinforce importance of follow-up care by rehabilitation team, e.g., physical, occupational, speech, vocational therapists, cognitive retrainers.	Diligent work (often as long as 3 years with these providers) may eventually overcome residual neurologic deficits and enable patient to resume desired/productive lifestyle.

Cerebrovascular Accident/Stroke _____

Cerebrovascular disease refers to any functional or structural abnormality of the central nervous system caused by a pathologic condition of the cerebral vessels or of the entire cerebral vascular system. It either causes hemorrhage from a tear in the vessel wall or impairs the cerebral circulation by a partial or complete occlusion of the vessel lumen with transient or permanent effects.

PATIENT ASSESSMENT DATA BASE

Data collected will be determined by location, severity and duration of pathology.

ACTIVITY/REST

May report: Difficulties with activity due to weakness, loss of sensation, or paralysis (hemiplegia).
Tiring easily; difficulty resting (pain or muscle twitchings).

May exhibit: Altered level of consciousness.
Altered muscle tone (flaccid or spastic); paralysis (hemiplegia); generalized weakness.
Visual disturbances.

CIRCULATORY

May report: History of cardiac disease (e.g., myocardial infarction, valvular heart disease, dysrhythmias, congestive heart failure, bacterial endocarditis), polycythemia.

May exhibit: Arterial hypertension (frequently found unless the CVA is due to embolism or vascular malformation).
Pulse: rate may vary (preexisting heart conditions, medications, effect of stroke on vasomotor center).
Bruit in carotid, femoral, and iliac arteries or abdominal aorta.

EGO INTEGRITY

May report: Feelings of helplessness, hopelessness.

May exhibit: Emotional lability and inappropriate response to anger, sadness, happiness.
Difficulty expressing self.

ELIMINATION

May exhibit: Change in voiding patterns, e.g., incontinence, anuria.
Distended abdomen (overdistended bladder); absent bowel sounds (paralytic ileus).

FOOD/FLUID

May report: History of diabetes.
Lack of appetite.
Nausea/vomiting initial event (increased intracranial pressure).
Loss of sensation in tongue, cheek, and throat; dysphagia.

May exhibit: Mastication/swallowing problems (palatal and pharyngeal reflex involvement).
Obesity (risk factor).

NEUROSENSORY

May report: Dizziness/syncope (before CVA/transient during TIA).
Headaches: severe with intracerebral or subarachnoid hemorrhage.

Tingling/numbness/weakness (commonly reported during TIAs, found in varying degrees in other types of stroke); involved side seems "dead."

Visual deficits, e.g., blurred vision, partial loss of vision (monocular blindness), double vision (diplopia), or other disturbances in visual fields.

Touch: sensory loss on contralateral side (opposite side) in extremities and sometimes in ipsilateral side (same side) of face.

Disturbance in senses of taste, smell.

May exhibit: Mental status/LOC: coma usually present in the initial stages of hemorrhagic disturbances; consciousness is usually preserved when the etiology is thrombotic in nature; altered behavior (e.g., lethargy, apathy, combativeness); altered cognitive function (e.g., memory, problem-solving sequencing).

Extremities: weakness/paralysis (contralateral with all kinds of stroke), unequal hand grasp; diminished deep tendon reflexes (contralateral).

Facial paralysis or paresis (ipsilateral).

Aphasia: defect or loss of language function may be expressive (difficulty producing speech), receptive (difficulty comprehending speech), and global (combination of the two).

Loss of ability to recognize or appreciate import of visual, auditory, tactile stimuli (agnosia), e.g., altered body image awareness, neglect or denial of contralateral side of body, disturbances in perception.

Loss of ability to execute purposeful motor acts despite physical ability and willingness to do so (apraxia).

Pupil size/reaction: inequality; dilated and fixed pupil on the ipsilateral side (hemorrhage/herniation).

Nuchal rigidity (common in hemorrhagic etiology).

Seizures (common in hemorrhagic etiology).

PAIN/COMFORT

May report: Headache of varying intensity (carotid artery involvement).

May exhibit: Guarding/distraction behaviors, restlessness, muscle/facial tension.

RESPIRATION

May report: Smoking (risk factor).

May exhibit: Inability to swallow/cough/protect airway.

Labored and/or irregular respirations.

Noisy respirations/rhonchi (aspiration of secretions).

SAFETY

May exhibit: Motor/sensory: problems with vision.

Changes in perception of body spatial orientation (RCVA).

Difficulty seeing objects on left side (RCVA).

Being unaware of affected side.

Inability to recognize familiar objects, colors, words, faces.

Diminished response to heat and cold/altered body temperature regulation.

Swallowing difficulty, inability to meet own nutritional needs.

Impaired judgment, little concern for safety, impatience/lack of insight (RCVA).

SOCIAL INTERACTION

May exhibit: Speech problems, inability to communicate.

TEACHING/LEARNING

May report: Family history of hypertension, strokes.

Use of oral contraceptives.

Discharge Plan Considerations: May require medication regimen/therapeutic treatments.

Assistance with transportation, shopping, food preparation, self-care and homemaker tasks.

Changes in physical layout of home; transition placement before return to home setting.

DIAGNOSTIC STUDIES

Cerebral angiography: helps determine specific lesion causing CVA.

CT: demonstrates edema, hematomas, infarctions.

Lumbar puncture: normal pressure and usually clear in cerebral thrombosis, embolism and TIA. Pressure elevation and grossly bloody fluid suggests subarachnoid and intracerebral hemorrhage. Total protein level may be elevated in cases of thrombosis due to inflammatory process.

MRI: shows areas of infarction, hemorrhage, arteriovenous malformations.

Cerebral blood flow studies: identifies deficiencies in cerebral circulation, e.g., hemorrhage, vasospasm, or other types of cerebral vascular disease.

Doppler ultrasonography: identifies arteriovenous disease, e.g., problems with carotid system (blood flow/ presence of atherosclerotic plaques).

EEG: identifies problems based on brain waves and may demonstrate specific areas of lesions.

X-rays (skull): may show shift of pineal gland to the opposite side from an expanding mass; calcifications of the internal carotid may be visible in cerebral thrombosis; partial calcification of walls of an aneurysm may be noted in subarachnoid hemorrhage.

NURSING PRIORITIES

1. Promote adequate cerebral oxygenation and perfusion.
2. Prevent/minimize complications and permanent disabilities.
3. Assist patient to gain independence in daily living activities.
4. Support coping process and integration of changes into self-concept.
5. Provide information about disease process/prognosis and treatment/rehabilitation needs.

DISCHARGE CRITERIA

1. Cerebral function improved, neurologic deficits resolving/stabilized.
2. Complications prevented or minimized.
3. ADL needs met by self or with assistance of other(s).
4. Coping with situation in positive manner, planning for the future.
5. Disease process/prognosis, and therapeutic regimen understood.

NURSING DIAGNOSIS:	TISSUE PERFUSION, ALTERED: CEREBRAL
May be related to:	**Interruption of blood flow: occlusive disorder, hemorrhage; cerebral vasospasm, cerebral edema**
Possibly evidenced by:	**Altered level of consciousness; memory loss**
	Changes in motor/sensory responses; restlessness
	Sensory, language, intellectual and emotional deficits
	Changes in vital signs

PATIENT OUTCOMES/
EVALUATION CRITERIA:

Maintains usual/improved level of consciousness, cognition and motor/sensory function. Demonstrates stable vital signs and absence of signs of IICP. Displays no further deterioration/recurrence.

ACTIONS/INTERVENTIONS	RATIONALE

Independent

Determine factors related to individual situation/cause for coma/decreased cerebral perfusion, and potential for IICP.

Influences choice of interventions. Deterioration in neurologic signs/symptoms or failure to improve after initial insult may require surgical intervention and/or that the patient be transferred to critical care area for monitoring of intracranial pressure.

Monitor/document neurologic status frequently and compare with baseline. (Refer to CP: Craniocerebral Trauma, ND: Tissue Perfusion, Altered: Cerebral, p. 228, for complete neurologic evaluation.)

Assesses trends in LOC and potential for IICP and is useful in determining location, extent, and progression/resolution of CNS damage.

Monitor vital signs, note hypertension/hypotension, compare blood pressure readings in both arms;

Variations may occur because of cerebral pressure/injury in vasomotor area of the brain; hypertension may have been a precipitating factor; hypotension may occur because of shock (circulatory collapse); IICP may occur. Subclavian artery blockage may be revealed by difference in pressure readings between arms.

Heart rate and rhythm, auscultate for murmurs;

Changes in rate, especially bradycardia, can occur because of the brain damage. Dysrhythmias and murmurs may reflect cardiac disease, which may have precipitated CVA (e.g., stroke after MI or from valve dysfunction).

Respiration, noting patterns and rhythm, e.g., periods of apnea after hyperventilation, Cheyne–Stokes breathing.

Irregularities can suggest location of cerebral insult/increasing ICP and need for further intervention, including possible respiratory support. (Refer to CP: Craniocerebral Trauma, ND: Breathing Pattern, Ineffective [Potential], p. 231.)

Evaluate pupils, noting size, shape, equality, light reactivity.

Pupil reactions are regulated by the oculomotor (III) cranial nerve and are useful in determining whether the brainstem is intact. Pupil size/equality is determined by balance between parasympathetic and sympathetic enervation. Response to light reflects combined function of the optic (II) and oculomotor (III) cranial nerves.

Assess for changes in vision, e.g., blurred vision, alterations in visual field/depth perception.

Specific visual alterations reflect area of brain involved, indicate safety concerns and influence choice of interventions.

Assess higher functions, including speech, if patient is alert. (Refer to ND: Communication, Impaired: Verbal, p. 249.)

Changes in cognition/speech content are an indicator of location/degree of cerebral involvement and may indicate deterioration/IICP.

Position with head slightly elevated and in neutral position.

Reduces arterial pressure by promoting venous drainage and may improve cerebral circulation/perfusion.

Maintain bedrest; provide quiet environment; restrict visitors/activities as indicated. Provide rest periods between care activities, limit duration of procedures.

Continual stimulation/activity can increase ICP. Absolute rest and quiet may be needed to prevent rebleeding in the case of hemorrhage.

Prevent straining at stool, holding breath.

Valsalva maneuver increases ICP and potentiates risk of rebleeding.

ACTIONS/INTERVENTIONS	RATIONALE

Independent

Assess for nuchal rigidity, twitching, increased restlessness, irritability, onset of seizure activity.

Indicative of meningeal irritation, especially in hemorrhagic disorders. Seizures may reflect IICP/cerebral injury, requiring further evaluation and interventions. (Refer to CP: Seizure Disorders, p. 218.)

Collaborative

Administer supplemental oxygen as indicated.

Reduces hypoxemia which can cause cerebral vasodilation and increase pressure/edema.

Administer medications as indicated:

Anticoagulants, e.g., warfarin sodium (Coumadin), heparin, antiplatelet agents (ASA), dipyridamole (Persantine);

May be used to improve cerebral blood flow and prevent further clotting when embolus/thrombosis is the problem. Contraindicated in hypertensive patients because of increased risk of hemorrhage.

Antifibrolytics, e.g., aminocaproic acid (Amicar);

Used with caution in hemorrhagic disorder to prevent lysis of formed clots and subsequent rebleeding.

Antihypertensives (based on preinsult therapy);

Preexisting/chronic hypertension requires cautious treatment, because aggressive management increases the risk of extension of tissue damage. Transient hypertension often occurs during acute stroke and resolves often without therapeutic intervention.

Peripheral vasodilators, e.g., cyclandelate (Cyclospasmol), papaverine (Pavabid/Vasospan), isoxsuprine (Vasodilan);

Used to improve collateral circulation or decrease vasospasm.

Steroids, dexamethasone (Decadron);

Use is controversial in control of cerebral edema.

Phenytoin (Dilantin), phenobarbital.

May be used to control seizures and/or for sedative action. Note: Phenobarbital enhances action of antiepileptics.

Monitor laboratory studies as indicated, e.g., prothrombin/PTT time, Dilantin level.

Provides information about drug effectiveness/therapeutic level.

NURSING DIAGNOSIS: MOBILITY, IMPAIRED PHYSICAL

May be related to: Neuromuscular involvement: weakness, parathesia; flaccid/hypotonic paralysis (initially); spastic paralysis

Perceptual/cognitive impairment

Possibly evidenced by: Inability to purposefully move within the physical environment; impaired coordination; limited range of motion; decreased muscle strength/control

PATIENT OUTCOMES/ EVALUATION CRITERIA: Maintains optimal position of function as evidenced by absence of contractures, footdrop. Maintains/increases strength and function of affected or compensatory body part. Demonstrates techniques/behaviors that enable resumption of activities. Maintains skin integrity.

247

ACTIONS/INTERVENTIONS

Independent

Assess functional ability/extent of impairment initially and on a regular basis. Classify according to 0–4 scale. (Refer to CP: Craniocerebral Trauma, ND: Mobility, Impaired, Physical, p. 236.)

Change positions at least every 2 hours (prone, supine, side-lying) and possibly more often if placed on affected side.

Position in prone position once or twice a day if patient can tolerate.

Begin active/passive range of motion (ROM) to all extremities (including splinted) on admission. Encourage exercises such as quadriceps/gluteal exercise, squeezing rubber ball, extension of fingers and legs/feet.

Prop extremities in functional position, use footboard during the period of flaccid paralysis. Maintain neutral position of head.

Use arm sling when patient in upright position as indicated.

Evaluate use of/need for positional aids and/or splints during spastic paralysis:

    Place pillow under axilla to abduct arm;

    Elevate arm and hand;

    Place hard hand rolls in the palm with fingers and thumb opposed;

    Place knee and hip in extended position;

    Maintain leg in neutral position with a trochanter roll;

    Discontinue use of footboard.

Assist to develop sitting balance (e.g., raise head of bed; assist to sit on edge of bed, having patient use the strong arm to support body weight and strong leg to move affected leg; increase sitting time) and standing balance (e.g., put flat walking shoes on patient; support patient's lower back with hands while positioning knees outside patient's knees; assist in using parallel bars/walkers).

Assess affected side for color, edema, or other signs of compromised circulation.

Inspect skin particularly over bony prominences regularly. Gently massage any reddened areas and provide aids such as sheepskin pads as necessary.

RATIONALE

Indentifies strengths/deficiencies and may provide information regarding recovery. Assists in choice of interventions, because different techniques are used for flaccid and spastic paralysis.

Reduces risk of tissue ischemia/injury. Affected side has poorer circulation and reduced sensation and is more predisposed to skin breakdown/decubitus.

Helps maintain functional hip extension; however, may increase anxiety, especially about ability to breathe.

Minimizes muscle atrophy, promotes circulation, helps prevent contractures. Reduces risk of hypercalciuria and osteoporosis if underlying problem is hemorrhage. Note: Excessive/imprudent stimulation can predispose to rebleeding.

Prevents contractures/footdrop and facilitates use when/if function returns. Flaccid paralysis may interfere with ability to support head, whereas spastic paralysis may lead to deviation of head to one side.

During flaccid paralysis, use of sling may reduce risk of shoulder subluxation and shoulder–hand syndrome.

Flexion contractures occur because flexor muscles are stronger than extensors.

Prevents adduction of shoulder and flexion of elbow.

Promotes venous return and helps prevent edema formation.

Hard cones decrease the stimulation of finger flexion, maintaining finger and thumb in a functional position.

Maintains functional position.

Prevents external hip rotation.

Continued use (after change from flaccid to spastic paralysis) can cause excessive pressure on the ball of the foot, enhance spasticity, and actually increase plantar flexion.

Aids in retraining neuronal pathways, enhancing proprioception and motor response.

Edematous tissue is more easily traumatized and heals more slowly.

Pressure points over bony prominences are most at risk for decreased perfusion/ischemia. Circulatory stimulation and padding helps prevent skin breakdown and decubitus development.

ACTIONS/INTERVENTIONS	RATIONALE
Independent	
Get up in chair as soon as vital signs are stable except following cerebral hemorrhage.	Helps stabilize blood pressure (restores vasomotor tone), promotes maintenance of extremities in a functional position and emptying of bladder/kidneys, reducing risk of urinary stones and infections from stasis.
Pad chair seat with foam or waterfilled cushion and assist patient to shift weight at frequent intervals.	Prevents/reduces risk of coccyx skin breakdown.
Set goals with patient/SO, e.g., for exercise and position changes.	Promotes sense of expectation of progress/improvement and provides some sense of control/independence.
Encourage patient to assist with movement and exercises using unaffected extremity to support/move weaker side.	May respond as if affected side is no longer part of body and needs encouragement and active training to "reincorporate" it as a part of own body.
Collaborative	
Provide egg crate mattress or other flotation device as indicated.	Promotes even weight distribution decreasing pressure on bony points and helping to prevent skin breakdown/decubitus formation.
Consult with physical therapist regarding active, resistive exercises and patient ambulation.	Individualized program can be developed to meet particular needs/deal with deficits in balance, coordination, strength.
Assist with electrical stimulation, e.g., TENS as indicated.	May assist with muscle restrengthening and increase voluntary muscle control.
Determine need for water bed, flotation mattress, or other specialized beds (kinetic) as indicated.	Specialized beds help with positioning the extremely obese patient, enhances circulation, and reduces venous stasis to decrease risk of tissue injury and complications such as orthostatic pneumonia.
Administer muscle relaxants, antispasmodics as indicated.	May be required to relieve spasticity in affected extremities.

NURSING DIAGNOSIS:	**COMMUNICATION, IMPAIRED: VERBAL [AND/OR WRITTEN]**
May be related to:	**Impaired cerebral circulation; neuromuscular impairment, loss of facial/oral muscle tone/control; generalized weakness/fatigue**
Possibly evidenced by:	**Impaired articulation; does not/cannot speak (dysarthria)**
	Inability to modulate speech, find words, name words, identify objects; inability to comprehend written/spoken language
PATIENT OUTCOMES/ EVALUATION CRITERIA:	**Indicates an understanding of the communication problems. Establishes method of communication in which needs can be expressed. Uses resources appropriately.**

ACTIONS/INTERVENTIONS	RATIONALE

Independent

Assess type/degree of dysfunction: e.g., patient does not seem to understand words or has trouble speaking or making self understood.	Helps determine area and degree of brain involvement and difficulty patient has with any or all steps of the communication process. Patient may have trouble understanding spoken words (receptive aphasia/damage to Wernicke's speech area), speaking words correctly (expressive aphasia/damage to Broca's speech areas) or experience damage to both areas.
Differentiate aphasia from dysarthria;	Choice of interventions is dependent on type of impairment. Aphasia is a defect in using and interpreting symbols of language and may involve sensory and/or motor components, e.g., inability to comprehend written/spoken words or write, make signs, speak. A dysarthric person can understand, read, and write language but has difficulty forming/pronouncing words due to weakness, paralysis of oral musculature.
Listen for errors in conversation and provide feedback;	Patient may lose ability to monitor verbal output and be unaware that communication is not sensible. Feedback helps patient realize why care givers are not understanding/responding appropriately and provides opportunity to clarify content/meaning.
Ask patient to follow simple commands (e.g., "Shut your eyes," "Point to the door") repeat simple words/sentences;	Tests for receptive aphasia.
Point to objects and ask patient to name them;	Tests for expressive aphasis; e.g., patient may recognize item but not be able to name it.
Have patient produce simple sounds, e.g., "Sh," "Cat";	Identifies dysarthria as motor components of speech (tongue, lip movement, breath control) can affect articulation and may/may not be accompanied by expressive aphasia.
Ask the patient to write name and/or a short sentence. If unable to write, have patient read a short sentence.	Tests for writing disability (agraphia) and deficits in reading comprehension (alexia), which are also part of receptive and expressive aphasia.
Post note at nurses' station and patient's room about speech impairment. Provide special call bell if necessary.	Allays anxiety related to inability to communicate and fear that needs will not be met promptly. Call bell that is activated by minimal pressure is useful when patient is unable to use regular call system.
Provide alternative methods of communication, e.g., writing or felt board, pictures. Provide visual clues (gestures, pictures, "needs" list, demonstration).	Provides for communication of needs/desires based on individual stiuation/underlying deficit.
Anticipate and provide for patient's needs.	Helpful in decreasing frustration when dependent on others and unable to communicate desires.
Talk directly to patient, speaking slowly and distinctly. Use yes/no questions to begin with, progressing in complexity as patient responds.	Reduces confusion/anxiety at having to process and respond to large amount of information at one time. As retraining progresses, advancing complexity of communication stimulates memory and further enhances work/idea association.
Speak in normal tones and avoid talking too fast. Give patient ample time to respond. Talk without pressing for a response.	Patient is not usually hearing-impaired, and raising voice may anger patient/cause irritation. Forcing responses can result in frustration and may cause patient to resort to "automatic" speech, e.g., garbled speech, obscenities, etc.

ACTIONS/INTERVENTIONS

Independent

Encourage SO/visitors to persist in efforts to communicate with patient, e.g., reading mail, discussing family happenings.

Discuss familiar topics, e.g., job, family, hobbies.

Respect patient's preinjury capabilities; avoid "speaking down" to patient or making patronizing remarks.

Collaborative

Consult with speech therapist.

RATIONALE

Reduces patient's social isolation and promotes establishment of effective communication.

Promotes meaningful conversation and provides opportunity to practice skills.

Enables patient to feel esteemed, because intellectual abilities often remain intact.

Assesses individual verbal capabilities and sensory, motor, and cognitive functioning and develops therapy plan for rehabilitation.

NURSING DIAGNOSIS: SENSORY-PERCEPTUAL ALTERATION

May be related to:

Altered sensory reception, transmission, integration (neurologic trauma or deficit)

Psychologic stress (narrowed perceptual fields caused by anxiety)

Possibly evidenced by:

Disorientation to time, place, persons

Change in behavior pattern/usual response to stimuli; exaggerated emotional responses

Poor concentration, altered thought processes/bizarre thinking

Reported/measured change in sensory acuity: hypoparesthesia; altered sense of taste/smell

Inability to tell position of body parts (proprioception)

Inability to recognize/attach meaning to objects (visual agnosia)

Altered communication patterns

Motor incoordination

PATIENT OUTCOMES/ EVALUATION CRITERIA

Regains/maintains usual level of consciousness and perceptual functioning. Acknowledges changes in ability and presence of residual involvement. Demonstrates behaviors to compensate for/overcome deficits.

ACTIONS/INTERVENTIONS

Independent

Review pathology of individual condition.

RATIONALE

Awareness of type/area of involvement aids in assessing for/anticipating specific deficits and planning care.

ACTIONS/INTERVENTIONS	RATIONALE

Independent

Evaluate for visual deficits. Note loss of visual field, changes in depth perception (horizontal/vertical planes), presence of diplopia (double vision).

Presence of visual disorders can negatively affect patient's ability to perceive environment and relearn motor skills, and increases risk of accident/injury.

Approach patient from visually intact side. Leave light on; position objects to take advantage of intact visual fields. Patch affected eye if indicated.

Provides for recognition of the presence of persons/objects; may help with depth perception problems; prevents patient from being startled. Patching may decrease the sensory confusion of double vision.

Simplify environment, removing excess equipment, furniture.

Decreases/limits amount of visual stimuli that may confuse interpretation of environment, reduces risk of accidental injury.

Assess sensory awareness, e.g., differentiation of hot/cold, dull/sharp; of position of body parts/muscle, joint sense.

Diminished sensory awareness and impairment of kinesthetic sense negatively affects balance/positioning and appropriateness of movement, which interferes with ambulation, increasing risk of trauma.

Stimulate remaining sense of touch; e.g., give patient objects to touch, grasp. Have patient practice touching walls/other boundaries.

Aids in retraining sensory pathways to integrate reception and interpretation of stimuli. Helps patient orient self spatially and strengthens use of affected side.

Protect from temperature extremes; assess environment for hazards. Teach to test warm water with unaffected hand.

Promotes patient safety, reducing risk of injury.

Note inattention to body parts, segments of environment; lack of recognition of familiar objects/persons.

Presence of agnosia (loss of comprehension of auditory, visual, or other sensations, although sensory sphere is intact) may lead to/result in unilateral neglect, inability to recognize environmental cues/meaning of commonplace objects, considerable self-care deficits, and disorientation or bizarre behavior.

Encourage patient to watch feet when appropriate, and consciously position body parts. Make the patient aware of all neglected body parts, e.g., sensory stimulation to affected side, exercises that bring affected side across midline, reminding person to dress/care for affected ("blind") side.

Use of visual and tactile stimuli assists in reintegration of affected side and allows patient to experience forgotten sensations of normal movement patterns.

Observe behavioral responses, e.g., hostility, crying, inappropriate affect, agitation, hallucination. (Refer to CP: Craniocerebral Trauma, ND: Thought Processes, Altered, p. 234.)

Individual responses may be variable, but commonalities such as emotional lability, lowered frustration level, apathy, impulsiveness may exist, complicating care.

Eliminate extraneous noise/stimuli as necessary.

Reduces anxiety and exaggerated emotional responses/confusion associated with sensory overload.

Speak in calm, quiet voice, using short sentences. Maintain eye contact.

Patient may have limited attention span, problems with comprehension, and these measures can help patient to attend to communication.

Ascertain/validate patient's perceptions. Reorient patient frequently to environment, staff, procedures.

Assists patient to identify inconsistencies in reception and integration of stimuli, and may reduce perceptual distortion of reality.

NURSING DIAGNOSIS:	**SELF-CARE DEFICIT: (SPECIFY)**
May be related to:	**Neuromuscular impairment, decreased strength and endurance, loss of muscle control/coordination**

Perceptual/cognitive impairment

Pain/discomfort

Depression

Possibly evidenced by: **Impaired ability to perform ADLs, e.g., inability to bring food from receptacle to mouth; inability to wash body part(s), regulate temperature of water; impaired ability to put on/take off clothing; difficulty completing toileting tasks**

PATIENT OUTCOMES/ EVALUATION CRITERIA: **Demonstrates techniques/lifestyle changes to meet self-care needs. Performs self-care activities within level of own ability. Identifies personal/community resources that can provide assistance as needed.**

ACTIONS/INTERVENTIONS

Independent

Assess abilities and level of deficit (0–4 scale) for performing activities of daily living (ADL).

Avoid doing things for the patient that the patient can do, but provide assistance as necessary.

Be aware of impulsive behavior/actions suggestive of impaired judgment.

Maintain a supportive, firm attitude. Allow patient sufficient time to accomplish tasks.

Provide positive feedback for efforts/accomplishments.

Create plan for visual deficits that are present, e.g.:

Place food and utensils on the tray related to the patient's unaffected side;

Situate the bed so that the patient's unaffected side is facing the room with the affected side to the wall;

Position furniture against wall/out of travel path.

Use self-help devices, e.g., knife–fork combinations, long-handled brushes, extensions for picking things up from floor, toilet riser, shower chair.

Assess patient's ability to communicate the need to void and/or ability to use urinal, bedpan. Take to the bathroom at frequent/periodic intervals for voiding if appropriate.

RATIONALE

Aids in anticipating/planning for meeting individual needs.

These patients may become fearful and dependent; and although assistance is helpful in preventing frustration, it is important for the patient to do as much as possible for self to maintain self-esteem and promote recovery.

May indicate need for additional assessment/ interventions and supervision to promote patient safety.

Patients will need empathy but need to know care givers will be consistent in their assistance.

Enhances sense of self-worth, promotes independence, and encourages patient to continue endeavors.

Patient will be able to see to eat the food.

Will be able to see when getting in/out of bed, observe anyone who comes into the room.

Provides for safety when patient is able to move around the room reducing risk of tripping/falling over furniture.

Enables patient to manage for self, enhancing independence and self-esteem.

May have neurogenic bladder, be inattentive, or be unable to communicate needs in acute recovery phase, but usually able to regain independent control of this function as recovery progresses.

ACTIONS/INTERVENTIONS

Independent

Identify previous bowel habits, and reestablish normal regimen. Increase bulk in diet; encourage fluid intake, increased activity.

Collaborative

Administer suppositories and stool softeners.

Consult with physical/occupational therapist.

RATIONALE

Assists in development of retraining program (independence) and aids in preventing constipation and impaction (long-term effects).

May be necessary at first to aid in establishing regular bowel function.

Provides expert assistance for developing a therapy plan and identifying special equipment needs.

NURSING DIAGNOSIS:	SELF-CONCEPT, DISTURBANCE IN: (SPECIFY)
May be related to:	**Biophysical, psychosocial, cognitive perceptual changes**
Possibly evidenced by:	**Actual change in structure and/or function**
	Change in usual patterns of responsibility/physical capacity to resume role
	Verbal/nonverbal response to actual or perceived change:
	Negative feelings about body, feelings of help-lessness/hopelessness
	Focus on past strength, function or appearance
	Preoccupation with change or loss
	Not touching/looking at involved body part
PATIENT OUTCOMES/ EVALUATION CRITERIA:	**Talking with SO about situation and changes that have occurred. Verbalizes acceptance of self in situation. Recognizes and incorporates change into self-concept in accurate manner without negating self-esteem.**

ACTIONS/INTERVENTIONS

Independent

Assess extent of altered perception and related degree of disability.

Identify meaning of the loss/dysfunction/change to the patient.

Encourage patient to express feelings including hostility or anger.

Note whether patient refers to affected side as "it" or denies affected side and says it is "dead."

Acknowledge statement of feelings about betrayal of body; remain matter-of-fact about reality that patient can still use unaffected side and learn to control af-

RATIONALE

Determination of individual factors aids in developing plan of care/choice of interventions.

Some patients accept and manage altered function effectively with little adjustment, while others have considerable difficulty recognizing and adjusting to deficits.

Demonstrates acceptance of/assists patient to recognize and begin to deal with these feelings.

Suggests rejection of body part/negative feelings about body image and abilities, indicating need for intervention and emotional support.

Helps patient to see that the nurse accepts both sides as part of the whole individual. Allows patient to feel hopeful and begin to accept current situation.

ACTIONS/INTERVENTIONS

Independent

fected side. Use words (e.g., weak, affected, right-left) that incorporate that side as part of the whole body.

Emphasize small gains either in recovery of function or independence.

Assist and encourage good grooming and makeup habits.

Encourage SO to allow patient to do as much as possible for self.

Support behaviors/efforts such as increased interest/ participation in rehabilitation activities.

Reinforce use of adaptive devices, e.g., cane, walker, button/zipper hook, leg bag for catheter, etc.

Monitor for sleep disturbance, increased difficulty concentrating, statements of inability to cope, lethargy, withdrawal.

Collaborative

Refer for psychologic and/or vocational testing and counseling if indicated.

RATIONALE

Consolidates gains, helps reduce feelings of anger and helplessness, and conveys sense of progress.

Helps enhance sense of self-esteem and control over one area of life.

Reestablishes sense of independence and fosters self-worth.

Suggests possible adaptation to changes and understanding about own role in future lifestyle.

Increases independence, reduces reliance on others for meeting physical needs, and enables patient to be more socially active.

May indicate onset of depression (common after-effect of stroke) which may require further evaluation and intervention.

May facilitate adaptation to role changes that are necessary to a sense of feeling/being a productive person.

NURSING DIAGNOSIS:	SWALLOWING, IMPAIRED [POTENTIAL]
May be related to:	Neuromuscular/perceptual impairment
Possibly evidenced by:	[Not applicable; presence of signs and symptoms establishes an *actual* diagnosis.]
PATIENT OUTCOMES/ EVALUATION CRITERIA:	Demonstrates feeding methods appropriate to individual situation and aspiration is prevented. Maintains desired body weight.

ACTIONS/INTERVENTIONS

Independent

Review individual pathology/ability to swallow, noting extent of paralysis, facial, tongue involvement, ability to protect airway. Weigh as indicated.

Promote effective swallowing, e.g.:

Assist patient with head control/support;

Place patient in upright position during and after feeding;

Stimulate lips to close, or manually open mouth by light pressure on lips/under chin, if needed;

RATIONALE

Nutritional interventions/choice of feeding route is determined by these factors.

Counteracts hyperextension, aiding in prevention of aspiration and enhancing ability to swallow.

Uses gravity to facilitate swallowing and reduce risk of aspiration.

Aids in sensory retraining and promotes muscular control.

ACTIONS/INTERVENTIONS

Independent

Place food in unaffected side of mouth;

Touch parts of the cheek with tongue blade/apply ice to weak tongue.

Feed slowly in quiet environment.

Begin oral feedings with semiliquid, soft foods when patient can swallow water.

Select/assist patient to select foods that require little or no chewing, are easy to swallow, e.g., custard, applesauce, eggs, soft finger foods. Encourage use of drinking straw for liquids.

Encourage SO to bring favorite foods.

Maintain accurate I&O; weigh as indicated.

Encourage participation in exercise/activity program.

Collaborative

Administer IV fluids.

RATIONALE

Provides sensory stimulation (including taste) that may trigger swallowing efforts and enhance intake.

Can improve tongue movement and control (necessary for swallowing) and inhibits tongue protrusion.

Enables patient to concentrate on mechanics of eating without external distraction.

Soft foods/thick fluids are easier to control in mouth, reducing risk of choking/aspiration.

Strengthens facial and swallowing muscles and reduces risk of choking.

Stimulates feeding efforts and may enhance swallowing/intake.

If swallowing efforts are not sufficient to meet fluid/nutrition needs, alternate methods of feeding must be pursued. (Refer to CP: Total Nutritional Support, p. 894.)

May increase release of endorphins in the brain, promoting a sense of general well-being and increasing appetite.

May be necessary for fluid replacement the first 24–48 hours if unable to take anything orally.

NURSING DIAGNOSIS:	KNOWLEDGE DEFICIT [LEARNING NEED] (SPECIFY)
May be related to:	Lack of exposure
	Cognitive limitation, information misinterpretation, lack of recall
	Unfamiliarity with information resources
Possibly evidenced by:	Request for information
	Statement of misconception
	Inaccurate follow-through of instructions
	Development of preventable complications
PATIENT OUTCOMES/ EVALUATION CRITERIA:	Participates in learning process. Verbalizes understanding of condition/prognosis and therapeutic regimen. Initiates necessary lifestyle changes.

ACTIONS/INTERVENTIONS

Independent

Evaluate type/degree of sensory-perceptual involvement.

RATIONALE

Deficits affect the choice of teaching methods and content/complexity of instruction.

ACTIONS/INTERVENTIONS	RATIONALE
Independent	
Discuss specific pathology and individual potentials.	Aids in establishing realistic expectations and promotes understanding of current situation and needs.
Review current restrictions/limitations and discuss planned/potential resumption of activities (including sexual relations).	Promotes understanding, provides hope for future, and creates expectation of resumption of more "normal life."
Review/reinforce current therapeutic regimen. Identify ways of continuing program after discharge.	Recommended activities, limitations, medication/therapy needs have been established on the basis of a coordinated interdisciplinary approach, and follow-through is essential to progression of recovery/prevention of complications.
Discuss plans for meeting self-care needs.	Varying levels of assistance may be required/need to be planned for, based on individual situation.
Provide written instructions, and schedules for activity, medication, important facts.	Provides visual reinforcement and reference source after discharge.
Encourage patient to refer to lists/written communications or notes instead of depending on memory.	Provides aids to support memory and promotes improvement in cognitive skills.
Suggest patient reduce/limit environmental stimuli, especially during cognitive activities.	Multiple/concomitant stimuli may aggravate alteration of thought processes.
Recommend patient seek assistance in problem-solving process, and validate decisions as indicated.	Some patients (especially those with right CVA) may display impaired judgment and impulsive behavior, compromising ability to make sound decisions.
Identify individual risk factors (e.g., hypertension, obesity, smoking, atherosclerosis, use of oral contraceptives) and necessary lifestyle changes.	Promotes general well-being and may reduce risk of recurrence.
Identify signs/symptoms requiring further follow-up, e.g., changes/decline in visual, motor, sensory functions; alteration in mentation or behavioral responses.	Prompt evaluation and intervention reduces risk of complications/further loss of function.
Collaborative	
Refer to Discharge Planner/Home Care supervisor.	Home environment may require evaluation and modifications to meet individual needs.
Identify community resources, e.g., stroke support clubs, senior services, Meals-on-Wheels, adult day care/respite program, and VNA.	Enhances coping abilities and promotes home management and adjustment to impairments.
Refer to/reinforce importance of follow-up care by rehabilitation team, e.g., physical, occupational, speech, vocational therapists.	Diligent work may eventually overcome/minimize residual deficits.

Intracranial Infections: Meningitis, Encephalitis, Brain Abscess

Intracranial infections can involve brain tissue (encephalitis) or the coverings of the brain (meningitis) or be an accumulation of free or encapsulated pus within the brain (abscess). The causative agent can be bacterial, viral, or fungal; and sequelae can range from complete recovery to residual neurologic deficit or to death.

PATIENT ASSESSMENT DATA BASE

ACTIVITY/REST

May report:	Limitations imposed by condition.
May exhibit:	Ataxia, gait problems, palsies, involuntary movement.
	Generalized weakness, limited range of motion.
	Hypotonia.

CIRCULATION

May report:	History of underlying cardiopathology, e.g., infective endocarditis, some congenital heart diseases (brain abscess).
May exhibit:	Blood pressure elevation, decreased pulse and widening pulse pressure (correlates with IICP and effects on the vasomotor center).
	Tachycardia, dysrhythmias (acute episode).

ELIMINATION

May exhibit:	Incontinence and/or retention.

FOOD/FLUID

May report:	Loss of appetite.
	Difficulty swallowing (acute episode).
May exhibit:	Anorexia; vomiting.
	Poor skin turgor, dry mucous membranes.

HYGIENE

May exhibit:	Dependence for all self-care needs (acute phase).

NEUROSENSORY

May report:	Headaches (may be first symptom and is usually severe).
	Paresthesia, itching, tingling along course of nerve.
	Hyperalgesia/increased sensitivity to pain (meningitis).
	Loss of sensation (damage to cranial nerves).
	Seizure activity (bacterial meningitis or brain abscesses).
	Disturbances in vision (initial phase of any of the infections).
	Photophobia (meningitis).
	Deafness (meningitis or encephalitis) or may be hypersensitive to noise.
	Olfactory/gustatory hallucinations.
May exhibit:	Mental status/LOC: altered level of consciousness (mild confusion to delirium to coma).
	Memory loss, lack of judgment (can be initial symptoms of developing communicating hydrocephalus following bacterial meningitis).

Aphasia/difficulty communicating.

Eyes: Pupil size/reaction: inequality of size or response to light (increased intracranial pressure).

Nystagmus (continuous movement of eyeballs).

Ptosis (drooping of the eyelid).

Facial characteristics: changes in motor or sensory function (V or VII cranial nerve involvement).

Focal seizures (abscesses), temporal lobe seizures.

Muscle hypotonia/flaccid paralysis (acute phase meningitis) or spasticity (encephalitis).

Hemiparesis or hemiplegia on occasion (encephalitis/meningitis).

Positive Brudzinski's sign and/or a positive Kernig's sign indicative of meningeal irritation (acute phase).

Nuchal rigidity (meningeal irritation).

Deep tendon reflexes: altered/accentuated, positive Babinski.

Abdominal reflexes diminished/absent and absence of cremasteric reflex in male (meningitis).

PAIN/COMFORT

May report: Headaches (severe throbbing, frontal), stiff neck; pain with ocular movement, photosensitivity, aches, sore throat.

May exhibit: Guarding.

Distraction behaviors/restlessness.

Crying/moaning.

RESPIRATION

May report: History of lung or sinus infection (brain abscess).

May exhibit: Work of breathing increased (initial episode).

Changes in mentation (lethargy to coma) and restlessness.

SAFETY

May report: History of upper respiratory/other infections, including mastoiditis, middle ear, sinus; recent lumbar puncture, surgery, skull fracture/ head injury; sickle cell anemia.

Recent immunizations; exposure to meningitis; measles, mumps, chickenpox, herpes simplex, mononucleosis; animal bites; foreign travel.

Visual/hearing impairment.

May exhibit: Temperature elevation, diaphoresis.

Petechial rashes, generalized purpura, subcutaneous bleeding.

Generalized weakness; flaccid or spastic muscle tone; paralysis or paresis.

Impaired sensation.

TEACHING/LEARNING

May report: History of drug use (brain abscess).

Drug hypersensitivity (nonbacterial meningitis).

Previous illness/concurrent medical problems, e.g., chronic condition/general debility, alcoholism, diabetes mellitus, splenectomy, implantation of ventricular shunt.

Discharge Plan Considerations: May require assistance in all areas, including self-care and homemaker tasks.

DIAGNOSTIC STUDIES

Lumbar puncture analysis of cerebrospinal fluid:
    Bacterial meningitis: pressure elevated, fluid cloudy, increased white cell count and protein; decreased glucose; smear and culture shows presence and type of bacteria.
    Viral meningitis: pressure varies, fluid usually clear, increased white cells; usually normal protein and glucose; Gram stain shows no bacteria, virus cultured only with special procedures.
    Encephalitis: increased white cells, normal glucose, slightly elevated protein; slight increase in pressure unless ICP elevated and then a marked elevation in cerebrospinal pressure.
    Brain abscess: elevated pressure, elevated WBC count and protein, and normal glucose.

Serum glucose: elevated (meningitis).

Serum LDH: elevated (bacterial meningitis).

Serum WBC: marked elevation with increased neutrophils (bacterial infection).

ESR: elevated (meningitis).

Blood/nose/throat cultures: may indicate area of "seeding" of infection or indicate type of infectious agent.

CT scan: may help localize lesion.

EEG: may show focal or generalized slowing (encephalitis) or increased voltage (abscess).

Chest, skull, and sinus x-rays: may indicate infection or source of intracranial infection.

NURSING PRIORITIES

1. Maximize cerebral function and tissue perfusion.
2. Prevent complications/injury.
3. Alleviate anxiety/provide emotional support to patient/SO.
4. Reduce/minimize pain.
5. Provide information about disease process/prognosis and treatment needs.

DISCHARGE CRITERIA

1. Infectious process(es) resolving/absent.
2. Complications/injury prevented or minimized.
3. Discomfort relieved/controlled.
4. ADL needs met by self or with assistance of other(s).
5. Disease process/prognosis and therapeutic regimen understood.

NURSING DIAGNOSIS:	**INFECTION, POTENTIAL FOR [SPREAD]**
May be related to:	**Hematogenous dissemination of pathogen**
	Stasis of body fluids
	Suppressed inflammatory response (medication-induced)
	Exposure of others to pathogens
Possibly evidenced by:	**[Not applicable; presence of signs and symptoms establishes an *actual* diagnosis.]**
PATIENT OUTCOMES/ EVALUATION CRITERIA:	**Achieves timely healing, with no evidence of endogenous spread of infection or involvement of others.**

ACTIONS/INTERVENTIONS	RATIONALE
Independent	
Provide isolation precautions as indicated.	During early stage of meningococcal meningitis or some encephalitis infections, isolation may be required until organism is known/sufficient doses of antibiotic have been administered to reduce risk of spread to others.
Maintain aseptic techniques and good hand washing by patient/visitors/staff. Monitor visitors/staff and restrict exposure of patient to those with upper respiratory infection.	Reduces patient's risk of acquiring secondary infection.
Monitor temperature regularly. Note persistence of clinical signs of infectious process.	Drug therapy is usually continued for 5 days after temperature returns to normal and clinical signs clear. Continuation of symptoms may indicate development of acute meningococcemia which can last weeks/months or sepsis/hematogenous dissemination of pathogens. (Refer to CP: Sepsis/Septicemia, p. 763.)
Investigate complaints of chest pain, development of irregular pulse/dysrhythmias, or persistent fever.	Secondary infection such as myocarditis/pericarditis may develop requiring further intervention. (Refer to CP: Inflammatory Cardiac Conditions, p. 109.)
Auscultate breath sounds. Monitor respiratory rate and effort.	Presence of rhonchi/wheezes, tachypnea, and increased work of breathing may reflect accumulation of secretions with risk of respiratory infection.
Reposition/turn frequently and encourage deep breathing.	Mobilizes secretions and promotes expectoration, reducing risk of respiratory complications.
Note urine characteristics, e.g., color, clarity, odor.	Urine stasis, dehydration and general debility increases risk of bladder/kidney infection/onset of sepsis.
Identify contacts at risk for development of cerebral infectious process and encourage them to seek medical attention.	Those with intimate respiratory contact may require antimicrobial prophylactic therapy to prevent spread of infection.
Collaborative	
Administer IV/intrathecal antibiotic therapy as indicated, e.g., penicillin G (Biotic-T), ampicillin (Amcill), chloramphenicol (Chloromycetin), gentamycin (Garamycin), amphotericin B (Fungizone);	Choice of drug is dependent on type of infection and individual sensitivity. Note: Intrathecal administration may be indicated for gram-negative bacilli, fungi, amoebae.
viderabine (Vira-A);	Useful for treatment of Herpes simplex encephalitis.
Prepare for surgical intervention, as indicated.	May require drainage of encapsulated brain abscess or removal of infected ventricular shunt to prevent rupture/control spread of infection.

NURSING DIAGNOSIS:	**TISSUE PERFUSION, ALTERED: CEREBRAL [POTENTIAL]**
May be related to:	**Cerebral edema altering/interrupting cerebral arterial/venous blood flow**
	Hypovolemia
	Exchange problems at cellular level (acidosis)
Possibly evidenced by:	**[Not applicable; presence of signs and symptoms establishes an *actual* diagnosis.]**

PATIENT OUTCOMES/ EVALUATION CRITERIA:	Maintains usual/improved level of consciousness and motor/sensory function. Demonstrates stable vital signs. Reports absence of/diminished severity of headache. Demonstrates improved cognition and absence of signs of IICP.

ACTIONS/INTERVENTIONS	RATIONALE

Refer to CP: Craniocerebral Trauma, ND: Tissue Perfusion, p. 228, for a more in-depth discussion.

Independent

Maintain bedrest with head flat and monitor vital signs as indicated after lumbar puncture.	Alteration of cerebrospinal fluid (CSF) pressure may potentiate risk of brainstem herniation, requiring immediate medical intervention.
Monitor/document neurologic status frequently and compare with baseline, such as Glasgow Coma Scale.	Assesses trends in LOC and potential for IICP and is useful in determining location, extent, and progression/resolution of CNS damage.
Assess for nuchal rigidity, twitching, increased restlessness, irritability, onset of seizure activity.	Indicative of meningeal irritation and may occur in acute and recovery period of brain injury.
Monitor vital signs, e.g.:	
BP, noting onset of/continuing systolic hypertension and widening pulse pressure;	Normally, autoregulation maintains constant cerebral blood flow despite fluctuations in systemic BP. Loss of autoregulation may follow local or diffuse cerebral vascular damage, resulting in IICP. This phenomenon may be manifested by elevated systolic BP, accompanied by decreasing diastolic BP (widening pulse pressure).
Heart rate/rhythm;	Changes in rate (most often bradycardia) and dysrhythmias may develop, reflecting brainstem pressure/injury in the absence of underlying cardiac disease.
Respirations, noting patterns and rhythm, e.g., periods of apnea after hyperventilation, Cheyne–Stokes breathing.	Type of respiratory pattern suggests severity of IICP/cerebral involvement and may indicate need for intubation with ventilatory support.
Monitor temperature and regulate environmental temperature as indicated. Limit use of blankets; administer tepid sponge bath in presence of fever. Wrap extremities in blankets when hypothermia blanket is used.	Fever is usually due to inflammatory process but may be complicated by damage to hypothalamus. Increased metabolic needs and oxygen consumption occur (especially with shivering), which can increase ICP.
Monitor intake and output. Note urine characteristics, skin turgor, status of mucous membranes.	Hyperthermia increases insensible losses and increases risk of dehydration, especially if level of consciousness/presence of nausea reduces oral intake. Note: SIADH may occur, potentiating fluid retention with edema formation and decreased urinary output.
Help patient avoid/limit coughing, vomiting, straining at stool/bearing down. Encourage patient to exhale during turning/movement in bed.	These activities increase intrathoracic and intrabdominal pressures, which can increase ICP. Exhaling during repositioning can prevent Valsalva effect.
Provide comfort measures, e.g., back massage, quiet environment, soft voice, gentle touch.	Promotes rest and decreases excessive sensory stimulation.
Provide rest periods between care activities and limit duration of procedures.	Prevents excessive fatigue/exhaustion. Continual activity can increase ICP by producing a cumulative stimulant effect.

ACTIONS/INTERVENTIONS	RATIONALE

Independent

Encourage SO to talk to patient if appropriate.

Hearing familiar voices of family/SO appears to have a relaxing effect on many patients and may reduce ICP.

Collaborative

Elevate head of bed 15–45 degrees as tolerated/indicated.

Promotes venous drainage from head, thereby decreasing ICP.

Administer IV fluids with control device. Restrict fluid intake and administer hypertonic/electrolyte solutions as indicated.

Minimizes fluctuations in vascular load and ICP. Fluid restriction may be needed to lower total body water and thereby reduce cerebral edema, especially in presence of SIADH.

Monitor ABGs. Provide supplemental oxygen as indicated.

Development of acidosis may inhibit release of oxygen at cellular level worsening cerebral ischemia.

Use hypothermia blanket.

Aids in control/stabilization of extreme temperature elevation, reducing metabolic demands/risk of seizures and promoting patient safety.

Administer medications as indicated, e.g.:

Steroids, dexamethasone (Decadron), methylprednisolone (Medrol);

May reduce capillary permeability to limit cerebral edema formation; may also reduce risk of rebound phenomena when mannitol is used.

Chlorpromazine (Thorazine);

Drug of choice in treating posturing and shivering, which can increase ICP. Note: This drug can lower the seizure threshold or precipitate Dilantin toxicity.

Acetaminophen (Tylenol), rectally or orally.

Reduces cellular metabolic/oxygen consumption, and risk of seizure activity.

NURSING DIAGNOSIS:	INJURY, POTENTIAL FOR: TRAUMA
May be related to:	**Irritation of cerebral cortex predisposing to neural discharge and generalized seizure activity**
	Involvement of localized area (focal seizure)
	Generalized weakness, paralysis, paresthesia
	Ataxia, vertigo
Possibly evidenced by:	**[Not applicable; presence of signs and symptoms establishes an *actual* diagnosis.]**
PATIENT OUTCOMES/ EVALUATION CRITERIA:	**Demonstrates absence of seizures/concomitant injury.**

ACTIONS/INTERVENTIONS	RATIONALE

Independent

Monitor for twitching of hands, feet, mouth or other facial muscles.

Reflects generalized CNS irritability, requiring further evaluation and possible intervention to prevent complications.

ACTIONS/INTERVENTIONS

RATIONALE

Independent

Provide for patient safety by padding side rails, keeping side rails up, and having a bite block and suction machine available.

Protects the patient if seizure occurs. (Refer to CP: Seizure Disorders, p. 218.)

Maintain bedrest during acute phase. Ambulate with assistance as condition improves.

Reduces risk of falls/injury when vertigo, syncope, ataxia present.

Collaborative

Administer medications as indicated, e.g., phenytoin (Dilantin), phenobarbital (Luminal).

Indicated for treatment and prevention of seizure activity. Note: Phenobarbital may cause respiratory depression and sedation and mask the signs/symptoms of IICP.

NURSING DIAGNOSIS:	COMFORT, ALTERED: PAIN, ACUTE
May be related to:	Biologic injuring agents: presence of infectious, inflammatory process, circulating toxins
Possibly evidenced by:	Complaints of headache, photophobia, muscle pain/backache
	Distraction behaviors: crying, moaning, restlessness
	Guarding behaviors, assumption of a characteristic position
	Muscular tension; facial mask of pain, pallor
	Changes in vital signs
PATIENT OUTCOMES/ EVALUATION CRITERIA:	Reports pain is relieved/controlled. Displays relaxed posture and able to sleep/rest appropriately.

ACTIONS/INTERVENTIONS

RATIONALE

Independent

Provide quiet environment; darken room as indicated.

Reduces reaction to external stimuli/sensitivity to light and promotes rest/relaxation.

Promote bedrest, assist with necessary self-care activities.

Reduces movement that may increase pain.

Place ice bag to head, cool cloth over eyes.

Promotes vasoconstriction; numbs sensory reception, thereby reducing pain.

Support assumption of position of comfort, e.g., curled up with head slightly extended in meningitis.

Reduces meningeal irritation, resultant discomfort.

Provide gentle active/passive ROM and massage to neck/shoulder muscles.

May help relax tension of muscles, promoting reduction of pain/discomfort.

Use moist heat for neck/back pain if afebrile.

Promotes muscle relaxation and reduces aches/discomfort.

Collaborative

Administer analgesics, e.g., codeine.

May be needed to relieve severe pain.

NURSING DIAGNOSIS:	MOBILITY, IMPAIRED PHYSICAL
May be related to:	Neuromuscular impairment, decreased strength/endurance
	Perceptual/cognitive impairment
	Pain/discomfort
	Restrictive therapies (bedrest)
Possibly evidenced by:	Reluctance to attempt movement
	Impaired coordination and decreased muscle strength/control
	Limited range of motion
	Inability to purposefully move within the physical environment
PATIENT OUTCOMES/ EVALUATION CRITERIA:	Regains/maintains optimal position of function as evidenced by absence of contractures, footdrop. Maintains/increases general strength and function. Maintains skin integrity, bladder and bowel function.

Refer to CP: Craniocerebral Trauma, ND: Mobility, Impaired Physical, p. 236.

NURSING DIAGNOSIS:	SENSORY-PERCEPTUAL ALTERATION: (SPECIFY)
May be related to:	Altered sensory reception, transmission, or integration
Possibly evidenced by:	Photosensitivity
	Paresthesia, hyperalgesia
	Change in usual response to stimuli
	Poor concentration, irritability, restlessness, disorientation
	Exaggerated emotional responses
PATIENT OUTCOMES/ EVALUATION CRITERIA:	Regains usual level of consciousness and perceptual functioning. Acknowledges changes in ability and presence of residual involvement. Demonstrates behaviors/lifestyle changes to compensate for/overcome deficits.

Refer to CP: Craniocerebral Trauma, ND: Sensory-Perceptual Alteration (Specify), p. 232.

NURSING DIAGNOSIS:	ANXIETY/FEAR
May be related to:	Situational crisis; interpersonal transmission and contagion

	Threat of death/change in health status (involvement of brain) Separation from support system (hospitalization)
Possibly evidenced by:	Increased tension/helplessness Apprehension/uncertainty of outcome, focus on self Sympathetic stimulation Restlessness
PATIENT OUTCOMES/ EVALUATION CRITERIA:	Acknowledges and discusses fears. Verbalizes accurate knowledge of the situation. Appears relaxed and reports anxiety is reduced to a manageable level.

ACTIONS/INTERVENTIONS	RATIONALE
Independent	
Assess patient's mentation and level of anxiety of patient/SO. Note both verbal and nonverbal cues.	Altered LOC may affect expression of fears but does not negate their presence. Degree of anxiety will affect how information is received by the individual.
Provide explanation of relationship between disease process and symptoms.	Promotes understanding, lessens fear of unknown, and may help reduce anxiety.
Answer questions honestly and give information about favorable prognosis.	Important to the establishing of trust as the diagnosis of meningitis may be frightening, and honesty and accurate information can provide reassurance.
Explain and prepare for procedures beforehand.	May alleviate apprehension when testing involves the brain.
Allow time to verbalize thoughts and fears.	Brings fears out into the open, where they can be addressed.
Involve patient/SO in care, daily planning, decision-making as much as possible.	Increases feeling of control and encourages independence.
Support planning for realistic lifestyle after illness within limitations but fully using capabilities.	Promotes sense of hope/expectation of recovery.
Explore sources of support; SO, clergy, professional counselor.	Provides reassurance that needed assistance is available to enhance/support coping. (Refer to CP: Psychosocial Aspects of Acute Care, p. 773.)
Let SO/patient know that uncharacteristic/inappropriate behavior is related to cerebral involvement and is usually self-limiting.	Bizarre behaviors, as may be seen with temporal lobe involvement in herpes encephalitis, can be very frightening, escalating anxiety and potentiating sense of helplessness/loss of control.
Protect patient's privacy if seizure activity occurs.	Consideration of the patient's need for privacy preserves and conveys a sense of dignity and self-worth, protecting the patient from embarrassment.
Provide explanation to patient/SO, e.g., unless permanent damage to the cerebrum occurs, seizure activity will likely subside as the patient recovers.	Seizure activity may be equated with the stigma of epilepsy, and an explanation of what is happening in relationship to the current illness may reduce anxiety, promote understanding of the condition.

NURSING DIAGNOSIS:	KNOWLEDGE DEFICIT [LEARNING NEED] (SPECIFY)
May be related to:	Lack of exposure
	Information misinterpretation
	Lack of recall, cognitive limitation
Possibly evidenced by:	Questions, statement of misconception
	Request for information
	Inaccurate follow-through of instruction
	Inappropriate or exaggerated behaviors (hostile, agitated, apathetic)
PATIENT OUTCOMES/ EVALUATION CRITERIA:	Verbalizes understanding of condition/disease process and treatment. Correctly performs necessary procedures and explains reasons for the actions.

ACTIONS/INTERVENTIONS

Independent

Provide information in short/brief segments.

Discuss anticipated length of convalescence.

Provide information about need for high protein/carbohydrate diet that should be offered in small/frequent meals.

Instruct in progressive ROM exercises, using warm bath to promote muscle relaxation.

Discuss importance of adequate rest, scheduling rest periods balanced with activities. Advance activity level as tolerated.

Promote development of diversional activities.

Review medication regimen and stress consulting health care provider before taking other medications/OTC drugs.

Discuss prevention of disease as appropriate, e.g., obtaining appropriate vaccinations, swimming only in chlorinated water, environmental control of mosquitoes, preventing/treating herpes infections.

Review signs/symptoms requiring physician notification, e.g., nausea/vomiting, recurrence of headache, problems with balance, or changes in mentation.

RATIONALE

Deceased attention span may reduce ability to process and retain information.

May be several weeks to months and accurate information about expectations will help patient to cope with enforced inactivity/deal with continued discomfort.

Promotes healing process. Frequent eating of small amounts of food uses less energy, reduces gastric irritation, and may enhance total intake.

Assists in regaining muscle strength/function.

Fatigue often persists beyond usual expectations of patient/SO. Extra rest is needed to help in healing process and enhance coping abilities.

Prevents boredom and helps to maintain sense of purpose in life during recuperation period.

Completion of scheduled drug program is necessary for complete resolution of infectious process. Other medications/OTC drugs may be incompatible with medication regimen.

Acute viral meningitis is often due to such viruses as mumps, herpes. A variety of encephalitic diseases are transmitted by the bite of infective mosquitoes.

Prompt evaluation and intervention may prevent relapse/development of complications.

Herniated Nucleus Pulposus (Ruptured Intervertebral Disk)

HNP is a major cause of severe, chronic, and recurrent low back pain. Herniation, either complete/partial, of the nuclear material in the areas of L4-5, L5-S1, or C6-7 is common.

PATIENT ASSESSMENT DATA BASE

Data are dependent on site, severity, whether acute/chronic, and effects of surrounding structures.

ACTIVITY/REST

May report: History of occupation requiring heavy lifting, sitting, driving for long periods of time.
Must sleep on bedboard/firm mattress.
Decreased ROM of extremities on one side.

May exhibit: Atrophy of muscles on the affected side.
Gait disturbances.

ELIMINATION

May report: Constipation, difficulty in defecation.
Urinary incontinence/retention.

EGO INTEGRITY

May report: Fear of paralysis.

May exhibit: Anxiety, depression, withdrawal from family/SO.

NEUROSENSORY

May report: Tingling, numbness, weakness, of arm/leg.

May exhibit: Hypotonia; decreased deep tendon reflexes; muscle weakness.
Tenderness/spasm of paravertebral muscles.
Decreased pain perception (sensory).

PAIN/COMFORT

May report: Pain knifelike, aggravated by coughing, sneezing, bending, lifting, defecation, straight leg raising; constant or intermittent episodes that are more severe; radiation to leg, buttocks area (lumbar); or shoulder, occiput with stiff neck (cervical).
Heard "snapping" sound at time of initial pain/trauma or felt "back giving way."
Limited mobility/forward bending.

May exhibit: Stance: leans away from affected area.
Altered gait, walking with a limp, elevated hip on affected side.
Pain on palpation.

SAFETY

May report: History of previous back problems.

TEACHING/LEARNING

May report: Lifestyle: sedentary or overactive.

Discharge Plan Considerations: May require assistance with transportation, self-care, and homemaker tasks.

DIAGNOSTIC STUDIES

Myelogram: may be normal or show "narrowing" of disk space.

MRI: noninvasive study for validation of disk herniation.

Spinal x-rays: may show degenerative changes in spine/intervertebral space; rule out other suspected pathology, e.g., tumors, osteomyelitis.

Electromyography: may localize lesion to level of particular nerve root involved.

Epidural venogram: may be done for cases where myelogram accuracy is limited.

Lumbar puncture: rule out other related conditions, infection, presence of blood.

Lasèque sign (straight leg raise test): initial confirmation of diagnosis prior to x-rays/myelograms.

CT scan: may reveal spinal canal narrowing.

NURSING PRIORITIES

1. Reduce spinal stress, muscle spasm, and pain.
2. Promote optimal functioning.
3. Support patient/SO in rehabilitation process.
4. Provide information concerning condition/prognosis and treatment needs.

DIAGNOSTIC CRITERIA

1. Pain relieved/controlled.
2. Motor function/sensation restored to optimal level.
3. Proper lifting, posture, exercises demonstrated.
4. Disease/injury process, prognosis, and therapeutic regimen understood.

NURSING DIAGNOSIS:	**COMFORT, ALTERED: PAIN, ACUTE/CHRONIC**
May be related to:	**Physical injury agents: nerve compression**
Possibly evidenced by:	**Complaints of back pain, stiff neck, muscle spasms**
	Walking with a limp, inability to walk
	Guarding behavior, leans toward affected side when standing
	Decreased tolerance for activity
	Preoccupation with pain, self/narrowed focus
	Altered muscle tone
	Facial mask of pain
	Distraction
	Autonomic responses (when pain is acute)
	Changes in sleep patterns
	Physical/social withdrawal
PATIENT OUTCOMES/ EVALUATION CRITERIA:	**Reports pain is relieved/controlled. Verbalizes methods that provide relief. Demonstrates use of therapeutic interventions (e.g., relaxation skills, behavior modification) to relieve pain.**

ACTIONS/INTERVENTIONS	RATIONALE

Independent

Assess complaints of pain, noting location, duration, precipitating/aggravating factors. Ask patient to rate on scale of 1–10.	Helps determine choice of interventions and provides basis for comparison and evaluation of therapy.
Maintain bedrest during acute phase. Place patient in semi-Fowler's with spine, hips, knees flexed; supine with/without head elevated 10–30 degrees; or lateral position.	Bedrest in position of comfort allows for decrease of muscle spasm, reduces stress on structures, and facilitates reduction of disk protrusion.
Logroll for position change.	Reduces flexion, twisting, and strain on back.
Assist with application of back brace/corset.	Useful during acute phase of ruptured lumbar disk to provide support and limit flexion/twisting. Prolonged use can increase muscle weakness and cause further degeneration.
Limit activity during acute phase as indicated.	Decreases forces of gravity and motion which can relieve muscle spasms, and reduce edema and stress on structures above affected disk.
Place needed items, call bell within easy reach.	Reduces risk of straining to reach.
Instruct in relaxation/visualization techniques.	Refocuses attention, aids in reducing muscle tension and promotes healing.
Instruct in/encourage proper body mechanics/body posture.	Alleviates stress on muscles and prevents further injury.
Provide opportunities to talk/listen to concerns.	Ventilation of worries can help to decrease stress factors present in illness/hospitalization. Provides opportunity to give information/correct misinformation.

Collaborative

Place board under mattress or provide orthopedic bed.	Provides support and reduces spinal flexion, decreasing spasms.
Administer medications as indicated:	
Muscle relaxants, e.g., diazepam (Valium), carisoprodol (Soma);	Relaxes muscles, decreasing pain.
Nonsteroidal antiinflammatory agents (NSAID), e.g., ibuprofen (Motrin, Advil), phenylbutazone (Butazolidin);	Decreases edema and pressure on nerve root(s). Note: Epidural or facet joint injection of antiinflammatory drugs may be tried if other interventions fail to alleviate pain.
Analgesics, e.g., acetaminophen (Tylenol); with codeine; narcotics, e.g., meperidine (Demerol).	May be required for relief of moderate to severe pain.
Apply physical supports, e.g., lumbar braces, cervical collar.	Support of structures decreases muscle stress/spasms and reduces pain.
Maintain traction if indicated.	Removes weight bearing from affected disk area, increasing intravertebral separation and allowing disk bulge to move away from nerve root.
Consult with physical therapist.	Developing individual stretching/exercise program can relieve muscle spasm; strengthen back, extensor, abdominal, and quadriceps muscles to increase support to lumbar area.
Apply/monitor use of moist hot packs, diathermy, ultrasound.	Increases circulation to affected muscles, promotes relief of spasms and enhances patient's relaxation.

ACTIONS/INTERVENTIONS

Collaborative

Instruct in postmyelogram procedures, e.g., force fluids and lie flat or at 30-degree elevation as indicated for specific number of hours.

Assist with/prepare for application of transcutaneous electrical stimulator (TENS).

Refer to pain clinic.

RATIONALE

Decreases risk of postprocedure headache/spinal fluid leak.

Decreases stimuli by blocking pain transmission.

Coordinated team efforts may include physical as well as psychologic therapy to deal with all aspects of chronic pain and allow patient to increase activity and productivity.

NURSING DIAGNOSIS:	MOBILITY, IMPAIRED PHYSICAL
May be related to:	Pain and discomfort, muscle spasms
	Restrictive therapies, e.g., bedrest, traction
	Neuromuscular impairment
Possibly evidenced by:	Complaints of pain on movement
	Reluctance to attempt/difficulty with purposeful movement
	Impaired coordination, limited range of motion, decreased muscle strength.
PATIENT OUTCOMES/ EVALUATION CRITERIA:	Verbalizes understanding of situation/risk factors and individual treatment regimen. Demonstrates techniques/behaviors that enable resumption of activities. Maintains or increases strength and function of affected and/or compensatory body part.

ACTIONS/INTERVENTIONS

Independent

Provide for safety measures as indicated by individual situation.

Note emotional/behavioral responses to immobility. Provide diversional activities.

Follow activity/procedures with rest periods. Encourage participation in ADLs within individual limitations.

Provide/assist with passive and active ROM exercises.

Encourage lower leg/ankle exercises. Evaluate for edema, erythema of lower extremities, presence of Homans' sign.

RATIONALE

Dependent on area of involvement/type of procedure, imprudent activity increases chance of spinal injury. (Refer to CP: Disk Surgery, ND: Injury, Potential for: Trauma, p. 276.)

Forced immobility may heighten restlessness, irritability. Diversional activity aids in refocusing attention and promotes coping with limitations.

Enhances healing and builds muscle strength and endurance. Patient participation promotes independence and sense of control.

Strengthens abdominal muscles and flexors of spine; promotes good body mechanics.

Stimulates venous circulation/return decreasing venous stasis and possible thrombus formation.

ACTIONS/INTERVENTIONS

Independent

Assist with activity/progressive ambulation.

Demonstrate use of adjunctive devices, e.g., walker, cane.

Provide good skin care; massage pressure points after each position change. Check skin under brace periodically.

Collaborative

Administer medication for pain approximately 30 minutes prior to turning patient/ambulation, as indicated.

Apply antiembolism stockings as indicated.

RATIONALE

Activity is limited, is dependent on individual situation, and progresses slowly, according to tolerance.

Provides stability and support to compensate for altered muscle tone/strength and balance.

Reduces risk of skin irritation/breakdown.

Anticipation of pain can increase muscle tension. Medication can relax patient, enhance comfort and cooperation during activity.

Promotes venous return.

NURSING DIAGNOSIS:	ANXIETY [SPECIFY LEVEL]/COPING, INEFFECTIVE INDIVIDUAL [CHRONIC]
May be related to:	Situational crisis
	Threat to/change in health status, socioeconomic status, role functioning
	Recurrent disorder with continuing pain
	Inadequate relaxation, little or no exercise
	Inadequate coping methods
Possibly evidenced by:	Apprehension, uncertainty, helplessness
	Expressed concerns regarding changes in life events
	Verbalization of inability to cope
	Muscular tension, general irritability, restlessness; insomnia/fatigue
	Inability to meet role expectations
PATIENT OUTCOMES/ EVALUATION CRITERIA:	Appears relaxed and reports anxiety is reduced to a manageable level. Identifies ineffective coping behaviors and consequences. Assesses the current situation accurately. Demonstrates problem-solving skills. Develops plan for necessary lifestyle changes.

ACTIONS/INTERVENTIONS

Independent

Assess level of anxiety. Determine how patient is coping with current situation as well as how individual has dealt with past problems.

RATIONALE

Aids in identifying strengths and skills that may help patient deal with current situation and/or enable others to provide appropriate assistance.

ACTIONS/INTERVENTIONS

Independent

Provide accurate information and honest answers.

Provide opportunity for expression of concerns, e.g., possible paralysis; effect on sexual ability; changes in employment/finances; altered role responsibilities.

Assess presence of secondary gains that may interfere with the wish to recover and may impede recovery.

Note behaviors of SO that promote "sick role" for the patient.

Collaborative

Refer to community support groups, social services, financial/vocational counselor, marriage/psychotherapy.

RATIONALE

Enables patient to make decisions based on knowledge.

Most patients have concerns that need to be expressed and responded to with accurate information in order to promote coping with situation.

The patient may experience advantages such as relief from responsibilities, attention and control of others that are not within the conscious realm and need to be dealt with positively to promote recovery.

SO may unconsciously enable patient to remain dependent by doing things that patient should do for self. (Refer to CP: Psychosocial Aspects of Acute Care, p. 773.)

Provides support for adapting to changes and provides resources to deal with problems.

NURSING DIAGNOSIS:	KNOWLEDGE DEFICIT [LEARNING NEED] (SPECIFY)
May be related to:	Misinformation/lack of knowledge
	Information misinterpretation, lack of recall
	Unfamiliarity with information resources
Possibly evidenced by:	Verbalization of problems
	Statement of misconception
	Inaccurate return demonstration
PATIENT OUTCOMES/ EVALUATION CRITERIA:	Verbalizes understanding of condition, prognosis, and treatment. Initiates necessary lifestyle changes and participates in treatment regimen.

ACTIONS/INTERVENTIONS

Independent

Review disease/injury process and prognosis and activity restrictions/limitations; e.g., avoid riding in car for long periods of time, refrain from participation in aggressive sports.

Give information about and discuss importance of proper body mechanics and exercise routine. Include proper posture/body mechanics for standing, sitting, lifting; use of low-heeled shoes.

RATIONALE

Helpful in clarifying and developing understanding and acceptance of necessary lifestyle changes. When patient has full knowledge base, choices can be made to assist with adherence to treatment program and achievement of optimal recovery.

Reduces risk of reinjuring back/neck area by using muscles of thighs/buttocks. Changing old habits is more easily accomplished when patient has sufficient information and understands how change will be helpful.

ACTIONS/INTERVENTIONS	RATIONALE

Independent

Discuss medications and side effects: e.g., some medications cause drowsiness (analgesics, muscle relaxants); others can aggravate ulcer disease (NSAID).	With accurate information, patient can make informed decisions and reduce risk of complications/injury.
Discuss sleep patterns (e.g., sleep on side with knees flexed, avoid prone position), use of bedboards/firm mattress, small flat pillow under neck.	May decrease muscle strain through structural support and prevention of hyperextension of spine.
Discuss dietary needs/goals.	High-fiber diet can limit constipation; calorie restrictions promote weight control/reduction, which can decrease pressure on disk.
Avoid prolonged heat application.	Can increase local tissue congestion; decreased sensing of heat can result in burn.
Review use of soft cervical collar.	Maintaining slight flexion of head (allows maximal opening of intervertebral foramina) may be useful for relieving pressure in mild to moderate cervical disk disease. Hyperextension should be avoided.
Stress necessity of medical follow-up.	Evaluates resolution/progression of degenerative process; monitors development of side effects/complications of drug therapy; may indicate need for change in therapeutic regimen.
Provide information about what symptoms need to be reported for further evaluation, e.g., sharp pain, loss of sensation/ability to walk.	Progression of the process may necessitate further treatment/surgery.
Review treatment alternatives, e.g.:	
Chemonucleolysis;	As an alternative to surgery, the enzyme chymopapain may be injected into the disk (dissolves the mucoprotein disk material without effect on surrounding structure). Although many patients experience relief, side effects include allergic reaction to the enzyme.
Surgical interventions.	Laminectomy may be performed when conservative treatment is ineffective or when neurologic deficits increase. (Refer to CP: Disk Surgery, p. 275.)

Disk Surgery

PATIENT ASSESSMENT DATA BASE

Refer to CP: Herniated Nucleus Pulposis, p. 268.

TEACHING/LEARNING

Discharge Plan Considerations: May require assistance with transportation and, depending on degree of limitation, may need assistance with homemaker tasks; vocational counseling; possible changes in layout of home.

DIAGNOSTIC STUDIES

Refer to CP: Herniated Nucleus Pulposis, p. 268.

NURSING PRIORITIES

1. Maintain tissue perfusion/neurologic function.
2. Promote comfort and healing.
3. Prevent/minimize complications.
4. Assist with return to normal mobility.
5. Provide information about condition/prognosis, treatment needs and limitations.

DISCHARGE CRITERIA

1. Neurologic function maintained/improved.
2. Complications prevented.
3. Limited mobility achieved with potential for increasing mobility.
4. Condition/prognosis, therapeutic regimen and behavior/lifestyle changes are understood.

Refer to CP: Surgical Intervention, p. 789, for general surgical considerations.

NURSING DIAGNOSIS:	TISSUE PERFUSION, ALTERED: (SPECIFY)
May be related to:	**Diminished/interrupted blood flow (e.g., edema of operative site, hematoma formation)**
	Hypovolemia
Possibly evidenced by:	**Paresthesia; numbness**
	Decreased range of motion, muscle strength
PATIENT OUTCOMES/ EVALUATION CRITERIA:	**Reestablishes normal sensations and movement.**

ACTIONS/INTERVENTIONS	RATIONALE
Independent	
Check neurologic signs periodically and compare with baseline. Assess movement/sensation of lower extremities and feet (lumbar) plus hands/arms (cervical).	Although some degree of prior sensory impairment is often present, changes may reflect development/ resolution of edema and inflammation of the tissues secondary to manipulation during surgery or operative damage to motor nerve roots, requiring prompt medical evaluation.

275

ACTIONS/INTERVENTIONS	RATIONALE

Independent

Keep patient flat on back for several hours.

Monitor vital signs. Note color, warmth, capillary refill.

Monitor intake/output and Hemovac drainage (if used).

Palpate operative site for swelling. Inspect dressing for excess drainage and test for glucose if indicated.

Collaborative

Administer IV fluids/blood as indicated.

Monitor Hb, Hct, and RBC.

Pressure to operative site reduces risk of hematoma.	
Hypotension (especially postural) with corresponding changes in pulse rate may reflect hypovolemia from blood loss, restriction of oral intake, nausea/vomiting.	
Provides information about circulatory status and replacement needs.	
Change in contour of operative site suggests hematoma/edema formation. Inspection may reveal frank bleeding or dura leak of CSF (will test glucose-positive), requiring prompt intervention.	
Fluid replacement is dependent on the degree of hypovolemia and duration of oozing/bleeding/spinal fluid leaking.	
Aids in establishing blood replacement needs and monitors effectiveness of therapy.	

NURSING DIAGNOSIS:	**INJURY, POTENTIAL FOR: TRAUMA [SPINAL]**
May be related to:	**Temporary weakness of spinal column**
	Balancing difficulties, changes in muscle coordination
Possibly evidenced by:	**[Not applicable; presence of signs and symptoms establishes an *actual* diagnosis.]**
PATIENT OUTCOMES/ EVALUATION:	**Maintains proper alignment of spine. Recognizes need for/seeks assistance with activity.**

ACTIONS/INTERVENTIONS	RATIONALE

Independent

Post sign at bedside regarding prescribed position.

Provide bedboard/firm mattress.

Maintain cervical collar postoperatively with cervical laminectomy procedure.

Limit activities when patient has had a spinal fusion.

Logroll patient from side to side. Have patient fold arms across chest, tighten long back muscles, keeping shoulders and pelvis straight. Use pillows between knees during position change and when on side. Use turning sheet and sufficient personnel when turning, especially on the first postoperative day.

Reduces risk of inadvertent strain/flexion of operative area.	
Aids in stabilizing back.	
Decreases muscle spasm and supports the surrounding structures, allowing normal sensory stimulation to occur.	
Movement in the involved vertebral area is eliminated when fusion has been done and recuperation is longer.	
Maintains body alignment while turning, because twisting motion may interfere with healing process.	

ACTIONS/INTERVENTIONS

Independent

Assist out of bed: logroll to side of bed, splint back, and raise to sitting position. Avoid prolonged sitting. Move to standing position in one smooth motion.

Avoid sudden stretching, twisting, flexing, or jarring of spine.

Check blood pressure; note complaints of dizziness or weakness. Change position slowly.

Wear firm/flat walking shoes when ambulating.

Collaborative

Apply lumbar brace/cervical collar as appropriate.

Refer to physical therapy.

RATIONALE

Avoids twisting and flexing of back while arising from bed, protecting surgical area.

May cause vertebral collapse, shifting of bone graft, delayed hematoma formation, or subcutaneous wound dehiscence.

Presence of postural hypotension may result in fainting/fall and possible injury to surgical site.

Reduces risk of falls.

May be needed while patient is ambulating to give support to spine and surrounding structures until muscle strength improves. Brace is applied while patient is in bed and before ambulation.

Strengthening exercises may be indicated during the rehabilitative phase to decrease muscle spasm and strain on the vertebral disk area.

NURSING DIAGNOSIS:	BREATHING PATTERN, INEFFECTIVE [POTENTIAL]
May be related to:	Tracheal bronchial obstruction/edema
	Decreased lung expansion, pain
Possibly evidenced by:	[Not applicable; presence of signs and symptoms establishes an *actual* diagnosis.]
PATIENT OUTCOMES/ EVALUATION CRITERIA:	Maintains a normal/effective respiratory pattern, free of cyanosis and other signs of hypoxia, with ABGs within patient's normal range.

ACTIONS/INTERVENTIONS

Independent

Inspect for edema of face/neck (cervical laminectomy).

Listen for hoarseness.

Auscultate breath sounds, note presence of wheezes/rhonchi.

Assist with cough, turn and deep breathing.

RATIONALE

Tracheal edema/compression or nerve injury can compromise respiratory function.

May indicate laryngeal nerve injury, which can negatively affect cough (ability to clear airway).

Suggests accumulation of secretions/ineffective airway clearance.

Facilitates movement of secretions, clearing of lungs and reduces risk of respiratory complications (pneumonia).

ACTIONS/INTERVENTIONS

Collaborative

Administer supplemental oxygen, humidified if indicated.

Monitor/graph ABGs/pulse oximetry.

RATIONALE

May be necessary for periods of respiratory distress or evidence of hypoxia.

Monitors effectiveness of breathing pattern/therapy.

NURSING DIAGNOSIS:	COMFORT, ALTERED: PAIN, ACUTE
May be related to:	Physical agent (surgical manipulation, edema, inflammation)
Possibly evidenced by:	Complaints of pain
	Autonomic responses (diaphoresis, changes in vital signs, pallor)
	Alteration in muscle tone
	Guarding, distraction behaviors/restlessness
PATIENT OUTCOMES/ EVALUATION CRITERIA:	Reports pain is relieved/controlled. Verbalizes methods that provide relief. Demonstrates use of relaxation skills and diversional activities.

ACTIONS/INTERVENTIONS

Independent

Assess intensity, description and location/radiation of pain, changes in sensation.

Review expected manifestations/changes in intensity of pain.

Allow patient to assume position of comfort if indicated. Use logroll for position change.

Provide backrub/massage avoiding operative site.

Demonstrate/encourage use of relaxation skills, e.g., deep breathing, visualization.

Provide soft diet, room humidifier and encourage voice rest following cervical laminectomy.

RATIONALE

May be mild to severe with radiation to shoulders/ occipital area (cervical) or hips/buttocks (lumbar). If bone graft has been taken from the iliac crest, pain may be more severe at the donor site. Numbness/ tingling discomfort may reflect return of sensation after nerve root decompression or result from developing edema of compressed nerve/operative site.

Development/resolution of edema and inflammation in the immediate postoperative phase can affect pressure on various nerves and cause changes in degree of pain (especially 3 days after operation, when muscle spasms/improved nerve root sensation intensify pain).

Positioning is dictated by physical preference, type of operation (e.g., head of bed may be slightly elevated after cervical laminectomy). Readjustment of position aids in relieving muscle fatigue and discomfort. Log-rolling avoids tension in the operative areas, maintains straight spinal alignment.

Relieves/reduces pain by alteration of sensory neurons, muscle relaxation.

Refocuses attention, reduces muscle tension, promotes sense of well-being, and controls/decreases discomfort.

Reduces discomfort associated with sore throat and difficulty swallowing.

278

ACTIONS/INTERVENTIONS

Independent

Note patient reports of return of radicular pain.

Collaborative

Administer medications, as indicated:

    Narcotics, e.g., meperidine (Demerol), analgesics, e.g., acetaminophen (Tylenol) with codeine;

    Diazepam (Valium).

Assist with patient-controlled analgesia (PCA).

Provide throat sprays/lozenges, viscous xylocaine.

Apply TENS unit as needed.

RATIONALE

Suggests complications (collapsing of disk space, shifting of bone graft or arachnoiditis with adhesions), requiring further medical evaluation and intervention. Note: Sciatica and muscle spasms often recur after laminectomy but should resolve within several days or weeks.

Given for pain relief/control.

Narcotics may be needed the first few postoperative days; then nonnarcotic agents are incorporated as intensity of pain diminishes.

May be used to relieve muscle spasms of back/thighs resulting from intraoperative nerve irritation.

Allows patient control of administration of medication (usually narcotics) to enhance level of comfort. Monitoring by the nurse is essential for avoiding over/underdosing of the patient.

Sore throat may be a major complaint following cervical laminectomy.

May be used for incisional pain or when nerve involvement continues after discharge.

NURSING DIAGNOSIS:	MOBILITY, IMPAIRED PHYSICAL
May be related to:	Neuromuscular impairment
	Limitations imposed by condition
	Pain
Possibly evidenced by:	Impaired coordination, limited range of motion
	Reluctance to attempt movement
	Decreased muscle strength/control
PATIENT OUTCOMES/ EVALUATION CRITERIA:	Demonstrates techniques/behaviors that enable resumption of activities. Maintains or increases strength and function of body. Verbalizes understanding of situation, treatment regimen, and safety measures.

ACTIONS/INTERVENTIONS

Independent

Schedule activity/procedures with rest periods. Encourage participation in ADLs within individual limitations.

Provide/assist with passive and active ROM exercises dependent on surgical procedure.

RATIONALE

Enhances healing and builds muscle strength and endurance. Patient participation promotes independence and sense of control.

Strengthens abdominal muscles and flexors of spine; promotes good body mechanics.

279

ACTIONS/INTERVENTIONS

Independent

Assist with activity/progressive ambulation.

(Refer to CP: Herniated Nucleus Pulposus, ND: Mobility, Impaired Physical, p. 271, for further considerations.)

RATIONALE

Until healing occurs, activity is limited, and progressed slowly according to individual tolerance.

NURSING DIAGNOSIS: BOWEL ELIMINATION, ALTERED: CONSTIPATION

May be related to:

Pain and swelling in surgical area

Immobilization, decreased physical activity

Altered nerve stimulation, ileus

Emotional stress, lack of privacy

Ch⌐ restriction of dietary intake

Possibly evidenced by:

⌐vel sounds

⌐ninal girth

⌐bdominal/rectal fullness, nausea

⌐ncy, consistency and amount of stool

PATIENT O⌐
EVALUA⌐.

⌐nal patterns of bowel functioning.
⌐ft/semiformed consistency without

ACTIONS/INTER⌐

Independent

Note abdominal distention, and listen bowel sounds.

Use fracture or child size bedpan until allowed out of bed.

Provide privacy.

Encourage ambulation as able.

Collaborative

Begin progressive diet as tolerated.

Provide rectal tube, suppositories and enemas as needed.

Administer laxatives, stool softeners as indicated.

RATIONALE

⌐istention and lack of bowel sounds indicate the bowel is not functioning possibly due to sudden loss of parasympathetic enervation of the bowel.

Promotes comfort, reduces muscle tension.

Promotes psychologic comfort.

Stimulates peristalsis facilitating passage of flatus.

Solid foods are not started until bowel sounds have returned/flatus has been passed and danger of ileus formation has abated.

May be necessary to relieve abdominal distention, promote resumption of normal bowel habits.

Given to soften stool, promote normal bowel habits, decrease straining.

NURSING DIAGNOSIS:	URINARY ELIMINATION, ALTERED PATTERNS [POTENTIAL]
May be related to:	Pain and swelling in operative area Need for remaining flat in bed
Possibly evidenced by:	[Not applicable; presence of signs and symptoms establishes an *actual* diagnosis.]
PATIENT OUTCOMES/ EVALUATION CRITERIA:	Empties bladder adequately according to individual need.

ACTIONS/INTERVENTIONS

RATIONALE

Independent

Observe and record amount/time of voiding.	Determines whether bladder is being emptied and when interventions may be necessary.
Palpate for bladder distention.	May indicate urine retention.
Force fluids.	Maintains kidney function.
Stimulate autonomic nervous system by running water, pouring warm water over perineum, placing hand in warm water.	Promotes urination by relaxing urinary sphincter.

Collaborative

Catheterize as indicated. Insert/maintain indwelling catheter as needed.	Intermittent or continuous catheterization may be necessary for several days postoperatively, until swelling is decreased.

NURSING DIAGNOSIS:	KNOWLEDGE DEFICIT [LEARNING NEED] (SPECIFY)
May be related to:	Lack of exposure Information misinterpretation; lack of recall Unfamiliarity with information resources
Possibly evidenced by:	Request for information Statement of misconception Inaccurate follow-through of instruction
PATIENT OUTCOMES/ EVALUATION CRITERIA:	Verbalizes understanding of condition, prognosis, and therapeutic regimen. Participates in treatment regimen. Initiates necessary lifestyle changes.

ACTIONS/INTERVENTIONS

RATIONALE

Independent

Review particular condition/prognosis.	Individual needs dictate tolerance levels/limitations of activity.

ACTIONS/INTERVENTIONS	RATIONALE
Independent	
Discuss return to activities, stressing importance of increasing as tolerated after hospitalization.	Although the recuperative period may be lengthy, following prescribed activity program promotes muscle and tissue circulation, healing and strengthening.
Encourage development of regular exercise program, e.g., walking.	Promotes healing, strengthens abdominal and erector muscles to provide support to the spinal column, and enhances general physical and emotional well-being.
Discuss importance of good posture and avoidance of prolonged standing/sitting. Recommend sitting in straight-backed chair with feet on a footstool or flat on the floor.	Prevents further injuries/stress by maintaining proper alignment of spine.
Stress importance of avoiding activities that increase the flexion of the spine, e.g., climbing stairs, automobile driving/riding, bending at the waist with knees straight, lifting more than 5 lbs, engaging in strenuous exercise/sports. Discuss limitations on sexual relations.	Flexing/twisting of the spine aggravates the healing process and increases risk of injury to spinal cord.
Encourage lying down rest periods, balanced with activity.	Reduces general and spinal fatigue and assists in the healing/recuperative process.
Discuss possibility of unrelieved/renewed pain.	Some pain may continue for several months as activity level increases and scar tissue stretches. Pain relief from surgical procedure could be temporary if other disks have similar amount of degeneration.
Discuss use of heat, e.g., warm packs, heating pad, or showers.	Increased circulation to the back/surgical area transports nutrients for healing to the area and resolution of pathogens/exudates out of the area. Decreases muscle spasms that may result from nerve root irritation during healing process.
Discuss judicious use of cold packs before/after stretching activity if indicated.	May decrease muscle spasm in some instances more effectively than heat.
Avoid tub baths for 3–4 weeks, depending on physician recommendation.	Tub baths increase risk of flexing/twisting of spine as well as danger of falls.
Review dietary/fluid needs.	Should be tailored to reduce risk of constipation and avoid excess weight gain while meeting nutrient needs to facilitate healing.
Review/reinforce incisional care.	Correct care promotes healing, reduces risk of wound infection.
Identify signs/symptoms requiring notification of health-care provider, e.g., fever, increased incisional pain, inflammation, wound drainage; decreased sensation/motor activity in extremities.	Prompt evaluation and intervention may prevent complications/permanent injury.
Discuss necessity of follow-up care.	Long term medical supervision may be needed to manage problems/complications and to reincorporate individual into desired/altered lifestyle and activities.
Assess current lifestyle/job, finances, activities at home and leisure.	Knowledge of current situation allows nurse to highlight areas for possible intervention, such as referral for occupational/vocational testing and counseling.
Listen/communicate with patient regarding alternatives of lifestyle changes. Be sensitive to patient's needs.	Laminectomy and low back pain are a frequent cause of chronic disability. Many patients may have to stop work, creating marital/financial crises. Often the concern that the patient is a malingerer creates further problems in social relationships.

ACTIONS/INTERVENTIONS	RATIONALE

Independent

Note overt/covert expressions of concern about sexuality.

Although patient may not ask directly, there may be concerns about the effect of this surgery on not only ability to cope with usual role in the family/community but also ability to perform sexually.

Explore limitations/abilities.

Placing limitations into perspective with abilities allows the patient to understand own situation and exercise choice.

Provide written copy of all instructions.

Useful as a reference after discharge.

Collaborative

Instruct patient not to resume heavy work until physician approves.

Allows time for sufficient healing before resumption of strenuous activity.

Review need for/use of immobilization device, as indicated.

Correct application and wearing time is important to gaining the most benefit from the brace.

Refer to resources as indicated, e.g., social services, counseling, sex therapy, rehabilitation/vocational counseling services.

A team effort can be helpful in providing support during recuperative period.

Refer for psychotherapy as indicated.

Depression is common in illness where lengthy recuperative time (2–9 months) is expected. Therapy may alleviate further anxiety, assist patient to cope effectively, and enhance healing process.

Spinal Cord Injury (Acute Rehabilitative Phase) _____

Spinal cord lesions are classified as complete (total loss of sensation and voluntary motor function) and incomplete (mixed loss of sensation and voluntary motor function).

Physical findings will vary, depending on the level of injury, degree of spinal shock, and phase and degree of recovery:

C1-3: Quadriplegia with total loss of muscular/respiratory function
C4-5: Quadriplegia with impairment, poor pulmonary capacity, complete dependency for ADLs
C6-7: Quadriplegia with some arm/hand movement allowing some independence in ADLs
C7-8: Quadriplegia with limited use of thumb/fingers, increasing independence
T1-L1: Paraplegia with intact arm function and varying function of intercostal and abdominal muscles
L1-2 or below: Mixed motor-sensory loss; bowel and bladder dysfunction

PATIENT ASSESSMENT DATA BASE

ACTIVITY/REST

May exhibit: Paralysis of muscles (flaccid during spinal shock) at/below level of lesion.

Muscle/generalized weakness (cord contusion and compression).

CIRCULATION

May report: Palpitations.

Dizziness with position changes.

May exhibit: Low blood pressure, postural blood pressure changes, bradycardia.

Cool, pale extremities.

Absence of perspiration in affected area.

ELIMINATION

May exhibit: Incontinence of bladder and bowel.

Abdominal distention; loss of bowel sounds.

Melena, coffee-ground emesis/hematemesis.

EGO INTEGRITY

May report: Denial, disbelief, sadness, anger.

May exhibit: Fear, anxiety, irritability, withdrawal.

FOOD/FLUID

May exhibit: Abdominal distention; loss of bowel sounds (paralytic ileus).

NEUROSENSORY

May report: Numbness, tingling, burning, twitching of arms/legs.

May exhibit: Flaccid paralysis (spasticity may develop as spinal shock resolves, dependent on area of cord involvement).

Loss of sensation (varying degrees may return after spinal shock resolves).

Loss of muscle/vasomotor tone.

Loss of/asymmetric reflexes, including deep tendon.

Changes in pupil reaction, ptosis of upper eyelid.

Loss of sweating in affected area.

PAIN/COMFORT

May report: Pain/tenderness in back, neck.
Hyperesthesia immediately above level of injury.

May exhibit: Vertebral tenderness, deformity.

RESPIRATION

May report: Shortness of breath, air hunger, inability to breathe.

May exhibit: Shallow/labored respirations; periods of apnea.
Pallor, cyanosis.

SAFETY

May exhibit: Temperature fluctuations (taking on temperature of environment).

SEXUALITY

May report: Expressions of concern about return to normal functioning.

May exhibit: Uncontrolled erection (priapism).

TEACHING/LEARNING

**Discharge Plan
Considerations:**   Will require varying degrees of assistance with transportation, shopping, food preparation, self-care, finances, medications/treatment, and homemaker tasks.
May require changes in physical layout of home and/or placement in a rehabilitative center.

DIAGNOSTIC STUDIES

Spinal x-rays: locates level and type of bony injury (fracture, dislocation), determines alignment and reduction after traction or surgery.

CT scan: locates injury, evaluates structural alterations.

Myelogram: may be done to visualize spinal column if pathology is unclear or occlusion of spinal subarachnoid space is suspected (not usually done after penetrating injuries).

MRI: identifies spinal cord lesions, edema and compression.

Chest x-ray: demonstrates pulmonary status (e.g., changes in level of diaphragm, atelectasis).

Pulmonary function studies (vital capacity, tidal volume): measures maximum volume of inspiration and expiration; especially important in patients with low cervical lesions or thoracic lesions with possible phrenic nerve and intercostal muscle involvement.

ABGs: indicates effectiveness of gas exchange and ventilatory effort.

NURSING PRIORITIES

1. Maximize respiratory function.
2. Prevent further injury to spinal column.
3. Promote mobility/independence.
4. Prevent or minimize complications.
5. Support psychologic adjustment of patient/SO.
6. Provide information about injury/prognosis, treatment needs and expectations, possible and preventable complications.

DISCHARGE CRITERIA

1. Ventilatory effort adequate for individual needs.
2. Spinal injury stabilized.

3. Complications prevented/controlled.
4. Self-care needs met by self/with assistance dependent on specific situation.
5. Beginning to cope with current situation and planning for future.
6. Condition/prognosis, therapeutic regimen, and possible complications understood.

NURSING DIAGNOSIS:	BREATHING PATTERN, INEFFECTIVE [POTENTIAL]
May be related to:	Impairment of innervation of diaphragm (lesions at or above C-5)
	Complete or mixed loss of intercostal muscle function
	Reflex abdominal spasms; gastric distension
Possibly evidenced by:	[Not applicable; presence of signs and symptoms establishes an *actual* diagnosis.]
PATIENT OUTCOMES/ EVALUATION CRITERIA:	Maintains adequate ventilation as evidenced by absence of respiratory distress and ABGs within acceptable limits. Demonstrates appropriate behaviors to support respiratory effort.

ACTIONS/INTERVENTIONS

Independent

Maintain patent airway: keep head in neutral position; elevate head of bed slightly if tolerated; use airway adjuncts as indicated.

Suction as necessary. Document quality and quantity of secretions.

Assess respiratory function, by asking patient to take a deep breath. Note presence or absence of spontaneous effort and quality of respirations, e.g., labored, using accessory muscles.

Auscultate breath sounds. Note areas of absent or decreased breath sounds or development of adventitious sounds (e.g., rhonchi).

Assess strength/effectiveness of cough.

Assist with coughing (when indicated) by placing hands below diaphragm and pushing upward as patient exhales.

Observe skin color for developing cyanosis, duskiness.

Assess for abdominal distension, and muscle spasm.

RATIONALE

Patients with high cervical injury and impaired gag/cough reflexes will require assistance in preventing aspiration/maintaining patent airway.

If cough is ineffective, suctioning may be needed to remove secretions, enhance gas distribution, and reduce risk of respiratory infections.

C1-C3 injuries result in complete loss of respiratory function. C4-C5 can result in variable loss of respiratory function, depending on phrenic nerve involvement and diaphragmatic function but generally have decreased vital capacity and inspiratory effort. Injuries below C6-C7 have respiratory muscle function preserved; however, weakness/impairment of intercostal muscles may impair effectiveness of cough, sigh, deep breathing ability.

Hypoventilation is common and leads to accumulation of secretions, atelectasis and pneumonia (frequent complications).

Level of injury determines function of intercostal muscles and ability to cough spontaneously/move secretions.

"Quad coughing" is performed to add volume to cough, to facilitate expectoration of secretions or to move them high enough to be suctioned out.

May reveal impending respiratory failure, need for immediate medical evaluation and intervention.

May impede diaphragmatic excursion, reducing lung expansion and further compromising respiratory function.

ACTIONS/INTERVENTIONS	RATIONALE

Independent

Reposition/turn periodically. Avoid/limit prone position when necessary.

Enhances ventilation of all lung segments, mobilizes secretions, reducing risk of complications, e.g., atelectasis and pneumonia. Note: Prone position significantly decreases vital capacity, increasing risk of respiratory compromise, failure.

Encourage fluids (at least 2000 ml/day).

Aids in liquefying secretions, promoting mobilization/expectoration.

Monitor/limit visitors as indicated.

General debilitation and respiratory compromise places patient at increased risk for acquiring URI.

Elicit concerns/questions regarding mechanical ventilation devices. Acknowledge reality of situation. Provide honest answers.

Future respiratory function/support needs will not be totally known until spinal shock resolves and acute rehabilitative phase is completed. Even though respiratory support may be required, alternative devices/techniques may be used to enhance mobility and promote independence.

Assist patient in "taking control" of respirations as indicated. Encouraging deep breathing, focusing of attention on steps of respiration, etc.

Breathing may no longer be a totally voluntary activity, but require conscious effort, depending on level of injury/involvement of respiratory muscles.

Monitor diaphragmatic movement when phrenic pacemaker implanted.

Stimulation of phrenic nerve may enhance respiratory effort, decreasing dependency on mechanical ventilator.

Collaborative

Measure/graph:

Vital capacity, tidal volume, inspiratory force;

Determines level of respiratory muscle function. Serial measurements may be done to predict impending respiratory failure (acute injury) or determine level of function after spinal shock phase and/or while weaning from ventilatory support.

Serial ABGs and/or pulse oximetry.

Documents status of ventilation and oxygenation, identifies respiratory problems, e.g., hypoventilation (low PaO_2/elevated $PaCO_2$), and pulmonary complications.

Administer oxygen by appropriate method, e.g., nasal prongs, mask, intubation/ventilator. (Refer to CP: Ventilatory Assistance [Mechanical], p. 191.)

Method is determined by level of injury, degree of respiratory insufficiency, and amount of recovery of respiratory muscle function after spinal shock phase.

Refer to/consult with respiratory and physical therapists.

Helpful in identifying exercises individually appropriate to stimulate and strengthen respiratory muscles/effort.

Assist with aggressive chest physiotherapy (e.g., chest percussion) and use of respiratory adjuncts (e.g., incentive spirometer, blow bottles).

Preventing retained secretions is essential to maximize gas diffusion and to reduce risk of pneumonia.

NURSING DIAGNOSIS:	INJURY, POTENTIAL FOR: [ADDITIONAL SPINAL] TRAUMA
May be related to:	Temporary weakness/instability of spinal column
Possibly evidenced by:	[Not applicable; presence of signs and symptoms establishes an *actual* diagnosis.]

ACTIONS/INTERVENTIONS	RATIONALE
Independent	
Maintain bedrest and immobilization device(s), e.g., traction, halo, sandbags, hard/soft cervical collars.	Prevents vertebral column instability and aids healing.
Check skeletal traction apparatus to ensure that frames are secure, pulleys aligned, weights hanging free.	Necessary for maintenance of specified traction for reduction and stabilization of vertebral column and prevention of further spinal cord injury.
Check weights for ordered traction pull (usually 10–20 lb).	Weight pull depends on patient's size and amount of reduction needed to maintain vertebral column alignment.
Elevate head of traction frame or bed as indicated.	Creates counterbalance to maintain both patient's position and traction pull.
Reposition at intervals, using adjuncts for turning and support, e.g., turn sheets, foam wedges, blanket rolls, pillows. Use several staff members when turning/logrolling patient. Follow special instructions for traction equipment, kinetic bed, and frames.	Maintains proper spinal column alignment reducing risk of further trauma.
Collaborative	
Maintain skeletal traction via tongs, calipers; halo/vest as indicated.	Reduces vertebral fracture/dislocation.
Prepare for surgery, e.g., spinal laminectomy or fusion if indicated. (Refer to CP: Disk Surgery, p. 275.)	Surgery may be indicated for spinal decompression or removal of bony fragments.

NURSING DIAGNOSIS:	MOBILITY, IMPAIRED PHYSICAL
May be related to:	**Neuromuscular impairment**
	Immobilization by traction
Possibly evidenced by:	**Inability to purposefully move; paralysis**
	Muscle atrophy; contractures
PATIENT OUTCOMES/ EVALUATION CRITERIA:	**Maintains position of function as evidenced by absence of contractures, footdrop. Increases strength of unaffected/compensatory body parts. Demonstrates techniques/behavior that enable resumption of activity.**

ACTIONS/INTERVENTIONS	RATIONALE
Independent	
Continually assess motor function (as spinal shock/edema resolves) by requesting that patient perform actions, e.g., shrug shoulders, spread fingers, squeeze/release examiner's hands.	Evaluates status of individual situation (motor-sensory impairment may be mixed and/or not clear) for a specific level of injury affecting type and choice of interventions.
Provide means to summon help, e.g., special sensitive call light.	Enables patient to have a sense of control and reduces fear of being left alone. Note: Quadriplegic on

ACTIONS/INTERVENTIONS	RATIONALE
Independent	
	ventilator requires continuous observation in early management.
Perform/assist with full range of motion exercises on all extremities and joints, using slow smooth movements. Hyperextend hips periodically.	Enhances circulation, restores/maintains muscle tone and joint mobility and prevents disuse contractures and muscle atrophy.
Position arms at 90 degree angle at regular intervals.	Prevents frozen shoulder contractures.
Maintain ankles at 90 degrees with footboard, high-top tennis shoes, etc. Use trochanter rolls along thighs when in bed.	Prevents footdrop and external rotation of hips.
Elevate lower extremities at intervals when in chair, or raise foot of bed when permitted in individual situation. Assess for edema of feet/ankles.	Loss of vascular tone and ''muscle action'' results in pooling of blood and venous stasis in lower extremities with increased risk of thrombus formation.
Measure/monitor blood pressure before and after activity in acute phases or until stable. Change position slowly. Use cardiac bed or tilt table/circoelectric bed as activity level is advanced.	Orthostatic hypotension may occur as a result of venous pooling (secondary to loss of vascular tone). Side-to-side movement or elevation of head can aggravate hypotension and cause syncope.
Reposition periodically even when sitting in chair.	Reduces pressure areas, promotes peripheral circulation.
Inspect skin daily. Observe for pressure areas, and provide meticulous skin care.	Altered circulation, loss of sensation, and paralysis potentiate pressure sore formation. This is a life-long consideration. (Refer to ND: Skin Integrity, Impaired: Potential, p. 298.)
Assist with/encourage pulmonary hygiene, e.g., deep breathing, cough, suction. (Refer to ND: Breathing Pattern, Ineffective, p. 286.)	Immobility/bedrest increases risk of pulmonary infection.
Assess for redness, swelling/muscle tension of calf tissues. Record calf and thigh measurements if indicated. (Refer to CP: Thrombophlebitis, p. 117.)	In a high percentage of patients with cervical cord injury, thrombi develop because of altered peripheral circulation, immobilization and flaccid paralysis.
Investigate sudden onset of dyspnea, cyanosis and/or other signs of respiratory distress. (Refer to CP: Pulmonary Embolism, p. 148.)	Development of pulmonary emboli may be ''silent'' because pain perception is altered and/or deep vein thrombosis is not readily recognized.
Collaborative	
Place patient in kinetic therapy bed when appropriate.	Effectively immobilizes unstable spinal column, and improves systemic circulation, which is thought to decrease complications associated with immobility.
Apply antiembolic hose/leotard.	Limits pooling of blood in lower extremities or abdomen, thus improving vasomotor tone and reducing incidence of thrombus formation and pulmonary emboli.
Consult with physical/occupational therapists.	Helpful in planning and implementing individualized exercise program and identifying/developing assistive devices to maintain function, enhance mobility and independence.

NURSING DIAGNOSIS:	**SENSORY-PERCEPTUAL ALTERATION: (SPECIFY)**
May be related to:	**Destruction of sensory tracts with altered sensory reception, transmission and integration**
	Reduced environmental stimuli

289

	Psychologic stress (narrowed perceptual fields caused by anxiety)
Possibly evidenced by:	Measured change in sensory acuity, including position of body parts/proprioception
	Change in usual response to stimuli
	Motor incoordination
	Anxiety, disorientation, bizarre thinking
	Exaggerated emotional responses
PATIENT OUTCOMES/ EVALUATION CRITERIA:	Recognizes sensory impairments. Identifies behaviors to compensate for deficits. Verbalizes awareness of sensory needs and potential for deprivation/overload.

ACTIONS/INTERVENTIONS

Independent

Assess/document sensory function or deficit (by means of touch, pinprick, hot/cold, etc.) progressing from area of deficit to neurologically intact area.

Protect from bodily harm, e.g., falls, positioning on arm or object, burns.

Assist the patient to recognize expected alterations in sensation.

Explain procedures prior to and during care, identifying the body part involved.

Provide tactile stimulation, touching patient in intact sensory areas, e.g., shoulders, face, head.

Position patient to see surroundings and activities. Provide prism glasses when prone on turning frame. Talk to patient frequently.

Provide diversional activities, e.g., television, radio, music, liberal visitation. Use clocks, calendars, etc.

Encourage uninterrupted sleep and rest periods.

Note presence of exaggerated emotional responses, altered thought processes, e.g., disorientation, bizarre thinking.

RATIONALE

Changes may not occur during acute phase; but as spinal shock resolves, changes should be documented by dermatome charts or anatomic land marks, e.g., "2 inches above nipple line."

Patient may not sense pain or be aware of body position.

May help reduce anxiety of the unknown.

Enhances patient perception of body as a whole.

Touching conveys caring and fulfills a normal physiologic and psychologic need.

Provides sensory input, which may be severely limited, especially when patient is in prone position.

Aids in maintaining reality orientation and provides some sense of normality in daily passage of time.

Reduces sensory overload, enhances orientation and coping abilities, and aids in reestablishing natural sleep patterns.

Indicative of damage to sensory tracts and/or psychologic stress, requiring further assessment and intervention.

NURSING DIAGNOSIS:	COMFORT, ALTERED: PAIN, ACUTE
May be related to:	Physical injury
	Traction apparatus
Possibly evidenced by:	Hyperesthesia immediately above level of injury
	Burning pain below level of injury (paraplegia)

Muscle spasm/spasticity

Phantom pain; headaches

PATIENT OUTCOMES/ EVALUATION CRITERIA:	Reports relief of pain/discomfort. Identifies ways to manage pain. Demonstrates use of relaxation skills and diversional activities as individually indicated.

ACTIONS/INTERVENTIONS

Independent

Assess for presence of pain. Help patient identify and quantify pain, e.g., location, type of pain, intensity on scale of 1–10.

Evaluate increased irritability, muscle tension, restlessness, unexplained vital sign changes.

Assist patient in identifying precipitating factors.

Provide comfort measures, e.g., position changes, massage, warm/cold packs as indicated.

Encourage use of relaxation techniques, e.g., guided imagery, visualization, deep breathing exercises. Provide diversional activities, e.g., television, radio, telephone, unlimited visitors.

Collaborative

Administer medications as indicated: muscle relaxants, e.g., dantrolene (Dantrium); analgesics; sedatives, e.g., diazepam (Valium).

RATIONALE

Patient may initially report pain above the level of injury, e.g., chest/back or headache possibly from stabilizer apparatus. After spinal shock phase, patient may report muscle spasms and phantom pain below level of injury.

Nonverbal cues indicative of pain/discomfort requiring intervention.

Burning pain and muscle spasms can be precipitated/aggravated by multiple factors, e.g., anxiety, tension, sitting for long periods of time, bladder distention.

Alternate measures for pain control are desirable for their emotional benefit, in addition to reducing pain medication needs/undesirable effects on respiratory function.

Refocuses attention, promotes sense of control, and may enhance coping abilities.

May be desired to relieve muscle spasm/pain or to alleviate anxiety and promote rest.

NURSING DIAGNOSIS:	GRIEVING, ANTICIPATORY
May be related to:	Perceived/actual loss of physiopsychosocial well-being
Possibly evidenced by:	Altered communication patterns
	Expression of distress, choked feelings, e.g., denial, guilt, fear, sadness; altered affect
	Alterations in sleep patterns
PATIENT OUTCOMES/ EVALUATION CRITERIA:	Expressing feelings and beginning to progress through recognized stages of grief, focusing on one day at a time.

ACTIONS/INTERVENTIONS	RATIONALE

Independent

Identify signs of grieving (e.g., shock, denial, anger, depression).

Patient experiences many emotional reactions to the injury and its impact on life. These stages are not static, and the rate at which the patient progresses through them is variable.

Shock

Note lack of communication or emotional response, absence of questions.

Shock is the initial reaction associated with overwhelming injury. Primary concern is to maintain life, and patient may be too ill to express feelings.

Provide simple, accurate information to patient and SO regarding diagnosis and care. Be honest; do not give false reassurance while providing emotional support.

Patient's awareness of surroundings and activity may be blocked initially, and attention span may be limited. Little is actually known about the final outcome of the patient's injuries during acute phase, and indeed knowledge may add to frustration and grief of family. Therefore, early focus of emotional support may be directed toward SO.

Encourage expressions of sadness, grief, guilt and fear among patient/SO/friends.

Knowledge that these are appropriate feelings that should be expressed may be very supportive to patient/SO.

Incorporate SO into problem-solving and planning for patient's care.

Assists in establishing therapeutic nurse–patient–SO relationships. Provides sense of control in face of so many losses/forced changes and promotes feeling of contributing to well-being of patient.

Denial

Assist patient/SO to verbalize feelings about situation, avoiding judgment about what is expressed.

Important beginning step to deal with what has happened. Helpful in identifying patient's coping mechanisms.

Note comments indicating that patient expects to walk shortly and/or is making a bargain with God. Do not confront these comments.

Patient may not deny entire disability but may deny its permanency. Situation is compounded by actual uncertainty of outcome, and denial may be useful for coping at this time.

Focus on present needs (e.g., range of motion exercises, skin care).

Attention on "here and now" reduces frustration and hopelessness of uncertain future and may make dealing with today's problems more manageable.

Anger

Identify use of manipulative behavior and reactions to care givers.

Patient may express anger verbally or physically (e.g., spitting, biting). Patient may say that nothing is done right by care givers/SO or may pit one care giver against another.

Encourage patient to take control when possible; for example, establishing care routines, dietary choices, diversional activities.

Helps reduce anger associated with powerlessness and provides patient with some sense of control and expectation of responsibility for own behavior.

Accept expressions of anger and hopelessness. Avoid arguing. Show concern for the patient.

Patient is acknowledged as a worthwhile individual, and nonjudgmental care is provided.

Set limits on acting-out and unacceptable behavior when necessary (e.g., abusive language, sexually aggressive or suggestive behavior).

Although it is important to express negative feelings, patient and staff need to be protected from violence and embarrassment. This phase is traumatic for all involved, and support of family is essential.

ACTIONS/INTERVENTIONS	RATIONALE
Independent	
Depression	
Note loss of interest in living, sleep disturbance, suicidal thoughts, hopelessness. Listen to but do not confront these expressions. Let patient know nurse is available for support.	Phase may last weeks, months, or even years. Acceptance of these feelings and consistent support during this phase is important to a satisfactory resolution.
Collaborative	
Consult with/refer to psychiatric nurse, social worker, psychiatrist, pastor.	Patient/SO will need assistance to work through feelings of alienation, guilt, and resentment concerning lifestyle and role changes. The family (required to make adaptive changes to a member who may be permanently "different") will benefit from supportive, long-term assistance and/or counseling in coping with these changes and the future. Patient and SO may suffer great spiritual distress, including feelings of guilt, deprivation of peace, and anger at God, which may interfere with resolution of grief process.

NURSING DIAGNOSIS: SELF-CONCEPT, DISTURBANCE IN: (SPECIFY)

May be related to: Traumatic injury; situational crisis; forced crisis

Possibly evidenced by:

Verbalization of forced change in lifestyle

Fear of rejection/reaction by others

Focus on past strength, function, or appearance

Negative feelings about body

Feelings of helplessness, hopelessness, or powerlessness

Actual change in structure and/or function

Lack of eye contact

Change in physical capacity to resume role

Confusion about self, purpose or direction of life

PATIENT OUTCOMES/ EVALUATION CRITERIA: Verbalizes acceptance of self in situation. Recognizes and incorporates changes into self-concept in accurate manner without negating self-esteem. Developing realistic plans for adapting to new role/role changes.

ACTIONS/INTERVENTIONS	RATIONALE
Independent	
Acknowledge difficulty in determining degree of functional incapacity and/or chance of functional improvement.	During acute phase of injury, long-term effects are unknown, which delays the patient's ability to integrate situation into self-concept.
Listen to patient's comments and responses to situation.	Provides clues to view of self, role changes, and needs and is useful for providing information at patient's level of acceptance.

ACTIONS/INTERVENTIONS	RATIONALE

Independent

Assess dynamics of patient and SOs (e.g., patient's role in family, cultural factors).

Patient's previous role in family unit is disrupted or altered by injury, adding to difficulty in integrating self-concept. In addition, issues of independence/dependence need to be addressed.

Encourage SO to treat patient as normally as possible (e.g., discussing home situations, family news).

Involving patient in family unit reduces feelings of social isolation, helplessness, and uselessness and provides opportunity for SO to contribute to patient's welfare.

Provide accurate information. Discuss concerns about prognosis and treatment honestly at patient's level of acceptance.

Focus of information should be on present and immediate needs initially and incorporated into long-term rehabilitation goals. Information should be repeated until patient has assimilated or integrated information.

Discuss meaning of loss or change with patient/SO. Assess interactions between patient and SO.

Actual change in body image may be different from that perceived by patient. Distortions may be unconsciously reinforced by SO.

Accept patient, show concern for individual as a person. Encourage patient, identify strengths, give positive reinforcement for progress noted.

Establishes therapeutic atmosphere for patient to begin self-acceptance.

Include patient/SO in care, allowing patient to make decisions and to participate in self-care activities as possible.

Recognizes that patient is still responsible for own life and provides some sense of control over situation. Sets stage for future lifestyle, pattern and interaction required in daily care. Note: Patient may reject all help or may be completely dependent during this phase.

Be alert to sexually oriented jokes/flirting or aggressive behavior. Elicit concerns, fears, feelings about current situation/future expectations.

Anxiety develops as a result of perceived loss/change in masculine/feminine self-image and role. Forced dependency is often devastating especially in light of change in function/appearance.

Be aware of own feelings/reaction to patient's sexual anxiety.

Behavior may be disruptive, creating conflict between patient/staff, further reinforcing negative feelings and possibly eliminating patient's desire to work through situation/participation in rehabilitation.

Arrange visit by similarly affected person if patient desires and/or situation allows.

May be helpful to patient by providing hope for the future/role model.

Collaborative

Refer to counseling/psychotherapy as indicated, e.g., psychiatric nurse/clinical specialist, psychiatrist, social worker, sex therapist.

May need additional assistance to adjust to change in body image/life.

NURSING DIAGNOSIS:	**BOWEL ELIMINATION, ALTERED: (SPECIFY)**
May be related to:	**Disruption of innervation to bowel and rectum**
	Altered dietary and fluid intake
Possibly evidenced by:	**Loss of ability to evacuate bowel voluntarily**
	Constipation
	Gastric dilatation, ileus

PATIENT OUTCOMES/ EVALUATION CRITERIA:	Establishes bowel program and reestablishes satisfactory bowel elimination pattern.

ACTIONS/INTERVENTIONS	RATIONALE
Independent	
Auscultate bowel sounds, noting location and characteristics.	May be absent during spinal shock phase. High tinkling sounds may indicate presence of ileus.
Assess for abdominal distention if bowel sounds are decreased or absent.	Loss of peristalsis (related to impaired innervation) paralyzes the bowel, creating ileus and bowel distention. Note: Overdistention of the bowel is a precipitator of autonomic dysreflexia once spinal shock subsides. (Refer to ND: Dysreflexia, p. 297.)
Note complaints of nausea, onset of vomiting. Check vomitus or gastric secretions (if tube in place) and stools for occult blood.	GI bleeding may occur in response to injury (Cushing's ulcer) or as a side effect of certain therapies (steroids or anticoagulants). (Refer to CP: Upper Gastrointestinal/Esophageal Bleeding, p. 397.)
Record frequency, characteristics and amount of stool.	Identifies degree of impairment/dysfunction and level of assistance required.
Recognize signs of impaction, check for presence of impaction, e.g., no formed stool for several days, semiliquid stool, restlessness, increased feelings of fullness in abdomen.	Early intervention is necessary in order to treat constipation/retained stool effectively and reduce risk of complications.
Establish regular bowel program when indicated.	This lifelong program is necessary to routinely evacuate the bowel, and usually includes digital stimulation and use of stool softeners/suppositories at set intervals. Ability to control bowel evacuation is important to the patient's physical independence and social acceptance.
Encourage well-balanced diet that includes bulk and roughage as well as increased fluid intake (at least 2000 ml/day), including fruit juices.	Improves consistency of stool for transit through the bowel.
Observe for incontinence and help patient relate incontinence to change in diet or routine.	Patient can eventually achieve fairly normal routine bowel habits, which enhances independence, self-esteem, and socialization.
Provide meticulous skin care.	Loss of sphincter control and innervation in the area potentiates risk of skin irritation/breakdown.
Collaborative	
Insert/maintain nasogastric tube and attach to suction if appropriate.	May be used initially to reduce gastric distention and prevent vomiting (reduces risk of aspiration).
Consult with dietician/nutritional support team.	Aids in creating dietary plan to meet individual nutritional needs with consideration of state of digestion/bowel function.
Insert rectal tube as needed.	Reduces bowel distention, which may precipitate autonomic responses.
Administer medications as indicated:	
Stool softeners, laxatives, suppositories, enemas;	Stimulates peristalsis and routine bowel evacuation when necessary.
Antacids, cimetidine (Tagamet), ranitidine (Zantac).	Reduces or neutralizes gastric acid to prevent gastric irritation, or potential for bleeding.

NURSING DIAGNOSIS:	URINARY ELIMINATION: ALTERED PATTERNS
May be related to:	Disruption in bladder innervation Bladder atony
Possibly evidenced by:	Bladder distention; incontinence/overflow Urinary tract infections Bladder, kidney stone formation Renal dysfunction
PATIENT OUTCOMES/ EVALUATION CRITERIA:	Verbalizes understanding of condition. Maintains balanced intake/output with clear, odor-free urine. Verbalizes/demonstrates behaviors and techniques to prevent retention/urinary infection.

ACTIONS/INTERVENTIONS

Independent

Assess voiding pattern, e.g., frequency and amount. Compare urine output with fluid intake. Note specific gravity.

Palpate for bladder distention and observe for overflow.

Encourage fluid intake (2–4 liters/day), including acid ash juices (e.g., cranberry).

Begin bladder retraining when appropriate, e.g., fluids between certain hours, digital stimulation of trigger area, contraction of abdominal muscles, Credé maneuver.

Observe for cloudy or bloody urine, foul odor.

Cleanse perineal area and keep dry.

Collaborative

Keep bladder deflated by means of indwelling catheter initially. Begin intermittent catheterization program when appropriate.

Monitor BUN, creatinine, WBC.

Administer medications as indicated, e.g., vitamin C, and/or urinary antiseptics, e.g., methenamine mandelate (Mandelamine).

RATIONALE

Identifies characteristics of bladder function (e.g., effectiveness of bladder emptying, renal function, and fluid balance).

Bladder dysfunction is variable, but may include loss of bladder contraction/inability to relax urinary sphincter, resulting in urine retention and reflux incontinence. Note: Bladder distention can precipitate autonomic dysreflexia. (Refer to ND: Dysreflexia, p. 297.)

Helps maintain renal function, prevents infection and formation of urinary stones. Note: Fluid may be restricted for a period of time during initiation of intermittent catheterization.

Timing and type of bladder program is dependent on type of injury (upper or lower neuron involvement). Note: Credé maneuver should be used with caution because it may precipitate autonomic dysreflexia.

Signs of urinary tract or kidney infection that can potentiate sepsis.

Decreases risk of skin irritation/breakdown and development of ascending infection.

Indwelling catheter is used during acute phase for prevention of urinary retention, reducing risk of infection, and monitoring output more carefully. Intermittent emptying may reduce complications usually associated with long-term use of indwelling catheters. Suprapubic catheter may also be inserted for long-term management.

Reflects renal function, identifies complications.

Maintains acidic environment and discourages bacterial growth.

NURSING DIAGNOSIS:	DYSREFLEXIA
May be related to:	**Altered nerve function (spinal cord injury at T-6 and above)**
	Bladder/bowel/skin stimulation
Possibly evidenced by:	**Changes in vital signs, paroxysmal hypertension, tachycardia, or bradycardia**
	Autonomic responses: sweating, flushing above level of lesion, pallor below injury, chills, gooseflesh, nasal stuffiness, diffuse headache
PATIENT OUTCOMES/ EVALUATION CRITERIA:	**Minimize/prevent occurrence.**

ACTIONS/INTERVENTIONS	RATIONALE

Independent

Be aware of/monitor precipitating risk factors, e.g., bladder/bowel distention or manipulation; bladder spasms, stones, infection; skin/tissue pressure areas, prolonged sitting position; temperature extremes/drafts.

Visceral distention is most common cause of autonomic hyperreflexia (AD). Treatment of acute episode must be carried out (removing stimulus, treating unresolved symptoms); then interventions and rationale must be geared toward prevention.

Observe for associated complaints/symptoms, e.g., chest pains, blurred vision, nausea, metallic taste, Horner's syndrome.

Early detection and immediate intervention is essential to prevention of serious complications.

Monitor blood pressure frequently (3–5 minutes) during acute AD, and take action to eliminate stimulus. Continue to monitor blood pressure at intervals after symptoms subside.

Aggressive therapy/removal of stimulus may drop blood pressure too rapidly resulting in a hypotensive crisis especially in those patients who routinely have a low blood pressure. In addition, autonomic dysreflexia may recur, particularly if stimulus is not eliminated.

Elevate head of bed to 45-degree angle or place in sitting position.

Lowers blood pressure to prevent intracranial hemorrhage, seizures or even death. Note: placing quadriplegic in sitting position automatically lowers blood pressure.

Correct/eliminate causative stimulus, e.g., bladder, bowel, skin pressure, temperature extreme.

Removing noxious stimulus usually terminates episode and may prevent more serious AD.

Inform patient/SO of warning signals, and how to avoid onset of syndrome.

This lifelong problem can be largely controlled by the avoidance of pressure from overdistention of visceral organs or pressure on the skin.

Collaborative

Administer medications as indicated and monitor response:

Ganglion blockers, e.g., trimethaphan camsylate (Arfonad);

Blocks excessive autonomic nerve transmission.

Atropine sulfate;

Increases heart rate if bradycardia occurs.

Diazoxide (Hyperstat), hydralazine (Apresoline);

Reduces blood pressure if severe/sustained hypertension occurs.

Adrenergic blockers, e.g., methysergide maleate (Sansert).

May be used prophylactically if problem persists, recurs frequently.

ACTIONS/INTERVENTIONS

Collaborative

Apply local anesthetic ointment to rectum; remove impaction if indicated after symptoms subside.

Prepare patient for pelvic/pudendal nerve block or posterior rhizotomy if indicated.

RATIONALE

Ointment blocks further autonomic stimulation and eases later removal of impaction without aggravating symptoms.

Procedures may be considered if AD does not respond to other therapies.

NURSING DIAGNOSIS:	SKIN INTEGRITY, IMPAIRED: POTENTIAL
May be related to:	Altered/inadequate peripheral circulation; sensation
	Presence of edema; pressure
	Altered metabolic state
	Immobility, traction apparatus
Possibly evidenced by:	[Not applicable; presence of signs and symptoms establishes an *actual* diagnosis.]
PATIENT OUTCOMES/ EVALUATION CRITERIA:	Identifies individual risk factors. Verbalizes understanding of treatment needs. Participates to level of ability to prevent skin breakdown.

ACTIONS/INTERVENTIONS

Independent

Inspect all skin areas, noting capillary blanching/refill, redness, swelling. Pay particular attention to skin under halo frame or vest, and folds where skin continuously touches.

Observe halo and tongs insertion sites. Note swelling, redness, drainage. Cleanse routinely and apply antibiotic ointment per protocol.

Massage skin and protect pressure points by use of lamb's wool, foam padding, egg crate mattress; and use skin hardening agents, e.g., tincture of benzoin, Karaya, Sween cream.

Reposition frequently whether in bed or in sitting position. Place in prone position periodically.

Wash and dry skin, especially in high moisture areas such as perineum.

Keep bedclothes dry and free of wrinkles, crumbs.

Encourage continuation of regular exercise program.

Elevate lower extremities periodically, if tolerated.

Collaborative

Provide kinetic therapy or alternating-pressure mattress as indicated.

RATIONALE

Skin is especially prone to breakdown because of changes in peripheral circulation, inability to sense pressure, immobility, altered temperature regulation.

These sites are prone to inflammation and infection and provide route for pathologic microorganisms to enter cranial cavity.

Enhances circulation and protects skin surfaces, reducing risk of ulceration. Quadriplegic and paraplegic patients require lifelong protection from decubiti formation, which can cause extensive tissue necrosis and sepsis.

Improves skin circulation and reduces pressure time on bony prominences.

Clean, dry skin is less prone to excoriation/ breakdown.

Reduces/prevents skin irritation.

Stimulates circulation, enhancing cellular nutrition/ oxygenation to improve tissue health.

Enhances venous return. Reduces edema formation.

Improves systemic and peripheral circulation and decreases pressure on skin, reducing risk of breakdown.

NURSING DIAGNOSIS:	KNOWLEDGE DEFICIT [LEARNING NEED] (SPECIFY)
May be related to:	Lack of exposure
	Information misinterpretation
	Unfamiliarity with information resources
Possibly evidenced by:	Questions; statement of misconception; request for information
	Inadequate follow-through of instruction
	Inappropriate or exaggerated behaviors, e.g., hostile, agitated, apathetic
	Development of preventable complication(s)
PATIENT OUTCOMES/ EVALUATION CRITERIA:	Participates in learning process. Verbalizes understanding of condition, prognosis, and treatment. Correctly performs necessary procedures and explains reasons for the actions. Initiates necessary lifestyle changes and participates in treatment regimen.

ACTIONS/INTERVENTIONS	RATIONALE
Independent	
Discuss injury process, current prognosis, and future expectations.	Provides common knowledge base necessary for making informed choices and commitment to the therapeutic regimen.
Provide information and demonstrate:	
Positioning;	Promotes circulation, reduces tissue pressure and risk of complications.
Use of pillows/supports, splints;	Keeps spine aligned and prevents/limits contractures for improving function and independence.
Exercise all extremities, encourage continued participation in daily exercise/conditioning program and avoidance of fatigue/chills.	Reduces spasticity, risk of thromboemboli (common complication). Increases mobility, muscle strength/tone for improving organ/body function, e.g., tightening/contracting rectum or vaginal muscles to improve bladder control; or pushing abdomen up, bearing down, contracting abdomen to strengthen trunk and improve GI function (paraplegic).
Have SO/care givers participate in patient care and demonstrate proper procedures, e.g., applications of splints, braces, suctioning, positioning, skin care, transfers, bowel/bladder program, checking temperature of bath water and food.	Allows home care givers to become adept and more comfortable with the care tasks they are called on to provide and reduces risk of injury/complications.
Recommend applying abdominal binder before arising (quad) and remind to change position slowly. Use safety belt during bed to wheelchair transfers and adequate number of people.	Reduces pooling of blood in abdomen/pelvis minimizing postural hypotension. Protects the patient from falls, and/or injury to care givers.
Instruct in proper skin care, inspection of all skin areas daily, use of adequate padding (foam, silicone gel, water pads) in bed and chair, and keep skin dry.	Reduces skin irritation decreasing incidence of decubitus (patient must manage this throughout life).

299

Independent

Discuss necessity of preventing excessive diaphoresis by using tepid bathwater, providing comfortable environment (fans, etc.), removing excess clothes.

Reduces skin irritation/possible breakdown.

Review dietary needs. Problem-solve solutions to alterations in muscular strength/tone and GI function.

Provides adequate nutrition to meet energy needs and promote healing, prevent complications (e.g., constipation).

Discuss ways to identify and manage autonomic dysreflexia.

Patient may be able to recognize signs, but care givers need to understand how to prevent precipitating factors and know what to do when AD occurs. (Refer to ND: Dysreflexia, p. 297.)

Identify symptoms to report immediately to health care provider, e.g., infection of any kind, especially urinary, respiratory; skin breakdown; unresolved AD; suspected pregnancy.

Early identification allows for intervention to prevent/minimize complications.

Stress importance of continuing with rehabilitation team to achieve specific functional goals.

No matter what the level of injury, individual may ultimately be able to exercise some independence, e.g., manipulate electric wheelchair with mouth stick (C3-4); be independent for dressing, transfers to bed, car, toilet (C-7); total wheelchair independence (C8-T4).

Evaluate home layout and make recommendations for necessary changes.

Physical changes may be required to accommodate both patient and support equipment.

Collaborative

Identify community resources, e.g., health agencies, VNA, financial counselor; service organizations, Spinal Cord Injury Foundation.

Assists with home management, respite for care givers.

Coordinate cooperation among community/rehabilitation resources.

Various agencies/therapists/individuals in community may be involved in the long-term care and safety of the patient, and coordination can ensure that needs are not overlooked and optimal level of rehabilitation is achieved.

Arrange for transmitter/emergency call system.

Provides for safety and access to emergency assistance and equipment.

Plan for alternate care givers as needed.

May be needed to provide respite if regular care givers are ill or other unplanned emergencies arise.

Guillain–Barré Syndrome (Polyradiculitis) _____

PATIENT ASSESSMENT DATA BASE

ACTIVITY/REST

May report: Weakness, progressive paralysis usually beginning in lower extremities.
Tripping, falling.
Loss of fine motor control of hands.

May exhibit: Muscle weakness, flaccid paralysis (symmetric).
Unsteady gait.

CIRCULATION

May exhibit: Changes in blood pressure (hypertension or hypotension).
Dysrhythmias.

EGO INTEGRITY

May report: Feelings of anxiety, concern.

May exhibit: Fear, confusion.

ELIMINATION

May report: Changes in usual pattern of elimination.

May exhibit: Weakness of abdominal muscles.
Loss of anal/bladder sensation and sphincter reflex.

FOOD/FLUID

May report: Difficulty chewing, swallowing.

May exhibit: Impaired gag, swallow reflex.

NEUROSENSORY

May report: Numbness, tingling beginning in toes or fingers and ascending upward (stocking or glove distribution).
Impaired sense of position.

May exhibit: Diminished/absent deep tendon reflexes.
Loss of muscle tone.
Loss of ability to speak.

PAIN/COMFORT

May report: Muscle tenderness, aching, pain (especially in shoulders, pelvis, thighs, back, buttocks).
Hypersensitivity to touch.

RESPIRATION

May report: Difficulty breathing, shortness of breath.

May exhibit: Shallow respirations, use of accessory muscles, apnea.
Decreased/absent breath sounds.
Reduced vital capacity.

Pallor/cyanosis.
Impaired gag, swallow, cough reflexes.

SOCIAL INTERACTION

May exhibit: Loss of ability to speak/communicate.

SAFETY

May exhibit: Fluctuation in body temperature (takes on temperature of the environment).

TEACHING/LEARNING

May report: Recent illness (URI, gastroenteritis), vaccinations (smallpox, influenza), chronic conditions (lupus erythematosus, Hodgkin's/malignant process), surgery, trauma.

Discharge Plan Considerations: May require assistance with transportation, food preparation, self-care, and homemaker tasks.

DIAGNOSTIC STUDIES

Serial lumbar puncture: demonstates classic phenomenon of normal pressure and normal number of white cells, with elevating protein levels that peak in 4–6 weeks. Because protein elevation may not appear in first 4–5 days, serial lumbar punctures may be indicated.

Electromyelography: results depend on stage and progression of syndrome. Nerve conduction velocity may be slowed. Fibrillations (repetitive firing of the same motor unit) are more common in later stage.

CBC: may reveal leukocytosis during early stage.

Chest x-ray: may demonstrate progressive signs of respiratory involvement, e.g., atelectatic areas, pneumonia.

Pulmonary function studies: may reveal decreased vital capacity, tidal volume and inspiratory force.

NURSING PRIORITIES

1. Maintain/support respiratory function.
2. Minimize/prevent complications.
3. Provide emotional support to patient/SO.
4. Control/eliminate pain.
5. Provide information about disease process/prognosis and treatment needs.

DISCHARGE CRITERIA

1. Respiratory function adequate for individual needs.
2. ADL needs met by self or with assistance of others.
3. Complications prevented/controlled.
4. Anxiety/fear reduced to manageable level.
5. Pain minimized/controlled.
6. Disease process/prognosis, therapeutic regimen and possible complications understood.

NURSING DIAGNOSIS:	SENSORY-PERCEPTUAL ALTERATION: (SPECIFY)
May be related to:	Altered sensory reception, transmission, and/or integration
	Altered status of sense organs
	Inability to communicate, to speak, or to respond
	Chemical alteration (hypoxia, electrolyte imbalance)

Possibly evidenced by:	Hypo/hyperesthesias; pain
	Change in usual response to stimuli
	Motor incoordination
	Restlessness, irritability, anxiety
	Altered communication patterns
PATIENT/CARE GIVER OUTCOMES/EVALUATION CRITERIA:	Verbalizes awareness of sensory deficits. Maintains usual mentation/orientation. Identifies interventions to minimize sensory impairments/complications.

ACTIONS/INTERVENTIONS	RATIONALE

Independent

Monitor neurologic status periodically (e.g., ability to speak, respond to simple commands and painful stimuli; awareness of hot and cold, dull and sharp). Record serial findings on flow sheets.	Progression and regression of symptoms may vary greatly. Progression is often quite rapid and may peak in a few days/weeks. Onset of recovery usually begins 2–4 weeks after disease progression stops and is much slower. Flow charts are helpful in alerting nurses to impending complications requiring further evaluation/intervention.
Provide alternate means of communication if patient cannot speak, e.g., "blink method," alphabet/picture boards, etc.	If syndrome develops slowly, patient can help establish preferred method of communication. If process is sudden (hours/days), consistent and constant effort on the part of the staff is required to establish effective communication.
Provide safe environment (side rails, protection from thermal injury). Note deficits on chart in room to alert all care givers, e.g., "absence of sensation below . . . ."	Loss of sensation, as well as motor control, leaves patient at the mercy of all care givers, who must maintain a therapeutic environment and prevent injury.
Allow for undisturbed periods of rest and provide diversional activities within patient ability.	Reduces excessive stimuli, which can greatly increase anxiety and diminish coping abilities.
Reorient patient to environment and staff, as indicated.	Helps reduce anxiety and is especially helpful if visual deficit is present.
Provide appropriate sensory stimulation, including familiar sounds (music), clocks (time), television (news/entertainment), conversation.	Patient (who is usually conscious) can feel completely isolated as paralysis progresses and during lengthy recovery phase.
Encourage SO to talk to and touch patient and to keep abreast of family events.	Helps SO to feel involved in patient's life (reduces helpless/hopeless feelings) and may reduce patient's anxiety regarding family during separation.
Patch eyes on a rotating basis if ptosis is present.	Maintains visual input while decreasing risk of corneal abrasions.

Collaborative

Refer to multiple resources for assistance, e.g., physical/occupational/speech therapists, pastoral care, social service, rehabilitation departments.	All services/departments coordinate efforts to promote recovery/minimize residual neurologic deficits.
Assist with plasmapheresis as indicated.	Removes antibodies/other factors that may relate to Guillain–Barré syndrome, possibly relieving symptoms for weeks/months.

NURSING DIAGNOSIS:	BREATHING PATTERN, INEFFECTIVE [POTENTIAL]
May be related to:	Weakness/paralysis of respiratory muscles
	Impaired gag and swallow reflexes
Possibly evidenced by:	[Not applicable: presence of signs and symptoms establishes an *actual* diagnosis.]
PATIENT OUTCOMES/ EVALUATION CRITERIA:	Demonstrates adequate ventilation with absence of signs of respiratory distress, breath sounds clear, and ABGs within acceptable limits.

ACTIONS/INTERVENTIONS	RATIONALE
Independent	
Monitor respiratory rate, depth, symmetry. Note increased work of breathing, and observe color of skin and mucous membranes.	Increased respiratory distress and cyanosis indicate advancing muscular weakness and/or paralysis, which can result in respiratory failure.
Assess sensation especially noting diminished response at T-8, or upper arm/shoulder area.	Decreased sensation often precedes motor weakness; e.g., loss at T-8 level can affect use of intercostal muscles, whereas arm/shoulder involvement often precedes respiratory failure.
Note breathlessness while talking.	Good indicator of interference with respiratory function/diminishing vital capacity.
Auscultate breath sounds, noting absence/development of adventitious sounds, e.g., rhonchi, wheezes.	Increased airway resistance and/or accumulation of secretions will impede gas diffusion and lead to pulmonary complications (e.g., pneumonia).
Elevate head of bed, or place patient in supported sitting position.	Enhances lung expansion and cough efforts, decreases work of breathing, and limits risk of aspiration of secretions.
Evaluate gag, swallow, cough reflexes periodically. Suction oral secretions, noting color and amount of secretions. Keep NPO if necessary.	Loss of muscle strength and function may result in inability to maintain and/or clear airway, preventing adequate ventilation. Note: Once muscles of head and neck are involved, frequent reevaluation of reflexes must be carried out for prevention of aspiration, pulmonary infections, and respiratory failure. Muscular weakness may impede cough/gag, requiring mechanical means to clear airway.
Investigate complaints of dyspnea, chest pain, increased restlessness.	These patients are at risk for pulmonary embolus (as a result of vascular pooling and immobility), requiring prompt interventions and respiratory support to prevent serious complications/death. May require transfer to critical care area for mechanical ventilatory support. (Refer to CP: Pulmonary Embolism, p. 148.)
Collaborative	
Monitor serial vital capacity, tidal volume, and inspiratory force.	Detects worsening of muscle paralysis and declining respiratory effort.
Monitor/graph serial ABGs, pulse oximetry.	Determines effectiveness of current ventilation and need for/effectiveness of interventions.
Review chest x-rays.	Reveals changes indicative of pulmonary congestion and/or atelectasis.

ACTIONS/INTERVENTIONS

Collaborative

Administer supplemental humidified oxygen as indicated, using appropriate route, e.g., cannula, mask, mechanical ventilator.

Administer/assist with pulmonary hygiene measures, e.g., breathing exercises/adjuncts, chest percussion, vibration and postural drainage.

Provide kinetic therapy as indicated.

Prepare for/maintain intubation, mechanical ventilation as indicated. (Refer to CP: Ventilatory Assistance [Mechanical], p. 191.)

Provide tracheostomy care when present.

Administer corticosteroids if indicated.

RATIONALE

Treats hypoxemia. Humidity loosens secretions and keeps mucous membranes moist, thereby reducing irritation of airways.

Improves ventilation and reduces atelectasis by mobilizing secretions and enhancing expansion of alveoli.

May be used to enhance circulation and oxygenation of lung segments and to promote mobilization of secretions to reduce atelectasis and risk of pulmonary infection and/or emboli.

Ten to twenty percent of patients suffer significant respiratory involvement requiring aggressive interventions/support.

May be needed for airway and secretion management. "Talking" tracheostomy may be inserted to facilitate communication, although muscle weakness and copious secretions can limit its effectiveness.

Use is controversial, may improve acute symptoms but not overall outcome.

NURSING DIAGNOSIS:	TISSUE PERFUSION, ALTERED [POTENTIAL]
May be related to:	Autonomic nervous system dysfunction, causing vascular pooling with decreased venous return
	Hypovolemia
	Interruption of venous blood flow (thrombosis)
Possibly evidenced by:	[Not applicable; presence of signs and symptoms establishes an *actual* diagnosis.]
PATIENT OUTCOMES/ EVALUATION CRITERIA:	Maintains perfusion with stable vital signs, cardiac dysrhythmias controlled/absent.

ACTIONS/INTERVENTIONS

Independent

Auscultate blood pressure, noting wide fluctuations. Observe for postural hypotension. Exercise care when changing patient's position.

Monitor heart rate and rhythm. Document dysrhythmias.

RATIONALE

Changes in BP (severe hyper/hypotension) occur because of loss of sympathetic outflow to maintain peripheral vascular tone (autonomic dysfunction). Reflexes to adjust BP during position changes (side to side) may be impaired, causing postural hypotension.

Sinus tachycardia/bradycardia may develop because of impaired sympathetic innervation or unopposed vagal stimulation, leading to cardiac arrest. Dysrhythmias can also occur because of hypoxemia, electrolyte imbalance, or reduced cardiac output (secondary to altered vascular tone and venous return).

ACTIONS/INTERVENTIONS	RATIONALE

Independent

Monitor body temperature. Provide comfortable environmental temperature, add or remove blankets, use room fans, etc.

Changes in vasomotor tone create difficulties with temperature regulation (e.g., inability to perspire), and patient may take on temperature of surrounding environment. Warming and cooling should be done with caution to prevent hot or cold injury inasmuch as the patient may have impaired sensation.

Document intake and output.

Relaxation of vascular tone, fluid shifts, and reduced oral intake can decrease circulating volume, negatively affecting BP and urine output.

Change position frequently. Observe skin for signs of irritation. Massage skin over bony prominences. Keep linens dry, wrinkle-free. Wash and dry skin with mild soap, and apply emollients. Provide sheepskin pads as indicated.

Changes in circulation/vascular pooling impair cellular perfusion, increasing risk of tissue ischemia/breakdown.

Elevate foot of bed slightly. Provide passive exercise for ankle/foot. Observe calf for edema, erythema, positive Homans' sign.

Loss of vascular tone and venous stasis increases risk of thrombus formation. Note: Deep vein thrombosis (which may go unrecognized because the patient cannot sense discomfort) can lead to pulmonary emboli if not detected and promptly treated.

Collaborative

Administer:

IV fluids with caution as indicated;

May be needed to correct/prevent hypovolemia/hypotension, but should be used cautiously because patient with impaired vascular tone may be sensitive to even small increases in circulating volume.

Medications: short-acting antihypertensive drugs;

Occasionally used to alleviate persistent hypertension.

Heparin.

May be used to reduce risk of thrombophlebitis.

Monitor laboratory studies, e.g., CBC or Hb/Hct, serum electrolytes.

Hct is useful in determining hypo/hypervolemia. Hyponatremia may develop, suggesting complication of SIADH.

Provide alternating pressure mattress, kinetic therapy bed, flotation mattress, as indicated.

Enhances circulation and prevents skin complications. Note: Kinetic therapy is widely thought to enhance organ perfusion/function and to reduce complications of immobility.

Apply antiembolic stockings and remove at scheduled intervals.

Promotes venous return, reduces venous stasis, lessens risk of thrombus formation.

NURSING DIAGNOSIS:	MOBILITY, IMPAIRED PHYSICAL
May be related to:	Neuromuscular impairment
Possibly evidenced by:	Loss of coordination; partial/complete paralysis Decreased muscle tone/strength
PATIENT OUTCOMES/ EVALUATION CRITERIA:	Maintains position of function with absence of complications (contractures, decubiti). Increases strength and function of affected parts. Demonstrates techniques/behaviors that enable resumption of desired activities.

ACTIONS/INTERVENTIONS

Independent

Assess functional ability on a scale of 0–4. Perform assessments on a regular basis and compare with baseline.

Position for optimum comfort. Reposition on a regular schedule as individually indicated.

Support extremities and joints with pillows, trochanter rolls, footboards.

Perform passive range of motion exercises. Avoid active exercise during acute phase.

Coordinate care to allow frequent rest periods.

Provide lubrication/artificial tears as needed.

Encourage activity progression, depending on individual tolerance, e.g., sitting on bedside with support, up in chair, then ambulating as able.

Collaborative

Refer to physical/occupational therapy.

RATIONALE

Determines progression/regression of syndrome, aiding in establishing goals/patient expectations. Note: Quadriplegia (symmetric paralysis) commonly occurs, requiring multiple interventions.

Reduces fatigue, promotes relaxation, decreases risk of skin ischemia/breakdown.

Maintains extremities in functional position; prevents contractures and loss of joint function.

Stimulates circulation, improves muscle tone, and promotes joint mobility. Note: Vigorous exercise may exacerbate symptoms, causing physiologic and emotional regression.

Overtaxing muscles can increase time needed for remyelination, thereby prolonging recovery time.

Prevents drying of delicate tissues when patient is unable to close/blink eyes appropriately.

Gradual/programmed resumption of activity denotes improvement, promotes normalization of organ function, and has a positive psychologic effect.

Useful in creating individualized muscle strengthening/conditioning exercises and gait training program; identifying assistive devices/braces to maintain mobility and independence in ADLs.

NURSING DIAGNOSIS:	BOWEL ELIMINATION, ALTERED: (SPECIFY) [POTENTIAL]
May be related to:	**Neuromuscular impairment (loss of anal sensation and reflexes)**
	Immobility
Possibly evidenced by:	**[Not applicable: presence of signs and symptoms establishes an *actual* diagnosis.]**
PATIENT OUTCOMES/ EVALUATION CRITERIA:	**Maintains usual pattern of bowel elimination with absence of ileus.**

ACTIONS/INTERVENTIONS

Independent

Auscultate bowel sounds, noting presence, absence, or change.

Monitor for nausea, vomiting, cessation of stool.

RATIONALE

Decreased or absent sounds may indicate onset of ileus owing to loss of intestinal motility and/or electrolyte imbalance. Hyperactive bowel sounds may be noted if diarrhea occurs as a side effect of tube feeding or kinetic therapy.

Rate of progression to complete ileus is variable but can be expected.

ACTIONS/INTERVENTIONS	RATIONALE

Independent

Assess for abdominal distention, tenderness. Measure abdominal girth as indicated.	May reflect developing ileus or fecal impaction.
Encourage fluid intake of at least 2000 ml/day (if patient able to swallow) in frequent small amounts, including fruit juices.	Promotes softer stool and facilitates elimination.
Check for rectal impaction.	Gentle manual removal of stool may be necessary, along with other interventions, to stimulate bowel evacuation.
Provide privacy and upright positioning on bedside commode (if possible) at regularly scheduled times.	Enhances bowel evacuation efforts.

Collaborative

Administer stool softeners, suppositories, laxatives, or use rectal tube as indicated.	Prevents constipation, reduces abdominal distention, and assists in regulation of bowel function.
Increase dietary intake of fiber and bulk or change rate and type of tube feedings when indicated.	Aids in regulating fecal consistency and reduces complications (diarrhea, constipation).
Insert/maintain nasogastric tube if indicated.	Reduces nausea and vomiting and decompresses abdominal distention associated with loss of peristalsis, presence of ileus.

NURSING DIAGNOSIS:	**URINARY ELIMINATION: ALTERED PATTERNS [POTENTIAL]**
May be related to:	**Neuromuscular impairment (loss of sensation and sphincter reflex)**
	Immobility
Possibly evidenced by:	**[Not applicable; presence of signs and symptoms establishes an *actual* diagnosis.]**
PATIENT OUTCOMES/ EVALUATION CRITERIA:	**Demonstrates adequate/timely bladder emptying with absence of urinary retention or infection.**

ACTIONS/INTERVENTIONS	RATIONALE

Independent

Record frequency and amount of voidings.	Provides information for assessment of bladder functioning.
Palpate abdomen for bladder distention.	If sphincter reflex is absent, the bladder will fill and become distended.
Encourage fluid intake (to 2000 ml/within cardiac tolerance) and include acidifying fruit juices (e.g., cranberry).	Maintains glomerular filtration rate, reduces risk of infection and formation of urinary tract stones.

Collaborative

Catheterize for residual urine, as indicated.	Monitors effectiveness of bladder emptying.

ACTIONS/INTERVENTIONS	RATIONALE
Collaborative	
Insert/maintain indwelling catheter if necessary.	May be needed if urinary retention occurs or until resolution of Guillain-Barré syndrome and restoration of bladder control.

NURSING DIAGNOSIS: **NUTRITION, ALTERED: LESS THAN BODY REQUIREMENTS [POTENTIAL]**

May be related to: **Neuromuscular impairment affecting gag, cough, swallow reflexes and GI dysfunction**

Possibly evidenced by: **[Not applicable; presence of signs and symptoms establishes an *actual* diagnosis.]**

PATIENT OUTCOMES/ EVALUATION CRITERIA: **Demonstrates stable weight, normalization of laboratory values, and free of signs of malnutrition.**

ACTIONS/INTERVENTIONS	RATIONALE
Independent	
Assess ability to chew, swallow, cough, on a regular basis.	Muscle weakness and hypo/hyperactive reflexes can indicate need for alternative methods of feeding, e.g., tube feeding.
Auscultate bowel sounds, evaluate abdominal distention.	Disturbance of gastric function often occurs because of paralysis/immobility.
Record daily caloric intake.	Identifies nutrient deficiencies and needs.
Note patient's food likes/dislikes and involve in dietary choices when oral feedings resume.	Promotes sense of control and may enhance feeding efforts.
Encourage self-feeding if possible. Allow plenty of time for self-directed efforts. Feed/assist patient as needed.	Degree of loss of motor control affects ability to feed self. Self-esteem and sense of control may be enhanced by self-directed efforts even when very limited.
Encourage SO to participate at mealtime, e.g., feeding and bringing food from home.	Provides socialization time which may enhance patient's food intake.
Weigh periodically.	Assesses effectiveness of dietary regimen.
Collaborative	
Provide high-calorie/high-protein beverages, e.g., eggnog, commercial preparations (Ensure).	Supplemental feedings can increase nutritional intake.
Insert/maintain feeding tube. Administer enteral/parenteral feedings.	May be indicated if patient cannot swallow (or if gag/swallow reflexes are impaired) to assure proper nutrient, caloric, electrolyte and mineral intake. (Refer to CP: Total Nutritional Support, p. 894.)

NURSING DIAGNOSIS: **ANXIETY/FEAR**

May be related to: **Situational crisis**

Threat of death/change in health status

Possibly evidenced by:	Increased tension, restlessness, helplessness
	Apprehension, uncertainty, fearfulness
	Focus on self
	Sympathetic stimulation
PATIENT OUTCOMES/ EVALUATION CRITERIA:	Acknowledges and discusses fears. Verbalizes accurate knowledge of the situation. Demonstrates appropriate range of feelings and lessened fear. Appears relaxed and reports anxiety is reduced to a manageable level.

ACTIONS/INTERVENTIONS	RATIONALE

Independent

Place close to nurses' station, check on patient frequently. Reassess ability to use call light regularly.	Provides reassurance that help is readily available if the patient suddenly becomes incapacitated.
Provide alternate means of communication, if necessary.	Reduces feelings of helplessness.
Discuss body image changes, fears of permanent disability, loss of function, dying, concerns regarding discharge needs/placement.	Bringing fears out into the open provides opportunity to assess patient perceptions/information/misinformation and to problem-solve ways to deal with situation.
Provide simple explanations of care; plan care with patient, involving SO.	Understanding can enhance cooperation in needed activities. Involving patient/SO in care planning restores some sense of control over life, enhancing self-esteem.

NURSING DIAGNOSIS:	COMFORT, ALTERED: PAIN, ACUTE
May be related to:	Neuromuscular impairment (paresthesia, dysesthesia)
Possibly evidenced by:	Painful sensations induced by gentle touch on skin
	Aching, tenderness of muscles/joints
	Altered muscle tone (flaccid, spastic)
	Guarding behavior
PATIENT OUTCOMES/ EVALUATION CRITERIA:	Reports pain is relieved/controlled. Verbalizes methods that provide relief. Demonstrates use of relaxation skills as indicated for individual situation.

ACTIONS/INTERVENTIONS	RATIONALE

Independent

Evaluate degree of pain/discomfort using 1–10 scale. Observe for nonverbal cues (e.g., facial mask of pain, withdrawal/crying).	Encourages patient to "localize"/quantify pain, recognizing changes, improvement.
Encourage verbalization of feelings about pain.	Reduces feelings of isolation, anger, and anxiety that may enhance pain.

ACTIONS/INTERVENTIONS

Independent

Provide heat or cold applications, warm baths, massage, or touch as individually tolerated.

Reposition frequently. Provide support by means of pillows, foam inserts, blankets.

Provide passive range of motion exercises.

Instruct in/encourage use of relaxation techniques, e.g., visualization, progressive relaxation exercises, guided imagery, biofeedback.

Collaborative

Provide moist heat packs, warm tub bath.

Administer analgesics as indicated. Avoid use of narcotics.

Assist with alternate therapies, e.g., ultrasound, diathermy, and TENS.

RATIONALE

Helps patient gain control over the constant discomfort caused by the paresthesias and decreases muscle stiffness/pain.

Helps alleviate fatigue and muscle tension. Note: Some patients prefer to lie on their backs in a "frog leg" position.

Decreases joint stiffness.

Redirects focus of attention/perception and enhances coping, which may help alleviate pain.

May help relieve muscle aches/stiffness.

Useful for alleviating pain when other methods do not help. Narcotics (except codeine, which has a lesser effect) should be avoided when possible because of their respiratory depressant and GI side effects.

Sometimes useful in relieving muscle discomfort.

NURSING DIAGNOSIS:	KNOWLEDGE DEFICIT [LEARNING NEED] (SPECIFY)
May be related to:	Lack of exposure Information misinterpretation Unfamiliarity with information resources Lack of recall, cognitive limitation
Possibly evidenced by:	Request for information Statement of misconception Development of preventable complications
PATIENT OUTCOMES/ EVALUATION CRITERIA:	Participates in learning process. Initiates necessary lifestyle changes and participates in rehabilitation efforts as individually able.

ACTIONS/INTERVENTIONS

Independent

Determine patient's level of knowledge and ability to participate in rehabilitation.

Review disease process and prognosis.

RATIONALE

Influences choice of interventions.

Knowledge base necessary to make informed choices and participate in rehabilitation efforts. Although the syndrome is transient, the residual effects may persist for weeks, months, or longer.

ACTIONS/INTERVENTIONS	RATIONALE

Independent

Encourage verbalization, socialization and independence.	Promotes return to sense of normality and developing a life around present circumstances.
Identify safety measures to meet individual sensorimotor deficits.	Reduces risk of injury/preventable complications.
Work with SO to have necessary equipment in the home before patient is discharged.	If patient is able to return home, care may be facilitated by assistive devices for mobilization, feeding, and bathing.
Stress importance of avoiding persons with infections, especially upper respiratory.	Patient is immunosuppressed and at risk for development of infections.
Instruct and assist patient/SO in learning ROM exercises, transfer techniques, good body techniques, breathing/speech exercises, use of assistive devices.	Promotes independence and continued recovery. Process often takes 4–6 months for remyelination and up to 2 years if quadriplegia developed.
Review signs/symptoms requiring medical follow-up, e.g., infectious process (UTI, URI), urinary retention, constipation.	Prompt intervention can prevent/minimize complications.
Discuss need for continued follow-up.	Necessary to monitor improvement, identify treatment needs and promote optimal recovery. Recovery is usually good, with varying degrees of weakness/atrophy remaining, although one third have permanent residual deficits (hyperreflexia, atrophy, distal muscle weakness, facial paresis).

Collaborative

Refer to community resources, e.g., VNA, home health agencies, social services.	Support may permit/sustain patient in home setting.

Alzheimer's Disease (Non-Substance-Induced Organic Mental Disorders)

Alzheimer's disease is a specific degenerative process occurring primarily in the cells located at the base of the forebrain which send information to the cerebral cortex and hippocampus. The affected cells first lose their capacity to secrete acetylcholine (ACh), then degenerate. Once this degeneration begins, nothing can be done to revive or replace them. The cause remains unknown, although research is being done in several areas, such as genetic factors and "slow" viruses.

Multi-infarct dementia reflects a pattern of intermittent deterioration in the brain. Symptoms fluctuate, are focal, or progress in a stepwise fashion, compared with the steady and global decline in Alzheimer's. Deterioration is thought to occur in response to repeated infarcts of the brain.

PATIENT ASSESSMENT DATA BASE

ACTIVITY/REST

May report:	Feeling tired.
May exhibit:	Day/night reversal; wakefulness/aimless wandering.
	Lethargy; decreased interest in usual activities, hobbies.
	Impaired motor skills.

CIRCULATION

May report:	History of systemic/cerebral vascular disease, hypertension, embolic episode (predisposing factors).

EGO INTEGRITY

May report:	Suspicion or fear of imaginary persons/situations.
	Misperception of environment, misidentification of objects and people, hoarding of objects; belief that misplaced objects are stolen.
May exhibit:	Concealing of inabilities (makes excuses not to perform task; may thumb through a book without reading it).
	Content sitting and watching others.
	Main activity may be hoarding inanimate objects, repetitive motions (fold–unfold–refold linen), hiding articles, or wandering.
	Emotional lability: cries easily, laughs inappropriately; variable mood changes (apathy, lethargy, restlessness, short attention span, irritability); sudden angry outbursts (catastrophic reactions); sleep disturbances.
	Multiple losses, perceived changes in body image, self-esteem; may show strong, depressive overlay.
	Clinging to significant other(s).

ELIMINATION

May report:	Urgency (may indicate loss of muscle tone).
May exhibit:	Incontinence of urine/feces; prone to constipation.
	May forget to go to bathroom, forget steps involved in toileting self, or be unable to find the bathroom.

FOOD/FLUID

May report:	History of hypoglycemic episodes (predisposing factor).
	Changes in taste, appetite.

| **May exhibit:** | Forgetting of mealtime; dependence on others for meals. |
| | Loss of ability to chew, feed self, use utensils; or may conceal lost skills by refusing to eat. |

NEUROSENSORY

May report:	Denial of symptoms, especially cognitive changes, and/or describe vague, hypochondriacal complaints of fatigue, diarrhea, dizziness, or occasional headache.
	Insidious decline in cognitive abilities, judgment, recent memory, behavior (observed by SOs).
	History of cerebral/systemic vascular disease, embolic/hypoxic episodes (predisposing factors).
	Seizure activity (secondary to the brain damage in Alzheimer's disease).
May exhibit:	Impaired communication: aphasic and dysphasic; difficulty with finding correct words (especially nouns); repetitive or scattered conversation with substituted meaningless words; fragmented, inaudible speech.
	Gradual loss of ability to read or write (fine motor skills).
	Neurologic status:
	May laugh at or feel threatened by these exams; may change answers during the interview.
	Usually oriented to person until late in the disease.
	Impaired recent memory, intact remote memory (early Alzheimer's).
	Inability to do simple calculations or repeat names of three objects.
	Impaired motor skills with tremors, rigidity, unsteady gait.
	Primitive reflexes (e.g., positive snout, suck, palmar).

SAFETY

May report:	History of serious head injury (may be a predisposing factor).
	Incidental trauma (falls, burns, etc.).
May exhibit:	Ecchymosis; lacerations.

SOCIAL INTERACTION

| **May report:** | Forced retirement. |
| | Prior psychosocial factors; individuality and personality influence present altered behavioral patterns. |

TEACHING/LEARNING

May report:	Familial history of Alzheimer's (four times greater than general population).
	Use/misuse of medications.
Discharge Plan Considerations:	May require alteration in medication regimen.
	Assistance in all areas; safety concerns; possible changes in physical layout of home or placement out of home.

DIAGNOSTIC STUDIES

Note: while no diagnostic studies are specific for Alzheimer's, they are used to rule out reversible problems that may be confused with these dementias.

Antibodies: abnormally high levels may be found (leading to a theory of an immunologic defect).

CBC, RPR, electrolytes, thyroid studies: may determine and/or eliminate treatable/reversible dysfunctions, e.g., metabolic disease processes, fluid/electrolyte imbalance, neurosyphilis.

B_{12}: may disclose a nutritional deficit.

Dexamethasone suppression test (DST): to rule out treatable depression.

ECG: may be normal; need to rule out cardiac insufficiency.

EEG: may be normal or show some slowing (aids in establishing treatable brain dysfunctions).

Skull x-rays: usually normal.

Vision/hearing tests: to rule out deficits that may be the cause of/contribute to disorientation, mood swings, or altered sensory perceptions (rather than cognitive impairment).

PET scan, BEAM, MRI: may show areas of decreased brain metabolism characteristic of Alzheimer's.

CT scan: may show widening of ventricles, cortical atrophy.

CSF: presence of abnormal protein from the brain cells is 90% indicative of Alzheimer's.

NURSING PRIORITIES

1. Provide safe environment, prevent injury.
2. Promote socially acceptable responses; limit inappropriate behavior.
3. Maximize reality orientation/prevent sensory deprivation/overload.
4. Encourage participation in self-care within individual limitations.
5. Promote coping mechanisms of patient/SO.
6. Support patient/SO in grieving process.
7. Provide information about disease process, prognosis and resources available for assistance.

DISCHARGE CRITERIA

1. Adequate supervision/support systems available.
2. Maximal level of independent functioning achieved.
3. Coping skills developed/strengthened, and SOs using available resources.
4. Disease process/prognosis and patient expectations/needs understood by SO.

NURSING DIAGNOSIS:	**INJURY, POTENTIAL FOR: (SPECIFY)**
May be related to:	**Inability to recognize/identify danger in environment**
	Disorientation, confusion, impaired judgment
	Weakness, muscular incoordination; seizure activity
Possibly evidenced by:	**[Not applicable; presence of signs and symptoms establishes an *actual* diagnosis.]**
PATIENT OUTCOMES/ EVALUATION CRITERIA:	**Injury is prevented. Care giver(s) recognizes potential risks in the environment and identifies steps to correct them.**

ACTIONS/INTERVENTIONS	RATIONALE
Independent	
Assess for degree of impairment in ability/competence. Assist SO to identify risks/potential hazards that may be present.	Identifies potential risks in environment and heightens awareness so care givers are more alert to dangers.
Eliminate/minimize identified hazards in the environment.	A person with cognitive impairment and perceptual disturbances is prone to accidental injury because of the inability to take responsibility for basic safety needs or to evaluate the unforeseen consequences, e.g., may light a stove/cigarette and forget it, attempt to eat plastic fruit, misjudge placement of chairs, stairs.
Provide with an identification bracelet showing name, phone number and diagnosis.	Facilitates safe return if lost. Because of poor verbal ability and confusion, may be unable to state address,

315

Independent

phone number, etc. Patient may wander and be detained by police, appearing confused, irritable; may have violent outbursts and exhibit poor judgment.

Dress according to physical environment/individual need.

The general slowing of metabolic processes results in lowered body heat. The hypothalamus is affected by the disease process, causing person to feel cold. Patient may have seasonal disorientation and may wander out in the cold. Note: Leading causes of death are pneumonia/accidents.

Use "child proof" locks; secure medications, poisonous substances, tools, sharp objects, etc. Remove stove knobs, burners.

As the disease worsens, the patient may fidget with objects/locks (hypermetamorphosis) or put small items in mouth (hyperorality), which potentiates accidental injury/death.

Monitor for medication side effects, signs of overmedication, e.g., extrapyramidal signs, orthostatic hypotension, visual disturbances, GI upsets.

Patient may not be able to report signs/symptoms and drugs can easily build up to toxic levels in the elderly. Dosages/drug choice may need to be altered.

Avoid continuous use of restraints. Have SO/others stay with patient during periods of acute agitation.

Endangers the individual who succeeds in partial removal of restraints. May increase agitation and potentiate fractures in the elderly (due to reduced calcium in the bones).

NURSING DIAGNOSIS: **THOUGHT PROCESSES, ALTERED**

May be related to:
     Irreversible neuronal degeneration
     Loss of memory
     Sleep deprivation
     Psychologic conflicts

Possibly evidenced by:
     Inability to interpret stimuli accurately and evaluate reality

     Disorientation and difficulty in grasping ideas/commands

     Paranoia, delusions, confusion/frustration and changes in behavioral responses

PATIENT OUTCOMES/ EVALUATION CRITERIA:
     Recognizes changes in thinking/behavior and causative factors when able. Demonstrates a decrease in undesired behaviors, threats, and confusion.

Independent

Assess degree of cognitive impairment, e.g., changes in orientation to person, place, time; attention span, thinking ability. Talk with SO about changes from usual behavior/length of time problem has existed.

Provides baseline for future evaluation/comparison and choice of interventions.

Maintain a pleasant, quiet environment.

Crowds, clutter, and noise generate sensory overload that stresses the impaired neurons.

ACTIONS/INTERVENTIONS	RATIONALE
Independent	
Approach in a slow, calm manner.	Hurried approaches can startle/threaten the confused patient who misinterprets or feels threatened by imaginary people and/or situations.
Face the individual when conversing.	Arouses attention, particularly in persons with perceptual disturbances.
Call by name.	Names form self-identity, establish reality and individual recognition. Patient may respond to own name long after failing to recognize SO.
Use lower voice register and speak slowly to patient.	Increases the chance for comprehension. High-pitched, loud tones convey stress/anger, which may trigger memory of previous confrontations and provoke an angry response.
Use short words and simple sentences and give simple directions (step-by-step instructions).	As the disease progresses, the communication centers in the brain are impaired, hindering the individual's ability to process and comprehend complex messages.
Pause between phrases or questions. Give hints and use open-ended phrases when possible.	Invites a verbal response and may increase comprehension. Hints stimulate communication and give the person a chance for a positive experience.
Listen with regard in spite of speech content. Interpret statements, meanings, and words. If possible, supply the correct word.	Conveys interest and worth to the individual. Assisting the patient with word processing aids in decreasing frustration.
Avoid negative criticism, arguments, confrontations (provocative stimuli).	Provocation decreases self-esteem and may be interpreted as a threat that triggers agitation or increases inappropriate behavior.
Use distraction. Talk about real people and real events when patient begins ruminating about false ideas, unless it increases anxiety/agitation.	Rumination serves to promote disorientation. Reality orientation increases patient's sense of reality, self-worth, and personal dignity.
Refrain from forcing activities and communications.	Force decreases cooperation and may increase suspiciousness, delusions.
Use humor with interactions.	Laughter can assist in communication and help reverse emotional lability.
Focus on appropriate behavior. Give positive reinforcement, e.g., a pat on the back, applaud. Use touch judiciously. Respect individual's personal space/response.	Reinforces correctness, appropriate behavior. While touch frequently transcends verbal interchange (conveying warmth, acceptance, and reality), the individual may misinterpret the meaning of touch. Intrusion into personal space may threaten the patient's distorted world.
Respect individuality and evaluate specific needs.	Persons experiencing a cognitive decline deserve respect, dignity, and worth as an individual. Patient's past and background are important in maintaining self-concept, planning activities, communicating, etc.
Allow personal belongings.	Familiarity enhances security, sense of self, and decreases increased feelings of loss/deprivation.
Permit hoarding of safe objects.	An activity that preserves security and counterbalances irrevocable losses.
Create simple, noncompetitive activities paced to the individual's abilities.	Motivates patient in ways that will reinforce usefulness and self-worth and stimulate reality.
Make useful activities out of hoarding and repetitive motions, e.g., collecting junk mail, scrapbook, folding/	May decrease restlessness and provide option for pleasurable activity.

Independent

unfolding linen, bouncing balls, dusting, sweeping floors.

Assist with finding misplaced items. Label drawers/belongings. Do not challenge patient.

May decrease defensiveness when patient believes he or she is being accused of stealing a misplaced, hoarded, or hidden item. To refute the accusation will not change the belief and may invite anger.

Monitor phone use closely. Post significant phone numbers in prominent place. Secure long-distance numbers.

Can be used as reality orientation, but impaired judgment does not allow for distinguishing long-distance numbers and makes client easy prey for phone sale pitches.

Evaluate sleep/rest pattern and adequacy. Note lethargy, increasing irritability/confusion, frequent yawning, dark circles under eyes.

Lack of sleep can impair thought processes and coping abilities. (Refer to ND: Sleep Pattern Disturbance, p. 320.)

Collaborative

Administer medications as individually indicated:

Antipsychotics, e.g., haloperidol (Haldol), thioridazine (Mellaril);

May be used to control agitation, delusions, hallucinations. Mellaril is often preferred because there are fewer extrapyramidal side effects (e.g., dystonia, akathisia), increased confusion; visual problems; and especially gait disturbances. Note: Phenathiazines may cause oversedation/excitation or bizarre reactions.

Vasodilators, e.g., cyclandelate (Cyclospasmol) and

May improve mental alertness but requires further research.

Ergoloid mesylates (Hydergine LC);

A metabolic enhancer (increases the brain's ability to metabolize glucose and use oxygen) that has few side effects. Although it does not increase cognition and memory, it may make patient more alert, less anxious/depressed. However, it may be of little value in dementia therapy because there is usually a limited degree of improvement. Note: This is an expensive drug, and families need accurate information in order to make informed therapy decisions, avoiding false hopes and disappointment due to lack of dramatic results.

Anxiolytic agents, e.g., diazepam (Valium), lorazepam (Librium), oxazepam (Serax).

More useful in early/mild stages for relief of anxiety. Can increase confusion in the elderly. Note: Serax may be preferred because it is shorter acting.

NURSING DIAGNOSIS:	SENSORY-PERCEPTUAL ALTERATION: (SPECIFY)
May be related to:	**Altered sensory reception, transmission, and/or integration (neurologic disease/deficit)**
	Socially restricted environment (homebound/institutionalized)
Possibly evidenced by:	**Changes in usual response to stimuli, e.g., spatial disorientation, confusion**
	Exaggerated emotional responses, e.g., anxiety, paranoia, and hallucinations

Inability to tell position of body parts

Diminished/altered sense of taste

**PATIENT OUTCOMES/
EVALUATION CRITERIA:** Demonstrates improved/appropriate response to stimuli. Care givers identify/control external factors that contribute to alterations in sensory-perceptual abilities.

ACTIONS/INTERVENTIONS	RATIONALE

Independent

Assess degree of sensory or perceptual impairment and how it affects the individual, including hearing/visual deficits.

While brain involvement is usually global, a small percentage may exhibit asymmetrical involvement which may cause the patient to neglect one side of the body (unilateral neglect). Individual may not be able to locate internal cues, recognize hunger/thirst, perceive external pain, or locate body within the environment.

Maintain a reality-oriented relationship and environment. Provide clues (around the clock) to reality orientation with calendars, clocks, notes, cards, signs, music, seasonal hues/color-code rooms, scenic pictures.

Reduces confusion and promotes coping with the frustrating struggles of misperception, being disoriented/confused. Dysfunction in visual/spatial perception interferes with the ability to recognize direction/patterns, and the patient may become lost, even in familiar surroundings. Clues are tangible reminders that aid recognition and may permeate memory gaps and increase independence.

Provide quiet, nondistracting environment when indicated, e.g., soft music, plain but colorful wallpaper/paint, etc.

Helps to avoid visual/auditory overload by emphasizing qualities of calmness, consistency. Note: Patterned wallpaper may be disturbing to some patients.

Provide touch in a caring way.

May enhance perception of self/body boundaries.

Use sensory games to stimulate reality, e.g., smell Vick's and tell of the time mother used it on you; use spring–fall nature boxes.

Communicates reality through multiple channels.

Indulge in periodic reminiscence (old music, historic events, photos, mementos).

Stimulates recollections, awakens memories, aids in the preservation of self/individuality via past accomplishments. Increases feelings of security while easing adaptation to a changed environment.

Provide simple outings, short walks.

Outings refresh reality and provide pleasurable sensory stimuli, which may reduce suspiciousness, hallucinations caused by feelings of imprisonment. Motor functioning may be decreased, because nerve degeneration results in weakness, decreasing stamina.

Promote balanced physiologic functions, using colorful Nerf/beach balls, arm dancing with music.

Preserves mobility (reducing the potential for bone and muscle atrophy) and provides diversional opportunity for interaction with others.

Involve in activities with others as dictated by individual situation, e.g., one-to-one visitors, socialization groups at Alzheimer center, occupational therapy.

Provides opportunity for the stimulation of participation with others and may maintain some level of social interaction.

NURSING DIAGNOSIS: **FEAR**

May be related to: Sensory impairment, physical deterioration

Separation from support systems

Public disclosure of disabilities

**PATIENT OUTCOMES/
EVALUATION CRITERIA:** Demonstrates more appropriate range of feelings and lessened fear.

ACTIONS/INTERVENTIONS

Independent

Note change of behavior, presence of suspiciousness, irritability, defensiveness.

Identify strengths the individual had previously.

Deal with aggressive behavior by imposing calm, firm limits.

Provide clear, honest information about actions/events.

Encourage hugging and use of touch unless patient is paranoid or agitated at the moment.

RATIONALE

Change in moods may be one of the first signs of cognitive decline. The patient who is aware of deterioration and/or who may be aware of diagnosis can fear helplessness and try to hide the increasing inability to remember/accomplish normal activities.

Facilitates assistance with communication and management of current deficits.

Acceptance can reduce fear and aggressive response.

Assists in maintaining trust and orientation as long as possible. When the patient knows the truth about what is happening, coping is often enhanced and guilt over what is imagined is decreased.

Provides reassurance, reduces stress, and enhances quality of life.

NURSING DIAGNOSIS:	SLEEP PATTERN DISTURBANCE
May be related to:	Neurologic impairment
Possibly evidenced by:	Changes in behavior and performance
	Disorientation (day/night reversal)
	Irritability
	Wakefulness/interrupted sleep, increased aimless wandering; inability to identify need/time for sleeping
	Lethargy, dark circles under eyes, frequent yawning
PATIENT OUTCOMES/ EVALUATION CRITERIA:	Establishes adequate sleep pattern, and wandering is reduced. Patient reports/appears rested.

ACTIONS/INTERVENTIONS

Independent

Provide for rest/naps; reduce physical/mental activity late in the day.

Avoid use of continuous restraints (particularly when in room alone).

RATIONALE

Prolonged physical and mental activity results in fatigue, which can increase confusion.

Potentiates sensory deprivation, increases agitation, and restricts rest.

ACTIONS/INTERVENTIONS	RATIONALE
Independent	
Evaluate level of stress/orientation as day progresses.	Increasing confusion, disorientation, and uncooperative behaviors (Sundowner's syndrome) may interfere with attaining restful sleep pattern.
Adhere to regular bedtime schedule and rituals. Tell patient that it is time to sleep.	Reinforces that it is bedtime and maintains stability of environment. Note: Later than normal bedtime may be indicated to allow patient to dissipate excess energy and facilitate falling asleep.
Provide evening snack, warm milk, backrub.	Promotes relaxation. L-Tryptophan (found in milk) induces drowsiness.
Reduce fluid intake in the evening.	Decreases need to get up to go to the bathroom/incontinence during the night.
Provide soft music or "white noise."	Reduces sensory stimulation by blocking out other environmental sounds that could interfere with restful sleep.
Collaborative	
Administer medications as indicated for sleep:	
Antidepressants, e.g., amitriptyline (Elavil), doxepin, and trazolone (Desyrel);	May be effective in treating pseudodementia, depression, improving ability to sleep. However, the anticholinergic properties can induce confusion or worsen cognition, and side effects (e.g., orthostatic hypotension) may limit usefulness.
Chloral hydrate, oxazepam (Serax), triazolam (Halcion);	Used sparingly, low-dose hypnotics may be effective in treating insomnia or Sundowner's syndrome.
Avoid use of diphenhydramine (Benadryl).	Once used for sleep, this drug is now contraindicated because it interferes with the production of acetylcholine, which is already inhibited in the brains of patients with Alzheimer's.

NURSING DIAGNOSIS: HOME MAINTENANCE MANAGEMENT, IMPAIRED/ HEALTH MAINTENANCE, ALTERED

May be related to:

Progressively impaired cognitive functioning

Complete or partial lack of gross and/or fine motor skills

Significant alteration in communication skills

Ineffective individual/family coping

Insufficient family organization/planning

Unfamiliarity with resources; inadequate support systems

Possibly evidenced by:

Home surroundings appear disorderly/unsafe

Household members express difficulty and request help in maintaining home in safe/comfortable fashion

Overtaxed family members, e.g., exhausted/anxious

Reported or observed inability to take responsibility for meeting basic health practices

321

	Reported or observed lack of equipment, financial or other resources; impairment of personal support system
CARE GIVER OUTCOMES/ EVALUATION CRITERIA:	**Identifies and corrects factors related to difficulty in maintaining a safe environment for the patient. Demonstrates appropriate, effective use of resources, e.g., respite care, homemakers, Alzheimer groups. Assumes responsibility for and adopts lifestyle changes supporting patient health care goals. Verbalizes ability to cope adequately with existing situation.**

ACTIONS/INTERVENTIONS	**RATIONALE**
Independent	
Evaluate level of cognitive/emotional/physical functioning (level of independence).	Identifies strengths/areas of need and how much responsibility the patient may be expected to assume. (Refer to ND: Self-Care Deficit, following.)
Assess environment, noting unsafe factors and ability of patient to care for self.	Determines what changes need to be made to accommodate disabilities. (Refer to ND: Injury, Potential for: (Specify), p. 315.)
Assist patient/SO to develop plan for keeping track of/ dealing with health needs.	Scheduling can be helpful in managing routine care.
Identify support systems available to patient/SO, e.g., other family members, friends.	Planning and constant care is necessary to maintain patient at home. If family system is unavailable/ unaware, patient needs, e.g., nutrition, dental care, eye exams can be neglected. Primary care giver may benefit from assistance, e.g., someone to come in and provide relief/respite from constant care.
Evaluate coping abilities, effectiveness, commitment of care giver(s)/support persons.	Progressive debilitation taxes care giver(s) and may alter ability to meet patient/own needs. (Refer to ND: Coping, Ineffective Family: Compromised/Disabling, p. 326.)
Collaborative	
Identify alternate care sources (such as sitter/day care facility), or senior care services, e.g., Meals on Wheels/respite care.	As patient's condition worsens, SO may need additional help from several sources or may eventually be unable to maintain patient at home.
Refer to supportive services as need indicates.	Consultant such as VNA may be helpful to developing ongoing plan/identifying resources as needs change.

NURSING DIAGNOSIS:	**SELF-CARE DEFICIT: (SPECIFY)**
May be related to:	**Cognitive decline; physical limitations**
	Frustration over loss of independence; depression
Possibly evidenced by:	**Impaired ability to perform ADLs, e.g., inability to bring food from receptacle to mouth; inability to wash body part(s), regulate temperature of water; impaired ability to put on/take off clothing; difficulty completing toileting tasks**

PATIENT OUTCOMES/ EVALUATION CRITERIA:	Performs self-care activities within level of own ability. Identifies and uses personal/community resources that can provide assistance.

ACTIONS/INTERVENTIONS	RATIONALE

Independent

Identify reason for difficulty in dressing/self-care, e.g., physical limitations in motion, apathy/depression, cognitive decline (such as apraxia) or room temperature ("too cold" to get dressed).	Underlying cause affects choice of interventions/strategies. Problem may be minimized by changes in environment or adaptation of clothing or may require consultation from other specialists.
Identify hygienic needs and provide assistance as needed with care of hair/nails/skin, cleaning glasses, brushing teeth.	As the disease progresses, basic hygienic needs may be forgotten. Harm, infection, or exhaustion may occur when patient/care givers become frustrated, irritated, or intimidated by these problems.
Be attentive to nonverbal physiologic symptoms.	Sensory loss and language dysfunction may cause patient to express self-care needs in nonverbal manner, e.g., thirst by panting; need to void by holding self/fidgeting.
Be alert to underlying meaning of verbal statements.	May direct a question to another, such as "Are you cold?" meaning "I am cold and need additional clothing," etc.
Supervise but allow as much autonomy as possible.	Eases the frustration over lost independence.
Allot plenty of time to perform tasks.	Tasks once easy (e.g., dressing, bathing) are now complicated by decreased motor skills or cognitive and physical change. Time and patience reduce chaos.
Assist with neat dressing/provide colorful clothes.	Enhances esteem, may diminish sense of sensory loss and convey aliveness.
Offer one item of clothing at a time, in sequential order. Talk through each step one at a time.	Simplicity reduces frustration and the potential for rage and despair. Guidance reduces confusion and allows autonomy.
Allow to sleep in shoes/clothing or to wear two sets of clothing if patient demands.	Providing no harm is done, altering the "normal" lessens the rebellion and allows rest.
Wait and/or change the time to approach dressing/hygiene if a problem arises.	Because anger is quickly forgotten, another time or approach may be successful.

NURSING DIAGNOSIS:	NUTRITION, ALTERED: LESS/MORE THAN BODY REQUIREMENTS [POTENTIAL]
May be related to:	Sensory changes
	Impaired judgment and coordination
	Agitation
	Forgetfulness, regressed habits and concealment
Possibly evidenced by:	[Not applicable; presence of signs and symptoms establishes an *actual* diagnosis.]

<table>
<tr><td>PATIENT OUTCOMES/
EVALUATION CRITERIA:</td><td>Ingests nutritionally balanced diet. Maintains/regains
appropriate weight.</td></tr>
</table>

ACTIONS/INTERVENTIONS	RATIONALE

Independent

Assess SO/patient's knowledge of nutritional needs.	Identifies needs to assist in formulating individual teaching plan. A role reversal situation can occur (e.g., child now taking care of parent, husband taking over duties of wife), increasing the need for information.
Determine amount of exercise/pacing patient does.	Nutritional intake may need to be adjusted to meet needs related to individual energy expenditure.
Offer/provide assistance in menu selection.	Patient may be indecisive/overwhelmed by choices or unaware of the need to maintain elemental nutrition.
Provide privacy, when eating habits become an insoluble problem. Accept eating with hands, tolerate spills without scolding, and expect whimsical mixtures, e.g., salad dressing in milk, or salt and pepper in ice cream. (Note: Avoid separating patient from other people too soon or too frequently.)	Socially unacceptable and embarrassing eating habits develop as the disease progresses. Acceptance preserves esteem, decreases frustration or not wanting to eat as a result of anger, frustration. Early separation can result in patient feeling upset and rejected and can actually decrease food intake.
Offer small feedings and/or snacks around the clock as indicated.	Large feedings may overload the patient, resulting either in complete abstinence or gorging. Small feedings may enhance appropriate intake.
Provide ample time for eating.	A leisurely approach aids digestion, decreases the chance of anger precipitated by rushing, and allows time for chewing when motor functioning is impaired.
Simplify steps of eating, e.g., serve food in courses. Anticipate needs, cut foods, provide soft/finger foods.	Promotes autonomy and independence. Decreases potential frustration/anger over lost abilities.
Avoid baby food and excessively hot foods.	Baby foods lack adequate nutritional content, fiber, and taste for adults and can add to patient's humiliation. Hot foods may result in mouth burns and/or refusal to eat.
Stimulate oral-suck reflex by gentle stroking of the cheeks or stimulating the mouth with a spoon.	As the disease progresses, the patient may clench teeth and refuse to eat. Stimulating the reflex may increase cooperation/intake.

Collaborative

Refer to dietician.	Assistance may be needed to develop a nutritionally balanced diet individualized to meet patient needs/food preferences.

NURSING DIAGNOSIS:	**BOWEL ELIMINATION, ALTERED: (SPECIFY) AND/OR URINARY ELIMINATION, ALTERED PATTERNS**
May be related to:	**Disorientation** **Lost neurologic functioning/muscle tone** **Inability to locate the bathroom/recognize need** **Changes in dietary/fluid intake**

Possibly evidenced by:	Inappropriate toileting behaviors
	Urgency/incontinence/constipation
PATIENT OUTCOMES/ EVALUATION CRITERIA:	Establishes adequate/appropriate pattern of elimination.

ACTIONS/INTERVENTIONS	RATIONALE
Independent	
Assess prior pattern and compare with current.	Provides information about changes that may require further assessment/intervention.
Locate near a bathroom; make signs for/color-code door. Provide adequate lighting particularly at night.	Promotes orientation/finding bathroom. Incontinence may be attributed to inability to find a toilet.
Take to the toilet at regular intervals. Dictate each step one at a time and use positive reinforcement.	Adherence to a daily and regular schedule may prevent accidents. Frequently the problem is forgetting what to do, e.g., pushing pants down, position, etc.
Establish bowel/bladder training program. Promote patient participation to level of ability.	Stimulates awareness, enhances regulation of body function and helps to avoid accidents.
Encourage adequate fluid intake during the day, diet high in fiber and fruit juices; limit intake during the late evening and at bedtime.	Reduces risk of dehydration/constipation. Restricting intake in evening may reduce frequency/incontinence during the night.
Avoid a sense of hurrying.	Hurrying may be perceived as intrusion, which leads to anger and lack of cooperation with activity.
Be alert to nonverbal cues, e.g., restlessness, holding self or picking at clothes.	May signal urgency, inattention to cues and/or inability to locate bathroom.
Be discreet.	Although the patient is confused, a sense of modesty is often retained.
Convey acceptance when incontinence occurs. Change promptly, provide good skin care.	Acceptance is important to decrease the embarrassment and feelings of helplessness that may occur during the changing process. Reduces risk of skin irritation/breakdown.
Monitor appearance/color of urine; note consistency of stool.	Detection of changes provides opportunity to alter interventions to prevent complications or acquire treatment as indicated (e.g., constipation/urinary infection).
Collaborative	
Administer stool softeners, Metamucil, glycerin suppository, as indicated.	May be necessary to facilitate/stimulate regular bowel movement.

NURSING DIAGNOSIS:	SEXUAL DYSFUNCTION [POTENTIAL]
May be related to:	Confusion, forgetfulness and disorientation to place or person
	Altered body function, decrease in habit/control of behavior
	Lack of intimacy/sexual rejection by SO
	Lack of privacy

Possibly evidenced by:	[Not applicable; presence of signs and symptoms establishes an *actual* diagnosis.]
PATIENT OUTCOMES/ EVALUATION CRITERIA:	Meeting sexuality needs in an acceptable manner.

ACTIONS/INTERVENTIONS	RATIONALE
Independent	
Assess individual needs/desires/abilities.	Alternative methods need to be designed for the individual situation to fulfill the need for intimacy and closeness.
Encourage partner to show affection/acceptance.	The cognitively impaired person retains the basic needs for affection, love, acceptance, and sexual expression.
Assure privacy.	Sexual expression or behavior may differ, and privacy allows sexual expression without embarrassment and/or the objections of others.
Use distraction, as indicated. Remind patient that this is a public area and current behavior is unacceptable.	Useful tool when there is inappropriate/objectionable behavior, e.g., self-exposure.
Provide time to listen/discuss concerns of SO.	May need information and/or counseling about alternatives for sexual activity/aggression.

NURSING DIAGNOSIS:	**COPING, INEFFECTIVE FAMILY: COMPROMISED/ DISABLING**
May be related to:	**Disruptive behavior of patient**
	Family grief about their helplessness watching loved one deteriorate
	Prolonged disease/disability progression that exhausts the supportive capacity of SO
	Highly ambivalent family relationships
Possibly evidenced by:	**Family becoming embarrassed and socially immobilized**
	Home maintenance becomes extremely difficult and leads to difficult decisions with legal/financial considerations
FAMILY OUTCOMES/ EVALUATION CRITERIA:	**Identifies/verbalizes resources within themselves to deal with the situation. Acknowledges loved one's condition and demonstrates positive coping behaviors in dealing with situation. Uses outside support systems effectively.**

ACTIONS/INTERVENTIONS	RATIONALE

Independent

Include all SO in teaching and planning for home care.

Can ease the burden of home management and adaptation. Comfortable and familiar lifestyle at home is helpful in preserving the affected individual's need for belonging.

Focus on specific problems as they occur, the "here and now."

Disease progression follows no set pattern. A premature focus on the possibility of long-term care can impair the ability to cope with present issues.

Establish priorities.

Helps to create a sense of order and facilitates problem solving.

Be realistic and honest in all matters.

Decreases stress that surrounds false hopes, e.g., that individual may regain past level of functioning from advertised or unproven medication.

Continually reassess family's ability to care for patient at home.

Behaviors like hoarding, clinging, unjust accusations, angry outbursts, etc., can precipitate family burnout and interfere with ability to provide effective care.

Help SO/family understand the importance of maintaining psychosocial functioning.

Embarrassing behavior, the demands of care, etc., may cause psychosocial withdrawal.

Provide time/listen with regard to concerns/anxieties.

SOs require constant support with the multifaceted problems that arise during the course of this illness to ease the process of adaptation and grieving.

Provide positive feedback for efforts.

Reassures individuals that they are doing their best.

Encourage unlimited visitation.

Contact with familiarity forms a base of reality and can provide a reassuring freedom from loneliness. Recurrent contact helps family members realize and accept situation.

Support concerns generated by consideration/decision to place in LTC facility.

Constant care requirements may be more than can be managed by SO. Support is needed for this difficult guilt-producing decision, which may create a financial burden as well.

Collaborative

Refer to local resources, e.g., adult day care, respite care, homemaker services, or a local chapter of Alzheimer's Disease and Related Disorders Association (ADRDA).

Coping with this individual is a full time, frustrating task. Respite/day care may lighten the burden, reduce potential social isolation, and prevent family burnout. ADRDA provides group support, family teaching, and promotes research. Local groups provide a social outlet for sharing grief and promotes problem solving with such matters as financial/legal advice, home care, etc.

NURSING DIAGNOSIS:	**GRIEVING, ANTICIPATORY**
May be related to:	**Patient awareness of something "being wrong" with changes in memory/family reaction, physiopsychosocial well-being**
	Family perception of potential loss of loved one
Possibly evidenced by:	**Expressions of distress/anger at potential loss**
	Choked feelings, crying

PATIENT/FAMILY OUTCOMES/ EVALUATION CRITERIA:	Alteration in activity level, communication patterns, eating habits, and sleep patterns Expresses concerns openly. Discusses loss and participates in planning for the future.

ACTIONS/INTERVENTIONS

Independent

Assess degree of deterioration/level of coping.

Review past life experiences, role changes, and coping skills.

Provide open environment for discussion. Use therapeutic communication skills of active listening, acknowledgment, etc.

Note statements of despair, hopelessness, "nothing to live for," expressions of anger.

Respect desire not to talk.

Be honest, do not give false reassurances or dire predictions about the future.

Discuss with patient/SO ways they can plan together for the future.

Assist patient/SO to identify positive aspects of the situation.

Identify strengths patient/SO see in self/situation and support systems available.

Collaborative

Refer to other resources, counseling, clergy, etc.

RATIONALE

Information is helpful to understand how much the patient is capable of doing to maintain highest level of independence and to provide encouragement to help individuals deal with losses.

Opportunity to identify skills that may help individuals cope with grief of current situation more effectively.

Encourages patient/SO to discuss feelings and concerns realistically.

May be indicative of suicidal ideation. Angry behavior may be patient's way of dealing with feelings of despair.

May not be ready to deal with grief.

Honesty promotes a trusting relationship. Expressions of gloom, such as "You'll spend the rest of your life in a nursing home" are not helpful. (No one knows what the future holds.)

Having a part in problem solving/planning can provide a sense of control over anticipated events.

Ongoing research, possibility of slow progression may offer some hope for the future.

Recognizing these resources provides opportunity to work through feelings of grief.

May need additional support/assistance to resolve feelings.

Myasthenia Gravis/Myasthenic Crisis _____

PATIENT ASSESSMENT DATA BASE

ACTIVITY/REST

May report: Excessive muscular weakness and extreme fatigue (hallmarks of the disease), which may fluctuate from hour to hour or from day to day.

May exhibit: Weakness with repetitive muscle activity and as a result of crisis.

CARDIOVASCULAR

May report: Palpitations.

May exhibit: Tachycardia, cardiac dysrhythmias (may be life-threatening).
Diaphoresis, pallor, cold and clammy skin, cyanosis.

EGO INTEGRITY

May report: Multiple stress factors, financial concerns.
Changes in relationship status; negative reactions by others.
Alteration in lifestyle.
Feelings of helplessness/hopelessness; forced losses; frustration/anger, e.g., misdiagnoses (being told they are crazy, hypochondriacal, etc.).

May exhibit: Emotional reactions of anxiety, fear, apathy, irritability.

ELIMINATION

May report: Stress incontinence.
Difficulty in getting to the bathroom/using bedpan.

May exhibit: Decreased urine output.

FOOD/FLUID

May report: Difficulty chewing/swallowing.
Choking.

May exhibit: Dysphagia, inability to chew (may have more difficulty swallowing fluids than solids).
Weight loss.
Poor skin turgor, dry mucous membranes/tongue (reflecting dehydration).

NEUROMUSCULAR

May report: Double vision.
Weakness in moving jaw/facial muscles.
Difficulty walking, climbing stairs, bending, lifting heavy objects, raising arms above head, etc. (weakness usually begins proximally).

May exhibit: Facial weakness/expressionless mask.
Ptosis, gaze paralysis.
Speech impairment (mushy, slurred, with nasal tone).

RESPIRATION

May report: Shortness of breath, breathlessness.

May exhibit: Tachypnea, dyspnea, shallow respirations.
Impaired coughing ability.

Rhonchi.
Hoarseness, stridor, crowing respirations.
Reduced tidal volume and vital capacity.

SAFETY

May exhibit: Temperature elevation.

TEACHING/LEARNING

May report: Recent infection, surgery, or trauma exacerbating symptoms.

Discharge Plan Considerations: May require changes in medication regimen and physical layout of home; assistance with transportation, shopping, food preparation, self-care, or homemaker tasks.

DIAGNOSTIC STUDIES

Tensilon test: a very rapid-acting cholinergic drug of short duration that inactivates acetylcholinesterase at the sites of cholinergic transmission. A significant increase in muscle strength denotes a positive Tensilon test, confirming diagnosis. (Also used in evaluating dosage needs of cholinergic drugs.)

Electromyography: as a muscle is repetitively electrically stimulated, the patient with MG has a decrease in the evoked potential (if the disease is confined to the eyes, this response may be absent).

Single-fiber electromyography: specialized electromyography that picks up electrical activity from one or two muscle fibers. An increase in the time of transmission of electrical activity is seen in MG.

Chest x-ray and CT scan: used to evaluate the status of the thymus. (There is an increased incidence of thymoma and thymic hyperplasia in patients with MG.)

Serum antibody levels: about 90% of patients with MG have acetylcholine receptor antibodies (AChRAb) which prevent adequate transmission of the electrical impulse across the synapse. Antistriational antibodies are found in approximately one third of patients with myasthenia gravis, and approximately three fourths of patients with MG who have thymoma.

Other studies are done as indicated to rule out conditions with similar symptoms, e.g., amyotrophic lateral sclerosis (ALS), botulism, tick fever, peripheral neuropathy, polymyositis, hysterical weakness, and hypothyroidism.

NURSING PRIORITIES

1. Maintain/improve respiratory effort.
2. Enhance neuromuscular function.
3. Prevent/minimize complications.
4. Assist patient/SO to cope with current situation and long-term implications.
5. Provide information about disease/prognosis, treatment needs, and potential complications.

DISCHARGE CRITERIA

1. Respiratory function adequate for individual needs.
2. Neuromuscular functioning/activity level improved.
3. Complications prevented/controlled.
4. Anxiety reduced to manageable level with problem solving initiated.
5. Disease process/prognosis, therapeutic regimen, and potential complications understood.

NURSING DIAGNOSIS:	AIRWAY CLEARANCE, INEFFECTIVE
May be related to:	**Neuromuscular weakness, decreased energy, fatigue**
Possibly evidenced by:	**Dyspnea**
	Changes in rate/depth of respiration

Adventitious breath sounds (crackles, wheezes)

Ineffective cough

PATIENT OUTCOMES/ EVALUATION CRITERIA:	Maintains patency of airway with breath sounds clear. Expectorates secretions effectively.

ACTIONS/INTERVENTIONS

RATIONALE

Independent

Monitor respiratory rate/rhythm/depth and vital signs.

Retained secretions may increase work of breathing potentiating risk of respiratory failure.

Auscultate breath sounds. Observe sputum color, consistency and amount.

Presence of wheezes, rhonchi indicates pooling of secretions (resulting from poor/weak cough effort) and increases risk of respiratory infections.

Suction airway as needed.

Aids in clearing airway when cough is ineffective; reduces risk of aspiration.

Elevate head of bed, support head/neck in neutral position as necessary.

Raising head reduces risk of oral pooling of secretions/regurgitation with aspiration. However, severe muscle weakness can interfere with ability to support head, mobilize and clear secretions and thus compromise airway.

Encourage coughing and deep breathing exercises/ "quad cough" techniques. Turn/reposition periodically.

Allows patient to use available muscle strength to promote mobilization/expectoration of secretions and reminds patient to be aware of optimal respiratory excursion.

Encourage fluid intake of at least 2000 ml/day.

Aids in liquefying secretions to enhance mobilization/ expectoration.

Collaborative

Monitor chest x-ray.

May signal early bronchitis/pneumonia.

Monitor/graph serial ABGs.

Decreased PO_2 may indicate inadequate pulmonary toilet.

Assist with bronchoscopy when indicated.

May be done to clear bronchial tree of pooled secretions when cough effort is ineffective.

NURSING DIAGNOSIS:	BREATHING PATTERN, INEFFECTIVE
May be related to:	Neuromuscular impairment, decreased lung expansion Muscular and general fatigue
Possibly evidenced by:	Changes in rate/depth of respirations, nasal flaring, use of accessory muscles Restlessness, changes in mentation Tachycardia Cyanosis; abnormal ABGs
PATIENT OUTCOMES/ EVALUATION CRITERIA:	Maintains/reestablishes normal, effective respiratory pattern, free of cyanosis and other signs of distress and with ABGs within patient's normal range.

331

ACTIONS/INTERVENTIONS	RATIONALE

Independent

Note rate/character of respirations; skin color and temperature, level of consciousness/mentation.

Indicators of adequacy of ventilation although cyanosis is generally a late sign. Note: Use of intercostal muscles or nasal flaring suggesting respiratory compromise could be absent because of muscle weakness.

Be aware of signs of respiratory muscle fatigue; assumption of "three-point" posture; changes in speech pattern (e.g., frequent pauses to catch a breath between words).

Suggests decreased respiratory reserve/developing failure.

Assess/record vital capacity periodically.

Direct measure of respiratory function and provides early indication of progressing failure.

Suction airway as needed. (Refer to ND: Airway Clearance, p. 330.)

Muscle weakness may impair airway patency, increasing respiratory distress.

Monitor vital signs and cardiac rhythm.

Elevated BP and tachycardia may reflect progressing respiratory failure. Decreased oxygenation and cardiac ischemia can lead to ventricular dysrhythmias.

Elevate head of bed.

Gravity aids in lowering diaphragm to enhance lung expansion.

Maintain calm attitude/approach.

Anxiety is contagious and may increase patient's emotional stress, exacerbating muscle weakness/respiratory compromise.

Assist patient in "taking control" of respirations.

Promotes slower/deeper respirations, maximizing respiratory effort.

Monitor dietary needs. Avoid ingestion of gas-forming foods, sipping through a straw, and carbonated beverages.

Abdominal distention can restrict diaphragmatic excursion and depth of respiration.

Collaborative

Administer medications as indicated:

    Edrophonium chloride (Tensilon), neostigmine methylsulfate (Prostigmin);

Drugs of choice to correct myasthenic crisis.

    Atropine.

Used to reduce symptoms of cholinergic crisis.

Provide supplemental oxygen as necessary.

Maximizes oxygen available in presence of decreased ventilation.

Monitor and chart serial ABGs.

Provides information about respiratory function, therapy needs/effectiveness.

Assist with respiratory adjuncts, e.g., blow bottles, incentive spirometer.

Periodic use enhances respiratory depth, reducing atelectasis and mobilizing secretions.

Prepare/assist with intubation.

In crisis, a patient may suffer respiratory arrest, because neuromuscular weakness is so pronounced that patient is unable to breathe unassisted.

NURSING DIAGNOSIS:	ACTIVITY INTOLERANCE/MOBILITY, IMPAIRED PHYSICAL
May be related to:	**Neuromuscular weakness (excessive fatigability)**
	Decreased strength and endurance

Possibly evidenced by:	Exertional fatigue/weakness
	Decreased muscle strength, control, impaired coordination, gait disturbances
PATIENT OUTCOMES/ EVALUATION CRITERIA:	Identifies factors affecting activity tolerance. Increases strength/function of affected muscles. Demonstrates techniques/behaviors that enable resumption of activities.

ACTIONS/INTERVENTIONS	RATIONALE
Independent	
Identify activity needs and desires. Evaluate degree of deficit in light of current needs/expectations.	Helps to set realistic goals. Identifies areas of life that may require changing/assistance, e.g., vocational retraining.
Reposition periodically. Inspect skin/bony prominences. Massage with lotion.	Prevents/minimizes complications of immobility.
Provide passive/active range of motion exercises.	Maintains muscle strength/joint mobility and prevents contractures/atrophy.
Encourage patient to be out of bed when able or in chair if fatigued.	Helps patient maintain muscle tone, prevents atrophy and promotes sense of normality in a restricted environment.
Help patient to identify peak effect of anticholinesterase medications.	Provides opportunity to plan activities to take advantage of medication effects.
Assess ability to stand/move about.	Helps to identify degree of assistance required/need for devices to support activity/reduce risk of injury.
Encourage patient to participate in care at level of ability. Avoid/limit repetitive activities (e.g., prolonged brushing of hair/teeth, and use shower chair, sitting during care tasks).	Enhances self-esteem, promotes sense of control, and prevents excessive fatigue. Note: Repetitive activity exhausts ability of neurons to transmit impulses, resulting in loss of muscle function.
Schedule adequate rest periods to balance activities. Allow extra time to complete tasks.	Reduces fatigue, which can increase muscle weakness.
Collaborative	
Refer to physical/occupational therapy.	Can devise activity programs within individual's physical limitations and help patient/SO alter the home environment to accommodate patient needs.
Administer medications as indicated:	
Cholinergic drugs, e.g., pyridostigmine bromide (Mestinon), neostigmine bromide (Prostigmin);	Anticholinesterase agents prevent destruction of acetylcholine, thereby facilitating transmission of impulses across the myoneural junction.
Ephedrine sulfate;	May be added to medication regimen when anticholinesterase drugs do not maintain adequate muscle strength within safe dosage range.
Steroids, e.g., prednisone (Deltasone);	Suppresses immune response to inhibit formation of AChRAb, which may improve muscle strength, especially during acute episodes/exacerbations.
Cytotoxic drugs, e.g., cyclophosphamide (Cytoxan), azathioprine (Imuran).	May be used to suppress immune response/antibody formation, but increased risk of side effects may negate benefits.

ACTIONS/INTERVENTIONS

Collaborative

Assist with plasmapheresis as needed.

Prepare for surgical intervention if indicated.

RATIONALE

May be tried during acute episode to remove free antibodies/abnormal factors that interfere with neuromuscular function when other therapies have been unsuccessful. Note: Pheresis can affect serum drug levels (e.g., plasma-bound drugs are removed), requiring alteration in drug dosage/administration times.

Thymectomy may be done in an attempt to decrease production of AChRAb and thereby to improve muscle strength.

NURSING DIAGNOSIS:	SWALLOWING, IMPAIRED [POTENTIAL]
May be related to:	**Neuromuscular impairment** **Fatigue**
Possibly evidenced by:	**[Not applicable; presence of signs and symptoms establishes an *actual* diagnosis.]**
PATIENT OUTCOMES/ EVALUATION CRITERIA:	**Verbalizes understanding of disease process. Identifies individually appropriate actions to promote intake and to prevent aspiration. Demonstrates emergency measures in the event of choking.**

ACTIONS/INTERVENTIONS

Independent

Observe for signs of choking/fluids regurgitating from nose.

Time medication dosage 30–60 minutes before meals as indicated.

Suggest restricting conversation before and during meals.

Provide small feedings, multiple meals; semisolid foods; cold beverages/foods to start meal. Add bulk/roughage as patient is able to manage.

Encourage high calorie, high-protein beverages between meals, e.g., eggnogs, prepared supplements.

Collaborative

Consult with dietician/nutritional support team.

Monitor chest x-ray.

RATIONALE

Muscular weakness creates swallowing difficulty and risk of nasal regurgitation/aspiration.

Peak drug effect enhances muscle strength/swallowing efforts.

Talking can exhaust some of the same muscles used in chewing/swallowing.

Difficulty in chewing increases as meal progresses, and fatigue can develop. Hot foods can increase muscle weakness/swallowing difficulties. Semisolids may be easier for patient to control than fluids. Increased roughage helps control drug-induced diarrhea.

Increases nutritional intake without additional fatigue.

Useful in creating an adequate dietary program to meet individual needs/limitations.

Aspiration pneumonia may indicate need to use nasogastric/tube feedings until infection cleared/swallowing ability improves.

NURSING DIAGNOSIS:	ANXIETY [SPECIFY]/FEAR
May be related to:	Situational crisis; threat to self-concept
	Change in health/socioeconomic status, role functioning
	Separation from support systems
	Lack of knowledge
	Inability to communicate
Possibly evidenced by:	Expressed concerns
	Increased tension, restlessness, apprehension
	Sympathetic stimulation
	Crying, focus on self
	Uncooperative behavior, withdrawal, anger
	Noncommunication
PATIENT OUTCOMES/ EVALUATION CRITERIA:	Appears relaxed, reports anxiety/fear reduced to manageable levels. Verbalizes feelings and healthy ways to deal with them. Demonstrates problem solving skills. Uses resources effectively.

ACTIONS/INTERVENTIONS	RATIONALE
Independent	
Encourage verbalization of fears and concerns. Note behavioral cues, e.g., restlessness, crying, uncooperativeness, lack of communication.	Although facial weakness may limit nonverbal cues, any discussion should be taken seriously as patient often fears lack of control over the disease/possibility of death. Note: If patient unable to express concerns (e.g., intubation with mechanical ventilation), staff should *anticipate* or expect presence of concerns.
Acknowledge the fear inherent in this situation and normality of these feelings.	Patient needs to know others care about what is happening. Providing opportunity for patient to express fears and concerns can enhance resolution of same.
Assist patient to identify and use positive coping behaviors. Discuss importance of dealing positively with emotional stress.	Patient has coping mechanisms available but may need assistance in identifying/implementing them. Stress can be cumulative and can potentiate muscle weakness.
Provide accurate information about procedures, treatments, machinery.	Decreases the fear of the unknown and promotes sense of control. Provides information necessary to make informed decisions/choices about own treatment plan.
Obtain call system that patient is able to operate. Respond to call signal quickly.	Muscle weakness may preclude use of regular call system. Patient needs to know staff is close at hand.
Arrange for someone to stay with patient as desired/indicated.	Presence of another person can reduce fear of being alone, provides assistance if a crisis occurs and distraction for the patient. Note: If patient prefers to be alone, wishes should be respected within safety concerns.

ACTIONS/INTERVENTIONS	RATIONALE

Independent

Give patient choices whenever possible.	Providing as much control over the situation as possible enhances self-esteem and promotes effective coping in the patient who has lost control over many aspects of life.
Get patient out of bed in wheelchair, recliner, etc., if medically able.	Taking patient off the unit for a change of scenery/to visit children not allowed on the unit provides diversion, promotes feelings of "normality," and strengthens hope of eventual discharge.
Have telephone, radio, tape recorder at the bedside.	Connects patient to the outside world, provides nonphysical diversion, refocuses attention, and may enhance coping abilities.
Help patient/SO identify signs of improvement.	Sustains hope of achieving remission, decreases feelings of helplessness/hopelessness, enhances own sense of power/control.

Collaborative

Refer to social services, pastoral care.	May help patient deal with present situation and plan for the future.
Refer to the Myasthenia Gravis Foundation.	Can provide information about MG treatment and research. Interaction with others in similar circumstances reduces sense of isolation, provides role models for problem solving and effecting coping behaviors.

NURSING DIAGNOSIS:	**COMMUNICATION, IMPAIRED: VERBAL**
May be related to:	**Neuromuscular weakness, fatigue**
	Physical barrier, e.g., intubation
Possibly evidenced by:	**Facial weakness; impaired articulation (mushy, nasal, slurred speech)**
	Hoarseness; inability to speak
PATIENT OUTCOMES/ EVALUATION CRITERIA:	**Verbalizes or indicates an understanding of the communication problems and ways of handling. Establishes method of communication in which needs can be expressed.**

ACTIONS/INTERVENTIONS	RATIONALE

Independent

Listen with regard. Maintain eye contact. Provide sufficient time for patient to respond.	Speech may be mushy, slurred, have a nasal twang, requiring close attention for understanding context. Caring listening conveys message that individual/ needs are important, and can enhance self-esteem and promote continued efforts at communication.
Provide alternatives to verbal communication, e.g., magic slate, spelling board, hand signals, yes/no signals with eye blink, pressure-sensitive call button.	Staff may need to be creative to find ways to meet the needs of the patient who may be too weak/fatigued to communicate verbally.

ACTIONS/INTERVENTIONS

Collaborative

Consult with physical, occupational, and speech therapists.

Refer to local telephone company as indicated.

RATIONALE

May be able to provide specific muscle retraining program to improve enunciation or tailor a specific device for the patient to use in communication.

Will work with patient to develop emergency communication system.

NURSING DIAGNOSIS:	KNOWLEDGE DEFICIT [LEARNING NEED] (SPECIFY)
May be related to:	Lack of exposure, misinterpretation
	Unfamiliarity with resources; lack of recall
Possibly evidenced by:	Request for information; statement of misconceptions
	Inaccurate follow-through of instructions
	Development of preventable complications
PATIENT OUTCOMES/ EVALUATION CRITERIA:	Verbalizes understanding of disease process and its implications. Identifies aggravating factors and specific actions to deal with them. Assumes responsibility for own learning.

ACTIONS/INTERVENTIONS

Independent

Review information about disease process/prognosis, treatment modalities, including alternatives, e.g., radiation.

Recommend patient keep diary of symptoms, response to medication and precipitating/contributing factors (e.g., temperature extremes, hot tub bath, exposure to household pesticides).

Identify factors that may increase muscular weakness, e.g., emotional stress, exposure to infection, repetitive muscle actions, menstruation, or some drugs, e.g., gentamicin, tobramycin, procainamide, quinine, streptomycin.

Identify fatigue-preventing techniques for postdischarge use, e.g., shower chair, sitting during homemaker tasks such as ironing (alternate arms) or food preparation.

Review medication regimen, necessity of maintaining time schedule.

Identify situations that may require increased medication dosage, e.g., stress, exertion, infection, menstruation.

Review drug side effects and nutritional considerations. Recommend restricting intake of diarrhea-

RATIONALE

Provides accurate information to the patient while allowing patient to ask pertinent questions/make informed choices.

Provides information to aid in establishing/tailoring medication needs. Promotes self-management and independence.

Provides opportunity to problem-solve solutions in advance, reducing risk factors/potential for complications.

Promotes independence, conserves strength.

Delaying drug may result in increased/debilitating muscle weakness.

Promotes patient control and independence, reduces risk of crisis.

Ingesting bread or crackers with oral drugs may reduce occurrence of nausea; bananas may decrease

ACTIONS/INTERVENTIONS	RATIONALE

Independent

producing foods (e.g., prunes, chili, corn) and tonic water or OTC cold remedies.

diarrhea. Tonic water and some cold products contain quinine, which may decrease muscle strength. Note: Hyperactivity of intestinal tract can impair drug absorption. If diarrhea is not controlled by dietary measures, may require addition of Pro-Banthine or Lomotil to decrease peristaltic action (these drugs should be used with caution because they may mask cholinergic crisis).

Stress importance of avoiding alcoholic beverages for minimum of 1 hour after taking medications.

Alcohol can increase drug absorption in the stomach, affecting both peak effect and duration.

Encourage intake of potassium-rich foods (e.g., bananas, oranges, tomatoes, whole grains) and restriction of sodium as indicated.

Development of hypokalemia can increase severity of muscle weakness, especially when patient is taking steroids, and sodium/water retention may lead to circulatory congestion.

Demonstrate/encourage use of relaxation techniques, e.g., deep breathing, guided imagery, biofeedback.

Helps patient to reduce/manage stress situations, aiding in control of exacerbations.

Stress importance of carrying/wearing medical identification.

Provides important information to health care workers in emergency situations.

Review need to notify health care providers of condition/medication regimen.

Reduces risk of developing complications, e.g., Novocain is often poorly tolerated and therefore is contraindicated for dental work.

Identify visual/eye deficits and problem-solve.

Patching one eye for double vision or use of "crutches" for drooping lids may improve vision/independence.

Review signs/symptoms requiring medical attention, e.g., increased dyspnea, difficulty swallowing and clearing secretions, or muscle twitching and increased weakness when peak effect of medication is expected.

Impending crisis or cholinergic overdose requires prompt evaluation and intervention to prevent serious complications.

Discuss avoidance of unnecessary exposure to infection, especially when using steroids/immunosuppressive agents.

Patient faces increased risk of URI, which may lead to myasthenic crisis/respiratory compromise.

Help patient recognize signs and symptoms of infection.

Early recognition of infection can lead to prompt treatment, which may avoid serious complications; e.g., infection may precipitate myasthenic crisis.

Collaborative

Refer to community resources, e.g., Myasthenia Gravis Foundation/Pill Bank, Muscular Dystrophy Association, VNA, social service, psychologic/financial resources.

Support groups/resources can provide assistance to enhance patient independence and aid in meeting health and home maintenance needs.

Refer to CP: Multiple Sclerosis, NDs: Self-concept, Disturbance in, p. 344; Powerlessness/Hopelessness, p. 345; Coping, Ineffective Individual [Potential], p. 346.

Multiple Sclerosis

Multiple sclerosis is the most common of the demyelinating disorders. It is a chronic disorder in which irregular demyelination of both the central and peripheral portions of the nervous system result in varying degrees of motor, sensory, and cognitive dysfunction.

PATIENT ASSESSMENT DATA BASE

Degree of symptomatology is dependent on the stage of disease and the neuronal involvement.

ACTIVITY/REST

May report:
Increased fatigue/weakness, exaggerated intolerance to activity, needing to rest after activities such as shaving/showering, intolerance to temperature extremes.
Difficult time with employment because of excessive fatigue/cognitive dysfunction.
Complaints of numbness, tingling in the extremities.
Sleep disturbances, may awaken early or frequently; nocturia.
Loss of position sense (may complain of uneasiness around small children or moving objects, fear of falling).

May exhibit:
Generalized weakness, decreased muscle tone/mass (disuse).
Balance interference.

CIRCULATION

May report:
Dependent edema (steroid therapy or inactivity).

May exhibit:
Blue/mottled, puffy extremities (inactivity).
Capillary fragility (especially on face).

EGO INTEGRITY

May report:
Statements reflecting loss of self-esteem/body image.
Expressions of grief.
Anxiety/fear of rejection, pity.
Keeping illness confidential.
Feelings of helplessness.
Personal tragedies (divorce, abandonment by SO/friends).

May exhibit:
Denial, rejection.
Mood changes, irritability, restlessness, lethargy, euphoria, depression, anger.
Memory loss, difficulty with incidental memory, retrieving/recalling, sorting out information (cerebral involvement).
Difficulty making decisions.

ELIMINATION

May report:
Nocturia.
Retention with overflow.
Urinary/bowel incontinence (cerebral/spinal lesions).
Constipation

May exhibit:
Loss of sphincter control.

FOOD/FLUID

May report: Difficulty chewing, swallowing (weak throat muscles).

Problems getting food to mouth (related to tremors).

Frequent hiccups, lasting extended periods.

May exhibit: Difficulty feeding self.

NEUROSENSORY

May report: Weakness, paralysis of muscles, numbness, tingling (prickling sensations in parts of the body).

Change in visual acuity (diplopia).

Moving head back and forth while watching television, difficulty driving (distorted visual field), blurred vision.

Communication difficulties, such as coining words.

Rapid or insidious progression of symptoms (which may be noted by SO rather than patient).

May exhibit: Mental status: mood swings, depression, euphoria, irritability, apathy; lack of judgment; slow hesitant speech; disorientation/confusion, impairment of short-term memory.

Partial/total loss of vision one eye; vision disturbances.

Positional/vibration sense impaired or absent.

Impaired touch/pain sensation.

Facial/trigeminal nerve involvement, nystagmus, diplopia (brainstem involvement).

Loss of motor skills, muscle tone, spastic paresis/total immobility (advanced stages).

Ataxia, loss of coordination, tremors (may be originally misinterpreted as intoxication).

Hyperreflexia, positive Babinski, absent superficial reflexes.

Intention tremor.

PAIN/DISCOMFORT

May report: Painful spasms, burning pain along nerve path (some patients do not experience normal pain sensations).

Facial neuralgia (central lesion).

Dull back pain (peripheral lesion).

Frequency: varying, may be sporadic/intermittent (possibly once a day) or may be constant.

Duration: lightninglike, repetitive, intermittent; painful spasms of persistent long-term back pain.

SAFETY

May report: History of falls/accidental injuries.

Use of ambulatory devices.

Vision impairment.

Suicidal ideation.

SEXUALITY

May report: Nocturnal erections.

Impotence/ejaculatory difficulties.

Disturbances in sexual relationships.

Enhanced sexual desire.

Problems with positioning.

SOCIAL INTERACTION

May report: Lack of social activities/involvement.

Withdrawal from interactions with others.

Feelings of isolation (increased divorce rate/loss of friends).

May exhibit: Speech impairment.

TEACHING/LEARNING

May report: Use of prescription/OTC medications.

Difficulty retaining information.

Family history of disease (possibly due to common environmental/inherited factors).

Use of "holistic"/natural products/health care practices, "trying out cures."

Discharge Plan Considerations: May require assistance in any or all areas, depending on individual situation.

May eventually need total care/placement in long-term care facility.

DIAGNOSTIC STUDIES

EEG: may be mildly abnormal in some cases.

CT scan: demonstrates brain lesions.

MRI: determines presence of plaques characteristic of MS (along with clinical symptoms, these findings are conclusive).

NURSING PRIORITIES

1. Maintain optimal mobility.
2. Assist with/provide for maintenance of ADLs.
3. Support acceptance of changes in body image/self-esteem and role performance.
4. Provide information about disease process/prognosis, therapeutic needs and available resources.

DISCHARGE CRITERIA

1. Remains mobile within limits of individual situation.
2. ADLs are managed by patient/care givers.
3. Changes in self-concept are acknowledged and being dealt with.
4. Disease process/prognosis, therapeutic regimen are understood and resources identified.

NURSING DIAGNOSIS:	MOBILITY, IMPAIRED PHYSICAL
May be related to:	**Neuromuscular impairment, heat/cold intolerance, decreased strength/endurance, fatigue**
	Perceptual/cognitive deficits
	Pain/discomfort
	Poor nutrition
	Sleep disturbances, depression
	Medication side effects
Possibly evidenced by:	**Statements of concern about ability to perform expected activities**
	Ataxia, paralysis, loss of sensation to limbs

Impaired coordination

Deconditioned status, decreased muscle strength/control

PATIENT OUTCOMES/EVALUATION CRITERIA:	**Identifies risk factors and individual strengths affecting activity tolerance. Identifies alternatives to help maintain current activity level. Participates in conditioning/rehabilitation programs to enhance ability to perform. Demonstrates techniques/behaviors that enable resumption/continuation of activities.**

ACTIONS/INTERVENTIONS	RATIONALE
Independent	
Determine current activity level/physical condition. Assess degree of functional impairment using 0–4 scale.	Provides information to develop plan of care for rehabilitation. Note: Motor symptoms are less likely to improve than sensory ones.
Identify/review factors affecting ability to be active, e.g., temperature extremes, inadequate food intake, insomnia, use of medications.	Provides opportunity to problem-solve to maintain/improve mobility.
Encourage patient to perform self-care to the maximum of ability as defined by the patient. Do not rush patient.	Promotes independence and sense of control, may decrease feelings of helplessness. (Refer to ND: Self-Care Deficit, p. 343.)
Accept when patient is unable to do activities.	Ability can vary from moment to moment. Nonjudgmental acceptance of the patient's evaluation of capabilities provides opportunity to build trust with care givers and maintain feeling of control, enhancing self-esteem.
Evaluate ability to ambulate safely. Provide walking aids, e.g., Canadian canes, wheelchair; review safety considerations.	Walking exercises improve gait/control. However, individual may display poor judgment about ability to safely engage in activity. Mobility aids can decrease fatigue, enhancing independence and comfort, as well as safety.
Plan care with consistent rest periods between activities.	Reduces fatigue, aggravation of muscle weakness.
Reposition frequently when patient is immobile (bed/chairbound). Position/encourage to sleep prone as tolerated.	Reduces continued pressure on same areas, prevents skin breakdown. Minimizes flexor spasms at knees and hips.
Perform active/passive range of motion exercises on a regular schedule. Encourage use of splints/footboards as indicated.	Prevents problems associated with disuse, helps to maintain muscle tone/strength and joint mobility, decrease risk of loss of calcium from bones and problems such as footdrop.
Encourage stretching exercises and use of cold packs, splints when indicated.	Helps decrease spasticity.
Collaborative	
Consult with physical/occupational therapists.	Useful in developing individual exercise program and identifying devices/equipment needs to relieve spastic muscles, improve motor functioning, prevent/reduce muscular atrophy and contractures. Can also provide structured activities to involve specific areas of deficit (e.g., cognitive, kinesthetic), and therapy (e.g., expressive) to improve sense of self-esteem.

ACTIONS/INTERVENTIONS

Collaborative

Recommend groups such as fitness/exercise, research-oriented, and Multiple Sclerosis Society.

Administer medications as indicated, e.g.:

    Diazepam (Valium), baclofen (Lioresal);

    Steroids, e.g., prednisone (Deltasone), dexamethasone (Decadron); pituitary hormones, (ACTH);

    Vitamin B;

    Immunosuppressives, e.g., cyclophosphamide (Cytoxin).

Assist with alternate therapies, e.g., hyperbaric oxygenation.

RATIONALE

Can help patient to stay motivated to remain active within the limits of the disability/condition. Group activities need to be selected carefully to meet the patient's need(s) and prevent discouragement or anxiety, which may occur when patient in early stages sees those in advanced stages.

May be used to decrease spasticity and to assist with mobility and maintenance of activity.

Reduces spasticity by inhibiting spinal cord reflexes. Note: Used with caution because may exacerbate general weakness, further reducing mobility.

May be used during acute exacerbations to prevent edema at the sclerotic plaques; however, long-term therapy seems to have little effect on progression of symptoms.

Supports nerve-cell replication and enhances metabolic functions.

May be tried in effort to slow progression of disease, promote remission.

Used experimentally (in early stages) to promote re-myelinization.

NURSING DIAGNOSIS:	SELF-CARE DEFICIT: (SPECIFY)
May be related to:	**Neuromuscular/perceptual impairment; intolerance to activity; decreased strength and endurance; motor impairment, tremors**
	Pain, discomfort, fatigue
	Memory loss
	Depression
Possibly evidenced by:	**Frustration; inability to perform tasks of self-care**
PATIENT OUTCOMES/ EVALUATION CRITERIA:	**Identifies individual areas of weakness/needs. Demonstrates techniques/lifestyle changes to meet self-care needs. Performs self-care activities within level of own ability. Identifies personal/community resources that provide assistance.**

ACTIONS/INTERVENTIONS

Independent

Assist according to degree of disability, allow as much autonomy as possible. Encourage patient input in planning schedule.

RATIONALE

Participation in own care can ease the frustration over loss of independence. Patient's quality of life is enhanced when desires/likes are considered in daily activities.

ACTIONS/INTERVENTIONS

Independent

Allot sufficient time to perform task(s) and display patience when movements are slow.

Anticipate hygienic needs and assist as necessary, e.g., care of nails, skin, and hair; mouth care; shaving (use electric razor).

Provide assistive devices/aids as indicated, e.g., shower chair.

Problem-solve ways to meet nutritional/fluid needs, e.g., wrap fork handle with tape, cut food, and show patient how to hold cup with both hands.

Collaborative

Consult with occupational therapist.

RATIONALE

Decreased motor skills/spasticity may interfere with ability to manage even simple activities.

Example by care giver can set a matter-of-fact tone for acceptance of handling mundane needs that may be embarrassing to patient/repugnant to SO.

Reduces fatigue, enhancing participation in self-care.

Provides for adequate intake and enhances patient's feelings of independence/self-esteem.

Useful in identifying devices/equipment to meet individual's needs, promoting independence and increasing sense of self-worth.

NURSING DIAGNOSIS:	**SELF-CONCEPT, DISTURBANCE IN: (SPECIFY)**
May be related to:	**Changes in structure/function**
	Disruption in how patient perceives own body
	Role reversal; dependence
Possibly evidenced by:	**Confusion about sense of self, purpose, direction in life**
	Denial, withdrawal, anger
	Negative/self-destructive behavior
	Using ineffective coping methods
	Change in self/others' perception of role/physical capacity to resume role
PATIENT OUTCOMES/ EVALUATION CRITERIA:	**Verbalizes realistic view and acceptance of body as it is. Views self as a capable person. Participates in and assumes responsibility for meeting own needs. Recognizes and incorporates changes in self-concept/role without negating self-esteem. Developing realistic plans for adapting to role changes.**

ACTIONS/INTERVENTIONS

Independent

Establish/maintain a therapeutic nurse–patient relationship, discussing fears/concerns.

RATIONALE

Conveys an attitude of caring and develops a sense of trust between patient and care giver in which the patient is free to express fears of rejection, loss of previous functioning/appearance, feelings of helplessness, powerlessness about changes that may occur. Promotes a sense of well-being for the patient.

ACTIONS/INTERVENTIONS	RATIONALE
Independent	
Note withdrawn behaviors/use of denial, or overconcern with body/disease process.	Initially may be a normal protective response, but if prolonged may prevent dealing appropriately with reality and may lead to ineffective coping.
Support use of defense mechanisms, allowing patient to deal with information in own time and way.	Confronting patient with reality of situation may result in increased anxiety, lessened ability to cope with changed self-concept/role.
Acknowledge reality of grieving process related to actual/perceived changes. Help patient deal realistically with feelings of anger and sadness.	Nature of the disease leads to ongoing losses and changes in all aspects of life, blocking resolution of grieving process.
Review information about course of disease, possibility of remissions, prognosis.	When patient learns about disease, and becomes aware that own behavior can significantly affect course/remission, the patient may feel more in control, enhancing sense of self-esteem. Note: Some patients may never have a remission.
Provide accurate verbal and written information about what is happening, and discuss with patient/SO.	Helps patient to stay in the here and now, reduces fear of the unknown, provides reference source for future use.
Explain that labile emotions are not unusual. Problem-solve ways to deal with these feelings.	Relieves anxiety and assists with efforts to manage unexpected emotional display.
Note presence of depression/impaired thought processes, expressions of suicidal ideation (evaluate on a scale of 1–10).	Adaptation to a long-term, progressively debilitating disease with a fatal outcome is a difficult emotional adjustment. In addition, brain damage may affect adaptation to these life changes. Individual may believe that suicide is the best way to deal with what is happening.
Assess interaction between patient and SO. Note changes in relationship(s).	SO may unconsciously/consciously reinforce negative attitudes and beliefs of the patient; or issues of secondary gain may interfere with progress and ability to manage situation.
Provide open environment for patient/SO to discuss concerns about sexuality.	Physical and psychologic changes often create stressors within the relationship, affecting usual roles/expectations, further impairing self-concept.

NURSING DIAGNOSIS:	POWERLESSNESS [SPECIFY DEGREE]/HOPELESSNESS
May be related to:	**Illness-related regimen**
	Lifestyle of helplessness
Possibly evidenced by:	**Verbal expressions of having no control or influence over the situation**
	Depression over physical deterioration that occurs despite patient compliance with regimen
	Nonparticipation in care or decision-making when opportunities are provided
	Passivity, decreased verbalization/affect
	Verbal cues (despondent content, "I can't . . . ," sighing)
	Lack of involvement in care/passively allowing care

Identifies and verbalizes feelings. Uses coping mechanisms to counteract feelings of hopelessness. Identifies
areas over which individual has control. Involved in and
controlling own self-care and ADLs within limits of the
individual situation.

ACTIONS/INTERVENTIONS	RATIONALE
Independent	
Note behaviors indicative of powerlessness/hopelessness, e.g., statements of despair, "They don't care," "It won't make any difference."	The degree to which the patient believes own situation is hopeless, that he or she is powerless to change what is happening, affects how patient handles life situation.
Acknowledge reality of situation, at the same time expressing hope for the patient.	While the prognosis may be discouraging, remissions may occur; and because the future cannot be predicted, hope for some quality of life should be encouraged.
Determine degree of mastery patient has exhibited in life to the present. Note locus of control, e.g., internal/external.	The patient who has assumed responsibility in life previously will tend to do the same during difficult times of exacerbation of illness. However, if locus of control has been focused outward, patient may blame others, not take control over own circumstances.
Assist patient to identify factors that are under own control, e.g., list things which can or cannot be controlled.	Knowing and accepting what is beyond individual control can reduce helpless/acting out behaviors, promote focusing on areas individual can control.
Encourage patient to assume control over as much of own care as possible.	Even when unable to do much physical care, individual can help to plan care, having a voice in what is/is not desired.
Discuss needs openly with the patient/SO, setting up agreed-upon routines for meeting identified needs.	Helps to deal with manipulative behavior, when patient feels powerless and not listened to.
Incorporate patient's daily routine into hospital stay as possible.	Maintains sense of control/self-determination and independence.
Discuss plans for the future. Suggest visiting alternate care facilities, taking a look at the possibilities for care as condition changes.	When options are considered and plans are made for any eventuality, patient has a sense of control over own circumstances.

NURSING DIAGNOSIS:	COPING, INEFFECTIVE INDIVIDUAL [POTENTIAL]
May be related to:	Physiologic changes (cerebral and spinal lesions)
	Psychologic conflicts; anxiety; fear
	Impaired judgment, short-term memory loss; confusion; unrealistic perceptions/expectations
	Personal vulnerability; inadequate support systems
	Multiple life changes
	Inadequate coping methods
Possibly evidenced by:	[Not applicable; presence of signs and symptoms establishes an *actual* diagnosis.]

PATIENT OUTCOMES/ EVALUATION CRITERIA:	Recognizes relationship between disease process (cerebral lesions) and emotional responses, changes in thinking/behavior. Verbalizes awareness of own capabilities/strengths. Displays effective problem-solving skills. Demonstrates behaviors/lifestyle changes to prevent/minimize changes in mentation and maintain reality orientation.

ACTIONS/INTERVENTIONS	RATIONALE

Independent

Assess current functional capacity/limitations; note presence of distorted thinking processes, labile emotions, cognitive dissonance and how these affect the individual's coping abilities.

Organic or psychologic effects may cause patient to be easily distracted, display difficulties with concentration, problem-solving, dealing with what is happening, being responsible for own care.

Determine patient's understanding of current situation and previous methods of dealing with life's problems.

Provides a clue to how the patient may deal with what is currently happening and helps identify individual resources and need for assistance.

Maintain an honest, reality-oriented relationship.

Reduces confusion and minimizes painful, frustrating struggles associated with adaptation to altered environment/lifestyle.

Encourage verbalization of feelings/fears, accepting what patient says in a nonjudgmental manner. Note statements reflecting powerlessness, inability to cope. (Refer to ND: Powerlessness/Hopelessness, p. 345.)

May diminish patient's fear, establish trust, and provide an opportunity to identify problems/begin the problem-solving process.

Observe nonverbal communication, e.g., posture, eye contact, movements, gestures, and use of touch. Compare with verbal content and verify meaning with patient as appropriate.

May provide significant information about what the patient is feeling; however, verification is important to ensure accuracy of communication. Discrepancy between feelings and what is being said can interfere with ability to cope, problem-solve.

Provide clues for orientation, e.g., calendars, clocks, notecards, organizers.

These serve as tangible reminders that aid recognition and permeate memory gaps and enable patient to cope with situation.

Encourage patient to tape-record important information and listen to periodically.

Repetition will put information in long-term memory, where it is more easily retrieved and can support decision-making/problem-solving process.

Collaborative

Refer to cognitive retraining program.

Improving cognitive abilities can help patient improve lifestyle by enhancing basic thinking skills when attention span is short, ability to process information is impaired, patient is unable to learn new tasks, or insight, judgment, and problem-solving skills are impaired.

Refer to counseling, psychiatric nurse clinical specialist/psychiatrist as indicated.

May need additional help to resolve issues of self-esteem and regain effective coping skills.

NURSING DIAGNOSIS:	COPING, INEFFECTIVE FAMILY: COMPROMISED/ DISABLING
May be related to:	Temporary family disorganization and role changes Situational crisis

Patient providing little support in turn for SO

Prolonged disease/disability progression that exhausts the supportive capacity of SO

SO with chronically unexpressed feelings of guilt, anxiety, hostility, despair

Highly ambivalent family relationships

Possibly evidenced by: Patient expresses/confirms concern or complaint about SO response to patient's illness

SO withdraws or has limited personal communication with patient or displays protective behavior disproportionate to patient's abilities or need for autonomy

SO preoccupied with own personal reactions

Intolerance, abandonment

Neglectful care of the patient

Distortion of reality regarding patient's illness

FAMILY OUTCOMES/ EVALUATION CRITERIA: Identifies/verbalizes resources within themselves to deal with the situation. Expresses more realistic understanding and expectations of the patient. Interacts appropriately with the patient/staff, providing support and assistance as indicated. Verbalizes knowledge and understanding of disability/disease.

ACTIONS/INTERVENTIONS	RATIONALE
Independent	
Note length/severity of illness. Determine patient's role in family and how illness has changed the family organization.	Chronic/unresolved illness, accompanied by changes in role performance/responsibility, often exhausts supportive capacity and coping abilities of SO.
Evaluate SO's understanding of disease process and expectations for the future.	Inadequate information/misconception regarding disease process, and/or unrealistic expectations affect ability to cope with current situation.
Assess other factors that are affecting abilities of family members to provide needed support, e.g., own emotional problems, work concerns.	Individual members, preoccupation with own needs/ concerns can interfere with providing needed care/ support for stresses of long-term illness.
Discuss underlying reasons for patient's behaviors.	Helps SO understand and accept/deal with behaviors that may be triggered by emotional or physical effects of MS.
Encourage patient/SO to develop and strengthen problem-solving skills to deal with situation.	Family may/may not have handled conflict well before illness and stress of long-term debilitating condition can create additional problems (including unresolved anger).
Encourage free expression of feelings, including frustration, anger, hostility, and hopelessness.	Individual members may be afraid to express "negative" feelings, believing it will discourage the patient. Free expression promotes awareness and can help with resolution of feelings and problems (especially when done in a caring manner). (Refer to CP: Psychosocial Aspects of Acute Care, p. 773.)

NURSING DIAGNOSIS:	URINARY ELIMINATION, ALTERED PATTERNS
May be related to:	Neuromuscular impairment (spinal cord lesions/neurogenic bladder)
Possibly evidenced by:	Incontinence; nocturia Retention with overflow
PATIENT OUTCOMES/ EVALUATION CRITERIA:	Verbalizes understanding of condition. Demonstrates behaviors/techniques to prevent/minimize infection.

ACTIONS/INTERVENTIONS

Independent

Note frequency, urgency, burning, incontinence, nocturia, size of/force of urinary stream. Palpate bladder after voiding.

Institute bladder training program.

Encourage adequate fluid intake, limiting intake during late evening and at bedtime. Recommend use of cranberry juice/vitamin C.

Promote continued mobility.

Recommend good handwashing/perineal care.

Encourage patient to observe for sediment/blood in urine, foul odor, fever.

Collaborative

Catheterize as indicated.

Teach self-catheterization.

Obtain urine culture and sensitivity as indicated.

Administer medications as necessary, e.g., antimicrobial agent, nitrofurantoin macrocrystals (Macrodantin).

RATIONALE

Provides information about degree of interference with elimination or may indicate bladder infection. Fullness over bladder following void is indicative of inadequate emptying and requires intervention.

Helps to restore adequate bladder functioning, lessens occurrence of bladder infection.

Sufficient hydration promotes urinary output and aids in preventing infection. Note: When patient is taking sulfa drugs, sufficient fluids are necessary to ensure adequate excretion of drug, reducing risk of cumulative effects.

Decreases risk of developing bladder and urinary tract infection.

Reduces skin irritation and risk of ascending infection.

Indicative of infection requiring further evaluation/treatment.

May be necessary if patient is unable to empty the bladder or retains residual urine.

Helps patient to maintain autonomy and encourages self-care.

Colony count over 100,000 indicates presence of infection requiring treatment.

Bacteriostatic agent that inhibits bacterial growth. Prompt treatment of infection is necessary to prevent serious complications of sepsis/shock.

NURSING DIAGNOSIS:	KNOWLEDGE DEFICIT [LEARNING NEED] (SPECIFY)
May be related to:	Lack of exposure; information misinterpretation Unfamiliarity with information resources Cognitive limitation, lack of recall

Possibly evidenced by:	Statement of misconception
	Request for information
	Inaccurate follow-through of instruction
	Inappropriate or exaggerated behaviors (e.g., hysterical, hostile, agitated, apathetic)
PATIENT OUTCOMES/ EVALUATION CRITERIA:	Participates in learning process. Assumes responsibility for own learning and begins to look for information and to ask questions. Verbalizes understanding of condition/disease process and treatment. Initiates necessary lifestyle changes and participates in treatment regimen.

ACTIONS/INTERVENTIONS	RATIONALE
Independent	
Evaluate desire/readiness to learn.	Determines amount/level of information to provide patient at any given moment.
Note signs of emotional lability or that patient is in dissociative state (loss of affect, inappropriate emotional responses).	Patient will not process/retain information and will have difficulty learning during this time.
Review disease process/prognosis.	Clarifies patient/SO understanding of individual situation.
Discuss importance of daily routine of rest, exercise, activity, eating, focusing on current capabilities. Instruct in use of appropriate devices to assist with ADLs, e.g., eating utensils, walking aids.	Helps patient to maintain current level of physical independence.
Discuss necessity of weight control.	Excess weight can interfere with balance and motor abilities and make care more difficult.
Stress need for stopping exercise/activity just short of fatigue.	Pushing self beyond physical limits can result in excessive fatigue and discouragement. Patient can become very adept at knowing where this limit is.
Review possible problems that may arise such as decreased perception of heat and pain, susceptibility to skin breakdown; infections, especially UTI.	These effects of demyelination and complications may compromise patient's safety and/or precipitate an exacerbation of symptoms.
Identify actions that can be taken to avoid injury: e.g., avoid hot baths, inspect skin regularly, take care with transfers, wheelchair/walker mobility, forcing fluids, and getting adequate nutrition.	Review of these factors can help patient take measures to maintain physical state at optimal level.
Discuss/encourage options for enhancing/developing remaining skills, using diversional activities, continuing with usual concerns as able.	Enables patient to maintain "active" quality of life.
Encourage patient to set goals for the future while focusing on the here-and-now, what can be done today.	Having a plan for the future helps to retain hope as well as provide opportunity for patient to see that although today is to be lived, one can plan for tomorrow even in the worst of circumstances.
Collaborative	
Refer for vocational rehabilitation.	May need assessment of capabilities/job retraining as indicated by individual limitations/disease progression.

CHAPTER 7

OPHTHALMOLOGY

Ocular Disorders: Cataracts (Postoperative), Glaucoma

PATIENT ASSESSMENT DATA BASE

ACTIVITY/REST

May report: Change in usual activities/hobbies due to altered vision.

FOOD/FLUID

May report: Nausea/vomiting (acute glaucoma).

NEUROSENSORY

May report: Visual distortions (blurred/hazy), bright light causing a glare with a gradual loss of peripheral vision, difficulty focusing on close work/adjusting to darkened room (cataracts).

Cloudy/blurred vision, appearance of halos/rainbows around lights, loss of peripheral vision (glaucoma).

Glasses/treatment change does not improve vision.

May exhibit: Pupil appears gray or milky white (cataract). Fixed pupil and red/hard eye with cloudy cornea (glaucoma emergency). Increased tearing.

PAIN/COMFORT

May report: Mild discomfort/tired eyes (chronic glaucoma).

Sudden/persistent severe pain in and around eyes, headache (acute glaucoma).

SAFETY

May report: History of hemorrhage, trauma, ocular disease, tumor (glaucoma).

Difficulty seeing, managing ADLs.

TEACHING/LEARNING

May report: Family history of glaucoma, diabetes, systemic vascular disorders.

History of stress, allergy, vasomotor disturbances, endocrine imbalance, diabetes (glaucoma).

Exposure to radiation; steroid/phenothiazine toxicity.

Discharge Plan Considerations: May require assistance with transportation, meal preparation, self-care/homemaker tasks.

DIAGNOSTIC STUDIES

Snellen eye chart/telebinocular machine: tests visual acuity and central vision; may be impaired by defects in cornea, lens, aqueous or vitreous humor, refractive error, or disease of the nervous system supplying the retina or optic pathway.

Visual fields: reduction may be caused by cerebrovascular accident (CVA), pituitary/brain tumor mass, carotid or cerebral artery pathology.

Tonography measurement: assesses intraocular pressure (IOP) (normal: 12–25 mmHg).

Gonioscopy measurement: helps differentiate open angle from angle-closure glaucoma.

Ophthalmoscopy examination: assess internal ocular structures, noting optic disk atrophy, papilledema, retinal hemorrhage, and microaneurysms: Dilation and slit-lamp examination confirms diagnosis of cataract.

CBC, sedimentation rate (ESR): rule out systemic anemia/infection.

ECG, serum cholesterol and lipid studies: rule out atherosclerosis, coronary artery disease.

Glucose tolerance test/FBS: determine presence/control of diabetes.

NURSING PRIORITIES

1. Prevent further visual deterioration.
2. Promote adaptation to changes in/reduced visual acuity.
3. Prevent complications.
4. Provide information about disease process/prognosis and treatment needs.

DISCHARGE CRITERIA

1. Vision maintained at highest possible level.
2. Patient coping with situation in a positive manner.
3. Complications prevented/minimized.
4. Disease process/prognosis and therapeutic regimen understood.

DEGENERATIVE CATARACT (POSTOPERATIVE CARE)

An opacity of the lens that develops in about half of all people over 65.

NURSING DIAGNOSIS:	INJURY, POTENTIAL FOR
May be related to:	Increased intraocular pressure
	Intraocular hemorrhage, vitreous loss
Possibly evidenced by:	[Not applicable; presence of signs and symptoms establishes an *actual* diagnosis.]
PATIENT OUTCOMES/ EVALUATION CRITERIA:	Verbalizes understanding of factors that contribute to possibility of injury. Demonstrates behaviors, lifestyle changes to reduce risk factors and to protect self from injury. Modifies environment as indicated to enhance safety.

ACTIONS/INTERVENTIONS	RATIONALE
Independent	
Discuss postoperative expectations concerning pain, activity restrictions, appearance, eye bandaging.	Can be helpful in allaying fears and enhancing cooperation with necessary restrictions.
Transfer from stretcher to bed in horizontal position. Patient may assist while nurse supports head.	Neutral position avoids pressure/strain on new suture line.
Place patient on chair/bedrest, in quiet environment, and elevate head of bed. Limit activities such as sudden movement of the head, rubbing eyes.	Rest may be required for only a few minutes to an hour with outpatient surgery or may be required overnight when complications are present. Reduces stress on operative area/decreases IOP.
Position patient on back, turn on side not operated upon (initially).	Reduces pressure in affected eye, minimizing risk of hemorrhage or suture stress/dehiscence.
Ambulate with assistance; provide regular bathroom facilities if required.	Requires less strain than use of bedpan, which could increase IOP.
Encourage deep breathing, instead of coughing for pulmonary hygiene.	Coughing increases IOP.
Recommend use of stress management techniques, e.g., guided imagery, visualization, deep breathing, and relaxation exercises.	Promotes relaxation, reduces IOP, and may enhance coping.
Maintain protective eye patch as indicated.	Used during sleep to protect from accidental injury and to reduce eye movement.
Evaluate eye at each dressing change and when eyedrops are instilled.	Early recognition of developing complications enhances opportunity for prompt medical evaluation and intervention.
Avoid putting pressure on eye during examination.	External pressure can raise IOP enough to rupture sutures.
Observe for bulging of wound, flat anterior chamber, pear-shaped pupil.	Denotes prolapse of iris or wound rupture caused by loosened sutures or pressure on the eye.
Have patient differentiate between discomfort and sudden sharp eye pain. Investigate restlessness, disorientation, disturbance of dressing. Observe for hyphema (bleeding in the eye) by inspecting the eye with a flashlight as indicated.	Discomfort is to be expected from the surgical procedure; however, acute pain suggests developing IOP and/or hemorrhage, which may occur due to strain or for no apparent reason (healing tissue is highly vascular, and capillaries are fragile).
Collaborative	
Administer medication as indicated:	
Antiemetics, e.g., prochlorperazine (Compazine);	Nausea/vomiting can increase IOP, necessitating prompt treatment to prevent ocular injury.
Acetazolamide (Diamox);	May be given to decrease IOP if elevation occurs, restricts enzymatic action in production of aqueous humor.
Cycloplegics;	May be given to paralyze ciliary muscle to dilate and rest iris after surgery if IOL is not implanted.
Analgesics, e.g., Empirin with codeine, acetaminophen (Tylenol).	May be used for mild discomfort to promote rest/prevent restlessness, which may affect IOP. Note: Use of aspirin is contraindicated because of increased bleeding tendencies.

NURSING DIAGNOSIS:	INFECTION, POTENTIAL FOR
May be related to:	Invasive procedure (surgical cataract removal)
Possibly evidenced by:	[Not applicable; presence of signs and symptoms establishes an *actual* diagnosis.]
PATIENT OUTCOMES/ EVALUATION CRITERIA:	Achieves timely wound healing, free of purulent drainage, erythema, and fever. Identifies interventions to prevent/reduce risk of infection.

ACTIONS/INTERVENTIONS	RATIONALE
Independent	
Discuss with patient/staff importance of handwashing before touching/treating eye.	Diminishes number of bacteria on hands, preventing contamination of operative area.
Use/demonstrate proper technique for cleaning eye from inner to outer corner with fresh tissue/cotton ball for each wipe, changing dressings and inserting contact lens if used.	Aseptic technique reduces risk of spread of bacteria and cross-contamination.
Stress importance of not touching/rubbing operated eye.	Prevents contamination and disruption of operative site.
Observe for/discuss signs of developing infection, e.g., redness, lid swelling, purulent drainage. Identify precautions to take if upper respiratory infection occurs.	Eye infection is most likely to develop 2–3 days after procedure and requires prompt intervention. Presence of URI increases risk of cross-contamination.
Collaborative	
Administer medications as indicated:	
Antibiotics (topical, parenteral or subconjunctival);	Topical preparations may be used prophylactically while more aggressive therapy is required if infection develops. Note: Steroids may be added to topical antibiotic when patient has intraocular lens implant.
Steroids.	May be used to decrease inflammation.

NURSING DIAGNOSIS:	SENSORY-PERCEPTUAL ALTERATION: VISUAL
May be related to:	Altered sensory reception/status of sense organs
	Therapeutically restricted environment
Possibly evidenced by:	Diminished acuity, visual distortions
	Change in usual response to stimuli
PATIENT OUTCOMES/ EVALUATION CRITERIA:	Regains visual acuity within limitations of individual situation. Recognizes sensory impairments and compensates for changes. Identifies/corrects potential hazards in the environment.

ACTIONS/INTERVENTIONS	RATIONALE
Independent	
Determine visual acuity, note whether one or both eyes are involved.	Individual needs and choice of interventions will vary because loss of vision is a slow, progressive process. If bilateral, each eye can progress at a different rate, but usually only one eye is corrected per procedure.
Orient patient to surroundings, staff, others in the area.	Provides for increased comfort level and familiarity, reducing anxiety and postoperative disorientation.
Observe for signs of disorientation; keep side rails up and bed in low position when indicated.	Unfamiliar place, visual limitations may result in confusion in the elderly person. Decreases risk of falling when patient is confused/unfamiliar with size of bed.
Approach from unoperated side, speak and touch often; encourage SO to stay with patient as much as possible.	Provides appropriate sensory stimulation to offset isolation and reduce confusion.
Caution about dim or blurred vision, irritation of eye, which may occur when using eye drops.	Visual disturbance/irritation may last for 1–2 hours after instillation of eyedrops but gradually decreases with use. Note: Local irritation should be reported to physician, but do not stop use of drug in interim.
Encourage diversional activities such as radio, conversation, television viewing in moderation.	Provides sensory input, maintains sense of normality, passes time more easily when unable to use vision sense fully. Note: Moderate watching of television requires less eye movement and is less stressful than reading.
Remind patient using cataract glasses that objects are magnified approximately 25%, peripheral vision is lost, and blind spots may be noted.	Changes in acuity and depth perception can cause visual confusion/increase risk of injury until patient learns to compensate.
Place needed items/position call bell within easy reach on side not operated on and orient patient to its position.	Allows patient to see objects more easily and facilitates calling for help when needed.
Position doors so they are completely opened or closed. Position furniture out of the travel pathways.	Decreased peripheral vision or altered depth perception may cause patient to walk into partially opened door, trip over footstools, and so forth.
Assist patient with locating food on plate. Encourage patient to check temperature of food with fingers. Describe food when patient cannot see; feed slowly with small bites.	Enhances taste perceptions/food intake, decreases chance of injury, e.g., burns, choking/vomiting.

NURSING DIAGNOSIS:	**KNOWLEDGE DEFICIT [LEARNING NEED] (SPECIFY)**
May be related to:	**Unfamiliarity with information resources, information misinterpretation**
	Lack of exposure/recall
	Cognitive limitation
Possibly evidenced by:	**Questions/statement of misconception**
	Inaccurate follow-through of instruction
	Development of preventable complications
PATIENT OUTCOMES/ EVALUATION CRITERIA:	**Verbalizes understanding of condition/disease process and treatment. Correctly performs necessary procedures and explains reasons for the actions.**

ACTIONS/INTERVENTIONS	RATIONALE
Independent	
Review information about individual condition, prognosis, type of procedure/lens.	Enhances understanding and promotes cooperation with postoperative regimen.
Stress importance of routine follow-up care. Report clouding of vision.	Periodic monitoring reduces risk of serious complications. In some patients the posterior capsule may thicken or become hazy within 2 weeks to several years postoperatively, requiring laser therapy to correct visual deficit.
Inform patient to avoid OTC eyedrops.	May counteract/interact with prescribed medications.
Discuss possible effects/interactions between eye medications and patient's medical problems, e.g., increase in hypertension, COPD, diabetes. Instruct in proper method of instilling eyedrops to minimize systemic effects.	Use of topical eye medications, e.g., sympathomimetic agents, beta-blockers, anticholinergic agents can cause BP to rise in hypertensive patients; precipitate dyspnea in patients with COPD; mask the symptoms of a hypoglycemic crisis in insulin-dependent diabetics. Correct application can limit absorption into systemic circulation, minimizing problems such as drug interactions and unwanted/untoward systemic effects.
Instruct patient to avoid reading, squinting; heavy lifting, straining at stool, excessive bending at the waist, blowing nose; use of sprays, dusting powder, smoking (self/others).	Activities that cause eye fatigue/strain, Valsalva maneuver, or IOP may compromise surgical results, precipitate hemorrhage. Note: Respiratory irritants that cause coughing/sneezing can increase IOP.
Recommend patient check with doctor about resumption/modifications of sexual activities.	May increase IOP, cause accidental injury to eye.
Stress need for wearing protective glasses during day/patching operative eye at night.	Prevents accidental injury to eye and reduces risk of increased IOP due to squinting or position of head.
Suggest patient sleep on back, regulate the intensity of light and wear dark glasses when outside/in bright lighting, shampoo with head slightly tilted back (not forward), cough with mouth/eyes open.	Prevents accidental injury to eye.
Encourage adequate intake of fluids, bulk/roughage; use of OTC stool softeners, if indicated.	Maintains consistency of stool to avoid straining at stool.
Recommend keeping extra bottle of eyedrops on hand.	Prevents inadvertent discontinuation of medication in the event of loss, and so forth.
Identify signs/symptoms requiring prompt medical evaluation, e.g., sharp sudden pain, decreased vision, lid swelling, purulent discharge, redness, watering of eyes, photophobia.	Early intervention can prevent development of serious complications, possible loss of vision.

GLAUCOMA

NURSING DIAGNOSIS:	**SENSORY-PERCEPTUAL ALTERATION: VISUAL**
May be related to:	**Altered sensory reception: altered status of sense organ**
Possibly evidenced by:	**Progressive loss of visual field**
PATIENT OUTCOMES/ EVALUATION CRITERIA:	**Maintains current visual field/acuity without further loss.**

ACTIONS/INTERVENTIONS	RATIONALE

Independent

Ascertain degree/type of visual loss.

Affects patient's future expectations and choice of interventions.

Encourage expression of feelings about loss/possibility of loss of vision.

While early intervention may prevent blindness, the patient faces the possibility or may have already experienced partial or complete loss of vision. Although vision loss that has already occurred cannot be restored (even with treatment), further loss can be prevented.

Demonstrate administration of eyedrops, e.g., counting drops, adhering to schedule, not missing doses.

Controls IOP, preventing further loss of vision.

Implement measures to assist patient to manage visual limitations, e.g., reduce clutter, arrange furniture out of travel path; remind to turn head to view subjects; correct for dim light, problems of night vision.

Reduces safety hazards related to changes in visual fields/loss of vision, and papillary accommodation to environmental light.

Collaborative

Administer medications as indicated:

Chronic, simple, open-angle type

Pilocarpine hydrochloride (IsoptoCarpine, Ocusert Pilo, Pilopine HS Gel);

These topical myotic drugs cause pupillary constriction, facilitating the outflow of aqueous humor.

Timolol maleate (Timoptic).

Decreases formation of aqueous humor without changing pupil size, vision or accommodation.

Acetazolamide (Diamox);

Decrease the rate of production of aqueous humor.

Narrow angle (angle closure)

Myotics (until pupil is constricted);

Creates contraction of sphincter muscles of the iris, deepens anterior chamber, and dilates vessels of outflow tract during acute attack/prior to surgery.

Carbonic anhydrase inhibitors, e.g., acetazolamide (Diamox); hyperosmotic agents, e.g., mannitol (Osmitrol), glycerine.

Decreases secretion of aqueous humor and lowers IOP. Used to decrease general fluid level which will decrease production of aqueous humor if other treatments have not been successful.

Provide sedation, analgesics as necessary.

Acute glaucoma attack is associated with sudden pain, which can precipitate anxiety/agitation, further elevating IOP. Note: Medical management may require 4–6 hours before IOP decreases and pain subsides.

Prepare for surgical intervention as indicated:

Iridectomy:

Surgical removal of a portion of the iris to facilitate drainage of aqueous humor. Upper iris usually is covered with upper eyelid, and flow of tears washes bacteria downward. Note: Bilateral iridectomy is performed because glaucoma usually develops in the other eye.

Trabeculectomy/trephination;

Filtering operations that create an opening between the anterior chamber and the subjunctival spaces so that aqueous humor can bypass the trabecular mesh block.

Malteno valve implantation;

Experimental device used to correct or prevent scarring over/closure of drainage sac created by trabeculectomy.

ACTIONS/INTERVENTIONS

Collaborative

Cyclodialysis;

Aqueous-venous shunt;

Diathermy/cryosurgery.

RATIONALE

Separates ciliary body from the sclera to facilitate out-flow of aqueous humor.

Used in intractable glaucoma.

If other treatments fail, destruction of the ciliary body will reduce formation of aqueous humor.

NURSING DIAGNOSIS:	ANXIETY [SPECIFY LEVEL]
May be related to:	**Physiologic factors, change in health status: presence of pain; possibility/reality of loss of vision**
	Unmet needs
	Negative self-talk
Possibly evidenced by:	**Apprehension, uncertainty**
	Expressed concern regarding changes in life events
PATIENT OUTCOMES/ EVALUATION CRITERIA:	**Appears relaxed and reports anxiety is reduced to a manageable level. Demonstrates problem-solving skills. Uses resources effectively.**

ACTIONS/INTERVENTIONS

Independent

Assess anxiety level, degree of pain experienced/suddenness of onset of symptoms, and current knowledge of condition.

Provide accurate, honest information.

Encourage patient to acknowledge concerns and express feelings.

Identify helpful resources/people.

RATIONALE

These factors affect patient perception of threat to self, potentiate the cycle of anxiety, and may interfere with medical attempts to control IOP.

Reduces anxiety related to unknown/future expectations and provides factual basis for making informed choices about treatment.

Provides opportunity for patient to deal with reality of situation, clarify misconception, and problem-solve concerns.

Provides reassurance that patient is not alone in dealing with problem.

NURSING DIAGNOSIS:	KNOWLEDGE DEFICIT [LEARNING NEED] (SPECIFY)
May be related to:	**Lack of exposure/unfamiliarity with resources**
	Lack of recall, information misinterpretation
Possibly evidenced by:	**Questions; statement of misconception**
	Inaccurate follow-through of instruction
	Development of preventable complications

PATIENT OUTCOMES/ EVALUATION CRITERIA:	Verbalizes understanding of condition/prognosis and treatment. Identifies relationship of signs/symptoms to the disease process. Correctly performs necessary procedures and explains reasons for the actions.

ACTIONS/INTERVENTIONS	RATIONALE

Independent

ACTIONS/INTERVENTIONS	RATIONALE
Discuss importance of wearing identification, e.g., Medi-Alert bracelet.	Vital to provide information for care givers in case of emergency to reduce risk of receiving contraindicated drugs (e.g., atropine).
Discuss importance of maintaining drug schedule, e.g., eye drops. Discuss medications that should be avoided, e.g., mydriatic drops (atropine/propantheline bromine), overuse of topical steroids.	This disease can be controlled, not cured, and maintaining consistent medication regimen is vital to control. Some drugs cause pupil dilation, increasing IOP and potentiating additional loss of vision.
Review potential side effects of treatment, e.g., nausea/vomiting, fatigue, "drugged" feeling, decreased libido, impotence, cardiac irregularities, syncope, congestive failure.	Drug side effects range from uncomfortable to severe/health-threatening. Approximately 50% of patients will develop sensitivity/alergy to parasympathomimetics (e.g., pilocarpine) or anticholinesterase drugs. These problems require medical evaluation and possible change in therapeutic regimen.
Encourage patient to make necessary changes in lifestyle.	A tranquil lifestyle decreases the emotional response to stress preventing ocular changes that push the iris forward which may precipitate an acute attack.
Reinforce avoidance of activities, such as heavy lifting/pushing, snow shoveling, wearing tight/constricting clothing.	May increase IOP, precipitating acute attack. Note: If patient is not experiencing pain, cooperation with drug regimen and acceptance of lifestyle changes are often difficult to sustain.
Discuss dietary considerations, e.g., adequate fluid, bulk/fiber intake.	Measures to maintain consistency of stool to avoid constipation/straining during defecation.
Stress importance of periodic checkups.	Important to monitor progression/maintenance of disease to allow for early intervention and prevent further loss of vision.
Advise patient to immediately report severe eye pain, inflammation, increased photophobia, increased lacrimation, changes in visual field/veillike curtain, blurred vision, flashes of light/particles floating in visual field.	Prompt action may be necessary to prevent further vision loss/other complications, e.g., detached retina.

CHAPTER 8

GASTROENTEROLOGY

Eating Disorders: Anorexia Nervosa/ Bulimia Nervosa _____

Anorexia nervosa is an illness of starvation, brought on by severe disturbance of body image and a morbid fear of obesity.

Bulimia nervosa is an eating disorder (binge–purge syndrome) characterized by extreme overeating, followed by self-induced vomiting and may include abuse of laxatives and diuretics.

PATIENT ASSESSMENT DATA BASE

ACTIVITY/REST

May report: Disturbed sleep patterns, e.g., early morning insomnia; fatigue.
Feeling "hyper" and/or anxious.
Increased activity/participation in high-energy sports.

May exhibit: Periods of hyperactivity, constant vigorous exercising.

CIRCULATION

May report: Feeling cold even when room is warm.

May exhibit: Low blood pressure.
Tachycardia.
Bradycardia.

EGO INTEGRITY

May report: Powerlessness/helplessness.
Distorted (unrealistic) body image—reports self as fat regardless of weight and sees thin body as fat; persistent overconcern with body shape and weight—fears gaining weight.
High self-expectations.
Holding back anger.

May exhibit: Emotional states of depression, anger, anxiety.

ELIMINATION

May report:
Diarrhea/constipation.
Vague abdominal pain and distress, bloating.
Laxative/diuretic use.

FOOD/FLUID

May report:
Constant hunger (may deny hunger), normal or exaggerated appetite (rarely vanishes until late in the disorder).
Preoccupation with food, e.g., calorie counting, gourmet cooking.
An unrealistic pleasure in weight loss, while denying self pleasure in other areas.
Recurrent episodes of binge eating, a feeling of lack of control over behavior during eating binges. A minimum average of two binge eating episodes a week for at least 3 months.
Regularly engaging in either self-induced vomiting or strict dieting or fasting.
Intense fear of gaining weight; may have prior history of being overweight.
Refusal to maintain body weight over minimal norm for age/height.

May exhibit:
Weight loss/maintenance of body weight 15% or more below that expected, or weight may be normal or slightly below (bulimia).
No medical illness evident to account for weight loss.
Cachectic appearance; skin may be dry, yellowish/pale, with poor turgor.
Hiding food, cutting food into small pieces, rearranging food on plate.
Irrational thinking about eating, food, and weight.
Binge–purge syndrome (bulimia) independently or as a complication of anorexia.
Peripheral edema.
Swollen salivary glands, sore inflamed buccal cavity, continuous sore throat.
Vomiting, bloody vomitus (may indicate esophageal tearing, Mallory–Weiss).

HYGIENE

May exhibit:
Increased hair growth on body (lanugo); hair loss (axillary/pubic).
Brittle nails.
Teeth show signs of erosion, gums in poor condition.

NEUROSENSORY

May exhibit:
Mental changes (apathy, confusion, memory impairment) brought on by malnutrition/starvation.
Depressive affect; may be depressed.
Appropriate affect, except in regard to body and eating.
High academic achievement.
Hysterical or obsessive personality style; no other psychiatric illness or evidence of a psychiatric thought disorder (although a significant number may show evidence of an affective disorder).

PAIN/COMFORT

May report:
Headaches.

SAFETY

May exhibit:
Decreased body temperature.
Recurrent infectious processes (indicative of depressed immune system).
Eczema.

SOCIAL INTERACTION

May report: Altered relationships or problems with relationships (not married, divorced), sexual abuse, promiscuity.

Middle-class or upper-class family background.

Passive father/dominant mother, family members closely fused, togetherness prized, personal boundaries not respected.

History of being a quiet, cooperative child.

Evidence of an emotional crisis of some sort, such as the onset of puberty or a family move.

Withdrawal from friends/social contacts.

Sense of helplessness.

SEXUALITY

May report: Absence of at least three consecutive menstrual cycles.

Denial/loss of sexual interest.

May exhibit: Breast atrophy, amenorrhea.

TEACHING/LEARNING

May report: Family history of higher than normal incidence of depression.

Onset of the illness usually between the ages of 10 and 18.

Health beliefs/practice, e.g., certain foods have "too many" calories, use of "health" foods.

Discharge Plan Considerations: Assistance with maintenance of treatment plan.

DIAGNOSTIC STUDIES

CBC with differential: to determine presence of anemia, leukopenia, lymphocytosis.

Electrolytes: imbalances may include decreased potassium, sodium, and chloride.

Endocrine studies:

Thyroid function: thyroxine (T_4) levels usually normal; however, circulating triiodothyronine (T_3) levels may be low.

Pituitary function: Thyroid stimulating hormone (TSH) response to thyrotropin-releasing factor (TRF) is abnormal in anorexia nervosa. Propranolol–glucagon stimulation test (studies the response of human growth hormone): depressed level of GH in anorexia nervosa. Gonadotropic hypofunction is noted.

Cortisol metabolism: may be elevated.

Dexamethasone suppression test (DST): evaluates hypothalamic–pituitary function; dexamethasone resistance indicates cortisol suppression, suggesting malnutrition and/or depression.

Luteinizing hormone secretions test: pattern often resembles those of prepubertal girls.

Estrogen: decreased.

Blood sugar and basal metabolism (BMR): may be low.

Other chemistries: SGOT elevated. Hypercarotenemia, hypoproteinemia, hypocholesterolemia. Blood platelets show significantly less than normal activity by the enzyme monoamine oxidase, which is thought to be a marker for depression.

MHP 6 levels: decreased, suggestive of malnutrition/depression.

Urinalysis and renal function: BUN may be elevated; ketones present reflecting starvation; decreased urinary 17-ketosteroids.

ECG: abnormal with low voltage, T-wave inversion.

NURSING PRIORITIES

1. Reestablish adequate/appropriate nutritional intake.
2. Correct fluid and electrolyte imbalance.
3. Assist patient to develop realistic body image/improve self-esteem.
4. Provide support/involve SO, if available, in treatment program.
5. Coordinate total treatment program with other disciplines.
6. Provide information about disease, prognosis, and treatment to patient/SO.

DISCHARGE CRITERIA

1. Adequate nutrition and fluid intake maintained.
2. Maladaptive coping behaviors and stressors that precipitate anxiety recognized.
3. Adaptive coping strategies and techniques for anxiety reduction and self-control implemented.
4. Self-esteem increased.
5. At least 90% of expected body weight achieved and maintained.
6. Disease process, prognosis, and treatment regimen understood.

NURSING DIAGNOSIS:	NUTRITION, ALTERED: LESS THAN BODY REQUIREMENTS
May be related to:	**Inadequate food intake; self-induced vomiting**
	Laxative use
Possibly evidenced by:	**Body weight 15% (or more) below expected or may be within normal range (bulimia)**
	Pale conjunctiva and mucous membranes; poor skin turgor/muscle tone
	Excessive loss of hair; increased growth of hair on body (lanugo)
	Amenorrhea
	Electrolyte imbalances
	Hypothermia
	Bradycardia; cardiac irregularities; hypotension
	Edema
PATIENT OUTCOMES/ EVALUATION CRITERIA:	**Verbalizes understanding of nutritional needs. Establishes a dietary pattern with caloric intake adequate to regain/maintain appropriate weight. Demonstrates weight gain toward individually expected range.**

ACTIONS/INTERVENTIONS	RATIONALE
Independent	
Establish a minimum weight goal, and daily nutritional requirements.	Malnutrition is a mood-altering condition leading to depression and agitation and affecting cognitive function/decision-making. Improved nutritional status enhances thinking ability, and psychologic work can begin.

363

ACTIONS/INTERVENTIONS	RATIONALE

Independent

Use a consistent approach. Sit with patient while eating; present and remove food without persuasion and/or comment. Promote pleasant environment and record intake.

Patient detects urgency and reacts to pressure. Any comment that might be seen as coercion provides focus on food. When staff responds in a consistent manner, patient can begin to trust their responses. The one area in which the patient has exercised power and control is food/eating and may experience guilt if forced to eat. Structuring meals and decreasing discussions about food will decrease power struggles with patient and avoid manipulative games.

Maintain a regular weighing schedule, such as Monday, Wednesday, Friday before breakfast in same attire, and graph results.

Provides accurate ongoing record of weight loss and/or gain. Also diminishes obsessing about gains and/or losses.

Weigh with back to scale (dependent on program protocols).

Forces issue of trust in patient who usually does not trust others.

Make selective menu available, and allow patient to control choices as much as possible.

Patient needs to gain confidence in self and feel in control of environment and is more likely to eat preferred foods.

Be alert to choices of low-calorie foods/beverages; hoarding food; disposing of food in various places such as pockets or wastebaskets.

Patient will try to avoid taking in what is viewed as excessive calories and may go to great lengths to avoid eating.

Provide one-to-one supervision, and have the patient remain in the room with no bathroom privileges for a specified period (e.g., ½ hour) following eating.

Prevents vomiting during/after eating. Patient may desire food and use a binge–purge syndrome to maintain weight. Note: Purging may occur for the first time in a patient as a response to establishment of a weight-gain program.

Avoid room checks and other control devices.

Reinforces feelings of powerlessness and are usually not helpful.

Monitor exercise program and set limits on physical activities. Chart activity/level of work (pacing, etc.).

Moderate exercise helps in maintaining muscle tone/weight and combatting depression. However, patient may exercise excessively to burn calories.

Maintain matter-of-fact, nonjudgmental attitude if giving tube feedings, hyperalimentation, etc.

Perception of punishment is counterproductive to patient's self-confidence and faith in own ability to control destiny.

Be alert to possibility of patient disconnecting tube and emptying hyperalimentation if used. Check measurements, and tape tubing snugly.

Sabotage behavior is common in attempt to prevent weight gain.

Collaborative

Administer nutritional therapy within a hospital treatment program as indicated.

Cure of the underlying problem cannot happen without improved nutritional status. Hospitalization provides a controlled environment in which food intake, vomiting/elimination, medications, and activities can be monitored. It also separates the patient from SO (who may be contributing factor) and provides exposure to others with the same problem, creating an atmosphere for sharing.

Involve patient in setting up/carrying out program of behavior modification. Provide reward for weight gain as individually determined; ignore loss.

Provides structured eating situation while allowing patient some control in choices. Behavior modification may be effective in mild cases or for short-term weight gain.

Provide diet and snacks with substitutions of preferred foods when available.

Having a variety of foods available will enable the patient to have a choice of potentially enjoyable foods.

ACTIONS/INTERVENTIONS	RATIONALE
Collaborative	
Administer liquid diet and/or tube feedings/hyperalimentation if needed.	When caloric intake is insufficient to sustain metabolic needs, nutritional support can be used to prevent malnutrition/death while therapy is continuing. High-calorie liquid feedings may be given as medication, at preset times separate from meals, as an alternative means of increasing caloric intake.
Blenderize and tube feed anything left on the tray after a given period of time if indicated.	May be used as part of behavior modification program to provide total intake of needed calories.
Avoid giving laxatives.	Use is counterproductive because they may be used by patient to rid body of food/calories.
Administer medications as indicated:	
Cyropheptadine (Periactin);	A serotonin and histamine antagonist that may be used in high doses to stimulate the appetite, decrease preoccupation with food, and combat depression. Does not appear to have serious side effects, although decreased mental alertness may occur.
Tricyclic antidepressants, e.g., amitriptyline (Elavil, Endep);	Lifts depression and stimulates appetite.
Antianxiety agents, e.g., alprazolam (Xanax);	Reduces tension, anxiety/nervousness and may help patient to participate with treatment.
Major tranquilizers, e.g., chlorpromazine (Thorazine).	Promotes weight gain and cooperation with psychotherapeutic program. Major tranquilizers are used only when absolutely necessary, because of extrapyramidal side effects.
Prepare for/assist with electroconvulsive therapy (ECT). Help patient understand this is not punishment.	In difficult cases where malnutrition is severe and may be life-threatening, a short-term ECT series may enable the patient to begin eating and become accessible to psychotherapy.

NURSING DIAGNOSIS:	**FLUID VOLUME DEFICIT, POTENTIAL/ACTUAL**
May be related to:	**Inadequate intake of food and liquids**
	Consistent self-induced vomiting
	Laxative/diuretic use
Possibly evidenced by:	**Dry skin and mucous membranes, decreased skin turgor**
	Increased pulse rate, body temperature, decreased BP
	Output greater than input (diuretic use); concentrated urine/decreased urine output (dehydration)
	Weakness
	Change in mental state
	Hemoconcentration, altered electrolyte balance
PATIENT OUTCOMES/ EVALUATION CRITERIA:	**Maintains/demonstrates improved fluid balance, as evidenced by adequate urine output, stable vital signs, moist mucous membranes, good skin turgor. Verbalizes**

understanding of causative factors and behaviors necessary to correct fluid deficit.

ACTIONS/INTERVENTIONS	RATIONALE
Independent	
Monitor vital signs, capillary refill, moisture of mucous membranes, skin turgor.	Indicators of adequacy of circulating volume. Orthostatic hypotension may occur with risk of falls/injury following sudden changes in position.
Monitor amount and types of fluid intake. Measure urine output accurately.	Patient may abstain from all intake resulting in dehydration or substitute fluids for caloric intake, affecting electrolyte balance. Note: Reduced urinary output may be a direct result of reduced food intake.
Discuss strategies to stop vomiting and laxative/diuretic use.	Helping patient deal with anxious feelings that lead to vomiting and/or laxative/diuretic use will prevent continued fluid loss.
Identify actions necessary to regain/maintain optimal fluid balance, e.g., specific fluid intake schedule.	Involving patient in plan to correct fluid imbalances improves chances for success.
Collaborative	
Review electrolyte/renal function test results.	Fluid/electrolyte shifts, decreased renal function can adversely affect patient's recovery/prognosis and may require additional intervention.
Administer/monitor IV, hyperalimentation;	Used as an emergency measure to correct fluid/electrolyte imbalance.
Potassium supplements, oral or IV, as indicated.	May be required to prevent cardiac dysrhythmias.

NURSING DIAGNOSIS:	THOUGHT PROCESSES, ALTERED
May be related to:	Severe malnutrition/electrolyte imbalance
	Psychologic conflicts, e.g., sense of low self-worth, perceived lack of control
Possibly evidenced by:	Impaired ability to make decisions, problem-solve
	Non-reality-based verbalizations
	Ideas of reference
	Altered sleep patterns, e.g., may go to bed late (stays up to binge/purge) and get up early
	Altered attention span/distractibility
	Perceptual disturbances with failure to recognize hunger; fatigue, anxiety, and depression
PATIENT OUTCOMES/ EVALUATION CRITERIA:	Verbalizes understanding of causative factors and awareness of impairment. Demonstrates behaviors to change/prevent malnutrition. Displays improved ability to make decisions, problem-solve.

ACTIONS/INTERVENTIONS	RATIONALE
Independent	
Be aware of patient's distorted thinking ability.	Allows the care giver to lower expectations and provide appropriate information and support.
Listen to and do not challenge irrational, illogical thinking. Present reality concisely and briefly.	It is not possible to respond logically when thinking ability is physiologically impaired. The patient needs to hear reality, but challenging leads to distrust and frustration.
Adhere strictly to nutrition regimen.	Improved nutrition is essential to improved brain functioning. (Refer to ND: Nutrition, Altered: Less than Body Requirements, p. 363.)
Collaborative	
Review electrolyte/renal function tests.	Imbalances negatively affect cerebral functioning and may require correction before therapeutic interventions can begin.

NURSING DIAGNOSIS:	**SELF-CONCEPT, DISTURBANCE IN: BODY IMAGE/SELF-ESTEEM**
May be related to:	**Morbid fear of obesity**
	Perceived loss of control in some aspect of life
	Unmet dependency needs
	Dysfunctional family system
Possibly evidenced by:	**Distorted body image (views self as fat even in the presence of normal body weight or severe emaciation)**
	Expresses little concern, uses denial as a defense mechanism, and feels powerless to prevent/make changes
PATIENT OUTCOMES/ EVALUATION CRITERIA:	**Establishes a more realistic body image. Acknowledges self as an individual who has responsibility for own actions.**

ACTIONS/INTERVENTIONS	RATIONALE
Independent	
Establish a therapeutic nurse/patient relationship.	Within a helping relationship, patient can begin to trust and try out new thinking and behaviors.
Promote self-concept without moral judgment.	Patient sees self as weak-willed, even though part of person may feel sense of power and control (e.g., dieting/weight loss).
Have patient draw picture of self.	Provides opportunity to discuss patient's perception of self/body image and realities of individual situation.
State rules re: weighing schedule, remaining in sight during medication and eating times, and consequences of not following the rules. Be consistent in carrying out rules without undue comment.	Consistency is important in establishing trust. As part of the behavior modification program, patient knows risks involved in not following established rules (e.g., decrease in privileges). Failure to follow rules is viewed as the patient's choice and accepted by staff in matter-

367

ACTIONS/INTERVENTIONS	RATIONALE
Independent	of-fact manner so as not to provide reinforcement for the undesirable behavior.
Respond (confront) with reality when patient makes unrealistic statements such as "I'm gaining weight; so there's nothing really wrong with me."	Patient needs to be confronted because he or she denies the psychologic aspects of own situation and is often expressing a sense of inadequacy and depression.
Be aware of own reaction to patient's behavior. Avoid arguing.	Feelings of disgust, hostility, and infuriation are not uncommon when caring for these patients. Prognosis often remains poor even with a gain in weight, because other problems may remain. Many patients continue to see themselves as fat, and there is also a high incidence of affective disorders, social phobias, obsessive–compulsive symptoms, drug abuse, and psychosexual dysfunction. Nurse needs to deal with own response/feelings so they do not interfere with care of patient.
Assist the patient to assume control in areas other than dieting/weight loss, e.g., management of own daily activities, work/leisure choices.	Feelings of personal ineffectiveness, low self-esteem, and perfectionism are often part of the problem. Patient feels helpless to change and requires assistance to problem-solve methods of control in life situations.
Help the patient formulate goals for self (not related to eating) and create a manageable plan to reach those goals, one at a time, progressing from simple to more complex.	Patient needs to recognize ability to control other areas in life and may need to learn problem-solving skills in order to achieve this control. Setting realistic goals fosters success.
Assist patient to confront sexual fears. Provide sex education as necessary.	Major physical/psychologic changes in adolescence can contribute to development of this problem. Feelings of powerlessness and loss of control of feelings (in particular sexual sensations) lead to an unconscious desire to desexualize themselves. Patient often believes that these fears can be overcome by taking control of bodily appearance/development/function.
Encourage patient to take charge of own life in a more healthful way by making own decisions and accepting self as is. Encourage acceptance of inadequacies as well as strengths. Let patient know that it is acceptable to be different from family, particularly mother.	Patient often does not know what he or she may want for self. Parents (mother) usually make decisions for patient. Patient may also believe he or she has to be the best in everything and holds self responsible for being perfect. Developing a sense of identity separate from family and maintaining sense of control in other ways besides dieting and weight loss is a desirable goal of therapy/program.
Involve in personal development program.	Learning about proper application of make-up, methods of enhancing personal appearance may be helpful to long-range sense of self-esteem/image.
Use interpersonal psychotherapy approach, rather than interpretive therapy.	Interaction between persons is more helpful for the patient to discover feelings/impulses/needs from within own self. Patient has not learned this internal control as a child and may not be able to interpret/attach meaning to behavior.
Encourage patient to express anger and acknowledge when it is verbalized.	Important to know that anger is part of self and as such is acceptable. Expressing anger may need to be taught to patient, because anger is generally considered unacceptable in the family, and therefore patient does not express it.

ACTIONS/INTERVENTIONS	RATIONALE

Independent

Assist patient to learn strategies other than eating for dealing with feelings. Have patient keep a diary of feelings, particularly when thinking about food.

Feelings are the underlying issue, and patient often uses food instead of dealing with feelings appropriately. Patient needs to learn to recognize feelings and how to express them clearly.

Assess feelings of helplessness/hopelessness.

Lack of control is a common/underlying problem for this patient and may be accompanied by more serious emotional disorders. Note: Fifty-four percent of patients with anorexia have a history of major affective disorder, and 33% have a history of minor affective disorder.

Be alert to suicidal ideation/behavior.

Intense anxiety/panic about weight gain, depression, hopeless feelings may lead to suicidal attempts, particularly if patient is impulsive.

Collaborative

Involve in group therapy.

Provides an opportunity to talk about feelings and try out new behaviors.

NURSING DIAGNOSIS:	SKIN INTEGRITY, IMPAIRED: POTENTIAL/ACTUAL
May be related to:	Altered nutritional/metabolic state; edema
	Dehydration/cachectic changes (skeletal prominence)
Possibly evidenced by:	Dry/scaly skin with poor turgor
	Tissue fragility
	Brittle/dry hair
	Complaints of itching
PATIENT OUTCOMES/ EVALUATION CRITERIA:	Verbalizes understanding of causative factors and relief of itching. Identifies and demonstrates behaviors to maintain soft, supple, intact skin.

ACTIONS/INTERVENTIONS	RATIONALE

Independent

Observe for reddened, blanched, excoriated areas.

Indicators of increased risk of breakdown requiring more intense treatment.

Encourage bathing every other day.

Frequent baths contribute to dryness of the skin.

Use skin cream twice a day and after bathing.

Lubricates skin and decreases itching.

Massage skin, especially over bony prominences.

Improves circulation to the skin and skin tone.

Discuss importance of frequent change of position, need for remaining active.

Enhances circulation and perfusion to skin by preventing prolonged pressure on tissues.

Stress importance of adequate nutrition/fluid intake. (Refer to ND: Nutrition, Altered: Less than Body Requirements, p. 363.)

Improved nutrition and hydration will improve skin condition.

NURSING DIAGNOSIS:	FAMILY PROCESS, ALTERED
May be related to:	Issues of control in family
	Situational/maturational crises
	History of inadequate coping methods
Possibly evidenced by:	Dissonance among family members
	Family developmental tasks not being met
	Focus on "identified patient" (IP)
	Family needs not being met
	Family member(s) acting as "enablers" for IP
	Ill-defined family rules, function, and roles
FAMILY OUTCOMES/ EVALUATION CRITERIA:	Demonstrates individual involvement in problem-solving processes directed at encouraging patient toward independence. Expresses feelings freely and appropriately. Demonstrates more autonomous coping behaviors with individual family boundaries more clearly defined. Recognizes and resolves conflict appropriately with the individuals involved.

ACTIONS/INTERVENTIONS

Independent

Identify patterns of interaction. Encourage each family member to speak for self. Do not allow two members to discuss a third without that member's participation.

Discourage members from asking for approval from each other. Be alert to verbal or nonverbal checking with others for approval. Acknowledge competent actions of patient.

Listen with regard when the patient speaks.

Encourage individuals not to answer to everything.

Communicate message of separation, that it is acceptable for family members to be different from one another.

Encourage and allow expression of feelings (e.g., crying, anger) by individuals.

Prevent intrusion in dyads by other members of the family.

Reinforce importance of parents as a couple who have rights of their own.

RATIONALE

Helpful information for planning interventions. The enmeshed, overinvolved family members often speak for each other and need to learn to be responsible for their own words and actions.

Each individual needs to develop own internal sense of self-esteem. Individual often is living up to others' (family's) expectations rather than making own choices. Provides recognition of self in positive ways.

Sets an example and provides a sense of competence and self-worth, in that the patient has been heard and attended to.

Reinforces individualization and return to privacy.

Individuation needs reinforcement. Such a message confronts rigidity and opens options for different behaviors.

Often these families have not allowed free expression of feelings and will need help and permission to learn and accept this.

Inappropriate interventions in family subsystems prevent individuals from working out problems successfully.

The focus on the child with anorexia is very intense and often is the only area around which the couple interact. The couple needs to explore their own rela-

ACTIONS/INTERVENTIONS

Independent

Prevent patient from intervening in conflicts between parents. Assist parents in identifying and solving their marital differences.

Be aware and confront sabotage behavior on the part of family members.

Collaborative

Refer to community resources, such as family therapy groups, parents' groups as indicated, and parent effectiveness classes.

RATIONALE

tionship and restore the balance within it in order to prevent its disintegration.

Triangulation occurs in which a parent–child coalition exists. Sometimes the child is openly pressed to ally self with one parent against the other. The symptom (anorexia) is the regulator in the family system, and the parents deny their own conflicts.

Feelings of blame, shame, and helplessness may lead to unconscious behavior designed to maintain the status quo.

May help reduce overprotectiveness, support/facilitate the process of dealing with unresolved conflicts and change.

NURSING DIAGNOSIS:	KNOWLEDGE DEFICIT [LEARNING NEED] (SPECIFY)
May be related to:	**Lack of exposure to/unfamiliarity with information about condition**
	Learned maladaptive coping skills
Possibly evidenced by:	**Verbalization of misconception of relationship of current situation and behaviors**
	Preoccupation with extreme fear of obesity and distortion of own body image
	Refusal to eat; binging and purging
	Abuse of laxatives and diuretics
	Excessive exercising
	Verbalization of need for new information
	Expressions of desire to learn more adaptive ways of coping with stressors
PATIENT OUTCOMES/ EVALUATION CRITERIA:	**Verbalizes awareness of and plans for lifestyle changes to maintain normal weight. Identifies relationship of signs/symptoms (weight loss, tooth decay) to behaviors of not eating/binge–purging. Assumes responsibility for own learning. Seeks out sources/resources to assist with making identified changes.**

ACTIONS/INTERVENTIONS

Independent

Determine level of knowledge and readiness to learn.

RATIONALE

Learning is easier when it begins where the learner is.

ACTIONS/INTERVENTIONS	RATIONALE
Independent	
Note blocks to learning, e.g., physical/intellectual/emotional.	Malnutrition, family problems, drug abuse, affective disorders, obsessive–compulsive symptoms can be blocks to learning requiring resolution before effective learning can occur.
Review dietary needs, answering questions as indicated. (Refer to ND: Nutrition, Altered: Less than Body Requirements, p. 363.)	Patient/family may need assistance with planning for new way of eating.
Encourage the use of relaxation and other stress management techniques, e.g., visualization, guided imagery, biofeedback.	New ways of coping with feelings of anxiety and fear will help patient to manage these feelings in more effective ways, assisting in giving up maladaptive behaviors of not eating/binging–purging.
Assist with establishing a sensible exercise program. Caution regarding overexercise.	Exercise can assist with developing a positive body image and combats depression (release of endorphins in the brain enhances sense of well-being). Patient may use excessive exercise as a way of controlling weight.
Provide written information for patient/significant other(s).	Helpful as reminder of and reinforcement for learning.
Discuss need for information about sex and sexuality.	Because avoidance of own sexuality is an issue for this patient, realistic information can be helpful in beginning to deal with self as a sexual being.
Collaborative	
Refer to therapist trained in dealing with sexuality.	May need professional assistance to accept self as a sexual adult.
Refer to National Association of Anorexia Nervosa and Associated Disorders.	May be a helpful source of support and information for patient/SO.

Eating Disorders: Obesity _____

PATIENT ASSESSMENT DATA BASE

ACTIVITY/REST

May report: Fatigue, constant drowsiness.

Inability/lack of desire to be active or engage in regular exercise.

Dyspnea with exertion.

CIRCULATION

May exhibit: Hypertension, edema.

EGO INTEGRITY

May report: History of cultural/lifestyle factors affecting food choice.

Weight may/may not be perceived as a problem.

Eating relieves unpleasant feelings, e.g., loneliness, frustration, boredom.

Perception of body image as undesirable.

SO resistant to weight loss (may sabotage patient's efforts).

FOOD/FLUID

May report: Normal/excessive ingestion of food.

Experimentation with numerous types of diets (yo-yo dieting) with varied/shortlived results.

History of recurrent weight loss and gain.

May exhibit: Weight disproportionate to height.

Endomorphic body type (soft/round).

Failure to adjust food intake to diminishing requirements (e.g., change in lifestyle from active to sedentary, aging).

PAIN/COMFORT

May report: Pain/discomfort on weight-bearing joints or spine.

RESPIRATION

May report: Dyspnea.

May exhibit: Cyanosis, respiratory distress (Pickwickian syndrome).

SEXUALITY

May report: Menstrual disturbances, amenorrhea.

TEACHING/LEARNING

May report: Problem may be lifetime or related to life event.

Family history of obesity.

Concomitant health problems may be present, e.g., hypertension, diabetes, gallbladder and cardiovascular disease, hypothyroidism.

Discharge Plan Considerations: May require support with therapeutic regimen.

DIAGNOSTIC STUDIES

Metabolic/endocrine studies: may reveal abnormalities, e.g., hypothyroidism, hypopituitarism, hypogonadism, Cushing's syndrome (increased insulin levels), hyperglycemia, hyperlipidemia, hyperuricemia, hyperbilirubinemia. It is also suggested that the cause of these disorders may arise out of neuroendocrine abnormalities within the hypothalamus, which result in various chemical disturbances.

Body measurements (including skinfold): estimates fat/muscle mass.

NURSING PRIORITIES

1. Assist patient to identify a pattern of weight control containing needed nutrients.
2. Promote improved self-concept, including body image, self-esteem.
3. Encourage health practices to provide for weight control throughout life.

DISCHARGE CRITERIA

1. Healthy patterns for nutrition and weight control identified.
2. Weight loss toward desired goal established.
3. Positive perception of self verbalized.
4. Plans for future control of weight made.

NURSING DIAGNOSIS:	NUTRITION, ALTERED: MORE THAN BODY REQUIREMENTS
May be related to:	Food intake which exceeds body needs
	Psychosocial factors
Possibly evidenced by:	Weight of 20% or more over optimum body weight; excess body fat by skinfold measurements
	Reported/observed dysfunctional eating patterns, intake more than body requirements
PATIENT OUTCOMES/ EVALUATION CRITERIA:	Identifies inappropriate behaviors and consequences associated with weight gain or overeating. Demonstrates change in eating patterns and involvement in individual exercise program. Displays weight loss with optimal maintenance of health.

ACTIONS/INTERVENTIONS	RATIONALE
Independent	
Review individual cause for obesity, e.g., organic or nonorganic.	Identifies/influences choice of interventions.
Implement/review daily food diary, e.g., caloric intake, types of food, and eating habits.	Provides realistic picture of amount of food ingested and corresponding eating habits/feelings. Identifies patterns requiring change and/or a base upon which to tailor the dietary program.
Discuss emotions/events associated with eating.	Helps to identify when patient is eating to satisfy an emotional need, rather than physiologic hunger.
Formulate a diet plan in consultation with the patient.	While there is no basis for recommending one diet over another, a good reducing diet should contain foods from all basic food groups and be as similar to

374

ACTIONS/INTERVENTIONS	RATIONALE

Independent

	patient's usual eating pattern as possible. A plan developed with and agreed to by the patient is more apt to be successful. Note: It is important to maintain adequate protein intake to prevent loss of muscle mass.
Use knowledge of individual's height, body build, age, gender, and individual patterns of eating, energy, and nutrient requirements.	Standard tables are subject to error when applied to individual situations, and circadian rhythms/lifestyle patterns need to be considered.
Stress the importance of avoiding fad diets.	Elimination of needed components can lead to metabolic imbalances, e.g., excessive reduction of carbohydrates can lead to fatigue, headache, instability and weakness, metabolic acidosis (ketosis) interfering with effectiveness of weight loss program.
Discuss realistic increment goals for weekly weight loss.	Reasonable weight loss (1–2 lb per week) achieves a more lasting loss. Excessive/rapid loss may result in fatigue and irritability and lead to failure in meeting ultimate goals for weight loss. Motivation is more easily sustained by meeting "stair-step" goals.
Weigh periodically as individually indicated, and obtain appropriate body measurements.	Provides information about effectiveness of therapeutic regimen, and visual evidence of success of patient's efforts. During hospitalization, for controlled fasting, daily weight may be required. Weekly weight is more appropriate after discharge.
Determine current activity levels and plan progressive exercise program (e.g., walking) tailored to the individual's goals and choice.	Exercise furthers weight loss by reducing appetite, increasing energy, toning muscles, and enhancing sense of well-being and accomplishment. Commitment on the part of the patient enables the setting of more realistic goals and adherence to the plan.
Develop an appetite reeducation plan with patient.	Signals of hunger and fullness often are not recognized, have become distorted, or are ignored.
Stress the importance of avoiding tension at mealtimes as well as not eating too quickly.	Reducing tension provides a more relaxed eating atmosphere and encourages more leisurely eating patterns. This is important because a period of time is required for the appestat mechanism to know the stomach is full.
Encourage patient to eat only at a table or designated eating place and to avoid standing while eating.	Techniques that modify behavior may be helpful in avoiding diet failure.
Discuss restriction of salt intake and diuretic drugs if used.	Water retention may be a problem because of increased fluid intake, as well as the result of fat metabolism.

Collaborative

Consult with dietician to determine caloric requirements for individual weight loss.	Individual intake can be calculated by several different formulas but is based on the basal caloric requirement for 24 hours, depending on patient's sex, age, current/desired weight, and length of time estimated to achieve desired weight.
Administer medications as indicated:	
Appetite-suppressant drugs, e.g., diethylpropion (Tenuate), mazindol (Sanorex);	Used with caution/supervision at the beginning of a weight loss program to support patient during stress of behaviorial/lifestyle changes. They are only effective for a few weeks and may cause problems of addiction in some people.

375

ACTIONS/INTERVENTIONS

Collaborative

Hormonal therapy, e.g., thyroid (Euthroid);

Vitamin, mineral supplements.

Maintain fasting regime and/or stabilization of medical problems, when indicated.

Refer for surgical interventions, e.g., gastric bypass, partitioning, if indicated.

RATIONALE

May be necessary when hypothyroidism is present. Replacement when no deficiency is present is not helpful and may actually be harmful. Note: Other hormonal treatments, such as human chorionic gonadotropin (HCG), although widely publicized, have no documented evidence of value.

Although obese individuals have large fuel reserves, this does not hold true for vitamins and minerals.

Aggressive therapy/support may be necessary to initiate weight loss, although fasting is not generally a treatment of choice. Patient can be monitored more effectively in a controlled setting, to minimize complications such as postural hypotension, anemia, cardiac irregularities, decreased uric acid excretion with hyperuricemia.

These interventions may be necessary to assist the client lose weight when obesity is life-threatening. (Refer to CP: Obesity: Surgical Interventions, p. 380.)

NURSING DIAGNOSIS:	**SELF-CONCEPT, DISTURBANCE IN: BODY IMAGE/SELF-ESTEEM**
May be related to:	**Biophysical/psychosocial factors: patient's view of self; slimness is valued in this society, and mixed messages are received when thinness is stressed**
	Family/subculture encouragement of overeating
	Control, sex and love issues
Possibly evidenced by:	**Verbalization of negative feelings about body (mental image often does not match physical reality); fear of rejection/reaction by others; feelings of hopelessness/powerlessness**
	Preoccupation with change (attempts to lose weight)
	Lack of follow through with diet plan
	Verbalization of powerlessness to change eating habits
PATIENT OUTCOMES/ EVALUATION CRITERIA:	**Verbalizes a more realistic self-image and demonstrates acceptance of self as is rather than an idealized image. Acknowledges self as an individual who has responsibility for self. Seeks information and actively pursues appropriate weight loss.**

ACTIONS/INTERVENTIONS

Independent

Discuss with the patient view of being fat and what it does for the individual. Be sure to provide privacy dur-

RATIONALE

Mental image includes our ideal and is usually not up to date. Fat and compulsive eating behaviors may

ACTIONS/INTERVENTIONS	RATIONALE
Independent	
ing care activities.	have deep-rooted psychologic implications, e.g., compensating for lack of love and nurturing, or be a defense against intimacy. In addition, individual often is sensitive/self-conscious about body.
Have patient recall coping patterns related to food in family of origin and how these affect current situation.	Parents act as role models for the child. Maladaptive coping patterns (overeating) are learned within the family system and are supported through positive reinforcement. Food may be substituted by the parent for affection and love, and eating is associated with a feeling of satisfaction, becoming the primary defense.
Determine the patient's motivation for weight loss and assist with goal setting.	The individual may harbor repressed feelings of hostility, which may be expressed inward on the self. Because of a poor self-concept, the person often has difficulty with relationships. Note: When losing weight for someone else, the patient is less likely to be successful/maintain weight loss.
Be alert to myths the patient/SO may have about weight and weight loss.	Beliefs about what an ideal body looks like or unconscious motivations (such as the feminine thought of "If I become thin, men will pursue me, or rape me," the masculine counterpart "I don't trust myself to stay in control of my sexual feelings"), as well as issues of strength, power, and "good cook" image, can sabotage efforts at weight loss.
Assist patient to identify feelings which lead to compulsive eating. Develop strategies for doing something besides eating for dealing with these feelings, e.g., talking with a friend.	Awareness of emotions that lead to overeating can be the first step in behavior change, e.g., people often eat because of depression, anger and guilt.
Graph weight on a weekly basis.	Provides ongoing visual evidence of weight changes (reality oriented).
Promote open communication avoiding criticism/judgment about patient's behavior.	Supports patient's own responsibility for weight loss; enhances sense of control and promotes willingness to discuss difficulties/setbacks and problem-solve. Note: Distrust and accusations of "cheating" on caloric intake are not helpful.
Outline and clearly state responsibilities of patient and nurse.	It is helpful for each individual to understand area of own responsibility in the program so misunderstandings do not arise.
Be alert to binge-eating and develop strategies for dealing with these episodes, e.g., substituting other actions for eating.	The patient who binges experiences guilt about it, which is also counterproductive, because negative feelings may sabotage further weight loss efforts.
Encourage patient to use imagery to visualize self as desired weight and to practice handling of new behaviors.	Mental rehearsal is very useful to help the patient plan for and deal with anticipated change in self-image or deal with occasions that may arise (family gatherings, special dinners) where confrontations with food will occur.
Provide information about the use of makeup, hairstyles, and ways of dressing to maximize figure assets.	Enhances feelings of self-esteem; promotes improved body image.
Encourage buying clothes as a reward for weight loss instead of food treats.	Properly fitting clothes enhance the body image as small losses are made and the individual feels more positive. Waiting until the desired weight loss is reached can become discouraging.

377

ACTIONS/INTERVENTIONS

Independent

Suggest the patient dispose of "fat clothes."

Help staff be aware of and deal with own feelings when caring for this patient.

Collaborative

Refer to support and/or therapy group.

RATIONALE

Removes the "safety valve" of having clothes available "in case" the weight is regained. Retaining "fat clothes" can convey the message that the weight loss will not occur/be maintained.

Judgmental attitudes, feelings of disgust, anger, weariness can interfere with care/be transmitted to patient, reinforcing negative self-esteem/image.

Support groups can provide companionship, enhance motivation, decrease loneliness and social ostracism, and give practical solutions to common problems. Group therapy can be helpful in dealing with underlying psychologic concerns.

NURSING DIAGNOSIS:	SOCIAL INTERACTION, IMPAIRED
May be related to:	Verbalized or observed discomfort in social situations
	Self-concept disturbance
Possibly evidenced by:	Reluctance to participate in social gatherings
	Verbalization of a sense of discomfort with others
PATIENT OUTCOMES/ EVALUATION CRITERIA:	Verbalizes awareness of feelings that lead to poor social interactions. Involved in achieving positive changes in social behaviors and interpersonal relationships.

ACTIONS/INTERVENTIONS

Independent

Review family patterns of relating and social behaviors.

Encourage patient to express feelings and perceptions of problems.

Assess patient's use of coping skills and defense mechanisms.

Have patient list behaviors that cause discomfort.

Involve in role-playing new ways to deal with identified behaviors/situations.

Discuss negative self-concepts, note negative self-talk, e.g., "No one wants to be with a fat person," "Who would be interested in talking to me?"

RATIONALE

Social interaction is primarily learned within the family of origin; when inadequate patterns are identified, actions for change can be instituted.

Helps to identify and clarify reasons for difficulties in interacting with others, e.g., may feel unloved/unlovable or insecure about sexuality.

May have developed coping skills in some areas of life that can be transferred to social settings. Defense mechanisms used to protect the individual may contribute to feelings of aloneness/isolation.

Identifies specific concerns and suggests actions that can be taken to effect change.

Practicing these new behaviors enables the individual to become comfortable with them in a safe situation.

May be impeding positive social interactions.

ACTIONS/INTERVENTIONS

Independent

Encourage use of positive self-talk such as telling one-self "I am OK," "I can enjoy social activities and do not need to be controlled by what others think or say."

Collaborative

Encourage ongoing family or individual therapy as indicated.

RATIONALE

Positive strategies enhance feelings of comfort and support efforts for change.

Patient benefits from involvement of SO to provide support and encouragement.

NURSING DIAGNOSIS:	KNOWLEDGE DEFICIT [LEARNING NEED] (SPECIFY)
May be related to:	**Lack of/misinterpretation of information**
	Lack of interest in learning, lack of recall
	Inaccurate/incomplete information presented
Possibly evidenced by:	**Statements of lack of and request for information about obesity and nutritional requirements**
	Verbalization of problem with weight reduction
	Inadequate follow through with previous diet and exercise instruction
PATIENT OUTCOMES/ EVALUATION CRITERIA:	**Assumes responsibility for own learning and begins to look for information about nutrition and ways to control weight. Verbalizes understanding of need for lifestyle changes to maintain/control weight.**

ACTIONS/INTERVENTIONS

Independent

Determine level of nutritional knowledge and what patient believes is most urgent need.

Provide information about ways to maintain satisfactory food intake in settings away from home.

Identify other sources of information, e.g., books, tapes, community classes, groups.

Stress necessity of continued follow-up care/counseling, especially when plateaus occur.

Reassess caloric requirements every 2–4 weeks.

Identify alternatives to chosen activity program to accommodate weather, travel, etc. Discuss use of mechanical devices for reducing.

RATIONALE

Necessary to know what additional information to provide. When patient's views are listened to, trust is enhanced.

"Smart" eating when dining out or when traveling helps individual to manage weight while still enjoying social outlets.

Using different avenues of accessing information will further patient's learning. Involvement with others who are also losing weight can provide support.

As weight is lost, changes in metabolism occur, interfering with further loss, creating a plateau as the body activates a survival mechanism, attempting to prevent "starvation." This requires new strategies and aggressive support to continue weight loss.

Changes in weight and exercise may necessitate changes in reducing diet.

Promotes continuation of program. Note: Fat loss occurs on a generalized overall basis, and there is no evidence that spot reducing or mechanical devices aid in weight loss in specific areas.

Obesity: Surgical Interventions (Gastric Partitioning, Gastric Bypass)

Gastric partitioning: small pouch created across stomach just distal to the gastroesophageal junction leaving a small opening through which food passes into stomach.

Gastric bypass: anastomosis of jejunum to upper portion of stomach, bypassing rest of stomach.

Refer to CPs: Eating Disorders: Obesity, p. 373; Intestinal Surgery, p. 436.

PATIENT ASSESSMENT DATA BASE

ACTIVITY/REST

May report:	Difficulty sleeping.
	Exertional discomfort, inability to participate in strenuous (possibly even moderate) activity/sports.

EGO INTEGRITY

May report:	Motivated to lose weight for oneself (not for gratification of others).
	Repressed feelings of hostility toward authority figures.
	History of psychiatric illness.
May exhibit:	Symptoms of emotional/psychiatric illness.

FOOD/FLUID

May report:	Weight exceeding ideal body weight by 100 lb or more (morbid obesity).
	Adequate trials and failure of other treatment approaches.
	Desire to lose weight.

TEACHING/LEARNING

May report:	Presence of chronic conditions (hypertension, diabetes, and arthritis, pickwickian syndrome, infertility).
Discharge Plan Considerations:	May require support with therapeutic regimen, assistance with self-care, homemaker tasks.

DIAGNOSTIC STUDIES

Studies are dependent on individual situations, to rule out underlying disease, in addition to preoperative workup, including psychiatric evaluation.

NURSING PRIORITIES

1. Support respiratory function.
2. Prevent/minimize complications.
3. Provide appropriate nutritional intake.
4. Provide information regarding surgical procedure, postoperative expectations, and treatment needs.

DISCHARGE CRITERIA

1. Ventilation and oxygenation adequate for individual needs.
2. Complications prevented/controlled.
3. Nutritional intake modified for specific procedure.
4. Procedure, prognosis, and therapeutic regimen understood.

Refer to CP: Intestinal Surgery (ostomy not anticipated), p. 436, for general considerations. Special problems and interventions are highlighted here.

NURSING DIAGNOSIS:	BREATHING PATTERNS, INEFFECTIVE
May be related to:	**Decreased lung expansion**
	Pain, anxiety
	Decreased energy, fatigue
	Tracheobronchial obstruction
Possibly evidenced by:	**Shortness of breath, dyspnea**
	Tachypnea, respiratory depth changes, reduced vital capacity
	Wheezes, rhonchi
	Abnormal ABGs
PATIENT OUTCOMES/ EVALUATION CRITERIA:	**Maintains adequate ventilation, free of cyanosis and other signs of hypoxia, with ABGs within patient's normal range.**

ACTIONS/INTERVENTIONS

Independent

Monitor respiratory rate/depth. Auscultate breath sounds. Investigate presence of pallor/cyanosis, increased restlessness or confusion.

Elevate head of bed 30 degrees.

Encourage deep breathing exercises. Assist with coughing and splint incision.

Turn periodically and ambulate as early as possible.

Pad siderails and teach patient to use them as armrests.

Use small pillow under head when indicated.

Avoid use of abdominal binders.

Collaborative

Administer supplemental oxygen.

Assist in use of IPPB and/or respiratory adjuncts, e.g., incentive spirometer, blow bottles.

Monitor/graph serial ABGs/pulse oximetry when indicated.

RATIONALE

Shallow respirations/effects of anesthesia decrease ventilation, potentiate atelectasis, and may result in hypoxia.

Encourages optimal diaphragmatic excursion/lung expansion and minimizes pressure of abdominal contents on the thoracic cavity.

Promotes maximal lung expansion and aids in clearing airways, thus reducing risk of atelectasis, pneumonia.

Promotes aeration of all segments of the lung, mobilizing and aiding in expectoration of secretions.

Using the siderail as an armrest allows for greater chest expansion.

Many obese patients have large, thick necks, and use of large, fluffy pillows may obstruct the airway.

Can restrict lung expansion.

Maximizes available oxygen for exchange and reduces work of breathing.

Enhances lung expansion; reduces potential for atelectasis.

Reflects ventilation/oxygenation and acid–base status. Used as a basis for evaluating need for/effectiveness of respiratory therapies.

381

NURSING DIAGNOSIS:	TISSUE PERFUSION, ALTERED: PERIPHERAL [POTENTIAL]
May be related to:	Diminished blood flow, hypovolemia
	Immobility/bedrest
	Interruption of venous blood flow (thrombosis)
Possibly evidenced by:	[Not applicable; presence of signs and symptoms establishes an *actual* diagnosis.]
PATIENT OUTCOMES/ EVALUATION CRITERIA:	Maintains perfusion as individually appropriate, e.g., skin warm/dry, peripheral pulses present/strong, vital signs within patient's normal range. Identifies causative/risk factors. Demonstrates behaviors to improve/maintain circulation.

ACTIONS/INTERVENTIONS	RATIONALE
Independent	
Monitor vital signs. Palpate peripheral pulses routinely; evaluate capillary refill and changes in mentation. Note 24-hour fluid balance.	Indicators of circulatory adequacy. (Refer to ND: Fluid Volume Deficit, Potential, following.)
Provide range of motion exercises for legs and ankles frequently.	Stimulates circulation in the lower extremities; reduces venous stasis.
Assess for Homans' sign, redness and edema of calf.	Indicators of thrombus formation but may not always be present in obese individual.
Encourage early ambulation; discourage sitting and/ or dangling at the bedside.	Sitting constricts venous flow, whereas walking encourages venous return.
Provide adequate/appropriate equipment and sufficient staff for handling patient.	Helpful in dealing with the bulk of the patient for moving, bowel care, and ambulating. Reduces risk of traumatic injury.
Collaborative	
Administer heparin therapy, as indicated.	May be used prophylactically to reduce risk of thrombus formation or to treat thromboemboli.
Monitor Hb/Hct and coagulation studies.	Provides information about circulatory volume/ alterations in coagulation and indicates therapy needs/ effectiveness.

NURSING DIAGNOSIS:	FLUID VOLUME DEFICIT, POTENTIAL
May be related to:	Excessive gastric losses: nasogastric suction, diarrhea
	Reduced intake
Possibly evidenced by:	[Not applicable; presence of signs and symptoms establishes an *actual* diagnosis.]
PATIENT OUTCOMES/ EVALUATION CRITERIA:	Maintains adequate fluid with balanced I&O and absence of signs reflecting dehydration.

ACTIONS/INTERVENTIONS	RATIONALE

Independent

Assess vital signs, noting changes in blood pressure (postural), tachycardia, fever. Assess skin turgor, capillary refill, and moisture of mucous membranes.

Indicators of dehydration/hypovolemia.

Monitor I&O, noting/measuring diarrhea and NG suction losses.

Changes in gastric capacity/intestinal motility and nausea greatly influence intake and fluid needs, increasing risk of dehydration.

Evaluate muscle strength/tone. Observe for muscle tremors.

Large gastric losses may result in decreased magnesium and calcium, leading to neuromuscular weakness/tetany.

Establish individual needs/replacement schedule.

Determined by amount of measured losses/estimated insensible losses and dependent on gastric capacity.

Encourage increased oral intake when able.

Permits discontinuation of invasive fluid support measures and contributes to return of normal bowel functioning.

Collaborative

Administer supplemental IV fluids as indicated.

Replaces fluid losses, restores fluid balance in immediate postoperative phase and/or until patient is able to take sufficient oral fluids.

Monitor electrolytes and replace as indicated.

Use of NG tube, and/or vomiting, onset of diarrhea can deplete electrolytes that affect organ functioning.

NURSING DIAGNOSIS:	NUTRITION, ALTERED: LESS THAN BODY REQUIREMENTS [POTENTIAL]
May be related to:	Decreased intake, dietary restrictions, early satiety Increased metabolic rate/healing Malabsorption of nutrients/impaired absorption of vitamins
Possibly evidenced by:	[Not applicable; presence of signs and symptoms establishes an *actual* diagnosis.]
PATIENT OUTCOMES/ EVALUATION CRITERIA:	Identifies individual nutritional needs. Demonstrates appropriate weight loss with normalization of laboratory values. Displays behaviors to maintain adequate nutritional intake.

ACTIONS/INTERVENTIONS	RATIONALE

Independent

Establish hourly intake schedule. Instruct in measuring fluids/foods and sipping or eating slowly.

After partitioning, gastric capacity is reduced to approximately 50 ml, necessitating frequent/small feedings.

Weigh daily. Establish regular schedule after discharge.

Monitors losses and aids in assessing nutritional needs/effectiveness of therapy.

Stress importance of being aware of satiety and stopping intake.

Overeating may cause nausea/vomiting or damage partitioning.

ACTIONS/INTERVENTIONS

Independent

Require that patient sit up to drink/eat.

Determine foods that are gas-forming.

Discuss food preferences with patient and include in diet.

Collaborative

Provide liquid diet, advancing to soft, high in protein and bulk, and low in fat, with liquid supplements as needed.

Refer to dietitian.

Administer vitamin supplements as well as B$_{12}$ injections, folate and calcium as indicated.

RATIONALE

Prevents possibility of aspiration.

May interfere with appetite/digestion and restrict nutritional intake.

May enhance intake when foods are puréed, promote sense of participation/control.

Provides nutrients without additional calories. Note: Liquid diet is usually maintained for 8 weeks after partitioning procedure.

May need assistance in planning a diet that meets nutritional needs.

Supplements may be needed to prevent anemia as absorption is impaired. Increased intestinal motility following bypass procedure lowers calcium level and increases absorption of oxalates, which can lead to urinary stone formation.

NURSING DIAGNOSIS:	SKIN INTEGRITY, IMPAIRED: ACTUAL/POTENTIAL
May be related to:	Reduced vascularity, altered circulation
	Altered nutritional state: obesity
	Trauma/surgery; difficulty in approximation of suture line of fatty tissue
Possibly evidenced by:	Disruption of skin surface, altered healing
PATIENT OUTCOMES/ EVALUATION CRITERIA:	Displays timely wound healing without complication. Demonstrates behaviors to reduce tension on suture line.

ACTIONS/INTERVENTIONS

Independent

Support incision when turning, coughing, deep breathing, and ambulating.

Observe incisions periodically, noting approximation of wound edges, hematoma formation and resolution, bleeding/drainage.

Provide routine incisional care, being careful to keep dressings dry and sterile. Assess patency of drains.

Encourage frequent position change, inspect pressure points, and massage as indicated.

Provide meticulous skin care; pay particular attention to skin folds.

RATIONALE

Reduces possibility of dehiscence and later incisional hernia.

Influences choice of interventions.

Promotes healing. Accumulation of serosanguinous drainan subcutaneous layers increases tension on suture line, may delay wound healing, and serves as a medium for bacterial growth.

Reduces pressure on skin promoting peripheral circulation and reducing risk of skin breakdown.

Moisture or excoriation enhances growth of bacteria that can lead to postoperative infection.

ACTIONS/INTERVENTIONS	RATIONALE

Collaborative

Provide foam/air mattress or kinesthetic therapy as indicated.

Reduces skin pressure and enhances circulation.

NURSING DIAGNOSIS: INFECTION, POTENTIAL FOR

May be related to: Inadequate primary defenses: broken/traumatized tissues; decreased ciliary action; stasis of body fluids

Invasive procedures

Possibly evidenced by: [Not applicable; presence of signs and symptoms establishes an *actual* diagnosis.]

PATIENT OUTCOMES/ EVALUATION CRITERIA: Achieves timely wound healing, free of signs of local or generalized infectious process.

ACTIONS/INTERVENTIONS	RATIONALE

Independent

Stress proper handwashing technique.

Prevents spread of bacteria, cross-contamination.

Maintain aseptic technique in dressing changes, invasive procedures.

Reduces risk of nosocomial infection.

Inspect surgical incisions/invasive sites for erythema, purulent drainage.

Early detection of developing infection provides for prevention of more serious complications.

Encourage frequent position changes; deep breathing, coughing, use of respiratory adjuncts, e.g., incentive spirometer.

Promotes mobilization of secretions, reducing risk of pneumonia.

Provide routine catheter care/encourage good perineal care.

Prevents ascending bladder infections.

Encourage patient to drink acid-ash juices, such as cranberry.

Maintain urine acidity to retard bacterial growth.

Observe for complaints of abdominal pain, elevated temperature, increased white count.

Suggest possibility of developing peritonitis. (Refer to CP: Peritonitis, p. 449.)

Collaborative

Apply topical antimicrobials/antibiotics as indicated.

Reduces bacterial colonization on skin; prevents infection in wound.

NURSING DIAGNOSIS: BOWEL ELIMINATION, ALTERED: DIARRHEA

May be related to: Rapid transit of food through shortened small intestine

Changes in dietary fiber and bulk

Inflammation, irritation and malabsorption of bowel

Possibly evidenced by: Loose, liquid stools, increased frequency

Increased/hyperactive bowel sounds

ACTIONS/INTERVENTIONS	**RATIONALE**
Independent	
Observe/record stool frequency, characteristics, and amount.	Diarrhea often develops after resumption of diet.
Encourage diet high in fiber/bulk within dietary limitations, with moderate fluid intake as diet resumes;	Increases consistency of the effluent. Although fluid is necessary for optimal body function, excessive amounts contribute to diarrhea.
Restriction of fat intake as indicated.	Low-fat diet reduces risk of steatorrhea and limits laxative effect of decreased fat absorption.
Observe for signs of "dumping syndrome," e.g., sweating, nausea, and weakness after eating.	Rapid emptying of food from the stomach may result in gastric distress and alter bowel function.
Assist with frequent perianal care, using ointments as indicated.	Anal irritation, excoriation, and pruritus occur because of diarrhea. The patient often cannot reach the area for proper cleansing and may be embarrassed to ask for help.
Collaborative	
Administer medications as indicated, e.g., diphenoxylate with atropine (Lomotil).	May be necessary to control frequency of stools until body readjusts to surgical changes in function.
Monitor serum electrolytes.	Increased gastric losses potentiate the risk of electrolyte imbalance, which can lead to more serious/life-threatening complications.

NURSING DIAGNOSIS:	KNOWLEDGE DEFICIT [LEARNING NEED] (SPECIFY)
May be related to:	**Lack of exposure, unfamiliarity with resources**
	Information misinterpretation
	Lack of recall
Possibly evidenced by:	**Questions, request for information**
	Statement of misconceptions
	Inaccurate follow through of instructions
	Development of preventable complications
PATIENT OUTCOMES/ EVALUATION CRITERIA:	**Verbalizes understanding of surgical procedure, potential complications, treatment regimen, and postoperative expectations. Initiates necessary lifestyle changes and participates in treatment regimen.**

ACTIONS/INTERVENTIONS	**RATIONALE**
Independent	
Review specific surgical procedure and postoperative expectations.	Provides knowledge base on which informed choices can be made and goals formulated.

ACTIONS/INTERVENTIONS	RATIONALE
Independent	
Address concerns about altered body size/image.	Anticipation of problems can be helpful in dealing with situations that arise. (Refer to CP: Eating Disorders: Obesity, ND: Self-Concept, Disturbance in: Body Image/Self-esteem, p. 376.)
Review medication regimen, dosage, and side effects.	Knowledge may enhance cooperation with therapeutic regimen and in maintenance of schedule.
Recommend avoidance of alcohol.	May contribute to liver/pancreatic dysfunction.
Discuss responsibility for self-care with patient/SO.	Full cooperation is important for successful outcome after procedure.
Stress importance of regular medical follow-up, including laboratory studies, and discuss possible health problems.	Periodic assessment/evaluation (e.g., over 3 months) promotes early recognition/prevention of such complications as liver dysfunction, malnutrition, electrolyte imbalances, and kidney stones, which may develop after bypass.
Encourage progressive exercise/activity program balanced with adequate rest periods.	Promotes weight loss, enhances muscle tone, and minimizes postoperative complications while preventing undue fatigue.
Review proper eating habits; e.g., eat small amounts of food slowly and chew well; sit at table in calm/relaxed environment; eat only at prescribed times; avoid between-meal snacking; do not "make up" skipped feedings;	Focuses attention on eating, increasing awareness of intake and feelings of satiety.
Avoid fluid intake half hour before/after meals and use of carabonated beverages.	May cause gastric fullness/gaseous distention, limiting intake.
Identify signs of hypokalemia, e.g., diarrhea, muscle cramps/weakness of lower extremities, weak/irregular pulse, dizziness with position changes.	Increasing dietary intake of potassium (e.g., milk, coffee, cola, potatoes, carrots, bananas, oranges) may correct deficit, preventing serious respiratory/cardiac complications.
Discuss symptoms that may indicate "dumping syndrome," e.g., weakness, profuse perspiration, nausea, vomiting, faintness, flushing, epigastric discomfort or palpitations, occurring during or immediately following meals. Problem-solve.	Generally occurring in early postoperative period (1–3 weeks), syndrome is usually self-limiting but may become chronic, requiring medical intervention.
Review symptoms requiring medical evaluation, e.g., persistent nausea/vomiting; abdominal distention, tenderness; change in pattern of bowel elimination; fever, purulent wound drainage; excessive weight loss or plateauing/weight gain.	Early recognition of developing complications allows for prompt intervention, preventing serious outcome.
Collaborative	
Refer to community support groups.	Involvement with others who have dealt with same problems enhances coping, may promote cooperation with therapeutic regimen and long-term positive recovery.

Reconstructive Facial Surgery (Intermaxillary Fixation, Facial Fractures)

PATIENT ASSESSMENT DATA BASE

EGO INTEGRITY

May report: Fear of outcome/appearance.

May exhibit: Increased tension; sympathetic stimulation.

FOOD/FLUID

May exhibit: Misalignment, asymmetry of jaw; malocclusion of teeth.
Facial edema.
Mastication, swallowing problems.

NEUROSENSORY

May report: Changes in vision, e.g., double vision (diplopia) if fracture extends into orbit.

May exhibit: Unequal eye movement, loss of peripheral vision.

PAIN/COMFORT

May report: Facial discomfort/pain.

May exhibit: Guarding affected area.
Altered facial muscle tone, generalized muscle tension.

RESPIRATION

May exhibit: Tachypnea; shallow, rapid or labored respirations.
Interference with airway patency (misalignment of mandible, swelling of oral tissues).
Presence of foreign materials, e.g., broken dentures/teeth, vomitus, external debris.
Crepitus in face/neck.

SAFETY

May report: Trauma deformities: recent injury to bony framework, cartilaginous structures, and soft tissues (bruising, lacerations, edema).

TEACHING/LEARNING

May report: Family/personal history of diabetes, keloid formation.

Discharge Plan Considerations: May require assistance with food preparation/dietary intake.

DIAGNOSTIC STUDIES

Facial x-rays: reveal extent of fracture(s).

NURSING PRIORITIES

1. Assure patent airway.
2. Prevent complications.
3. Assist patient to develop realistic expectations/adjust to altered appearance.
4. Provide information about procedure(s)/prognosis and treatment needs.

DISCHARGE CRITERIA

1. Airway patent.
2. Complications/infection minimized/prevented.
3. Anxiety reduced and patient dealing realistically with situation.
4. Surgical procedure/prognosis and therapeutic regimen understood.

Refer to CP: Surgical Intervention, p. 789, for general considerations and additional nursing diagnoses as indicated.

NURSING DIAGNOSIS:	AIRWAY CLEARANCE, INEFFECTIVE [POTENTIAL]
May be related to:	Trauma to soft tissues/airway (surgery and/or injuries)
Possibly evidenced by:	[Not applicable; presence of signs and symptoms establishes an *actual* diagnosis.]
PATIENT OUTCOMES/ EVALUATION CRITERIA:	Maintains/regains patency of airway with normal respiratory pattern, breath sounds clear and noiseless, and aspiration prevented. Demonstrates behaviors to improve/maintain patent airway/dispose of secretions.

ACTIONS/INTERVENTIONS	RATIONALE
Independent	
Elevate head of bed.	Promotes drainage of secretions, reduces edema formation, enhances venous/lymphatic drainage and risk of aspiration.
Observe respiratory rate, rhythm. Note use of accessory muscles, nasal flaring, crowing respirations/stridor, hoarseness.	May indicate impending respiratory failure. Trauma to soft tissue and bone usually produces marked edema of facial tissue, which may develop to its maximum 24 hours after the trauma/surgery.
Examine mouth for swelling, discoloration, accumulation of oral secretions or blood. Encourage patient to "push" secretions through clamped jaw. Suction as necessary/teach patient self-suctioning techniques.	Careful examination is required because bleeding may be "hidden" in the loose tissue in this area. Removal of material keeps the airway clear, reduces risk of aspiration.
Note patient's complaint of increasing dysphagia, high-pitched cough, wheezing, facial tissue edema.	May indicate soft tissue swelling in the posterior pharynx.
Monitor vital signs and changes in mentation.	Tachycardia, increasing restlessness may indicate developing hypoxia/respiratory compromise.
Auscultate breath sounds.	Presence of wheezes/rhonchi suggests retained secretions, indicating need for more aggressive intervention.
Assess color of nailbeds, fingers/toes.	Helpful in determining adequacy of oxygenation. Note: Face may appear dusky because of venous congestion, rather than hypoxia.
Apply ice bags to operative area as indicated.	Reduces edema/tissue congestion.
Reposition periodically and encourage deep breathing.	Promotes ventilation of all lung segments and mobilization of secretions, reducing risk of atelectasis, pneumonia.
Let patient know he or she will be carefully observed and needs will be met promptly.	May feel fearful about choking or suffocating because of wires.

Independent

Encourage fluid intake of at least 2–3 l/day as possible. Avoid carbonated beverages.

Liquefies oral/respiratory secretions to enhance expectoration. Carbonated beverages "foam" in the oropharynx area and may be difficult for patient to handle, compromising airway.

Tend closely when patient is vomiting or taking fluids/food.

Provides reassurance and allows for prompt intervention if problems arise.

Keep wirecutters/scissors at bedside. Be sure care giver knows which wires to cut.

When the jaw is wired, there are usually two to six major wires/bands that may need cutting to release the jaw and open the airway.

Collaborative

Provide humidified air or oxygen by face tent.

Reduces congestion, moisturizes mucous membranes, liquefies secretions. Supplemental oxygen may improve oxygenation/correct hypoxia.

Maintain NPO and patency of NG tube if used.

Reduces risk of vomiting/regurgitation and aspiration.

Administer antiemetics, e.g., hydroxyzine (Vistaril) as indicated.

Used to prevent vomiting, which may obstruct the airway/cause aspiration.

Assist with procedures as needed:

    Insertion/maintenance of Penrose drains/Hemovacs;

Hematoma/drainage in area may need evacuation if swelling is compromising airway.

    Tracheostomy.

May be needed when airway is threatened by swelling/major facial reconstruction.

NURSING DIAGNOSIS:	TISSUE INTEGRITY, IMPAIRED
May be related to:	Tissue trauma/damage, preexisting injury/intraoperative manipulation
	Mechanical factors (fixation devices)
	Altered circulation
	Nutritional deficit
Possibly evidenced by:	Edema
	Hematoma, ecchymotic areas
	Erythema, inflammation
	Delayed healing
PATIENT OUTCOMES/ EVALUATION CRITERIA:	Displays timely healing of incisional areas without complications.
	Demonstrates behaviors to promote healing.

Independent

Remind patient (in immediate postoperative period) about fixation devices and that mouth cannot be

Individual coming out of anesthesia may feel panic when cannot open mouth, and struggle to do so can

ACTIONS/INTERVENTIONS	RATIONALE

Independent

opened.

Monitor facial edema. Assess skin/tissue color and temperature around/under dressings. Observe for oral and facial bleeding, drainage. Apply ice packs, maintain pressure dressings to face (when used).

be damaging.

Vascular nature of tissues increases risk of hemorrhage. Ice packs, pressure dressings may be used (12–24 hours) to limit edema formation, but dressings may need to be loosened to prevent compromising circulation to tissues.

Cleanse mouth frequently with lukewarm saline or dilute peroxide solutions, especially after each feeding.

Promotes healing by reducing risk of infection, keeping suture line intact.

Use WaterPik (low-pressure spray) or soft bristled, child sized toothbrush to cleanse area. Brush teeth and gums, around arch bars, other fixation devices.

Removes debris, food particles, reducing risk of inflammation/tissue deterioration, especially of gums.

Avoid use of sponge/cotton-tipped applicators for mouth care and use of lemon–glycerine or commercial mouthwash preparations.

Fibers may lodge under wires, between teeth and irritate fragile tissues. Products containing alcohol are drying to mucous membranes.

Apply bees/dental wax to ends of wires. Instruct patient to remove wax before eating or mouth care.

Protects buccal tissue from injury.

Provide local wound/pin site care if indicated.

Reduces risk of infection/osteomyelitis when wire or pin fixation is used to stabilize facial fractures.

Inspect mouth/sutures. Observe for development of erythema, inflammation, and drainage/ulcerations around gum/suture line. Avoid disturbing sutures.

Early identification and treatment of localized infection can prevent more serious complications, e.g., bacteremia, osteomyelitis, brain infection.

Note continuance or increase in pain, development of throbbing pain; presence of opaque/odoriferous drainage.

May indicate infection. Any jaw fracture involving a tooth-bearing portion is considered a compound fracture, even when there is no break in the soft tissue, because a tooth acts to allow communication between the mouth and the fracture that may lead to infection. This may lead to the development of gangrene (even gas gangrene) or abscess formation that may involve the oropharynx and endanger airway patency.

Do neurologic checks as indicated, noting changes in mentation, increased complaints of headache, onset of fever. Note rhinorrhea, otorrhea. (Refer to CP: Craniocerebral Trauma, p. 226.)

May indicate meningeal irritation/brain infection as a complication of facial fractures or localized infection. When head injuries have occurred concurrently with facial injuries, cerebrospinal fluid leak indicates communication between brain and outside, predisposing to meningitis.

Collaborative

Monitor Hct/Hb, clotting studies.

Influences healing; abnormalities encourage bleeding and hematoma formation.

Apply topical ointments to suture lines if indicated, maintaining sterile technique.

May be used to reduce topical bacteria, which interfere with fine-line suture healing.

Administer IV/oral antimicrobials as indicated.

Reduces risk of/prevents local and systemic infection.

NURSING DIAGNOSIS:	COMMUNICATION, IMPAIRED: VERBAL
May be related to:	Wiring of jaws
	Edema of mouth and surrounding structures
	Pain of tissue/muscle movement

Possibly evidenced by:	Inability/reluctance to talk
PATIENT OUTCOMES/ EVALUATION CRITERIA:	Establishes method of communication in which needs can be expressed.

ACTIONS/INTERVENTIONS	RATIONALE

Independent

Determine extent of inability to communicate.	Type of injuries/individual situation will dictate needs for assistance.
Provide alternate means of communication, e.g., pencil and pad, magic slate, picture board. Place call light/bell where patient can reach it; answer promptly.	Enables patient to communicate needs/concerns, and reduces anxiety associated with being alone/unable to summon help.
Validate meaning of attempted communication. Maintain eye contact. Use "Yes" and "No," blink, etc.	Conveys interest in individual and desire to communicate, encouraging continued attempts.
Anticipate needs. Stop in frequently to check on patient.	Reduces anxiety and feelings of powerlessness.
Place notice at nurses' station and at bedside concerning communication needs and how they are met. Answer summons promptly.	Patient may not be able to enunciate clearly or obtain emergency/needed assistance.

NURSING DIAGNOSIS:	NUTRITION, ALTERED: LESS THAN BODY REQUIREMENTS [POTENTIAL]
May be related to:	Biologic factors (structural changes)
	Facial/tissue edema
	Inability to chew/swallow
	Anorexia
Possibly evidenced by:	[Not applicable; presence of signs and symptoms establishes an *actual* diagnosis.]
PATIENT OUTCOMES/ EVALUATION CRITERIA:	Maintains usual weight as individually appropriate with timely healing and free of signs of malnutrition.

ACTIONS/INTERVENTIONS	RATIONALE

Independent

Weigh as indicated.	Monitors weight loss and effectiveness of dietary program.
Provide ice chips, water, other beverages as soon as nausea subsides.	Maintains adequate fluid intake to prevent dehydration.
Recommend patient lean forward when ingesting food/fluid. Suggest serving each food in an individual container. Instruct patient in use of straw/feeding syringe as indicated. Provide small/frequent "meals" of acceptable consistency, such as puréed or semiliquid.	Facilitates swallowing and reduces risk of aspiration. Being able to identify various flavors adds to the pleasure of eating when patient is unable to masticate.
Avoid temperature extremes of "foods"/fluids.	Reduces risk of burning tender mucosal areas.

ACTIONS/INTERVENTIONS

Collaborative

Consult with dietitian to provide diet high in calories, vitamins, proteins, and dietary supplements as indicated.

Provide commercial supplements as indicated, e.g., Ensure.

RATIONALE

Adequate nutrition is important to promote healing and combat excessive weight loss (can reach 10–20 lb in short period of time). Patient/SO may need assistance in food choices/menu planning to meet individual dietary needs in view of difficulty with ingestion of nutrients.

Decreased energy/easy fatigability may lead to difficulty ingesting adequate nutrients, and use of these specially formulated products can enhance nutritional intake.

NURSING DIAGNOSIS:	COMFORT, ALTERED: PAIN, ACUTE
May be related to:	Presence of tissue and bone trauma, wires, edema
	Nasal congestion/inability to breathe through nose
	Immobility (jaw fixation)
Possibly evidenced by:	Complaints of pain
	Narrowed focus, grimacing, facial tension
	Sympathetic stimulation
PATIENT OUTCOMES/ EVALUATION CRITERIA:	Reports pain is relieved/controlled. Follows prescribed pharmacologic regimen. Demonstrates use of relaxation techniques.

ACTIONS/INTERVENTIONS

Independent

Assess type/location of pain on a 1–10 scale. Note response to medication.

Provide information about anticipated discomforts and relieving interventions.

Provide frequent oral hygiene, lubricate lips.

Examine mouth for loose or protruding wires. Apply dental wax to wire ends.

Maintain immobilization of facial fractures by appropriate means, e.g., nasal packing, wires, pins, etc.

Perform passive/active ROM to extremities/joints. Encourage position changes even when up in chair.

Provide routine comfort measures, e.g., backrub, diversional activities.

Allow time for expression of feelings, within level of ability to communicate.

RATIONALE

Useful in differentiating postoperative discomfort from developing complications, and in evaluating effectiveness of interventions.

Knowing what to expect can prevent surprises and resultant anxiety.

Reduces discomfort associated with dry mouth/pooled secretions.

May irritate or damage surrounding tissues. Wax protects buccal surface.

Maintains proper positioning and prevents undue stress on supporting musculature.

Reduces discomfort and stiffness, stimulates circulation that may be sluggish due to bedrest and areas of tissue edema.

Promotes relaxation and refocuses attention.

Expression of concerns/fears reduces anxiety/pain cycle.

ACTIONS/INTERVENTIONS

Independent

Encourage use of stress management techniques, e.g., deep breathing, visualization, diversional activities.

Collaborative

Administer medications as indicated:

    Analgesics;

    Nasal decongestants;

    Steroids, e.g., dexamethasone (Decadron).

Apply cold/warm compresses.

Provide supplemental humidification.

RATIONALE

Promotes relaxation, refocuses attention, may enhance coping ability, relieving pain.

May be needed to provide relief for pain/discomfort.

Helps relieve upper airway congestion/feeling of suffocation. Note: Must be used with caution or may be contraindicated because can reduce local blood supply needed for healing.

Reduces inflammatory response and tissue edema.

Cold is used initially to prevent/minimize edema formation. Heat enhances circulation, promoting resolution of edema.

Relieves discomfort of dry mucous membranes.

NURSING DIAGNOSIS:	**ANXIETY/FEAR [SPECIFY LEVEL]**
May be related to:	**Situational crisis**
	Perceived threat to self-concept/body image
	Perceived threat of death (choking/suffocation)
Possibly evidenced by:	**Increased tension, apprehension**
	Expressed concern regarding changes
	Fearfulness
	Sympathetic stimulation/restlessness
PATIENT OUTCOMES/ EVALUATION CRITERIA:	**Appears relaxed and reports anxiety reduced to manageable level. Acknowledges and discusses fears. Demonstrates appropriate range of feelings.**

ACTIONS/INTERVENTIONS

Independent

Discuss safety measures, e.g., suctioning secretions, use of wire cutters, suture cleansing. Place necessary articles within reach.

Encourage expression of fears, concerns.

Acknowledge reality/normality of feelings, including anger.

Give realistic explanation about altered facial appearance, possible nerve involvement, facial droop, un-

RATIONALE

Provides reassurance and reduces anxiety associated with unknown and/or fear of being alone (unsupervised).

Defines problem and influences choice of interventions.

Provides emotional support which can help patient through the initial adjustment as well as throughout recovery.

Providing honest information about what to expect will help patient/SO to accept and deal with situation more

ACTIONS/INTERVENTIONS

Independent

even smile, presence of circumoral numbness/tingling, altered taste sensation. Provide patient with mirror on request.

Encourage use of stress management, e.g, deep breathing, guided imagery, visualization.

RATIONALE

effectively. As edema resolves and healing occurs, alterations in facial nerve function may disappear.

Assists in refocusing attention, promotes relaxation, and may enhance coping ability.

NURSING DIAGNOSIS:	KNOWLEDGE DEFICIT [LEARNING NEED] (SPECIFY)
May be related to:	Lack of exposure/recall; information misinterpretation
	Unfamiliarity with information resources
Possibly evidenced by:	Questions, request for information, statement of misconception
	Inaccurate follow-through of instruction
	Development of preventable complications
PATIENT OUTCOMES/ EVALUATION CRITERIA:	Verbalizes understanding of condition/disease process, prognosis and treatment. Correctly performs necessary procedures and explains reasons for the actions.

ACTIONS/INTERVENTIONS

Independent

Review surgical procedure/prognosis and potential complications.

Instruct patient/SO to carry wire cutters at all times and to know which wire(s) to cut.

Review prescribed medications, e.g., vitamin supplements, stool softeners/mild laxatives, use of and cautions about decongestants as indicated.

Stress importance of medical follow-up.

Discuss signs/symptoms to report to health care giver, e.g., increased pain, edema, fever, halitosis/foul odor from mouth.

Recommend progressing diet as tolerated.

Review dietary needs. Identify high-calorie, low-fiber foods. Provide recipes for blenderized balanced meals. Suggest addition of spices after oral mucosa heals.

RATIONALE

Provides knowledge base on which informed choices about future care and outcome can be made.

Permits immediate intervention to maintain airway in case of emergency.

Reinforces information patient needs to promote optimal recuperation, and prevent untoward occurrences (including constipation from lack of dietary fiber). Decongestants may occasionally be used to decrease nasal congestion but are contraindicated in some facial fractures.

Necessary for evaluation of healing/jaw stabilization as well as presence of complications, e.g., oral fistula formation, jaw malalignment.

Prompt evaluation and intervention of developing infection reduces risk of more serious complications, e.g., sepsis, osteomyelitis, brain infection.

Muscle stiffness, dental malocclusion may delay capability for eating normal foods for a period of time (usually 5–6 weeks).

Promotes intake of adequate nutrients to meet metabolic needs, especially during time when weight loss is prevalent. Low-fiber foods reduce risk of materials lodging under fixation devices/between teeth and becoming a medium for growth of pathogenic micro-

ACTIONS/INTERVENTIONS	RATIONALE
Independent	
	organisms. Addition of spices, new recipes may improve appetite and make food more palatable.
Stress importance of good oral hygiene. Demonstrate use of WaterPik, dental wax.	Fixation devices usually remain in place 6–8 weeks and are associated with risk of local irritation, inflammation, and local/systemic infection.
Recommend avoidance of alcohol and alcohol-containing products, e.g., mouthwash, liquid decongestants.	Alcohol is drying and may cause irritation to oral mucosa. In addition, alcoholic beverages dull oral sensation and reflexes necessary to protect the airway.
Discuss activity limitations, e.g., swimming, boating, fishing, etc., until wires are removed.	Jaw fixation increases risk of aspiration/drowning, as well as potential for infection by bacteria in untreated water or tissue irritation from chlorine.
Suggest restricting/stopping smoking.	Can irritate mucosa and cause vasoconstriction, which may further impair circulation to involved tissues.

Upper Gastrointestinal/Esophageal Bleeding _____

Bleeding duodenal ulcer is the most frequent cause of massive upper GI hemorrhage, but bleeding may also occur because of gastric ulcers, gastritis, and esophageal varices. Severe vomiting can precipitate gastric bleeding due to a tear of the mucosa at the gastroesophageal junction (Mallory–Weiss syndrome). Stress ulcer can occur owing to severe burns, major trauma/surgery, or severe systemic disease. Esophagitis, esophageal/gastric carcinoma, hiatal hernia, hemophilia, leukemia, and DIC are less common causes of upper GI bleeding.

Generally, a patient with severe, active bleeding will be admitted directly to the critical care unit; however, a patient may develop GI bleeding on the medical/surgical unit or be admitted there with subacute bleeding.

PATIENT ASSESSMENT DATA BASE

ACTIVITY/REST

May report: Weakness, fatigue.

May exhibit: Tachycardia, tachypnea/hyperventilation (response to activity).

CIRCULATION

May exhibit: Hypotension (including postural).

Tachycardia, dysrhythmias (hypovolemia/hypoxemia).

Weak/thready peripheral pulse.

Capillary refill slow/delayed (vasoconstriction).

Skin color: pallor, cyanosis (depending on the amount of blood loss).

Skin/mucous membrane moisture: diaphoresis (reflecting shock state, acute pain, psychological response).

EGO INTEGRITY

May report: Acute or chronic stress factors (financial, relationship, job-related).

Feelings of helplessness.

May exhibit: Signs of anxiety, e.g., restlessness, pallor, diaphoresis, narrowed focus, trembling, quivering voice.

ELIMINATION

May report: History of previous hospitalizations for GI bleeding or related GI problems, e.g., peptic/gastric ulcer, gastritis, gastric surgery; irradiation of gastric area.

Change in usual bowel patterns/characteristics of stool.

May exhibit: Abdominal tenderness, distention.

Bowel sounds: often hyperactive during bleed, hypoactive after bleeding subsides.

Character of stool: diarrhea; dark bloody, tarry, or bright red stools; frothy, foul-smelling (steatorrhea).

Urine output: may be decreased.

FOOD/FLUID

May report: Anorexia, nausea, vomiting.

Problems swallowing; hiccups.

Heartburn, burping with sour taste, nausea/vomiting.

Food intolerances, e.g., spicy food, chocolate; special diet for preexisting ulcer disease.

May exhibit: Vomitus coffee ground, or bright red, with or without clots.

Mucous membranes dry, decreased mucous production, poor skin turgor (chronic bleeding).

Urine output decreased, concentrated, with increased specific gravity (hypovolemia).

NEUROSENSORY

May report: Fainting, dizziness/lightheadedness, weakness.

Mental status: level of consciousness may be altered, ranging from slight drowsiness, disorientation/confusion, to stupor and coma (dependent on circulating volume/oxygenation).

PAIN/COMFORT

May report: Pain sharp, sudden, excruciating or chronic, dull, burning, gnawing, occurring 1 or 2 to 4 hours after meals; more intense during night; excruciating pain can accompany perforation.

Heartburn, substernal burning relieved by eating, use of antacids, vomiting, etc.

Location: varies, depending on underlying cause, e.g., gastric ulcers: left to mid epigastric pain with radiation to back; duodenal ulcers: associated with right epigastric pain.

Precipitating factors: may be foods, smoking, ingestion of alcohol, use of certain drugs (salicylates, reserpine, antibiotics, motrin), psychologic stressors.

May exhibit: Facial grimacing, guarding of affected area, pallor, diaphoresis, narrowed focus.

SAFETY

May report: Drug allergies/sensitivities, e.g., acetylsalicylic acid (ASA).

May exhibit: Temperature elevation.

Spider angiomas, palmar erythema (reflecting cirrhosis/portal hypertension).

TEACHING/LEARNING

May report: Presence of risk factors:

Recent use of drugs: prescription/nonprescription/OTC drugs containing ASA, alcohol, steroids.

Current complaint may reveal admission for related (e.g., anemia) or unrelated (e.g., head trauma) diagnosis; intestinal flu or severe vomiting episode.

Longstanding health problems, e.g., cirrhosis, alcoholism, hepatitis; eating disorders.

Discharge Plan Considerations: May require changes in therapeutic/medication regimen.

DIAGNOSTIC STUDIES

Endoscopy: of esophagus, stomach, duodenum: key diagnostic test for upper GI bleeding, done to visualize site of bleeding/degree of tissue ulceration/injury.

Barium swallow with x-ray: done for differential diagnosis of cause/site of lesion.

Gastric analysis: may be done to determine presence of blood, assess secretory activity of gastric mucosa: e.g., increased hydrochloric acid indicative of duodenal ulcer; decreased or normal amount suggests gastric ulcer; enormous hypersecretion and acidity may reflect Zollinger–Ellison syndrome.

Angiography: GI vasculature may be reviewed if endoscopy is inconclusive or impractical.

Stools: testing for blood will be positive.

CBC: Hb/Hct: decreased levels occur within 6–24 hours after bleed.

WBC: may elevate, reflecting body's response to injury.

BUN: elevates within 24–48 hours as blood proteins are broken down in the gastrointestinal tract and kidney filtration is decreased.

Creatinine: usually not elevated if renal perfusion is maintained.

Ammonia: may be elevated when severe liver dysfunction disrupts the metabolism and proper excretion of urea or when massive whole blood transfusions have been given.

Coagulation profile: increased platelets and decreased clotting times may be noted, reflecting the body's attempt to restore hemostasis. Severe abnormalities may reveal coagulopathy, e.g., DIC, as cause of bleed.

ABGs: may reveal initial respiratory alkalosis (compensating for diminished blood flow through lungs). Later, metabolic acidosis develops in response to sluggish liver flow/accumulation of metabolic waste products.

Sodium: may be elevated as a hormonal compensation to conserve body fluid.

Potassium: may initially be depleted because of massive gastric emptying or bloody diarrhea. Elevated potassium levels may occur after multiple transfusions of stored blood or with acute renal impairment.

NURSING PRIORITIES

1. Control hemorrhage.
2. Achieve/maintain hemodynamic stability.
3. Promote stress reduction.
4. Provide information about disease process/prognosis, treatment needs, and potential complications.

DISCHARGE CRITERIA

1. Hemorrhage curtailed.
2. Hemodynamic stability maintained.
3. Anxiety/fear reduced to manageable level.
4. Disease process/prognosis, therapeutic regimen, and potential complications understood.

NURSING DIAGNOSIS:	FLUID VOLUME DEFICIT, ACTUAL 2
May be related to:	**Active loss (hemorrhage)**
Possibly evidenced by:	**Hypotension, tachycardia, delayed capillary refill**
	Changes in mentation, restlessness
	Concentrated/decreased urine, pallor, diaphoresis
PATIENT OUTCOMES/ EVALUATION CRITERIA:	**Demonstrates improved fluid balance as evidenced by individually adequate urinary output with normal specific gravity, stable vital signs, moist mucous membranes, good skin turgor, prompt capillary refill.**

ACTIONS/INTERVENTIONS	RATIONALE

Independent

Note characteristics of vomitus and/or drainage.	May be helpful in differentiating cause of gastric distress. Yellow-green (bile content) implies that the pylorus is open. Fecal content indicates bowel obstruction. Bright red blood signals recent or acute arterial bleeding, perhaps due to gastric ulceration; dark red blood may be old blood (retained in intestine) or venous bleeding from varices. Coffee-ground appearance is suggestive of partially digested blood from slowly oozing area. Undigested food indicates obstruction or gastric tumor.
Monitor vital signs; compare with patient's normal/previous readings. Take BP in sitting, lying, standing position when possible.	Changes in BP and pulse may be used for rough estimate of blood loss, (e.g., BP <90 mmHg, and pulse <110 suggests a 25% decrease in volume or approx-

ACTIONS/INTERVENTIONS	RATIONALE

Independent

Note patient's individual physiologic response to bleeding, e.g., changes in mentation, weakness, restlessness, anxiety; pallor, diaphoresis; tachypnea; temperature elevation.

Measure CVP, if available.

Monitor intake and output, and correlate with weight changes. Measure blood/fluid losses via emesis, gastric suction/lavage, and stools.

    Keep accurate record of subtotals of solutions/blood during replacement therapy.

Maintain bedrest; prevent vomiting and straining at stool. Schedule activities/provide undisturbed rest periods. Eliminate noxious stimuli.

Elevate head of bed during antacid gavage.

Note signs of renewed bleeding after cessation of initial bleeding.

Observe for secondary bleeding, e.g., nose/gums, oozing from puncture sites, appearance of ecchymotic areas following minimal trauma.

Provide clear/bland fluids when intake resumed. Avoid caffeinated beverages.

Collaborative

Administer fluids/blood as indicated:

    Fresh whole blood/packed red cells;

    Fresh frozen plasma (FFP) and/or platelets.

Insert/maintain large-bore NG tube in acute bleeding.

---

imately 1000 ml). Postural hypotension reflects a decrease in circulating volume.

Symptomatology may be useful in gauging severity/length of bleeding episode. Worsening of symptoms may reflect continued bleeding or inadequate fluid replacement.

Reflects circulating volume and cardiac response to bleeding and fluid replacement; e.g., CVP values between 5 and 20 cm H_2O usually reflect adequate volume.

Provides guidelines for fluid replacement.

Potential exists for overtransfusion of fluids, especially when volume expanders are given before blood transfusions.

Activity/vomiting increases intraabdominal pressure and can predispose to further bleeding.

Prevents gastric reflux, because aspiration of antacids can cause serious pulmonary complications.

Increased abdominal fullness/distention, nausea or renewed vomiting, and bloody diarrhea may indicate rebleeding.

Loss of/inadequate replacement of clotting factors may precipitate development of DIC.

More easily tolerated by irritated gastric mucosa. Caffeine stimulates hydrochloric acid production, possibly potentiating rebleeding.

Fluid replacement is dependent on degree of hypovolemia and duration of bleeding (acute or chronic). Volume expanders (albumin) may be infused until type and cross-match can be completed and blood transfusions begun. Approximately 80–90% of gastric bleeding is controlled by fluid resuscitation and medical management.

Fresh whole blood is indicated for acute bleeding (with shock), because stored blood may be deficient in clotting factors. Packed cells may be adequate for stable patients with subacute/chronic bleeding and are required for patients with CHF, to prevent fluid overload.

Clotting factors/components are depleted by two mechanisms: hemorrhagic loss and the clotting process at the site of bleeding. Fresh frozen plasma is an excellent source of clotting factors. Platelet replacement may potentiate formation of platelet plug at injury sites.

Removes irritating gastric secretions, blood, and clots; reduces nausea/vomiting; and facilitates diagnostic

ACTIONS/INTERVENTIONS

Collaborative

Perform gastric lavage with cold or room-temperature saline until aspirate is light pink or clear and free of clots.

Administer medications, as indicated:

    Cimetidine (Tagamet), ranitidine (Zantac);

    Antacids, e.g., Amphojel, Maalox, Mylanta, Riopan;

    Belladonna; atropine;

    Vasopressin (Pitressin);

    Phenobarbital;

    Antiemetics, e.g., metoclopramide (Reglan), prochlorperazine (Compazine);

    Supplemental vitamin B_{12};

    Antibiotics.

Monitor laboratory studies, e.g.:

    Hb, Hct, RBC count;

    BUN/creatinine levels.

Assist with/prepare for:

    Sclerotherapy:

    Electrocoagulation or photocoagulation (laser) therapy;

RATIONALE

endoscopy. Note: Blood remaining in the stomach/intestines will be broken down into ammonia, which can produce a toxic CNS effect, e.g., encephalopathy.

Removes clots and may reduce bleeding by local vasoconstriction. Facilitates visualization by endoscopy to locate bleeding source. Note: Some research suggests that iced saline may not be any more effective than room temperature solution in controlling bleeding, and may actually damage gastric mucosa.

Histamine H_2-blockers reduce gastric acid production, increase gastric pH, and reduce irritation to gastric mucosa.

Antacids (administered orally or by gavage) may be given to maintain gastric pH level at 4.5 or higher to reduce risk of rebleeding. Antacids block the gastric absorption of oral histamine antagonists and therefore should not be administered within 1 hour after oral administration of histamine blockers.

Anticholinergics may be used to decrease gastric motility, particularly in peptic ulcer disease after acute bleeding has subsided.

Administration of intraarterial vasocontrictors may be needed in severe, prolonged bleeding (varices).

Mild sedatives may be given to promote rest, reduce intensity of bleeding, and alleviate pain. Note: Use with caution to avoid masking signs of developing hypovolemia.

Alleviates nausea and prevents vomiting.

In diffuse atrophic gastritis, the intrinsic factor necessary for B_{12} absorption from the GI tract is not secreted and individual may develop pernicious anemia.

May be used when infection is the cause of gastritis.

Aids in establishing blood replacement needs and monitoring effectiveness of therapy, e.g., 1 unit of whole blood should raise Hct 2–3%. Levels may initially remain stable, due to loss of both plasma and RBCs.

BUN > 40 with normal creatinine level indicates major bleeding. BUN should return to patient's normal level approximately 12 hours after bleeding has ceased.

Injection of an irritating (sclerosing) agent into esophageal varices (to create thrombosis) may be performed to prevent recurrence after initial bleed is controlled.

Provides direct coagulation of bleeding sites.

Collaborative

Surgical intervention.

Total/partial gastrectomy, pyloroplasty, and/or vagotomy may be required to control/prevent future gastric bleeding. Shunt procedures may be done to divert blood flow and reduce pressure within esophageal vessels when other measures fail. (Refer to CP: Cirrhosis, p. 479.)

NURSING DIAGNOSIS:	TISSUE PERFUSION, ALTERED: (SPECIFY) [POTENTIAL]
May be related to:	Hypovolemia
Possibly evidenced by:	[Not applicable; presence of signs and symptoms establishes an *actual* diagnosis.]
PATIENT OUTCOMES/ EVALUATION CRITERIA:	Maintains/improves tissue perfusion as evidenced by stabilized vital signs, warm skin, palpable peripheral pulses, ABGs within patient norms, adequate urine output.

Independent

Investigate changes in level of consciousness, complaints of dizziness/headache.

Changes may reflect inadequate cerebral perfusion as a result of reduced arterial blood pressure. Note: Changes in sensorium may also reflect elevated ammonia levels/hepatic encephalophathy in patient with liver disease. (Refer to CP: Cirrhosis of the Liver, p. 479.)

Investigate complaints of chest pain. Note location, quality, duration, and what relieves pain.

May reflect cardiac ischemia related to decreased perfusion. Note: Impaired oxygenation status resulting from blood loss can bring on MI in patient with cardiac disease.

Auscultate apical pulse. Monitor cardiac rate/rhythm if continuous ECG available.

Dysrhythmias and ischemic changes can occur as a result of hypotension, hypoxia, acidosis, electrolyte imbalance, or cooling near the heart if cold saline lavage is used to control bleeding.

Assess skin for coolness, pallor, diaphoresis, delayed capillary refill, and weak, thready peripheral pulses.

Vasoconstriction is a sympathetic response to lowered circulating volume and/or may occur as side effect of vasopressin administration.

Note urinary output and specific gravity.

Decreased systemic perfusion may cause kidney ischemia/failure manifested by decreased urine output. Acute tubular necrosis (ATN) may develop if hypovolemic state is prolonged. (Refer to CP: Renal Failure: Acute, p. 544.)

Note complaints of abdominal pain, especially sudden, severe pain, or pain radiating to shoulder.

Pain caused by gastric ulcer is often relieved after acute bleeding because of buffering effects of blood. Continued severe or sudden pain may reflect ischemia due to vasoconstrictive therapy, bleeding into biliary tract (hematobilia), or indicate perforation/onset of peritonitis. (Refer to CP: Peritonitis, p. 449.)

ACTIONS/INTERVENTIONS

Independent

Observe skin for pallor, redness. Massage with lotion. Change position frequently.

Collaborative

Provide supplemental oxygen if indicated.

Monitor ABGs/pulse oximetry.

Administer IV fluids as indicated.

RATIONALE

Compromised peripheral circulation increases risk of skin breakdown.

Treats hypoxemia and lactic acidosis during acute bleed.

Identifies hypoxemia, effectiveness of/need for therapy.

Maintains circulating volume and perfusion. Note: Use of Ringer's lactate may be contraindicated in presence of hepatic failure because metabolism of lactate is impaired, and lactic acidosis may develop.

NURSING DIAGNOSIS:	FEAR/ANXIETY [SPECIFY LEVEL]
May be related to:	Change in health status, threat of death
Possibly evidenced by:	Increased tension, restlessness, irritability, fearfulness
	Trembling, tachycardia, diaphoresis
	Lack of eye contact, focus on self
	Withdrawal, panic or attack behavior
PATIENT OUTCOMES/ EVALUATION CRITERIA:	Verbalizes appropriate range of feelings. Appears relaxed and reports anxiety is reduced to a manageable level.

ACTIONS/INTERVENTIONS

Independent

Monitor physiologic responses, e.g., tachypnea, palpitations, dizziness, headache, tingling sensations.

Note behavioral clues, e.g., restlessness, irritability, lack of eye contact, combativeness/attack behavior.

Encourage verbalization of fear and anxiety; provide feedback.

Acknowledge that this is a fearful situation and that others have expressed similar fears. Assist patient in expressing feelings by active listening.

Provide accurate, concrete information about what is being done, e.g., sensations to expect, usual procedures undertaken.

Provide a calm, restful environment.

RATIONALE

May be indicative of the degree of fear patient is experiencing, but may also be related to physical condition/ shock state.

Indicators of degree of fear patient is experiencing; e.g., patient may feel out of control of the situation or reach a state of panic.

Establishes a therapeutic relationship. Assists the patient in dealing with feelings and provides opportunity to clarify misconceptions.

When patient is expressing own fear, the validation that these feelings are normal can help patient to feel less isolated.

Involves patient in plan of care and decreases unnecessary anxiety about unknowns.

Removing patient from outside stressors promotes relaxation, may enhance coping skills.

ACTIONS/INTERVENTIONS

Independent

Make arrangements for SO to be with patient. Respond to call signal promptly. Use touch and eye contact as appropriate.

Encourage SO to project caring, concerned attitude and maintain communication with patient.

Demonstrate relaxation techniques, e.g., visualization, deep breathing exercises, guided imagery.

Help the patient to identify and initiate positive coping behaviors used successfully in past.

Encourage and support patient in evaluation of lifestyle.

Collaborative

Administer medications as indicated, e.g.:

Diazepam (Valium), clorazepate (Tranxene), alprazolam (Xanax).

Refer to psychiatric nurse/social services/spiritual advisor.

RATIONALE

Helps reduce fear of going through a frightening experience alone.

Supportive manner is helpful and does not add to the stress of the patient. A significant support system assists in maintaining healthful behaviors.

Learning ways to relax can be helpful in reducing fear and anxiety. As the patient with GI bleeding is often a person with type A personality who has difficulty relaxing, learning these skills can be important to recovery and prevention of recurrence.

Successful behaviors can be fostered in dealing with current fear, enhancing patient's sense of self-control, and providing reassurance.

Changes may be necessary to avoid recurrence of ulcer condition.

Sedatives/tranquilizers may be used on occasion to reduce anxiety and promote rest, particularly in the ulcer patient.

May need additional assistance during recovery to deal with consequences of emergency situation/adjustments to required/desired changes in lifestyle. (Refer to CP: Psychosocial Aspects of Acute Care, p. 773.)

NURSING DIAGNOSIS:	COMFORT, ALTERED: PAIN, ACUTE/CHRONIC
May be related to:	Chemical burn of gastric mucosa, oral cavity
	Physical response, e.g., reflex muscle spasm in the stomach wall
Possibly evidenced by:	Communication of pain descriptors
	Abdominal guarding, rigid body posture, facial grimacing
	Autonomic responses, e.g., changes in vital signs (acute pain)
PATIENT OUTCOMES/ EVALUATION CRITERIA:	Verbalizes relief of pain. Demonstrates relaxed body posture and is able to sleep/rest appropriately.

ACTIONS/INTERVENTIONS

Independent

Note complaints of pain, including location, duration, intensity (1–10 scale).

RATIONALE

Pain is not always present, but if present, should be compared with patient's previous pain symptoms,

ACTIONS/INTERVENTIONS	RATIONALE

Independent

which may assist in diagnosis of etiology of bleeding, development of complications.

Review factors that aggravate or alleviate pain.

Helpful in establishing diagnosis and treatment needs.

Note nonverbal pain cues, e.g., restlessness, reluctance to move, abdominal guarding, tachycardia, diaphoresis. Investigate discrepancies between verbal and nonverbal cues.

Nonverbal cues may be both physiologic and psychologic and may be used in conjunction with verbal cues to identify extent/severity of the problem.

Provide small frequent meals as indicated for individual patient. Identify and limit foods that create discomfort.

Has an acid neutralizing effect, as well as diluting the gastric contents. Small meals prevent distention and the release of gastrin.

Assist with active/passive ROM exercises.

Reduces joint stiffness, minimizing pain/discomfort.

Provide frequent oral care and routine comfort measures, e.g., backrub, position change.

Halitosis from stagnant oral secretions are unappetizing and aggravate nausea. Gingivitis and dental problems may arise.

Collaborative

Provide and implement prescribed dietary modifications.

Patient may be NPO initially. When oral intake is allowed, food choices will depend on the diagnosis and etiology of the bleed.

Use regular rather than skim milk, if milk and antacid regimen is used.

Fat in regular milk decreases gastric secretions while the calcium in skim milk increases them.

Administer medications, as indicated, e.g.:

Analgesics, e.g., morphine sulfate,

May be narcotic of choice to relieve acute/severe pain and reduce peristaltic activity. Note: Demerol has been associated with increased incidence of nausea/vomiting.

Acetaminophen (Tylenol);

Promotes comfort and rest.

Antacids;

Decreases gastric acidity by absorption or by chemical neutralization. Evaluate type of antacid in regard to total health picture, e.g., sodium restriction.

Anticholinergics, e.g., belladonna, atropine.

May be given at bedtime to decrease gastric motility, suppress acid production, delay gastric emptying, and alleviate nocturnal pain associated with gastric ulcer.

NURSING DIAGNOSIS:	**KNOWLEDGE DEFICIT [LEARNING NEED] (SPECIFY)**
May be related to:	**Lack of information/recall**
	Unfamiliarity with information resources
	Information misinterpretation
Possibly evidenced by:	**Verbalization of the problem, request for information, statement of misconceptions**
	Inaccurate follow-through of instructions
	Development of preventable complications
PATIENT OUTCOMES/ EVALUATION CRITERIA:	**Verbalizes understanding of cause of own bleeding episode (if known) and treatment modalities used. Begins**

to discuss own role in preventing recurrence. Identifies necessary lifestyle changes and participates in treatment regimen.

ACTIONS/INTERVENTIONS	RATIONALE
Independent	
Determine patient perception of cause of bleeding.	Establishes knowledge base and provides some insight into how the teaching plan needs to be constructed for this individual.
Provide/review information regarding etiology of bleeding, cause/effect relationship of lifestyle behaviors and ways to reduce risk/contributing factors. Encourage questions.	Provides knowledge base on which patient can make informed choices/decisions about future and control of health problems.
Assist patient to identify relationship of food intake and precipitation of/or relief from epigastric pain, including avoidance of gastric irritants, e.g., caffeine, alcohol, fruit juices, carbonated beverages, smoking, extremely hot, cold, or spicy foods.	Caffeine and smoking stimulate gastric acidity. Alcohol contributes to erosion of gastric mucosa. Individuals may find that certain foods/fluids increase gastric secretion and pain.
Recommend small frequent meals/snacks, chew food slowly, eating at regular time and avoid "skipping" meals.	Frequent eating keeps HCl neutralized, dilutes stomach contents to minimize action of acid on gastric mucosa.
Stress importance of reading labels on OTC drugs and avoiding drugs containing aspirin or switching to enteric-coated aspirin.	Aspirin damages the protective mucosa, permitting gastric erosion, ulceration, and bleeding to occur.
Review significance of signs/symptoms such as coffee-ground emesis, tarry stools, abdominal distention, severe epigastric/abdominal pain radiating to shoulder/back.	Prompt immediate medical evaluation/intervention is required to prevent more serious complications, e.g., perforation, Zollinger–Ellison syndrome.
Support use of stress management techniques, avoidance of emotional stress.	Decreases extrinsic stimulation of HCl, reducing risk of recurrence of bleeding.
Review drug regimen and possible side effects.	Helpful to patient's understanding of reason for taking drugs, and what symptoms are important to report to health care giver.
Collaborative	
Refer to support groups/counseling for lifestyle/behavior changes/reduction of associated risk factors, e.g., substance abuse/stop smoking clinics.	Alcohol users have a higher incidence of gastritis/esophageal varices, and cigarette smoking is associated with peptic ulcers and delayed healing.

Subtotal Gastrectomy/Gastric Resection _____

Indicated for gastric hemorrhage/intractable ulcers, pyloric obstruction, perforation, cancer.
Refer to CPs: Upper Gastrointestinal/Esophageal Bleeding, p. 397; Intestinal Surgery, p. 436; Surgical Intervention, p. 789.

NURSING PRIORITIES

1. Promote healing and adequate nutritional intake.
2. Prevent complications.
3. Provide information about surgical procedure/prognosis, treatment needs and concerns.

DISCHARGE CRITERIA

1. Nutritional intake adequate for individual needs.
2. Complications prevented/minimized.
3. Surgical procedure/prognosis, therapeutic regimen and long-term needs understood.

NURSING DIAGNOSIS:	NUTRITION, ALTERED: LESS THAN BODY REQUIRE-MENTS [POTENTIAL]
May be related to:	Restriction of fluids and food
	Change in digestive process/absorption of nutrients
Possibly evidenced by:	[Not applicable; presence of signs and symptoms establishes an *actual* diagnosis.]
PATIENT OUTCOMES/ EVALUATION CRITERIA:	Maintains stable weight/demonstrates progressive weight gain toward goal with normalization of laboratory values and free of signs of malnutrition. Verbalizes understanding of functional changes. Identifies necessary interventions/behaviors to maintain appropriate weight.

ACTIONS/INTERVENTIONS	RATIONALE
Independent	
Maintain patency of NG tube. *Do not* reposition tube if it becomes dislodged.	Provides rest for gastrointestinal tract during acute postoperative phase until return of normal function. Note: Even though gastric distention may cause stress on the sutures/possible rupture of stump (Billroth II), the tube needs to be repositioned by the physician to prevent injury to the operative area.
Note character and amount of gastric drainage.	Will be bloody for first 12 hours, and then should clear/turn greenish. Continued/recurrent bleeding suggests complications. Decline in output may reflect progression of fluid through the GI tract, suggesting return of function.
Caution the patient to limit the intake of ice chips.	Excessive intake of ice will increase washout of electrolytes via the NG tube.
Provide oral hygiene on a regular, frequent basis, including petroleum jelly for lips.	Prevents discomfort of dry mouth and cracked lips caused by fluid restriction and the NG tube.

ACTIONS/INTERVENTIONS	RATIONALE

Independent

Auscultate for bowel sounds and note passage of flatus.

Peristalsis can be expected to return about the third postoperative day, signaling readiness to resume oral intake.

Monitor tolerance to fluid and food intake, note abdominal distention, complaints of pain/cramping, nausea, vomiting.

Complications of paralytic ileus, obstruction and gastric dilatation may occur, possibly requiring reinsertion of NG tube.

Avoid the use of milk (high-carbohydrate foods) in the diet.

May trigger dumping syndrome. (Refer to ND: Knowledge Deficit [Learning Need] (Specify), following.)

Weigh regularly and continue after discharge.

Provides information about adequacy of dietary intake/determination of nutritional needs.

Collaborative

Administer IV fluids, hyperalimentation as indicated.

Meets fluid/nutritional needs until oral intake can be resumed. (Refer to CP: Total Nutritional Support, p. 789.)

Monitor laboratory studies, e.g., Hb/Hct and electrolytes.

Indicators of fluid/nutritional needs, effectiveness of therapy and detects developing complications.

Progress diet as tolerated, advancing from clear liquid to bland diet with several small feedings.

Usually NG tube is clamped for specified periods of time when peristalsis returns, to determine tolerance. Often NG tube is removed, intake is advanced gradually to prevent gastric irritation/distention.

Administer medications as indicated:

Anticholinergics, e.g., atropine, propantheline bromide (Pro-Banthine);

Controls dumping syndrome, enhancing digestion and absorption of nutrients.

Fat-soluble vitamin supplements, including B_{12}, calcium;

Removal of the stomach prevents absorption (due to loss of intrinsic factor) and can lead to pernicious anemia. In addition, rapid emptying of the stomach reduces absorption of calcium.

Iron preparations;

Corrects/prevents iron deficiency anemia.

Protein supplements;

Additional protein may be helpful for tissue repair and healing.

Pancreatic enzymes, bile salts;

Enhances digestive process.

Medium chain triglycerides (MCT).

Promotes absorption of fats and fat-soluble vitamins.

NURSING DIAGNOSIS:	KNOWLEDGE DEFICIT [LEARNING NEED] (SPECIFY)
May be related to:	Lack of exposure/recall, information misinterpretation
	Unfamiliarity with information resources
Possibly evidenced by:	Questions, statement of misconception
	Inaccurate follow-through of instruction
	Development of preventable complications
PATIENT OUTCOMES/ EVALUATION CRITERIA:	Verbalizes understanding of procedure, disease process/ prognosis, treatment. Correctly performs necessary procedures, explaining reasons for actions.

ACTIONS/INTERVENTIONS	RATIONALE

Independent

Review surgical procedure and long-term expectations.

Provides knowledge base from which informed choices can be made. Recovery following gastric surgery is often slower than may be anticipated with similar types of surgery. Improved strength and partial normalization of dietary pattern may not be evident for up to 3 months, and full return to usual intake (3 "normal" meals/day) may take up to 12 months. This prolonged convalescence may be difficult for the patient/SO to deal with if they have not been prepared.

Discuss and identify stress situations and how to avoid them. Investigate job-related issues.

Can alter gastric motility interfering with optimal digestion. Note: Patient may require vocational counseling if change in employment is indicated. (Refer to CP: Psychosocial Aspects of Acute Care, p. 773.)

Review dietary needs/regimen (e.g., low carbohydrate, high-fat, high-protein) and importance of maintaining vitamin supplementation.

May prevent deficiencies, enhances healing and promotes cooperation with therapy. Note: Low-fat diet may be required to reduce risk of alkaline reflux gastritis.

Discuss the importance of eating small frequent meals, slowly and in a relaxed atmosphere, resting after meals; avoiding temperature extremes of food; restricting high-fiber foods, caffeine, milk products and alcohol, high intake of sugars and salt; taking fluids between meals, rather than with food.

These measures can be helpful in avoiding gastric distention/stress on surgical repair, occurrence of dumping syndrome and hypoglycemic reactions as well as preventing gastric irritation to reduce incidence of recurrence of peptic ulcers. Note: Ice-cold fluids/foods can cause gastric spasms.

Instruct in avoiding fibrous foods and necessity of chewing food well.

Remaining gastric tissue may not be able to digest such foods as citrus skins and seeds and these may collect and form a mass (phytobezoar formation), which is not excreted.

Recommend foods containing pectin, e.g., citrus fruits, bananas, apples, yellow vegetables and beans.

Increased intake of these foods may reduce incidence of dumping syndrome.

Identify foods that can cause gastric irritation, increased gastric acid production, e.g., chocolate, spicy foods, whole grains, raw vegetables.

Limiting/avoiding these foods reduces risk of gastric bleeding/ulceration based on individual response/tolerance. Note: Ingestion of fresh fruits to reduce risk of dumping syndrome should be tempered with adverse effect of gastric irritation.

Identify symptoms that may indicate dumping syndrome, e.g., weakness, profuse perspiration, epigastric fullness, nausea/vomiting, abdominal cramping, faintness, flushing, explosive diarrhea and palpitations occurring within 15 minutes to 1 hour after eating.

Can cause severe discomfort even shock and reduces absorption of nutrients. Usually self-limiting (1–3 weeks after surgery) but may become chronic.

Discuss signs of hypoglycemia and corrective interventions, e.g., ingestion of cheese and crackers, orange/grape juice, candy.

Awareness helps patient to take actions to prevent progression of symptoms.

Review medications, purpose, dosage and schedule as well as possible side effects.

Understanding rationale/therapeutic needs can reduce risk of complications, e.g., anticholinergics/pectin powder may be given to reduce incidence of dumping syndrome; antacids/histamine antagonists reduce gastric irritation.

Caution patient to read labels and avoid products containing acetylsalicylic acid.

Can cause gastric irritation/bleeding.

Discuss reasons and importance of stopping smoking.

Smoking stimulates gastric acid production and may cause vasoconstriction compromising mucous membranes, increasing risk of gastric irritation/ulceration.

ACTIONS/INTERVENTIONS

Independent

Identify signs/symptoms requiring medical evaluation, e.g., persistent nausea/vomiting or abdominal fullness, weight loss, diarrhea, foul-smelling fatty or tarry stools; bloody or coffee-ground vomitus/presence of bile; fever. Instruct patient to report changes in pain characteristics.

Stress importance of regular checkup with health care provider.

RATIONALE

Prompt recognition and intervention may prevent serious consequences of potential complications such as pancreatitis, peritonitis, afferent loop syndrome.

Necessary to detect developing complications, e.g., anemia, problems with nutrition, and/or recurrence of disease.

Inflammatory Bowel Disease: Ulcerative Colitis, Crohn's Disease (Regional Enteritis, Ileocolitis) _____

Ulcerative colitis and regional enteritis share common symptoms but differ in the degree of severity and complications. Therefore, separate data bases are provided.

PATIENT ASSESSMENT DATA BASE

Ulcerative colitis (UC) usually starts in the rectum and distal portions of the colon and may spread upward to involve the sigmoid and descending colon or the entire colon. It is usually intermittent (acute exacerbation with long remissions), but some people have continuous symptoms (30–40%).

ACTIVITY/REST

May report: Weakness, fatigue, malaise, exhaustion.

Insomnia, not sleeping through the night because of diarrhea.

Feeling restless and anxious

CIRCULATION

May exhibit: Tachycardia (response to fever, dehydration, inflammatory process, and pain).

Bruising, ecchymotic areas (insufficient vitamin K).

Blood pressure: hypotension, including postural.

Skin/mucous membranes: poor turgor, dry; cracking of tongue (dehydration/malnutrition).

EGO INTEGRITY

May report: Anxiety, apprehension, emotional upsets, e.g., feelings of helplessness/hopelessness.

Acute/chronic stress factors, e.g., family/job-related, expense of treatment.

May exhibit: Withdrawal, narrowed focus, depression.

ELIMINATION

May report: Stool texture varying from soft-formed to mushy or watery.

Unpredictable, intermittent, frequent, uncontrollable episodes of diarrhea; sense of urgency/cramping (tenesmus), passing blood/pus/mucus with/without passing feces.

Rectal bleeding.

May exhibit: Diminished bowel sounds, absence of peristalsis or presence of visible peristalsis.

Hemorrhoids, anal fissures (25%); perianal fistula (less frequently than with Crohn's).

Oliguria.

FOOD/FLUID

May report: Anorexia; nausea/vomiting.

Weight loss.

Dietary intolerances/sensitivities, e.g., dairy products, fatty foods

May exhibit: Decreased subcutaneous fat/muscle mass.

Weakness, poor muscle tone and skin turgor.

Mucous membrane pale; sore, inflamed buccal cavity.

HYGIENE

May exhibit: Inability to maintain self-care.

Stomatitis reflecting vitamin deficiency.
Body odor.

PAIN/COMFORT

May report: Pain/tenderness in lower left quadrant (may be relieved with defecation).
Migratory joint pain, tenderness (arthritis).
Eye pain, photophobia (iritis).

May exhibit: Abdominal tenderness/distention.

SAFETY

May report: History of lupus erythematosus, hemolytic anemia, vasculitis.
Arthritis (worsening of symptoms with exacerbations in bowel disease).
Temperature elevation 104–105°F (acute exacerbation).
Skin lesions may be present; e.g., erythema nodosum (raised, tender, red, and swollen) on arms/legs.
Eye lesions, e.g., conjunctivitis/iritis with blurred vision.

SOCIAL INTERACTION

May report: Relationship/role problems related to condition.
Inability to be active socially.

TEACHING/LEARNING

May report: Family history of disease.

Discharge Plan Considerations: Assistance with dietary requirements, medication regimen, equipment (ostomy), psychologic support.

DIAGNOSTIC STUDIES

Stool specimens: mainly composed of mucus, blood, pus, and intestinal organisms, especially Entamoeba histolytica (active stage). (Stool examinations are used in initial diagnosis and in following disease progression.)

Proctosigmoidoscopy: visualizes ulcerations, edema, hyperemia, and inflammation (result of secondary infection of the mucosa and submucosa). Friability and hemorrhagic areas caused by necrosis and ulceration occur in 85% of these patients.

Cytology and rectal biopsy: differentiates between infectious process and carcinoma (occurs 10–20 times more often than in general population). Neoplastic changes can be detected, as well as characteristic inflammatory infiltrates called crypt abscesses.

Barium enema: may be performed after visual examination has been done, though rarely done during acute, relapsing stage, because it can exacerbate condition.

Colonoscopy: identifies adhesions, changes in luminal wall (narrowing/irregularity); rules out bowel obstruction.

CBC: may show hyperchromic anemia (active disease generally present due to blood loss and iron deficiency); leukocytosis may occur, especially in fulminating or complicated cases and in patients on steroid therapy.

Serum iron level: lowered due to blood loss.

Prothrombin time: prolonged in severe cases from altered factors VII and X caused by vitamin K deficiency.

Sedimentation rate (ESR): increased according to severity of disease.

Thrombocytosis: may occur due to inflammatory disease process.

Electrolytes: decreased potassium is common in severe disease.

Albumin level: decreased because of loss of plasma proteins/disturbed liver function.

Alkaline phosphatase: increased, along with serum cholesterol and hypoproteinemia, indicating disturbed liver function.

Bone marrow: a generalized depression is common in fulminating types/after a long inflammatory process.

PATIENT ASSESSMENT DATA BASE

Crohn's disease (regional enteritis; ileocolitis) may be found in portions of the alimentary tract from the mouth to the anus but is most commonly found in the small intestine (terminal ileum). It is a slowly progressive chronic disease with intermittent acute episodes.

ACTIVITY/REST

May report: Weakness, fatigue, malaise, exhaustion.
Feeling restless and anxious.

EGO INTEGRITY

May report: Anxiety, apprehension, emotional upsets, feelings of helplessness/hopelessness.
Acute/chronic stress factors, e.g., family/job-related, expense of treatment.

May exhibit: Withdrawal, narrowed focus, depression.

ELIMINATION

May report: Unpredictable, intermittent, frequent, uncontrollable episodes of diarrhea, soft or semi-liquid with flatus; foul-smelling and fatty (steatorrhea) stools; melena.

May exhibit: Hyperactive bowel sounds with gurgling, splashing sound (borborygmus).
Visible paristalsis.

FOOD/FLUID

May report: Anorexia; nausea/vomiting.
Weight loss.
Dietary intolerance/sensitivity, e.g., dairy products, fatty foods.

May exhibit: Decreased subcutaneous fat/muscle mass.
Weakness, poor muscle tone and skin turgor.
Mucous membrane pale.

HYGIENE

May exhibit: Inability to maintain self-care.
Body odor.

PAIN/COMFORT

May report: Tender abdomen with cramping pain in lower right quadrant; pain in mid lower abdomen (jejunal involvement).
Referred tenderness to periumbilical region.
Migratory joint pain, tenderness (arthritis).
Eye pain, photophobia (iritis).

May exhibit: Abdominal tenderness/distention.

SAFETY

May report: History of arthritis, lupus erythematosus, hemolytic anemia, vasculitis.
Temperature elevation (low-grade fever).
Perianal fissures, anorectal fistula.
Skin lesions may be present; erythema nodosum (raised tender, red swelling) on arms/legs.
Eye lesions, e.g., conjunctivitis/iritis with blurred vision.

SOCIAL INTERACTION

May report: Relationship/role problems related to condition.

Inability to be active socially.

TEACHING/LEARNING

May report: Family history of disease.

Discharge Plan Considerations: Assistance with dietary requirements, medication regimen, equipment (ostomy), psychologic support.

DIAGNOSTIC STUDIES

Stool examination: occult blood may be positive (mucosal erosion); steatorrhea and bile salts may be found.

X-rays: barium swallow may demonstrate luminal narrowing in the terminal ileum, stiffening of the bowel wall, mucosal irritability or ulceration.

Barium enema: Small bowel is nearly always involved but the rectal area is affected only 50% of the time. Fistulas are frequent and are usually found in the terminal ileum but may be present in segments throughout the GI tract.

Sigmoidoscopic examination: can demonstrate edematous hyperemic colon mucosa, transverse fissures, or longitudinal ulcers.

Endoscopy: provides visualization of involved areas.

CBC: anemia (hypochromic, occasionally macrocytic) may occur due to malnutrition or malabsorption or depressed bone marrow function (chronic inflammatory process); increased WBCs.

Sedimentation rate (ESR): increased reflecting inflammation.

Albumin/total protein: decreased.

Cholesterol: elevated (may have gallstones).

Serum iron-binding folic acid capacity: decreased due to chronic infection or secondary to blood loss.

Clotting studies: alterations may occur due to poor vitamin B_{12} absorption.

Electrolytes: decreased potassium chloride, calcium, and magnesium, with increased sodium.

Urine: hyperoxaluria (can cause kidney stones).

Urine culture: if Escherichia coli organisms are present, suspect fistula formation into the bladder.

NURSING PRIORITIES

1. Control diarrhea/promote optimal bowel function.
2. Minimize/prevent complications.
3. Minimize mental/emotional stress.
4. Provide information about disease process, treatment needs, and long-term aspects/potential complications of recurrent disease.

DISCHARGE CRITERIA

1. Bowel function stabilized.
2. Complications prevented/controlled.
3. Dealing positively with condition.
4. Disease process/prognosis, therapeutic regimen, and potential complications understood.

NURSING DIAGNOSIS:	BOWEL ELIMINATION, ALTERED: DIARRHEA
May be related to:	**Inflammation, irritation or malabsorption of the bowel**
	Toxins; segmental narrowing of the lumen
Possibly evidenced by:	**Increased bowel sounds/peristalsis**

Frequent, and often severe, watery stools (acute phase)

Changes in stool color

Abdominal pain; urgency (sudden painful need to defecate), cramping

**PATIENT OUTCOMES/
EVALUATION CRITERIA:** Reports reduction in frequency of stools, return to more normal stool consistency. Verbalizes understanding of causative factors and treatment rationale.

ACTIONS/INTERVENTIONS	RATIONALE
Independent	
Observe and record stool frequency, characteristics, amount, and precipitating factors.	Helps differentiate individual disease and assesses severity of episode.
Promote bedrest, provide bedside commode.	Rest decreases intestinal motility as well as reducing the metabolic rate when infection or hemorrhage is a complication. Defecation urges may occur without warning and be uncontrollable, increasing risk of incontinence/falls if facilities are not close at hand.
Remove stool promptly. Provide room deodorizers.	Reduces noxious odors to avoid undue patient embarrassment.
Identify foods and fluids that precipitate diarrhea, e.g., raw vegetables and fruits, whole-grain cereals, condiments, and carbonated drinks.	Avoidance of intestinal irritants promotes intestinal rest.
Restart oral fluid intake gradually. Offer clear liquids hourly; avoid cold fluids.	Provides colon rest by omitting or decreasing the stimulus of foods/fluids. Gradual resumption of liquids may prevent cramping and recurrence of diarrhea; however, cold fluids can increase intestinal motility.
Provide opportunity to vent frustrations related to disease process.	Presence of disease with unknown cause that is difficult to cure and surgical alternatives can lead to stress reactions that may aggravate condition.
Observe for fever, tachycardia, lethargy, leukocytosis, decreased serum protein, anxiety, and prostration.	May signify that toxic megacolon or perforation and peritonitis are imminent/have occurred necessitating immediate medical intervention.
Collaborative	
Administer medications as indicated:	
Anticholinergics, e.g., tincture of belladonna, atropine, diphenoxylate (Lomotil), anodyne suppositories;	Decreases GI motility/propulsion (peristalsis) and diminishes digestive secretions to relieve cramping and diarrhea.
Sulfasalazine (Azulfidine);	Prolongs remission and is used to treat mild/acute exacerbations.
Psyllium (Metamucil);	Absorbs water to increase bulk in stools, thereby decreasing diarrhea.
Cholestyramine (Questran);	Binds bile salts, reducing diarrhea that results from excess bile acid.
Steroids, e.g., ACTH, hydrocortisone, prednisolone (Delta-Cortef), prednisone (Deltasone);	Given to decrease inflammatory process. Note: Contraindicated in Crohn's if intraabdominal abscesses are suspected.
Azathioprine (Imuran);	Immunosuppressant may be given to block inflammatory response. May be given in conjunction with sulfasalazine.

415

Collaborative

Antacids;

Decreases gastric irritation, preventing inflammation and reducing risk of infection in colitis.

Enema (hydrocortisone), with/without suppository;

Steroid enemas may be given to aid absorption of the drug (may be given with atropine sulfate or belladonna suppository).

Antibiotics.

Treats local suppurative infections.

Assist with/prepare for surgical intervention.

May be necessary if perforation or bowel obstruction occurs or disease is unresponsive to medical treatment. (Refer to CP: Intestinal Surgery, p. 436.)

NURSING DIAGNOSIS:	FLUID VOLUME DEFICIT, POTENTIAL
May be related to:	**Excessive losses through normal routes (severe frequent diarrhea, vomiting)**
	Hypermetabolic state (inflammation, fever)
Possibly evidenced by:	**[Not applicable; presence of signs and symptoms establishes an *actual* diagnosis.]**
PATIENT OUTCOMES/ EVALUATION CRITERIA:	**Maintains adequate fluid volume as evidenced by moist mucous membranes, good skin turgor, and capillary refill; stable vital signs; balanced I&O with urine of normal concentration/amount.**

ACTIONS/INTERVENTIONS   RATIONALE

Independent

Monitor intake and output. Note number, character, and amount of stools; estimate insensible fluid losses, e.g., diaphoresis. Measure urine specific gravity; observe for oliguria.

Provides information about overall fluid balance, renal function, and bowel disease control, as well as guidelines for fluid replacement.

Assess vital signs changes, e.g., blood pressure, pulse, temperature.

Hypotension (including postural), tachycardia, fever can indicate response to and/or effect of fluid loss.

Observe for excessively dry skin and mucous membranes, decreased skin turgor, slowed capillary refill.

Indicates excessive fluid loss/resultant dehydration.

Weigh daily.

Indicator of overall fluid and nutritional status.

Maintain oral restrictions, bedrest; avoid exertion.

Colon is placed at rest for healing and to decrease intestinal fluid losses.

Observe for overt or occult bleeding.

Inadequate diet and decreased absorption may lead to vitamin K deficiency and defects in coagulation, potentiating risk of hemorrhage.

Note generalized muscle weakness or cardiac dysrhythmias.

Excessive intestinal loss may lead to electrolyte imbalance, e.g., potassium which is necessary for proper skeletal and cardiac muscle function. Minor alterations in serum levels can result in profound and/or life-threatening symptoms. (Refer to CP: Fluid and Electrolyte Imbalances, p. 907.)

ACTIONS/INTERVENTIONS	RATIONALE
Collaborative	
Administer parenteral fluids as indicated.	Maintenance of bowel rest will require alternate fluid replacement to correct losses.
Monitor laboratory studies, e.g., electrolytes (especially potassium) and ABGs (acid–base balance).	Determines replacement needs and effectiveness of therapy.
Administer medications as indicated:	
Antidiarrheals (Refer to ND: Bowel Elimination, Altered: Diarrhea, p. 414);	Reduces fluid losses from intestines.
Antiemetics, e.g., trimethobenzamide (Tigan), hydroxyzine (Vistaril), prochlorperazine (Compazine);	Used to control nausea and vomiting in acute exacerbations.
Antipyretics, e.g., acetaminophen (Tylenol);	Controls fever, reducing insensible losses.
Electrolytes, e.g., potassium supplement (K-lyte, Slow-K);	Electrolytes are lost in large amounts, especially in bowel with denuded, ulcerated areas and diarrhea can also lead to metabolic acidosis through loss of bicarbonate (HCO_3).
Vitamin K (Mephyton).	Stimulates hepatic formation of prothrombin, stabilizing coagulation, reducing risk of hemorrhage.

NURSING DIAGNOSIS:	**NUTRITION, ALTERED: LESS THAN BODY REQUIREMENTS**
May be related to:	**Altered absorption of nutrients**
	Hypermetabolic state
	Medically restricted intake; fear that eating may cause diarrhea
Possibly evidenced by:	**Weight loss; decreased subcutaneous fat/muscle mass; poor muscle tone**
	Hyperactive bowel sounds; steatorrhea
	Pale conjunctiva and mucous membranes
	Aversion to eating
PATIENT OUTCOMES/ EVALUATION CRITERIA:	**Demonstrates stable weight or progressive gain toward goal with normalization of laboratory values and absence of signs of malnutrition.**

ACTIONS/INTERVENTIONS	RATIONALE
Independent	
Weigh daily.	Provides information about dietary needs/effectiveness of therapy.
Encourage bedrest and/or limited activity during acute phase of illness.	Decreasing metabolic needs aid in preventing caloric depletion and conserves energy.

ACTIONS/INTERVENTIONS	RATIONALE

Independent

Recommend rest before meals.

Provide oral hygiene.

Serve foods in well-ventilated, pleasant surroundings, with unhurried atmosphere, congenial company.

Limit foods that might cause abdominal cramping, flatulence (e.g., milk products).

Record intake and changes in symptomatology.

Promote patient participation in dietary planning as possible.

Encourage patient to verbalize feelings concerning resumption of diet.

Collaborative

Keep patient NPO as indicated.

Resume/advance diet as indicated, e.g., clear liquids progressing to bland, low residue; then high in protein, high-calorie, and low-fiber as indicated.

Administer medications as indicated, e.g.:

    Donnatal, barbital sodium with belladonna (Butibel), propanthelene bromide (Pro-Banthine);

    Iron (Imferon injectable);

    Vitamin B_{12} (Crystimin, Rubisol);

    Vitamin C (Ascorbicap).

Provide total parenteral nutrition (TPN), IV therapy as indicated.

Quiets peristalsis and increases available energy for eating.

A clean mouth can enhance the taste of food.

Pleasant environment aids in reducing stress and is more conducive to eating.

Prevents acute attack/exacerbation of symptoms.

Useful in identifying specific deficiencies and determining GI response to foods.

Provides sense of control for patient and opportunity to select food desired/enjoyed, which may increase intake.

Hesitation to eat may be result of fear that food will cause exacerbation of symptoms.

Resting the bowel decreases peristalsis and diarrhea, which causes malabsorption/loss of nutrients.

Allows the intestinal tract to readjust to the digestive process. Protein is necessary for tissue healing integrity. Low bulk decreases peristaltic response to meal.

Anticholinergics given 15–30 minutes prior to eating provide relief from cramping pain and diarrhea, decreasing gastric motility and enhancing time for absorption of nutrients.

Prevent/treat anemia. Oral route for iron supplement is ineffective because of intestinal alterations that severely reduce absorption.

Malabsorption of B_{12} is a result of marked loss of functional ileum. Replacement reverses bone marrow depression caused by prolonged inflammatory process, promoting RBC production/correction of anemia.

Promotes tissue healing/regeneration.

This regimen rests the GI tract while providing essential nutrients. (Refer to CP: Total Nutritional Support, p. 894.)

NURSING DIAGNOSIS:	**ANXIETY [SPECIFY LEVEL]**
May be related to:	**Physiologic factors/sympathetic stimulation (inflammatory process)**
	Threat to self-concept (perceived or actual)
	Threat to/change in health status, socioeconomic status, role functioning, interaction patterns

Possibly evidenced by:	Exacerbation of acute stage of disease
	Increased tension, distress, apprehension
	Expressed concern regarding changes in life
	Somatic complaints
	Focus on self
PATIENT OUTCOMES/ EVALUATION CRITERIA:	Appears relaxed and reports anxiety reduced to a manageable level. Verbalizes awareness of feelings of anxiety and healthy ways to deal with them.

ACTIONS/INTERVENTIONS	RATIONALE
Independent	
Note behavioral clues, e.g., restlessness, irritability, withdrawal, lack of eye contact, demanding behavior.	Indicators of degree of anxiety/stress, e.g., patient may feel out of control at home, work/personal problems.
Encourage verbalization of feelings. Provide feedback.	Establishes a therapeutic relationship. Assists the patient/SO in identifying problems causing stress. Patient with severe diarrhea may hesitate to use/ask for help for fear of becoming a burden to the staff.
Acknowledge that the anxiety and problems are similar to those expressed by others. Active-listen patient's concerns.	Validation that feelings are normal can help to reduce stress/isolation and belief that "I am the only one."
Provide accurate, concrete information about what is being done, e.g., reason for bedrest, restriction of oral intake, and procedures.	Involving patient in plan of care provides sense of control and helps to decrease anxiety.
Provide a calm, restful environment.	Removing patient from outside stressors helps to reduce anxiety.
Encourage staff/SO to project caring, concerned attitude.	A supportive manner can help the patient feel less stressed, allowing energy to be directed toward healing.
Help patient to identify/initiate positive coping behaviors used in the past.	Successful behaviors can be fostered in dealing with current problems/stress, enhancing patient's sense of self-control.
Assist patient to learn new coping mechanisms, e.g., stress management techniques, organizational skills.	Learning new ways to cope can be helpful in reducing stress and anxiety, enhancing disease control.
Collaborative	
Administer medications as indicated:	
Sedatives, e.g., barbiturates (Luminal); tranquilizers, e.g., diazepam (Valium).	May be used to reduce anxiety and to facilitate rest, particularly in the patient with ulcerative colitis.
Refer to psychiatric nurse/social services/spiritual advisor.	May require additional assistance to regain control and cope with acute episodes/exacerbation as well as learning to deal with the chronicity and consequences of the disease and therapeutic regimen.

NURSING DIAGNOSIS:	COMFORT, ALTERED: PAIN, ACUTE
May be related to:	Hyperperistalsis, prolonged diarrhea, skin/tissue irrita-

	tion, perirectal excoriation, fissures; fistulas
Possibly evidenced by:	Complaints of colicky/cramping abdominal pain/referred pain
	Guarding/distraction behaviors, restlessness
	Facial mask of pain
	Self-focusing
PATIENT OUTCOMES/ EVALUATION CRITERIA:	Reports pain is relieved/controlled. Appears relaxed and able to sleep/rest appropriately.

ACTIONS/INTERVENTIONS

Independent

Encourage patient to report pain.

Assess complaints of abdominal cramping or pain, noting location, duration, intensity (1–10 scale).

Note nonverbal clues, e.g., restlessness, reluctance to move, abdominal guarding, withdrawal, and depression. Investigate discrepancies between verbal and nonverbal clues.

Review factors that aggravate or alleviate pain.

Permit patient to assume position of comfort, e.g., knees flexed.

Provide routine comfort measures (e.g., backrub, reposition) and diversional activities.

Cleanse rectal area with mild soap and water/wipes after each stool and provide skin care, e.g., A & D ointment, Sween ointment, karya gel, Desitin, petroleum jelly.

Observe for ischiorectal and perianal fistulas.

Observe/record abdominal distention, increased temperature, decreased BP.

Collaborative

Implement prescribed dietary modifications, e.g., commence with liquids and increase to solid foods as tolerated.

Administer medications as indicated:

Analgesics;

RATIONALE

May try to tolerate pain, rather than request analgesics.

Colicky intermittent pain occurs with Crohn's. Predefecation pain frequently occurs with UC with urgency, which may be severe and continuous. Changes in pain characteristics may indicate spread of disease/developing complications.

Body language/nonverbal clues may be both physiologic and psychologic and may be used in conjunction with verbal cues to identify extent/severity of the problem.

May pinpoint precipitating or aggravating factors (such as stressful events, food intolerance) or identify developing complications.

Reduces abdominal tension and promotes sense of control.

Promotes relaxation, refocuses attention, and may enhance coping abilities.

Protects skin from undigested bowel contents, preventing excoriation.

Fistulas may develop from erosion and weakening of intestinal bowel wall.

May indicate developing intestinal obstruction from inflammation, edema, and scarring.

Complete bowel rest can reduce pain, cramping.

Pain varies from mild to severe and necessitates management to facilitate adequate rest and recovery. Note: Opiates should be used with caution, because they may precipitate toxic megacolon.

ACTIONS/INTERVENTIONS

Collaborative

Anticholinergics;

Anodyne suppositories.

Assist with sitz bath as indicated.

RATIONALE

Relieves spasms of GI tract and resultant colicky pain.

Relaxes rectal muscle, decreasing painful spasms.

Provides local soothing and comfort to irritated rectal area.

NURSING DIAGNOSIS:	COPING, INEFFECTIVE INDIVIDUAL
May be related to:	Multiple stressors, repeated over period of time
	Unpredictable nature of disease process
	Personal vulnerability
	Severe pain
	Lack of sleep, rest
	Situational crisis
	Inadequate coping method; lack of support systems
Possibly evidenced by:	Verbalization of inability to cope, discouragement, anxiety
	Preoccupation with physical self, chronic worry, emotional tension, poor self-esteem
	Depression and dependency
PATIENT OUTCOMES/ EVALUATION CRITERIA:	Identifies ineffective coping behaviors and consequences. Acknowledges own coping abilities. Assesses the current situation accurately. Demonstrates necessary lifestyle changes to limit/prevent recurrent episodes.

ACTIONS/INTERVENTIONS

Independent

Assess patient/SO understanding and previous methods of dealing with disease process.

Determine outside stresses, e.g., family, social or work environment.

Help patient identify individually effective coping skills.

Provide emotional support as needed by:

Active-listening in a nonjudgmental manner;

RATIONALE

Enables the nurse to deal more realistically with current problems. Anxiety and other problems may have interfered with previous health teaching/patient learning.

Stress can alter autonomic nervous response and contribute to exacerbation of disease. Even the goal of independence in the dependent patient can be an added stressor.

Use of previously successful behaviors can help patient deal with current situation/plan for future.

Aids in communication and understanding the patient's viewpoint. Adds to patient's feelings of self-worth.

ACTIONS/INTERVENTIONS

Independent

Use of nonjudgmental body language when caring for patient;

Assigning same staff.

Provide uninterrupted sleep/rest periods.

Encourage use of stress management skills, e.g., relaxation techniques, visualization, guided imagery, deep breathing exercises.

Collaborative

Include patient/SO in team conferences to develop individualized program.

Administer tranquilizers, as indicated: antipsychotics, e.g., thioridazine (Mellaril); antianxiety agents, e.g., lorazepam (Ativan), alprazolam (Xanax).

Refer to resources as indicated, e.g., social worker, psychiatric nurse, spiritual advisor.

RATIONALE

Prevents reinforcing patient's feelings of being a burden, e.g., frequent need to empty bedpan.

Provides a more therapeutic environment and lessens the stress of constant adjustments.

Exhaustion brought on by the disease tends to magnify problems, interfering with ability to cope.

Refocuses attention, promotes relaxation, and enhances coping abilities.

Promotes continuity of care and enables patient/SO to feel a part of the plan, giving them a sense of control and increasing cooperation with therapeutic regimen.

Aids in psychological/physical rest. Conserves energy and may strengthen coping abilities.

Additional support and counseling can assist patient/SO in dealing with specific stress/problem areas.

NURSING DIAGNOSIS:	KNOWLEDGE DEFICIT [LEARNING NEED] (SPECIFY)
May be related to:	Information misinterpretation, lack of recall
	Unfamiliarity with resources
Possibly evidenced by:	Questions, request for information, statements of misconceptions
	Inaccurate follow-through of instructions
	Development of preventable complications
PATIENT OUTCOMES/ EVALUATION CRITERIA:	Verbalizes understanding of disease processes, treatment, and own ability to cope with situation. Initiates necessary lifestyle changes and participates in treatment regimen.

ACTIONS/INTERVENTIONS

Independent

Determine patient's perception of disease process.

Review disease process, cause/effect relationship of factors which precipitate symptoms and identify ways to reduce contributing factors. Encourage questions.

RATIONALE

Establishes knowledge base and provides some insight into individual learning needs.

Precipitating factors are individual; therefore, the patient needs to be aware of what foods, fluids, and lifestyle factors can precipitate episodes of diarrhea/symptoms. Accurate knowledge base provides opportunity for patient to make informed decisions/choices about future and control of chronic disease. Although most patients know about their own disease

ACTIONS/INTERVENTIONS	RATIONALE

Independent

process, they may have outdated information or misconceptions.

Review medications, purpose, frequency, dosage and possible side effects.

Promotes understanding and may enhance cooperation with regimen.

Remind patient to observe for side effects if steroids are given on a long-term basis, e.g., GI upset, edema, muscle weakness.

Steroids may be used to control inflammation to effect a remission of the disease; however, drug may lower resistance to infection and cause fluid retention.

Stress good handwashing techniques and perineal skin care.

Reduces spread of bacteria, reduces risk of skin irritation/infection.

Recommend cessation of smoking.

Can increase intestinal motility, aggravating symptoms.

Collaborative

Refer to appropriate community resources, e.g., Public Health Nurse, Ostomy Association, dietitian, support groups, and social services.

Patient may benefit from the services of these agencies in coping with chronicity of the disease.

Fecal Diversions: Postoperative Care of Ileostomy and Colostomy

Ileostomy: diversion of the effluent of the small intestines, usually permanent.

Colostomy: diversion of the effluent of the colon, which may be temporary or permanent.

PATIENT ASSESSMENT DATA BASE

The data are dependent on the underlying problem, duration, and severity (e.g., obstruction, perforation, inflammation, congenital defects).

Refer to appropriate CP, e.g., Inflammatory Bowel Disease, p. 411.

TEACHING/LEARNING

Discharge Plan Considerations: Assistance with dietary concerns, management of ostomy, and acquisition of supplies.

NURSING PRIORITIES

1. Assist patient/SO in psychosocial adjustment.
2. Prevent complications.
3. Support independence in self-care.
4. Provide information about procedure/prognosis, treatment needs, potential complications, and community resources.

DISCHARGE CRITERIA

1. Adjusting to perceived/actual changes.
2. Complications prevented/minimized.
3. Self-care needs met by self/with assistance dependent on specific situation.
4. Procedure/prognosis, therapeutic regimen, potential complications understood and sources of support identified.

NURSING DIAGNOSIS:	SKIN INTEGRITY, IMPAIRED: POTENTIAL
May be related to:	**Absence of sphincter at stoma**
	Character/flow of effluent and flatus from stoma
	Reaction to product/chemicals; improper fitting of appliance or removal of adhesive
Possibly evidenced by:	**[Not applicable; presence of signs and symptoms establishes an *actual* diagnosis.]**
PATIENT OUTCOMES/ EVALUATION CRITERIA:	**Maintains skin integrity. Identifies individual risk factors. Demonstrates behaviors/techniques to promote healing/prevent skin breakdown.**

ACTIONS/INTERVENTIONS	RATIONALE
Independent	
Inspect stoma/peristomal skin area. Clean with water and pat dry. Note irritation, bruises (dark, bluish color),	Monitors healing process/effectiveness of appliances, and identifies areas of concern, need for further

ACTIONS/INTERVENTIONS	RATIONALE
Independent	
rashes.	evaluation/intervention. Maintaining a clean/dry area helps to prevent skin breakdown. Early identification of stomal necrosis/ischemia or fungal infection provides for timely interventions to prevent serious complications.
Measure stoma periodically, e.g., each appliance change for first 6 weeks, then monthly times 6.	As postoperative edema resolves (during first 6 weeks), size of appliance must be altered to ensure proper fit so that effluent is collected as it flows from the ostomy, and contact with the skin is prevented.
Make sure opening on adhesive backing of pouch is only ⅛ inch larger than the base of the stoma with adequate adhesiveness left to apply pouch.	Prevents trauma to the stoma tissue and protects the peristomal skin. Adequate adhesive area is important to maintain a seal. Note: Too tight a fit may cause stomal edema or stenosis.
Use a transparent, odor-proof drainable pouch.	A transparent appliance during first 4–6 weeks allows easy observation of stoma without necessity of removing pouch/irritating skin.
Apply effective skin barrier, e.g., Stomahesive (Squibb), karaya gum, Reliaseal (Davol), or similar products.	Protects skin from pouch adhesive, enhances adhesiveness of pouch and facilitates removal of pouch when necessary. Note: Sigmoid colostomy may not require use of a skin barrier once stool becomes formed and elimination is regulated through irrigation.
Empty and cleanse ostomy pouch on a routine basis, using appropriate equipment.	Frequent pouch changes are irritating to the skin and should be avoided. Emptying and rinsing the pouch with the proper solution not only removes bacteria and odor-causing stool and flatus but also deodorizes the pouch.
Remove appliance (when necessary) gently while supporting skin. Use adhesive removers as indicated and wash off completely.	Prevents tissue irritation/destruction associated with "pulling" pouch off.
Investigate complaints of burning/itching around stoma.	Suggests leakage of effluent with peristomal irritation requiring intervention or possibly Candida infections.
Apply antacids to the skin if indicated.	Occasionally may be used to neutralize the digestive enzymes and lessens risk of irritation.
Evaluate adhesive product and appliance fit on ongoing basis.	Provides opportunity for problem solving. Determines need for further intervention.
Collaborative	
Consult with enterostomal nurse.	Helpful in choosing products appropriate for patient's needs, considering type of effluent, patient's physical/mental status, and financial resources. In the presence of persistent or recurring problems, the ostomy nurse will have a wider range of knowledge.
Apply corticosteroid aerosol spray and nystatin powder.	Assists in healing if peristomal irritation persists/fungal infection develops. Note: These products can have potent side effects and should be used sparingly.

NURSING DIAGNOSIS:	SELF-CONCEPT, DISTURBANCE IN: (SPECIFY)
May be related to:	**Biophysical: presence of stoma; loss of control of bowel elimination**

	Psychosocial: altered body structure
	Disease process and associated treatment regimen, e.g., cancer, colitis
Possibly evidenced by:	Verbalization of change in body image, fear of rejection/reaction of others, and negative feelings about body
	Actual change in structure and/or function (ostomy)
	Not touching/looking at stoma, refusal to participate in care
PATIENT OUTCOMES/ EVALUATION CRITERIA:	Verbalizes acceptance of self in situation, incorporating change into self-concept without negating self-esteem. Demonstrates beginning acceptance by viewing/touching stoma and participating in self-care. Verbalizes feelings about stoma/illness; begins to deal constructively with situation.

ACTIONS/INTERVENTIONS	RATIONALE

Independent

Ascertain whether counseling was initiated when the possibility and/or necessity of ostomy was first discussed.

Provides information about patient's/SO's level of knowledge about individual situation and process of acceptance.

Encourage patient/SO to verbalize feelings regarding the ostomy. Acknowledge normality of feelings of anger, depression, and grief over loss. Discuss daily "ups and downs" that can occur after discharge.

Helps the patient to realize that feelings experienced are not unusual and that feeling guilty for them is not necessary/helpful. Patient needs to recognize feelings before they can be dealt with effectively.

Review reason for surgery and future expectations.

Patient may find it easier to accept/deal with an ostomy done for chronic/long-term disease than for traumatic injury, even if ostomy is only temporary. Also, the patient who will be undergoing a second procedure (to convert ostomy to a continent or anal reservoir) may possibly encounter lesser degree of self-image problems because body function will be "more normal."

Note behaviors of withdrawal, increased dependency, manipulation, or noninvolvement in care.

Suggestive of problems in adjustment that may require further evaluation and more extensive therapy.

Provide opportunities for patient/SO to view and touch stoma, using the moment to point out positive signs of healing, normal appearance, etc.

Although integration of stoma into body image can take months or even years, looking at the stoma and hearing comments (made in a normal, matter-of-fact manner) can help patient with this acceptance. Touching stoma reassures patient/SO that it is not fragile and that slight movements of stoma actually reflect normal peristalsis.

Provide opportunity for patient to deal with ostomy through participation in self-care.

Independence in self-care helps to improve self-esteem.

Plan/schedule care activities with patient.

Promotes sense of control and gives message that patient can handle this, enhancing self-esteem.

Maintain positive approach, during care activities, avoiding expressions of disdain or revulsion. Do not take angry expressions personally.

Assists patient/SO to accept body changes and feel all right about self. Anger is most often directed at the situation and lack of control individual has over what

ACTIONS/INTERVENTIONS

Independent

Discuss possibility of contacting ostomy visitor, and make arrangements for visit if desired.

RATIONALE

has happened (powerlessness), not with the individual care giver.

Can provide a good support system. Helps to reinforce teaching (shared experiences) and facilitates acceptance of change as patient realizes "life does go on" and can be relatively normal.

NURSING DIAGNOSIS:	COMFORT, ALTERED: PAIN, ACUTE
May be related to:	Physical factors: e.g., disruption of skin/tissues (incisions/drains) Biologic: activity of disease process (cancer, trauma) Psychologic factors: e.g., fear, anxiety
Possibly evidenced by:	Complaints of pain, self-focusing Guarding/distraction behaviors, restlessness Autonomic responses, e.g., changes in vital signs
PATIENT OUTCOMES/ EVALUATION CRITERIA:	Verbalizes/displays relief of pain. Demonstrates ability to assist with general comfort measures and able to sleep/rest appropriately.

ACTIONS/INTERVENTIONS

Independent

Assess pain, noting location, characteristics, intensity (1–10 scale).

Encourage patient to verbalize concerns. Active-listen these concerns, and provide support by acceptance, remaining with patient, and giving appropriate information.

Provide routine comfort measures, e.g., mouth care, backrub, repositioning (use proper support measures as needed). Assure patient that position change will not injure stoma.

Encourage use of relaxation techniques, e.g., guided imagery, visualization. Provide diversional activities.

Assist with ROM exercises and encourage early ambulation. Avoid prolonged sitting position.

RATIONALE

Helps evaluate degree of discomfort and effectiveness of analgesia or may reveal developing complications; e.g., because abdominal pain usually subsides gradually by the 3rd or 4th postoperative day, continued or increasing pain may reflect delayed healing or peristomal skin irritation. Note: Pain in anal area associated with abdominal-perineal resection may persist for months.

Reduction of anxiety/fear can promote relaxation/comfort.

Prevents drying of oral mucosa and associated discomfort. Reduces muscle tension, promotes relaxation, and may enhance coping abilities.

Helps patient to rest more effectively and refocuses attention, thereby reducing pain and discomfort.

Reduces muscle/joint stiffness. Ambulation returns organs to normal position and promotes return of usual level of functioning. Note: Presence of edema, packing, and drains (if perineal resection has been done) increases discomfort and creates a sense of needing

427

ACTIONS/INTERVENTIONS	RATIONALE
Independent	
	to defecate. Ambulation and frequent position changes reduce perineal pressure.
Investigate and report abdominal muscle rigidity, involuntary guarding, and rebound tenderness.	Suggestive of peritoneal inflammation, requiring prompt medical intervention.
Collaborative	
Administer medication as indicated, e.g., narcotics, analgesics, PCA.	Relieves pain, enhances comfort and promotes rest. Patient control of analgesia may be more beneficial, especially following AP repair.
Provide sitz baths.	Relieves local discomfort, reduces edema, and promotes healing of perineal wound.
Apply/monitor effects of TENS unit.	Cutaneous stimulation may be used to block transmission of pain stimulus.

NURSING DIAGNOSIS:	SKIN/TISSUE INTEGRITY, IMPAIRED: ACTUAL
May be related to:	Invasion of body structure (perineal resection)
	Stasis of secretions/drainage
	Altered circulation, edema; malnutrition
Possibly evidenced by:	Disruption of skin/tissue: presence of incision, and sutures, drains
PATIENT OUTCOMES/ EVALUATION CRITERIA:	Achieves timely wound healing free of signs of infection.

ACTIONS/INTERVENTIONS	RATIONALE
Independent	
Observe wounds, note characteristics of drainage.	Postoperative hemorrhage is most likely to occur during first 48 hours, whereas infection may develop at any time. Dependent on type of wound closure (e.g., first or second intention), complete healing may take 6–8 months.
Change dressings as needed using aseptic technique.	Large amounts of serous drainage require that dressings be changed frequently to reduce skin irritation and potential for infection.
Encourage side-lying position with head elevated. Avoid prolonged sitting.	Promotes drainage from perineal wound/drains reducing risk of pooling. Prolonged sitting increases perineal pressure, reducing circulation to wound, and may delay healing.
Collaborative	
Irrigate wound as indicated, using normal saline, dilute hydrogen peroxide, or antibiotic solution.	May be required to treat preoperative inflammation/ infection or intraoperative contamination.
Provide sitz baths.	Promotes cleanliness and facilitates healing especially after packing is removed (usually day 3–5).

<table>
<tr><td>NURSING DIAGNOSIS:</td><td>FLUID VOLUME DEFICIT, POTENTIAL</td></tr>
<tr><td>May be related to:</td><td>Excessive losses through normal routes, e.g., preoperative emesis and diarrhea</td></tr>
<tr><td></td><td>Losses through abnormal routes, e.g., nasogastric/intestinal tube, perineal wound drainage tubes</td></tr>
<tr><td></td><td>Medically restricted intake</td></tr>
<tr><td></td><td>Altered absorption of fluid, e.g., loss of colon function</td></tr>
<tr><td></td><td>Hypermetabolic states, e.g., inflammation, healing process</td></tr>
<tr><td>Possibly evidenced by:</td><td>[Not applicable; presence of signs and symptoms establishes an actual diagnosis.]</td></tr>
<tr><td>PATIENT OUTCOMES/ EVALUATION CRITERIA:</td><td>Maintains adequate hydration as evidenced by moist mucous membranes, good skin turgor and capillary refill, stable vital signs, and individually appropriate urinary output.</td></tr>
</table>

ACTIONS/INTERVENTIONS	RATIONALE
Independent	
Monitor I&O carefully, measure liquid stool. Weigh regularly.	Provides direct indicators of fluid balance. Greatest fluid losses occur with ileostomy but generally do not exceed 500–800 ml/day.
Monitor vital signs noting postural hypotension, tachycardia. Evaluate skin turgor, capillary refill and mucous membranes.	Reflects hydration status/possible need for increased fluid replacement.
Limit intake of ice chips during period of gastric intubation.	Stimulates gastric secretions and washes out electrolytes.
Collaborative	
Monitor laboratory results, e.g., Hct and electrolytes.	Detects homeostasis or imbalance and aids in determining replacement needs.
Administer IV fluid and electrolytes as indicated.	May be necessary to maintain adequate tissue perfusion/organ function.

<table>
<tr><td>NURSING DIAGNOSIS:</td><td>NUTRITION, ALTERED: LESS THAN BODY REQUIREMENTS [POTENTIAL]</td></tr>
<tr><td>May be related to:</td><td>Prolonged anorexia/altered intake preoperatively</td></tr>
<tr><td></td><td>Hypermetabolic state (preoperative inflammatory disease; healing process)</td></tr>
<tr><td></td><td>Presence of diarrhea/altered absorption</td></tr>
<tr><td></td><td>Restriction of bulk and residue-containing foods</td></tr>
</table>

Possibly evidenced by:	**[Not applicable; presence of signs and symptoms establishes an *actual* diagnosis.]**
PATIENT OUTCOMES/ EVALUATION CRITERIA:	**Maintains weight/demonstrates progressive weight gain toward goal with normalization of laboratory values and free of signs of malnutrition. Plans diet to meet nutritional needs/limit gastrointestinal disturbances.**

ACTIONS/INTERVENTIONS	RATIONALE
Independent	
Do a thorough nutritional assessment.	Identifies deficiencies/needs to aid in choice of interventions.
Auscultate bowel sounds. Observe for ostomy drainage.	Return of intestinal function indicates readiness to resume intake.
Resume solid foods slowly.	Reduces incidence of abdominal cramps, nausea.
Identify offensive foods (flatus/odor, etc.) and temporarily restrict from diet. Gradually reintroduce one food at a time.	Sensitivity to certain foods is not uncommon following intestinal surgery. Patient can experiment with food several times before determining whether it is creating a problem.
Recommend patient increase use of yogurt and buttermilk.	May help decrease odor.
Suggest patient with ileostomy exercise caution in the use of prunes, dates, stewed apricots, strawberries, grapes, bananas, cabbage family, beans, and nuts and avoidance of cellulose products, e.g., peanuts.	These products increase ileal effluent. Digestion of cellulose requires colon bacteria.
Discuss mechanics of swallowed air as a factor in the formation of flatus and some ways the patient can exercise control.	Drinking through a straw, snoring, anxiety, smoking, ill-fitting dentures, and gulping down food increase the production of flatus. Too much flatus not only necessitates frequent emptying but can be a causative factor in leakage from too much pressure within the pouch.
Collaborative	
Consult with dietician.	Helpful in assessing patient's nutritional needs in light of changes in digestion and intestinal function.
Advance diet from liquids to low-residue food when oral intake is resumed.	Low-residue diet may be maintained during first 6–8 weeks to provide adequate time for intestinal healing.
Administer TPN when indicated. (Refer to CP: Total Nutritional Support, p. 894.)	In the presence of severe debilitation/intolerance of oral intake, hyperalimentation may be used to supply needed components for healing and prevention of catabolic state.

NURSING DIAGNOSIS:	**SLEEP PATTERN DISTURBANCE**
May be related to:	**External factors: necessity of ostomy care, excessive flatus/ostomy effluent**
	Internal factors: psychologic stress, fear of leakage of pouch/injury to stoma
Possibly evidenced by:	**Verbalizations of interrupted sleep, not feeling well rested**

Changes in behavior, e.g., irritability, listlessness/
lethargy

PATIENT OUTCOMES/ EVALUATION CRITERIA:	Sleeping/resting between disturbances. Reports increased sense of well-being and feeling rested.

ACTIONS/INTERVENTIONS

Independent

Explain necessity for monitoring intestinal function.

Provide adequate pouching system. Empty pouch before retiring and, if necessary, on a preagreed schedule.

Let patient know that stoma will not be injured when sleeping.

Restrict intake of caffeine-containing foods/fluids.

Support continuation of usual bedtime rituals.

Collaborative

Determine cause of excessive flatus or effluent, e.g, confer with dietician regarding restriction of foods if diet-related.

Administer analgesics, sedatives at bedtime as indicated.

RATIONALE

Patient is more apt to be tolerant of disturbances if he or she understands the reasons for them and the importance of care.

Excessive flatus/effluent can occur despite interventions. Emptying on a regular schedule minimizes threat of leakage.

Patient will be able to rest better if feeling secure about stoma and ostomy.

Caffeine may delay patient's falling asleep and interfere with REM sleep, resulting in patient not feeling well rested.

Promotes relaxation and readiness for sleep.

Identification of cause enables institution of corrective measures that may promote sleep/rest.

Pain pathways in the brain lie near the sleep center and may interfere with patient's ability to fall/remain asleep. Timely medication can enhance rest/sleep during initial postoperative period.

NURSING DIAGNOSIS:	**BOWEL ELIMINATION, ALTERED: CONSTIPATION [POTENTIAL]**
May be related to:	**Placement of ostomy in descending or sigmoid colon** **Inadequate diet/fluid intake**
Possibly evidenced by:	**[Not applicable; presence of signs and symptoms establishes an *actual* diagnosis.]**
PATIENT OUTCOMES/ EVALUATION CRITERIA:	**Establishes an elimination pattern suitable to physical needs and lifestyle with effluent of appropriate amount and consistency.**

ACTIONS/INTERVENTIONS

Independent

Ascertain patient's previous bowel habits and lifestyle.

Investigate delayed onset/absence of effluent. Auscultate bowel sounds.

RATIONALE

Assists in formulation of an effective schedule.

Postoperative paralytic/adynamic ileus usually resolves within 48–72 hours and ileostomy should begin

ACTIONS/INTERVENTIONS

Independent

Inform the patient with an ileostomy that initially the effluent will be liquid and if constipation occurs, to report it to enterostomal nurse or physician.

Review dietary pattern and amount/type of fluid intake.

Review physiology of the colon and discuss irrigation management of sigmoid ostomy, if appropriate.

Demonstrate use of irrigation equipment to inject normal saline per protocol until relief is obtained. Irrigations may be used on a daily basis, or for special occasions.

Instruct patient in the use of closed-end pouch or a patch, dressing/Bandaid when irrigation is successful and the sigmoid colostomy effluent becomes more manageable, with stool expelled every 24 hours.

Involve the patient in care of the ostomy on an increasing basis.

Collaborative

Provide TENS unit if indicated.

RATIONALE

draining within 12–24 hours. Delay may indicate persistent ileus or stomal obstruction, which may occur postoperatively because of edema, improperly fitting pouch (too tight), prolapse, or stenosis of the stoma.

Although the small intestine eventually begins to take on water-absorbing functions to permit a more semi-solid, pasty discharge, constipation may indicate an obstruction. Absence of stool requires emergency medical attention.

Adequate intake of fiber and roughage provides bulk, while fluid is an important factor in determining the consistency of the stool.

This knowledge helps the patient understand care.

May be used to relieve constipation when immediate relief is desired. There are differing views on the use of daily irrigations. Some believe cleaning the bowel on a regular basis is helpful. Others believe that this interferes with normal functioning. Most authorities agree that occasional irrigating is useful for emptying the bowel to avoid leakage when special events are planned.

Enables patient to feel more comfortable socially and is less expensive than regular ostomy pouches.

Rehabilitation can be facilitated by encouraging patient independence and control.

Electrical stimulation has been used in some patients to stimulate peristalsis and relieve postoperative ileus.

NURSING DIAGNOSIS:	SEXUAL DYSFUNCTION [POTENTIAL]
May be related to:	Altered body structure/function; radical resection/treatment procedures
	Vulnerability/psychologic concern about response of SO
	Disruption of sexual response pattern, e.g., erection difficulty
Possibly evidenced by:	[Not applicable; presence of signs and symptoms establishes an *actual* diagnosis.]
PATIENT OUTCOMES/EVALUATION CRITERIA:	Verbalizes understanding of relationship of physical condition to sexual problems. Identifies satisfying/acceptable sexual practices, and explores alternate methods. Resumes sexual relationship as appropriate.

ACTIONS/INTERVENTIONS	RATIONALE

Independent

Assess the patient's/SO sexual relationships prior to the disease and/or surgery. Identify future expectations and desires.

Mutilation and loss of privacy/control of a bodily function can affect patient's view of personal sexuality. When coupled with the fear of rejection by SO, the desired level of intimacy can be greatly impaired. Sexual needs are very basic, and the patient will be rehabilitated more successfully when a satisfying sexual relationship is continued/developed.

Review with the patient/SO anatomy and physiology of sexual functioning in relation to own situation.

Understanding normal physiology helps patient/SO to understand the mechanisms of nerve damage and need for exploring alternate methods of satisfaction.

Reinforce information given by the physician. Encourage questions. Provide additional information as needed.

Reiteration of data previously given assists the patient/SO to hear and process the knowledge again, moving toward acceptance of individual limitations/restrictions and prognosis (e.g., that it may take up to 2 years to regain potency after a radical procedure or that a penile prosthesis may be necessary).

Discuss resumption of sexual activity approximately 6 weeks after discharge, beginning slowly and progressing (e.g., cuddling/caressing until both partners are comfortable with body image/function changes). Include alternate methods of stimulation as appropriate.

Knowing what to expect in progress of recovery helps patient avoid performance anxiety/reduce risk of "failure." If the couple is willing to try new ideas, this can assist with adjustment and may help to achieve sexual fulfillment.

Encourage dialogue between patient/SO. Suggest wearing pouch cover, T-shirt, or shortie nightgown.

Disguising ostomy appliance may aid in reducing feelings of self-consciousness, embarrassment during sexual activity.

Stress awareness of factors that might be distracting (e.g., unpleasant odors and pouch leakage). Encourage use of sense of humor.

Promotes resolution of solvable problems. Laughter can help individuals to deal more effectively with difficult situation, promote positive sexual experience.

Problem-solve alternative positions for coitus.

Minimizing awkwardness of appliance and physical discomfort can enhance satisfaction.

Discuss/role-play possible interactions or approaches when dealing with new sexual partners.

Rehearsal is helpful in dealing with actual situations when they arise, preventing self-consciousness about "different" body image.

Provide birth control information as appropriate and stress that impotence does not mean the patient is sterile.

Confusion may exist that can lead to an unwanted pregnancy.

Collaborative

Arrange meeting with an ostomy visitor if appropriate.

Sharing of how these problems have been resolved by others can be helpful and reduce sense of isolation.

Refer to counseling/sex therapy as indicated.

If problems persist longer than several months after surgery, a trained therapist may be required to facilitate communication between patient and SO.

NURSING DIAGNOSIS:	KNOWLEDGE DEFICIT [LEARNING NEED] (SPECIFY)
May be related to:	**Lack of exposure; information misinterpretation; lack of recall**
	Unfamiliarity with information resources

	Inaccurate follow-through of instruction/performance of ostomy care
	Inappropriate or exaggerated behaviors (e.g., hostile, agitated, apathetic withdrawal)
PATIENT OUTCOMES/ EVALUATION CRITERIA:	Verbalizes understanding of condition/disease process and treatment and prognosis. Correctly performs necessary procedures, explains reasons for the action. Initiates necessary lifestyle changes.

ACTIONS/INTERVENTIONS	RATIONALE
Independent	
Evaluate patient's emotional and physical capabilities.	These factors affect patient's ability to master tasks and willingness to assume responsibility for ostomy care.
Review anatomy, physiology and implications of surgical intervention. Discuss future expectations, including anticipated changes in character of effluent.	Provides knowledge base on which patient can make informed choices and an opportunity to clarify misconceptions regarding individual situation. (Temporary ileostomy may be converted to ileoanal reservoir at a future date; ileostomy and ascending colostomy cannot be regulated by diet, irrigations, or medications, etc.)
Include written/picture resources.	Provides references post discharge to support patient efforts for independence in self-care.
Instruct patient/SO in stomal care. Allot time for return demonstrations and provide positive feedback for efforts.	Promotes positive management and reduces risk of improper ostomy care.
Recommend increased fluid intake during warm weather months.	Loss of normal colon function of conserving water and electrolytes can lead to dehydration.
Discuss possible need to decrease salt intake.	Increases ileal output, potentiating risk of dehydration and increasing frequency of ostomy care needs/ patient's inconvenience.
Identify symptoms of electrolyte depletion, e.g., anorexia, abdominal muscle cramps, feelings of faintness or "cold" in arms/legs; general fatigue/weakness, bloating, decreased sensations in arms/legs.	Loss of colon function with altered fluid/electrolyte absorption may result in sodium/potassium deficits requiring dietary correction with foods/fluids high in sodium (e.g., bouillon, Gatorade) or potassium (e.g., orange juice, prunes, tomatoes, bananas, or Gatorade).
Stress importance of chewing food well, adequate intake of fluids with/following meals, and only moderate use of high-fiber foods, avoidance of cellulose.	Reduces risk of bowel obstruction, especially in patient with ileostomy.
Review foods that are/may be a source of flatus (e.g., carbonated drinks, beer, beans, cabbage family, onions, fish, and highly seasoned foods) or odor (e.g., onions, cabbage family, eggs, fish, and beans).	These foods may be restricted or eliminated for better ostomy control, or it may be necessary to empty the pouch more frequently if they are ingested.
Discuss resumption of presurgery level of activity and possibility of sleep disturbance, anorexia, loss of interest in usual activities.	Patient should be able to manage same degree of activity as previously enjoyed and in some cases increase activity level. "Homecoming depression" may occur, lasting for up to 3 months after surgery, requiring patience/support and ongoing evaluation.

ACTIONS/INTERVENTIONS	RATIONALE

Independent

Explain necessity of notifying health care providers and pharmacists of type of ostomy and avoidance of sustained-release medications.

Presence of ostomy may alter rate/extent of absorption of oral medications and increase risk of drug-related complications, e.g., diarrhea/constipation or peristomal excoriation.

Identify community resources, e.g., United Ostomy Association, and local ostomy support group, enterostomal therapist, VNA, pharmacy/medical supply house.

Continued support post discharge is essential to facilitate the recovery process and patient's independence in care. Enterostomal nurse can be very helpful in solving appliance problems, identifying alternatives to meet individual patient needs.

Intestinal Surgery (Without Ostomy) _____

PATIENT ASSESSMENT DATA BASE

The data are dependent on the underlying disease process.
Refer to specific CPs where available, e.g., Cancer, p. 872; Inflammatory Bowel Disease, p. 411.

NURSING PRIORITIES

1. Maintain adequate circulating volume.
2. Control/minimize pain.
3. Prevent complications.
4. Promote proper GI functioning.
5. Provide information about surgical procedure/prognosis, complications, and treatment needs.

DISCHARGE CRITERIA

1. Fluid intake adequate to maintain circulating volume.
2. Pain relieved/controlled.
3. Complications prevented/minimized.
4. GI function returned, intake adequate to meet nutritional needs.
5. Procedure/prognosis, possible complications, and therapeutic regimen understood.

Refer to CP: Surgical Intervention, p. 789, for general considerations and additional nursing diagnoses as indicated.

NURSING DIAGNOSIS:	FLUID VOLUME DEFICIT, POTENTIAL
May be related to:	**Excessive losses through normal routes, e.g., vomiting, diarrhea**
	Loss of fluid through abnormal routes, e.g., indwelling drains, nasogastric/intestinal suctioning, hemorrhage, insufficient replacement, fever
Possibly evidenced by:	**[Not applicable; presence of signs and symptoms establishes an *actual* diagnosis.]**
PATIENT OUTCOMES/ EVALUATION CRITERIA:	**Maintains adequate hydration as evidenced by moist mucous membranes, good skin turgor and capillary refill, stable vital signs, and individually appropriate urinary output.**

ACTIONS/INTERVENTIONS	RATIONALE
Independent	
Monitor vital signs frequently, noting increased pulse, postural BP changes, tachypnea, and apprehension. Check dressings and wound frequently during first 24 hours for signs of bright blood or excessive incisional swelling.	Early signs of hemorrhage and/or hematoma formation, which may contribute to hypovolemic shock.
Palpate peripheral pulses. Evaluate capillary refill, skin turgor, and status of mucous membranes. Note pres-	Provides information about general circulating volume and level of hydration. Note: Edema may occur due to

ACTIONS/INTERVENTIONS	RATIONALE
Independent	
ence of edema.	fluid shifts associated with decreased serum albumin/protein levels.
Monitor I&O, noting urine output, specific gravity. Calculate 24-hour balance, and weigh daily.	Direct indicators of hydration/organ perfusion and function. Provides guidelines for replacement.
Observe/record quantity, amount and character of NG drainage. Test pH as indicated. Encourage and assist with frequent changes of position.	Excessive fluid output may cause electrolyte imbalance and metabolic alkalosis with further loss of potassium by the kidneys attempting to compensate. Hyperacidity, as indicated by a pH of less than 5, may identify patients at risk, such as those with previous history of ulcers and/or those with potential for stress ulcer formation. Repositioning prevents formation of magenstrasse in the stomach, which can channel gastric fluid and air past tip of NG tube into duodenum.
Monitor temperature.	Low grade fever is common during the first 24–48 hours and can add to insensible fluid losses.
Review cause for surgery and possible effects on fluid balance. Observe for complications, e.g., intestinal obstruction, paralytic ileus, and fistula formation.	Exacerbates fluid and electrolyte losses.
Do guaiac test on stool.	Microscopic/subacute bleeding may not be readily evident.
Collaborative	
Maintain patency of nasogastric/intestinal suction. Maintain low, intermittent suction, as indicated.	Promotes bowel decompression to reduce distention/pressure on suture lines and to reduce nausea and vomiting, which can accompany anesthesia, manipulation of the bowel, or preexisting conditions, e.g., cancer.
Monitor laboratory studies, e.g., Hb/Hct, electrolytes, BUN/Cr.	Provides information about hydration and replacement needs and organ function.
Administer fluids, blood, albumin, electrolytes as indicated.	Maintains circulating volume and electrolyte balance.

NURSING DIAGNOSIS:	**COMFORT, ALTERED: PAIN, ACUTE**
Related to:	**Physical agents, e.g., surgical incisions, abdominal distention, presence of nasogastric/intestinal tube**
Possibly evidenced by:	**Complaints of pain**
	Guarding/distraction behaviors, self-focus
	Autonomic responses, e.g., changes in BP, pulse, respirations
PATIENT OUTCOMES/ EVALUATION CRITERIA:	**Reports pain relieved/controlled. Appears relaxed, able to rest/sleep appropriately.**

ACTIONS/INTERVENTIONS	RATIONALE

Independent

Investigate complaints of pain, noting location, intensity (1–10 scale), and aggravating/relieving factors. Note nonverbal cues, e.g., muscle guarding, shallow breathing, emotional responses.

Incisional pain can be significant in early postoperative phase, aggravated by movement, coughing, abdominal distention, nausea. Having patient rate own discomfort helps identify appropriate interventions and evaluate effectiveness of analgesia.

Encourage patient to report pain as soon as it begins.

Early intervention in pain control facilitates muscle/tissue healing by reducing muscle tension and improving circulation.

Monitor vital signs.

Autonomic responses can include changes in blood pressure, pulse and respirations, which should correlate with complaints/relief of pain. Continuation of abnormal vital signs requires further evaluation.

Assess surgical incisions, noting edema, changes in contour of wound (hematoma formation) or inflammation, drying of wound edges.

Bleeding into tissues, swelling, local inflammation, or development of infection can cause an increased incisional pain.

Provide routine comfort measures, e.g., backrub; splinting incision during position changes and coughing/breathing exercises; calm, quiet environment. Encourage use of guided imagery, relaxation techniques. Provide diversional activities.

Provides support (physical, emotional), reduces muscle tension, enhances relaxation. Continuation of abnormal vital signs requires further evaluation. Refocuses attention, enhances sense of control and coping abilities.

Give frequent oral care, use water-soluble lubricant to the nares. Tape tube so there is no pressure on the nares.

Irritation of mucous membranes causes patient to swallow more frequently and results in abdominal distention (increased ingestion of air).

Maintain patency of NG/intestinal drainage tubes, irrigating as indicated. Note presence of "gas pain," passage of flatus.

Obstruction of tubes can increase abdominal distention (retention of gas), stress internal suture lines, and greatly increase pain.

Palpate bladder for distention when voiding is delayed. Promote privacy and use nursing measures to promote relaxation when patient is attempting to void. Place in semi-Fowler's or standing position as appropriate.

Psychologic factors and pain may increase muscle tension. Upright position increases intraabdominal pressure, which may aid in micturition.

Ambulate patient as soon as possible.

Decreases problems that occur because of immobility, e.g., muscle tension, retained flatus.

Collaborative

Administer analgesics, narcotics as indicated.

Controls/relieves pain to promote rest and enhance cooperation with therapeutic regimen.

Catheterize as necessary.

Single/multiple straight catheterization as well as indwelling insertion may be used to empty the bladder until function returns.

NURSING DIAGNOSIS:	INFECTION, POTENTIAL FOR
May be related to:	Inadequate primary defenses, e.g., chronic disease, invasive procedures, malnutrition
	Opening of the abdominal cavity/bowel with possible contamination, stasis of body fluids, altered peristalsis

Possibly evidenced by:	[Not applicable; presence of signs and symptoms establishes an *actual* diagnosis.]
PATIENT OUTCOMES/ EVALUATION CRITERIA:	Achieves timely wound healing; free of purulent drainage or erythema and fever.

ACTIONS/INTERVENTIONS	RATIONALE

Independent

Monitor vital signs, noting temperature elevation.	Evening temperature spike that returns to normal level in the morning is characteristic of infection. Fever of 38°C (100°F) soon after surgery may indicate pulmonary/urinary/wound infection or thrombophlebitis formation. Fever 38.3°C (101°F) of sudden onset and accompanied by chills, fatigue, weakness, tachypnea, tachycardia, hypotension indicates septic shock. Temperature elevation 4–7 days after surgery is often indicative of wound abscess or fluid leak from anastomosis site.
Observe wound approximation, character of drainage, presence of inflammation.	Development of infection can delay healing.
Monitor respirations, breath sounds. Keep head of bed elevated 35–45 degrees. Turn, cough, help deep-breathe, assist with incentive spirometer, blow bottles.	Pulmonary infections may occur because of respiratory depression (anesthesia, narcotics), ineffective cough (abdominal incision), abdominal distention (decreased lung expansion).
Observe for signs/symptoms of peritonitis, e.g., fever, increasing pain, abdominal distention. (Refer to CP: Peritonitis, p. 449.)	Although bowel preparation is done before elective surgery, peritonitis can occur when intestine is interrupted, e.g., preoperative rupture, leaking anastomosis (postoperative), or when surgery is an emergency/result of an accidental wound.
Maintain aseptic wound care and frequent dressing changes with use of Montgomery straps to secure dressings, if indicated.	Protects patient from cross-contamination. Wet dressings act as a retrograde wick, drawing in external contaminants. Frequent removal of tape (especially when drains are present) may cause skin abrasion, which can also become a site of infection.

Collaborative

Culture suspicious drainage/secretions; if wound, culture both center and outer edges of wound and obtain anaerobic cultures as well.	Multiple organisms may be present in open wounds and after bowel surgery. Anaerobic bacteria, e.g., Bacteroides fragilis, can only be detected by anaerobic cultures. Identifying all organisms involved allows for more specific antibiotic therapy.
Administer medications as indicated:	
Antibiotics, e.g., cefazolin (Ancef).	Given prophylactically and to combat infection.
Do wound irrigations, as needed.	Combats infection when present.

NURSING DIAGNOSIS:	NUTRITION, ALTERED: LESS THAN BODY REQUIREMENTS [POTENTIAL]
May be related to:	Inability to ingest/digest food or absorb sufficient nutrients to meet metabolic demands
	NPO status; nasogastric/intestinal aspiration

439

Possibly evidenced by:	[Not applicable; presence of signs and symptoms establishes an *actual* diagnosis.]
PATIENT OUTCOMES/ EVALUATION CRITERIA:	Demonstrates maintenance of/progressive weight gain toward goal with normalization of laboratory values and no signs of malnutrition.

ACTIONS/INTERVENTIONS	RATIONALE

Independent

Review individual factors that affect ability to ingest/ digest food, e.g., NPO status, nausea, paralytic ileus after tube removal.	Influences choice of interventions.
Weigh as indicated. Record intake and output.	Identifies fluid status as well as ascertaining current metabolic needs.
Palpate abdomen and auscultate for bowel sounds. Record passage of flatus.	Determines return of peristalsis (usually within 2–4 days).
Identify dietary likes/dislikes of patient. Encourage choice of foods high in protein and vitamin C.	Increases patient cooperation with dietary regimen. Proteins/vitamin C are prime contributors to tissue maintenance and repair. Malnutrition is a factor in lowered resistance to infection.
Observe for development of diarrhea; "greasy," foul-smelling stools.	Malabsorption syndrome may develop after surgery of small intestine, requiring further evaluation and dietary modifications, e.g., low-fat diet.

Collaborative

Maintain patency of NG/intestinal tube.	Maintains decompression of stomach/bowel; promotes bowel rest/healing.
Administer IV fluids, albumin, electrolytes;	Corrects fluid and electrolyte imbalances. Bowel inflammation, mucosal erosion, infection, or neoplasm may lead to anemia or malabsorption, reducing delivery of nutrients at the cellular level. Restricted diet gastric/intestinal suction, preoperative bowel preparation may result in electrolyte imbalance, especially sodium and potassium. Loss of plasma, decreased serum albumin (edema, ascites formation, or effusion), and immunodeficiency can prolong wound healing.
Vitamin supplements, with particular attention to vitamin K, parenterally.	Preoperative use of cathartics (bowel preparation) may deplete vitamin supply and/or intestinal problems may have blocked absorption of vitamins. Note: Sterilized bowel cannot synthesize vitamin K, decreasing coagulation potential).
Administer medications as indicated:	
Antiemetics, e.g., prochlorperazine (Compazine);	Prevents vomiting.
Antacids and/or histamine inhibitors, e.g., cimetidine (Tagamet).	Neutralizes or decreases acid formation to prevent mucosal erosion and possible ulceration.
Consult with dietician, nutritional support team. Provide TPN as indicated.	Useful in evaluating and establishing individual dietary needs. Many patients present with marked weight loss and are generally debilitated, thus being at greater risk for postoperative complications. (Refer to CP: Total Nutritional Support, p. 894.)

ACTIONS/INTERVENTIONS

Collaborative

Give liquids, progressing to clear liquid, full diet as tolerated after NG tube is removed.

RATIONALE

Resumption of fluids and diet is essential to return of normal intestinal functioning and promotes adequate nutritional intake.

NURSING DIAGNOSIS:	SKIN/TISSUE INTEGRITY, IMPAIRED: ACTUAL
May be related to:	External factors; surgical incision, radiation
	Internal factors: medication, altered nutritional state, altered circulation, immunologic deficit
	Mechanical factors: pressure, friction
Possibly evidenced by:	Disruption of integumentary and subcutaneous tissues, invasion of body structures
PATIENT OUTCOMES/ EVALUATION CRITERIA:	Achieves timely wound healing without complications.

ACTIONS/INTERVENTIONS

Independent

Monitor vital signs frequently noting fever, tachypnea, tachycardia, and apprehension. Check wound frequently for excessive incisional swelling, inflammation, drainage.

Splint incision during coughing and breathing exercises. Apply binder/support for elderly and obese patients if indicated.

Use paper tape/montgomery straps for dressings as indicated.

Be aware of further risk factors, i.e., malignancies, such as lymphosarcoma and multiple myeloma; radiation therapy of operative site.

If dehiscence occurs:

Maintain calm attitude. Notify physician.

Keep patient on complete bedrest. Position with knees bent.

If evisceration occurs:

Cover exposed intestines with sterile moist dressings. Prepare for surgical repair of wound.

RATIONALE

May be indicative of hematoma formation/developing infection, which contributes to delayed wound healing and increases risk of wound separation/dehiscence.

Minimizes stress/tension on healing wound edges. The aging process and atherosclerosis contribute to diminished circulation to the wound. Fatty tissue is difficult to approximate, and suture line is more easily disrupted.

Frequent dressing changes may result in damage to skin from regular tape.

Reduces immunocompetence thus interfering with wound healing and resistance to infection. Promotes vasculitis and fibrosis in connective tissue, interfering with delivery of oxygen and nutrients necessary for healing.

Stressful situation in which it is extremely important to prevent panic in both the patient and the nurse.

Reduces intraabdominal tension. May prevent evisceration from occurring.

Prevents drying of mucosal tissue.

ACTIONS/INTERVENTIONS

Collaborative

Review laboratory values for evidence of anemia and decreased serum albumin. Note leukocyte count.

RATIONALE

Anemia and edema formation can interfere with healing. Steroid therapy and anticancer drugs reduce leukocyte count and suppress capillary formation and fibrogenesis.

NURSING DIAGNOSIS:	**BOWEL ELIMINATION, ALTERED: (SPECIFY)**
May be related to:	**Effects of anesthesia, surgical manipulation**
	Less than adequate dietary intake and bulk
	Physical inactivity, immobility
	Inflammation, irritation, malabsorption of bowel
	Pain, medication effects
Possibly evidenced by:	**Absence of stool (immediately postoperatively); constipation; diarrhea**
PATIENT OUTCOMES/ EVALUATION CRITERIA:	**Reestablishes normal pattern of bowel functioning.**

ACTIONS/INTERVENTIONS

Independent

Auscultate bowel sounds.

Investigate complaints of abdominal pain.

Observe bowel movements, noting color, consistency and amount.

Encourage nonirritating foods/fluids when oral intake is resumed.

Collaborative

Provide stool softener, glycerine suppository as indicated.

RATIONALE

Return of GI function may be delayed by depressant effects of anesthesia, paralytic ileus, intraperitoneal inflammation, medications.

May be related to gas distention as intestinal function resumes or developing complications, e.g., ileus.

Indicator of return of GI function, identifies appropriate interventions.

Reduces risk of mucosal irritation/diarrhea.

May be necessary to gently stimulate peristalsis/stool evacuation.

NURSING DIAGNOSIS:	**KNOWLEDGE DEFICIT [LEARNING NEED] (SPECIFY)**
May be related to:	**Lack of exposure/recall**
	Information misinterpretation
	Unfamiliarity with information resources
Possibly evidenced by:	**Questions; request for information**
	Statement of misconception

Inaccurate follow-through of instruction

PATIENT OUTCOMES/ EVALUATION CRITERIA:	Verbalizes understanding of disease process and treatment. Identifies relationship of signs/symptoms to the disease process and correlates symptoms with causative factors. Correctly performs necessary procedures and explains reasons for actions.

ACTIONS/INTERVENTIONS	RATIONALE
Independent	
Review surgical procedure and postoperative expectations.	Provides knowledge base on which patient can make informed choices.
Discuss importance of adequate fluid intake, dietary needs.	Promotes healing and normalization of bowel function.
Demonstrate appropriate wound care/dressing change. Encourage showering and use of mild soap to clean wound.	Promotes healing, reduces risk of infection, provides opportunity to observe wound healing.
Identify signs/symptoms requiring medical evaluation, e.g., persistent fever, swelling, erythema, or opening of wound edges.	Early recognition of complications and prompt intervention may prevent progression to serious, life-threatening situation.
Review activity limitations/restrictions, e.g., no heavy lifting for 6–8 weeks, avoidance of strenuous exercise/ sports.	Reduces risk of incisional strain/trauma.
Encourage progressive advancement of activity as tolerated and balance with adequate rest periods.	Prevents fatigue, stimulates circulation and normalization of organ function, promotes healing.

Appendectomy

Refer to CP: Surgical Intervention, p. 789, for general considerations.

PATIENT ASSESSMENT DATA BASE (Preoperative)

CIRCULATION

May exhibit: Tachycardia.

ELIMINATION

May report: Constipation of recent onset.
Diarrhea (occasional).

May exhibit: Abdominal distention, tenderness/rebound tenderness, rigidity.
Decreased or absent bowel sounds.

FOOD/FLUID

May report: Anorexia.
Nausea and vomiting.

PAIN/COMFORT

May report: Abdominal pain around the epigastrium and umbilicus, which becomes increasingly severe and localizes at McBurney's point (halfway between umbilicus and crest of right ileum), aggravated by walking, sneezing, coughing, or deep respiration (sudden cessation of pain suggests perforation).
Varied complaints of pain/vague symptoms (due to location of appendix, e.g., retrocecally or next to ureter).

May exhibit: Guarding behavior; lying on side or back with knees flexed; increased RLQ pain with extension of right leg/upright position.

SAFETY

May exhibit: Fever (usually low-grade).

RESPIRATION

May exhibit: Tachypnea; shallow respirations.

TEACHING/LEARNING

May report: History of acute pyelitis, ureteral stone, acute salpingitis, regional ileitis.
May occur at any age.

Discharge Plan Considerations: May need brief assistance with transportation, home management.

DIAGNOSTIC STUDIES

WBC: leukocytosis above 10,000/cu mm, neutrophil count elevated to 75%.
Urinalysis: normal but erythrocytes/leukocytes may be present.
Abdominal x-rays: may reveal hardened bit of fecal material in appendix (fecalith), localized ileus.

NURSING PRIORITIES

1. Promote comfort.
2. Prevent complications.
3. Provide information about surgical procedure/prognosis, treatment needs, and potential complications.

DISCHARGE CRITERIA

1. Complications prevented/minimized.
2. Pain alleviated/controlled.
3. Surgical procedure/prognosis, therapeutic regimen, and possible complications understood.

NURSING DIAGNOSIS:	INFECTION, POTENTIAL FOR
May be related to:	Inadequate primary defenses; perforation/rupture of the appendix; peritonitis; abscess formation
	Invasive procedures, surgical incision
Possibly evidenced by:	[Not applicable; presence of signs and symptoms establishes an *actual* diagnosis.]
PATIENT OUTCOMES/ EVALUATION CRITERIA:	Achieves timely wound healing; free of signs of infection/inflammation, purulent drainage, erythema, and fever.

ACTIONS/INTERVENTIONS	RATIONALE
Independent	
Monitor vital signs. Note onset of fever, chills, diaphoresis, changes in mentation, complaints of increasing abdominal pain.	Suggestive of presence of infection/developing sepsis, abscess, peritonitis.
Practice good handwashing and aseptic wound care. Provide peri-care.	Reduces risk of spread of bacteria.
Inspect incision and dressings. Note characteristics of drainage from wound/drains (if inserted), presence of erythema.	Provides for early detection of developing infectious process, and/or monitors resolution of pre-existing peritonitis.
Provide accurate, honest information to patient/SO.	Being informed about progress of situation, provides emotional support, helping to decrease anxiety.
Collaborative	
Obtain drainage specimens if indicated.	Gram stain, culture and sensitivity are useful in identifying causative organism and choice of therapy.
Administer antibiotics as indicated.	May be given prophylactically or to reduce number of multiplying organisms in the presence of infection to decrease spread and seeding of the abdominal cavity. (Refer to CP: Peritonitis, p. 449.)
Assist with incision and drainage (I&D) if indicated.	May be necessary to drain contents of localized abscess.

```
┌─────────────────────────────────────────────────────────────────────────────┐
│  NURSING DIAGNOSIS:          FLUID VOLUME DEFICIT, POTENTIAL                  │
│                                                                               │
│     May be related to:       Preoperative vomiting                           │
│                                                                               │
│                              Postoperative restrictions (e.g., NPO)          │
│                                                                               │
│                              Hypermetabolic state (e.g., fever, healing      │
│                              process)                                         │
│                                                                               │
│                              Inflammation of peritoneum with sequestration   │
│                              of fluid                                         │
│                                                                               │
│     Possibly evidenced by:   [Not applicable; presence of signs and symptoms │
│                              establishes an actual diagnosis.]                │
│                                                                               │
│  PATIENT OUTCOMES/           Maintains adequate fluid balance as evidenced   │
│  EVALUATION CRITERIA:        by moist mucous membranes, good skin turgor,    │
│                              stable vital signs, and individually adequate    │
│                              urinary output.                                  │
└─────────────────────────────────────────────────────────────────────────────┘
```

ACTIONS/INTERVENTIONS	RATIONALE
Independent	
Monitor blood pressure, pulse, central venous pressure (CVP).	Variations help identify fluctuating intravascular volumes, e.g., low CVP is an early indicator of hypovolemia.
Inspect mucous membranes; assess skin turgor and capillary refill.	Indicators of adequacy of peripheral circulation and cellular hydration.
Monitor intake and output; note urine color/concentration, specific gravity.	Decreasing output of concentrated urine with increasing specific gravity suggests dehydration/need for increased fluids.
Provide clear liquids in small amounts when oral intake is resumed and progress diet as tolerated.	Reduces risk of gastric irritation/vomiting to minimize fluid loss.
Give frequent mouth care with special attention to protection of the lips.	Dehydration results in drying and painful cracking of the lips and mouth.
Collaborative	
Maintain gastric/intestinal suction.	An NG tube is usually inserted preoperatively and maintained in immediate postoperative phase to decompress the bowel, promote intestinal rest, prevent vomiting (reduce fluid loss).
Administer IV fluids and electrolytes.	The peritoneum reacts to irritation/infection by producing large amounts of fluid that may reduce the circulating blood volume, resulting in hypovolemia. Dehydration and relative electrolyte imbalances (e.g., hypoproteinemia) may occur.

```
┌─────────────────────────────────────────────────────────────────────────────┐
│  NURSING DIAGNOSIS:          COMFORT, ALTERED: PAIN, ACUTE                    │
│                                                                               │
│     May be related to:       Distention of intestinal tissues by            │
│                              inflammation                                     │
│                                                                               │
│                              Presence of surgical incision                   │
│                                                                               │
│     Possibly evidenced by:   Complaints of pain                              │
│                                                                               │
│                              Facial grimacing, muscle guarding; distraction  │
│                              behaviors                                        │
```

Autonomic responses

| PATIENT OUTCOMES/ EVALUATION CRITERIA: | Reports pain is relieved/controlled. Appears relaxed, able to sleep/rest appropriately. |

ACTIONS/INTERVENTIONS

Independent

Assess pain, noting location, characteristics, severity (1–10 scale).

Keep at rest in semi-Fowler's position.

Encourage early ambulation.

Provide diversional activities.

Collaborative

Keep NPO/maintain NG suction initially.

Administer analgesics as indicated, e.g., oxycodone (Tylox); propoxyphene napsylate and acetaminophen (Darvocet-N).

Place ice bag on abdomen.

RATIONALE

Useful in monitoring effectiveness of medication, progression of healing. Changes in characteristics of pain may indicate developing abscess/peritonitis, requiring prompt medical evaluation and intervention.

Gravity localizes inflammatory exudate into lower abdomen or pelvis, relieving abdominal tension, which is accentuated by supine position.

Promotes normalization of organ function, e.g., stimulates peristalsis and passing of flatus, reducing abdominal discomfort.

Refocuses attention, promotes relaxation, and may enhance coping abilities.

Decreases discomfort of early intestinal peristalsis and gastric irritation/vomiting.

Relief of pain facilitates cooperation with other therapeutic interventions, e.g., ambulation, pulmonary toilet.

Soothes and relieves pain through desensitization of nerve endings. Note: Do not use heat, because it may cause tissue congestion.

NURSING DIAGNOSIS:	KNOWLEDGE DEFICIT [LEARNING NEED] (SPECIFY)
May be related to:	Lack of exposure/recall; information misinterpretation
	Unfamiliarity with information resources
Possibly evidenced by:	Questions; request for information; verbalization of the problem/concerns
	Statement of misconception
	Inaccurate follow-through of instruction
	Development of preventable complications
PATIENT OUTCOMES/ EVALUATION CRITERIA:	Verbalizes understanding of disease process, treatment, and potential complications. Participates in treatment regimen.

ACTIONS/INTERVENTIONS	RATIONALE

Independent

Review postoperative activity restrictions, e.g., heavy lifting, exercise (sex/sports).

Provides information for patient to plan for return to usual routines without untoward incidence.

Encourage progressive activities as tolerated with periodic rest periods.

Prevents fatigue, promotes healing and feeling of well-being and facilitates resumption of normal activities.

Recommend use of mild laxative/stool softeners as necessary and avoidance of enemas.

Assists with return to usual bowel function; prevents undue straining for defecation.

Discuss care of incision, including dressing changes, bathing restrictions, and return to physician for suture removal.

Understanding promotes cooperation with therapeutic regimen, enhancing healing and recovery process.

Identify symptoms requiring medical evaluation, e.g., increasing pain; edema/erythema of wound; presence of drainage, fever.

Prompt intervention reduces risk of serious complications, e.g., delayed wound healing, peritonitis.

Peritonitis

Inflammation of the peritoneal cavity can be primary or secondary, acute or chronic. Major sources of inflammation are from the GI tract, ovaries/uterus, urinary system, or the bloodstream. Surgical intervention may be curative in localized peritonitis, e.g., appendicitis/appendectomy, ulcer plication, and bowel resection. If peritonitis is diffuse, medical management is necessary before or in place of surgical treatment.

PATIENT ASSESSMENT DATA BASE

ACTIVITY/REST

May report: Weakness.

May exhibit: Difficulty ambulating.

CIRCULATION

May exhibit: Tachycardia, diaphoresis, pallor, hypotension (signs of shock).
Tissue edema.

ELIMINATION

May report: Inability to pass stool or flatus.

May exhibit: Hiccups; abdominal distention; quiet abdomen.
Decreased urinary output, dark color.
Decreased/absent bowel sounds (ileus); intermittent loud, rushing bowel sounds (obstruction); abdominal rigidity, distention, rebound tenderness.
Hyperresonance/tympany (ileus); loss of dullness over liver (free air in abdomen).

FOOD/FLUID

May report: Anorexia, nausea, vomiting; thirst.

May exhibit: Projectile vomiting.
Dry mucous membranes, poor skin turgor.

PAIN/COMFORT

May report: Abdominal pain, generalized or localized, referred to shoulder, intensified by movement.

May exhibit: Distention, rigidity, rebound tenderness.
Muscle guarding (abdomen), distraction behaviors, restlessness, self-focus.

RESPIRATION

May exhibit: Shallow respirations, tachypnea.

SAFETY

May report: Fever, chills.

SEXUALITY

May report: History of pelvic organ inflammation (salpingitis), puerperal infection, septic abortion; retroperitoneal abscess.

May report:	History of recent trauma with abdominal penetration, e.g., gunshot/stab wound or blunt trauma to the abdomen; bladder perforation/rupture; illness of GI tract, e.g., appendicitis with perforation, gangrenous/ruptured gallbladder, perforated carcinoma of the stomach, perforated gastric/duodenal ulcer, gangrenous obstruction of the bowel, perforation of diverticulum, ulcerative colitis, regional ileitis; strangulated hernia.
Discharge Plan Considerations:	Assistance with homemaker tasks

DIAGNOSTIC STUDIES

CBC: WBCs elevated, sometimes greater than 20,000. Red blood cell count may be increased, indicating hemoconcentration.

Serum protein/albumin: may be decreased owing to fluid shifts.

Serum amylase: usually elevated.

ABGs: respiratory alkalosis and metabolic acidosis may be noted.

Cultures: causative organism may be identified from blood, exudate/secretions, or ascitic fluid.

Abdominal x-ray examination: may reveal gas distention of bowel/ileus. If a perforated viscera is the etiology, free air will be found in the abdomen.

Paracentesis: peritoneal fluid samples may contain blood, pus/exudate, amylase, bile, and creatinine.

NURSING PRIORITIES

1. Control infection.
2. Restore/maintain circulating volume.
3. Promote comfort.
4. Maintain nutrition.
5. Provide information about disease process, possible complications and treatment needs.

DISCHARGE CRITERIA

1. Infection resolved.
2. Complications prevented/minimized.
3. Pain relieved.
4. Disease process, potential complications, and therapeutic regimen understood.

NURSING DIAGNOSIS:	**INFECTION, POTENTIAL FOR [SEPTICEMIA]**
May be related to:	**Inadequate primary defenses (broken skin, traumatized tissue, altered peristalsis)**
	Inadequate secondary defenses (immunosuppression)
	Invasive procedures
Possibly evidenced by:	**[Not applicable; presence of signs and symptoms establishes an *actual* diagnosis.]**
PATIENT OUTCOMES/ EVALUATION CRITERIA:	**Achieves timely healing; free of purulent drainage or erythema; and afebrile. Verbalizes understanding of the individual causative/risk factor(s).**

ACTIONS/INTERVENTIONS	RATIONALE

Independent

Note individual risk factors, e.g., abdominal trauma, acute appendicitis, peritoneal dialysis.

Influences choice of interventions.

Assess vital signs frequently, noting unresolved or progressing hypotension, decreased pulse pressure, tachycardia, fever, tachypnea.

Signs of impending septic shock. Circulating endotoxins eventually produce vasodilation, loss of fluid from circulation, and a low cardiac output state.

Note changes in mental status (e.g., confusion, stupor).

Hypoxemia, hypotension, and acidosis can cause deteriorating mental status.

Note skin color, temperature, moisture.

Warm, flushed, dry skin is early sign of septicemia. Later manifestations include cool, clammy pale skin and cyanosis as shock becomes refractory. (Refer to CP: Sepsis/Septicemia, p. 763.)

Monitor urine output.

Oliguria develops as a result of decreased renal perfusion and circulating toxins.

Maintain strict aseptic technique in care of abdominal drains, incisions/open wounds, dressings and invasive sites. Cleanse with Betadine or other appropriate solution.

Prevents access or limits spread of infecting organisms/cross-contamination.

Observe drainage from wounds/drains.

Provides information about resolution of infection.

Maintain sterile technique when catheterizing patient, and provide catheter care/perineal cleansing on a routine basis.

Prevents access, limits bacterial growth in urinary tract.

Provide protective isolation if indicated.

Reduce risk of secondary infection in immunosuppressed patient.

Collaborative

Obtain specimens/monitor results of serial blood, urine, wound cultures.

Identifies causative microorganisms and helps in assessing effectiveness of antimicrobial regimen.

Administer antimicrobials, e.g., gentamicin (Garamycin), amikacin (Amikin), clindamycin (Cleocin), IV/peritoneal lavage.

Therapy is directed at anaerobic bacteria and aerobic gram-negative bacilli. Lavage may be used to remove necrotic debris and treat inflammation which is poorly localized/diffuse.

Assist with peritoneal aspiration, if indicated.

May be done to remove fluid and to identify infecting organisms(s) so appropriate antibiotic therapy can be instituted.

Prepare for surgical intervention if indicated. (Refer to CPs: Surgical Intervention, p. 789; Intestinal Surgery, p. 436; Subtotal Gastrectomy, p. 407.)

May be treatment of choice (curative) in acute, localized peritonitis, e.g., to drain localized abscess, remove peritoneal exudates, remove ruptured appendix/gallbladder, plicate perforated ulcer, or resect bowel.

NURSING DIAGNOSIS:	FLUID VOLUME DEFICIT, ACTUAL 2
May be related to:	**Active loss, e.g., fluid shifts from extracellular, intravascular, and interstitial compartments into intestines and/ or peritoneal space; vomiting; nasogastric/intestinal aspiration; fever**
	Medically restricted intake

Possibly evidenced by:	Dry mucous membranes, poor skin turgor, delayed capillary refill, weak peripheral pulses
	Diminished urinary output, dark/concentrated urine
	Hypotension, tachycardia
PATIENT OUTCOMES/ EVALUATION CRITERIA:	Demonstrates improved fluid balance as evidenced by adequate urinary output with normal specific gravity, stable vital signs, moist mucous membranes, good skin turgor, prompt capillary refill, and weight within acceptable range.

ACTIONS/INTERVENTIONS	RATIONALE
Independent	
Monitor vital signs, noting presence of hypotension (including postural changes), tachycardia, tachypnea, fever. Measure CVP if available.	Aids in evaluating degree of fluid deficit/effectiveness of fluid replacement therapy and response to medications.
Maintain accurate intake/output and correlate with daily weights. Include measured/estimated losses, e.g., gastric suction, drains, dressings, hemovacs, diaphoresis, abdominal girth.	Reflects overall hydration status. Urine output may be diminished owing to hypovolemia and decreased renal perfusion, but weight may still increase, reflecting tissue edema/ascites accumulation. Gastric suction losses may be large, and a great deal of fluid can be sequestered in the bowel and peritoneal space (ascites).
Measure urine specific gravity.	Reflects hydration status and changes in renal function, which may warn of developing acute renal failure in response to hypovolemia, effect of toxins. Note: Many antibiotics also have nephrotoxic effects which may further affect kidney function/urine output.
Observe skin/mucous membrane dryness, turgor. Note peripheral/sacral edema.	Hypovolemia, fluid shifts, nutritional deficits contribute to poor skin turgor, taut edematous tissues.
Eliminate noxious sights/smells from environment. Limit intake of ice chips.	Reduces gastric stimulation and vomiting response. Note: Excess use of ice chips during gastric aspiration can increase gastric washout of electrolytes.
Change position frequently, provide frequent skin care, and maintain dry/wrinkle free bedding.	Edematous tissue with compromised circulation is prone to breakdown.
Collaborative	
Monitor laboratory studies, e.g., Hb/Hct, electrolytes, protein, albumin, BUN, Cr.	Provides information about hydration, organ function. Varied alterations with significant consequences to systemic function are possible as a result of fluid shifts, hypovolemia, hypoxemia, circulating toxins, and necrotic tissue products.
Administer plasma, fluids, electrolytes, diuretics as indicated.	Replenishes/maintains circulating volume and electrolyte balance. Colloids help move water back into intravascular compartment by increasing osmotic pressure gradient. Diuretics may be used to assist in excretion of toxins and to enhance renal function.
Maintain NPO with nasogastric/intestinal aspiration.	Reduces hyperactivity of bowel and diarrhea losses.

NURSING DIAGNOSIS:	COMFORT, ALTERED: PAIN, ACUTE
May be related to:	Injuring agents: stimulation of the parietal peritoneum by toxins; trauma to tissues; accumulation of fluid in abdominal/peritoneal cavity (abdominal distention)
Possibly evidenced by:	Verbalizations of pain
	Muscle guarding, rebound tenderness
	Facial mask of pain, self-focus
	Distraction behavior, autonomic/emotional responses (anxiety)
PATIENT OUTCOMES/ EVALUATION CRITERIA:	Reports pain is relieved/controlled. Demonstrates use of relaxation skills, other methods to promote comfort.

ACTIONS/INTERVENTIONS	RATIONALE
Independent	
Investigate pain complaints, noting location, duration, intensity (1–10 scale), and characteristics (dull, sharp, constant).	Changes in location/intensity are not uncommon but may reflect developing complications. Pain tends to become constant, more intense, and diffuse over the entire abdomen as inflammatory process accelerates; or pain may localize if an abscess develops.
Maintain semi-Fowler's position as indicated.	Facilitates fluid/wound drainage by gravity, reducing diaphragmatic irritation/abdominal tension, and thereby reduces pain.
Move patient slowly and deliberately, splinting painful area.	Reduces muscle tension/guarding, which may help minimize pain of movement.
Provide routine comfort measures, e.g., massage, backrubs, deep breathing, relaxation/visualization exercises.	Promotes relaxation and may enhance patient's coping abilities by refocusing attention.
Provide frequent oral care. Remove noxious environmental stimuli.	Reduces nausea/vomiting, which can increase intraabdominal pressure/pain.
Collaborative	
Administer medications as indicated:	
Analgesics, narcotics;	Reduces metabolic rate and intestinal irritation from circulating/local toxins, which aids in pain relief and promotes healing. Note: Pain is usually severe and may require narcotic pain control.
Antiemetics, e.g., hydroxyzine (Vistaril);	Reduces nausea, vomiting, which can increase abdominal pain.
Antipyretics, e.g., acetaminophen (Tylenol).	Reduces discomfort associated with fever/chills

NURSING DIAGNOSIS:	NUTRITION, ALTERED: LESS THAN BODY REQUIRE-MENTS [POTENTIAL]
May be related to:	Nausea, vomiting, intestinal dysfunction

	Metabolic abnormalities; increased metabolic needs
Possibly evidenced by:	[Not applicable; presence of signs and symptoms establishes an *actual* diagnosis.]
PATIENT OUTCOMES/ EVALUATION CRITERIA:	Maintains usual weight and positive nitrogen balance.

ACTIONS/INTERVENTIONS

Independent

Monitor NG tube output. Note presence of vomiting/diarrhea.

Auscultate bowel sounds, noting absent/hyperactive sounds.

Measure abdominal girth.

Weigh regularly.

Assess abdomen frequently for return to softness, reappearance of normal bowel sounds, and passage of flatus.

Collaborative

Monitor BUN, protein, albumin, glucose as indicated.

Advance diet as tolerated, e.g., clear liquid to soft.

Administer hyperalimentation (TPN) as indicated. (Refer to CP: Total Nutritional Support, p. 894.)

RATIONALE

Large amounts of gastric aspirant, vomiting/diarrhea suggest bowel obstruction, requiring further evaluation.

Although bowel sounds are frequently absent, inflammation/irritation of the intestine may be accompanied by intestinal hyperactivity, diminished water absorption, and diarrhea.

Provides quantitative evidence of changes in gastric/intestinal distention and/or accumulation of ascites.

Initial losses/gains reflect changes in hydration but sustained losses suggest nutritional deficit.

Indicates return of normal bowel function and ability to resume oral intake.

Reflects organ function and nutritional status/needs.

Careful progression of diet when intake is resumed reduces risk of gastric irritation.

Promotes nutrient utilization and positive nitrogen balance in patients who are unable to assimilate nutrients in a normal fashion.

NURSING DIAGNOSIS:	**ANXIETY [SPECIFY]/FEAR**
May be related to:	**Situational crisis**
	Threat of death/change in health status
	Physiologic factors, hypermetabolic state
Possibly evidenced by:	**Increased tension/helplessness**
	Apprehension, uncertainty, worry
	Sense of impending doom
	Sympathetic stimulation; restlessness; focus on self
PATIENT OUTCOMES/ EVALUATION CRITERIA:	**Appears relaxed and reports anxiety is reduced to a manageable level. Verbalizes awareness of feelings and healthy ways to deal with them.**

ACTIONS/INTERVENTIONS

Independent

Evaluate anxiety level, noting patient's verbal and non-verbal response. Encourage free expression of emotions.

Provide information regarding disease process and anticipated treatment.

Schedule adequate rest and uninterrupted periods for sleep.

(Refer to CP: Psychosocial Aspects of Acute Care, p. 773.)

RATIONALE

Apprehension may be escalated by severe pain, increasingly ill feeling, urgency of diagnostic procedures, and possibility of surgery.

Knowing what to expect can reduce anxiety.

Limits fatigue, conserves energy and can enhance coping ability.

NURSING DIAGNOSIS:	KNOWLEDGE DEFICIT [LEARNING NEED] (SPECIFY)
May be related to:	**Lack of exposure/recall**
	Information misinterpretation
	Unfamiliarity with information resources
Possibly evidenced by:	**Questions; request for information**
	Statement of misconception
	Inaccurate follow-through of instruction
PATIENT OUTCOMES/ EVALUATION CRITERIA:	**Verbalizes understanding of disease process and treatment. Identifies relationship of signs/symptoms to the disease process and correlates symptoms with causative factors. Correctly performs necessary procedures and explains reasons for actions.**

ACTIONS/INTERVENTIONS

Independent

Review underlying disease process and recovery expectations. (Refer to CP: Upper Gastrointestinal/ Esophageal Bleeding, p. 397; Inflammatory Bowel Disease, p. 411.)

Discuss medication regimen, schedule, and possible side effects.

Recommend gradual resumption of usual activities as tolerated, allowing for adequate rest.

Review activity restrictions/limitations, e.g., avoid heavy lifting, constipation.

Demonstrate aseptic dressing change, wound care.

Identify signs/symptoms requiring medical evaluation, e.g., recurrent abdominal pain/distention, vomiting, fever, chills; or presence of purulent drainage, swelling/ erythema of surgical incision (if present).

RATIONALE

Provides knowledge base on which patient can make informed choices.

Antibiotics may be continued after discharge dependent on length of stay.

Prevents fatigue, enhances feeling of well-being.

Avoids unnecessary increase of intraabdominal pressure and muscle tension.

Reduces risk of contamination. Provides opportunity to evaluate healing process.

Early recognition and treatment of developing complications may prevent more serious illness/injury.

Herniorrhaphy (Uncomplicated)

Refer to CPs: Intestinal Surgery, p. 436, for concerns regarding gangrenous bowel; Surgical Intervention, p. 789.

PATIENT ASSESSMENT DATA BASE

The data are dependent on location and severity.

ACTIVITY/REST

May report: Limitation of desired activity.

Occupation, usual activity, lifting or straining activities, and body mechanics.

CIRCULATION

May exhibit: Tachycardia.

ELIMINATION

May report: Constipation.

May exhibit: Abdominal distention/rigidity (incarcerated/irreducible hernia).

Palpable abdominal mass.

Bowel sounds may be high-pitched/hyperactive in mechanical obstruction, progressing to decreased/absent.

FOOD/FLUID

May report: Nausea/vomiting (intestinal obstruction).

PAIN/COMFORT

May report: Complaints of localized pain (may be colicky in nature), increasing with cough/straining.

RESPIRATION

May report: Recent/current upper respiratory infection with coughing.

Chronic cough (smoking); sneezing (allergies).

SAFETY

May exhibit: Fever.

Lump or swelling that has been previously reducible.

Palpation of herniated area revealing contents of the sac.

Elevated WBC.

TEACHING/LEARNING

May report: Onset of occurrence of increase in size of previous hernia (directly related to an increase in intraabdominal pressure, e.g., pregnancy, lifting heavy objects).

Discharge Plan Considerations: Assistance with strenuous homemaker/maintenance tasks; vocational counseling.

DIAGNOSTIC STUDIES

CBC with differential: elevated WBC reflects inflammatory process.

Chest x-ray: may reveal presence of respiratory problems which may affect healing.

NURSING PRIORITIES

1. Maximize incisional healing.
2. Prevent complications.
3. Provide information about occurrence/prognosis, treatment needs, and possible complications.

DISCHARGE CRITERIA

1. Optimal incisional healing.
2. Complications prevented/minimized.
3. Condition/prognosis, therapeutic regimen, and potential complications understood.

NURSING DIAGNOSIS:	SKIN/TISSUE INTEGRITY, IMPAIRED: ACTUAL
May be related to:	Surgical intervention
	Altered circulation, nutritional state (obesity)
Possibly evidenced by:	Disruption of integumentary, subcutaneous tissues
PATIENT OUTCOMES/ EVALUATION CRITERIA:	Achieves timely wound healing without recurrence of hernia.

ACTIONS/INTERVENTIONS	RATIONALE
Independent	
Promote good handwashing techniques, aseptic wound care.	Prevents cross contamination, promotes healing.
Inspect incision, note presence of erythema, purulent drainage.	Development of infection can delay healing and increase risk of recurrence of hernia.
Palpate bladder. Use appropriate nursing measures to encourage voiding. Stand male patient at side of bed as tolerated.	Urinary retention is a frequent complication, and bladder distention can result in stress on the abdominal incision.
Examine scrotum at regular intervals to note any occurrence of swelling.	After inguinal herniorrhaphy, swelling may occur because of inflammation, edema, or hemorrhage, stressing suture line, delaying healing.
Encourage deep breathing and turning instead of coughing. Splint incision if patient does cough/sneeze.	Aids in maintaining good respiratory function without increasing intraabdominal pressure and stressing the incision.
Assist with early ambulation.	Surgical procedure is often done as outpatient procedure, but initial activity may be hampered by changes in BP/syncope, residual effects of anesthesia, and postoperative discomfort.
Provide adequate hydration and return to full diet as tolerated.	Promoting normal bowel function minimizes straining during defecation, which could cause incisional stress.
Collaborative	
Apply ice bags to scrotum, and provide scrotal support as indicated.	Minimizes edema and swelling, prevents tension of spermatic cord, and relieves swelling and pain.
Administer medications as indicated, e.g.:	
Laxatives/stool softeners;	Prevents and/or relieves constipation.

457

ACTIONS/INTERVENTIONS

Collaborative

Analgesics;

Antibiotics.

Catheterize if unable to void.

RATIONALE

Promotes relaxation, relieves pain, and enhances co-operation with other therapeutic interventions.

Prevents the development of epididymitis.

Prevents bladder distention with subsequent pressure on operative area.

NURSING DIAGNOSIS:	KNOWLEDGE DEFICIT [LEARNING NEED] (SPECIFY)
May be related to:	**Lack of exposure/recall; information misinterpretation**
	Unfamiliarity with information resources
Possibly evidenced by:	**Questions; request for information; statement of misconception**
	Verbalization of problem
	Inaccurate follow-through of instruction
	Development of preventable complication
PATIENT OUTCOMES/ EVALUATION CRITERIA:	**Verbalizes understanding of condition/treatment, activities allowed after discharge. Initiates necessary lifestyle changes and participates in treatment regimen.**

ACTIONS/INTERVENTIONS

Independent

Review procedure and prognosis.

Discuss use of stool softeners/laxatives; prescribed medications.

Instruct patient in necessity of restricting lifting/strenuous activities, including a review of occupational duties. Recommend regular activity program, e.g., walking daily.

Review good body mechanics. Provide information as needed.

Encourage adequate fluid intake and high-residue/bulk diet.

Suggest weight reduction program if needed.

Give information about ability to return to normal sexual activity as soon as healing and pain allow.

Identify symptoms requiring medical evaluation, e.g., inflammation, erythema, drainage from wound, bulging of incision, presence of fever.

RATIONALE

Provides knowledge base on which patient can make informed choices.

Reduces risk of postoperative complications, e.g., recurrence of hernia or infection.

Restrictions may range from minimal to major, depending on the extent of the surgery. Occupational duties/manual labor may need to be curtailed for up to 6 weeks/until healing has progressed.

Prevent recurrence of hernia.

Prevention of constipation reduces risk of straining at stool with corresponding increase in abdominal pressure and resultant stress on incision.

Obesity increases risk of recurrence/surgical failure.

Sexual functioning should not be affected, but patient concerns/fears may interfere with resumption.

Prompt intervention may prevent more serious complications related to infection, delayed wound healing.

Cholecystitis With Cholelithiasis

PATIENT ASSESSMENT DATA BASE

Activity/Rest

May report:	Fatigue.
May exhibit:	Restlessness.

CIRCULATION

May exhibit:	Tachycardia.

ELIMINATION

May report:	Change in color of urine and stools.
May exhibit:	Abdominal distention.
	Palpable mass in upper right quadrant.
	Dark, concentrated urine.
	Clay-colored stool, steatorrhea.

FOOD/FLUID

May report:	Anorexia, nausea and vomiting.
	Intolerance of fatty and "gas-forming" foods; recurrent regurgitation, heartburn, indigestion, flatulence, bloating (dyspepsia).
	Belching (eructation).
May exhibit:	Obesity; recent weight loss.

PAIN/COMFORT

May report:	Severe upper abdominal pain, may radiate to shoulder.
	Midepigastric colicky pain associated with eating.
	Pain starting suddenly and usually peaking in 30 minutes.
May exhibit:	Rebound tenderness, muscle guarding or rigidity when RUQ is palpated; positive Murphy's sign.

RESPIRATION

May exhibit:	Increased respiratory rate.
	Splinted respiration marked by short, shallow breathing.

SAFETY

May exhibit:	Fever, chills.
	Jaundice, with dry, itching skin (pruritis).
	Bleeding tendencies (vitamin K deficiency).

TEACHING/LEARNING

May report:	Familial tendency for gallstones.
	Recent pregnancy/delivery; history of diabetes mellitus, inflammatory bowel disease, blood dyscrasias.
Discharge Plan Considerations:	May require support with dietary changes/weight reduction.

459

DIAGNOSTIC STUDIES

CBC: moderate leukocytosis (acute).

Serum bilirubin and amylase: elevated.

Serum liver enzymes (SGOT [AST], SGPT [ALT], LDH): slight elevation; alkaline phosphatase and 5-nucleotidase markedly elevates in biliary obstruction.

Prothrombin levels: reduced when obstruction to the flow of bile into the intestine decreases absorption of vitamin K.

Ultrasound: reveals calculi, with gallbladder and/or bile duct distention (frequently the initial diagnostic procedure).

CT scan: may reveal gallbladder cysts, dilation of bile ducts.

Liver scan (with radioactive dye): shows obstruction of the biliary tree.

Abdominal x-ray films (multipositional): reveal radiopaque (calcified) gallstones, calcification of the wall or enlargement of the gallbladder.

Cholecystograms (for chronic cholecystitis): reveal stones in the biliary system. Note: contraindicated in acute cholecystitis because the patient is too ill to take the dye by mouth.

Chest x-ray: rule out pneumonitis as a cause of pain.

NURSING PRIORITIES

1. Relieve pain and promote rest.
2. Maintain fluid and electrolyte balance.
3. Prevent complications.
4. Provide information about disease process, prognosis, and treatment needs.

DISCHARGE CRITERIA

1. Pain relieved.
2. Homeostasis achieved.
3. Complications prevented/minimized.
4. Disease process, prognosis, and therapeutic regimen understood.

NURSING DIAGNOSIS:	COMFORT, ALTERED: PAIN, ACUTE
May be related to:	**Biologic injuring agents: obstruction/ductal spasm, inflammatory process, tissue ischemia/necrosis**
Possibly evidenced by:	**Complaints of pain, biliary colic (waves of pain)**
	Facial mask of pain; guarding behavior
	Autonomic responses
	Self-focusing; narrowed focus
PATIENT OUTCOMES/ EVALUATION CRITERIA:	**Reports pain is relieved/controlled. Demonstrates use of relaxation skills and diversional activities as indicated for individual situation.**

ACTIONS/INTERVENTIONS	RATIONALE
Independent	
Observe and document location, severity (1–10 scale), and character of pain (steady, intermittent, col-	Assists in differentiating cause of pain and provides information about disease progression/resolution, de-

460

ACTIONS/INTERVENTIONS	RATIONALE

Independent

icky).

Note response to medication and report to physician if pain is not being relieved.

Promote bedrest, allowing patient to assume position of comfort.

Use soft/cotton linens, calamine lotion, oil (Alpha-Keri) bath, cool/moist compresses as indicated.

Control environmental temperature.

Encourage use of relaxation techniques, e.g., guided imagery, visualization, deep breathing exercises. Provide diversional activities.

Make time to listen to complaints and maintain frequent contact with the patient.

Collaborative

Maintain NPO status, insert/maintain NG suction.

Administer medications as indicated:

  Anticholinergics, e.g., atropine, propantheline (Pro-Banthine);

  Sedatives, e.g., phenobarbital; narcotics, e.g., meperidine hydrochloride (Demerol),

  Morphine sulfate;

  Smooth muscle relaxants, e.g., papaverine (Pavabid), nitroglycerin, amyl nitrate;

  Chenodeoxycholic acid (Chenic acid), chenodiol (Chenix);

  Antibiotics;

  Hyperlipidemic agents, e.g., cholestyramine (Questran).

Prepare for procedures, e.g., endoscopic papillotomy (removal of ductal stone), ultrasonic lithotripsy (noninvasive destruction of stones), or surgery.

---

velopment of complications, and effectiveness of interventions.

Severe pain not relieved by routine measures may indicate developing complications/need for further intervention.

Bedrest in low Fowler's position reduces intraabdominal pressures; however, patient will naturally assume least painful position.

Reduces irritation/dryness of the skin and itching sensation.

Cool surroundings aid in minimizing dermal discomfort.

Promotes rest, redirects attention, may enhance coping.

Helpful in alleviating anxiety and refocusing attention, which can relieve pain.

Removes gastric secretions that stimulate release of cholecystokinin and gallbladder contractions.

Relieves reflex spasm/smooth muscle contraction and assists with pain management.

Promotes rest and relaxes smooth muscle, relieving pain.

Given to reduce severe pain. Morphine is used with caution because it may increase spasms of the sphincter of Oddi, although nitroglycerin may be given to reduce morphine-induced spasms if they occur.

Relieves ductal spasm.

A natural bile acid that decreases cholesterol synthesis, reducing size of gallstones.

To treat infectious process reducing inflammation.

Reduces itching (pruritis) from bile salts in skin.

Choice of procedure is dictated by individual situation. (Refer to CP: Cholecystectomy, p. 465.)

NURSING DIAGNOSIS: **FLUID VOLUME DEFICIT, POTENTIAL**

May be related to: **Excessive losses through gastric suction; vomiting, distention, and gastric hypermotility**

Medically restricted intake

Altered clotting process

Possibly evidenced by:	[Not applicable; presence of signs and symptoms establishes an *actual* diagnosis.]
PATIENT OUTCOMES/ EVALUATION CRITERIA:	Demonstrates fluid balance evidenced by stable vital signs; moist mucous membranes; good skin turgor, capillary refill; individually adequate urinary output; and absence of vomiting.

ACTIONS/INTERVENTIONS	RATIONALE

Independent

Maintain accurate I&O, noting output less than intake, increased urine specific gravity. Assess skin/mucous membranes, peripheral pulses, and capillary refill.	Provides information about fluid status/circulating volume and replacement needs.
Monitor for signs/symptoms of increased/continued nausea/vomiting, abdominal cramps, weakness, twitching, seizures, irregular heart rate, paresthesia, hypoactive or absent bowel sounds, depressed respirations.	Prolonged vomiting, gastric aspiration, restricted oral intake can lead to deficits in sodium, potassium, and chloride. (Refer to CP: Fluid and Electrolyte Imbalances, p. 907.)
Eliminate noxious sights/smells from environment.	Reduces stimulation of vomiting center.
Perform frequent oral hygiene with mouthwash; apply lubricants.	Decreases dryness of oral mucous membranes; reduces risk of oral bleeding.
Use small gauge needles for injections and apply firm pressure for longer than usual after venipuncture.	Reduces trauma, risk of bleeding/hematoma.
Assess for unusual bleeding, e.g., oozing from injection sites, epistaxis, bleeding gums, ecchymosis, petechiae, hematemesis/melena.	Blood prothrombin is reduced and coagulation time prolonged when bile flow is obstructed, increasing risk of bleeding/hemorrhage.

Collaborative

Keep patient NPO as necessary.	Decreases gastrointestinal secretions and motility.
Insert NG tube, connect to suction, and maintain patency as indicated.	Provides rest for gastrointestinal tract.
Administer medications as indicated: antiemetics, e.g., prochlorperazine (Compazine).	Reduces nausea and prevents vomiting.
Review laboratory studies, e.g., Hb/Hct, electrolytes, ABGs (pH), clotting times.	Aids in evaluating circulating volume, identifies deficits, and influences choice of intervention for replacement/correction.
Administer IV fluids, electrolytes, and vitamin K.	Maintains circulating volume and corrects imbalance.

NURSING DIAGNOSIS:	NUTRITION, ALTERED: LESS THAN BODY REQUIRE-MENTS [POTENTIAL]
May be related to:	Self-imposed or prescribed dietary restrictions; nausea, vomiting, dyspepsia, pain
	Loss of nutrients; impaired fat digestion due to obstruction of bile flow
Possibly evidenced by:	[Not applicable; presence of signs and symptoms establishes an *actual* diagnosis.]

PATIENT OUTCOMES/ EVALUATION CRITERIA:	Achieves relief of nausea and vomiting. Demonstrates progression toward desired weight gain or maintains weight at an optimal level.

ACTIONS/INTERVENTIONS	RATIONALE
Independent	
Assess for abdominal distention, frequent belching, guarding, reluctance to move.	Nonverbal signs of discomfort associated with impaired digestion, gas pain.
Estimate/calculate caloric intake.	Identifies nutritional deficiencies/needs.
Consult with patient about likes/dislikes, foods that cause distress, and preferred meal schedule.	Involving patient in planning enables patient to have a sense of control and encourages patient to eat.
Keep comments about appetite to a minimum.	Focusing on problem creates a negative atmosphere and may interfere with intake.
Provide a pleasant atmosphere at mealtime; remove noxious stimuli.	Useful in promoting appetite/reducing nausea.
Provide oral hygiene before meals.	A clean mouth enhances appetite.
Offer effervescent drinks with meals, if tolerated.	May lessen nausea and relieve gas. Note: May be contraindicated if beverage causes gas formation/ gastric discomfort.
Ambulate and increase activity as tolerated.	Helpful in expulsion of flatus, reduction of abdominal distention. Contributes to overall recovery and sense of well-being and decreases possibility of secondary problems related to immobility (e.g., pneumonia, thrombophlebitis).
Weigh as indicated.	Monitors effectiveness of dietary plan.
Collaborative	
Consult with dietician/nutritional support team as indicated.	Useful in establishing individual nutritional needs via most appropriate route.
Begin low-fat liquid diet after NG tube is removed.	Limiting fat content reduces stimulation of gallbladder and pain associated with incomplete fat digestion and is helpful in preventing recurrence.
Advance diet as tolerated, usually low-fat, high-carbohydrate and protein. Restrict gas-producing foods (e.g., onions, cabbage, popcorn) and foods/ fluids high in fats (e.g., butter, fried foods, nuts).	Meets nutritional requirements while minimizing stimulation of the gallbladder.
Administer medications as indicated: bile salts, e.g., Bilron, Zanchol, dehydrocholic acid (Decholin).	Promotes digestion and absorption of fats, fat-soluble vitamins, cholesterol.
Monitor laboratory studies, e.g., BUN, serum albumin/ protein, transferrin levels.	Provides information about nutritional deficits/ effectiveness of therapy.
Provide TPN as needed. (Refer to CP: Total Nutritional Support, p. 894.)	Alternate feeding may be required dependent on degree of disability/gallbladder involvement and need for prolonged gastric rest.

NURSING DIAGNOSIS:	KNOWLEDGE DEFICIT [LEARNING NEED] (SPECIFY)
May be related to:	**Lack of knowledge/recall**
	Information misinterpretation

	Unfamiliarity with information resources
Possibly evidenced by:	Questions; request for information
	Statement of misconception
	Inaccurate follow-through of instruction
	Development of preventable complication
PATIENT OUTCOMES/ EVALUATION CRITERIA:	Verbalizes understanding of disease process, treatment, prognosis. Initiates necessary lifestyle changes and participates in treatment regimen.

ACTIONS/INTERVENTIONS

Independent

Provide explanations of/reasons for test procedures and preparation needed.

Review disease process/prognosis. Discuss hospitalization and prospective surgery as indicated. Encourage questions, expression of concern.

Review drug regimen, possible side effects.

Discuss weight reduction programs if indicated.

Instruct patient to avoid food/fluids high in fats (e.g., whole milk, ice cream, butter, fried foods, nuts, gravies, pork); gas-producers (e.g., cabbage, beans, onions, carbonated beverages) or gastric irritants (e.g., spicy foods, caffeine, citrus).

Review signs/symptoms requiring medical intervention, e.g., recurrent fever, persistent nausea, vomiting, or pain; jaundice of skin or eyes, itching; dark urine, clay-colored stools; blood in urine, stools, vomitus, or bleeding from mucous membranes.

Recommend resting in semi-Fowler's position after meals.

Suggest patient limit gum chewing, sucking on straw/hard candy, or smoking.

Discuss avoidance of aspirin-containing products, forceful blowing of nose, straining for bowel movement, contact sports. Recommend use of soft tooth brush, electric razor.

RATIONALE

Information can decrease anxiety, thereby reducing sympathetic stimulation.

Provides knowledge base on which patient can make informed choices. Effective communication and support at this time can diminish anxiety and promote healing.

Gallstones often recur, necessitating long-term therapy (up to 2 years). Development of diarrhea/cramps during chenodiol therapy may be dose related/correctable. Note: Women of childbearing age should be counseled regarding birth control to prevent pregnancy and risk of fetal hepatic damage.

Obesity is a risk factor associated with cholecystitis, and weight loss is beneficial in medical management of chronic condition.

Prevents/limits recurrence of gallbladder attacks.

Indicative of progression of disease process/development of complications requiring further intervention.

Promotes flow of bile and general relaxation during initial digestive process.

Promotes gas formation, which can increase gastric distention/discomfort.

Reduces risk of bleeding related to changes in coagulation time, mucosal irritation, and trauma.

Cholecystectomy

Refer to CP: Surgical Intervention, p. 789.

PATIENT ASSESSMENT DATA BASE/DIAGNOSTIC STUDIES

Refer to CP: Cholecystitis With Cholelithiasis, p. 459.

TEACHING/LEARNING

Discharge Plan Considerations: May require assistance with wound care/supplies, homemaker tasks.

NURSING PRIORITIES

1. Promote respiratory function.
2. Prevent complications.
3. Provide information about disease, procedure(s), prognosis, and treatment needs.

DISCHARGE CRITERIA

1. Ventilation/oxygenation adequate for individual needs.
2. Complications prevented/minimized.
3. Disease process, surgical procedure, prognosis, and therapeutic regimen understood.

NURSING DIAGNOSIS:	**BREATHING PATTERN, INEFFECTIVE**
May be related to:	**Pain**
	Muscular impairment
	Decreased energy/fatigue
Possibly evidenced by:	**Tachypnea**
	Respiratory depth changes, reduced vital capacity
	Holding breath; reluctance to cough
PATIENT OUTCOMES/ EVALUATION CRITERIA:	**Establishes effective breathing pattern; free of signs of respiratory compromise/complications.**

ACTIONS/INTERVENTIONS	RATIONALE
Independent	
Observe respiratory rate/depth.	Shallow breathing, splinting with respirations, holding breath may result in atelectasis/pneumonia.
Auscultate breath sounds.	Areas of decreased/absent breath sounds suggest atelectasis, whereas adventitious sounds (wheezes, rhonchi) reflect congestion.
Turn, cough, deep breath periodically. Assist patient to splint incision. Instruct in effective breathing techniques.	Promotes ventilation of all lung segments, mobilization and expectoration of secretions.

ACTIONS/INTERVENTIONS

Independent

Elevate head of bed, maintain low Fowler's position. Support abdomen when ambulating.

Collaborative

Assist with respiratory treatments, e.g., incentive spirometer.

Administer analgesics before breathing treatments/therapeutic activities.

RATIONALE

Facilitates lung expansion. Splinting provides incisional support/decreases muscle tension to promote cooperation with therapeutic regimen.

Maximizes expansion of lungs.

Facilitates more effective coughing, deep breathing, and activity.

NURSING DIAGNOSIS:	FLUID VOLUME DEFICIT, POTENTIAL
May be related to:	Losses from nasogastric aspiration, vomiting
	Medically restricted intake
	Altered coagulation, e.g., reduced prothrombin, prolonged coagulation time
Possibly evidenced by:	[Not applicable; presence of signs and symptoms establishes an *actual* diagnosis.]
PATIENT OUTCOMES/ EVALUATION CRITERIA:	Displays fluid balance as evidenced by stable vital signs, moist mucous membranes, good skin turgor/capillary refill, and individually adequate urinary output.

ACTIONS/INTERVENTIONS

Independent

Monitor I&O, including drainage from NG/T tube and wound. Weigh patient periodically.

Monitor vital signs. Assess mucous membranes, skin turgor, peripheral pulses, and capillary refill.

Observe for signs of bleeding, e.g., hematemesis, melena; petechiae, ecchymosis.

Use small-gauge needles for injections and apply firm pressure for longer than usual after venipuncture.

Have the patient use cotton/sponge swabs and mouthwash instead of a toothbrush.

Collaborative

Monitor laboratory studies, e.g., Hb/Hct, electrolytes, prothrombin level/clotting time.

Administer IV fluids, blood products, as indicated:

RATIONALE

Provides information about replacement needs and organ function. Initially, 200–500 ml of bile drainage is to be expected, decreasing as more bile enters the intestine. Continuing large amounts of bile drainage may be an indication of obstruction or, occasionally, a biliary fistula.

Indicators of adequacy of circulating volume/perfusion.

Blood prothrombin is reduced and coagulation time prolonged when bile flow is obstructed, increasing risk of bleeding/hemorrhage.

Reduces trauma, risk of bleeding/hematoma.

Avoids trauma and bleeding of the gums.

Provides information about circulating volume, electrolyte balance, and adequacy of clotting factors.

Maintains adequate circulating volume and aids in replacement of clotting factors.

ACTIONS/INTERVENTIONS

Collaborative

Electrolytes;

Vitamin K.

Administer patient's own bile, if indicated, either orally or through NG tube. If oral, chill, strain, and dilute in chilled fruit juice. Do not volunteer nature of the liquid.

RATIONALE

Corrects imbalances resulting from excessive gastric/wound losses.

Provides replacement of factors necessary for clotting process.

Used on rare occasion when excessive or chronic bile losses occur. Prevents the patient from losing the benefit of the constituents necessary for digestion. Note: Patient may be repulsed by thought of drinking own bile, affecting ability to ingest/retain it.

NURSING DIAGNOSIS:	SKIN/TISSUE INTEGRITY, IMPAIRED: ACTUAL
May be related to:	Chemical substance (bile), stasis of secretions
	Altered nutritional state (obesity)/metabolic state
	Invasion of body structure (T tube)
Possibly evidenced by:	Disruption of skin/subcutaneous tissues
PATIENT OUTCOMES/ EVALUATION CRITERIA:	Achieves timely wound healing without complications. Demonstrates behaviors to promote healing/prevent skin breakdown.

ACTIONS/INTERVENTIONS

Independent

Check the T tube and incisional drains; make sure they are free flowing.

Maintain T tube in closed collection system.

Observe the color and character of the drainage. Use a disposable ostomy bag over a stab wound drain.

Anchor drainage tube, allowing sufficient tubing to permit free turning, and avoid kinks and twists.

Place patient in low or semi-Fowler's position.

Observe for hiccups, abdominal distention, or signs of peritonitis, pancreatitis. (Refer to CPs: Peritonitis, p. 449; Pancreatitis, p. 491.)

Change dressings as often as necessary. Clean the skin with soap and water. Use sterile Vaseline gauze, zinc oxide, or karaya powder around the incision.

Apply Montgomery straps.

RATIONALE

T tube may remain in common bile duct for 7–10 days to remove retained stones. Incision site drains are used to remove any accumulated fluid and bile. Correct positioning prevents backup of the bile in the operative area.

Prevents skin irritation and facilitates measurement of output. Reduces risk of contamination.

Initially, may contain blood and blood-stained fluid, normally changing to greenish brown (bile color) after the first several hours. Ostomy appliance collects heavy drainage for more accurate measurement of output and protection of the skin.

Avoids dislodging tube and/or occlusion of the lumen.

Facilitates drainage of bile.

Dislodgment of the T tube can result in diaphragmatic irritation or more serious complications if bile drains into abdomen or pancreatic duct is obstructed.

Keeps the skin around the incision clean and provides a barrier to protect skin from excoriation.

Facilitates frequent dressing changes and minimizes skin trauma.

ACTIONS/INTERVENTIONS	RATIONALE

Independent

Observe skin, sclerae, urine for change in color.

Developing jaundice may indicate obstruction of bile flow.

Note color and consistency of stools.

Clay-colored stools result when bile is not present in the intestines.

Investigate increased/consistent RUQ pain; development of fever, tachycardia; leakage of bile drainage around tube/from wound.

Signs suggestive of abscess or fistula formation, requiring medical intervention.

Collaborative

Administer antibiotics if needed.

Necessary for treatment of abscess/infection.

Clamp the T tube per schedule.

Tests the patency of the common bile duct before tube is removed.

Prepare for surgical interventions as indicated.

Incision and drainage (I&D) or fistulectomy may be required to treat abscess/fistula.

Monitor laboratory studies, e.g., WBC.

Leukocytosis reflects inflammatory process, e.g., abcess formation or development of peritonitis/pancreatitis.

NURSING DIAGNOSIS:	KNOWLEDGE DEFICIT [LEARNING NEED] (SPECIFY)
May be related to:	**Lack of exposure; information misinterpretation**
	Unfamiliarity with information resources
	Lack of recall
Possibly evidenced by:	**Questions; statement of misconception**
	Request for information
	Inaccurate follow-through of instruction
PATIENT OUTCOMES/ EVALUATION CRITERIA:	**Verbalizes understanding of disease process, surgical procedure/prognosis and treatment. Correctly performs necessary procedures and explains reasons for the actions. Initiates necessary lifestyle changes and participates in treatment regimen.**

ACTIONS/INTERVENTIONS	RATIONALE

Independent

Review disease process, surgical procedure/prognosis.

Provides knowledge base on which patient can make informed choices.

Demonstrate care of incisions/dressings and drains (T tube).

Promotes independence in care and reduces risk of complications (e.g., infection, biliary obstruction).

Recommend periodic drainage of T tube collection bag and recording of output.

Reduces risk of reflux, strain on tube/appliance seal. Provides information about resolution of ductal edema/return of ductal function.

ACTIONS/INTERVENTIONS	RATIONALE

Independent

Stress importance of maintaining low-fat diet, eating frequent small meals, gradual reintroduction of foods/fluids containing fats over a 4–6-month period.

During initial 6 months after surgery, low-fat diet limits need for bile and reduces discomfort associated with inadequate digestion of fats.

Discuss use of florantyrone (Zanchol) or dehydrocholic acid (Decholin).

Oral replacement of bile salts may be required to facilitate fat absorption.

Avoid alcoholic beverages.

Minimizes risk of pancreatic involvement.

Inform patient that loose stools (up to three a day) may occur for several months.

Intestines require time to adjust to stimulus of continuous output of bile.

Advise patient to note and avoid foods that seem to aggravate the diarrhea.

Although dietary changes are not usually necessary, certain restrictions may be helpful; e.g., fats in small amounts are usually tolerated. After a period of adjustment, patient usually does not have problems with most foods.

Identify signs/symptoms requiring notification of physician, e.g., dark urine, jaundiced color of eyes/skin, clay-colored stools; or recurrent heartburn, bloating.

Indicators of obstruction of bile flow/altered digestion, requiring further evaluation and intervention.

Review activity limitations, dependent on individual situation.

Resumption of usual activities is normally accomplished within 4–6 weeks.

Hepatitis

Refer to CPs: Chemical Dependency, alcohol/toxic agent as appropriate.

PATIENT ASSESSMENT DATA BASE

Data are dependent on the cause and severity of liver involvement.

ACTIVITY/REST

May report: Fatigue, general malaise.

CIRCULATION

May exhibit: Bradycardia (severe hyperbilirubinemia).
Jaundiced sclera, skin, mucous membranes.

ELIMINATION

May report: Dark urine.
Diarrhea/constipation; clay-colored stools.

FOOD/FLUID

May report: Loss of appetite (anorexia), weight loss or gain (edema).
Nausea/vomiting.

May exhibit: Ascites.

NEUROSENSORY

May exhibit: Irritability, drowsiness, lethargy; asterixis.

PAIN/COMFORT

May report: Abdominal cramping; right upper quadrant tenderness.
Myalgias, arthralgia; headache.
Itching (pruritis).

May exhibit: Muscle guarding, restlessness.

RESPIRATION

May report: Distaste for/aversion to cigarettes in smokers.

SAFETY

May exhibit: Fever.
Urticaria, maculopapular lesions, irregular patches of erythema.
Exacerbation of acne.
Spider angiomas, palmar erythema, gynecomastia in men (reflects alcohol involvement).
Splenomegaly, posterior cervical node enlargement.

TEACHING/LEARNING

May report: History of known/possible exposure to virus, bacteria, or toxins (contaminated food, water, needles, surgical equipment or blood transfusion); or carriers (symptomatic or asymptomatic); recent surgical procedure with halothane anesthesia.

Street/IV drug use.

Concurrent diabetes, congestive heart failure, malignancy or renal disease.

Recent flulike upper respiratory infection.

Discharge Plan Considerations: May require assistance with homemaker tasks.

DIAGNOSTIC STUDIES

Liver function tests: abnormal (4–10 times normal values).

SGOT (AST)/SGPT (ALT): initially elevated (may rise 1–2 weeks before jaundice is apparent), then declines.

CBC: RBCs decreased due to decreased life of red blood cells (liver enzyme alterations), or result of hemorrhage. Leukopenia, thrombocytopenia may be present (splenomegaly).

Differential WBC: leukocytosis, monocytosis, atypical lymphocytes and plasma cells.

Alkaline phosphatase: slight elevation (unless severe cholestasis present).

Stools: clay-colored, steatorrhea (decreased hepatic function).

Serum albumin: decreased.

Blood sugar: transient hyper/hypoglycemia (altered liver function).

Anti-HAV IgM: positive in Type A.

HbsAG: may be positive (Type B) or negative (Type A). Note: may be diagnostic before clinical symptoms occur.

Prothrombin time: may be prolonged (liver dysfunction).

Serum bilirubin: above 2.5 mg/100 ml. (If above 200 mg/100 ml, poor prognosis is probable due to increased cellular necrosis.)

Bromsulphalein (BSP) excretion test: blood level elevated.

Liver biopsy: defines diagnosis and extent of necrosis.

Liver scan: aids in estimation of severity of parenchymal damage.

Urinalysis: elevated bilirubin levels; protein/hematuria may occur.

NURSING PRIORITIES

1. Reduce demands on liver while promoting physical well-being.
2. Prevent complications.
3. Enhance self-concept, acceptance of situation.
4. Provide information about disease process, prognosis, and treatment needs.

DISCHARGE CRITERIA

1. Meeting basic self-care needs.
2. Complications prevented/minimized.
3. Dealing with reality of current situation.
4. Disease process, prognosis, and therapeutic regimen understood.

NURSING DIAGNOSIS:	ACTIVITY INTOLERANCE
May be related to:	**Generalized weakness; decreased strength/endurance; pain**
	Imposed activity restrictions; depression
Possibly evidenced by:	**Complaints of fatigue, exertional discomfort**
	Decreased muscle strength
	Reluctance to attempt movement

471

PATIENT OUTCOMES/ EVALUATION CRITERIA:	Verbalizes understanding of situation/risk factors and individual treatment regimen. Demonstrates techniques/behaviors that enable resumption of activities.

ACTIONS/INTERVENTIONS

Independent

Promote bed/chair rest. Provide quiet environment; visitors may need to be limited.

Change position frequently. Provide good skin care.

Do necessary tasks quickly and at one time.

Increase activity as tolerated, assist with passive/active ROM exercises.

Encourage use of stress management techniques, e.g., progressive relaxation, visualization, guided imagery. Provide appropriate diversional activities, e.g., radio, TV, reading.

Monitor for recurrence of anorexia and liver tenderness/enlargement.

Collaborative

Administer medications as indicated: sedatives, antianxiety agents, e.g., diazepam (Valium), lorazepam (Ativan).

Monitor liver enzyme levels.

RATIONALE

Promotes rest and relaxation. Available energy is used for healing. Activity and an upright position are believed to decrease hepatic blood flow, which prevents optimal circulation to the liver cells.

Promotes optimal respiratory function and minimizes pressure areas to reduce risk of tissue breakdown.

Allows for extended periods of uninterrupted rest.

Prolonged bedrest can be debilitating. This can be offset by limited activity with rest periods.

Promotes relaxation and conserves energy, redirects attention and may enhance coping.

Indicates lack of resolution/exacerbation of the disease, requiring further rest, change in therapeutic regimen.

Assists in managing required rest. Note: Avoid the use of barbiturates and tranquilizers, such as Compazine and Thorazine, which are known to have hepatotoxic effects.

Aids in determining appropriate levels of activity as premature increase in activity potentiates risk of relapse.

NURSING DIAGNOSIS:	NUTRITION, ALTERED: LESS THAN BODY REQUIREMENTS
May be related to:	Insufficient intake to meet metabolic demands: anorexia, nausea and vomiting
	Altered absorption and metabolism of ingested foods: reduced peristalsis (visceral reflexes), bile stasis
	Increased calorie needs/hypermetabolic state
Possibly evidenced by:	Aversion to eating/lack of interest in food
	Altered taste sensation
	Abdominal pain/cramping
	Loss of weight; poor muscle tone

PATIENT OUTCOMES/ EVALUATION CRITERIA:	Demonstrates progressive weight gain toward goal with normalization of laboratory values and free of signs of malnutrition. Demonstrates behaviors, lifestyle changes to regain/maintain appropriate weight.

ACTIONS/INTERVENTIONS

Independent

Monitor dietary intake/calorie count. Give several small feedings and offer largest meal at breakfast.

Provide mouth care before meals.

Recommend eating in sitting position.

Encourage intake of fruit juices, carbonated beverages, and hard candy throughout the day.

Collaborative

Consult with dietician, nutritional support team to provide diet according to patient's needs, with fat and protein intake as tolerated.

Monitor blood glucose.

Administer medications as indicated:

Antiemetics, e.g., metalopramide (Reglan), trimethobenzamide (Tigan);

Antacids, e.g., Mylanta, Titralac;

Vitamins, e.g., B complex, C, other dietary supplements as indicated;

Steroid therapy, e.g., Prednisone (Deltasone), alone or in combination with azathioprine (Imuran).

Provide supplemental/TPN if needed.

RATIONALE

Large meals are difficult to manage when patient is anorexic. Anorexia may also worsen during the day, making intake of food difficult later in the day.

Eliminating unpleasant taste may enhance appetite.

Reduces abdominal tenderness and sensation of GI fullness and may enhance intake.

These supply extra calories and may be more easily digested/tolerated when other foods are not.

Useful in formulating dietary program to meet individual needs. Fat metabolism varies according to bile production and excretion and may necessitate restriction of fat intake if diarrhea develops. If tolerated, a normal or increased protein intake will help with liver regeneration. Protein restriction may be indicated in severe disease (e.g., fulminating hepatitis) because the accumulation of the end products of protein metabolism can potentiate hepatic encephalopathy.

Hyper/hypoglycemia may develop, necessitating dietary changes/insulin administration.

Given one-half hour before meals, may reduce nausea and increase food tolerance. Note: Compazine is contraindicated in hepatic disease.

Counteracts gastric acidity reducing irritation/risk of bleeding.

Corrects deficiencies and aids in the healing process.

Steroids often contraindicated as they may increase risk of relapse/development of chronic hepatitis in patients with viral hepatitis. However, antiinflammatory effect may be useful in chronic active hepatitis (especially idiopathic) to reduce nausea/vomiting and enable patient to retain food and fluids. May decrease serum aminotransferase and bilirubin levels, but has no effect on liver necrosis or regeneration. Combination therapy has fewer steroid-related side effects.

May be necessary to meet caloric requirements if marked deficits are present/symptoms are prolonged. (Refer to CP: Total Nutritional Support, p. 894.)

NURSING DIAGNOSIS:	FLUID VOLUME DEFICIT, POTENTIAL
May be related to:	Excessive losses through vomiting and diarrhea, third-space shift (ascites)
	Altered clotting process
Possibly evidenced by:	[Not applicable; presence of signs and symptoms establishes an *actual* diagnosis.]
PATIENT OUTCOMES/ EVALUATION CRITERIA:	Maintains adequate hydration, as evidenced by stable vital signs; good skin turgor, capillary refill; strong peripheral pulses; and individually appropriate urinary output.

ACTIONS/INTERVENTIONS	RATIONALE
Independent	
Monitor intake and output, compare with daily weight. Note enteric losses, e.g., vomiting and diarrhea.	Provides information about replacement needs/effects of therapy. Note: Diarrhea may be due to transient flu-like response to viral infection or represent a more serious problem of obstructed portal blood flow with vascular congestion in the GI tract.
Assess vital signs, peripheral pulses, capillary refill, skin turgor, and mucous membranes.	Indicators of circulating volume/perfusion.
Check for ascites or edema formation. Measure abdominal girth as indicated.	Useful in monitoring progression/resolution of fluid shifts (edema/ascites).
Use small gauge needles for injections, applying pressure for longer than usual after venipuncture.	Reduces possibility of bleeding into tissues.
Have patient use cotton/sponge swabs and mouthwash instead of toothbrush.	Avoids trauma and bleeding of the gums.
Observe for signs of bleeding, e.g., hematuria/melena, ecchymosis, oozing from gums/puncture sites.	Prothrombin levels are reduced and coagulation times prolonged when vitamin K absorption is altered in GI tract and synthesis of prothrombin is decreased in affected liver.
Collaborative	
Monitor laboratory values, e.g., Hb/Hct, Na^+, albumin, and clotting times.	Reflects hydration and identifies sodium retention/protein deficits which may lead to edema formation. Deficits in clotting potentiate risk of bleeding/hemorrhage.
Administer IV fluids (usually glucose), electrolytes;	Provides fluid and electrolyte replacement.
Protein hydrolysates;	Correction of albumin/protein deficits can aid in return of fluid from tissues to the circulatory system.
Vitamin K;	Because absorption is altered, supplementation may prevent coagulation problems, which may occur if clotting factors/prothrombin time is depressed.
Antacids or H_2-receptor antagonists, e.g., cimetadine (Tagamet);	Neutralizes/reduces gastric secretions to lower risk of gastric irritation/bleeding.
Antidiarrheal agents, e.g., diphenoxylate and atropine (Lomotil).	Reduces fluid/electrolyte loss from GI tract.

NURSING DIAGNOSIS:	SELF-CONCEPT, DISTURBANCE IN: (SPECIFY)
May be related to:	Annoying/debilitating symptoms, confinement/isolation, length of illness/recovery period
Possibly evidenced by:	Verbalization of change in lifestyle; fear of rejection/reaction of others, negative feelings about body; feelings of helplessness
	Depression; lack of follow-through; self-destructive behavior
PATIENT OUTCOMES/ EVALUATION CRITERIA:	Identifies feelings and methods for coping with negative perception of self. Verbalizes acceptance of self in situation, including length of recovery/need for isolation. Acknowledges self as worthwhile and responsible for self.

ACTIONS/INTERVENTIONS

Independent

Contract with patient regarding time for listening. Encourage discussion of feelings/concerns.

Avoid making moral judgments regarding lifestyle (alcohol use/sexual practices).

Discuss recovery expectations.

Assess effect of illness on economic factors of patient/SO.

Offer diversional activities based on energy levels.

Suggest patient wear bright reds or blues/blacks instead of yellows or greens.

Collaborative

Make appropriate referrals for help, as needed, e.g., discharge planners, social services, and/or other community agencies.

RATIONALE

Establishing time enhances trusting relationship. Opportunity to express feelings allows patient to feel more in control of the situation. Verbalization decreases anxiety and depression and facilitates positive coping behaviors. Patient may need to express feelings about being ill; length and cost of illness; possibility of infecting others; and in severe illness, fear of death. May have concerns regarding the stigma of the disease.

Patient may already feel upset/angry, and condemn self; judgments from others will further damage self-esteem.

Recovery period may be prolonged (up to 6 months), potentiating family/situational stress and necessitating need for planning, support, and follow-up.

Financial problems may exist because of loss of patient's role functioning in the family/prolonged recovery.

Enables patient to use time and energy in constructive ways that enhance self-esteem and minimizes anxiety and depression. (Refer to CP: Psychosocial Aspects of Acute Care, p. 773.)

Enhances appearance, because yellow skin tones are intensified by yellow/green colors. Jaundice usually peaks within 1–2 weeks, then gradually resolves over 2–4 weeks.

Can facilitate problem-solving and help involved individuals to cope more effectively with situation.

NURSING DIAGNOSIS:	INFECTION, POTENTIAL FOR
May be related to:	Inadequate secondary defenses (e.g., leukopenia, suppressed inflammatory response), and immunosuppression Malnutrition Insufficient knowledge to avoid exposure to pathogens
Possibly evidenced by:	[Not applicable; presence of signs and symptoms establishes an *actual* diagnosis.]
PATIENT OUTCOMES/ EVALUATION CRITERIA:	Verbalizes understanding of individual causative/risk factor(s). Demonstrates techniques, lifestyle changes to avoid reinfection/transmission to others.

ACTIONS/INTERVENTIONS

Independent

Establish isolation techniques for enteric and respiratory infections according to hospital policy; include effective handwashing.

Monitor/restrict visitors as indicated.

Explain isolation procedures to patient/SO.

Give information regarding availability of gamma globulin, ISG, HBIG, hepatitis B vaccine (Hepatovox-B) through health department or family physician.

RATIONALE

Prevents transmission of disease to others. Thorough handwashing is effective in preventing virus transmission. Type A (infectious) is transmitted by oral–fecal route, contaminated water, milk and food, especially inadequately cooked shellfish. Type B (serum) is transmitted by contaminated blood/blood products, needle punctures, open wounds, ingestion, saliva, urine, stool, and semen. Incidence of both has increased among hospital personnel and high-risk patients. Note: Toxic/alcoholic hepatitis are not communicable and do not require special measures/isolation.

Patient exposure to infectious processes (especially URI) potentiates risk of secondary complications.

Understanding of reasons for safeguarding themselves and others can lessen feelings of isolation and stigmatization. Isolation may last 2–3 weeks from onset of illness, depending on type/duration of symptoms.

May be effective in preventing hepatitis in those who have been exposed, depending on type of hepatitis and period of incubation.

NURSING DIAGNOSIS:	SKIN/TISSUE INTEGRITY, IMPAIRED: POTENTIAL
May be related to:	Chemical substance: bile salt accumulation in the tissues
Possibly evidenced by:	[Not applicable; presence of signs and symptoms establishes an *actual* diagnosis.]
PATIENT OUTCOMES/ EVALUATION CRITERIA:	Displays intact skin/tissues, free of excoriation. Reports absence/decrease of pruritis/scratching.

ACTIONS/INTERVENTIONS

Independent

Use cool showers and baking soda or starch baths. Avoid use of alkaline soaps. Apply calamine lotion as indicated.

Provide diversional activities.

Suggest use of knuckles if desire to scratch is uncontrollable. Keep fingernails cut short, apply gloves on comatose patient or during hours of sleep. Recommend loose-fitting clothing. Provide soft cotton linens.

Provide a soothing massage at bedtime.

Avoid comments regarding patient's appearance.

Collaborative

Administer medications as indicated:

    Antihistamines, e.g., methdilazine (Tacaryl), diphenhydramine (Benadryl);

    Antilipemics, e.g., cholestyramine (Questran).

RATIONALE

Prevents excessive dryness of skin. Provides relief from itching.

Aids in refocusing attention reducing tendency to scratch.

Reduces potential for dermal injury.

May be helpful in promoting sleep.

Minimizes psychologic stress associated with skin changes.

Relieves itching. Note: Used cautiously in hepatic disease.

May be used to bind bile acids in the intestine and prevent their absorption. Note side effects of nausea and constipation.

NURSING DIAGNOSIS:	KNOWLEDGE DEFICIT [LEARNING NEED] (SPECIFY)
May be related to:	Lack of exposure/recall; information misinterpretation
	Unfamiliarity with resources
Possibly evidenced by:	Questions; statement of misconception
	Request for information
	Inaccurate follow-through of instruction
PATIENT OUTCOMES/ EVALUATION CRITERIA:	Verbalizes understanding of disease process and treatment. Identifies relationship of signs/symptoms to the disease and correlates symptoms with causative factors. Initiates necessary lifestyle changes and participates in treatment regimen.

ACTIONS/INTERVENTIONS

Independent

Assess level of understanding of the disease process and expectations.

Provide specific information regarding prevention/transmission of disease: e.g., contacts may require gamma globulin; personal items should not be shared; strict handwashing and sanitizing of clothes, dishes, and toilet facilities while liver enzymes are ele-

RATIONALE

Identifies areas of lack of knowledge/misinformation and provides opportunity to give additional information as necessary.

Needs/recommendations will vary with type of hepatitis (causative agent) and individual situation.

ACTIONS/INTERVENTIONS	RATIONALE

Independent

vated. Avoid intimate contact, such as kissing and sexual contact, and exposure to infections, especially URI.

Plan resumption of activity as tolerated with adequate periods of rest. Discuss restriction of heavy lifting, strenuous exercise/contact sports.

It is not necessary to wait until serum bilirubin levels return to normal to resume activity (may take as long as 2 months), but strenuous activity needs to be limited until the liver returns to normal size. When patient begins to feel better, s/he needs to understand the importance of continued adequate rest in preventing relapse or recurrence. (Relapse occurs in 5–25% of adults.) Note: Energy level may take up to 3–6 months to return to normal.

Help patient identify diversional activities.

Enjoyable activities will help patient avoid focusing on prolonged convalescence.

Encourage continuation of balanced diet.

Promotes general well-being and enhances energy for healing process/tissue regeneration.

Identify ways to maintain usual bowel function, e.g., adequate intake of fluids/dietary roughage, moderate activity/exercise to tolerance.

Decreased level of activity, changes in food/fluid intake and slowed bowel motility may result in constipation.

Discuss the side effects and dangers of taking OTC/prescribed drugs (e.g., acetaminophen, aspirin, sulfonamides, some anesthetics) and necessity of notifying future health care givers of diagnosis.

Some drugs are toxic to the liver; others are metabolized by the liver and should be avoided in severe liver diseases because they may cause cumulative toxic effects/chronic hepatitis.

Discuss restrictions on donating blood.

Prevents spread of disease. Most state laws prevent accepting as donors those who have a history of any type of hepatitis.

Emphasize importance of follow-up physical examination and laboratory evaluation.

Disease process may take several months to resolve. If symptoms persist longer than 6 months, liver biopsy may be required to verify presence of chronic hepatitis.

Review necessity of avoidance of alcohol for a minimum of 6–12 months or longer based on individual tolerance.

Increases hepatic irritation and may interfere with recovery.

Collaborative

Refer to drug/alcohol treatment program as indicated.

May need additional assistance to withdraw from substance and maintain abstinence to avoid further liver damage.

Cirrhosis of the Liver

PATIENT ASSESSMENT DATA BASE

Refer to CP: Alcoholism (Acute), p. 825, for related observations, considerations.

ACTIVITY/REST

May report: Weakness, fatigue, exhaustion.

May exhibit: Decreased muscle mass/tone.

CIRCULATION

May report: History of chronic congestive heart failure (CHF), pericarditis, rheumatic heart disease, cancer (liver malfunction leading to liver failure).

May exhibit: Hypertension or hypotension (fluid shifts).
Dysrhythmias, extra heart sounds (S_3, S_4).
Jugular venous distention; distended abdominal veins.

ELIMINATION

May report: Flatulence.
Diarrhea or constipation; gradual abdominal enlargement.

May exhibit: Abdominal distention (hepatomegaly, splenomegaly, ascites).
Decreased/absent bowel sounds.
Clay-colored stools, melena.
Dark, concentrated urine.

FOOD/FLUID

May report: Anorexia, food intolerance.

May exhibit: Weight loss or gain (fluid).
Tissue wasting.
Edema generalized in tissues.
Dry skin, poor turgor.
Jaundice; spider angiomas.
Halitosis/fetor hepaticus.

NEUROSENSORY

May report: SO may report personality changes, depressed mentation.

May exhibit: Changes in mentation, confusion, hallucinations.
Slowed/slurred speech.
Asterixis (hepatic encephalopathy).

PAIN/COMFORT

May report: Abdominal tenderness/RUQ pain.
Pruritis.

May exhibit: Guarding/distraction behaviors.
Self-focus.

RESPIRATION

May report:	Dyspnea.
May exhibit:	Tachypnea, shallow respiration, adventitious breath sounds.
	Limited thoracic expansion (ascites).

SAFETY

May report:	Pruritis.
May exhibit:	Fever.
	Jaundice, ecchymosis, petechiae.
	Spider telangiectasis, palmar erythema.

SEXUALITY

May report:	Menstrual disorders.
May exhibit:	Testicular atrophy, gynecomastia, loss of hair (chest, underarm, pubic).

TEACHING/LEARNING

May report:	History of long-term alcohol use/abuse, alcoholic liver disease.
	History of biliary disease, hepatitis, exposure to toxins; liver trauma; upper GI bleeding; episodes of bleeding esophageal varices; use of drugs affecting liver function.
Discharge Plan Considerations:	May need assistance with homemaker/management tasks.

DIAGNOSTIC STUDIES

Serum bilirubin: elevated because of cellular disruption, inability of liver to conjugate, or biliary obstruction.

SGOT (AST), SGPT (ALT), LDH: increased owing to cellular damage and release of enzymes.

Alkaline phosphatase: elevated owing to reduced excretion.

Serum albumin: decreased owing to depressed synthesis.

Globulins (IgA and IgG): increased synthesis.

CBC: Hb/Hct and RBCs may be decreased because of bleeding. RBC destruction and anemia is seen with hypersplenism and iron deficiency. Leukopenia may be present as a result of hypersplenism.

Prothrombin time: prolonged (decreased synthesis of prothrombin).

Fibrinogen: decreased.

BUN: elevation indicates breakdown of blood/protein.

Serum ammonia: elevated owing to inability to convert ammonia to urea.

Serum glucose: hypoglycemia suggests impaired glycogenesis.

Electrolytes: hypokalemia may reflect increased aldosterone, although various imbalances may occur.

Calcium: may be decreased due to impaired absorption of vitamin D.

Urine urobilinogen: may/may not be present; serves as guide for differentiating liver disease, hemolytic disease and biliary obstruction.

Liver scans/biopsy: detects fatty infiltrates, fibrosis, destruction of hepatic tissues.

Esophagoscopy: may demonstrate presence of esophageal varices.

Percutaneous transhepatic portography: visualizes portal venous system circulation.

NURSING PRIORITIES

1. Maintain adequate nutrition.
2. Prevent complications.
3. Enhance self-concept, acceptance of situation.
4. Provide information about disease process/prognosis, potential complications and treatment needs.

DISCHARGE CRITERIA

1. Nutritional intake adequate for individual needs.
2. Complications prevented/minimized.
3. Dealing with current reality.
4. Disease process, prognosis, potential complications and therapeutic regimen understood.

NURSING DIAGNOSIS:	NUTRITION, ALTERED: LESS THAN BODY REQUIRE-MENTS
May be related to:	Inadequate diet; inability to process/digest nutrients
	Anorexia, nausea, vomiting, indigestion, early satiety (ascites)
	Abnormal bowel function
Possibly evidenced by:	Weight loss
	Changes in bowel sounds and function
	Poor muscle tone/wasting
PATIENT OUTCOMES/ EVALUATION CRITERIA:	Demonstrates progressive weight gain toward goal with normalization of laboratory values and free of signs of malnutrition.

ACTIONS/INTERVENTIONS	RATIONALE
Independent	
Measure dietary intake by calorie count.	Provides information about intake needs/deficiencies.
Assist and encourage patient to eat; explain reasons for the type of diet. Feed patient if tiring easily, or have SO assist patient. Consider food preferences in food choices.	Proper diet is vital to recovery. Patient may eat better if family is involved and preferred food is included as much as possible.
Encourage patient to eat all meals/supplementary feedings.	Patient may pick at food, eat only a few bites because of loss of interest in food, in addition to nausea, generalized weakness, malaise.
Serve small frequent meals.	Poor tolerance to larger meals may be due to increased intraabdominal pressure/ascites.
Provide mouth care frequently and prior to meals.	Patient is prone to sore and/or bleeding gums and bad taste in mouth, which adds to anorexia.
Weigh as indicated. Compare changes in fluid status, recent weight history, triceps skin measurement.	It may be difficult to use weight as a direct indicator of nutritional status in view of edema/ascites. Triceps skinfold measurement is useful in assessing changes in muscle mass and subcutaneous fat reserves.
Promote undisturbed rest periods, especially before meals.	Conserving energy reduces metabolic demands on the liver and promotes cellular regeneration.
Provide salt substitutes if allowed; avoid those containing ammonium.	Salt substitutes enhance the flavor of food and aid in increasing appetite; ammonia potentiates risk of encephalopathy.
Recommend cessation of smoking.	Reduces excessive gastric stimulation and risk of irritation/bleeding.

481

ACTIONS/INTERVENTIONS	RATIONALE

Collaborative

Monitor laboratory studies, e.g., serum glucose, albumin, total protein, ammonia.	Glucose may be decreased because of impaired glycogenesis, depleted glycogen stores, or inadequate intake. Protein may be low because of impaired metabolism, decreased hepatic synthesis, or loss into peritoneal cavity (ascites). Elevation of ammonia level may require restriction of protein intake to prevent serious complications.
Maintain nothing-by-mouth (NPO) status when indicated.	Initially, GI rest may be required to reduce demands on the liver and production of GI ammonia/urea.
Consult with dietician to provide diet that is high in calories and simple carbohydrates, low in fat, and moderate to high in protein; limit sodium and fluid as necessary. Provide liquid supplements as indicated.	High-calorie foods are desired inasmuch as patient intake is usually limited. Carbohydrates supply readily available energy. Fats are poorly absorbed because of liver dysfunction and may contribute to abdominal discomfort. Proteins are needed to improve serum protein levels to reduce edema and to promote liver cell regeneration. Note: Protein and foods high in ammonia (e.g., gelatin) are restricted if ammonia level is elevated or if patient has clinical signs of hepatic encephalopathy.
Restrict intake of caffeine, gas-producing or spicy and excessively hot or cold foods.	Aids in reducing gastric irritation/diarrhea and abdominal discomfort that may impair oral intake/digestion.
Administer tube feedings, hyperalimentation, lipids if indicated.	May be required to supplement diet or to provide nutrients when patient is too nauseated or anorexic to eat or esophageal varices interfere with oral intake.
Provide soft foods, avoid roughage if indicated.	Hemorrhage from esophageal varices may occur in advanced cirrhosis.
Administer medications as indicated, e.g.:	
Vitamin supplements, thiamine, iron, folic acid;	Patient is usually vitamin-deficient because of previous poor diet. Also the injured liver is unable to store vitamins A, B complex. There may also be an iron and folic acid-deficiency–induced anemia.
Zinc;	Enhances sense of taste/smell, which may stimulate appetite.
Digestive enzymes, e.g., pancreatin (Viokase).	Promotes digestion of fats and may reduce steatorrhea/diarrhea.

NURSING DIAGNOSIS:	FLUID VOLUME, ALTERED: EXCESS
May be related to:	Compromised regulatory mechanism (e.g., SIADH, decreased plasma proteins, malnutrition)
	Excess sodium/fluid intake
Possibly evidenced by:	Edema, anasarca, weight gain
	Intake greater than output, oliguria, changes in urine specific gravity
	Dyspnea, adventitious breath sounds, pleural effusion
	Blood pressure changes, including CVP

Jugular venous distention, positive hepatojugular reflex

Altered electrolytes

Change in mental status

PATIENT OUTCOMES/ EVALUATION CRITERIA:	Demonstrates stabilized fluid volume, with balanced intake and output, stable weight, vital signs within patient's normal range, and absence of edema.

ACTIONS/INTERVENTIONS	RATIONALE
Independent	
Measure intake/output (I&O), noting positive balance (intake in excess of output). Weigh daily, and note gain greater than 0.5 kg/day.	Reflects circulating volume status, developing/resolution of fluid shifts, and response to therapy. Positive balance/weight gain reflects continuing fluid retention. Note: Decreased circulating volume (fluid shifts) may directly affect renal function/urine output, resulting in hepatorenal syndrome. (Refer to CPs: Renal Failure: Acute, p. 544; Renal Dialysis, p. 567.)
Monitor blood pressure and CVP. Note jugular/abdominal vein distention.	Blood pressure elevations are usually associated with fluid volume excess, but may not occur because of fluid shifts out of the vascular space. Distention of external jugular and abdominal veins is associated with vascular congestion.
Assess respiratory status, noting increased respiratory rate, dyspnea.	Indicative of pulmonary congestion/edema.
Auscultate lungs, noting diminished/absent breath sounds and developing adventitious sounds (e.g., crackles).	Increasing pulmonary congestion may result in consolidation, impaired gas exchange, and complications, e.g., pulmonary edema.
Monitor for cardiac dysrhythmias. Auscultate heart sounds, noting development of S_3/S_4 gallop rhythm.	May be caused by CHF, decreased coronary arterial perfusion, and electrolyte imbalance.
Assess degree of peripheral/dependent edema.	Fluids shift into tissues as a result of sodium and water retention, decreased albumin, and increased ADH.
Measure abdominal girth.	Reflects accumulation of ascites resulting from loss of plasma proteins/fluid into peritoneal space.
Encourage bedrest when ascites is present.	May promote incumbency induced diuresis.
Provide frequent mouth care; occasional ice chips (if NPO).	Decreases thirst.
Collaborative	
Monitor serum albumin and electrolytes (particularly potassium and sodium).	Decreased serum albumin affects plasma colloid osmotic pressure, resulting in edema formation. Reduced renal blood flow accompanied by elevated ADH and aldosterone levels, and the use of diuretics (to reduce total body water) may cause various electrolyte shifts/imbalances. (Refer to CP: Fluid and Electrolyte Imbalances, p. 907.)
Monitor serial chest x-rays.	Vascular congestion, pulmonary edema, and pleural effusions frequently occur.
Restrict sodium and fluids as indicated.	Sodium may be restricted to minimize fluid retention in extravascular spaces. Fluid restriction may be necessary to correct/prevent dilutional hyponatremia.

ACTIONS/INTERVENTIONS	RATIONALE

Collaborative

Administer salt-free albumin/plasma expanders as indicated.

Albumin may be used to increase the colloid osmotic pressure in vascular compartment (pull fluid into vascular space), thereby increasing effective circulating volume and decreasing ascitic formation.

Administer medications as indicated:

Diuretics, e.g., spironolactone (Aldactone);

Used to control edema and ascites, block effect of aldosterone and increase water excretion while sparing potassium.

Potassium;

Serum and cellular potassium are usually depleted because of liver disease as well as urinary losses.

Positive inotropic drugs and arterial vasodilators.

Given to increase cardiac output/improve renal blood flow and function, thereby reducing excess fluid.

NURSING DIAGNOSIS:	SKIN INTEGRITY, IMPAIRED: POTENTIAL
May be related to:	**Altered circulation/metabolic state**
	Accumulation of bile salts in skin
	Poor skin turgor; skeletal prominence; presence of edema, ascites
Possibly evidenced by:	**[Not applicable; presence of signs and symptoms establishes an *actual* diagnosis.]**
PATIENT OUTCOMES/ EVALUATION CRITERIA:	**Maintains skin integrity. Identifies individual risk factors and demonstrates behaviors/techniques to prevent skin breakdown.**

ACTIONS/INTERVENTIONS	RATIONALE

Independent

Inspect skin surfaces/pressure points routinely. Massage reddened areas, bony prominence or areas of continued stress. Use emollient lotions; limit use of soap for bathing.

Edematous tissues are more prone to breakdown and to the formation of decubiti. Ascites may stretch the skin to the point of tearing in severe cirrhosis.

Reposition on a regular schedule, in bed/chair, assist with active/passive range of motion exercises.

Repositioning reduces pressure on edematous tissues to improve circulation. Exercises enhance circulation and improve/maintain joint mobility.

Elevate lower extremities.

Enhances venous return and reduces edema formation in extremities.

Keep linens dry and free of wrinkles.

Moisture aggravates pruritis and increases risk of skin breakdown.

Clip fingernails short; provide mittens/gloves if indicated.

Prevents the patient from inadvertently injuring the skin, especially while sleeping.

Provide perineal care following urination and bowel movement.

Prevents skin excoriation breakdown from bile salts.

ACTIONS/INTERVENTIONS	RATIONALE
Collaborative	
Use alternating pressure mattress, egg carton mattress, waterbed, sheepskins, as indicated.	Reduces dermal pressure increasing circulation and diminishing risk of tissue ischemia/breakdown.
Apply calamine lotion, baking soda baths. Administer cholestyramine (Questran) if indicated.	May be soothing for itching associated with jaundice, bile salts in skin.

NURSING DIAGNOSIS:	**BREATHING PATTERN, INEFFECTIVE [POTENTIAL]**
May be related to:	**Intraabdominal fluid collection (ascites)**
	Decreased lung expansion, accumulated secretions
	Decreased energy, fatigue
	Immunosuppression, immobility
Possibly evidenced by:	**[Not applicable; presence of signs and symptoms establishes an *actual* diagnosis.]**
PATIENT OUTCOMES/ EVALUATION CRITERIA:	**Establishes effective respiratory pattern; free of dyspnea and cyanosis, with ABGs and vital capacity within acceptable range.**

ACTIONS/INTERVENTIONS	RATIONALE
Independent	
Monitor respiratory rate, depth, and effort.	Rapid shallow respirations/dyspnea may be present due to hypoxia and/or fluid accumulation in abdomen.
Auscultate breath sounds, noting crackles, wheezes, rhonchi.	Indicates developing complications, e.g., presence of adventitious sounds reflects accumulation of fluid/ secretions; absent/diminished sounds suggest atelectasis.
Investigate changes in level of consciousness.	Changes in mentation may reflect hypoxemia and respiratory failure, which often accompany hepatic coma.
Keep head of bed elevated. Position on sides.	Facilitates breathing by reducing pressure on the diaphragm and minimizes risk of aspiration of secretions.
Reposition frequently; encourage deep breathing exercises and coughing.	Aids in lung expansion and mobilizing secretions.
Monitor temperature. Note presence of chills, increased coughing, changes in color/character of sputum.	Indicative of onset of infection, e.g., pneumonia.
Collaborative	
Monitor serial ABGs, pulse oximetry, vital capacity measurements, chest x-rays.	Reveals changes in respiratory status, developing pulmonary complications.
Administer supplemental oxygen as indicated.	May be necessary to treat/prevent hypoxia. If respirations/oxygenation inadequate, mechanical ventilation may be required.
Assist with respiratory adjuncts, e.g., incentive spirometer, blow bottles.	Reduces incidence of atelectasis, enhances mobilization of secretions.

485

ACTIONS/INTERVENTIONS	RATIONALE

Collaborative

Assist with paracentesis.

Occasionally done to remove ascites fluid when respiratory embarrassment is not corrected by other measures.

NURSING DIAGNOSIS:	INJURY, POTENTIAL FOR: [HEMORRHAGE]
May be related to:	**Abnormal blood profile: altered clotting factors (decreased production of prothrombin, fibrinogen and factors VIII, IX, and X; impaired vitamin K absorption and release of thromboplastin)**
	Portal hypertension, development of esophageal varices
Possibly evidenced by:	**[Not applicable; presence of signs and symptoms establishes an *actual* diagnosis.]**
PATIENT OUTCOMES/ EVALUATION CRITERIA:	**Maintains homeostasis with absence of bleeding. Demonstrates behaviors to reduce risk of bleeding.**

ACTIONS/INTERVENTIONS	RATIONALE

Independent

Assess for signs/symptoms of GI bleed; e.g., check all secretions for frank or occult blood. Observe color and consistency of stools and vomitus.

The GI tract (esophagus and rectum) is the most usual source of bleeding due to mucosal fragility and alterations in hemostasis associated with cirrhosis. (Refer to CP: Upper Gastrointestinal/Esophageal Bleeding, p. 397.)

Observe for presence of petechiae, ecchymosis, bleeding from one or more sites.

Subacute disseminated intravascular coagulation (DIC) may develop secondary to altered clotting factors.

Monitor pulse, blood pressure and CVP if available.

An increased pulse with decreased BP and CVP can indicate loss of circulating blood volume, requiring further evaluation.

Note changes in mentation/level of consciousness.

Changes may indicate decreased cerebral perfusion secondary to hypovolemia, hypoxemia.

Avoid rectal temperature; be gentle with GI tube insertions.

Rectal and esophageal vessels are most vulnerable to rupture.

Encourage use of soft toothbrush, electric razor, avoiding straining for stool, forceful nose blowing, etc.

In the presence of clotting factor disturbances, minimal trauma can cause mucosal bleeding.

Use small needles for injections. Apply pressure to small bleeding/venipuncture sites for longer than usual.

Minimizes damage to tissues, reducing risk of bleeding/hematoma.

Collaborative

Monitor Hb/Hct and clotting factors.

Indicators of anemia, active bleeding or impending complications (e.g., DIC).

Administer medications as indicated:

Supplemental vitamins (e.g., vitamins K, D);

Promotes prothrombin synthesis and coagulation if liver is functional. Vitamin C deficiencies increase susceptibility of GI system to irritation/bleeding.

ACTIONS/INTERVENTIONS

Collaborative

Stool softeners.

Provide gastric lavage with room temperature/cool saline solution as indicated.

Assist with insertion/maintenance of GI/esophageal tube (e.g., Sengstaken–Blakemore tube).

Avoid use of aspirin containing products.

Prepare for surgical procedures, e.g., direct ligation of varices, esophagogastric resection, splenorenal–portacaval anastomosis.

RATIONALE

Prevents straining for stool with resultant increase in intraabdominal pressure and risk of vascular rupture/hemorrhage.

Evacuation of blood from GI tract reduces ammonia production and risk of hepatic encephalopathy.

Temporarily controls bleeding of esophageal varices when control by other means (e.g., lavage) and hemodynamic stability cannot be achieved. (Refer to CP: Upper Gastrointestinal/Esophageal Bleeding, p. 397.)

Prolongs coagulation, potentiating risk of hemorrhage.

May be needed to control active hemorrhage, or decrease portal and collateral blood vessel pressure to minimize risk of recurrence of bleeding.

NURSING DIAGNOSIS:	THOUGHT PROCESSES, ALTERED [POTENTIAL]
May be related to:	**Physiologic changes: increased serum ammonia level, inability of liver to detoxify certain enzymes/drugs**
Possibly evidenced by:	**[Not applicable; presence of signs and symptoms establishes an *actual* diagnosis.]**
PATIENT OUTCOMES/ EVALUATION CRITERIA:	**Maintains usual level of mentation/reality orientation. Demonstrates behaviors/lifestyle changes to prevent/ minimize changes in mentation.**

ACTIONS/INTERVENTIONS

Independent

Observe for changes in behavior and mentation, e.g., lethargy, confusion, drowsiness, slowing/slurring of speech, and irritability (may be intermittent). Arouse patient at intervals.

Note development/presence of asterixis, fetor hepaticus, seizure activity.

Consult with SO about patient's usual behavior and mentation.

Have patient write name periodically and keep this record for comparison. Report deterioration of ability. Have patient do simple arithmetic computations.

Reorient to time, place, person as needed.

Maintain a pleasant, quiet environment and approach in a slow, calm manner. Provide uninterrupted rest periods.

Provide continuity of care. If possible, assign same nurse over a period of time.

RATIONALE

Ongoing assessment of behavior and mental status is important because of fluctuating nature of impending hepatic coma.

Suggests elevating serum ammonia levels, increased risk of progression to encephalopathy.

Provides baseline for comparison of current status.

Easy test of neurologic status and muscle coordination.

Assists in maintaining reality orientation, reducing confusion/anxiety.

Reduces excessive stimulation/sensory overload, promotes relaxation, and may enhance coping.

Familiarity provides reassurance, aids in reducing anxiety and provides a more accurate documentation of subtle changes.

ACTIONS/INTERVENTIONS	RATIONALE

Independent

Reduce provocative stimuli, confrontation. Refrain from forcing activities. Assess potential for violent behavior.

Avoids triggering agitated, violent responses; promotes patient safety.

Discuss current situation, future expectation.

Patient/SO may be reassured that intellectual (as well as emotional) function may improve as liver involvement resolves.

Maintain bedrest, assist with self-care activities.

Reduces metabolic demands on liver, prevents fatigue, promotes healing, lowering risk of ammonia buildup.

Leave siderails up and pad if necessary. Provide close supervision.

Reduces risk of injury when confusion, seizures, or violent behavior occurs.

Investigate temperature elevations. Monitor for signs of infection.

Infection may precipitate hepatic encephalopathy owing to tissue catabolism and release of nitrogen.

Avoid use of narcotics or sedatives, tranquilizers, and limit/restrict use of medications metabolized by the liver.

Certain drugs are toxic to the liver and other drugs may not be metabolized quickly because of cirrhosis, causing cumulative effects that affect mentation, mask signs of developing encephalopathy, or precipitate coma.

Collaborative

Monitor laboratory studies, e.g., ammonia, electrolytes, pH, BUN, glucose, CBC with differential.

Elevated ammonia levels, hypokalemia, metabolic alkalosis, hypoglycemia, anemia, and infection can precipitate or potentiate development of hepatic coma.

Eliminate or restrict protein in diet. Provide glucose supplements, adequate hydration.

Ammonia (product of the breakdown of protein in the GI tract) is responsible for mental changes in hepatic encephalopathy. Dietary changes may result in constipation, which also increases bacterial action and formation of ammonia. Glucose provides a source of energy, reducing need for protein catabolism.

Administer medications as indicated:

Electrolytes:

Corrects imbalances and may improve cerebral function/metabolism of ammonia.

Stool softeners, colonic purges (e.g., magnesium sulfate), enemas, Lactulose;

Removes protein and blood from intestines. Acidifying the intestine produces diarrhea and decreases production of nitrogenous substances, reducing risk/severity of encephalopathy.

Bactericidal agents, e.g., neomycin (Neobiotic), kanamycin (Kantrex).

Destroys intestinal bacteria, reducing production of ammonia, to prevent encephalopathy.

Administer supplemental oxygen.

Mentation is affected by oxygen concentration and utilization in the brain.

Assist with procedures as indicated, e.g., dialysis, plasmapheresis, or extracorporeal liver perfusion.

May be used to reduce serum ammonia levels if encephalopathy develops/other measures unsuccessful.

NURSING DIAGNOSIS: SELF-CONCEPT, DISTURBANCE IN: (SPECIFY)

May be related to: Biophysical changes/altered physical appearance

Uncertainty of prognosis, changes in role function

Self-destructive behavior (alcohol-induced disease)

	Need for behavior/lifestyle changes
Possibly evidenced by:	**Verbalization of change in lifestyle**
	Fear of rejection or of reaction by others
	Negative feelings about body
	Feelings of helplessness, hopelessness, or powerlessness
PATIENT OUTCOMES/ EVALUATION CRITERIA:	**Verbalizes understanding of changes and acceptance of self in the present situation. Identifies feelings and methods for coping with negative perception of self.**

ACTIONS/INTERVENTIONS

Independent

Discuss situation/encourage verbalization of fears/ concerns. Explain relationship between nature of disease and symptoms.

Support and encourage patient; provide care with a positive, friendly attitude.

Encourage family/SO to verbalize feelings, visit/ participate in care.

Assist patient/SO to cope with change in appearance; suggest clothing that does not emphasize altered appearance, e.g., use of red, blue, or black clothing.

Collaborative

Refer to support services, e.g., counselors, psychiatric resources, social service, clergy, and/or alcohol treatment program.

RATIONALE

The patient is very sensitive to body changes and may also experience feelings of guilt when cause is related to alcohol (80%) or drug use.

Care givers sometimes allow judgmental feelings to affect the care of the patient and need to make every effort to help the patient feel valued as a person.

Family members may feel guilty about the patient's condition and fearful of impending death. They need nonjudgmental emotional support and free access to the patient. Participation in care helps them feel useful and promotes trust between staff, patient, and SO.

Patient may present unattractive appearance due to jaundice, ascites, ecchymotic areas. Providing support can enhance self-esteem and promote patient sense of control.

Increased vulnerability/concerns associated with this illness may require services of professional resources. (Refer to CP: Psychosocial Aspects of Acute Care, p. 773.)

NURSING DIAGNOSIS:	**KNOWLEDGE DEFICIT [LEARNING NEED] (SPECIFY)**
May be related to:	**Lack of exposure/recall; information misinterpretation**
	Unfamiliarity with information resources.
Possibly evidenced by:	**Questions; request for information**
	Statement of misconception
	Inaccurate follow-through of instruction
PATIENT OUTCOMES/ EVALUATION CRITERIA:	**Verbalizes understanding of disease process/prognosis. Correlates symptoms with causative factors. Initiates necessary lifestyle changes and participates in care.**

ACTIONS/INTERVENTIONS	RATIONALE

Independent

Review disease process/prognosis and future expectations.	Provides knowledge base on which patient can make informed choices.
Stress importance of avoiding alcohol. Give information about community services available to aid in alcohol rehabilitation if indicated.	Alcohol is the leading cause in the development of cirrhosis.
Inform the patient of altered effects of medications with cirrhosis and the importance of using only drugs prescribed or cleared by a physician who is familiar with patient's history.	Some drugs are hepatotoxic (especially narcotics, sedatives, and hypnotics). In addition, the damaged liver has a decreased ability to metabolize drugs, potentiating cumulative effect and/or aggravation of bleeding tendencies.
Assist patient in identifying support person(s).	Because of length of recovery, potential for relapses, and slow convalescence, support systems are extremely important in maintaining behavior modifications.
Emphasize the importance of good nutrition. Provide written instructions. Recommend avoidance of onions, strong cheeses.	Proper dietary maintenance and avoidance of foods high in ammonia aids in remission of symptoms and helps prevent further liver damage. Written instructions will be helpful for patient to refer to at home.
Stress necessity of follow-up care and adherence to therapeutic regimen.	Chronic nature of disease has potential for life-threatening complications.
Discuss sodium and salt substitute restrictions and necessity of reading food/OTC drug labels.	Minimizes ascites and edema formation. Overuse of substitutes may result in other electrolyte imbalances. Food, OTC/personal care products (e.g., antacids, some mouthwashes) may contain high sodium levels.
Encourage scheduling activities with adequate rest periods.	Adequate rest decreases metabolic demands on the body and increases energy available for tissue regeneration.
Promote diversional activities that are enjoyable to the patient.	Prevents boredom and minimizes anxiety and depression.
Recommend avoidance of persons with infections, especially URI.	Decreased resistance and altered nutritional status and immune response (e.g., leukopenia may occur with splenomegaly) potentiate risk of infection.
Identify environmental dangers, e.g., carbon tetrachloride type cleaning agents, exposure to hepatitis.	Can precipitate recurrence.
Instruct patient/SO of signs/symptoms that warrant notification of health care provider, e.g., increased abdominal girth, rapid weight loss/gain, edema, fever, blood in stool or urine, excess bleeding of any kind, jaundice.	Prompt reporting of symptoms reduces risk of further hepatic damage and provides opportunity to treat complications before they become life-threatening.
Instruct SO to notify health care providers of any confusion, untidiness, night wandering, tremors, or personality change.	Changes (reflecting deterioration) may be more apparent to SO, although insidious changes may be noted by others with less frequent contact with patient.

Pancreatitis

PATIENT ASSESSMENT DATA BASE

Refer to CP: Alcoholism (Acute), p. 825, for related observations, considerations.

CIRCULATION

May exhibit: Hypertension (acute pain), hypotension and tachycardia (hypovolemic shock or toxemia).

Edema, ascites.

Skin pale, cold, mottled with diaphoresis (vasoconstriction/fluid shifts); jaundiced (inflammation/obstruction of common duct); blue–green–brown discoloration around umbilicus (Cullen's sign) from accumulation of blood (hemorrhagic pancreatitis).

EGO INTEGRITY

May exhibit: Agitation, restlessness, distress, apprehension.

ELIMINATION

May report: Diarrhea, vomiting.

May exhibit: Bowel sounds decreased/absent (reduced peristalsis/ileus).

Dark amber or brown, foamy urine (bile).

Frothy, foul-smelling, grayish, greasy, nonformed stool (steatorrhea).

Polyuria (developing diabetes mellitus).

FOOD/FLUID

May report: Food intolerance, anorexia, vomiting, retching, dry heaves.

Weight loss.

NEUROSENSORY

May exhibit: Confusion, agitation.

Coarse tremors of extremities (hypocalcemia).

PAIN/COMFORT

May report: Unrelenting abdominal pain, usually located in the epigastrium and periumbilical regions, may be of sudden onset and associated with consumption of alcohol or a large meal.

Radiation to chest and back, may increase in supine position.

May exhibit: Abdominal guarding, distention, and rebound tenderness; rigidity.

May curl up with both arms over abdomen.

RESPIRATION

May exhibit: Tachypnea, with/without dyspnea.

Decreased depth of respiration with splinting/guarding actions.

Bibasilar crackles (pleural effusion).

SAFETY

May exhibit: Low-grade fever.

SEXUALITY

May exhibit: Current pregnancy (third trimester) with shifting of abdominal contents and compression of biliary tract.

TEACHING/LEARNING

May report: Family history of pancreatitis.

History of cholelithiasis with partial or complete common bile duct obstruction; gastritis, duodenal ulcer, duodenitis; diverticulitis; Crohn's disease; recent abdominal surgery (e.g., procedures on the pancreas, biliary tract, stomach, or duodenum), external abdominal trauma.

Excessive alcohol intake.

Use of medications, e.g., antihypertensives, opiates, thiazides, steroids, some antibiotics, estrogens.

Discharge Plan Considerations: May require assistance with dietary program, homemaker tasks.

DIAGNOSTIC STUDIES

CT scan/ultrasound of abdomen: may be used to identify pancreatic inflammation, carcinoma, or obstruction of biliary tract.

Endoscopy: visualization of pancreatic ducts is useful to diagnose fistulas, obstructive biliary disease, and pancreatic duct strictures/anomalies. Note: This procedure is contraindicated in acute phase.

X-ray: may demonstrate dilated loop of small bowel adjacent to pancreas or other intraabdominal precipitator of pancreatitis; presence of free intraperitoneal air caused by perforation or abscess formation; pancreatic calcification.

Upper GI series: frequently exhibits evidence of pancreatic enlargement/inflammation.

Serum amylase: increased due to obstruction of normal outflow of pancreatic enzymes (normal level does not rule out disease).

Urine amylase: increased within 2 to 3 days after onset of attack.

Serum lipase: usually elevates along with amylase, but stays elevated longer.

Serum bilirubin: increase is common (may be caused by alcoholic liver disease or compression of common bile duct).

Alkaline phosphatase: usually elevated if pancreatitis is accompanied by biliary disease.

Serum albumin and protein: may be decreased (increased capillary permeability and transudation of fluid into extracellular space).

Serum calcium: hypocalcemia may appear 2–3 days after onset of illness (usually indicates fat necrosis and may accompany pancreatic necrosis).

Potassium: hypokalemia may occur because of gastric losses; hyperkalemia may develop secondary to tissue necrosis, acidosis, renal insufficiency.

Triglycerides: levels may exceed 1700 mg/dl and may be causative agent in acute pancreatitis.

LDH/SGOT (AST): may be elevated up to 15 times normal because of biliary and liver involvement.

CBC: WBC of 10,000–25,000 is present in 80% of patients. Hct is usually elevated (hemoconcentration associated with vomiting or from effusion of fluid into pancreas or retroperitoneal area).

Serum glucose: transient elevations are common, especially during initial/acute attacks. Sustained hyperglycemia reflects widespread beta cell damage and pancreatic necrosis and is a poor prognostic sign.

Prothrombin time: prolonged due to liver involvement and fat necrosis.

Urinalysis: hematuria and proteinuria may be present (glomerular damage).

Stool: increased fat content (steatorrhea) indicative of insufficient digestion of fats and protein.

NURSING PRIORITIES

1. Control pain and promote comfort.
2. Prevent/treat fluid and electrolyte imbalance.

3. Reduce pancreatic stimulation while maintaining adequate nutrition.
4. Prevent complications.
5. Provide information about disease process/prognosis and treatment needs.

DISCHARGE CRITERIA

1. Pain relieved/controlled.
2. Homeostasis maintained.
3. Complications prevented/minimized.
4. Disease process/prognosis, potential complications and therapeutic regimen understood.

NURSING DIAGNOSIS:	COMFORT, ALTERED: PAIN, ACUTE
May be related to:	**Obstruction of pancreatic, biliary ducts**
	Chemical contamination of peritoneal surfaces by pancreatic exudate/autodigestion of pancreas
	Extension of inflammation to the retroperitoneal nerve plexus
Possibly evidenced by:	**Complaints of pain**
	Self-focusing, grimacing, distraction/guarding behaviors
	Autonomic responses, alteration in muscle tone
PATIENT OUTCOMES/ EVALUATION CRITERIA:	**Reports pain is relieved/controlled. Follows prescribed therapeutic regimen. Demonstrates use of methods that provide relief.**

ACTIONS/INTERVENTIONS	RATIONALE
Independent	
Investigate verbal complaints of pain, noting specific location and intensity (1–10 scale). Note factors that aggravate and relieve pain.	Pain is often diffuse, severe, and unrelenting in acute or hemorrhagic pancreatitis and may be a chronic, dull aching in chronic pancreatitis. Localized pain may indicate development of pseudocysts or abscesses.
Maintain bedrest during acute attack. Provide quiet, restful environment.	Decreases metabolic rate and gastrointestinal stimulation/secretions, thereby reducing pancreatic activity.
Promote position of comfort, e.g., on one side with knees flexed.	Reduces abdominal pressure/tension, providing some measure of comfort and pain relief
Provide alternate comfort measures (e.g., backrub); encourage relaxation techniques (e.g., guided imagery, visualization), quiet diversional activities (e.g., television, radio).	Promotes relaxation and enables patient to refocus attention, may enhance coping.
Keep environment free of food odors.	Sensory stimulation can activate pancreatic enzymes, increasing pain.
Administer analgesics in timely manner (smaller, more frequent doses).	Severe/prolonged pain can aggravate shock and is more difficult to relieve, requiring larger doses of medication, which can mask underlying problems/complications and may contribute to respiratory depression.

ACTIONS/INTERVENTIONS	RATIONALE

Independent

Maintain meticulous skin care, especially in presence of draining abdominal wall fistulas.	Pancreatic enzymes can digest the skin and tissues of the abdominal wall, creating a chemical burn.

Collaborative

Administer medications as indicated:

Narcotic analgesics, e.g., meperidine (Demerol);	Meperidine is usually effective in relieving pain and may be preferred over morphine, which can display side effect of biliary–pancreatic spasms. Paravertebral block has been used to achieve prolonged pain control. Note: Patients who have recurrent pancreatitis episodes may be difficult to manage because they may become addicted to the narcotics given for pain control.
Sedatives, e.g., diazepam (Valium), antispasmodics, e.g., atropine;	Potentiates action of narcotic to promote rest and to reduce muscular/ductal spasm, thereby reducing metabolic needs, enzyme secretions.
Antacids, e.g., Mylanta;	Neutralizes gastric acid to reduce production of pancreatic enzymes and to reduce incidence of upper GI bleed.
Cimetidine (Tagamet), ranitidine (Zantac).	Decreasing secretion of hydrochloric acid (HCl) reduces stimulation of the pancreas and associated pain. Oral intake during acute phase, stimulates release of pancreatic enzymes, increasing pain.
Withhold food and fluid as indicated.	Limits/reduces release of pancreatic enzymes and resultant pain.
Maintain gastric suction when used.	Prevents accumulation of gastric secretions, which can stimulate pancreatic enzyme activity.
Prepare for surgical intervention if indicated.	Surgical exploration may be required in presence of intractable pain/complications involving the biliary tract.

NURSING DIAGNOSIS:	**FLUID VOLUME DEFICIT, POTENTIAL**
May be related to:	**Excessive losses: vomiting, gastric suctioning**
	Increase in size of vascular bed (vasodilation, effects of kinins)
	Third space fluid transudation, ascites formation
	Alteration of clotting process, hemorrhage
Possibly evidenced by:	**[Not applicable; presence of signs and symptoms establishes an *actual* diagnosis.]**
PATIENT OUTCOMES/ EVALUATION CRITERIA:	**Maintains adequate hydration as evidenced by stable vital signs; good skin turgor, capillary refill; strong peripheral pulses and individually appropriate urinary output.**

ACTIONS/INTERVENTIONS	RATIONALE

Independent

Monitor blood pressure and measure CVP if available.

Fluid shifts into third space, bleeding, and release of vasodilators (kinins) may result in severe hypotension. Reduced cardiac output/poor organ perfusion secondary to a hypotensive episode can precipitate widespread systemic complications.

Measure I & O including vomiting/gastric aspirate, diarrhea. Calculate 24-hour fluid balance.

Indicator of replacement needs/effectiveness of therapy.

Note decrease in urine output (less than 400 ml in 24 hours).

Oliguria may occur, signaling renal impairment/acute tubular necrosis (ATN), related to increase in renal vascular resistance, or reduced/altered renal blood flow.

Record color, and character of gastric drainage as well as noting pH and presence of occult blood.

Increased risk of gastric bleeding/hemorrhage.

Weigh as indicated. Correlate with calculated fluid balance.

Weight loss may suggest hypovolemia; however, edema, fluid retention, and ascites may be reflected by increased or stable weight.

Note poor skin turgor, dry skin/mucous membranes, complaints of thirst.

Further physiologic indicators of dehydration.

Observe/record peripheral and dependent edema. Measure abdominal girth if ascites present.

Edema/fluid shifts occur as a result of increased vascular permeability, sodium retention, and decreased colloid osmotic pressure in the intravascular compartment. Note: Fluid loss (sequestration) of greater than 6 liters in 48 hours is considered a poor prognostic sign.

Investigate changes in sensorium, e.g., confusion, slowed responses.

Changes may be related to hypovolemia, hypoxia, electrolyte imbalance, or impending delirium tremens (in the patient with acute pancreatitis secondary to excessive alcohol intake). Severe pancreatic disease may cause toxic psychosis.

Auscultate heart sounds, note rate and rhythm. Monitor/document rhythm changes.

Cardiac changes/dysrhythmias may reflect hypovolemia or electrolyte imbalance, commonly hypokalemia/hypocalcemia. Hyperkalemia may occur related to tissue necrosis, acidosis, and renal insufficiency and may precipitate lethal dysrhythmias if uncorrected. S_3 gallop in conjunction with jugular vein distention and crackles suggest heart failure/pulmonary edema. Note: Cardiovascular complications are common and include myocardial infarction, pericarditis, and pericardial effusion with/without tamponade. (Refer to appropriate care plans as needed.)

Inspect skin for petechiae, hematomas, and unusual wound or venipuncture bleeding. Note hematuria, mucous membrane bleeding, and bloody gastric contents.

Disseminated intravascular coagulation (DIC) may be initiated by release of active pancreatic proteases into the circulation. The most frequently affected organs are the kidneys, skin, and lungs.

Observe/report coarse muscle tremors, twitching, positive Chvostek's or Trousseau's sign.

Symptoms of calcium imbalance. Calcium binds with free fats in the intestine and is lost by secretion in the stool.

Collaborative

Administer fluid replacement as indicated, e.g., saline solutions, albumin, blood/blood products, dextran.

Choice of replacement solution may be less important than rapidity and adequacy of volume restoration. Saline solutions and albumin may be used to promote mobilization of fluid back into vascular space. Low-molecular-weight dextran is sometimes used to re-

ACTIONS/INTERVENTIONS	RATIONALE
Collaborative	
	duce risk of renal dysfunction and pulmonary edema associated with pancreatitis.
Monitor laboratory studies, e.g., Hb/Hct, protein, albumin, electrolytes, BUN, creatinine, urine osmolality and sodium/potassium, coagulation studies.	Identifies deficits/replacement needs and developing complications, e.g., acute tubular necrosis, DIC. (Refer to CP: Renal Failure: Acute, p. 544.)
Replace electrolytes, e.g., sodium, potassium, chloride, calcium as indicated.	Decreased oral intake and excessive losses greatly affect electrolyte/acid base balance, which is necessary to maintain optimal cellular/organ function.
Prepare for/assist with peritoneal lavage, hemoperitoneal dialysis.	Removes toxic chemicals/pancreatic enzymes and allows for more rapid correction of metabolic abnormalities in severe/unresponsive cases of acute pancreatitis.

NURSING DIAGNOSIS:	NUTRITION, ALTERED: LESS THAN BODY REQUIREMENTS
May be related to:	**Vomiting, decreased oral intake**
	Prescribed dietary restrictions
	Loss of digestive enzymes and insulin (related to pancreatic outflow obstruction or necrosis/autodigestion)
Possibly evidenced by:	**Reported inadequate food intake**
	Aversion to eating, reported altered taste sensation, lack of interest in food
	Weight loss
	Poor muscle tone
PATIENT OUTCOMES/ EVALUATION CRITERIA:	**Demonstrates progressive weight gain toward goal with normalization of laboratory values and free of signs of malnutrition. Demonstrates behaviors, lifestyle changes to regain and/or maintain appropriate weight.**

ACTIONS/INTERVENTIONS	RATIONALE
Independent	
Assess abdomen, noting presence/character of bowel sounds, abdominal distention, and complaints of nausea.	Gastric distention and intestinal atony are frequently present, resulting in reduced/absent bowel sounds. Return of bowel sounds and relief of symptoms signal readiness for discontinuation of gastric aspiration (NG tube).
Provide frequent oral care.	Decreases vomiting stimulus and inflammation/irritation of dry mucous membranes associated with dehydration and mouth breathing when nasogastric tube is in place.
Assist patient in selecting food/fluids that meet nutritional needs and restrictions when diet resumed.	Previous dietary habits may be unsatisfactory in meeting current needs for tissue regeneration and healing. Use of gastric stimulants, e.g., caffeine, alcohol, ciga-

ACTIONS/INTERVENTIONS	RATIONALE

Independent

Observe color/consistency/amount of stools. Note frothy consistency/foul odor.

Note signs of increased thirst and urination, or changes in mentation and visual acuity.

Test urine for sugar and acetone.

rettes, gas-producing foods, or ingestion of large meals may result in excessive stimulation of the pancreas/recurrence of symptoms.

Steatorrhea may develop from incomplete digestion of fats.

May warn of developing hyperglycemia associated with increased release of glucagon (damage to alpha cells) or decreased release of insulin (damage to beta cells).

Early detection of inadequate glucose utilization may prevent development of ketoacidosis.

Collaborative

Maintain NPO status and gastric suctioning in acute phase.

Prevents stimulation and release of pancreatic enzymes (secretin), released when chyme and HCl acid enter the duodenum.

Monitor serum glucose.

Indicator of insulin needs because hyperglycemia is frequently present but not usually in levels high enough to produce ketoacidosis.

Administer hyperalimentation and lipids, if indicated. (Refer to CP: Total Nutritional Support, p. 894.)

IV administration of calories, lipids, and amino acids should be instituted before nutrition/nitrogen depletion is advanced.

Resume oral intake with clear liquids and advance diet slowly to provide high protein, high carbohydrate diet, when indicated.

Oral feedings given too early in the course of illness may exacerbate symptoms. Loss of pancreatic function/reduced insulin production may require initiation of a diabetic diet.

Provide medium-chain triglycerides (e.g., Isocal).

MCTs provide supplemental calories/nutrients that do not require pancreatic enzymes for digestion/absorption.

Administer medications as indicated:

Vitamins, e.g., A, D, E, K;

Replacement required as fat metabolism is altered, reducing absorption/storage of fat-soluble vitamins.

Replacement enzymes, e.g., pancreatin (Viokase), pancrelipase (Cotazym);

Corrects deficiencies promoting digestion and absorption of nutrients.

Anticholinergics, e.g., methantheline bromide (Banthine);

Thought to reduce pancreatic and gastric secretions with depression of the vagal mechanisms and decrease of motility. The decrease in volume and concentration of enzymes provides rest for the inflamed area. Note: These drugs are contraindicated in the presence of shock/paralytic ileus, and current drug studies have not proven their efficiency.

Regular insulin;

Corrects persistent hyperglycemia caused by injury to beta cells and increased release of glucocorticoids. Insulin therapy is usually short-term unless permanent damage to pancreas occurs.

NURSING DIAGNOSIS: **INFECTION, POTENTIAL FOR**

May be related to: **Inadequate primary defenses: stasis of body fluids, altered peristalsis, change in pH secretions**

Immunosuppression

Nutritional deficiencies

Tissue destruction, chronic disease

Possibly evidenced by:	**[Not applicable; presence of signs and symptoms establishes an *actual* diagnosis.]**
PATIENT OUTCOMES/ EVALUATION CRITERIA:	**Achieves timely healing; free of signs of infection/ afebrile. Participates in activities to reduce risk of infection.**

ACTIONS/INTERVENTIONS	RATIONALE
Independent	
Use strict aseptic technique when changing surgical dressings or working with IV lines, indwelling catheters/tubes, drains. Change soiled dressings promptly.	Limits sources of infection, which can lead to sepsis in a compromised patient.
Stress importance of good handwashing.	Reduces risk of cross-contamination.
Observe rate and characteristics of respirations, breath sounds. Note occurrence of cough and sputum production.	Fluid accumulation and limited mobility predisposes to respiratory infections and atelectasis. Accumulation of ascites fluid may cause elevated diaphragm and shallow abdominal breathing.
Encourage frequent position changes, deep breathing and coughing. Assist with ambulation as soon as stable.	Enhances ventilation of all lung segments and promotes mobilization of secretions.
Observe for signs of infection, e.g.:	
Fever and respiratory distress in conjunction with jaundice:	Cholestatic jaundice and decreased pulmonary function may be first sign of sepsis involving gram-negative organisms.
Increased abdominal pain, rigidity/rebound tenderness, diminished/absent bowel sounds;	Suggestive of peritonitis. (Refer to CP: Peritonitis, p. 449.)
Increased abdominal pain/tenderness, recurrent fever (greater than 101°F), leukocytosis, hypotension, tachycardia, and chills.	Abscesses can occur 2 or more weeks after the onset of pancreatitis (mortality can exceed 50%) and should be suspected whenever the patient is deteriorating despite supportive measures.
Collaborative	
Obtain culture specimens, e.g., blood, wound, urine, sputum, or pancreatic aspirate.	Identifies presence of infection and causative organism.
Administer antibiotic therapy as indicated: cephalosporins, e.g., cefoxitin sodium (Mefoxin), plus aminoglycosides, e.g., gentamicin (Garamycin), tobramycin (Nebcin).	Broad spectrum antibiotics are generally recommended for sepsis. However, therapy will be based on the specific organisms cultured.
Prepare for surgical intervention as necessary.	Abscesses may be surgically drained with resection of necrotic tissue. Sump tubes may be inserted for antibiotic irrigation and drainage of pancreatic debris. Pseudocysts (persisting for several weeks) may be drained because of the risk and incidence of infection/ rupture.

NURSING DIAGNOSIS:	KNOWLEDGE DEFICIT [LEARNING NEED] (SPECIFY)
May be related to:	**Lack of exposure/recall**
	Information misinterpretation, unfamiliarity with information resources
Possibly evidenced by:	**Questions, request for information**
	Statement of misconception
	Inaccurate follow-through of instruction
	Development of preventable complication
PATIENT OUTCOMES/ EVALUATION CRITERIA:	**Verbalizes understanding of condition/disease process and treatment. Correctly performs necessary procedures and explains reasons for the actions. Initiates necessary lifestyle changes and participates in treatment regimen.**

ACTIONS/INTERVENTIONS	RATIONALE

Independent

Review specific cause of current episode and prognosis.

Provides knowledge base on which patient can make informed choices.

Discuss other causative/associated factors, e.g., excessive alcohol intake, gallbladder disease, duodenal ulcer, hyperlipoproteinenemias, some drugs (e.g., oral contraceptives, thiazides, Lasix, INH, glucocorticoids, sulfonamides).

Avoidance may help to limit damage and prevent development of a chronic condition.

Explore availability of treatment programs/ rehabilitation of chemical dependency if indicated.

Alcohol abuse is currently the most common cause of recurrence of or chronic pancreatitis. Drug usage is increasing as a factor, whether prescribed or illicit. Note: Pain of pancreatitis can be severe and prolonged and may lead to narcotic dependence, requiring need for referral to pain clinic.

Stress the importance of follow-up care, and review symptoms that need to be reported immediately to physician, e.g., recurrence of pain, persistent fever, nausea/vomiting, abdominal distention, frothy/foul-smelling stools, general intolerance of food.

Prolonged recovery period requires close monitoring to prevent recurrence/complications, e.g., infection, pancreatic pseudocysts.

Review importance of initially continuing bland, low-fat diet with frequent small feedings and restricted caffeine; then gradual resumption of a normal diet within individual tolerance.

Understanding the purpose of the diet in maximizing the use of available enzymes while avoiding overstimulation of the pancreas may enhance patient involvement in self-monitoring of dietary needs and responses to foods.

Instruct in use of pancreatic enzyme replacements and bile salt therapy as indicated, avoiding concomitant ingestion of hot foods/fluids.

If permanent damage has occurred to the pancreas, exocrine deficiencies will occur, requiring long-term replacement. Hot foods/fluids can inactivate enzymes.

Recommend cessation of smoking.

Nicotine stimulates gastric secretions and unnecessary pancreatic activity.

Discuss signs/symptoms of diabetes mellitus, i.e., polydipsia, polyuria, weakness, weight loss. (Refer to CP: Diabetes Mellitus/Diabetic Ketoacidosis, p. 645.)

Damage to the beta cells may result in a temporary or permanent alteration of insulin production.

499

Hemorrhoids/Hemorrhoidectomy

PATIENT ASSESSMENT DATA BASE

ACTIVITY/REST

May report: Occupation/recreation engaging in activities involving sitting/standing for long periods.

EGO INTEGRITY

May report: Fear, anxiety, embarrassment.

ELIMINATION

May report: Straining at stool, chronic constipation/use of laxatives.
Bleeding with defecation, mucus discharge.

May exhibit: Rectal/anal examination reveals presence of hemorrhoids.
Occult blood (positive guaiac) in stool.

FOOD/FLUID

May report: Low fiber intake.

May exhibit: Obesity.

PAIN/COMFORT

May report: Perianal pain; intense pain (related to thromboses of external hemorrhoids).
Itching (pruritis).

TEACHING/LEARNING

May report: History of cirrhosis/portal hypertension.
Problems with hemorrhoids during/after pregnancy.
Family history of hemorrhoids.

Discharge Plan Considerations: May require vocational counseling.

DIAGNOSTIC STUDIES

CBC: may indicate anemia due to chronic or acute rectal bleeding.
Serum iron: deficiency may be noted.
Proctoscopy: detects internal hemorrhoids.

NURSING PRIORITIES

1. Maintain patient comfort.
2. Prevent constipation.
3. Provide information about condition/prognosis and treatment needs.

DISCHARGE CRITERIA

1. Discomfort relieved/controlled.
2. Constipation corrected.
3. Condition, prognosis and therapeutic regimen understood.
Refer to CP: Surgical Intervention, p. 789, for general concerns, considerations.

NURSING DIAGNOSIS:	COMFORT, ALTERED: PAIN, ACUTE
May be related to:	Congestion and edema, thrombosis of vessels
Possibly evidenced by:	Complaints of pain
	Guarding behaviors, facial grimacing
PATIENT OUTCOMES/ EVALUATION CRITERIA:	Reports pain/discomfort is controlled. Identifies methods that provide relief.

ACTIONS/INTERVENTIONS	RATIONALE
Independent	
Assess amount, character, and threshold of discomfort/pain; use scale of 1–10.	Provides information about individual analgesic needs and effectiveness of therapy.
Allow patient to assume position of comfort. Turn side to side; avoid high-Fowler's position/prolonged sitting.	Patient will naturally choose position that provides most relief from pain, but prolonged sitting decreases tissue perfusion and may cause edema.
Provide flotation pad/cushion under buttocks; pad bottom of sitz tub. Avoid use of rubber doughnut ring.	Distributes pressure more evenly to reduce pain/discomfort, may enhance tissue circulation. Note: Use of rubber ring may increase anal pressure/discomfort.
Avoid use of soap for pericare/in sitz.	May be irritating/drying to tissues.
Prevent constipation. (Refer to ND: Bowel Elimination, Altered: Constipation, following.)	Reduces stress on tissues decreasing potential for injury/bleeding.
Investigate complaints of abdominal discomfort or continuous urge to defecate after surgical intervention.	May indicate developing complications such as urinary retention (localized swelling/anal packing) or hematoma formation.
Collaborative	
Apply ice pack/cold compresses to area initially.	Local application reduces congestion and edema formation.
Use warm compresses and sitz baths as indicated.	Promotes circulation, reduces tissue congestion and is soothing to the area.
Administer medications as indicated; topical cream/suppositories, analgesics/anesthetics, e.g., dibucaine hydrochloride (Nupercainal); steroidal ointment. Apply witch hazel pads (Tucks).	Relieves pain/itching, reduces inflammation. Note: Administration of analgesic half hour before patient attempts to defecate promotes perianal relaxation.
Discuss use of hypnosis.	Has been used with some success for pain control. Note: It is important to avoid the use of the word "pain" when talking to the patient.
Assist with procedures, e.g., manual reduction, sclerosing, incision/drainage of clots, ligation, surgical excision.	Nonsurgical interventions may provide temporary relief permitting time to accomplish medical management. Surgical removal may be required if hemorrhoids do not respond to other measures.

NURSING DIAGNOSIS:	BOWEL ELIMINATION, ALTERED: CONSTIPATION
May be related to:	Inadequate dietary intake (including bulk)
	Decreased physical activity

	Pain on defecation
Possibly evidenced by:	Decreased frequency/amount of stool
	Hard formed stool
	Straining at stool
	Chronic use of laxatives
PATIENT OUTCOMES/ EVALUATION CRITERIA:	Establishes/returns to normal pattern of bowel functioning with regular production of soft formed stool.

ACTIONS/INTERVENTIONS

Independent

Ascertain usual bowel habits.

Encourage minimum intake of 2000 ml of fluid per day, within cardiac tolerance.

Establish routine bowel habits and remind patient to heed defecation urge.

Discuss the importance of using high-fiber foods and low roughage in the diet, e.g., whole grain products.

Avoid the use of opiates and their derivatives.

Collaborative

Administer bulk laxatives, e.g., Metamucil; stool softeners and/or lubricants.

RATIONALE

Aids in identifying individual problem areas and appropriate interventions.

Improves consistency of stools to facilitate defecation without straining.

Regular evacuation helps maintain softer stool.

Helpful in maintaining adequate amount of soft formed stool.

These medications have a constipating effect.

Maintains soft stool by softening and adding bulk and moisture to stool to facilitate defecation.

NURSING DIAGNOSIS:	KNOWLEDGE DEFICIT [LEARNING NEED] (SPECIFY)
May be related to:	Lack of exposure/recall
	Information misinterpretation
	Unfamiliarity with information resources
Possibly evidenced by:	Questions; request for information
	Statement of misconception
	Inaccurate follow-through of instruction
PATIENT OUTCOMES/ EVALUATION CRITERIA:	Verbalizes understanding of condition and treatment. Correctly performs necessary procedures and explains reasons for the actions. Initiates necessary lifestyle changes and participates in treatment regimen.

ACTIONS/INTERVENTIONS

Independent

Review cause of condition and prognosis.

RATIONALE

Provides knowledge base on which patient can make informed choices.

ACTIONS/INTERVENTIONS	RATIONALE
Independent	
Encourage continuation of low-residue diet with addition of roughage as tolerated and adequate fluid intake.	Promotes formation of adequate amount/soft formed stool to reduce occurrence of constipation and straining at stool.
Discuss use of stool softeners, mild cathartics, suppositories, enemas.	Stimulates evacuation and should be used judiciously along with dietary, activity and fluid management in order to prevent dependence on laxatives or injury to incisional tissues.
Encourage patient to avoid use of strong laxatives.	Prevents liquid bowel movements (formed stool helps maintain lumen size of anal canal) and reduces painful peristalsis/cramping.
	May help to prevent recurrence of hemorrhoids.
Discuss activity limitations, e.g., avoidance of prolonged sitting/standing, heavy lifting, straining for stool.	
Review incisional care, e.g., perianal cleansing, sitz baths when appropriate.	Promotes healing, reduces risk of infection following hemorrhoidectomy.
Stress importance of exercising caution when exiting sitz bath.	Dilation of the pelvic blood vessels during sitz baths may result in hypotension and dizziness.
Identify symptoms requiring notification of health care provider, e.g., rectal bleeding, fever, local erythema, purulent drainage, ribbon-shaped stool, inability to pass stool.	Early intervention may prevent more serious complications, e.g., wound infection, anal stricture.

CHAPTER 9

DISEASES OF THE BLOOD/ BLOOD-FORMING ORGANS

Anemias (Iron Deficiency [ID], Pernicious, Aplastic) _____

Anemia is a symptom of an underlying condition, such as loss of blood components, inadequate elements, or lack of required nutrients for the formation of blood cells, that results in the decreased oxygen-carrying capacity of the blood.

PATIENT ASSESSMENT DATA BASE

ACTIVITY/REST

May report:	Fatigue, weakness, general malaise.
	Loss of productivity; diminished enthusiasm for work.
	Low exercise tolerance.
	Greater need for rest and sleep.
May exhibit:	Tachycardia/tachypnea; dyspnea on exertion or at rest.
	Lethargy, withdrawal, apathy, lassitude and lack of interest in surroundings.
	Muscle weakness and decreased strength.
	Ataxia, unsteady gait.
	Slumping of shoulders, drooping posture, slow walk, and other cues indicative of fatigue.

CIRCULATION

May report:	History of chronic blood loss, e.g., GI bleeding, heavy menses (ID); angina, CHF (due to increased workload of the heart).
	Palpitations (compensatory tachycardia).
May exhibit:	BP: increased systolic with stable diastolic and a widened pulse pressure; postural hypotension.
	Dysrhythmias; ECG abnormalities, e.g., ST segment depression and flattening or depression of the T wave; tachycardia.
	Throbbing carotid pulsations (compensatory mechanism to provide oxygen/nutrients to cells).
	Heart sounds: systolic murmur (ID).

Extremities (color): pallor of the skin and mucous membranes (conjunctiva, mouth, pharynx, lips) and nail beds (Note: In black patients, pallor may appear as a grayish cast); waxy, pale skin (aplastic, pernicious) or bright lemon yellow (pernicious).

Sclera: blue or pearl white (ID).

Capillary refill delayed (diminished blood flow to the periphery and compensatory vasoconstriction).

Nails: brittle, spoon-shaped (koilonychia) (ID).

Hair: dry, brittle, thinning; premature graying (pernicious).

EGO INTEGRITY

May report: Religious/cultural beliefs affecting treatment choices, e.g., blood transfusions.

May exhibit: Depression.

ELIMINATION

May report: Flatulence, malabsorption syndrome (ID).

Hematemesis, fresh blood in stool, melena.

Diarrhea or constipation.

Diminished urine output.

May exhibit: Abdominal distention.

FOOD/FLUID

May report: Decreased dietary intake, low intake of animal protein/high intake of cereal products.

Oral pain, difficulty swallowing (ulcerations in pharynx).

Nausea/vomiting, dyspepsia, anorexia.

Recent weight loss.

Insatiable craving or pica for ice, dirt, cornstarch, paint, clay, etc. (ID).

May exhibit: Beefy red/smooth appearance of tongue (pernicious, folic acid and vitamin B_{12} deficiencies).

Dry, pale mucous membranes.

Skin turgor: poor, with dry, shriveled appearance/loss of elasticity (ID).

Stomatitis and glossitis (deficiency states).

Lips: chelitis, inflammation of the lips with cracking at the corners of the mouth (ID).

HYGIENE

May exhibit: Debilitated, unkempt appearance.

NEUROSENSORY

May report: Headaches, fainting, dizziness, vertigo, tinnitus, inability to concentrate.

Insomnia, dimness of vision, and spots before eyes.

Weakness; paresthesias of hands/feet (pernicious); claudication.

Sensation of being cold.

May exhibit: Irritability, restlessness, depression, drowsiness, apathy.

Mentation: notable slowing and dullness in response.

Ophthalmic: retinal hemorrhages (aplastic, pernicious).

Epistaxis, bleeding from other orifices (aplastic).

Disturbed coordination, ataxia: decreased vibratory and position sense, positive Romberg's sign, paralysis (pernicious).

505

PAIN/COMFORT

May report: Vague abdominal pains; headache (ID).

RESPIRATION

May report: Shortness of breath at rest and with activity.

May exhibit: Tachypnea, orthopnea, and dyspnea.

SAFETY

May report: History of occupational exposure to chemicals, e.g., benzene, lead, insecticides, phenylbutazone, naphthalene.

History of exposure to radiation either as a treatment modality or by accident.

History of cancer, cancer therapies.

Cold and/or heat intolerance.

Previous blood transfusions.

Impaired vision.

Poor wound healing, frequent infections.

May exhibit: Low grade fever, chills, night sweats.

Generalized lymphadenopathy.

Petechiae and ecchymosis (aplastic).

SEXUALITY

May report: Changes in menstrual flow, e.g., menorrhagia or amenorrhea (ID).

Loss of libido (males and females).

Impotence.

May exhibit: Pale cervix and vaginal walls.

TEACHING/LEARNING

May report: Family tendency for iron deficiency anemia.

Past/present drug history of anticonvulsants, antibiotics, chemotherapeutic agents (bone marrow failure), aspirin, antiinflammatory drugs, or anticoagulants.

Chronic use of alcohol.

History of liver, renal disease; hematologic problems; celiac or other malabsorption disease; regional enteritis; tapeworm manifestations; polyendocrinopathies.

Prior surgeries, e.g., splenectomy; tumor excision; prosthetic valve replacement; surgical excision of duodenum or gastric resection, partial/total gastrectomy (ID/pernicious).

History of problems with wound healing or bleeding; chronic infections, rheumatoid arthritis, chronic granulomatous disease, or cancer (secondary anemias).

Discharge Plan Considerations: May require assistance with treatment (injections); self-care/homemaker tasks; changes in dietary plan.

DIAGNOSTIC STUDIES

CBC: decreased hemoglobin and hematocrit.

Erythrocyte count: decreased (pernicious); severely decreased (aplastic); MCV and MCH decreased and microcytic with hypochromic erythrocytes (ID), elevated (pernicious). Pancytopenia (aplastic anemia).

Reticulocyte count: varies, e.g., decreased (pernicious), elevated (bone marrow response to blood loss/hemolysis).

Stained red blood cell examination: detects changes in color and shape (may indicate particular type of anemia).

Erythrocyte sedimentation rate (ESR): elevation indicates presence of inflammatory reaction, e.g., increased red cell destruction or malignant disease.

Red blood cell survival time: useful in the differential diagnosis of the anemias, e.g., in certain types of anemias RBCs have shortened life spans.

Erythrocyte fragility test: decreased (ID).

WBCs: total cell count as well as specific white blood cells (differential) may be increased or decreased.

Platelet count: decreased (aplastic); elevated (ID).

Hemoglobin electrophoresis: identifies type of hemoglobin structure.

Serum bilirubin (unconjugated): elevated (pernicious).

Serum folate and vitamin B_{12}: aids in diagnosing anemias related to deficiencies in intake/absorption.

Serum iron: decreased (ID).

Serum total iron binding capacities: increased (ID).

Serum ferritin: decreased (ID).

Bleeding time: prolonged (aplastic).

Serum lactate dehydrogenase (LDH): may be elevated (pernicious).

Schilling test: decreased urinary excretion of vitamin B (pernicious).

Guaiac: may be positive for occult blood in urine, stools, and gastric contents, reflecting acute/chronic bleeding (ID).

Gastric analysis: decreased secretions with elevated pH and absence of free hydrochloric acid (pernicious).

Bone marrow aspiration/biopsy examination: cells may show changes in number, size and shape, helping to differentiate type of anemia, e.g., increased megaloblasts (pernicious), fatty marrow with diminished blood cells (aplastic).

Endoscopic and radiographic studies: checks for bleeding sites; gastrointestinal bleeding.

NURSING PRIORITIES

1. Enhance tissue perfusion.
2. Provide nutritional/fluid needs.
3. Prevent complications.
4. Provide information about disease process, prognosis, and treatment regimen.

DISCHARGE CRITERIA

1. ADLs met by self or with assistance of others.
2. Complications prevented/minimized.
3. Disease process/prognosis and therapeutic regimen understood.

NURSING DIAGNOSIS:	**TISSUE PERFUSION, ALTERED: (SPECIFY)**
May be related to:	**Reduction of cellular components necessary for delivery of oxygen/nutrients to the cells**
Possibly evidenced by:	**Palpitations, angina**
	Pallor of skin, mucous membranes; dry, brittle nails and hair
	Cold extremities
	Decreased urinary output
	Nausea/vomiting, abdominal distension
	Changes in blood pressure, delayed capillary refill

PATIENT OUTCOMES/ EVALUATION CRITERIA:	**Demonstrates increased perfusion as individually appropriate, e.g., stable vital signs; pinkish mucous membranes, good capillary refill; adequate urine output; usual mentation.**

ACTIONS/INTERVENTIONS	RATIONALE
Independent	
Monitor vital signs, assess capillary refill, color of skin/ mucous membranes, nailbeds.	Provides information about degree/adequacy of tissue perfusion and helps to determine needed interventions.
Elevate head of bed as tolerated.	Enhances lung expansion to maximize oxygenation for cellular uptake. Note: May be contraindicated if hypotension is present.
Monitor respiratory effort; auscultate breath sounds noting adventitious sounds.	Presence of dyspnea, crackles may reflect developing CHF due to prolonged cardiac strain/compensatory elevation of cardiac output.
Investigate complaints of chest pain, palpitations.	Cellular ischemia affects myocardial tissues/ potentiates risk of infarction.
Assess for slowed verbal response, irritability, agitation, impaired memory, confusion.	May indicate impaired cerebral function due to hypoxia or vitamin B_{12} deficiency.
Orient/reorient patient as needed. Write out schedule of activities for patient to refer to. Provide sufficient time for patient to complete thoughts, communication, activities.	Aids in improving thought processes, and ability to perform/maintain needed activities of daily living.
Observe for complaints of feeling cold. Maintain environmental temperature and body warmth as indicated.	Vasoconstriction (shunting of blood to vital organs) decreases peripheral circulation, impairing tissue perfusion. Patient's comfort/need for warmth needs to be balanced with need to avoid excessive heat with resultant vasodilation (reduces organ perfusion).
Avoid the use of heating pads or hot water bottles. Measure temperature of bath water with a thermometer.	Thermoreceptors in the dermal tissues may be dulled due to oxygen deprivation.
Collaborative	
Monitor laboratory studies, e.g., Hb/Hct and RBC count, ABGs.	Identifies deficiencies and treatment needs/response to therapy.
Administer whole blood/packed RBCs, blood products as indicated. Monitor closely for transfusion complications.	Increases number of oxygen-carrying cells; corrects deficiencies to reduce risk of hemorrhage.
Administer supplemental oxygen as indicated.	Maximizes oxygen transport to tissues.
Prepare for surgical intervention if indicated.	Bone marrow transplant may be done in presence of bone marrow failure/aplastic anemia.

NURSING DIAGNOSIS:	**ACTIVITY INTOLERANCE**
May be related to:	**Imbalance between oxygen supply (delivery) and demand**

Possibly evidenced by:	Weakness and fatigue
	Complaints of decreased exercise/activity tolerance
	Greater need for sleep/rest
	Palpitations, tachycardia, increased BP/respiratory response with minor exertion
PATIENT OUTCOMES/ EVALUATION CRITERIA:	Reports an increase in activity tolerance (including ADLs). Demonstrates a decrease in physiologic signs of intolerance, e.g., pulse, respirations, and BP remain within patient's normal range.

ACTIONS/INTERVENTIONS

Independent

Assess patient's ability to perform normal tasks/ADLs, noting complaints of weakness, fatigue, difficulty accomplishing tasks.

Assess for loss of balance/gait disturbance, muscle weakness.

Monitor BP, pulse, respirations, during and following activity. Note adverse responses to increased levels of activity (e.g., increased heart rate, dysrhythmias, increased BP, dizziness, dyspnea, tachypnea, etc.).

Provide quiet atmosphere. Maintain bedrest if indicated. Monitor and limit visitors, phone calls, and repeated unplanned interruptions.

Change patient's position slowly and monitor for dizziness.

Prioritize nursing care schedules to enhance rest. Alternate rest periods with activity periods.

Provide assistance with activities/ambulation as necessary allowing patient to do as much as possible.

Plan activity progression with patient, including activities that the patient views as essential. Increase activity levels as tolerated.

Use energy-saving techniques, e.g., shower chair, sitting to perform tasks.

Instruct patient to stop activity if palpitations, chest pain, shortness of breath, weakness or dizziness occur.

RATIONALE

Influences choice of intervention/needed assistance.

May indicate neurologic changes associated with vitamin B_{12} deficiency affecting patient safety/risk of injury.

Cardiopulmonary manifestations result from additional attempts by the heart and lungs to bring adequate amounts of oxygen to the tissues.

Enhances rest to lower body's oxygen requirements and reduces strain on the heart and lungs.

Indicative of postural hypotension or cerebral hypoxia that may cause nausea/vomiting, risk of injury.

Maintains energy level and alleviates additional strain on the cardiac and respiratory systems.

While help may be necessary, self-esteem is enhanced when patient does some things for self.

Promotes gradual return to normal activity level improved muscle tone/stamina without undue fa Increases self-esteem and sense of control.

Encourages patient to do as much as possible conserving limited energy and preventing fati

Excessive cardiopulmonary strain/stress may decompensation/failure.

NURSING DIAGNOSIS:	NUTRITION, ALTERED: LESS THAN BODY REC MENTS
May be related to:	Failure to ingest or inability to digest food/absor ents necessary for formation of normal red blo
Possibly evidenced by:	Weight loss/weight below normal for age, height, build

Decreased triceps skinfold measurement

Changes in gums, oral mucous membranes

Decreased tolerance for activity, weakness, loss of muscle tone

PATIENT OUTCOMES/ EVALUATION CRITERIA:	**Demonstrates progressive weight gain or stable weight, with normalization of laboratory values, free of signs of malnutrition. Demonstrates behaviors, lifestyle changes to regain and/or maintain appropriate weight.**

ACTIONS/INTERVENTIONS

Independent

Assess nutritional history, including food preferences.

Observe and record patient's food intake.

Weigh daily.

Provide attractive, appetizing meals in a pleasant atmosphere.

Provide small, frequent meals and/or between-meal nourishments.

Observe and record occurrence of nausea/vomiting, flatus, and other related symptoms.

Provide and assist with good oral hygiene; before and after meals, using soft-bristled toothbrush, gentle brushing. Provide dilute mouthwash if oral mucosa is ulcerated.

Collaborative

Consult with dietician.

Monitor laboratory studies, e.g., Hb/Hct, BUN, albumin, protein, transferrin, serum iron, B_{12}), folic acid, TIBC, serum electrolytes.

Administer medications as indicated:

Vitamin and mineral supplements, e.g, cyanocobalamin (vitamin B_{12}), folic acid (Folvite), ascorbic acid (vitamin C);

Iron dextran (IM/IV);

Oral iron supplements, e.g., ferrous sulfate (Feosol), ferrous gluconate (Fergon);

Hydrochloric acid (HCl);

Nutritional supplements, e.g., Ensure, Isocal;

RATIONALE

Identifies deficiencies, suggests possible interventions.

Monitors caloric intake or insufficient quality of food consumption.

Monitors weight loss or effectiveness of nutritional interventions.

May promote appetite, desire to eat and enhance intake.

Eating small meals may reduce fatigue and thus enhance intake, while preventing gastric distension.

GI symptoms may reflect effects of anemias (hypoxia) on organs.

Enhances appetite and/oral intake and diminishes bacterial growth, minimizing possibility of infection. Special mouth-care techniques may be needed if tissue fragile/ulcerated/bleeding and pain is severe.

Aids in establishing dietary plan to meet individual needs.

Evaluates effectiveness of treatment regimen, including dietary sources of needed nutrients.

Replacements needed depend on type of anemia and/or presence of poor oral intake and identified deficiencies.

Administered until estimated deficit is corrected and is reserved for those who cannot absorb or comply with oral iron therapy, or when blood loss is too rapid for oral replacement to be effective.

May be useful in some types of iron deficiency anemias. (Refer to ND: Knowledge Deficit, p. 513.)

Potentiates absorption of vitamin B_{12} during initial weeks of therapy.

Provides additional protein and calories.

ACTIONS/INTERVENTIONS

Collaborative

Antifungal or anesthetic mouthwash if indicated.

Provide bland diet, low in roughage, avoiding hot, spicy or very acid foods as indicated.

RATIONALE

May be needed in the presence of stomatitis, glossitis to promote oral tissue healing and facilitate intake.

When oral lesions are present, pain may restrict type foods patient can tolerate.

NURSI[ ] IMPAIRED: POTENTIAL

Ma[ ] neurologic changes (anemia)

[ ]

Pos[ ] [pr]esence of signs and symptoms estab-[ ] [di]agnosis.]

PATIENT [ ] [i]ntegrity. Identifies individual risk
EVALUA[ ] [t]o prevent dermal injury.

ACT[ ]

Independent

Assess skin integrity, noting changes in turgor, altered color, local warmth, erythema, excoriation.

Reposition periodically and massage bony surfaces when patient is sedentary or in bed.

Keep sk[ ]

Assist w[ ]
cises.

Collab[ ]

Use prote[ ]
ternating [ ]
tectors, a[ ]

RATIONALE

Condition of the skin is affected by circulation, nutrition, and immobility. Tissues may become fragile and prone to infection and breakdown.

Increases circulation to all skin areas limiting tissue ischemia/effects of cellular hypoxia.

Moist, contaminated areas provide excellent media for growth of pathogenic organisms. Soap may dry skin excessively and increase irritation.

[P]romotes circulation; prevents stasis.

[A]voids skin breakdown by preventing/reducing pressure against skin surfaces.

NURS[ ] [ELIMI]NATION, ALTERED: CONSTIPATION/

M[ ] [dieta]ry intake; changes in digestive processes

Drug therapy side effects

Possibly evidenced by: Changes in frequency, characteristics, and amount of stool

Nausea/vomiting, decreased appetite

511

Complaints of abdominal pain, urgency, cramping

Altered bowel sounds

| PATIENT OUTCOMES/ EVALUATION CRITERIA: | Establishes/returns to normal patterns of bowel functioning. Demonstrates changes in lifestyle, as necessitated by causative, contributing factors. |

ACTIONS/INTERVENTIONS

Independent

Observe stool color, consistency, frequency, and amount.

Auscultate bowel sounds.

Monitor/record oral food/fluid intake and output.

Encourage fluid intake of 2500–3000 ml/day within cardiac tolerance.

Avoid foods that are gas forming.

Assess perianal skin condition frequently, noting changes in skin condition or beginning breakdown. Perform pericare after each BM if diarrhea is present.

Collaborative

Consult with dietician to provide well-balanced diet high in fiber and bulk.

Administer stool softeners, mild stimulants, bulk-forming laxatives, or enemas as indicated. Monitor effectiveness.

Administer antidiarrheal medications, e.g., diphenoxylate hydrochloride with atropine (Lomotil) and water-absorbing drugs, e.g., Metamucil.

RATIONALE

Assists in identifying causative/contributing factors and appropriate interventions.

Bowel sounds are generally increased in diarrhea and decreased in constipation.

May identify dehydration, excessive loss of fluids or aid in identifying dietary deficiencies.

Assists in improving stool consistency if constipated. Will help to maintain hydration status if diarrhea is present.

Decreases gastric distress and abdominal distention.

Prevents skin excoriation and breakdown.

Fiber resists enzymatic digestion and absorbs liquids in its passage along the intestinal tract and thereby produces bulk, which acts as a stimulant to defecation.

Facilitates defecation when constipation is present.

Decreases intestinal motility when diarrhea is present.

NURSING DIAGNOSIS:	INFECTION, POTENTIAL FOR
May be related to:	Inadequate secondary defenses, e.g., decreased hemoglobin, leukopenia, or decreased granulocytes (suppressed inflammatory response)
	Inadequate primary defenses, e.g., broken skin, stasis of body fluids; invasive procedures; chronic disease, malnutrition
Possibly evidenced by:	[Not applicable; presence of signs and symptoms establishes an *actual* diagnosis.]

Identifies behaviors to prevent/reduce risk of infection. Achieves timely wound healing, free of purulent drainage or erythema, and is afebrile.

ACTIONS/INTERVENTIONS	RATIONALE
Independent	
Promote good hand washing by health care givers and patient.	Prevents cross-contamination/colonization. Note: Patient with severe/aplastic anemia may be at risk from normal skin flora.
Maintain strict aseptic techniques with procedures/wound care.	Reduces risk of bacterial colonization/infection.
Provide meticulous skin, oral, and perianal care.	Reduces risk of skin/tissue breakdown and infection.
Encourage frequent position changes/ambulation, coughing, and deep breathing exercises.	Promotes ventilation of all lung segments and aids in mobilizing secretions to prevent pneumonia.
Promote adequate fluid intake.	Assists in liquefying respiratory secretions to facilitate expectoration, and prevent stasis of body fluids (e.g., respiratory and renal).
Monitor/limit visitors. Provide isolation if appropriate. Restrict live plants/cut flowers.	Limits exposure to bacteria/infections. Protective isolation may be required in aplastic anemia, when immune response is most compromised.
Monitor temperature. Note presence of chills, tachycardia.	Reflective of inflammatory process/infection requiring treatment.
Observe for wound erythema/drainage.	Indicators of local infection. Note: Pus formation may be absent if granulocytes are depressed.
Collaborative	
Obtain specimens for culture/sensitivity as indicated.	Verifies presence of infection, identifies specific pathogen and influences choice of treatment.
Administer topical antiseptics; systemic antibiotics.	May be used prophylactically to reduce colonization or used to treat specific infectious process.

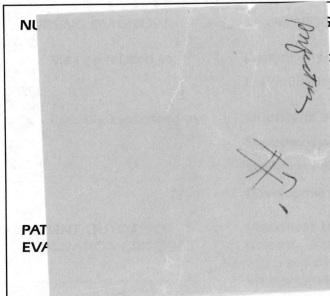

NU... ...GE DEFICIT [LEARNING NEED] (SPECIFY)

...osure/recall; information misinterpretation

...y with information resources

...equest for information

...f misconception

...llow-through of instruction

... of preventable complications

PAT... ...derstanding of the nature of the disease
EV... ...nostic procedures, treatment plan. Identi-
...e factors. Initiates necessary behaviors/
...ges.

ACTIONS/INTERVENTIONS	RATIONALE
Independent	
Provide information about specific anemia. Discuss the fact that therapy depends on the type and severity of the anemia.	Provides knowledge base upon which patient can make informed choices. Allays anxiety and may promote cooperation with therapeutic regimen.
Review purpose and preparations for diagnostic studies.	Anxiety/fear of the unknown increases stress level, which in turn increases the cardiac workload. Knowledge of what to expect can diminish anxiety.
Explain that blood taken for laboratory studies will not worsen anemia.	This is often an unspoken concern that can potentiate patient's anxiety.
Review required diet alterations to meet specific dietary needs (determined by type of anemia/deficiency).	Red meat, liver, egg yolks, green leafy vegetables, whole wheat bread, and dried fruits are sources of iron. Green vegetables, whole grains, liver and citrus fruits are sources of folic acid and vitamin C (enhances absorption of iron).
Assess resources (financial and cooking).	Inadequate resources may affect ability to purchase/prepare appropriate food items.
Encourage cessation of smoking.	Decreases available oxygen and causes vasoconstriction.
Instruct and demonstrate self-administration of oral iron preparations:	Iron replacement is usually 3–6 months, whereas vitamin B_{12} injections may be necessary for the rest of the patient's life.
Discuss importance of taking only prescribed dosages;	Overdose of iron medication can be toxic.
Advise taking with meals or immediately following meals;	Iron is best absorbed on an empty stomach. However, iron salts are gastric irritants and may cause dyspepsia, diarrhea, and abdominal discomfort if taken on an empty stomach.
Dilute liquid preparations (preferably with orange juice) and administer through a straw;	Undiluted liquid iron preparations may stain the teeth. Ascorbic acid promotes iron absorption.
Caution that BM may appear greenish black/tarry;	Excretion of excessive iron will change stool color.
Stress importance of good oral hygiene measures.	Certain iron supplements (e.g., Feosol) may leave deposits on teeth and gums.
Instruct patient/SO about parenteral iron administration:	
Z track administration of medication;	Prevents extravasation (leaking) with accompanying pain.
Use separate needles for withdrawing and injecting the medication;	Medication may stain the skin.
Caution regarding possible systemic reaction, (e.g., flushing, vomiting, nausea, myalgia) and discuss importance of reporting symptoms.	Possible side effects of therapy requiring reevaluation of drug and dosage.
Discuss increased susceptibility to infections, signs/symptoms requiring medical intervention, e.g., fever, sore throat; erythema/draining wound; cloudy urine, burning with urination.	Decreased leukocyte production potentiates risk of infection. Note: purulent drainage may not form in absence of granulocytes (aplastic anemia).
Identify safety concerns, e.g., avoidance of forceful blowing of nose, contact sports, constipation/straining for stool; use of electric razors, soft toothbrush.	Reduces risk of hemorrhage from fragile tissues.

514

ACTIONS/INTERVENTIONS	RATIONALE

Independent

Review good oral hygiene, necessity for regular dental care.

Instruct to avoid use of aspirin products.

Collaborative

Refer to appropriate community resources when indicated, e.g., Social Services for food stamps, Meals-on-Wheels.

Effects of anemia (oral lesions) and/or iron supplements increase risk of infection/bacteremia.

Increases bleeding tendencies.

May need assistance with groceries/meal preparation.

Sickle Cell Crisis

Vasoocclusive/thrombocytic crisis: Related to infection, dehydration, fever, hypoxia, and characterized by multiple infarcts of bones, joints, and other target organs, with tissue pain and necrosis caused by plugs of sickled cells in the microcirculation.

Hypoplastic/aplastic crisis: May be secondary to severe (usually viral) infection or folic acid deficiency, resulting in cessation of production of red blood cells, bone marrow.

Hyperhemolytic crisis: Reticulocytes increased in peripheral blood; bone marrow hyperplastic. Characterized by anemia and jaundice (effects of hemolysis).

Sequestration crisis: Massive, sudden erythrostasis with pooling of blood in the viscera (splenomegaly), resulting in hypovolemic shock/possible death. This crisis occurs in patients with intact splenic function.

PATIENT ASSESSMENT DATA BASE

ACTIVITY/REST

May report: Lethargy, fatigue, weakness, general malaise.

Loss of productivity; decreased exercise tolerance; greater need for sleep and rest.

May exhibit: Listlessness; severe weakness and increasing pallor (aplastic crisis).

Gait disturbances (pain, kyphosis, lordosis); inability to walk (pain).

Poor body posture (slumping of shoulders indicative of fatigue).

Decreased ROM (swollen, inflamed joints); joint, bone deformities.

Generalized retarded growth; tower-shaped skull with frontal bossing; disproportionately long arms and legs, short trunk, narrowed shoulders/hips, and long, tapered fingers.

CIRCULATION

May report: Palpitations or anginal chest pain (concomitant coronary artery disease/myocardial ischemia).

Intermittent claudication.

May exhibit: Apical pulse: PMI may be displaced to the left (cardiomegaly).

Tachycardia, dysrhythmias (hypoxia), systolic murmurs.

Blood pressure: widened pulse pressure.

Generalized symptoms of shock, e.g., hypotension, rapid thready pulse, and shallow respirations (sequestration crisis).

Peripheral pulses: throbbing upon palpation.

Bruits (compensatory mechanisms of anemia; may also be auscultated over the spleen due to multiple splenic infarcts).

Capillary refill delayed (anemia or hypovolemia).

Skin color: pallor or cyanosis of skin, mucous membranes and conjunctiva. Note: Pallor may appear as yellowish brown color in brown-skinned patients, and as ashen gray in black-skinned patients. Jaundice: scleral icterus, generalized icteric coloring (excessive RBC hemolysis).

Dry skin/mucous membranes.

Diaphoresis (either sequestration or vasoocclusive crisis; acute pain or shock).

ELIMINATION

May report: Frequent voiding, voiding in large amounts, nocturia.

May exhibit: RUQ tenderness, enlargement/distention (hepatomegaly); ascites.

LUQ fullness (enlarged spleen, or may be atrophic and nonfunctional in adults from repeated splenic infarcts and fibrosis).

Dilute, pale, straw-colored urine; hematuria or a smoky appearance (multiple renal infarcts).

Urine specific gravity decreased (may be fixed with progressive renal disease).

EGO INTEGRITY

May report: Resentment and frustration with disease, fear of rejection from others.

Generalized poor self-esteem/poor self-concept.

Concern regarding being a burden to SOs; financial concerns, possible loss of insurance/benefits; lost time at work/school, fear of genetic transmission of disease.

May exhibit: Anxiety, restlessness, irritability, apprehension, withdrawal, narrowed focus, self-focusing, unresponsive to questions, regression; depression, decreased self-esteem.

Dependent relationship with whoever can offer security and protection.

FOOD/FLUID

May report: Thirst.

Anorexia, nausea/vomiting.

May exhibit: Height/weight usually in the lower percentiles.

Poor skin turgor with visible tenting (crisis, infection, and dehydration).

Dry skin, mucous membranes.

JVD and general peripheral edema (concomitant CHF).

HYGIENE

May report: Difficulty maintaining ADL (pain or severe anemia).

May exhibit: Slovenly, unkempt appearance.

NEUROSENSORY

May report: Headaches or dizziness.

Transient visual disturbances (e.g., hymianopsia, nystagmus).

Tingling in the extremities.

Disturbances in pain and position sense.

May exhibit: Mental status: usually unaffected except in cases of severe sickling (cerebral infarction/intracranial hemorrhage).

Weakness of the mouth, tongue, and facial muscles; aphasia (in cerebral infarction when dominant hemisphere infarcted).

Abnormal reflexes, decreased muscle strength/tone; abnormal involuntary movements; hemiplegia or sudden hemiparesis, quadraplegia.

Ataxia, seizures.

Meningeal irritation (intracranial hemorrhage), e.g., decreasing level of consciousness, nuchal rigidity, focal neurologic deficits, vomiting, severe headache.

PAIN/COMFORT

May report: Pain as severe, throbbing, gnawing of varied location (localized, migratory, or generalized).

Recurrent, sharp, transient headaches.

Back pain (changes in vertebral column from recurrent infarctions); joint/bone pain accompanied by warmth, tenderness, erythema, and occasional effusions (vasoocclusive crisis). Note: Deep bone infarctions may have no apparent signs of irritation.

Gallbladder tenderness and pain (excessive accumulation of bilirubin due to increased erythrocyte destruction).

517

May exhibit:	Sensitivity to palpation over affected areas.
	Holding joints in position of comfort; decreased range of motion (result of pain and swollen joints).
	Maladaptive pain relief behavior, e.g., guilt for being ill, denial of any aspect of disease, indulgence in precipitating factors (overwork, overstrenuous exercise).

RESPIRATION

May report:	Dyspnea on exertion/or at rest.
	History of repeated pulmonary infections/or infarctions, pulmonary fibrosis, pulmonary hypertension or cor pulmonale.
May exhibit:	Acute respiratory distress, e.g., dyspnea, chest pain, and cyanosis (especially in crisis).
	Bronchial/bronchovesicular sounds in lung periphery; diminished breath sounds (pulmonary fibrosis).
	Crackles, rhonchi, wheezes, diminished breath sounds (CHF).
	Increased AP diameter of the chest (barrel chest).

SAFETY

May report:	History of transfusions.
May exhibit:	Low-grade fever.
	Impaired vision (sickle retinopathy), decreased visual acuity (temporary/permanent blindness).
	Leg ulcers (common in adult patients, especially found on the internal and external malleoli and the medial aspect of the tibia).
	Lymphadenopathy.

SEXUALITY

May report:	Loss of libido; amenorrhea; priapism, impotence.
May exhibit:	Delayed sexual maturity.
	Pale cervix and vaginal walls (anemia).

TEACHING/LEARNING

May report:	History of CHF (chronic anemic state); pulmonary hypertension or cor pulmonale (multiple pulmonary infections/infarctions); chronic leg ulcers, delayed healing.
Discharge Plan Considerations:	May need assistance with shopping, transportation, self-care/homemaker tasks.

DIAGNOSTIC STUDIES

CBC: reticulocytosis (count may vary from 5% to 30%); leukocytosis (especially in vasoocclusive crisis), decreased Hb/Hct/total red blood cells, thrombocytosis, and a normal to decreased mean corpuscular volume (MCV).

Stained RBC examination: demonstrates partially or completely sickled, crescent-shaped cells, anisocytosis, poikilocytosis, polychronasia, target cells, Howell–Jolly bodies, basophilic stippling, occasional nucleated red cells (normoblasts).

Sickle-turbidity tube test (Sickledex): routine screening test that determines the presence of hemoglobin S (HbS) but does not differentiate between sickle cell anemia and trait.

Hemoglobin electrophoresis: identifies any abnormal hemoglobin types and differentiates between sickle cell trait and sickle cell anemia. May obtain inaccurate results if patient has received a blood transfusion 3–4 months prior to testing.

Erythrocyte sedimentation rate (ESR): elevated.

Erythrocyte fragility: decreased (osmotic fragility or red cell fragility). *RBC survival time:* decreased (accelerated breakdown).

ABGs: may reflect decreased PO_2 (defects in gas exchange at the alveolar capillary level); acidosis (hypoxemia and acidic states in vasoocclusive crisis).

Serum bilirubin (total and indirect): elevated (increased RBC hemolysis).

Acid phosphatase: elevated (release of erythrocytic ACP into the serum).

Alkaline phosphatase: elevated during vasoocclusive crisis (bone and liver damage).

Lactic dehydrogenase (LDH): elevated (RBC hemolysis).

Serum potassium and uric acid: elevated during vasoocclusive crisis (RBC hemolysis).

Serum iron: may be elevated or normal (increased iron absorption due to excessive RBC destruction).

Total iron binding capacity (TIBC): normal or decreased.

Urine/fecal urobilinogen: increased (more sensitive indicators of RBC destruction than serum levels).

IVP: may be done to evaluate kidney damage.

Bone radiographs: may demonstrate skeletal changes, e.g., osteoporosis, osteosclerosis, osteomyelitis, or avascular necrosis.

X-rays: may indicate bone thinning, osteoporosis.

NURSING PRIORITIES

1. Promote adequate cellular oxygenation/perfusion.
2. Alleviate pain.
3. Prevent complications.
4. Provide information about disease, process/prognosis, and treatment needs.

DISCHARGE CRITERIA

1. Oxygenation/perfusion adequate to meet cellular needs.
2. Pain relieved/controlled.
3. Complications prevented/minimized.
4. Disease process, future expectations, potential complications, and therapeutic regimen understood.

NURSING DIAGNOSIS:	**GAS EXCHANGE, IMPAIRED**
May be related to:	**Decreased oxygen-carrying capacity of the blood, reduced red blood cell (RBC) life span/premature destruction, abnormal red cell structure; sensitivity to low oxygen tension (strenuous exercise, increase in altitude)**
	Increased blood viscosity (occlusions created by sickled cells packing together within the capillaries) and pulmonary congestion (impairment of surface phagocytosis)
	Predisposition to bacterial pneumonia, pulmonary infarcts
Possibly evidenced by:	**Dyspnea, use of accessory muscles**
	Restlessness, confusion
	Tachycardia
	Cyanosis (hypoxia)
PATIENT OUTCOMES/	**Demonstrates improved ventilation and oxygenation as**

EVALUATION CRITERIA:	evidenced by respiratory rate within normal limits and absence of cyanosis and use of accessory muscles; normal breath sounds; able to participate in ADLs without weakness and fatigue; pulmonary function tests improved/normal.

ACTIONS/INTERVENTIONS

RATIONALE

Independent

Monitor respiratory rate/depth, use of accessory muscles, areas of cyanosis.

Indicators of adequacy of respiratory function or degree of compromise, and therapy needs/effectiveness.

Auscultate breath sounds, noting presence/absence, and adventitious sounds.

Development of atelectasis and stasis of secretions can impair gas exchange.

Monitor vital signs; note changes in cardiac rhythm.

Compensatory changes in vital signs and development of dysrhythmias reflect effects of hypoxia on cardiovascular system.

Assess complaints of chest pain and increasing fatigue. Observe for signs of increased fever, cough, adventitious breath sounds.

Reflective of developing respiratory infection which increases the workload of the heart and oxygen demand.

Assist in turning, coughing, and deep breathing.

Promotes optimum chest expansion, mobilization of secretions, and aeration of all lung fields; reduces risk of stasis of secretions/pneumonia.

Assess level of consciousness/mentation regularly.

Brain tissue is very sensitive to decreases in oxygen and may be an early indicator of developing hypoxia.

Assess activity tolerance; limit activities to within patient tolerance or place patient on bedrest. Assist with ADLs and mobility as needed.

Reduction of the metabolic requirements of the body reduces the oxygen requirements/degree of hypoxia.

Encourage patient to alternate periods of rest and activity. Schedule rest periods as indicated.

Protects from overfatigue, reduces oxygen demands/degree of hypoxia.

Demonstrate and encourage use of relaxation techniques, e.g., guided imagery and visualization.

Relaxation decreases muscle tension and anxiety and hence the metabolic demand for oxygen.

Promote adequate fluid intake, e.g., 2–3 liters/day within cardiac tolerance.

Sufficient intake is necessary to provide for mobilization of secretions and to prevent hyperviscosity of blood/capillary occlusion.

Screen visitors/staff.

Protects from potential sources of respiratory infection.

Collaborative

Administer supplemental humidified oxygen as indicated.

Maximizes oxygen transport to tissues, particularly in presence of pulmonary insults/pneumonia.

Monitor laboratory studies, e.g., CBC, cultures, ABGs/ear oximetry, chest x-ray, pulmonary function tests.

Patients are particularly prone to pneumonia, which is potentially fatal due to its hypoxemic effect of increasing sickling.

Perform/assist with chest physiotherapy, IPPB, and incentive spirometer.

Done to mobilize secretions and increase aeration of lung fields.

Administer packed RBCs or exchange transfusions as indicated.

Increases number of oxygen carrying cells, dilutes the percentage of HbS (to prevent sickling), improves circulation, and dislodges sickled cells. Packed RBCs are usually used because they are less likely to create circulatory overload. Note: Partial transfusions are sometimes used prophylactically in high-risk individuals, e.g., chronic, severe leg ulcers, preparation for general anesthesia, third trimester of pregnancy.

ACTIONS/INTERVENTIONS

Collaborative

Administer medications as indicated:

Antipyretics, e.g., acetaminophen (Tylenol);

Antibiotics.

RATIONALE

Maintains normothermia to reduce metabolic oxygen demands without affecting serum pH, which may occur with aspirin.

A broad spectrum antibiotic is started immediately pending culture results of suspected infections, then may be changed when the specific pathogen is identified.

NURSING DIAGNOSIS:	TISSUE PERFUSION, ALTERED: DECREASED
May be related to:	Vasoocclusive nature of sickling, inflammatory response
	AV shunts in both pulmonary and peripheral circulation
	Myocardial damage from small infarcts, iron deposits and fibrosis
Possibly evidenced by:	Changes in vital signs; diminished peripheral pulses/capillary refill; general pallor
	Decreased mentation, restlessness
	Angina, palpitations
	Tingling in extremities, intermittent claudication, bone pain
	Transient visual disturbances
	Ulcerations of lower extremities, delayed healing
PATIENT OUTCOMES/ EVALUATION CRITERIA:	Demonstrates improved tissue perfusion as evidenced by stabilized vital signs, strong/palpable peripheral pulses, adequate urine output, absence of pain; alert and oriented; normal capillary refill; skin warm/dry; nailbeds, lips and ear lobes are natural pale, pink color; absence of paresthesias.

ACTIONS/INTERVENTIONS

Independent

Monitor vital signs carefully. Assess pulses for rate, rhythm and volume. Note hypotension; rapid, weak, thready pulse; and increased/shallow respirations.

Assess skin for coolness, pallor, cyanosis, diaphoresis, delayed capillary refill.

Note changes in level of consciousness; complaints of headaches, dizziness; development of sensory/motor

RATIONALE

Sludging and sickling in peripheral vessels may lead to complete or partial obliteration of a vessel with diminished perfusion to surrounding tissues. Sudden massive splenic sequestration of cells can lead to shock.

Changes reflect diminished circulation/hypoxia potentiating capillary occlusion. (Refer to ND: Gas Exchange, Impaired, p. 519.)

Changes may reflect diminished perfusion to the central nervous system due to ischemia or infarction.

ACTIONS/INTERVENTIONS	RATIONALE

Independent

deficits, (e.g., hemiparesis or paralysis) seizures.

Stagnant cells must be mobilized immediately to reduce further ischemia/infarction. (Refer to CPs: Cerebrovascular Accident/Stroke, p. 243; Seizure Disorders, p. 218.)

Maintain adequate fluid intake. (Refer to ND: Fluid Volume. Deficit, Potential, p. 523.) Monitor urine output.

Dehydration not only causes hypovolemia but increases sickling and occlusion of capillaries. Decreased renal perfusion/failure may occur due to vascular occlusion.

Assess lower extremities for skin texture, edema, ulcerations (especially of internal and external malleoli).

Reduced peripheral circulation often leads to dermal changes and delayed healing.

Investigate complaints of change in character of pain, or development of bone pain, angina, tingling of extremities, eye pain/vision disturbances.

Changes may reflect increased sickling of cells/diminished circulation with further involvement of organs, e.g., MI or pulmonary infarction, occlusion of vasculature of the eye.

Maintain environmental temperature and body warmth.

Prevents vasoconstriction, aids in maintaining circulation and perfusion.

Evaluate for developing edema (including genitals in males).

Vasoocclusion/circulatory stasis may lead to edema of extremities (and priapism in males) potentiating risk of tissue ischemia/necrosis.

Collaborative

Monitor laboratory studies, e.g.:

ABGs, CBC, LDH, SGOT (AST)/SGPT (ASL), CPK, BUN;

Decreased tissue perfusion may lead to gradual infarction of organ tissues such as the brain, liver, spleen, kidney, skeletal muscle, etc., with consequent release of intracellular enzymes.

Serum electrolytes. Provide replacements as indicated.

Electrolyte losses (especially sodium) are increased during crisis because of fever, diarrhea, vomiting, diaphoresis.

Administer hypo-osmolar solutions (e.g., 0.45 NS) via an infusion pump.

Hydration lowers the HbS concentration within the RBC which decreases the sickling tendency, and also reduces blood viscosity which helps to maintain perfusion. Infusion pump may prevent circulatory overload. Note: D5W or LR may cause RBC hemolysis and potentiate thrombus formation.

Administer experimental antisickling agents (e.g., sodium cyanate) carefully, observing for possible lethal side effects.

Antisickling agents (currently under investigational use) are aimed at prolonging erythrocyte survival and preventing sickling by effecting cell membrane changes. Note: Use of anticoagulants, plasma expanders, nitrates, vasodilators, and alkylating agents have proven essentially unsuccessful in the management of the vasoocclusive crisis.

Assist with/prepare for surgical diathermy or photocoagulation.

Direct coagulation of bleeding sites in the eye (resulting from vascular stasis/edema) may prevent progression of proliferative changes if initiated early.

Assist/prepare for needle aspiration of blood from corpora cavernosa;

Sickling within the penis can cause sustained erection (priapism) and edema. Removal of sludged sickled cells can improve circulation, decreasing psychologic trauma and risk of necrosis/infection.

Surgical intervention.

Direct incision and ligation of the dorsal arteries of the penis and saphenocavernous shunting may be necessary in severe cases of priapism to prevent tissue necrosis.

522

NURSING DIAGNOSIS:	FLUID VOLUME DEFICIT, POTENTIAL
May be related to:	Increased fluid needs, e.g., hypermetabolic state/fever, inflammatory processes
	Renal parenchymal damage/infarctions limiting the kidneys' ability to concentrate urine (hyposthenuria)
Possibly evidenced by:	[Not applicable; presence of signs and symptoms establishes an *actual* diagnosis.]
PATIENT OUTCOMES/ EVALUATION CRITERIA:	Maintains adequate fluid balance as evidenced by individually appropriate urine output with a near normal specific gravity, stable vital signs, moist mucous membranes, good skin turgor, and prompt capillary refill.

ACTIONS/INTERVENTIONS	RATIONALE
Independent	
Maintain accurate I&O. Weigh daily.	Patient may reduce fluid intake during periods of crisis because of malaise, anorexia, etc. Dehydration from vomiting, diarrhea, fever, may reduce urine output and precipitate a vasoocclusive crisis.
Note urine characteristics and specific gravity.	Kidney can lose its ability to concentrate urine, resulting in excessive losses of dilute urine.
Monitor vital signs, comparing with patient's normal/ previous readings. Take BP in lying, sitting, standing positions if possible.	Reduction of circulating blood volume can occur from increased fluid loss resulting in hypotension and tachycardia.
Observe for fever, changes in level of consciousness, poor skin turgor, dryness of skin and mucous membranes, pain.	Symptoms reflective of dehydration/hemoconcentration with consequent vasoocclusive state.
Monitor vital signs closely during blood transfusions and note presence of dyspnea, crackles, rhonchi, wheezes, JVD, diminished breath sounds, cough, frothy sputum, and cyanosis.	Patient's heart may already be weakened and prone to failure due to chronic demands placed on it by the anemic state. Heart may be unable to tolerate the added fluid volume from transfusions or rapid IV fluid administered to treat crisis/shock.
Collaborative	
Administer fluids as indicated.	Replaces losses/deficits; may reverse renal concentration of red blood cells/presence of failure. Fluids must be given immediately (especially in CNS involvement) to decrease hemoconcentration and prevent further infarction.
Monitor laboratory studies, e.g., Hb/Hct, serum and urine electrolytes.	Elevations may indicate hemoconcentration. Kidneys' loss of ability to concentrate urine may result in serum depletions of Na^+K^+, and Cl^-.

NURSING DIAGNOSIS:	COMFORT, ALTERED: PAIN, ACUTE/CHRONIC
May be related to:	Intravascular sickling with localized stasis, occlusion, and infarction/necrosis

523

	Activation of pain fibers due to deprivation of oxygen and nutrients, accumulation of noxious metabolites
Possibly evidenced by:	Localized, migratory, or more generalized pain, described as throbbing, gnawing, or severe and incapacitating, affecting peripheral extremities; bones, joints, back; abdomen; or head (headaches recurrent/transient)
	Decreased ROM, guarding of the affected areas
	Facial grimacing, narrowed/self-focus
PATIENT OUTCOMES/ EVALUATION CRITERIA:	Verbalizes relief/control of pain. Demonstrates relaxed body posture, has freedom of movement, able to sleep/ rest appropriately.

ACTIONS/INTERVENTIONS

Independent

Assess complaints of pain, including location, duration, and intensity (scale of 1–10).

Observe nonverbal pain cues, e.g., gait disturbances, body positioning, reluctance to move, facial expressions, and physiologic manifestations of pain (e.g., elevated BP, tachycardia, increased respiratory rate). Explore discrepancies between verbal and nonverbal cues.

Discuss with the patient/SO what pain relief measures were effective in the past.

Explore alternate pain relief measures, e.g., relaxation techniques, biofeedback, yoga, meditation, progressive relaxation techniques, distraction (e.g., visual/ auditory, tactile kinesthetic, guided imagery, and breathing techniques).

Provide support for and carefully position affected extremities.

Apply local massage gently to affected areas.

Encourage ROM exercises.

Plan activities during peak analgesic effects.

Maintain adequate fluid intake.

Collaborative

Apply warm, moist compresses to affected joints or other painful areas. Avoid use of ice or cold compresses.

Administer medications as indicated: narcotics, e.g., meperidine (Demerol), morphine; nonnarcotic analgesics, e.g., acetaminophen (Tylenol) or sedatives, e.g., hydroxyzine (Vistaril).

RATIONALE

Sickling of cells potentiates cellular hypoxia and may lead to infarction of tissue/resultant pain.

Pain is very unique to each patient; therefore, one may encounter varying descriptions due to individualized perceptions. Nonverbal cues may aid in evaluation of pain and effectiveness of therapy.

Involves patient/SO in care and allows for identification of remedies that have already been found to relieve pain. Helpful in establishing individualized treatment needs.

May reduce reliance on pharmacologic therapy and enhances patient's sense of control.

Reduces edema, discomfort, and risk of injury, especially if osteomyelitis is present.

Helps to reduce muscle tension.

Prevents joint stiffness and possible contracture formation.

Maximizes movement of joints, enhancing mobility.

Dehydration increases sickling/vasoocclusion and corresponding pain.

Warmth causes vasodilation and increases circulation to hypoxic areas. Cold causes vasoconstriction and compounds the crisis.

Reduces pain and promotes rest and comfort. Note: Tylenol can be used for control of headache, pain, and fever. Aspirin should be avoided because it alters blood pH and can make cells sickle more easily.

ACTIONS/INTERVENTIONS

Collaborative

Administer/monitor RBC transfusion.

RATIONALE

Frequency of painful crisis may be reduced by partial exchange transfusion to maintain population of normal RBCs.

NURSING DIAGNOSIS:	MOBILITY, IMPAIRED PHYSICAL
May be related to:	Multiple/recurrent bone infarctions or infections (weight-bearing bones)
	Pain/discomfort: kyphosis of upper back/lordosis of lower back, possible joint effusions
	Osteoporosis with fragmentation/collapse of femoral head or vertebra (compression deformities)
	Bacterial infections (osteomyelitis)
Possibly evidenced by:	Complaints of pain
	Limited joint ROM, reluctance to move, inability to walk/perform ADLs, guarding of joints, gait disturbances
	Generalized weakness, therapeutic restrictions (e.g., bedrest)
PATIENT OUTCOMES/ EVALUATION CRITERIA:	Able to assume ADLs and participate in activities with absence of/or improvement in gait disturbances, increased joint ROM, and absence of inflammatory signs.

ACTIONS/INTERVENTIONS

Independent

(Refer to CP: Long-Term Care, ND: Mobility, Impaired Physical, p. 820.)

RATIONALE

NURSING DIAGNOSIS:	SKIN INTEGRITY, IMPAIRED: POTENTIAL
May be related to:	Impaired circulation (venous stasis and vasoocclusion); altered sensation
	Decreased mobility/bedrest
Possibly evidenced by:	[Not applicable; presence of signs and symptoms establishes an *actual* diagnosis.]
PATIENT OUTCOMES/ EVALUATION CRITERIA:	Prevents dermal ischemia injury. Participates in behaviors to reduce risk factors/skin breakdown. Observed improvement in wound/lesion healing if present.

ACTIONS/INTERVENTIONS	RATIONALE
Independent	
Reposition frequently, even when sitting in chair.	Prevents prolonged tissue pressure where circulation is already compromised, reducing risk of tissue trauma/ischemia.
Inspect skin/pressure points regularly for redness, provide gentle massage.	Poor circulation may predispose to rapid skin breakdown.
Protect bony prominences with sheepskin, heel/elbow protectors, pillows, as indicated.	Decreases pressure on tissues, preventing skin breakdown.
Keep skin surfaces dry and clean; linens dry/wrinkle-free.	Moist, contaminated areas provide excellent media for growth of pathogenic organisms.
Monitor leg bruises, cuts, bumps, etc., closely for ulcer formation.	Potential entry sites for pathogenic organisms in presence of altered immune system increases risk of infection/delayed healing.
Elevate lower extremities when sitting.	Enhances venous return reducing venous stasis/edema formation.
Collaborative	
Provide egg-crate, alternating air pressure or water mattresses.	Reduces tissue pressure and aids in maximizing cellular perfusion to prevent dermal injury.
Monitor status of ischemic areas, ulcer. Note distribution, size, depth, character and drainage. Cleanse with H_2O_2, boric acid, or betadine solutions as indicated.	Improvement or delayed healing reflects adequacy of tissue perfusion and effectiveness of interventions. Note: These patients are at increased risk of serious complications because of lowered resistance to infection, and decreased nutrients for healing.
Prepare for/assist with hyperbaric oxygenation to ulcer sites.	Maximizes oxygen delivery to tissues enhancing healing.

NURSING DIAGNOSIS:	**INFECTION, POTENTIAL FOR**
May be related to:	Chronic disease process, tissue destruction, e.g., infarction, fibrosis, loss of spleen (autosplenectomy)
	Inadequate primary defenses (broken skin, stasis of body fluids, decreased ciliary action)
Possibly evidenced by:	[Not applicable; presence of signs and symptoms establishes an *actual* diagnosis.]
PATIENT OUTCOMES/ EVALUATION CRITERIA:	Verbalizes understanding of individual causative/risk factors. Identifies interventions to prevent/reduce risk of infection.

Refer to CPs: Bacterial Pneumonia, p. 138; Sepsis/Septicemia, p. 763; Fractures, ND: Infection, Potential for, p. 693.

NURSING DIAGNOSIS:	**KNOWLEDGE DEFICIT [LEARNING NEED] (SPECIFY)**
May be related to:	Lack of exposure/recall
	Information misinterpretation

	Unfamiliarity with resources
Possibly evidenced by:	**Questions; request for information**
	Statement of misconceptions
	Inaccurate follow-through of instructions; development of preventable complications
	Verbal/nonverbal cues of anxiety
PATIENT OUTCOMES/ EVALUATION CRITERIA:	**Verbalizes understanding of disease process, including symptoms of crisis. Initiates necessary behaviors/ lifestyle changes to prevent complications. Identifies need for continued medical follow-up; genetic counseling/family planning services.**

ACTIONS/INTERVENTIONS	RATIONALE
Independent	
Review disease process, and treatment needs.	Provides knowledge base on which patient can make informed choices.
Assess patient's knowledge of precipitating factors, e.g.:	
Travel to places over 7000 feet above sea level or flying in unpressurized aircraft;	Decreased oxygen tension present at higher altitudes causes hypoxia and potentiates sickling of cells.
Strenuous physical activity/or contact type sports, and extremely warm temperatures;	Increases metabolic demand for oxygen and increases insensible fluid losses (evaporation and perspiration), which may increase blood viscosity and tendency to sickle.
Cold environmental temperatures, failure to dress warmly when engaging in winter activities; wearing tight, restrictive clothing; stressful situations.	Causes peripheral vasoconstriction, which may result in sludging of the circulation, increased sickling and may precipitate a vasoocclusive crisis.
Encourage consumption of at least 4–6 quarts of fluid daily, during a steady state of the disease. Increase the amount to 6–8 quarts during a painful crisis or while engaging in activities that might precipitate dehydration.	Prevents dehydration and consequent hyperviscosity that can potentiate sickling/crisis.
Encourage ROM exercise and regular physical activity with a balance between rest and activity.	Prevents bone demineralization and may reduce risk of fractures. Aids in maintaining level of resistance and decreases oxygen needs.
Review patient's current diet, reinforcing the importance of diet including liver, green leafy vegetables, citrus fruits, and wheat germ. Provide necessary instruction regarding supplementary vitamins such as folic acid.	Sound nutrition is essential because of increased demands placed on bone marrow (e.g., folate and vitamin B_{12} are used in greater quantities than usual), and folic acid supplements are frequently ordered to prevent aplastic crisis.
Discourage smoking and alcohol consumption; identify community support groups.	Nicotine induces peripheral vasoconstriction and decreases oxygen tension, which may contribute to cellular hypoxia and sickling. Alcohol increases the possibility of dehydration (precipitating sickling). Maintaining these changes in behavior/lifestyle may require prolonged support.
Discuss principles of skin/extremity care and protection from injury. Encourage prompt treatment of cuts, insect bites, sores.	Due to impaired tissue perfusion, especially in the periphery, distal extremities are especially susceptible to altered skin integrity/infection.

527

ACTIONS/INTERVENTIONS	RATIONALE

Independent

Include instructions on care of any leg ulcers which might develop.	Fosters independence and maintenance of self-care at home.
Instruct patient to avoid persons with infections such as URI.	Altered immune response places patient at risk for infections, especially bacterial pneumonia.
Recommend patient avoid cold remedies and decongestants containing ephedrine. Stress the importance of reading labels on OTC drugs and consulting health care provider prior to consuming any drugs.	Those remedies containing vasoconstrictors may decrease peripheral tissue perfusion and cause sludging of sickled cells.
Discuss conditions for which medical attention should be sought, e.g.:	
Urine that appears blood tinged or smoky;	Symptoms suggestive of sickling in the renal medulla.
Indigestion, persistent vomiting, diarrhea, high fever, excessive thirst;	Dehydration may trigger a vasoocclusive crisis.
Severe joint or bone pain;	May signify a vasoocclusive crisis due to sickling in the bones or spleen (ischemia or infarction) or onset of osteomyelitis.
Severe chest pain, with or without cough;	May reflect angina, impending MI, or pneumonia.
Abdominal pain; gastric distress following meals;	High incidence of gallbladder disease/stone formation.
Fever, swelling, redness, increasing fatigue/pallor, leg ulcers, dizziness, drowsiness.	Suggestive of infections which may precipitate a vasoocclusive crisis if dehydration develops. Note: Severe infections are the most frequent cause of aplastic crisis.
Assist patient to strengthen coping abilities, e.g., deal appropriately with anxiety, get adequate information, use relaxation techniques.	Promotes patient's sense of control, may avert a crisis.
Suggest wearing a medical alert bracelet or carrying a card.	May prevent inappropriate treatment in emergency situation.
Discuss genetic implications of the disease. Encourage SO/family members to seek testing to determine presence of HbS.	Hereditary nature of the disease with the possibility of transmitting the mutation may have a bearing on the decision to have children.
Explore concerns regarding childbearing/family planning and refer to community resources as indicated.	Provides opportunity to correct misconceptions/present information necessary to make informed decisions. Pregnancy can precipitate a vasoocclusive crisis because the placenta's tortuous blood supply and low oxygen tension potentiates sickling, which in turn can lead to fetal hypoxia.
Encourage patient to have routine follow-ups, e.g.:	
Periodic laboratory studies, e.g., CBC;	Monitors changes in blood components, identifies need for changes in treatment regimen.
Biannual dental examination;	Sound oral hygiene limits opportunity for bacterial invasion/sepsis.
Annual ophthalmologic examination.	May develop sickle retinopathy with either proliferative or nonproliferative ocular changes.
Determine need for vocational/career guidance.	Sedentary career may be necessary because of the decreased oxygen-carrying capacity and diminished exercise tolerance.

ACTIONS/INTERVENTIONS	RATIONALE

Independent

Encourage participation in community support groups available to sickle cell patients/SO, such as The National Association for Sickle Cell Anemia, March of Dimes, Public Health/VNA nurse.

Helpful in adjustment to long-term situation, reduces feelings of isolation and enhances problem solving through sharing of common experiences. Note: Failure to resolve concerns/deal with situation may require more intensive therapy/psychologic support. (Refer to CP: Psychosocial Aspects of Acute Care, p. 773.)

Leukemias

The leukemias are a malignant disorder of the blood-forming organs of the body (spleen, lymphatic system, bone marrow). They are differentiated according to the leukocytic system that is involved. The common trait of all leukemias is the unregulated accumulation of a proliferation of white blood cells in the bone marrow that replaces the normal elements. There is an apparent lesion in the hematopoietic stem cell, which results in its inability to differentiate into normal cells. As the normal cells are replaced by leukemic cells, anemia, neutropenia, and thrombocytopenia occur.

PATIENT ASSESSMENT DATA BASE

The data are dependent on degree/duration of the disease and other organ involvement.

ACTIVITY/REST

May report:	Fatigue, malaise, weakness; inability to engage in usual activities.
May exhibit:	Muscle wasting.
	Increased need for sleep, rest, somnolence.

CIRCULATION

May report:	Palpitations.
May exhibit:	Tachycardia, heart murmurs.
	Pallor of skin, mucous membranes.
	Cranial nerve deficits and/or signs of cerebral hemorrhage.

ELIMINATION

May report:	Diarrhea; perianal tenderness, pain.
	Bright red blood on tissue paper, tarry stools.
	Blood in urine, decreased urine output.
May exhibit:	Perianal abscess; hematuria.

EGO INTEGRITY

May report:	Feelings of helplessness/hopelessness.
May exhibit:	Depression, withdrawal, anxiety, fear, anger, irritability.
	Mood changes, confusion.

FOOD/FLUID

May report:	Loss of appetite, anorexia, vomiting.
	Change in taste/taste distortions.
	Weight loss.
	Pharyngitis, dysphagia.
May exhibit:	Abdominal distention, decreased bowel sounds.
	Splenomegaly, hepatomegaly; jaundice.
	Stomatitis, oral ulcerations.
	Gum hypertrophy (gum infiltration may be indicative of acute monocytic leukemia).

NEUROSENSORY

May report:	Lack of coordination/decreased coordination.
	Mood changes, confusion, disorientation, lack of concentration.

Dizziness; numbness, tingling, paresthesias.

May exhibit: Muscle irritability, seizure activity.

PAIN/COMFORT

May report: Abdominal pain, headaches, bone/joint pain; sternal tenderness, muscle cramping.

May exhibit: Guarding/distraction behaviors, restlessness; self-focus.

RESPIRATION

May report: Dyspnea with minimal exertion.

May exhibit: Dyspnea, tachypnea.
Cough.
Crackles, rhonchi.
Decreased breath sounds.

SAFETY

May report: History of recent/recurrent infections; falls.
Visual disturbances/impairment.
Spontaneous uncontrollable bleeding with minimal trauma.

May exhibit: Fever.
Bruises, purpura, retinal hemorrhages, gum bleeding, or epistaxis.
Enlarged lymph nodes, spleen, or liver (due to tissue invasion).
Papilledema and exophthalmos.
Leukemic infiltrates in the dermis.

SEXUALITY

May report: Changes in libido.
Changes in menstrual flow, menorrhagia.
Impotence.

TEACHING/LEARNING

May report: History of exposure to chemicals, e.g., benzene, phenylbutazone, and chloramphenicol, or excessive levels of ionizing radiation.
Chromosomal disorder, e.g., Down's syndrome or Franconi's aplastic anemia.

Discharge Plan Considerations: May need assistance with therapy and treatment needs/supplies, shopping, food preparation, self-care/homemaker tasks, transportation.

DIAGNOSTIC STUDIES

CBC: indicates a normocytic, normochromic anemia. *Hemoglobin (Hb):* may be less than 10 g/100 ml. *Reticulocytes:* count is usually low. *Platelet count:* may be very low (<50,000/mm). *WBC:* may be more than 50,000/cm with increased immature WBC ("shift to left").

Prothrombin time/PTT: prolonged.

LDH: may be elevated.

Serum/urine uric acid: may be elevated.

Serum muramidase (a lysozyme): elevated in acute monocytic and myelomonocytic leukemias.

Serum copper: elevated.

Serum zinc: decreased.

Bone marrow biopsy: indicates 60–90% of the cells are blast cells, with erythroid precursors, mature cells, and megakaryocytes reduced.

Chest x-ray and lymph node biopsies: indicates degree of involvement.

NURSING PRIORITIES

1. Prevent infection during acute phases of disease/treatment.
2. Maintain circulating blood volume.
3. Alleviate pain.
4. Promote optimal physical functioning.
5. Provide psychologic support.
6. Provide information about disease process/prognosis and treatment needs.

DISCHARGE CRITERIA

1. Complications prevented/minimized.
2. Pain relieved/controlled.
3. Activities of daily living met by self or with assistance.
4. Dealing with disease realistically.
5. Disease process/prognosis and therapeutic regimen understood.

Refer to CP: Cancer, p. 872, for further discussion/expansion of interventions related to cancer care and for patient teaching.

NURSING DIAGNOSIS:	INFECTION, POTENTIAL FOR
May be related to:	**Inadequate secondary defenses: alterations in mature WBC (low granulocyte and abnormal lymphocyte count), increased number of immature lymphocytes; immunosuppression, bone marrow suppression (effects of therapy/transplant)**
	Inadequate primary defenses (stasis of body fluids, traumatized tissue)
	Invasive procedures
	Malnutrition; chronic disease
Possibly evidenced by:	**[Not applicable; presence of signs and symptoms establishes an *actual* diagnosis.]**
PATIENT OUTCOMES/ EVALUATION CRITERIA:	**Identifies actions to prevent/reduce risk of infection. Demonstrates techniques, lifestyle changes to promote safe environment, achieve timely healing.**

ACTIONS/INTERVENTIONS	RATIONALE
Independent	
Place in reverse isolation in private room. Screen/limit visitors as indicated. Restrict use of live plants/cut flowers.	Protects patient from potential sources of pathogens/infection.
Require good handwashing protocol for all personnel and visitors.	Prevents cross contamination/reduces risk of infection.

ACTIONS/INTERVENTIONS	RATIONALE

Independent

Monitor temperature. Note correlation between temperature elevations and chemotherapy treatments. Observe for fever associated with tachycardia, hypotension, subtle mental changes.

Progressive hyperthermia occurs in some types of infections, and fever (unrelated to drugs or blood products) occurs in most leukemia patients. Note: Septicemia may occur without fever.

Prevent chilling, force fluids. Administer tepid sponge bath.

Helps reduce fever, which contributes to fluid imbalance, discomfort, and CNS complications.

Encourage frequent turning; deep breathing, coughing.

Prevents stasis of respiratory secretions, reducing risk of atelectasis/pneumonia.

Auscultate breath sounds noting crackles, rhonchi; inspect secretions for changes in characteristics, e.g., increased sputum production or cloudy, foul-smelling urine with urgency or burning.

Early intervention is essential to prevent sepsis/septicemia in immunosuppressed person.

Handle patient carefully. Keep linens dry/wrinkle-free.

Prevents sheet burn/skin excoriation.

Inspect skin for tender, erythematous areas; open wounds. Cleanse skin with antibacterial solutions.

May indicate local infection. Note: Open wounds may not produce pus because of insufficient number of granulocytes.

Inspect oral mucous membranes. Provide good oral hygiene. Use a soft brush for frequent mouth care.

The oral cavity is an excellent medium for growth of organisms.

Promote good perianal hygiene. Provide sitz baths.

Promotes cleanliness, reducing risk of perianal abscess; enhances circulation and healing.

Provide uninterrupted rest periods.

Conserves energy for healing, cellular regeneration.

Avoid/limit invasive procedures (e.g., venipuncture and injections) if possible.

Break in skin could provide an entry for pathogenic/potentially lethal organisms.

Collaborative

Monitor laboratory studies, e.g.:

CBC, noting whether WBC falls or sudden changes occur in neutrophils;

Decreased numbers of normal/mature white blood cells can result from the disease process or chemotherapy, compromising the immune response and increasing risk of infection.

Gram stain cultures/sensitivity.

Verifies presence of infections, identifies specific organisms and appropriate therapy.

Review serial chest x-rays.

Indicator of development/resolution of respiratory complications.

Administer medications as indicated, e.g.:

Antibiotics;

May be given prophylactically or to treat specific infection.

Granulocyte transfusion.

May be given when WBC count is severely depleted (leukopenia) and patient has signs of infection or is unresponsive to antimicrobial therapy.

Avoid use of aspirin-containing antipyretics.

Aspirin can cause gastric bleeding.

Provide low-bacteria diet, e.g., cooked, processed foods.

Minimizes potential sources of bacterial contamination.

NURSING DIAGNOSIS:	FLUID VOLUME DEFICIT, POTENTIAL
May be related to:	Excessive losses, e.g., vomiting, hemorrhage, diarrhea

Decreased fluid intake: e.g., nausea, anorexia

Increased fluid need, e.g., hypermetabolic state, fever; predisposition for kidney stone formation

Possibly evidenced by: [Not applicable; presence of signs and symptoms establishes an *actual* diagnosis.]

PATIENT OUTCOMES/ EVALUATION CRITERIA: Demonstrates adequate fluid volume, as evidenced by stable vital signs; palpable pulses; urine output, specific gravity, and pH within normal limits. Identifies individual risk factors and appropriate interventions. Initiates behaviors/lifestyle changes to prevent development of fluid volume deficit.

ACTIONS/INTERVENTIONS	RATIONALE

Independent

Monitor intake/output. Calculate insensible losses and fluid balance. Note decreased urine in presence of adequate intake. Measure specific gravity and urine pH.

Decreased circulation secondary to destruction of RBCs and their precipitation in the kidney tubules and/ or development of kidney stones (related to elevated uric acid levels) may lead to urinary retention or renal failure.

Weigh daily.

Measure of adequacy of fluid replacement as well as kidney function. Continued intake greater than output may indicate renal insult/obstruction.

Monitor blood pressure and heart rate.

Changes may reflect effects of hypovolemia (bleeding/ dehydration).

Evaluate skin turgor, capillary refill and general condition of mucous membranes.

Indirect indicators of fluid status/hydration.

Note presence of nausea, fever, etc.

Affects intake, fluid needs and route of replacement.

Encourage fluids of up to 3–4 liters/day when oral intake is resumed.

Promotes urine flow, prevents uric acid precipitation and clearance of antineoplastic drugs.

Inspect skin/mucous membranes for petechiae, ecchymotic areas; note bleeding gums, frank or occult blood in stools and urine; oozing from invasive-line sites.

Suppression of bone marrow and platelet production places the patient at risk for spontaneous/uncontrolled bleeding.

Implement measures to prevent tissue injury/bleeding, e.g., gentle brushing of teeth or gums; avoiding sharp razors and forceful nose-blowing; sustained pressure on oozing puncture sites.

Fragile tissues and altered clotting mechanisms can result in hemorrhage following even minor trauma.

Limit oral care to mouthwash if indicated (a mixture of hydrogen peroxide and water may be preferred). Avoid mouth washes with alcohol.

When bleeding is present even gentle brushing may cause more tissue damage. Alcohol has a drying effect and may be painful to irritated tissues.

Provide soft diet.

May help reduce gum irritation.

Collaborative

Administer fluids as indicated.

Maintains fluid/electrolyte balance in the absence of oral intake, reduces risk of renal complications.

Monitor laboratory studies, e.g., platelets, Hb/Hct, clotting.

When the platelet count is less than 20,000/mm (proliferation of white blood cells and/or bone marrow suppression secondary to antineoplastic drugs), the pa-

ACTIONS/INTERVENTIONS

Collaborative

Administer RBCs, platelets, clotting factors.

Maintain external central vascular access device (Hickman/Broviac catheter).

Administer medications as indicated, e.g.:

Allopurinol (Zyloprim);

Potassium acetate or citrate, sodium bicarbonate;

Stool softeners.

RATIONALE

tient is prone to spontaneous life-threatening bleeding. Decreasing Hb/Hct is indicative of bleeding (may be occult).

Restores/normalizes red cell count and oxygen carrying capacity to correct anemia. Used to prevent/treat hemorrhage.

Eliminates peripheral venipuncture as source of infection and bleeding.

Although use is controversial, may be given to reduce the chances of nephropathy as a result of uric acid production.

May be used to alkalinize the urine preventing formation of kidney stones.

Helpful in reducing straining at stool with trauma to rectal tissues.

NURSING DIAGNOSIS:	COMFORT, ALTERED: PAIN, ACUTE
May be related to:	Physical agents, e.g., enlarged organs/lymph nodes, bone marrow packed with leukemic cells
	Chemical agents, e.g., antileukemic treatments
	Psychologic manifestations, e.g., anxiety, fear
Possibly evidenced by:	Complaints of pain (bone, nerve, headaches, etc.)
	Guarding/distraction behaviors, facial grimacing, alteration in muscle tone
	Autonomic responses
PATIENT OUTCOMES/ EVALUATION CRITERIA:	Reports pain is relieved/controlled. Demonstrates behaviors to manage pain.

ACTIONS/INTERVENTIONS

Independent

Investigate complaints of pain. Note changes in degree and site (use scale of 1–10).

Monitor vital signs, note nonverbal cues, e.g., muscle tension, restlessness.

Provide quiet environment and reduce stressful stimuli, e.g., noise, lighting, constant interruptions.

Place in position of comfort and support joints, extremities with pillows/padding.

Reposition periodically and provide/assist with gentle ROM exercises.

RATIONALE

Helpful in assessing need for intervention; may indicate developing complications.

May be useful in validating verbal comments and evaluating effectiveness of interventions.

Promotes rest and enhances coping abilities.

May decrease associated bone/joint discomfort.

Improves tissue circulation and joint mobility.

ACTIONS/INTERVENTIONS	RATIONALE

Independent

Provide routine comfort measures (e.g., massage, cool packs), and psychologic support (e.g., encouragement, presence).

Minimizes need for/enhances effects of medication.

Review/promote patient's own comfort interventions, position, physical activity/nonactivity, etc.

Successful management of pain requires patient involvement. Use of effective techniques provides positive reinforcement, promotes sense of control, and prepares patient for interventions to be used after discharge.

Evaluate and support patient's coping mechanisms.

Using own learned perceptions to manage pain can help the patient to cope more effectively.

Encourage use of stress management techniques, e.g., relaxation/deep breathing exercises, guided imagery, visualization; Therapeutic Touch.

Facilitates relaxation, augments pharmacologic therapy and enhances coping abilities.

Assist with/provide diversional, relaxation techniques.

Helps with pain management by redirecting attention.

Collaborative

Administer medications as indicated:

Analgesics, e.g., acetominaphen (Tylenol);

Given for mild pain not relieved by comfort measures. Note: Avoid aspirin-containing products as they may potentiate hemorrhage.

Narcotics, e.g., codeine, meperidine (Demerol); morphine; hydromorphone (Dilaudid);

Used when pain is severe. Use of patient-controlled analgesia (PCA) may be beneficial in preventing peaks and valleys of intermittent administration.

Tranquilizers, e.g., diazepam (Valium); lorazepam (Ativan).

May be given to enhance the action of analgesics/ narcotics.

NURSING DIAGNOSIS:	ACTIVITY INTOLERANCE
May be related to:	**Generalized weakness; reduced energy stores, increased metabolic rate from massive production of leukocytes**
	Imbalance between oxygen supply and demand (anemia/hypoxia)
	Therapeutic restrictions (isolation/bedrest)
Possibly evidenced by:	**Verbal report of fatigue or weakness**
	Exertional discomfort or dyspnea
	Abnormal heart rate or blood pressure response
PATIENT OUTCOMES/ EVALUATION CRITERIA:	**Reports a measurable increase in activity tolerance. Participates in ADLs to level of ability. Demonstrates a decrease in physiologic signs of intolerance; e.g., pulse, respiration, and blood pressure remain within patient's normal range.**

ACTIONS/INTERVENTIONS	RATIONALE

Independent

Evaluate complaints of fatigue, noting inability to participate in activities or ADLs.

Effects of leukemia, anemia, and chemotherapy may be cumulative (especially during acute and active treatment phase), necessitating assistance.

Provide quiet environment and uninterrupted rest periods. Encourage rest periods before meals.

Restores energy needed for activity and cellular regeneration/tissue healing.

Implement energy-saving techniques, e.g., sitting, rather than standing, use of shower chair. Assist with ambulation/other activities as indicated.

Maximizes available energy for self-care tasks.

Schedule meals around chemotherapy. Give oral hygiene before meals and administer antiemetics as indicated.

May enhance intake by reducing nausea. (Refer to CP: Cancer, ND: Nutrition, Altered: Less than Body Requirements, p. 880.)

Collaborative

Provide supplemental oxygen.

Maximizes oxygen available for cellular uptake.

Lymphomas

Lymphomas are a group of tumors with varying degrees of malignancy, characterized by progressive and painless enlargement of lymphoid tissue. They are categorized histologically according to the presence or absence of nodules as well as the degree of cellular differentiation, e.g., Hodgkin's disease, lymphosarcomas, Burkitt's lymphoma, mycosis fungoides, and the leukemias.

Hodgkin's Disease:
Contiguous node involvement is classified histologically into subgroups important in prognosis: lymphocyte predominant, nodular sclerosis, mixed cellularity, and lymphocytopenia. Lymphocyte predominant and nodular sclerosis have a good prognosis, whereas lymphocytopenia carries the worst prognosis of the three.

Non-Hodgkin's Disease:
Noncontiguous nodal spread with extranodal involvement comprised of many histologic variations.

PATIENT ASSESSMENT DATA BASE

Refer to CP: Anemias, p. 504.

ACTIVITY/REST

May report:	Fatigue, weakness, or general malaise.
	Complaints of loss of productivity and decreased exercise tolerance.
	Diminished strength, slumping of the shoulders, slow walk, and other cues indicative of fatigue.
	Need for more sleep and rest.
	Night sweats.

CIRCULATION

May report:	Palpitations, angina/chest pain.
May exhibit:	Tachycardia, dysrhythmias.
	Cyanosis of the face and neck (obstruction of venous drainage from enlarged lymph nodes) (rare).
	Scleral icterus and a generalized icteric coloring related to liver damage and consequent obstruction of bile ducts by enlarged lymph nodes (may be late).
	Pallor (anemia), diaphoresis, night sweats.

EGO INTEGRITY

May report:	Stress factors, e.g., school, job, family.
	Fear and anxiety related to diagnosis and possible fear of dying.
	Anxiety/fear related to diagnostic testing and treatment modalities (chemotherapy and radiation therapy).
	Financial concerns: hospital costs, treatment expenses, fear of losing job-related benefits due to lost time from work.
	Relationship status: fear and anxiety related to being a burden on the family.
May exhibit:	Varied behaviors, e.g., angry, withdrawn, passive.

ELIMINATION

May report:	Heaviness or discomfort in the LUQ/epigastrium with tenderness on palpation (enlarged spleen).
	History of ulcers/perforation, hemorrhage; intestinal obstruction, e.g., intussusception, or malabsorption syndrome (infiltration from retroperitoneal lymph nodes); kidney/bladder problems.

May exhibit: RUQ tenderness and enlargement on palpation (hepatomegaly).

LUQ tenderness and enlargement on palpation (splenomegaly).

Signs/symptoms of renal failure secondary to ureteral obstruction, e.g., decreased output, dark/concentrated urine, anuria.

Bowel and bladder dysfunction (spinal cord compression) (late).

FOOD/FLUID

May report: Anorexia/loss of appetite.

Dysphagia (pressure on the esophagus).

Recent unexplained weight loss equivalent to 10% or more of body weight in previous 6 months with no attempt at dieting.

May exhibit: Swelling of the face, neck, jaw or right arm (secondary to superior vena cava compression by enlarged lymph nodes).

Extremities: edema of the lower extremities related to inferior vena cava obstruction from intraabdominal lymph node enlargement (non-Hodgkin's).

Ascites (inferior vena cava obstruction related to intraabdominal lymph node enlargement).

NEUROSENSORY

May report: Nerve pain (neuralgias) reflecting compression of nerve roots by enlarged lymph nodes in the brachial, lumbar, and sacral plexuses.

Muscle weakness, paresthesia.

May exhibit: Mental status: lethargy, withdrawal, general lack of interest in surroundings.

Paraplegia (spinal cord compression from vertebral body, disk involvement with compression/degeneration, or compromised blood supply to the spinal cord).

PAIN/COMFORT

May report: Tenderness/pain over involved lymph nodes, e.g., in or around the mediastinum; back pain (vertebral compression); generalized bone pain (lymphomatous bone involvement).

Immediate pain in involved areas following injection of alcohol.

May exhibit: Self-focusing; guarding behaviors.

RESPIRATION

May report: Dyspnea on exertion or at rest; chest pain.

May exhibit: Dyspnea; tachypnea.

Dry, nonproductive cough.

Signs of respiratory distress, e.g, increased respiratory rate and depth, use of accessory muscles, stridor, cyanosis.

Hoarseness/laryngeal paralysis (pressure from enlarged nodes on the laryngeal nerve).

SAFETY

May report: History of frequent/recurrent infections (abnormalities in cellular immunity predispose the patient to systemic herpes virus infections, tuberculosis, toxoplasmosis, or bacterial infections).

Waxing and waning pattern of lymph node size.

Cyclical pattern of evening temperature elevations lasting a few days to weeks (Pel-Epstein fever) followed by alternate afebrile periods; drenching night sweats without chills.

539

	Generalized pruritus.
May exhibit:	Unexplained, persistent fever (greater than 38°C (100.4°F) without symptoms of infection).
	Asymmetric, painless, yet swollen/enlarged lymph nodes (cervical nodes most commonly involved, left side more than right; then axillary and mediastinal nodes).
	Nodes may feel rubbery and hard, discrete and movable.
	Tonsilar enlargement.
	Generalized pruritis.
	Patchy areas of loss of melanin pigmentation (vitiligo).

SEXUALITY

May report:	Concern about fertility/pregnancy (while disease does not affect either, treatment does).
	Decreased libido.

TEACHING/LEARNING

May report:	Familial risk factors (higher incidence among families of Hodgkin's patients than that of general population).
	History of mononucleosis (higher risk of Hodgkin's disease in patient with high titers of Epstein–Barr virus).
	Occupational exposure to herbicides (woodworkers/chemists).
Discharge Plan Considerations:	May need assistance with medical therapies/supplies, self-care/homemaker tasks, transportation, shopping.

DIAGNOSTIC STUDIES

These diseases are staged according to the microscopic appearance of involved lymph nodes and the extent and severity of the disorder. Accurate staging is most important in deciding on subsequent treatment regimens and prognosis.

Refer to CP: Anemias, p. 504.

Blood studies may vary from completely normal to marked abnormalities. In Stage I, few patients have abnormal blood findings.

Hematologic studies:
  CBC:

  WBC: variable, may be normal, decreased or markedly elevated.

  Differential WBC: neutrophilia, monocytosis, basophilia, and eosinophilia may be found. Complete lymphopenia (late symptom).

  RBC and Hb/Hct: decreased.

  Erythrocytes:

  Stained red cell examination: May demonstrate mild to moderate normocytic, normochromic anemia (hypersplenism).

  Erythrocyte sedimentation rate (ESR): elevated during active stages and indicates inflammatory or malignant disease. Useful to monitor patients in remission and to detect early evidence of recurrence of disease.

  Erythrocyte osmotic fragility: increased.

  Platelets: decreased (may be severely depleted; bone marrow replacement by the lymphoma and by hypersplenism).

  Coombs' test: positive reaction (hemolytic anemia) may occur; however, negative Coombs' usually occurs in advanced disease.

Serum iron and TIBC: decreased.

Bone marrow biopsy: determines bone marrow involvement. Bone marrow invasion is seen in advanced stages.

Blood chemistries:

Serum alkaline phosphatase: elevation may indicate either liver or bone involvement.

Serum copper: elevation may be seen in exacerbations.

Serum calcium: may be elevated when bone is involved.

Serum uric acid: elevated related to increased destruction of nucleoproteins, liver and kidney involvement.

Liver and kidney function studies: BUN may be elevated when kidney involvement is present. Creatinine clearance, serum creatinine, bilirubin, SGOT (ASL), etc., may be done to detect organ involvement.

Hypergammaglobulinemia is common; *hypogammaglobulinemia* may occur in advanced disease.

Chest x-ray: may reveal mediastinal or hilar adenopathy, nodular infiltrates or pleural effusions.

Whole lung tomography or chest CT scan: done if hilar adenopathy is present. Reveals possible involvement of mediastinal lymph nodes.

X-rays of thoracic, lumbar vertebrae, proximal extremities, pelvis, or areas of bone tenderness: determine areas of involvement and assist in staging.

Bipedal lymphangiography: detects involvement of abdominal retroperitoneal lymph nodes.

Inferior venacavography: permits visualization of right iliac vein, inferior vena cava and ureters. May demonstrate indentation of vena cava by enlarged lymph nodes (done 24–48 hours after lymphangiography).

Intravenous pyelography (IVP): may be done to detect renal involvement or ureteral deviation by involved nodes.

Abdominal CT scans: may be done to rule out diseased nodes in the abdomen and pelvis and in organs not accessible by physical examination.

Abdominal ultrasound: evaluates extent of involvement of retroperitoneal lymph nodes.

Bone scans: done to detect bone involvement.

Gallium-67 scintigraphy: proven useful for detecting recurrent nodal disease, especially above the diaphragm.

Lymph node biopsy: establishes the diagnosis of Hodgkin's disease based on the presence of the Reed–Sternberg cell.

Mediastinoscopy: may be performed to establish mediastinal node involvement.

Staging laparotomy: may be done to obtain specimens of retroperitoneal nodes, of both lobes of the liver, and/or remove the spleen. Splenectomy is controversial because it may increase the risk of infection and is currently not usually implemented unless the patient has clinical manifestations of stage IV disease. Laparoscopy sometimes done as an alternative approach to obtain specimens.

NURSING PRIORITIES

1. Provide physical and psychologic support during extensive diagnostic testing and treatment regimen.
2. Prevent complications.
3. Alleviate pain.
4. Provide information about disease process/prognosis and treatment needs.

DISCHARGE CRITERIA

1. Complications prevented/diminished.
2. Dealing with situation realistically.
3. Pain relieved/controlled.
4. Disease process/prognosis, possible complications, and therapeutic regimen understood.

Treatment for Hodgkin's disease includes extensive radiotherapy, a combination of radiotherapy and chemotherapy, or chemotherapy alone.

Refer to CPs: Cancer, p. 872, Leukemias, p. 530, for general nursing diagnoses and interventions.

NURSING DIAGNOSIS:	BREATHING PATTERN, INEFFECTIVE/AIRWAY CLEARANCE, INEFFECTIVE [POTENTIAL]
May be related to:	Tracheobronchial obstruction: enlarged mediastinal nodes and/or airway edema (Hodgkin's and non-Hodgkin's); superior vena cava syndrome (non-Hodgkin's)

Possibly evidenced by:	[Not applicable; presence of signs and symptoms establishes an *actual* diagnosis.]
PATIENT OUTCOMES/ EVALUATION CRITERIA:	Maintains a normal/effective respiratory pattern, free of dyspnea, cyanosis, or other signs of respiratory distress.

ACTIONS/INTERVENTIONS	RATIONALE
Independent	
Assess/monitor respiratory rate, depth, rhythm. Note complaints of dyspnea and/or use of accessory muscles, nasal flaring, altered chest excursion.	Changes (such as tachypnea, dyspnea, use of accessory muscles) may indicate progression of respiratory involvement/compromise requiring prompt intervention.
Place patient in position of comfort, usually with head of bed elevated or sitting upright leaning forward (weight supported on arms), feet dangling.	Maximizes lung expansion, decreases work of breathing, and reduces risk of aspiration.
Reposition and assist with turning periodically.	Promotes aeration of all lung segments and mobilizes secretions.
Instruct in/assist with deep breathing techniques and/or pursed lip or abdominal diaphragmatic breathing if indicated.	Helps promote gas diffusion and maintenance of small airways. Provides patient with some control over respiration, helping to reduce anxiety.
Monitor/evaluate skin color, noting pallor, development of cyanosis (particularly in nailbeds, earlobes, lips).	Proliferation of white blood cells can reduce oxygen-carrying capacity of the blood, leading to hypoxemia.
Assess respiratory response to activity. Note complaints of dyspnea/"air hunger," increased fatigue. Schedule rest periods between activities.	Decreased cellular oxygenation reduces activity tolerance. Rest reduces oxygen demands and prevents fatigue and dyspnea.
Identify/encourage energy-saving techniques, e.g., rest periods before and after meals, use of shower chair, sitting for care.	Aids in reducing fatigue and dyspnea and conserves energy for cellular regeneration and respiratory function.
Promote bedrest and provide care if indicated during acute/prolonged exacerbation.	Worsening respiratory involvement/hypoxia may necessitate cessation of activity to prevent more serious respiratory compromise.
Encourage expression of feelings. Acknowledge reality of situation and normality of feelings.	Anxiety increases oxygen demand and hypoxemia potentiates respiratory distress/cardiac symptoms, which in turn escalates anxiety.
Provide calm, quiet environment.	Promotes relaxation, conserving energy and reducing oxygen demand.
Observe for neck vein distension, headache, dizziness, periorbital/facial edema, dyspnea and stridor.	Non-Hodgkin's patients are at risk for superior vena cava syndrome, which may result in tracheal deviation and airway obstruction, representing an oncologic emergency.
Collaborative	
Provide supplemental oxygen.	Maximizes oxygen available for circulatory uptake; aids in reducing hypoxemia.
Monitor laboratory studies, e.g., ABGs, ear oximetry.	Measures adequacy of respiratory function and effectiveness of therapy.
Assist with respiratory treatments/adjuncts, e.g., IPPB, incentive spirometer.	Promotes maximal aeration of all lung segments, preventing atelectasis.
Administer analgesics, tranquilizers as indicated.	Reducing physiologic responses to pain/anxiety de-

ACTIONS/INTERVENTIONS

Collaborative

Assist with intubation, mechanical ventilation.

Prepare for emergency radiation therapy when indicated.

RATIONALE

creases oxygen demands and may limit respiratory compromise.

May be necessary to support respiratory function until airway edema is resolved.

Treatment of choice for superior vena cava syndrome.

Renal Failure: Acute

Causes of ARF can be categorized into three major areas:

Prerenal: Caused by interference with renal perfusion and manifested by decreased glomerular filtration rate (GFR), e.g.:

Volume depletion: hemorrhage, vomiting, diarrhea, excessive diuresis, burns, renal salt-wasting conditions, glycosuria, renal artery occlusion.

Volume shifts: "Third space" sequestration of fluid, vasodilating drugs, gram-negative sepsis.

Volume expansion: cardiac pump failure; hepatorenal syndrome; major vascular surgery; severe nephrotic syndrome.

Renal (or intrarenal): Parenchymal changes caused by ischemia or nephrotoxic substances.

Acute tubular necrosis (ATN) accounts for 90% of cases of acute oliguria. Destruction of tubular epithelial cells results from (1) ischemia/hypoperfusion (similar to prerenal hypoperfusion except that correction of the causative factor may be followed by continued oliguria for up to 30 days) and/or (2) direct damage from nephrotoxins. Causes of ATN include transfusion reactions with massive hemolysis, malignant hypertension, DIC, eclampsia, gram-negative septicemia, and glomerulonephritis; microvascular and large renal vascular occlusion (as in hemolytic-uremic syndrome), thrombosis, vasculitis, scleroderma, trauma/crush injuries, atherosclerosis, tumor invasion, and cortical necrosis (caused by prolonged vasospasm of the cortical blood vessels); heavy metals (e.g., pesticides); physical agents (electrical shock).

Postrenal: Obstruction in the urinary tract anywhere from the tubules to the urethral meatus, e.g., prostatic hypertrophy, calculi, invading tumors, surgical accidents, and retroperitoneal fibrosis.

Iatrogenically induced acute renal failure should be considered when other sources have been ruled out. The most common causative factors are administration of potentially nephrotoxic agents, e.g., antibiotics, anesthetics, and radiographic contrast media; failure to adjust the dosage of drugs whose primary site for excretion is the kidneys; failure to exercise adequate preventive measures, such as adequate hydration; and delay in recognizing and responding to the primary disease.

PATIENT ASSESSMENT DATA BASE

ACTIVITY/REST

May report:	Fatigue, weakness, malaise.
May exhibit:	Muscle weakness, loss of tone.

CIRCULATION

May exhibit:	Hypertension.

Cardiac dysrhythmias.

Weak/thready pulses, orthostatic hypotension (hypovolemia).

Jugular venous distention, full/bounding pulses (hypervolemia).

Generalized tissue edema (including periorbital area, ankles, sacrum).

Pallor.

Bleeding tendencies.

ELIMINATION

May report: Change in usual urination pattern: increased frequency, polyuria (early failure), or decreased frequency/oliguria (later phase).

Dysuria, hesitancy, urgency, and retention (inflammation/obstruction/infection).

Abdominal bloating, diarrhea, or constipation.

May exhibit: Change in urinary color, e.g., deep yellow, red, brown, cloudy.

Oliguria (usually 12–21 days); polyuria (2–6 liters/day).

FOOD/FLUID

May report: Weight gain (edema), weight loss (dehydration).

Nausea, anorexia, heartburn, vomiting.

Use of diuretics.

May exhibit: Changes in skin turgor/moisture.

Edema (generalized, dependent).

NEUROSENSORY

May report: Headache, blurred vision.

Muscle cramps/twitching; "restless leg" syndrome.

May exhibit: Altered mental state, e.g., decreased attention span, inability to concentrate, loss of memory, confusion, decreasing level of consciousness (azotemia, electrolyte/acid–base imbalance).

Twitching, muscle fasciculations, seizure activity.

PAIN/COMFORT

May report: Flank pain, headache.

May exhibit: Guarding/distraction behaviors, restlessness.

RESPIRATION

May report: Shortness of breath.

May exhibit: Tachypnea, dyspnea, increased rate/depth (Kussmaul's respiration); ammonia breath.

Cough productive of pink-tinged sputum (pulmonary edema).

SAFETY

May exhibit: Fever (sepsis, dehydration).

Petechiae, eccyhmotic areas on skin.

TEACHING/LEARNING

May report: Family history of polycystic disease, hereditary nephritis, urinary calculus, malignancy.

History of exposure to toxins, e.g., drugs, environmental poisons.

Current/recent use of nephrotoxic antibiotics.

Discharge Plan Considerations: May require alteration/assistance with medications, treatments, supplies; transportation, homemaker tasks.

DIAGNOSTIC STUDIES

Urine:

Volume: usually less than 400 ml per 24 hours (oliguric phase), which occurs within 24 to 48 hours after renal insult.

Color: dirty, brown sediment indicates presence of blood, hemoglobin, myoglobin, porphyrins.

Specific gravity: less than 1.020 reflects kidney disease, e.g., glomerulonephritis; pyelonephritis with loss of ability to concentrate; fixed at 1.010 reflects severe renal damage.

pH: greater than 7 found in urinary tract infections, renal tubular necrosis, and chronic renal failure.

Osmolality: less than 350 mOsm/kg is indicative of tubular damage, and urine/serum ratio is often 1:1.

Creatinine clearance: may be significantly decreased before BUN and serum creatinine show significant elevation.

Sodium: greater than 40 mEq/l because kidney is not able to resorb sodium.

HCO_3: elevated if metabolic acidosis present.

RBCs: may be present because of infection, stones, trauma, tumor, or altered glomerular filtration.

Protein: high-grade proteinuria (3–4+) strongly indicates glomerular damage when RBCs and casts are also present. Low-grade proteinuria (1–2+) and WBCs may be indicative of infection or interstitial nephritis. In ATN there is usually minimal proteinuria.

Casts: usually signal renal disease or infection. Cellular casts with brownish pigments and numerous renal tubular epithelial cells are diagnostic of ATN. Red casts suggest acute glomerular nephritis.

Blood:

Hb: decreased in presence of anemia.

RBCs: often decreased owing to increased fragility/decreased survival.

pH: metabolic acidosis (less than 7.2) may develop because of decreased renal ability to excrete hydrogen and end-products of metabolism.

BUN/creatinine: usually rise in proportion with ratio of 10:1.

Serum osmolality: greater than 285 mOsm/kg; often equal to urine.

Potassium: elevated related to retention as well as cellular shifts (acidosis) or tissue release (red cell hemolysis).

Protein: decreased serum level may reflect protein loss via urine, fluid shifts, decreased intake, or decreased synthesis owing to lack of essential amino acids.

Radiographic studies: may reveal calicectasis, hydronephrosis, narrowing, and delayed filling or emptying as a cause of ARF.

KUB (abdomen): demonstrates size of kidneys, ureters, and bladder and presence of obstruction (stones).

Retrograde pyelogram: outlines abnormalities of renal pelvis and ureters.

Renal arteriogram: assesses renal circulation and identifies extravascularities, masses.

Voiding cystourethrogram: shows bladder size, reflux into ureters, retention.

Renal ultrasound: determines kidney size; and presence of masses, cysts, obstruction in upper urinary tract.

ECG: may be abnormal reflecting electrolyte and acid/base imbalances.

NURSING PRIORITIES

1. Reestablish/maintain fluid and electrolyte balance.
2. Prevent complications.
3. Provide emotional support for patient/SO.
4. Provide information about disease process/prognosis and treatment needs.

DISCHARGE CRITERIA

1. Homeostasis achieved.
2. Complications prevented/minimized.

3. Dealing realistically with current situation.
4. Disease process/prognosis and therapeutic regimen understood.

NURSING DIAGNOSIS:	FLUID VOLUME, ALTERED: EXCESS
May be related to:	Compromised regulatory mechanism (renal failure) with retention of water
Possibly evidenced by:	Intake greater than output, oliguria; changes in urine specific gravity
	Venous distention; blood pressure/CVP changes
	Generalized tissue edema, weight gain
	Changes in mental status, restlessness
	Decreased Hb/Hct, altered electrolytes, pulmonary congestion on x-ray
PATIENT OUTCOMES/ EVALUATION CRITERIA:	Displays appropriate urinary output with specific gravity/laboratory studies near normal; stable weight, vital signs within patient's normal range; absence of edema.

ACTIONS/INTERVENTIONS

Independent

Monitor heart rate, blood pressure, and CVP.

Record accurate intake and output. Include "hidden" fluids such as antibiotic additives. Measure gastrointestinal losses, and estimate insensible losses, e.g., diaphoresis.

Monitor urine specific gravity.

Plan oral fluid replacement with patient, within multiple restrictions. Space desired beverages throughout 24 hours. Vary offerings, e.g., hot, cold, frozen.

Weigh daily on same scale with same equipment and clothing.

Assess skin, face, dependent areas for edema. Evaluate degree of edema (on scale of +1 to +4).

RATIONALE

Tachycardia and hypertension can occur because of (1) failure of the kidneys to excrete urine, (2) excessive fluid resuscitation during efforts to treat hypovolemia/ hypotension or convert oliguric phase of renal failure, and/or (3) changes in the renin–angiotension system. Note: Invasive monitoring may be needed for assessing intravascular volume, especially in patients with poor cardiac function.

Necessary for determining renal function, fluid replacement needs, and reducing risk of fluid overload.

Measures the kidney's ability to concentrate urine. In intrarenal failure, specific gravity is usually equal to/ less than 1.010, indicating loss of ability to concentrate the urine.

Helps avoid periods without fluids, minimizing boredom of limited choices and reducing sense of deprivation and thirst.

Daily body weight is best monitor of fluid status. A weight gain of more than 0.5 kg/day suggests fluid retention.

Edema occurs primarily in dependent tissues to the body, e.g., hands, feet, lumbosacral area. Patient can gain up to 10 pounds (4.5 kg) of fluid before pitting edema is detected. Periorbital edema may be a presenting sign of this fluid shift, because these fragile tis-

ACTIONS/INTERVENTIONS

Independent

Auscultate lung and heart sounds.

Assess level of consciousness; investigate changes in mentation, presence of restlessness.

Collaborative

Monitor laboratory studies, e.g.:

    BUN, creatinine;

    Urine sodium and creatinine;

    Serum sodium;

    Serum potassium;

    Hb/Hct;

    Serial chest x-rays.

Administer/restrict fluids as indicated.

Administer medications as indicated:

    Diuretics, e.g., furosemide (Lasix), mannitol (Osmitrol);

    Antihypertensives, e.g., clonidine (Catapres), methyldopa (Aldomet).

RATIONALE

sues are easily distended by even minimal fluid accumulation.

Fluid overload may lead to pulmonary edema and CHF evidenced by development of adventitious breath sounds, extra heart sounds. (Refer to ND: Cardiac Output, Altered: Decreased [Potential], p. 549.)

May reflect fluid shifts, accumulation of toxins, acidosis, electrolyte imbalances, or developing hypoxia.

Assesses progression and management of renal dysfunction/failure. Although both values may be increased, creatinine is a better indicator of renal function because it is not affected by hydration, diet, tissue catabolism.

In ATN, tubular functional integrity is lost and sodium resorption is impaired, resulting in increased sodium excretion. Urine creatinine is usually decreased as serum creatinine elevates.

Hyponatremia may result from fluid overload (dilutional) or inability of kidney to conserve sodium. Hypernatremia indicates deficit of total body water.

Lack of renal excretion and/or selective retention of potassium in order to excrete excess hydrogen ions (corrects acidosis) leads to hyperkalemia.

Decreased values may indicate hemodilution (hypervolemia); however, during prolonged failure anemia frequently develops as a result of red blood cell loss/decreased production. Other possible causes (active or occult hemorrhage) should also be evaluated.

Increased cardiac size, prominent pulmonary vascular markings, pleural effusion, infiltrates/congestion indicate acute responses to fluid overload, or chronic changes associated with renal and heart failure.

Fluid management is usually calculated to replace output from all sources plus estimated insensible losses (metabolism, diaphoresis). Prerenal failure (azotemia) is treated with volume replacement and/or vasopressors. The oliguric patient with adequate circulating volume or fluid overload who is unresponsive to fluid restriction and diuretics requires dialysis.

Given early in oliguric phase of ARF in an effort to convert to nonoliguric phase, to flush the tubular lumen of debris, reduce hyperkalemia, and promote adequate urine volume.

May be given to treat hypertension by counteracting effects of decreased renal blood flow, and/or circulating volume overload.

ACTIONS/INTERVENTIONS

Collaborative

Insert/maintain indwelling catheter, as indicated.

Prepare for dialysis as indicated. (Refer to CP: Renal Dialysis, p. 567.)

RATIONALE

Catheterization excludes lower tract obstruction and provides means of accurate monitoring of urine output during acute phase. However, catheterization is not always maintained because of increased risk of infection.

Done to correct volume overload, electrolyte, and acid–base imbalances and remove toxins.

NURSING DIAGNOSIS:	CARDIAC OUTPUT, ALTERED: DECREASED [POTENTIAL]
May be related to:	Fluid overload (kidney dysfunction/failure, overzealous fluid replacement)
	Fluid shifts, fluid deficit (excessive losses)
	Electrolyte imbalance (potassium, calcium); severe acidosis
	Uremic effects on cardiac muscle/oxygenation
Possibly evidenced by:	[Not applicable; presence of signs and symptoms establishes an *actual* diagnosis.]
PATIENT OUTCOMES/ EVALUATION CRITERIA:	Maintains cardiac output as evidenced by BP and heart rate/rhythm within patient's normal limits; peripheral pulses strong, equal with adequate capillary refill time.

ACTIONS/INTERVENTIONS

Independent

Monitor BP and heart rate.

Observe ECG or telemetry for changes in rhythm.

Auscultate heart sounds.

Assess color of skin, mucous membranes and nail beds. Note capillary refill time.

RATIONALE

Fluid volume excess, combined with hypertension (often occurs in renal failure) and effects of uremia, increases cardiac workload and can lead to cardiac failure. In acute renal failure, cardiac failure is usually reversible.

Changes in electromechanical function may become evident in response to progressing renal failure/ accumulation of toxins and electrolyte imbalance. For example, hyperkalemia is associated with peaked T wave, wide QRS, prolonged PR interval, flattened/ absent P wave. Hypokalemia is associated with flat T wave, peaked P wave and appearance of U waves. Prolonged QT interval may reflect calcium deficit.

Development of S_3/S_4 are indicative of failure. Pericardial friction rub may be only manifestation of uremic pericarditis, requiring prompt intervention/possibly acute dialysis.

Pallor may reflect vasoconstriction or anemia. Cyanosis may be related to pulmonary congestion and/or cardiac failure.

549

ACTIONS/INTERVENTIONS	RATIONALE

Independent

Note occurrence of slow pulse, hypotension, flushing, nausea/vomiting, and depressed level of consciousness (CNS depression).

Using drugs (antacids) containing magnesium can result in hypermagnesmia, potentiating neuromuscular dysfunction and risk of respiratory/cardiac arrest.

Investigate complaints of muscle cramps, numbness/tingling of fingers, with muscle twitching, hyperreflexia.

Neuromuscular indicators of hypocalcemia, which can also affect cardiac contractility and function.

Maintain bedrest or encourage adequate rest and provide assistance with care and desired activities.

Reduces oxygen consumption/cardiac workload.

Collaborative

Monitor laboratory studies, e.g.:

Potassium;

During oliguric phase, hyperkalemia may develop but shift to hypokalemia in diuretic or recovery phase. Any potassium value associated with ECG changes requires intervention. Note: Serum levels of 6.5 mEq or greater constitutes a medical emergency.

Calcium;

In addition to its own cardiac effects, calcium deficit enhances the toxic effects of potassium.

Magnesium.

Dialysis or calcium administration may be necessary to combat the CNS-depressive effects of elevated serum magnesium level.

Administer/restrict fluids as indicated. (Refer to NDs: Fluid Volume, Altered: Excess, p. 547, and Fluid Volume Deficit, Potential, p. 554.)

Cardiac output is dependent on circulating volume (affected by both fluid excess and deficit) and myocardial muscle function.

Provide supplemental oxygen if indicated.

Maximizes available oxygen for myocardial uptake to reduce cardiac workload and cellular hypoxia.

Administer medications as indicated:

Inotropic agents, e.g., digoxin (Lanoxin);

May be used to improve cardiac output by increasing myocardial contractility and stroke volume. Dosage is dependent on renal function and potassium balance to obtain therapeutic effect without toxicity.

Calcium gluconate;

May be given to treat hypocalcemia and to offset the effects of hyperkalemia by modifying cardiac irritability.

Aluminum hydroxide gels (Amphojel, Basaljel);

Increased phosphate levels may occur as a result of failure of glomerular filtration and require use of phosphate-binding antacids to limit phosphate absorption from the GI tract.

Glucose/insulin solution;

Temporary measure to lower serum potassium by driving potassium into cells when cardiac rhythm is endangered.

Sodium bicarbonate or sodium citrate;

May be used to correct acidosis or hyperkalemia (by increasing serum pH) if patient is severely acidotic and not fluid-overloaded.

Sodium polystyrene sulfonate (Kayexalate) with/without sorbitol.

Exchange resin which trades sodium for potassium in the GI tract to lower serum potassium level. Sorbitol may be included to cause osmotic diarrhea to help excrete potassium.

Prepare for/assist with dialysis as necessary. (Refer to CP: Renal Dialysis, p. 567.)

May be indicated for persistent dysrhythmias, progressive heart failure unresponsive to other therapies.

NURSING DIAGNOSIS:	NUTRITION, ALTERED: LESS THAN BODY REQUIRE-MENTS [POTENTIAL]
May be related to:	Protein catabolism; dietary restrictions to reduce nitrogenous waste products; increased metabolic needs
	Anorexia, nausea/vomiting; ulcerations of oral mucosa
Possibly evidenced by:	[Not applicable; presence of signs and symptoms establishes an *actual* diagnosis.]
PATIENT OUTCOMES/ EVALUATION CRITERIA:	Maintains/regains weight as indicated by individual situation, free of edema.

ACTIONS/INTERVENTIONS	RATIONALE
Independent	
Assess/document dietary intake.	Aids in identifying deficiencies and dietary needs. General physical condition, uremic symptoms (e.g., nausea, anorexia, altered taste), and multiple dietary restrictions affect food intake.
Provide frequent, small feedings.	Minimizes anorexia and nausea associated with uremic state/diminished peristalsis.
Give patient/SO a list of permitted foods, fluids; and encourage involvement in menu choices.	Provides patient with a measure of control within dietary restrictions. Food from home may enhance appetite.
Offer frequent mouth care/rinse with dilute (25%) acetic acid solution; provide gum, hard candy, breath mints between meals.	Mucous membranes may become dry and cracked. Mouth care soothes, lubricates, and helps freshen mouth taste, which is often unpleasant owing to uremia and restricted oral intake. Rinsing with acetic acid helps neutralize ammonia formed by conversion of urea.
Weigh daily.	The fasting/catabolic patient will normally lose 0.2 to 0.5 kg/day. Changes in excess of 0.5 kg may reflect shifts in fluid balance.
Collaborative	
Monitor laboratory studies, e.g., BUN, serum albumin, transferrin, sodium and potassium.	Indicators of nutritional needs, restrictions and necessity for/effectiveness of therapy.
Consult with dietician/nutritional support team.	Determines individual calorie and nutrient needs within the restrictions, and identifies most effective route, e.g., oral supplements, tube feedings, hyperalimentation. (Refer to CP: Total Nutritional Support, p. 894.)
Provide high calorie, low/moderate protein diet. Include complex carbohydrates and fat sources to meet caloric needs (avoiding concentrated sugar sources) and essential amino acids.	The amount of needed exogenous protein is less than normal unless the patient is on dialysis. Carbohydrates meet energy needs and limit tissue catabolism, preventing ketoacid formation from protein and fat oxidation. Carbohydrate intolerance mimicking diabetes mellitus may occur in severe renal failure. Essential amino acids improve nitrogen balance and nutritional status.

551

ACTIONS/INTERVENTIONS	RATIONALE

Collaborative

Restrict potassium, sodium, and phosphorus intake as indicated.	Restriction of these electrolytes may be needed to prevent further renal damage, especially if dialysis is not part of treatment, and/or during recovery phase of ARF.
Administer medications as indicated:	
Iron preparations;	Iron deficiency may occur if protein is restricted, patient is anemic or GI function is impaired.
Calcium;	Restores normal serum levels to improve cardiac and neuromuscular function, blood clotting, and bone metabolism.
Vitamin D;	Necessary to facilitate absorption of calcium from the GI tract.
B complex vitamins;	Vital as coenzyme in cell growth and actions. Intake is decreased owing to protein restrictions.
Antiemetics, e.g., prochlorperazine (Compazine), trimethozenzamide (Tigan).	Given to relieve nausea/vomiting and may enhance oral intake.

NURSING DIAGNOSIS:	**FATIGUE**
May be related to:	**Decreased metabolic energy production/dietary restrictions, anemia**
	Increased energy requirements, e.g., fever/inflammation, tissue regeneration
Possibly evidenced by:	**Overwhelming lack of energy**
	Inability to maintain usual activities, decreased performance
	Lethargy, disinterest in surroundings
PATIENT OUTCOMES/ EVALUATION CRITERIA:	**Reports improved sense of energy. Participates in desired activities.**

ACTIONS/INTERVENTIONS	RATIONALE

Independent

Evaluate complaints of fatigue, difficulty accomplishing tasks. Note ability to sleep/rest appropriately.	Determines degree of disabling effects.
Assess ability to participate in desired/required activities.	Identifies individual needs and aids in choosing appropriate interventions.
Identify stress/psychologic factors that may be contributory.	May have an accumulative effect (along with physiologic factors) that can be reduced when concerns and fears are acknowledged/addressed.
Plan care with adequate rest periods.	Prevents excessive fatigue, and conserves energy for healing, tissue regeneration.
Provide assistance with ADLs and ambulation.	Conserves energy, permits continuation of normal/ required activities, provides for patient safety.

ACTIONS/INTERVENTIONS	RATIONALE

Independent

Increase level of participation as patient tolerates.

Promotes sense of improvement/enhances well-being, and limits frustration.

Collaborative

Monitor electrolyte levels, including calcium, magnesium, and potassium.

Imbalances can impair neuromuscular function requiring increased energy expenditure to accomplish tasks and potentiating feelings of fatigue.

NURSING DIAGNOSIS:	INFECTION, POTENTIAL FOR
May be related to:	**Depression of immunologic defenses (secondary to uremia)**
	Invasive procedures/devices (e.g., urinary catheter)
	Changes in dietary intake/malnutrition
Possibly evidenced by:	**[Not applicable; presence of signs and symptoms establishes an *actual* diagnosis.]**
PATIENT OUTCOMES/ EVALUATION CRITERIA:	**Free of signs/symptoms of infection.**

ACTIONS/INTERVENTIONS	RATIONALE

Independent

Promote good handwashing by patient and staff.

Reduces risk of cross-contamination.

Use aseptic technique when caring for/manipulating intravenous/invasive lines. Change site/dressings per protocol. Note edema, purulent drainage.

Limits introduction of bacteria into body. Early detection/treatment of developing infection may prevent sepsis.

Provide routine catheter care and promote meticulous perianal care. Keep urinary drainage system closed and remove indwelling catheter as soon as possible.

Reduces bacterial colonization and risk of ascending urinary tract infection.

Encourage deep breathing, coughing, frequent position changes.

Prevents atelectasis and mobilizes secretions to reduce risk of pulmonary infections.

Assess skin integrity. (Refer to CP: Renal Failure: Chronic, ND: Skin Integrity, Impaired, Potential, p. 562.)

Excoriations from scratching may become secondarily infected.

Monitor vital signs.

Fever with increased pulse and respirations is typical of increased metabolic rate resulting from inflammatory process, although sepsis can occur without a febrile response.

Collaborative

Monitor laboratory studies, e.g., CBC with differential.

Although elevated WBCs may indicate generalized infection, leukocytosis is commonly seen in ARF and may reflect inflammation/injury within the kidney. A shifting of the differential to the left is indicative of infection.

Obtain specimen(s) for culture and sensitivity and administer appropriate antibiotics as indicated.

Verification of infection and identification of specific organism aids in choice of the most effective treatment.

553

NURSING DIAGNOSIS:	FLUID VOLUME DEFICIT, POTENTIAL
May be related to:	Excessive loss of fluid (diuretic phase of ARF, with rising urinary volume and delayed return of tubular reabsorption capabilities)
Possibly evidenced by:	[Not applicable; presence of signs and symptoms establishes an *actual* diagnosis.]
PATIENT OUTCOMES/ EVALUATION CRITERIA:	Displays intake/output near balance; good skin turgor, moist mucous membranes, palpable peripheral pulses, stable weight and vital signs, electrolytes within normal range.

ACTIONS/INTERVENTIONS

Independent

Measure intake and output accurately. Weigh daily. Calculate insensible fluid losses.

Provide allowed fluids throughout 24-hour period.

Monitor blood pressure (noting postural changes) and heart rate.

Note signs/symptoms of dehydration, e.g., dry mucous membranes, thirst, dulled sensorium, peripheral vasoconstriction.

Control environmental temperature; limit bed linens as indicated.

Collaborative

Monitor laboratory studies, e.g., sodium.

RATIONALE

Helps estimate fluid replacement needs. Fluid intake should approximate losses through urine, nasogastric/ wound drainage, and insensible losses (e.g., diaphoresis and metabolism). Note: Some sources believe that fluid replacement should not exceed two-thirds of the previous day's output to prevent prolonging the diuresis.

Diruetic phase of ARF may revert to oliguric phase if fluid intake is not maintained or nocturnal dehydration occurs.

Orthostatic hypotension and tachycardia suggests hypovolemia.

In diuretic phase of renal failure, urine output can exceed 3 liters/day. Extracellular fluid (ECF) volume depletion activates the thirst center, and sodium depletion causes persistent thirst, unrelieved by drinking water. Continued fluid losses/inadequate replacement may lead to hypovolemic state.

May reduce diaphoresis, which contributes to overall fluid losses.

In nonoliguric ARF or in diuretic phase of ARF, large urine losses may result in sodium wasting while elevated urinary sodium acts osmotically to increase fluid losses. Restriction of sodium may be indicated to break the cycle.

NURSING DIAGNOSIS:	KNOWLEDGE DEFICIT [LEARNING NEED] (SPECIFY)
May be related to:	Lack of exposure/recall
	Information misinterpretation
	Unfamiliarity with information resources

Possibly evidenced by:	Questions/request for information, statement of misconception
	Inaccurate follow-through of instructions, development of preventable complications
PATIENT OUTCOMES/ EVALUATION CRITERIA:	Verbalizes understanding of condition/disease process, prognosis, and treatment. Identifies relationship of signs/symptoms to the disease process and correlates symptoms with causative factors. Initiates necessary lifestyle changes and participates in treatment regimen.

ACTIONS/INTERVENTIONS	RATIONALE
Independent	
Review disease process, prognosis, and precipitating factors if known.	Provides knowledge base upon which patient can make informed choices.
Discuss dietary plan/restrictions. Include fact sheet listing food restrictions.	Adequate nutrition is necessary to promote healing/tissue regeneration while adherence to restrictions may prevent complications.
Encourage patient to observe characteristics of urine and amount/frequency of output.	Changes may reflect alterations in renal function/need for dialysis.
Establish regular schedule for weighing.	Useful tool for monitoring fluid and dietary status/needs.
Review fluid intake/restriction. Remind patient to spread fluids over entire day and to include all fluids (e.g., ice) in daily fluid counts.	Depending on the cause of ARF, patient may need to either restrict or increase intake of fluids.
Discuss activity restriction, and gradual resumption of desired activity. Encourage use of energy-saving, relaxation, and diversional techniques.	Patient with severe ARF may need to restrict activity and/or may feel weak for an extended period of time during lengthy recovery phase, requiring measures to conserve energy and reduce boredom/depression.
Discuss/review medication use. Encourage patient to discuss all medications (including OTC drugs) with physician.	Medications that are concentrated in/excreted by the kidneys can cause toxic cumulative reactions and/or permanent damage to kidneys.
Stress necessity of follow-up care, laboratory studies.	Renal function may be slow to return following acute failure (up to 12 months) and deficits may persist, requiring changes in therapy to avoid recurrence/complications.
Identify symptoms requiring medical intervention, e.g., decreased urinary output, sudden weight gain, presence of edema, lethargy, bleeding, signs of infection; altered mentation.	Prompt evaluation and intervention may prevent serious complications/progression to chronic failure.

Renal Failure: Chronic _____

PATIENT ASSESSMENT DATA BASE

ACTIVITY/REST

May report: Extreme fatigue, weakness, malaise.

Sleep disturbances (insomnia/restlessness or somnolence).

May exhibit: Muscle weakness, loss of tone, decreased range of motion.

CIRCULATION

May report: Palpitations; chest pain (angina).

May exhibit: Hypertension; jugular venous distention, full/bounding pulses, generalized tissue and pitting edema of feet, legs, hands (hypervolemia).

Cardiac dysrhythmias.

Weak/thready pulses, orthostatic hypotension (hypovolemia) (rare in end-stage).

Pericardial friction rub (response to accumulated wastes).

Pallor; bronze-gray, yellow skin.

Bleeding tendencies.

EGO INTEGRITY

May report: Stress factors, e.g., financial, relationship, etc.

Feelings of helplessness, hopelessness, powerlessness.

May exhibit: Denial, anxiety, fear, anger, irritability, personality changes.

ELIMINATION

May report: Decreased urinary frequency, oliguria, anuria (advanced failure).

Abdominal bloating, diarrhea, or constipation.

May exhibit: Change in urinary color, e.g., deep yellow, red, brown, cloudy.

Oliguria, may become anuric.

FOOD/FLUID

May report: Rapid weight gain (edema), weight loss (malnutrition).

Anorexia, heartburn, nausea/vomiting; unpleasant metallic taste in the mouth (ammonia breath).

Use of diuretics.

May exhibit: Abdominal distention/ascites, liver enlargement (end-stage).

Changes in skin turgor/moisture.

Edema (generalized, dependent).

Gum ulcerations, bleeding of gums/tongue.

Muscle wasting, decreased subcutaneous fat, debilitated appearance.

NEUROSENSORY

May report: Headache, blurred vision.

Muscle cramps/twitching; "restless leg" syndrome; burning numbness of soles of feet.

Numbness/tingling and weakness, especially of lower extremities (peripheral neuropathy).

May exhibit:	Altered mental state, e.g., decreased attention span, inability to concentrate, loss of memory, confusion, decreasing level of consciousness, stupor, coma. Diminished deep tendon reflexes. Positive Chvostek's and Trousseau's signs. Twitching, muscle fasciculations, seizure activity. Thin, brittle nails; thin hair.

PAIN/COMFORT

May report:	Flank pain; headache; muscle cramps/leg pain (worse at night).
May exhibit:	Guarding/distraction behaviors, restlessness.

RESPIRATION

May report:	Shortness of breath; paroxysmal nocturnal dyspnea; cough with/without thick, tenacious sputum.
May exhibit:	Tachypnea, dyspnea, increased rate/depth (Kussmaul's respiration). Cough productive of pink-tinged sputum (pulmonary edema).

SAFETY

May report:	Itching skin. Recent/recurrent infections.
May exhibit:	Pruritis. Fever (sepsis, dehydration); normothermia may actually represent an elevation in the patient who has developed a lower than normal body temperature (effect of chronic renal failure/depressed immune response). Petechiae, ecchymotic areas on skin. Bone fractures; calcium phosphate deposits (metastatic calcifications) in skin, soft tissues, joints; limited joint movement.

SEXUALITY

May report:	Decreased libido; amenorrhea; infertility.

SOCIAL INTERACTION

May report:	Difficulties imposed by condition, e.g., unable to work, maintain usual role function in family.

TEACHING/LEARNING

May report:	Family history of diabetes mellitus (high risk for renal failure), polycystic disease, hereditary nephritis, urinary calculus, malignancy. History of exposure to toxins, e.g., drugs, environmental poisons. Current/recent use of nephrotoxic antibiotics.
Discharge Plan Considerations:	May require alteration/assistance with medications, treatments, supplies; transportation, homemaker tasks.

DIAGNOSTIC STUDIES

Urine:

Volume: usually less than 400 ml/24 hr (oliguria) or urine is absent (anuria).

Color: dirty, brown sediment indicates presence of blood, hemoglobin, myoglobin, porphyrins.

Specific gravity: less than 1.015 (fixed at 1.010 reflects severe renal damage).

Osmolality: less than 350 mOsm/kg is indicative of tubular damage, and urine/serum ratio is often 1:1.

Creatinine clearance: may be significantly decreased.

Sodium: greater than 40 mEq/liter because kidney is not able to reabsorb sodium.

Protein: high-grade proteinuria (3–4 +) strongly indicates glomerular damage when RBCs and casts are also present.

Blood:

BUN/creatinine: usually rise in proportion. Creatinine level of 10 mg/dl suggests end stage (may be as low as 5).

CBC: Hct: decreased in presence of anemia. *Hb:* usually less than 7–8 g/dl. *RBCs:* lifespan decreased owing to erythropoietin deficiency as well as azotemia.

ABGs: pH: decreased metabolic acidosis (less than 7.2) occurs because of loss of renal ability to excrete hydrogen and ammonia or end products of protein catabolism. HCO_3 decreased. PCO_2 decreased.

Serum sodium: may be low (if kidney "wastes sodium") or normal (reflecting dilutional state of hypernatremia).

Potassium: elevated related to retention as well as cellular shifts (acidosis) or tissue release (red cell hemolysis). In end-stage, ECG changes may not occur until potassium is 6.5 mEq or greater.

Magnesium: elevated.

Phosphorus: elevated.

Protein: decreased serum level may reflect protein loss via urine, fluid shifts, decreased intake, or decreased synthesis owing to lack of essential amino acids.

Serum osmolality: greater than 285 mOsm/kg; often equal to urine.

KUB (abdomen): demonstrates size of kidneys, ureters, bladder and presence of obstruction (stones).

Retrograde pyelogram: outlines abnormalities of renal pelvis and ureters.

Renal arteriogram: assesses renal circulation and identifies extravascularities, masses.

Voiding cystourethrogram: shows bladder size, reflux into ureters, retention.

Renal ultrasound: determines kidney size; and presence of masses, cysts, obstruction in upper urinary tract.

ECG: may be abnormal reflecting electrolyte and acid/base imbalances.

X-rays of feet, skull, spinal column, and hands: may reveal demineralization, calcifications.

NURSING PRIORITIES

1. Maintain homeostasis.
2. Prevent complications.
3. Provide information about disease process/prognosis and treatment needs.
4. Support adjustment to lifestyle changes.

DISCHARGE CRITERIA

1. Fluid/electrolyte balance stabilized.
2. Complications prevented/minimized.
3. Disease process/prognosis and therapeutic regimen understood.
4. Dealing realistically with situation, initiating necessary lifestyle changes.

NURSING DIAGNOSIS:	CARDIAC OUTPUT, ALTERED: DECREASED [POTENTIAL]
May be related to:	Fluid imbalances affecting circulating volume, myocardial workload and systemic vascular resistance
	Alterations in rate, rhythm, cardiac conduction (electrolyte imbalances, hypoxia)

	Accumulation of toxins (urea), soft tissue calcification (deposition of calcium phosphate)
Possibly evidenced by:	**[Not applicable; presence of signs and symptoms establishes an *actual* diagnosis.]**
PATIENT OUTCOMES/ EVALUATION CRITERIA:	**Maintains cardiac output as evidenced by BP and heart rate within patient's normal range; peripheral pulses strong, equal with adequate capillary refill time.**

ACTIONS/INTERVENTIONS	RATIONALE

In addition to those in CP: Renal Failure: Acute, ND: Cardiac Output, Decreased [Potential], p. 549.

Independent

Auscultate heart and lung sounds. Evaluate presence of peripheral edema/vascular congestion and complaints of dyspnea.	S_3/S_4 heart sounds with muffled tones, tachycardia, irregular heart rate, tachypnea, dyspnea, crackles, wheezes, and edema/jugular distention suggest CHF. (Refer to CP: Congestive Heart Failure, p. 41.)
Monitor blood pressure; note postural changes, e.g., sitting, lying, standing.	Significant hypertension can occur because of disturbances in the renin-angiotensin aldosterone system (caused by renal dysfunction). Although hypertension is common, orthostatic hypotension may occur due to intravascular fluid deficit or in response to effects of antihypertensive medications.
Investigate complaints of chest pain, noting location, radiation, severity (1–10 scale) and if it is intensified by deep inspiration and supine position. Evaluate heart sounds (note friction rub), BP, peripheral pulses, capillary refill, vascular congestion, temperature, and sensorium/mentation.	While hypertension and chronic CHF may cause MI, approximately half of CRF patients on dialysis develop pericarditis, potentiating risk of pericardial effusion/ tamponade. Presence of sudden hypotension, paradoxical pulse, narrow pulse pressure, diminished/ absent peripheral pulses, marked jugular distention, pallor, and a rapid mental deterioration indicate tamponade, which is a medical emergency.
Assess activity level, response to activity.	Weakness can be attributed to CHF as well as anemia.

Collaborative

Monitor laboratory studies, e.g.:	
Electrolytes (potassium, sodium, calcium, magnesium), BUN;	Imbalances can alter electrical conduction and cardiac function.
Chest x-rays.	Useful in identifying developing cardiac failure or soft tissue calcification.
Administer antihypertensive drugs, e.g., propranolol (Inderal), metoprolol-tartrate (Lopressor), clonidine (Catapres), hydralazine (Apresoline).	Reduces systemic vascular resistance and/or renin release to decrease myocardial workload and aid in prevention of CHF and/or MI.
Assist with pericardiocentesis as indicated.	Accumulation of fluid within pericardial sac can compromise cardiac filling and myocardial contractility impairing cardiac output and potentiating risk of cardiac arrest.
Prepare for dialysis. (Refer to CP: Renal Dialysis, p. 567.)	Reduction of uremic toxins and correction of electrolyte imbalances and fluid overload may limit/prevent cardiac manifestations, including hypertension and pericardial effusion.

559

NURSING DIAGNOSIS:	INJURY, POTENTIAL FOR (ABNORMAL BLOOD PROFILE)
May be related to:	Suppressed erythropoietin production/secretion; decreased RBC production and survival; altered clotting factors; increased capillary fragility
Possibly evidenced by:	[Not applicable; presence of signs and symptoms establishes an *actual* diagnosis.]
PATIENT OUTCOMES/ EVALUATION CRITERIA:	Free of signs/symptoms of bleeding/hemorrhage. Maintains/demonstrates improvement in laboratory values.

ACTIONS/INTERVENTIONS

Independent

Note complaints of increasing fatigue, weakness. Observe for tachycardia, pallor of skin/mucous membranes, dyspnea, and chest pain.

Monitor level of consciousness and behavior.

Evaluate response to activity, ability to perform tasks. Assist as needed and develop schedule for rest.

Limit vascular sampling, combine laboratory tests when possible.

Observe for oozing from venipuncture sites, bleeding/ecchymotic areas following slight trauma, petechiae; joint swelling or mucous membrane involvement, e.g., bleeding gums, recurrent epistaxis, hematemesis, melena, and hazy/red urine.

Hematest GI secretions/stool for blood.

Provide soft tooth brush, electric razor; use smallest needle possible and apply prolonged pressure following injections/vascular punctures.

Collaborative

Monitor laboratory studies, e.g.:

CBC: RBCs, Hb/Hct;

Platelet count, clotting factors;

RATIONALE

May reflect effects of anemia, and cardiac response necessary to keep cells oxygenated.

Anemia may cause cerebral hypoxia manifested by changes in mentation, orientation, and behavioral responses.

Anemia decreases tissue oxygenation and increases fatigue, which may require intervention, changes in activity, and rest.

Recurrent/excessive blood sampling can worsen anemia.

Bleeding can occur easily because of capillary fragility/altered clotting functions and may worsen anemia.

Stress and hemostatic abnormalities may result in GI hemorrhage. (Refer to CP: Upper Gastrointestinal/Esophageal Bleeding, p. 397.)

Reduces risk of bleeding/hematoma formation.

Uremia (e.g., elevated ammonia, urea, other toxins) decreases production of erythropoietin and depresses RBC production and survival time. In chronic renal failure, hemoglobin and hematocrit are usually low but tolerated; e.g., patient may not be symptomatic until Hb is below 7.

Suppression of platelet formation and inadequate levels of factors III and VIII impair clotting and potentiate risk of bleeding. Note: Bleeding may become intractable in end-stage disease.

Prothrombin level.	Abnormal prothrombin consumption lowers serum levels and impairs clotting.
Administer fresh blood, packed red cells as indicated.	May be necessary when patient is symptomatic with anemia. Packed RBCs are usually given when patient is fluid-overloaded or being dialyzed. Washed RBCs are used to prevent hyperkalemia associated with stored blood.
Administer medications, as indicated, e.g.:	
Iron, folic acid (Folvite), cyanocobalamin (Betalin);	Useful in correcting symptomatic anemia related to nutritional/dialysis-induced deficits. Note: Iron should not be given with phosphate binders because they may decrease iron absorption.
Cimetadine (Tagamet), ranitidine (Zantac), antacids;	May be given prophylactically to reduce/neutralize gastric acid and thereby reduce the risk of GI hemorrhage.
Hemastatics/fibrinolysis inhibitors, e.g., aminocaproic acid (Amicar).	Inhibits bleeding that does not subside spontaneously/respond to usual treatment.

NURSING DIAGNOSIS:	**THOUGHT PROCESSES, ALTERED**
May be related to:	**Physiologic changes: accumulation of toxins (e.g., urea, ammonia), metabolic acidosis, hypoxia; electrolyte imbalances, metastatic calcifications in the brain**
Possibly evidenced by:	**Disorientation to person, place, time**
	Memory deficit
	Altered attention span, decreased ability to grasp ideas; impaired ability to make decisions, problem-solve
PATIENT OUTCOMES/ EVALUATION CRITERIA:	**Regains usual level of mentation. Identifies ways to compensate for cognitive impairment/memory deficits.**

ACTIONS/INTERVENTIONS

Independent

RATIONALE

ACTIONS/INTERVENTIONS	RATIONALE
Assess extent of impairment in thinking ability, memory, and orientation. Note attention span.	Uremic syndrome's effect can begin with minor confusion/irritability and progress to altered personality or inability to assimilate information and participate in care. Awareness of changes provides opportunity for evaluation and intervention.
Ascertain from SO, patient's usual level of mentation.	Provides comparison to evaluate progression/resolution of impairment.
Provide SO with information about patient's status.	Some improvement in mentation may be expected with restoration of more normal levels of BUN, electrolytes and serum pH.
Provide quiet/calm environment and judicious use of television, radio, and visitation.	Minimizes environmental stimuli to reduce sensory overload/increased confusion while preventing sen-

ACTIONS/INTERVENTIONS

Independent

Reorient to surroundings, person, etc. Provide calendars, clocks, outside window.

Present reality concisely, briefly, and do not challenge illogical thinking.

Communicate information/instructions in simple, short sentences. Ask direct, yes/no questions. Repeat explanations as necessary.

Establish a regular schedule for expected activities.

Promote adequate rest and undisturbed periods for sleep.

Collaborative

Monitor laboratory studies, e.g., BUN/creatinine, serum electrolytes, glucose level and ABGs (PO$_2$, pH).

Provide supplemental oxygen as indicated.

Avoid use of barbiturates and opiates.

Prepare for dialysis.

RATIONALE

sory deprivation.

Provides clues to aid in recognition of reality.

Confrontation potentiates defensive reactions and may lead to patient mistrust and heightened denial of reality.

May aid in reducing confusion and increases possibility that communications will be understood/remembered.

Aids in maintaining reality orientation and may reduce fear/confusion.

Sleep deprivation may further impair cognitive abilities.

Correction of elevations/imbalances can have profound effects on cognition/mentation.

Correction of hypoxia alone can improve cognition.

Drugs normally detoxified in the kidneys will have increased half-life/cumulative effects, worsening confusion.

Marked deterioration of thought processes may indicate worsening of azotemia and general condition, requiring prompt intervention to regain homeostasis.

NURSING DIAGNOSIS:	SKIN INTEGRITY, IMPAIRED: POTENTIAL
May be related to:	**Altered metabolic state, circulation (anemia with tissue ischemia) and sensation (peripheral neuropathy)**
	Alterations in skin turgor (edema/dehydration)
	Reduced mobility
	Accumulation of excretory waste products in the skin
Possibly evidenced by:	**[Not applicable; presence of signs and symptoms establishes an *actual* diagnosis.]**
PATIENT OUTCOMES/ EVALUATION CRITERIA:	**Maintains skin integrity. Demonstrates behaviors/ techniques to prevent skin breakdown/injury.**

ACTIONS/INTERVENTIONS

Independent

Inspect skin for redness, excoriation.

Change position frequently; move patient carefully; pad bony prominences with sheepskin, elbow/heel

RATIONALE

Indicates areas of poor circulation/breakdown which may lead to decubitus formation/infection.

Decreases pressure on edematous, poorly perfused tissues to reduce ischemia. Elevation promotes ve-

ACTIONS/INTERVENTIONS

Independent

protectors.

Provide soothing skin care. Restrict use of soaps.

Keep linens dry, wrinkle-free.

Investigate complaints of itching.

Recommend patient use cool, moist compresses to apply pressure (rather than scratch) pruritic areas. Keep fingernails short; provide gloves during sleep if needed.

Suggest wearing loose-fitting cotton garments.

Collaborative

Provide foam/flotation mattress.

RATIONALE

nous return limiting venous stasis/edema formation.

Baking soda, cornstarch baths decrease itching and are less drying than soaps. Lotions and ointments may be desired to relieve dry, cracked skin.

Reduces dermal irritation and risk of skin breakdown.

Although dialysis has largely eliminated skin problems associated with uremic frost, itching can occur because the skin is an excretory route for waste products, e.g., phosphate crystals (associated with hyperparathyroidism in end-stage disease).

Alleviates discomfort and reduces risk of dermal injury.

Prevents direct dermal irritation and promotes evaporation of moisture on the skin.

Reduces prolonged pressure on tissues, which can limit cellular perfusion potentiating ischemia/necrosis.

NURSING DIAGNOSIS:	ORAL MUCOUS MEMBRANE, ALTERED [POTENTIAL]
May be related to:	Lack of/or decreased salivation, fluid restrictions Chemical irritation, conversion of urea in saliva to ammonia
Possibly evidenced by:	[Not applicable; presence of signs and symptoms establishes an *actual* diagnosis.]
PATIENT OUTCOMES/ EVALUATION CRITERIA:	Maintains integrity of mucous membranes. Identifies/ initiates specific interventions to promote healthy oral mucosa.

ACTIONS/INTERVENTIONS

Independent

Inspect oral cavity; note moistness, character of saliva, presence of inflammation, ulcerations, leukoplakia.

Provide fluids throughout 24-hour period within prescribed limit.

Offer frequent mouth care/rinse with 25% acetic acid solution; provide gum, hard candy, breath mints between meals.

RATIONALE

Provides opportunity for prompt intervention and prevention of infection.

Prevents excessive oral dryness from prolonged period without oral intake.

Mucous membranes may become dry and cracked. Mouth care soothes, lubricates, and helps freshen mouth taste, which is often unpleasant owing to uremia and restricted oral intake. Rinsing with acetic acid helps neutralize ammonia formed by conversion of urea.

ACTIONS/INTERVENTIONS

Independent

Encourage good dental hygiene following meals and at bedtime. Recommend avoidance of dental floss.

Recommend patient stop smoking and avoid lemon-glycerine products/mouthwash containing alcohol.

Provide artificial saliva as needed, e.g., Ora-Lub.

RATIONALE

Reduces bacterial growth and potential for infection. Dental floss may cut gums, potentiating bleeding.

These substances are irritating to the mucosa and have a drying effect, potentiating discomfort.

Prevents dryness, buffers acids, and promotes comfort.

NURSING DIAGNOSIS:	KNOWLEDGE DEFICIT [LEARNING NEED] (SPECIFY)
May be related to:	Cognitive limitation
	Lack of exposure/recall, information misinterpretation
Possibly evidenced by:	Questions/request for information, statement of misconception
	Inaccurate follow-through of instruction/development of preventable complications
PATIENT OUTCOMES/ EVALUATION CRITERIA:	Verbalizes understanding of condition/disease process and treatment. Correctly performs necessary procedures and explains reasons for the actions. Demonstrates necessary lifestyle changes and participates in treatment regimen.

ACTIONS/INTERVENTIONS

Independent

In addition to interventions outlined in CP: Renal Failure: Acute, p. 544.

Review disease process/prognosis and future expectations.

Review dietary restrictions, including phosphorus (e.g., milk products, poultry, corn, peanuts) and magnesium (e.g., whole grain products, legumes).

Discuss drug therapy, including use of calcium supplements and phosphate binders, e.g., aluminum hydroxide antacids (amphojel, Basaljel) and avoidance of magnesium antacids (Mylanta, Maalox, Gelusil).

Stress importance of reading all product labels (drugs and food) and not taking medications without prior approval of health care provider.

RATIONALE

Provides knowledge base on which patient can make informed choices.

Retention of phosphorus stimulates the parathyroid glands to shift calcium from bones (renal osteodystrophy), and accumulation of magnesium can impair neuromuscular function and mentation.

Prevents serious complications, e.g., reducing phosphate absorption from the GI tract and supplying calcium to maintain normal serum levels, reducing risk of bone demineralization/fractures, tetany. Use of aluminum-containing products should be monitored, however, because accumulation in the bones potentiates osteodystrophy. Magnesium products potentiate risk of hypermagnesemia.

It is difficult to maintain electrolyte balance when exogenous intake is not factored into dietary restrictions, e.g., hypercalcemia, can result from routine supplement use in combination with increased dietary intake of calcium-fortified foods and medications containing calcium.

ACTIONS/INTERVENTIONS	RATIONALE

Independent

Review measures to prevent bleeding/hemorrhage, e.g., use of soft toothbrush, electric razor; avoidance of constipation, forceful blowing of nose, strenuous exercise/contact sports.

Reduces risks related to alteration of clotting factors/decreased platelet count.

Instruct in home monitoring of BP, including scheduling rest period before taking pressure, using same arm/position.

Incidence of hypertension is increased in CRF, often requiring management with antihypertensive drugs, necessitating close observation of treatment effects, e.g., vascular response to medication.

Caution against exposure to external temperature extremes, e.g., heating pad/snow.

Peripheral neuropathy may develop, especially in lower extremities (effects of uremia, electrolyte/acid–base imbalances), impairing peripheral sensation and potentiating risk of tissue injury.

Establish routine exercise program, within individual ability; intersperse adequate rest periods with activities.

Aids in maintaining muscle tone and joint flexibility. Reduces risks associated with immobility (including bone demineralization) while preventing fatigue.

Address sexual concerns.

Physiologic effects of uremia/antihypertensive therapy may impair sexual desire/performance.

Stress necessity of medical and laboratory follow-up.

Close monitoring of renal function and electrolyte balance is necessary to readjust treatment and/or make decisions about dialysis/transplantation.

Identify signs/symptoms requiring medical evaluation, e.g.:

Low-grade fever, chills, changes in characteristics of urine/sputum, tissue swelling/drainage, oral ulcerations;

Depressed immune system, anemia, malnutrition all contribute to increased risk of infection.

Numbness/tingling of digits, abdominal/muscle cramps, carpopedal spasms;

Decreased absorption of calcium may lead to hypocalcemia.

Joint swelling/tenderness, decreased range of motion, reduced muscle strength;

Hyperphosphatemia with corresponding calcium shifts from the bone may result in deposition of the excess calcium phosphate as calcifications in joints and soft tissues. Symptoms of skeletal involvement are often noted before impairment in organ function is evident.

Headaches, blurred vision, periorbital/sacral edema.

Suggestive of development/poor control of hypertension.

Review strategies to prevent constipation, including stool softeners (e.g., Colace) and bulk laxatives (e.g., Metamucil) but avoiding magnesium products (e.g., Milk of Magnesia).

Reduced fluid intake, changes in dietary pattern, and use of phosphate-binding products often results in constipation that is not responsive to nonmedical interventions. Use of products containing magnesium increases risk of hypermagnesemia.

NURSING DIAGNOSIS: **NONCOMPLIANCE [COMPLIANCE, ALTERED] (SPECIFY)**

May be related to: Patient value system: health beliefs, cultural influences

Changes in mentation; lack/refusal of support systems/resources

Complexities, costs, side effects of therapy

Possibly evidenced by:	Reported unwillingness to follow therapeutic regimen
	Failure to progress; exacerbation of symptoms; development of complications
	Denial of reality of the situation
PATIENT OUTCOMES/ EVALUATION CRITERIA:	Verbalizes accurate knowledge of disease and understanding of therapeutic regimen. Participates in the development of goals and treatment plan. Makes choices at level of readiness based on accurate information. Identifies/uses resources appropriately.

ACTIONS/INTERVENTIONS	RATIONALE
Independent	
Ascertain patient's/SO's perception/understanding of situation and consequences of behavior.	Provides insight into how the patient views own illness and treatment regimen and aids in understanding problems patient is encountering.
Determine value system (health care beliefs and cultural values).	Therapeutic regimen may be incongruent with patient's social/cultural lifestyle and perceived role/responsibilities.
Listen/Active-listen patient's complaints/comments.	Conveys message of concern, belief in individual's capability to resolve situation in a positive manner.
Identify behaviors indicative of failure to follow treatment program.	May give information about reasons for lack of cooperation and clarifies areas which need problem-solving.
Assess level of anxiety, locus of control, feelings of hopelessness/powerlessness.	Severe level of anxiety interferes with patient's ability to cope with situation. Even when patient is internally motivated (internal locus-of-control), patient tends to become passive/dependent in long-term, debilitating illness.
Determine psychologic meanings of behavior.	Patient may deny reality of physical condition/chronic irreversible disease process; stage of the grieving process may be reflected in angry, acting-out, or withdrawn behavior.
Evaluate support systems/resources used by the patient. Recommend alternatives as appropriate.	Presence of adequate support systems assists patient to handle difficulties of a long-term illness.
Assess attitudes of health care providers toward patient/behavior.	Judgmental approaches may create barriers/power struggles that alienate the patient, reducing likelihood of achieving compromise.
Accept patient's choice/point of view, even if it appears to be self-destructive.	Patient has the right to make own decisions/choices, and acceptance may give a sense of control, which will help patient to look more clearly at consequences of choice.
Establish graduated goals with patient; modify regimen as necessary/possible.	When patient has participated in setting of goals, a sense of investment encourages cooperation and willingness to adhere to/work with program as established.
Develop a system of self-monitoring, e.g., BP, weight, provide copies of laboratory reports.	Provides a sense of control, enables patient to follow own progress and to make informed choices.
Provide positive feedback for efforts/involvement in therapy.	Promotes sense of self-esteem, encourages continued participation in regimen.

Renal Dialysis

Dialysis is a process that substitutes functionally for impaired renal function by removing excess fluid and/or accumulated endogenous or exogenous toxins.

PATIENT ASSESSMENT DATA BASE

Refer to CP: Renal Failure: Acute, p. 544; Renal Failure: Chronic, p. 556.

DIAGNOSTIC STUDIES

Procedures and results are variable, depending on cause (e.g., removal of excess fluid or toxins/drugs), degree of renal involvement, and patient considerations (e.g., distance from treatment center, cognition, available support). Refer to CP: Renal Failure: Acute, p. 544; Renal Failure: Chronic, p. 556.

NURSING PRIORITIES

1. Promote homeostasis.
2. Maintain comfort.
3. Prevent complications.
4. Support patient independence/self-care.
5. Provide information about disease process/prognosis and treatment needs.

DISCHARGE CRITERIA

1. Fluid and electrolyte balance maximized.
2. Complications prevented/minimized.
3. Discomfort alleviated.
4. Dealing realistically with current situation; independent within limits of condition.
5. Disease process/prognosis and therapeutic regimen understood.

GENERAL CONSIDERATIONS

This section addresses the general nursing management issues of the patient receiving some form of dialysis.

NURSING DIAGNOSIS:	NUTRITION, ALTERED: LESS THAN BODY REQUIREMENTS
May be related to:	GI disturbances (result of uremia); anorexia, nausea/vomiting and stomatitis
	Dietary restrictions (bland, tasteless food)
	Loss of protein during dialysis (crosses the semipermeable membrane/peritoneum)
Possibly evidenced by:	Inadequate food intake, aversion to eating, altered taste sensation
	Poor muscle tone/weakness
	Sore, inflamed buccal cavity; pale conjunctiva/mucous membranes

PATIENT OUTCOMES/
EVALUATION CRITERIA:

**Demonstrates stable weight/gain toward goal with nor-
malization of laboratory values and free of signs of malnutrition.**

ACTIONS/INTERVENTIONS	RATIONALE
Independent	
Monitor food/fluid ingested and calculate daily caloric intake.	Identifies nutritional deficits/therapy needs.
Recommend patient keep a food diary, including estimation of ingested amounts of electrolytes (of individual concern, e.g., Na^+, K^+, Cl^-, Mg^{2+}), and protein.	Helps patient to realize "big picture" and allows opportunity to alter dietary choices to meet individual desires within identified restriction.
Measure muscle mass via triceps skinfold.	Assesses adequacy of nutrient utilization by measuring changes in fat deposits which may suggest presence/absence of tissue catabolism.
Note presence of nausea/anorexia.	Symptoms accompany accumulation of endogenous toxins which can alter/reduce intake and require intervention.
Encourage patient to participate in menu planning.	May enhance oral intake and promotes sense of control/responsibility.
Serve small, frequent meals. Schedule meals according to dialysis needs.	Smaller portions may enhance intake. Type of dialysis influences meal patterns, e.g., patients receiving hemodialysis might not be fed directly before/during procedure, because this can alter fluid removal; and patients undergoing peritoneal dialysis may be unable to ingest food while abdomen is distended with dialysate.
Promote visits by SO during meals.	Provides diversion and promotes social aspects of eating.
Provide frequent mouth care.	Reduces discomfort of oral stomatitis and undesirable/metallic taste in mouth, which can interfere with food intake.
Collaborative	
Refer to dietician.	Useful for individualizing dietary program to meet cultural/lifestyle needs enhancing patient cooperation.
Provide a high carbohydrate diet which includes ordered amount of high-quality protein and essential amino acids with restriction of sodium/potassium as indicated.	Provides sufficient nutrients to improve energy, prevent muscle wasting, promote tissue regeneration/healing, and electrolyte balance.
Administer multivitamins, including ascorbic acid, folic acid, vitamin D, and iron supplements, as indicated.	Replaces vitamins lost because of malnutrition/anemia or during dialysis.
Administer parenteral supplements as indicated. (Refer to CP: Total Nutritional Support, p. 894.)	Hyperalimentation may be needed to enhance renal tubular regeneration/resolution of underlying disease process and to provide nutrients if oral/enteral feeding is contraindicated.
Monitor serum protein/albumin levels.	Indicator of protein needs. Note: Peritoneal dialysis is associated with significant protein loss.
Administer antiemetics, e.g., prochlorperazine (Compazine).	Reduces stimulation of the vomiting center.
Insert/maintain nasogastric tube if indicated.	May be necessary when persistent vomiting occurs or when enteric feeding is desired.

NURSING DIAGNOSIS:	MOBILITY, IMPAIRED PHYSICAL
May be related to:	Restrictive therapies, e.g., lengthy dialysis procedure
	Fear of/real danger of dislodging dialysis lines/catheter
	Decreased strength/endurance; musculoskeletal impairment
	Perceptual/cognitive impairment
Possibly evidenced by:	Reluctance to attempt movement; inability to move within physical environment
	Decreased muscle mass/tone and strength; impaired co-ordination
	Pain, discomfort
PATIENT OUTCOMES/ EVALUATION CRITERIA:	Maintains optimal mobility/function, increases strength and is free of associated complications (contractures, decubiti).

ACTIONS/INTERVENTIONS	RATIONALE
Independent	
Assess activity limitations, noting presence/degree of restriction/ability.	Influences choice of interventions.
Change position frequently when on bedrest; support affected body parts/joints with pillows, rolls, sheepskin, elbow/heel pads as indicated.	Decreases discomfort, maintains muscle strength/joint mobility, enhances circulation, and prevents skin breakdown.
Provide skin massage. Keep skin clean and dry well. Keep linens dry and wrinkle-free.	Stimulates circulation, prevents skin irritation.
Encourage deep breathing and coughing. Elevate head of bed as allowed. Turn side to side.	Mobilizes secretions, improves lung expansion and reduces risk of respiratory complications, e.g., atelectasis, pneumonia.
Provide diversion as appropriate to patient's condition, e.g., visitors, radio/television, books.	Decreases boredom, promotes relaxation.
Assist with active/passive range of motion exercises.	Maintains joint flexibility, prevents contractures, and aids in reducing muscle tension.
Institute a planned activity program with patient's input.	Increases patient's energy and sense of well-being/control.
Collaborative	
Provide foam/flotation mattress.	Reduces tissue pressure, and may enhance circulation, thereby reducing risk of dermal ischemia/breakdown.

NURSING DIAGNOSIS:	SELF-CARE DEFICIT
May be related to:	Perceptual/cognitive impairment (accumulated toxins)
	Intolerance to activity; decreased strength and endur-

ance; pain/discomfort

Possibly evidenced by: Inability to carry out activities of daily living, e.g., bathing, feeding, grooming.

PATIENT OUTCOMES/ EVALUATION CRITERIA: Participates in activities of daily living within level of own ability/constraints of the illness.

ACTIONS/INTERVENTIONS	RATIONALE
Independent	
Determine patient's ability to participate in self-care activities (scale of 0–4).	Underlying condition will dictate level of deficit/needs.
Provide assistance with activities as necessary.	Meets needs while supporting patient participation and independence.
Encourage/use energy saving techniques, e.g., sitting, not standing; shower chair; doing tasks in small increments.	Conserves energy, prevents fatigue, enhances patient ability to perform tasks.
Schedule activities allowing patient sufficient time to accomplish tasks to fullest extent of ability.	Unhurried approach reduces frustration, promotes patient participation, enhancing self-esteem.

NURSING DIAGNOSIS: BOWEL ELIMINATION, ALTERED: CONSTIPATION [POTENTIAL]

May be related to: Decreased fluid intake, altered dietary pattern

Reduced intestinal motility, compression of bowel (peritoneal dialysate); electrolyte imbalances; decreased mobility

Possibly evidenced by: [Not applicable; presence of signs and symptoms establishes an *actual* diagnosis.]

PATIENT OUTCOMES/ EVALUATION CRITERIA: Restores/maintains normal patterns of bowel function.

ACTIONS/INTERVENTIONS	RATIONALE
Independent	
Auscultate bowel sounds. Note consistency/frequency of bowel movements, presence of abdominal distention.	Decreased bowel sounds, passage of hard formed/ dry stools suggests constipation and requires ongoing intervention to manage.
Review current medication regimen.	Side effects of some drugs (e.g., iron products, some antacids) may compound problem.
Ascertain usual dietary pattern/food choices.	Although restrictions may be present, thoughtful consideration of menu choices can aid in controlling problem.
Add fresh fruits, vegetables, and fiber to diet when indicated.	Provides bulk, which improves stool consistency.

ACTIONS/INTERVENTIONS

Independent

Encourage/assist with ambulation when able.

Provide privacy at bedside commode/bathroom.

Collaborative

Administer stool softeners (e.g., Colace), bulk-forming laxatives (e.g., Metamucil) as indicated.

Keep patient NPO; insert nasogastric tube as indicated.

RATIONALE

Activity may stimulate peristalsis, promoting return to normal bowel activity.

Promotes psychologic comfort needed for elimination.

Produces a softer/more easily evacuated stool.

Decompresses stomach when recurrent/unrelieved vomiting occurs. Large gastric output suggests ileus (common early complication of peritoneal dialysis) with accumulation of gas and intestinal fluid which cannot be passed rectally.

NURSING DIAGNOSIS:	THOUGHT PROCESSES, ALTERED
May be related to:	**Physiologic changes, e.g., presence of uremic toxins, electrolyte imbalances, hypervolemia/fluid shifts; hyperglycemia (infusion of a dialysate with a high glucose concentration)**
Possibly evidenced by:	**Changes in mentation/behavior, e.g., decreased concentration, memory; disorientation; altered sleep patterns; lethargy, confusion, stupor, dementia**
PATIENT OUTCOMES/ EVALUATION CRITERIA:	**Regains usual/improved level of mentation. Recognizes changes in thinking behavior and demonstrates behaviors to prevent/minimize changes.**

ACTIONS/INTERVENTIONS

Independent

Assess for behavioral change/change in level of consciousness, e.g., orientation to time, place, and person.

Keep explanations simple, reorient frequently. Provide "normal" day/night lighting patterns, clock, calendar.

Provide a safe environment, restrain as indicated, pad siderails.

Drain peritoneal dialysate promptly at end of specified equilibration period.

Investigate complaint of headache, associated with onset of nausea/vomiting, confusion/agitation, hypertension, tremors, or seizure activity.

RATIONALE

May indicate level of uremic toxicity, response or developing complication of dialysis, and requires further assessment/intervention.

Improves reality orientation.

Prevents patient trauma and/or inadvertent removal of dialysis lines/catheter.

Prompt outflow will decrease risk of hyperglycemia/hyperosmolar fluid shifts affecting cerebral function.

May reflect development of disequilibrium syndrome, which can occur near completion of/following hemodialysis and is thought to be caused by ultrafiltration or by the too rapid removal of urea from the bloodstream not accompanied by equivalent removal from brain tissue. The hypertonic cerebrospinal fluid causes a fluid shift into the brain, resulting in cerebral edema.

ACTIONS/INTERVENTIONS

Independent

Monitor changes in speech pattern, development of dementia, myoclonus activity during hemodialysis.

Collaborative

Monitor BUN/Cr serum glucose; alternate/change dialysate concentrations or add insulin as indicated.

Obtain aluminum level as indicated.

Administer medication, as indicated, e.g., phenytoin (Dilantin).

RATIONALE

Occasionally, accumulation of aluminum may cause dialysis dementia, progressing to death if untreated.

Follows progression/resolution of azotemia. Hyperglycemia may develop secondary to glucose crossing peritoneal membrane and entering circulation. May require initiation of insulin therapy.

Elevation may warn of impending cerebral involvement/dialysis dementia.

If disequilibrium syndrome occurs during dialysis, medication may be needed to control seizures in addition to a change in dialysis prescription, or discontinuation of therapy.

NURSING DIAGNOSIS:	ANXIETY [SPECIFY LEVEL]/FEAR
May be related to:	Situational crisis, threat to self-concept; change in health status/role functioning, socioeconomic status
	Threat of death, unknown consequences/outcome
PATIENT OUTCOMES/ EVALUATION CRITERIA:	Verbalizes awareness of feelings and reduction of anxiety/fear to a manageable level. Demonstrates problem-solving skills and effective use of resources. Appears relaxed, able to rest/sleep appropriately.

ACTIONS/INTERVENTIONS

Independent

Assess level of fear of both patient and SO. Note signs of denial, depression, or narrowed focus of attention.

Explain procedures/care as delivered. Repeat explanations frequently/as needed.

Acknowledge normalcy of feelings in this situation.

Encourage and provide opportunities for patient/SO to ask questions and verbalize concerns.

Encourage SO to participate in care, as indicated.

Acknowledge concerns of patient/SO. (Refer to CP: Psychosocial Aspects of Acute Care, p. 773.)

RATIONALE

Helps determine the kind of interventions required.

Fear of unknown is lessened by information/knowledge and may enhance acceptance of dialysis. Alteration in thought processes and high levels of anxiety/fear may reduce comprehension, requiring repetition of important information.

Knowing feelings are normal can allay fear that patient is losing control.

Creates feeling of openness and cooperation and provides information that will assist in problem identification/solving.

Involvement promotes sense of sharing, strengthens feelings of usefulness, provides opportunity to acknowledge individual capabilities, and may lessen fear of the unknown.

Prognosis/possibility of need for long-term dialysis and resultant lifestyle changes are a major concern for this patient and those who may be involved in future care.

ACTIONS/INTERVENTIONS	RATIONALE

Independent

Point out positive indicators of treatment, e.g., improvement in laboratory values, stable BP, lessened fatigue.

Promotes sense of success/progress.

NURSING DIAGNOSIS:	SELF-CONCEPT, DISTURBANCE IN: (SPECIFY)
May be related to:	Situational crisis, chronic illness with changes in usual roles
Possibly evidenced by:	Verbalization of changes in lifestyle; focus on past function, negative feelings about body; feelings of helplessness, powerlessness
	Extension of body boundary to incorporate environmental objects (e.g., dialysis machine)
	Change in social involvement
	Overdependence on others for care, not taking responsibility for self-care/lack of follow-through, self-destructive behavior
PATIENT OUTCOMES/ EVALUATION CRITERIA:	Identifies feelings and methods for coping with negative perception of self. Verbalizes acceptance of self in situation. Demonstrates adaptation to changes/events that have occurred, as evidenced by setting realistic goals and active participation in care/life.

ACTIONS/INTERVENTIONS	RATIONALE

Independent

Assess level of patient's knowledge about condition and treatment, and anxiety related to current situation.

Identifies extent of problem/concern and interventions necessary.

Discuss meaning of loss/change to the patient.

Some patients may view situation as a challenge, though many have difficulty dealing with changes in life/role performance and loss of ability to control own body.

Note withdrawn behavior, ineffective use of denial or behaviors indicative of overconcern with body and its functions.

Indicators of developing difficulty handling stress of what is happening.

Assess use of addictive substances (e.g., alcohol), self-destructive/suicidal behavior.

May reflect dysfunctional coping and attempt to handle problems in an ineffective manner.

Determine stage of grieving. Note signs of severe/ prolonged depression.

Identification of stage patient is experiencing provides guide to recognizing and dealing appropriately with behavior. Prolonged depression may indicate need for further intervention.

Acknowledge normalcy of feelings.

Recognition that feelings are to be expected helps patient to accept and deal with them more effectively.

Encourage verbalization of personal and work conflicts that may arise, and active-listen concerns.

Helps patient ot identify problems and problem-solve solutions.

ACTIONS/INTERVENTIONS

Independent

Determine patient's role in family constellation and patient's perception of expectation of self and others.

Recommend SO treat patient normally and not as an invalid.

Assist patient to incorporate disease management into lifestyle.

Identify strengths, past successes, previous methods patient has used to deal with life stressors.

Help patient identify areas over which they have some measure of control. Provide opportunity to participate in decision-making process.

Collaborative

Refer to health care/community resources, e.g., support groups, psychiatric nurse specialist, social service, vocational counselor.

RATIONALE

Long-term/permanent illness and disability alter patient's ability to fulfill usual role(s) in family/work setting. Unrealistic expectations can undermine self-esteem and affect outcome of illness.

Conveys expectation that patient is able to manage situation and helps to maintain sense of self-esteem and purpose in life.

Necessities of treatment assume a more normal aspect when they are a part of the daily routine.

Focusing on these reminders of own ability to deal with problems can help patient to deal with current situation.

Provides sense of control over uncontrollable situation, fostering independence.

Provides additional assistance for long-term management of chronic illness/change in lifestyle.

NURSING DIAGNOSIS:	KNOWLEDGE DEFICIT [LEARNING NEED] (SPECIFY)
May be related to:	Lack of exposure/recall
	Unfamiliarity with information resources
	Cognitive limitations
Possibly evidenced by:	Questions/request for information; statement of misconception
	Inaccurate follow-through of instruction; development of preventable complications
PATIENT OUTCOMES/ EVALUATION CRITERIA:	Verbalizes understanding of condition and relationship of signs/symptoms to the disease process. Correctly performs necessary procedures and explains reasons for actions.

ACTIONS/INTERVENTIONS

Independent

Note level of anxiety/fear and alteration of thought processes.

Review particular disease process, procedures, and purpose of dialysis in terms understandable to the patient. Repeat explanations.

Acknowledge that certain feelings/patterns of response are normal during course of therapy.

RATIONALE

These factors directly affect ability to participate/access and use knowledge.

Providing information at the level of the patient/SO understanding will reduce anxiety and misconceptions about what the patient is experiencing.

Patient/SO may initially be hopeful and postive about the future, but as treatment continues and progress is

ACTIONS/INTERVENTIONS	RATIONALE
Independent	
	less dramatic, they can become discouraged/depressed, and conflicts of dependence/independence may develop.
Encourage and provide opportunity for questions.	Enhances learning process, and reduces anxiety associated with the unknown.
Stress necessity of reading all product labels (food/beverage and OTC drugs) and not taking medications without prior approval of health care provider.	It is difficult to maintain electrolyte balance when exogenous intake is not factored into dietary restriction, e.g., hypercalcemia can result from routine supplement use in combination with increased dietary intake of calcium-fortified foods and medicines.
Discuss significance of maintaining nutritious eating habits; preventing wide fluctuation of fluid/electrolyte balance; avoidance of crowds/people with infectious processes.	Depressed immune system, presence of anemia, invasive procedures, and malnutrition potentiate risk of infection.
Instruct patient/SO in home dialysis as indicated:	
Purpose of dialysis;	Provides knowledge base on which patient can make informed observations/choices.
Operation and maintenance of equipment (including vascular shunt); sources of supplies;	Information diminishes anxiety of the unknown and provides opportunity for patient to be knowledgeable about own care.
Aseptic/clean technique;	Prevents contamination and reduces risk of infection.
Self-monitoring of effectiveness of procedure;	Provides information necessary to evaluate effects of therapy/need for change.
Management of potential complications;	Reduces concerns regarding personal well-being; supports efforts at self-care.
Contact person.	Readily available support person can answer questions, troubleshoot problems, and facilitate timely medical intervention when indicated.
Identify health care/community resources, e.g., dialysis support group, social services, mental health clinic.	Knowledge of availability of these resources assists patient/SO to manage own care more effectively.

PERITONEAL DIALYSIS

The peritoneum serves as the semipermeable membrane permitting transfer of nitrogenous wastes/toxins and fluid from the blood into a dialysate solution. Peritoneal dialysis is sometimes preferred because it uses a simpler technique and provides more gradual physiologic changes than hemodialysis.

Manual single bottle method is usually done as an inpatient procedure with short dwell times of only 30–60 minutes and is repeated until desired effects are achieved.

Continuous ambulatory peritoneal dialysis (CAPD) permits the patient to manage procedure at home with bag and gravity flow, using a prolonged dwell time at night and a total of three to five cycles daily, 7 days a week.

Continuous cycling peritoneal dialysis (CCPD) mechanically cycles shorter dwell times during night, with a longer dwell time during daylight hours, increasing the patient's independence.

NURSING DIAGNOSIS:	FLUID VOLUME, ALTERED: EXCESS [POTENTIAL]
May be related to:	**Inadequate osmotic gradient of dialysate**
	Fluid retention (malpositioned, kinked/clotted catheter, bowel distention; peritonitis, scarring of peritoneum)
	Excessive oral/IV intake

Possibly evidenced by:	[Not applicable; presence of signs and symptoms establishes an *actual* diagnosis.]
PATIENT OUTCOMES/ EVALUATION CRITERIA:	Demonstrates dialysate outflow exceeding/approximating infusion; free of rapid weight gain, edema, pulmonary congestion.

ACTIONS/INTERVENTIONS

Independent

Maintain a record of inflow/outflow volumes, and cumulative fluid balance.

Record serial weights, compare with intake/output balance. Weigh patient when abdomen is empty of dialysate (consistent reference point).

Assess patency of catheter, noting difficulty in drainage. Note presence of fibrin strings/plugs.

Check tubing for kinks; note placement of bottles/bags. Anchor catheter so that adequate inflow/outflow is achieved.

Turn from side to side, elevate the head of the bed, apply gentle pressure to the abdomen.

Note abdominal distention associated with decreased bowel sounds, changes in stool consistency, complaints of constipation.

Monitor BP, pulse, noting hypertension, bounding pulses, neck vein distention, peripheral edema; measure CVP, if available.

Assess heart and breath sounds, noting S_3 and/or crackles, rhonchi.

Evaluate development of tachypnea, dyspnea, increased respiratory effort. Drain dialysate, and notify physician.

Assess for headache, muscle cramps, mental confusion, disorientation.

Collaborative

Alter dialysate regime as indicated.

Monitor serum sodium.

Add heparin to initial dialysis runs, assist with irrigation of catheter with heparinized saline.

Maintain fluid restriction as indicated.

RATIONALE

In most cases, the amount drained should equal or exceed the amount instilled. A positive balance indicates need of further evaluation.

Serial body weights are an accurate indicator of fluid volume status. A positive fluid balance with an increase in weight indicates fluid retention.

Slowing of flow rate/presence of fibrin suggests partial catheter occlusion requiring further evaluation/intervention.

Improper functioning of equipment may result in retained fluid in abdomen, and insufficient clearance of toxins.

May enhance outflow of fluid when catheter is malpositional/obstructed by the omentum.

Bowel distention/constipation may impede outflow of effluent. (Refer to ND: Bowel Elimination, Altered: Constipation, p. 570.)

Elevations indicate hypervolemia.

Fluid overload may potentiate CHF/pulmonary edema.

Abdominal distention/diaphragmatic compression may cause respiratory distress.

Symptoms suggest hyponatremia or water intoxication.

Changes may be needed in the glucose or sodium concentration to facilitate efficient dialysis.

Hypernatremia may be present, although serum levels may reflect dilutional effect of fluid volume overload.

May be useful in preventing fibrin clot formation, which can obstruct peritoneal catheter.

Fluid restrictions may have to be continued to decrease fluid volume overload.

NURSING DIAGNOSIS:	FLUID VOLUME DEFICIT, POTENTIAL
May be related to:	Use of hypertonic dialysate with excessive removal of fluid from circulating volume
Possibly evidenced by:	[Not applicable; presence of signs and symptoms establishes an *actual* diagnosis.]
PATIENT OUTCOMES/ EVALUATION CRITERIA:	Achieves desired alteration in fluid volume and weight with blood pressure, electrolyte levels within acceptable range, free of symptoms of dehydration.

ACTIONS/INTERVENTIONS	RATIONALE
Independent	
Maintain record of inflow/outflow volumes and individual/cumulative fluid balance.	Provides information about the status of the patient's loss or gain at the end of each exchange.
Adhere to schedule for draining dialysate from abdomen.	Prolonged dwell times, especially when 4.5% glucose solution is used, may cause excess fluid loss.
Weigh when abdomen is empty, following initial 6–10 runs, then as indicated.	Detects rate of fluid removal by comparison with baseline body weights.
Monitor BP (lying and sitting) and pulse. Note level of jugular pulsation.	Decreased BP, postural hypotension, and tachycardia are early signs of hypovolemia.
Note complaints of dizziness, nausea, increasing thirst.	May indicate hypovolemia hyperosmolar syndrome.
Inspect mucous membranes, evaluate skin turgor, peripheral pulses, capillary refill.	Dry mucous membranes, poor skin turgor and diminished pulses/capillary refill are indicators of dehydration and need for increased intake/changes in strength of dialysate.
Collaborative	
Monitor laboratory studies as indicated, e.g.:	
Serum sodium and glucose levels;	Hypertonic solutions may cause hypernatremia by removing more water than sodium. In addition, dextrose may be absorbed from the dialysate, thereby elevating serum glucose.
Serum potassium levels.	Hypokalemia may occur and can cause cardiac dysrhythmias.

NURSING DIAGNOSIS:	INJURY, POTENTIAL FOR: TRAUMA
May be related to:	Catheter inserted into peritoneal cavity
	Site near the bowel/bladder with potential for perforation during insertion or by manipulation of the catheter
Possibly evidenced by:	[Not applicable; presence of signs and symptoms establishes an *actual* diagnosis.]

577

PATIENT OUTCOMES/ EVALUATION CRITERIA:	Injury does not occur to bowel or bladder.

ACTIONS/INTERVENTIONS

Independent

Have patient empty bladder prior to peritoneal catheter insertion if indwelling catheter not present.

Anchor catheter/tubing with tape. Stress importance of patient avoiding pulling/pushing on catheter. Restrain hands if indicated.

Note presence of fecal material in dialysate effluent, or strong urge to defecate, accompanied by severe, watery diarrhea.

Note complaints of intense urge to void, or large urine output following initiation of dialysis run. Test urine for sugar as indicated.

Stop dialysis if there is evidence of bowel/bladder perforation, leaving peritoneal catheter in place.

RATIONALE

An empty bladder is more distant from insertion site and reduces likelihood of being punctured during catheter insertion.

Reduces risk of trauma by manipulation of the catheter.

Suggests bowel perforation with mixing of dialysate and bowel contents.

Suggests bladder perforation with dialysate leaking into bladder. Dialysate contains glucose and if it is leaking into the bladder, the urine will have an elevated glucose level.

Prompt action will prevent further injury. Immediate surgical repair may be required. Leaving catheter in place facilitates diagnosing/locating the perforation.

NURSING DIAGNOSIS:	COMFORT, ALTERED: PAIN, ACUTE
May be related to:	Insertion of catheter through abdominal wall/catheter irritation, improper catheter placement
	Irritation/infection within the peritoneal cavity
	Infusion of cold or acidic dialysate, abdominal distention, rapid infusion of dialysate
Possibly evidenced by:	Complaints of pain
	Self-focusing
	Guarding/distraction behaviors, restlessness
PATIENT OUTCOMES/ EVALUATION CRITERIA:	Verbalizes decrease of pain/discomfort. Demonstrates relaxed posture/facial expression, able to sleep/rest appropriately.

ACTIONS/INTERVENTIONS

Independent

Investigate patient's complaints of pain; note intensity (1–10), location, and precipitating factors.

Explain that initial discomfort usually subsides after the first few exchanges.

Monitor for pain that begins during inflow and continues during equilibration phase. Slow infusion rate as indicated.

RATIONALE

Assists in identification of source of pain and appropriate interventions.

Explanation may reduce anxiety, and promote relaxation during procedure.

Pain will occur at these times if acidic dialysate causes chemical irritation of peritoneal membrane.

ACTIONS/INTERVENTIONS	RATIONALE

Independent

Note discomfort which is most pronounced near the end of inflow. Instill no more than 2000 ml of solution at one time.

Likely the result of abdominal distention from dialysate. Amount of infusion may have to be decreased initially.

Note complaint of pain in area of shoulder blade. Prevent air from entering peritoneal cavity during infusion.

Inadvertent introduction of air into the abdomen irritates the diaphragm and results in referred pain to shoulder blade. This type of discomfort may also be reported during initiation of therapy/during infusions and usually is related to stretching/irritation of the diaphragm with abdominal distention. Smaller exchange volumes may be required until patient adjusts.

Elevate head of bed at intervals. Turn patient from side to side. Provide back care and tissue massage.

Position changes may relieve abdominal and general muscle discomfort.

Warm dialysate to body temperature before infusing.

Warming the solution increases the rate of urea removal by dilating peritoneal vessels. Cold dialysate causes vasoconstriction, which can cause discomfort and/or excessively lower the core body temperature, precipitating cardiac arrest.

Monitor for severe/continuous abdominal pain, and temperature elevation (especially after dialysis has been discontinued).

May indicate developing peritonitis. (Refer to ND: Infection, Potential for, following.)

Encourage use of relaxation techniques, e.g., deep-breathing exercises, guided imagery, visualization. Provide diversional activities.

Redirects attention, promotes sense of control.

Collaborative

Administer analgesics.

Relieves pain and discomfort.

Add sodium hydroxide to dialysate, if indicated.

Occasionally used to alter pH if patient is not tolerating acidic dialysate.

NURSING DIAGNOSIS:	INFECTION, POTENTIAL FOR: [PERITONITIS]
May be related to:	Contamination of the catheter during insertion, changing the tubings/bottles/bags
	Skin contaminants at catheter insertion site
	Sterile peritonitis (response to the composition of dialysate)
Possibly evidenced by:	[Not applicable; presence of signs and symptoms establishes an *actual* diagnosis.]
PATIENT OUTCOMES/ EVALUATION CRITERIA:	Free of signs/symptoms of infection. Identifies interventions to prevent/reduce risk of infection.

ACTIONS/INTERVENTIONS	RATIONALE

Independent

Observe meticulous aseptic techniques and wear masks during catheter insertion, dressing changes

Prevents the introduction of organisms and airborne contamination which may cause infection.

ACTIONS/INTERVENTIONS

Independent

and whenever the system is opened. Change tubings per protocol.

Change dressings as indicated being careful not to dislodge the catheter. Note character, color, odor of drainage from around insertion site.

Observe color and clarity of effluent.

Apply Betadine barrier in distal, clamped portion of catheter when intermittent dialysis therapy used.

Investigate complaints of nausea/vomiting; increased/severe abdominal pain, rebound tenderness, fever, and leukocytosis.

Collaborative

Monitor WBC count of effluent.

Obtain specimens of blood, effluent and/or drainage from insertion site as indicated for culture/sensitivity.

Monitor renal clearance/BUN, creatinine.

Administer antibiotics systemically or in dialysate as indicated.

RATIONALE

Moist environment promotes bacterial growth. Purulent drainage at insertion site suggests presence of local infection.

Cloudy effluent is suggestive of peritoneal infection.

Reduces risk of bacterial entry through catheter between dialysis treatments when catheter is disconnected from closed system.

Signs/symptoms suggesting peritonitis, requiring prompt intervention.

Presence of WBCs initially may reflect normal response to a foreign substance; however, continued/new elevation suggests developing infection.

Identifies types of organism(s) present, choice of interventions.

Choice and dosage of antibiotics will be influenced by renal function.

Treats infection, prevents sepsis.

NURSING DIAGNOSIS:	BREATHING PATTERN, INEFFECTIVE [POTENTIAL]
May be related to:	Abdominal pressure/restricted diaphragmatic excursion; rapid infusion of dialysate; pain Inflammatory process (e.g., atelectasis/pneumonia)
Possibly evidenced by:	[Not applicable; presence of signs and symptoms establishes an *actual* diagnosis.]
PATIENT OUTCOMES/ EVALUATION CRITERIA:	Displays an effective respiratory pattern with clear breath sounds, ABGs within patient's normal range and free of dyspnea/cyanosis.

ACTIONS/INTERVENTIONS

Independent

Monitor respiratory rate/effort. Reduce infusion rate if dypsnea present.

Auscultate lungs, noting decreased, absent, or adventitious breath sounds, e.g., crackles/wheezes/rhonchi.

RATIONALE

Tachypnea, dyspnea, shortness of breath and shallow breathing during dialysis suggests diaphragmatic pressure from distended peritoneal cavity, or may indicate developing complications.

Decreased areas of ventilation suggest presence of atelectasis, whereas adventitious sounds may suggest fluid overload, retained secretions or infection.

ACTIONS/INTERVENTIONS	RATIONALE

Independent

Note character, amount and color of secretions.

Patient is susceptible to pulmonary infections as a result of depressed cough reflex and respiratory effort, increased viscosity of secretions, as well as altered immune response and chronic/debilitating disease.

Elevate head of bed. Promote deep-breathing exercises and coughing.

Facilitates chest expansion/ventilation and mobilization of secretions.

Collaborative

Review ABGs and serial chest x-rays.

Changes in PaO_2/$PaCO_2$ and appearance of infiltrates/congestion on chest x-ray suggests developing pulmonary problems.

Administer supplemental oxygen as indicated.

Maximizes oxygen for vascular uptake, preventing/lessening hypoxia.

Administer analgesics as indicated.

Alleviates pain, promotes comfortable breathing.

ACUTE HEMODIALYSIS

Blood is shunted through an artificial kidney (dialyzer) for removal of toxins/excess fluid and then returned to the venous circulation. Hemodialysis is a faster and more efficient method than peritoneal dialysis for removing urea and other toxic products, but requires permanent arteriovenous access.

NURSING DIAGNOSIS:	INJURY, POTENTIAL FOR: LOSS OF VASCULAR ACCESS
May be related to:	Clotting; hemorrhage related to accidental disconnection; infection
Possibly evidenced by:	[Not applicable; presence of signs and symptoms establishes an *actual* diagnosis.]
PATIENT OUTCOMES/ EVALUATION CRITERIA:	Maintains patent vascular access.

ACTIONS/INTERVENTIONS	RATIONALE

Independent

Clotting:

Monitor internal AV shunt patency at frequent intervals:

Palpate for distal thrill;

Thrill is caused by turbulence of high-pressure arterial blood flow entering low-pressure venous system and should be palpable above venous exit site.

Auscultate for a bruit,

Bruit is the sound caused by the turbulence of arterial blood entering venous system and should be audible by stethoscope, although may be very faint.

Note color of blood, and/or obvious separation of cells and serum;

Change of color from uniform medium red color to dark purplish red color suggests sluggish blood flow/early clotting. Separation in tubing is indicative of clotting. Very dark reddish black blood next to clear yellow fluid indicates full clot formation.

ACTIONS/INTERVENTIONS	RATIONALE

Independent

Palpate skin around shunt for warmth.	Diminished blood flow will result in "coolness" of shunt.
Notify physician and/or initiate declotting procedure if there is evidence of loss of shunt patency.	Rapid intervention may save access; however, declotting must be done by experienced personnel.
Evaluate complaints of pain, numbness/tingling; note extremity swelling distal to access.	May indicate inadequate blood supply.
Avoid trauma to shunt; e.g., handle tubing gently, maintain cannula alignment. Limit activity of extremity. Avoid taking BP or drawing blood samples in shunt extremity. Instruct patient not to sleep, or carry packages, books, purse on affected extremity.	Decreases risk of clotting/disconnection.

Hemorrhage:

Attach two cannula clamps to shunt dressing. Have tourniquet available. If cannulas separate, clamp first the arterial, then venous cannula. If tubing comes out of vessel, clamp cannula that is still in place and apply direct pressure to bleeding site. Place tourniquet above site or inflate BP cuff to pressure just above patient's systolic BP.	Prevents massive blood loss if cannula separates or shunt is dislodged while awaiting medical assistance.

Infection:

Assess skin around vascular access, noting redness, swelling, local warmth, exudate, tenderness.	Signs of local infection, which can progress to sepsis if untreated.
Avoid contamination of access site. Use aseptic technique and masks when giving shunt care, applying/changing dressings, and when starting/completing dialysis process.	Prevents introduction of organisms which can cause infection.
Monitor temperature. Note presence of fever, chills, hypotension.	Signs of infection/sepsis requiring prompt medical intervention.

Collaborative

Culture the site/obtain blood samples as indicated.	Determines presence of pathogens.
Administer medications as indicated, e.g.:	
Heparin (low-dose);	Infused on arterial side of filter to prevent clotting in the filter without systemic side effects.
Antibiotics (systemic and/or topical).	Prompt treatment of infection may save access, prevent sepsis.

NURSING DIAGNOSIS:	**FLUID VOLUME DEFICIT, POTENTIAL**
May be related to:	**Ultrafiltration**
	Fluid restrictions; actual blood loss (systemic heparinization or disconnection of the shunt)
Possibly evidenced by:	**[Not applicable; presence of signs and symptoms establishes an *actual* diagnosis.]**

PATIENT OUTCOMES/ EVALUATION CRITERIA:	Maintains fluid balance as evidenced by stable/ appropriate weight and vital signs, good skin turgor, moist mucous membranes, absence of bleeding.

ACTIONS/INTERVENTIONS	RATIONALE

Independent

Measure all sources of intake/output. Have patient keep diary.	Aids in evaluating fluid status, especially when compared with weights.
Weigh daily before/after dialysis run using bed scales.	Weight loss over precisely measured time is a measure of ultrafiltration and fluid removal.
Monitor BP, pulse, and hemodynamic pressures if available during dialysis.	Hypotension, tachycardia, falling hemodynamic pressures suggest volume depletion.
Note/ascertain whether diuretics and/or antihypertensives are to be withheld.	Dialysis potentiates hypotensive effects if these drugs have been ingested.
Monitor hourly outputs during continuous arteriovenous hemofiltration (CAVH) and compare with total intake to calculate net fluid balance.	Excess/rapid fluid removal may result in hypotension/ hypovolemia.
Verify continuity of shunt/access catheter.	Disconnected shunt/open access will permit exsanguination.
Apply external shunt dressing. Permit no puncture of shunt.	Minimizes stress on cannula insertion site to reduce inadvertent dislodgement and bleeding from site.
Place patient in a supine/Trendelenburg position as necessary.	Maximizes venous return when hypotension occurs.
Assess for oozing or frank bleeding at access site, mucous membranes, incisions/wounds. Hematest/ guaiac stools, gastric drainage.	Systemic heparinization during dialysis increases clotting times and places patient at risk for bleeding, especially first 4 hours after procedure.

Collaborative

Monitor laboratory studies as indicated:	
Hb and Hct;	May be reduced because of anemia, hemodilution, or actual blood loss.
Serum electrolytes and pH;	Imbalances may require changes in the dialysate solution or supplemental replacement to achieve balance.
Clotting times, e.g., ACT, PT/PTT, and platelet count.	Use of heparin to prevent clotting in blood lines and hemofilter (alters coagulation) may potentiate active bleeding.
Administer IV solutions (e.g., normal saline)/or volume expanders (e.g., albumin) during dialysis as indicated;	Volume expanders may be required during/following hemodialysis if sudden/marked hypotension occurs. Saline/dextrose solutions, electrolytes, and sodium bicarbonate may be infused in the venous side of CAV hemofilter when high ultrafiltration rates are used for removal of extracellular fluid and toxic solutes.
Blood/packed red cells if needed.	Destruction of red blood cells (hemolysis) by mechanical dialysis, hemorrhagic losses, decreased red cell production may result in profound/progressive anemia.
Reduce rate of ultrafiltration during dialysis as indicated.	Reduces the amount of water being removed and may correct hypotension/hypovolemia.
Administer protamine sulfate if indicated.	May be needed to return clotting times to normal or if heparin rebound occurs (up to 16 hours after hemodialysis).

583

NURSING DIAGNOSIS:	FLUID VOLUME, ALTERED: EXCESS [POTENTIAL]
May be related to:	Rapid/excessive fluid intake; IV blood, plasma expanders, saline given to support BP during dialysis
Possibly evidenced by:	[Not applicable; presence of signs and symptoms establishes an *actual* diagnosis.]
PATIENT OUTCOMES/ EVALUATION CRITERIA:	Maintains "dry weight" within patient's normal range; free of edema; breath sounds clear and serum sodium levels within normal limits.

ACTIONS/INTERVENTIONS	RATIONALE
Independent	
Measure all sources of intake/output. Weigh routinely.	Aids in evaluating fluid status especially when compared with weight. Weight gain between treatments should not exceed 0.5 kg/day.
Monitor BP, pulse.	Hypertension and tachycardia between hemodialysis runs may result from fluid overload and/or heart failure.
Note presence of peripheral/sacral edema, respiratory rales, dyspnea, orthopnea, distended neck veins, ECG changes indicative of ventricular hypertrophy. (Refer to CP: Congestive Heart Failure, p. 41.)	Fluid volume excess because of inefficient dialysis or repeated hypervolemia between dialysis treatments may cause/exacerbate heart failure, as indicated by signs/symptoms of respiratory and/or systemic venous congestion.
Note changes in mentation. (Refer to ND: Thought Processes, Altered, p. 571.)	Fluid overload/hypervolemia, may potentiate cerebral edema (disequilibrium syndrome).
Collaborative	
Monitor serum sodium levels. Restrict sodium intake as indicated.	High sodium levels are associated with fluid overload, edema, hypertension, and cardiac complications.
Restrict PO/IV fluid intake as indicated, spacing allowed fluids through 24-hour period.	The intermittent nature of hemodialysis results in fluid retention/overload between procedures and may require fluid restriction. Spacing fluids helps reduce thirst.

Urinary Diversions/Urostomy (Postoperative Care) _____

Ileal conduit: Ureters are anastomosed to a segment of ileum resected with the blood supply intact (usually 15–20 cm long). The proximal section is closed, and the distal end brought to skin opening to form a stoma (a passageway, not a storage reservoir).

Colonic conduit: This is a similar procedure using a segment of colon.

Ureterostomy: The ureter(s) is brought directly through the abdominal wall to form its own stoma.

PATIENT ASSESSMENT DATA BASE

Data are dependent on underlying problem, duration, and severity, e.g., malignant bladder tumor, congenital malformations, trauma, chronic infections, or intractable incontinence due to injury/disease of other body systems (e.g., multiple sclerosis). (Refer to appropriate CP.)

TEACHING/LEARNING

Discharge Plan Considerations: May require assistance with management of ostomy and acquisition of supplies.

DIAGNOSTIC STUDIES

IVP: visualizes size/location of kidneys and ureters and to rule out presence of tumors elsewhere in urinary tract.

Cystoscopy with biopsy: determines tumor location/degree of malignancy. Ultraviolet cystoscopy outlines bladder lesion.

Bone scan: determines presence of metastatic disease.

Bilateral pedal lymphangiogram: determines involvement of pelvic nodes, where bladder tumor easily seeds because of close proximity.

CT scan: defines size of tumor mass, degree of pelvic spread.

Urine cystology: detects tumor cells in urine (for determining presence and type of tumor).

Endoscopy: evaluates intestines for use as conduit.

Conduitogram: assesses length and emptying ability of the conduit and presence of stricture, obstruction, reflux, angulation, calculi, or tumor (may complicate or contraindicate use as a urinary diversion).

NURSING PRIORITIES

1. Assist patient/SO in physical/psychosocial adjustment.
2. Prevent complications.
3. Support independence in self-care.
4. Provide information about procedure/prognosis, treatment needs, potential complications, and resources.

DISCHARGE CRITERIA

1. Adjusting to perceived/actual changes.
2. Complications prevented/minimized.
3. Self-care needs met by self/with assistance as necessary.
4. Procedure/prognosis, therapeutic regimen, potential complications understood and sources of support identified.

NURSING DIAGNOSIS:	SKIN INTEGRITY, IMPAIRED: POTENTIAL
May be related to:	**Absence of sphincter at stoma (actual)**
	Character/flow of urine from stoma

Reaction to product/chemicals; improper fitting of appliance or removal of adhesive

Possibly evidenced by: [Not applicable; presence of signs and symptoms establishes an *actual* diagnosis.]

PATIENT OUTCOMES/ EVALUATION CRITERIA: Maintains skin integrity. Identifies individual risk factors. Demonstrates behaviors/techniques to promote healing/prevent skin breakdown.

ACTIONS/INTERVENTIONS	RATIONALE
Independent	
Inspect stoma/peristomal skin. Note irritation, bruises (dark, bluish color), rashes, status of sutures.	Monitors healing process/effectiveness of appliances, and identifies areas of concern, need for further evaluation/intervention. Stoma should be pink or reddish, similar to mucous membranes. Early identification of stomal necrosis/ischemia or fungal infection provides for timely interventions to prevent serious complications. Sutures may not adequately hold stoma in place to prevent prolapse, ischemia, or obstruction. Tension on mesenteric vessels may cause ischemia. Color changes may be temporary, but persistent changes may require surgical intervention.
Clean with water and pat dry.	Maintaining a clean/dry area helps to prevent skin breakdown.
Handle stoma gently to prevent irritation.	Mucosa has good blood supply and bleeds easily with rubbing or trauma.
Measure stoma periodically, e.g., each appliance change for first 6 weeks, then monthly times six.	As postoperative edema resolves (during first 6 weeks), size of appliance must be altered to ensure proper fit so that urine is collected as it flows from the ostomy, and contact with the skin is prevented.
Make sure opening on adhesive backing of pouch is only 1/6 to 1/8 inch larger than the base of the stoma with adequate adhesiveness left to apply pouch.	Prevents trauma to the stoma tissue and protects the peristomal skin. Adequate adhesive area is important to maintain a seal. Note: Too tight a fit may cause stomal edema or stenosis.
Use a transparent, odor-proof drainable pouch. Keep gauze square/wick over stoma while cleansing area, and have patient cough or strain before applying pouch.	A transparent appliance during first 4–6 weeks allows easy observation of stoma and stents (when used) without necessity of removing pouch and irritating skin. Covering stoma prevents urine from wetting the peristomal area. Coughing empties distal portion of conduit, followed by a brief pause in drainage to facilitate application of pouch.
Apply effective sealant barrier, e.g., Skin Prep/Gel or similar products.	Protects skin from pouch adhesive, enhances adhesiveness of pouch, and facilitates removal of pouch when necessary.
Avoid use of karaya type appliances.	Will not protect skin as urine melts karaya.
Apply waterproof tape around pouch edges if desired.	Reinforces anchoring.
Connect to continuous bedside drainage system.	Rate of urine formation is increased while IV fluids are administered. Weight of the urine will cause pouch to pull loose/leak when pouch becomes more than half full.
Empty and cleanse ostomy pouch on a routine basis, using vinegar solution.	Frequent pouch changes are irritating to the skin and should be avoided. Emptying and rinsing the pouch

ACTIONS/INTERVENTIONS	RATIONALE

Independent

	with the proper solution not only removes bacteria but also deodorizes the pouch.
Change pouch every 3–5 days, or sooner if needed because of leakage. Remove appliance gently while supporting skin. Use adhesive removers as indicated, and wash off completely.	Prevents tissue irritation/destruction associated with "pulling" pouch off.
Investigate complaints of burning/itching around stoma.	Suggests leakage of urine with peristomal irritation or possibly Candida infections both requiring intervention. Note: Continuous exposure of skin to urine can cause hyperplasia around stoma, affecting pouch fit and increasing risk of infection.
Evaluate adhesive product and appliance fit on ongoing basis.	Provides opportunity for problem solving. Determines need for further intervention.

Collaborative

Consult with enterostomal nurse.	Helpful in choosing products appropriate for patient needs, considering stoma placement, patient's physical/mental status, and financial resources. In the presence of persistent or recurring problems, the ostomy nurse will have a wider range of knowledge.
Apply antifungal spray or powder.	Assists in healing if peristomal irritation persists/fungal infection develops. Note: These products can have potent side effects and should be used sparingly, and creams/ointments are avoided because they interfere with adhesion of the appliance.

NURSING DIAGNOSIS:	SELF-CONCEPT, DISTURBANCE IN: (SPECIFY)
May be related to:	Biophysical: presence of stoma; loss of control of urine elimination
	Psychosocial: altered body structure
	Disease process and associated treatment regimen, e.g., cancer
Possibly evidenced by:	Verbalization of change in body image, fear of rejection/reaction of others, and negative feelings about body
	Actual change in structure and/or function (ostomy)
	Not touching/looking at stoma, refusal to participate in care
PATIENT OUTCOMES/ EVALUATION CRITERIA:	Verbalizes acceptance of self in situation, incorporating change into self-concept without negating self-esteem. Demonstrates beginning acceptance by viewing/touching stoma and participating in self-care. Verbalizes feelings about stoma/illness; begins to deal constructively with situation.

ACTIONS/INTERVENTIONS	RATIONALE

Independent

Review reason for surgery and future expectations.

Patient may find it easier to accept/deal with an ostomy done for chronic/long-term disease (e.g., intractable incontinence, infections) than for traumatic injury.

Ascertain whether counseling was initiated when the possibility and/or necessity of urinary diversion was first discussed.

Provides information about patient's/SO's level of knowledge about individual situation and process of acceptance.

Answer all questions concerning urostomy and its function.

Establishes rapport and adds further information for patient to consider. Conveys interest/concern of care giver.

Encourage the patient/SO to verbalize feelings. Acknowledge normality of feelings of anger, depression, and grief over loss. Discuss daily "ups and downs" that can occur after discharge.

Provides opportunity to deal with issues/misconceptions. Helps the patient/SO to realize that feelings experienced are not unusual and that feeling guilty for them is not necessary/helpful. Patient needs to recognize feelings before they can be dealt with effectively.

Note behaviors of withdrawal, increased dependency, manipulation or noninvolvement in care.

Suggestive of problems in adjustment that may require further evaluation and more extensive therapy. May reflect grief response to loss of body part/function and worry over acceptance by others as well as fear of further disability/loss of life from cancer.

Provide opportunities for patient/SO to view and touch stoma, using the moment to point out positive signs of healing, normal appearance, etc.

Although integration of stoma into body image can take months or even years, looking at the stoma and hearing comments (made in a normal, matter-of-fact manner) can help patient with this acceptance. Touching stoma reassures patient/SO that it is not fragile and that slight movements of stoma actually reflect normal peristalsis.

Provide opportunity for patient to deal with ostomy through participation in self-care.

Independence in self-care helps to improve self-esteem.

Maintain positive approach, during care activities, avoiding expressions of disdain or revulsion. Do not take patient's angry expressions personally.

Assists patient/SO to accept body changes and feel all right about self. Anger is most often directed at the situation and lack of control individual has over what has happened (powerlessness), not the individual care giver.

Plan/schedule care activities with patient.

Promotes sense of control, and gives message that the patient can handle this, enhancing self-esteem.

Discuss possibility of contacting ostomy/urostomy visitor and make arrangements for visit if desired.

Can provide a good support system. Helps to reinforce teaching (shared experiences) and facilitates acceptance of change as patient realizes "life does go on" and can be relatively normal.

Discuss sexual functioning and penile implant, if applicable, and alternate ways for sexual pleasuring. (Refer to ND: Sexual Dysfunction [Potential], p. 592.)

Patient may experience anticipatory anxiety, fear of failure in relation to sex after surgery, usually because of ignorance, lack of knowledge. Surgery that removes the bladder and prostate (removed with the bladder) may disrupt parasympathetic nerve fibers that control erection in the male, although newer techniques are available that may be used in individual cases to preserve these nerves.

NURSING DIAGNOSIS:	**COMFORT, ALTERED: PAIN, ACUTE**
May be related to:	**Physical factors, e.g., disruption of skin/tissues (incisions/drains)**

	Biologic: activity of disease process (cancer, trauma)
	Psychologic factors, e.g., fear, anxiety
Possibly evidenced by:	**Complaints of pain, self-focusing**
	Guarding/distraction behaviors, restlessness
	Autonomic responses, e.g., changes in vital signs
PATIENT OUTCOMES/ EVALUATION CRITERIA:	**Verbalizes/displays relief of pain. Demonstrates ability to assist with general comfort measures and able to sleep/rest appropriately.**

ACTIONS/INTERVENTIONS	RATIONALE
Independent	
Assess pain, noting location, characteristics, intensity (1–10 scale).	Helps evaluate degree of discomfort and effectiveness of analgesia or may reveal developing complications, e.g., because abdominal pain usually subsides gradually by the third or fourth postoperative day, continued or increasing pain may reflect delayed healing, peristomal skin irritation, infection, intestinal obstruction.
Auscultate bowel sounds, note passage of flatus.	Indicates reestablishment of bowel function, which may herald NG tube removal. Lack of return of bowel function within 72 hours may indicate presence of complication, e.g., peritonitis, hypokalemia, mechanical obstruction.
Note urine flow and characteristics.	Decreased flow may reflect urinary retention (due to edema) with increased pressure in upper urinary tract or leakage into peritoneal cavity (failure of anastomosis); cloudy urine may be normal (presence of mucus) or indicate infectious process.
Encourage patient to verbalize concerns. Active-listen these concerns and provide support by acceptance, remaining with patient and giving appropriate information.	Reduction of anxiety/fear can promote relaxation/ comfort.
Provide routine comfort measures, e.g., backrub, repositioning (use proper support measures as needed). Assure patient that position change will not injure stoma.	Reduces muscle tension, promotes relaxation and may enhance coping abilities.
Encourage use of relaxation techniques, e.g., guided imagery, visualization; diversional activities.	Helps patient to rest more effectively and refocuses attention, which may enhance coping ability, reducing pain and discomfort.
Assist with ROM exercises and encourage early ambulation.	Reduces muscle/joint stiffness. Ambulation returns organs to normal position and promotes return of peristalsis/passage of flatus and feelings of general well-being.
Investigate and report abdominal muscle rigidity, involuntary guarding, and rebound tenderness.	Suggestive of peritoneal inflammation, requiring prompt medical intervention. (Refer to CP: Peritonitis, p. 449.)
Collaborative	
Administer medications as indicated, e.g., narcotics, analgesics; PCA.	Relieves pain, enhances comfort and promotes rest. Patient control of analgesia may be more beneficial, especially following radical resection.

589

ACTIONS/INTERVENTIONS	RATIONALE
Collaborative	
Provide sitz baths, if indicated.	Relieves local discomfort, reduces edema, and promotes healing of perineal wound associated with radical procedure.
Apply/monitor effects of TENS unit.	Cutaneous stimulation may be used to block transmission of pain stimulus.
Maintain patency of NG tube.	Decompresses stomach/intestines, prevents abdominal distention when intestinal function impaired.

NURSING DIAGNOSIS:	INFECTION, POTENTIAL FOR
May be related to:	**Inadequate primary defenses (e.g., break in skin/ incision; reflux of urine into urinary tract)**
Possibly evidenced by:	**[Not applicable; presence of signs and symptoms establishes an *actual* diagnosis.]**
PATIENT OUTCOMES/ EVALUATION CRITERIA:	**Achieves timely wound healing, free of purulent drainage or erythema, and afebrile. Verbalizes understanding of individual causative/risk factors. Demonstrates techniques, lifestyle changes to reduce risk.**

ACTIONS/INTERVENTIONS	RATIONALE
Independent	
Empty urine pouch when it becomes one-third full once IV fluids and continuous drainage have been discontinued.	Reduces risk of urinary reflux and maintains integrity of appliance seal. Note: Urinary pouches are available with antireflux valve.
Document urine characteristics, and note whether changes are associated with complaints of flank pain.	Cloudy odorous urine indicates infection (possibly pyelonephritis); however, urine normally contains mucus after a conduit procedure.
Test urine pH with Nitrazine paper (use fresh specimen, not from pouch); notify physician if above 6.5.	Urine is normally acid, which discourages bacterial growth/urinary tract infections. Note: Presence of alkaline urine also creates favorable environment for stone formation in presence of hypercalciuria.
Report sudden cessation of urethral drainage.	Drainage usually subsides over 10 days. Abrupt cessation may indicate plugging and lead to abscess formation.
Note red rash around stoma.	Rash is most commonly caused by yeast. Urine leakage or allergy to appliance or products may also cause red, irritated areas.
Inspect incision line around stoma. Observe and document wound drainage, signs of incisional inflammation, systemic indicators of sepsis.	Provides baseline reference. Complications may include interrupted anastomosis of intestine/bowel or ureteral conduit, with leakage of bowel contents into abdomen or urine into peritoneal cavity.
Change dressings as indicated when used.	Moist dressings act as a wick to the wound and provide media for bacterial growth.
Monitor for distention of lower abdomen (with ileal conduit); assess bowel sounds.	May cause tension on suture line with possibility of rupture.

ACTIONS/INTERVENTIONS	RATIONALE

Independent

Monitor vital signs.

Elevation of temperature suggests incisional infection, UTI and/or respiratory complications.

Auscultate breath sounds.

Patient is at high risk for development of respiratory complications because of length of time under anesthesia. Often this patient is older and may already have a compromised immune system. Painful abdominal incisions cause patient to breath more shallowly than normal and to limit coughing. Accumulation of secretions in respiratory system predisposes to atelectasis and infections.

Collaborative

Provide pouch with antireflux valve.

Prevents backflow of urine into stoma, reducing risk of infection.

Obtain specimens of exudates, urine, sputum, blood as indicated.

Identifies source of infection/most effective treatment. Infected urine may cause pyelonephritis. Note: Urine specimen must be obtained from the conduit because the pouch is considered contaminated.

Administer antibiotics as indicated:

    Cephalosporins, e.g., cefoxitin (Mefoxin), cefazolin (Ancef);

Given to treat identified infection or may be given prophylactically, especially with history of recurrent pyelonephritis.

    Antifungal powder;

Used to treat yeast infections around stoma.

    Ascorbic acid/vitamin C.

Given to acidify urine, reduce bacterial growth/risk of infection. Note: Large doses of vitamin C can impair GI absorption of B_{12}, potentiating pernicious anemia.

Assist with injection of IV methylene blue.

If dye appears in wound drainage, signifies urine leakage into peritoneal cavity and need for surgical repair.

NURSING DIAGNOSIS:	URINARY ELIMINATION: ALTERED PATTERNS
May be related to:	**Surgical diversion; tissue trauma, postoperative edema**
Possibly evidenced by:	**Loss of continence**
	Changes in amount, character of urine; urinary retention
PATIENT OUTCOMES/ EVALUATION CRITERIA:	**Displays continuous flow of urine, with output adequate for individual situation.**

ACTIONS/INTERVENTIONS	RATIONALE

Independent

Assess for presence of stents/ureteral catheters. Label "right" and "left" and observe urine flow through each.

Maintains patency of ureters and assists in healing of anastomosis by keeping it urine free.

Record urinary output, investigate sudden reduction/cessation of urine flow.

Sudden decrease may indicate obstruction/dysfunction, e.g., blocked by edema or mucus. De-

ACTIONS/INTERVENTIONS	RATIONALE

Independent

	crease may also signify dehydration. Note: Reduced urine output (not related to hypovolemia) associated with abdominal distention, fever and clear/watery discharge from incision suggests urinary fistula also requiring prompt intervention.
Observe and record color of urine. Note hematuria, and/or bleeding from stoma.	Urine may be slightly pink, which should clear up in 2–3 days. Rubbing/washing stoma may cause temporary oozing due to vascular nature of tissues. Continued bleeding, frank blood in the pouch, or oozing around the base of stoma requires medical evaluation/intervention.
Position tubing and drainage pouch so that it allows unimpeded flow of urine. Monitor/protect placement of stents.	Blocking drainage allows pressure to build within urinary tract risking anastomosis leakage and damage to renal parenchyma. Also, because ostomy pouch is not sterile, urine allowed to collect may backflow into stoma, causing contamination if antireflux valve is not used. Note: Stents may be inserted to maintain patency of ureters during period of postoperative edema and may be inadvertently dislodged, compromising urine flow.
Encourage increased fluids and maintain accurate intake.	Should correlate with output.
Weigh daily.	Indicators of fluid balance.
Monitor vital signs. Assess peripheral pulses, skin turgor, capillary refill, and oral mucosa.	Reflects level of hydration and effectiveness of fluid replacement therapy.

Collaborative

Administer IV fluids as indicated.	Assists in maintaining hydration/adequate circulating volume and urinary flow.
Monitor electrolytes, ABGs, calcium.	Impaired renal function in patient with intestinal conduit increases risk of severe electrolyte/acid–base problems, e.g., hyperchloremic acidosis. Elevated calcium levels increase risk of crystal/stone formation, affecting both urinary flow and tissue integrity.
Prepare for diagnostic testing, procedures as indicated.	Retrograde ileogram may be done to evaluate patency of conduit; insertion of nephrostomy tube or stents may be required for maintaining urine flow until edema/obstruction is resolved.

NURSING DIAGNOSIS:	SEXUAL DYSFUNCTION [POTENTIAL]
May be related to:	**Altered body structure/function; radical resection/treatment procedures**
	Vulnerability/psychologic concern about response of SO
	Disruption of sexual response pattern, e.g., erection difficulty
Possibly evidenced by:	**[Not applicable; presence of signs and symptoms establishes an *actual* diagnosis.]**

PATIENT OUTCOMES/ EVALUATION CRITERIA:	Verbalizes understanding of relationship of physical condition to sexual problems. Identifies satisfying/acceptable sexual practices, and explores alternate methods. Resumes sexual relationship as appropriate.

ACTIONS/INTERVENTIONS

Independent

Ascertain the patient's/SO's sexual relationship prior to the disease and/or surgery. Identify future expectations and desires.

Review with the patient/SO anatomy and physiology of sexual functioning in relation to own situation.

Reinforce information given by the physician. Encourage questions. Provide additional information as needed.

Discuss resumption of sexual activity approximately 6 weeks after discharge, beginning slowly and progressing (e.g., cuddling/caressing until both partners are comfortable with body image/function changes). Include alternate methods of stimulation as appropriate.

Encourage dialogue between patient/SO. Suggest wearing pouch cover, T-shirt, or shortie nightgown.

Stress awareness of factors that might be distracting (e.g., unpleasant odors and pouch leakage).

Encourage use of a sense of humor.

Problem-solve alternative positions for coitus.

Discuss/role-play possible interactions or approaches when dealing with new sexual partners.

Provide birth control information as appropriate and stress that impotence does not mean the patient is necessarily sterile.

Collaborative

Arrange meeting with an ostomy visitor if appropriate.

Refer to counseling/sex therapy as indicated.

RATIONALE

Mutilation and loss of privacy/control of a bodily function can affect patient's view of personal sexuality. When coupled with the fear of rejection by SO, the desired level of intimacy can be greatly impaired. Sexual needs are very basic, and the patient will be rehabilitated more successfully when a satisfying sexual relationship is continued/developed.

Understanding normal physiology helps patient/SO understand the mechanisms of nerve damage and need for exploring alternative methods of satisfaction.

Reiteration of data previously given assists the patient/SO hear and process the knowledge again, moving toward acceptance of individual limitations/restrictions and prognosis (e.g., that it may take up to 2 years to regain potency after a radical procedure, or that a penile prosthesis may be necessary).

Knowing what to expect in progress of recovery helps patient avoid performance anxiety/reduce risk of "failure." If the couple is willing to try new ideas, this can assist with adjustment and may help to achieve sexual fulfillment.

Disguising urostomy appliance may aid in reducing feelings of self-consciousness, embarrassment during sexual activity.

Promotes resolution of solvable problems.

Laughter can help individuals to deal more effectively with difficult situation, promote positive sexual experience.

Minimizing awkwardness of appliance and physical discomfort can enhance satisfaction.

Rehearsal is helpful to dealing with actual situations when they arise, preventing self-consciousness about "different" body image.

Confusion about impotency and sterility may exist that can lead to an unwanted pregnancy.

Sharing of how these problems have been resolved by others can be helpful and reduce sense of isolation.

If problems persist longer than several months after surgery, a trained therapist may be required to facilitate communication between patient and SO.

593

NURSING DIAGNOSIS:	KNOWLEDGE DEFICIT [LEARNING NEED] (SPECIFY)
May be related to:	Lack of exposure/recall; information misinterpretation
	Unfamiliarity with information resources
Possibly evidenced by:	Questions; statement of misconception/misinformation
	Inaccurate follow-through of instruction/performance of urostomy care
	Inappropriate or exaggerated behaviors (e.g., hostile, agitated, apathetic withdrawal)
PATIENT OUTCOMES/ EVALUATION CRITERIA:	Verbalizes understanding of condition/disease process and treatment and prognosis. Correctly performs necessary procedures, explains reasons for the action. Initiates necessary lifestyle changes.

ACTIONS/INTERVENTIONS	RATIONALE
Independent	
Evaluate patient's emotional and physical capabilities.	These factors affect patient's ability to master tasks and willingness to assume responsibility for ostomy care.
Review anatomy, physiology and implications of surgical intervention. Discuss future expectations.	Provides knowledge base on which patient can make informed choices and an opportunity to clarify misconceptions regarding individual situation.
Include written/picture resources.	Provides references post discharge to support patient efforts for independence in self-care.
Instruct patient/SO in stomal care. Allot time for return demonstrations and provide positive feedback for efforts.	Promotes positive management and reduces risk of improper ostomy care.
Assure that stoma and appliance are odorless, non-leaking.	When patient feels confident about urostomy, energy/attention can be focused on other tasks.
Demonstrate padding to absorb urethral drainage; ask patient to report changes in amount, odor, character.	Small amount of leakage may continue for several weeks after prostate surgery with bladder left in place (temporary diversion procedure).
Encourage optimal nutrition.	Promotes wound healing, increases utilization of energy to facilitate tissue repair.
Discuss use of acid ash diet (e.g., cranberries, prunes, plums, cereals, rice, peanuts, noodles, cheese, poultry, fish), avoidance of salt substitutes, sodium bicarbonate, antacids and cautious use of products containing calcium.	May be useful in acidifying urine to decrease risk of infection and crystal/stone formation. Products containing bicarbonate/calcium potentiate risk of crystal/stone formation affecting both urinary flow and tissue integrity. Note: Use of sulfa drugs requires alkaline urine for optimal absorption; so acid ash diet/vitamin C supplements should be withheld.
Discuss importance of maintaining normal weight.	Changes in weight can affect size of stoma/appliance fit.
Stress necessity of increased fluid intake of at least 2–3 l/day, cranberry juice or ascorbic acid/vitamin C tablets.	Maintains urinary output and promotes acitic urine to reduce risk of infection and stone formation. Note: Oranges/citrus fruits make urine alkaline and therefore are contraindicated.

594

ACTIONS/INTERVENTIONS	RATIONALE

Independent

Discuss resumption of presurgery level of activity and possibility of sleep disturbance, anorexia, loss of interest in usual activities.

Patient should be able to manage same degree of activity as previously enjoyed and in some cases increase activity level except for contact sports. "Homecoming depression" may occur, lasting for up to 3 months after surgery, requiring patience/support and ongoing evaluation.

Encourage regular activity/exercise program.

Immobility/inactivity increases urinary stasis and calcium shift out of bones, potentiating risk of stone formation and resultant urinary obstruction, infection.

Identify signs/symptoms requiring medical evaluation, e.g., changes in character, amount and flow of urine, unusual drainage from wound; fatigue/muscle weakness, anorexia, abdominal distention, confusion.

Early detection and prompt intervention of developing problems such as UTI, stricture, intestinal fistula may prevent more serious complications. Urinary electrolytes (especially chloride) are resorbed in the intestinal conduit, which leads to compensatory bicarbonate loss, lowered serum pH (metabolic acidosis) and potassium deficit.

Stress importance of follow-up appointments.

Monitors healing, disease process, provides opportunity for discussion of mechanical fitting problems, generalized health, and adaptation to condition. Note: Extensive surgery requires prolonged recuperation for regaining strength and endurance.

Identify community resources, e.g., United Ostomy Association, and local ostomy support group, enterostomal therapist, VNA, pharmacy/medical supply house.

Continued support after discharge is essential to facilitate the recovery process and patient's independence in care. Enterostomal nurse can be very helpful in solving appliance problems, identifying alternatives to meet individual patient needs.

Benign Prostatic Hyperplasia _____

PATIENT ASSESSMENT DATA BASE

CIRCULATION

May exhibit: Elevated blood pressure (renal effects of advanced enlargement).

ELIMINATION

May report: Decreased force of urinary stream; dribbling.
Hesitancy in initiating voiding.
Inability to empty bladder completely; urgency and frequency of urination.
Nocturia, dysuria, hematuria.
Recurrent urinary tract infections.
Constipation (protrusion of prostate into rectum).

May exhibit: Firm mass in lower abdomen (distended bladder).
Bladder tenderness, distention.

FOOD/FLUID

May report: Anorexia; nausea, vomiting.
Recent weight loss.

PAIN/COMFORT

May report: Suprapubic, flank, or back pain; sharp, intense (in acute).
Low back pain.

SAFETY

May report: Fever.

SEXUALITY

May report: Concerns about effects of condition/therapy on sexual abilities.
Fear of incontinence/dribbling during intimacy.

May exhibit: Enlarged, tender prostate.

TEACHING/LEARNING

May report: Family history of cancer, hypertension, kidney disease.
Use of antihypertensive medications, urinary antibiotics or antibacterial agents.

Discharge Plan Considerations: May need assistance with management of therapy, e.g., catheter.

DIAGNOSTIC STUDIES

Urinalysis: Color yellow, dark brown, dark or bright red (bloody); appearance may be cloudy, pH 7 or above (suggests infection); bacteria, WBCs, RBCs may be present microscopically.

Urine culture: may reveal Staphylococcus aureus, Proteus, Klebsiella, Pseudomonas, or Escherichia coli.

BUN/creatinine: elevated if renal function is compromised.

Acid phosphatase: increased because of cellular growth and hormonal influences in cancer of the prostate (may indicate metastasis to the bone).

WBC: may be greater than 11,000, indicating infection if patient is not immunosuppressed.

IVP with postvoiding film: shows delayed emptying of bladder, varying degrees of urinary tract obstruction, and presence of prostatic enlargement.

Voiding cystourethrography: may be used instead of IVP to visualize bladder and urethra because it uses local dyes.

Cystourethroscopy: to view degree of prostatic enlargement and bladder wall changes (contraindicated in presence of acute urinary tract infection due to risk of gram-negative sepsis).

Cystometry: evaluates detrusor muscle function and tone.

NURSING PRIORITIES

1. Relieve acute urinary retention.
2. Promote comfort.
3. Prevent complications.
4. Assist patient to deal with psychosocial concerns.
5. Provide information about disease process/prognosis and treatment needs.

DISCHARGE CRITERIA

1. Voiding pattern normalized.
2. Pain/discomfort relieved.
3. Complications prevented/minimized.
4. Dealing with situation realistically.
5. Disease process/prognosis and therapeutic regimen understood.

NURSING DIAGNOSIS:	**URINARY RETENTION [ACUTE/CHRONIC]**
May be related to:	**Mechanical obstruction; enlarged prostate**
	Decompensation of detrusor musculature; inability of bladder to contract adequately
Possibly evidenced by:	**Frequency, hesitancy, inability to empty bladder completely; incontinence/dribbling**
	Bladder distention, residual urine
PATIENT OUTCOMES/ EVALUATION CRITERIA:	**Voiding in sufficient amounts with no palpable bladder distention, postvoid residuals are less than 50 ml; absence of dribbling/overflow.**

ACTIONS/INTERVENTIONS	RATIONALE
Independent	
Encourage patient to void every 2–4 hours and when urge is noted.	May minimize urinary retention/overdistention of the bladder.
Assess for stress/overflow incontinence.	High urethral pressure inhibits complete bladder emptying and/or can inhibit voiding until increased abdominal pressure causes urine to be involuntarily lost.
Observe urinary stream, noting size and force.	Useful in evaluating degree of obstruction and choice of intervention.
Monitor and document time and amount of each voiding. Note diminished urinary output and changes in specific gravity.	Urinary retention increases pressure within the upper urinary tract, which may compromise renal function. Any deficit in blood flow to the kidney impairs its ability to filter and concentrate substances.

597

ACTIONS/INTERVENTIONS	RATIONALE

Independent

Percuss/palpate suprapubic area.	A distended bladder can be felt in the suprapubic area.
Force fluids up to 3000 ml daily, within cardiac tolerance.	Increased circulating fluid maintains renal perfusion and flushes kidneys and bladder of bacterial growth.
Monitor vital signs closely. Observe for hypertension, peripheral/dependent edema, changes in mentation. Weigh daily. Maintain accurate intake and output.	Loss of kidney function results in decreased fluid elimination and accumulation of toxic wastes, may progress to complete renal shutdown. (Refer to CP: Renal Failure: Acute, p. 544.)
Provide/encourage meticulous catheter and perineal care.	Reduces risk of ascending infection.

Collaborative

Administer medications as indicated:	
Antispasmotics, e.g., oxybutynin chloride (Ditropan);	Spasms may occur due to irritation of the catheter.
Rectal suppositories (B & O);	Suppositories are absorbed easily through mucosa into bladder tissue to produce relaxation.
Antibiotics and antibacterials;	Given to combat infection. May be used prophylactically.
Phenoxybenzamine (Dibenzyline).	May be given to make urinating easier in some men with enlarged prostates. However, it is not in widespread use because it does not shrink the gland and has unpleasant side effects.
Catheterize for residual urine and leave indwelling catheter as indicated.	Relieves/prevents urinary retention and rules out presence of ureteral stricture. Note: Bladder decompression should be done in increments of 200 ml to prevent hematuria (rupture of blood vessels in the mucosa of the overdistended bladder) and syncope (excessive autonomic stimulation).
Irrigate catheter as indicated.	Maintains patency.
Monitor laboratory studies, e.g.:	
BUN, creatinine, electrolytes;	Prostatic enlargement (obstruction) eventually causes dilatation of upper urinary tract (ureters and kidneys), potentially impairing kidney function and leading to uremia.
Urinalysis and culture.	Urinary stasis potentiates bacterial growth increasing risk of urinary tract infection.
Provide sitz bath as indicated.	Promotes muscle relaxation, decreases edema, and may enhance voiding effort.
Prepare for/assist with urinary drainage, e.g.:	
Cystostomy;	May be indicated to drain bladder during acute episode with azotemia or when surgery is contraindicated because of patient's health status.
Experimental procedures, e.g.:	
Transurethral hyperthermia (TH);	Heating the central portion of the prostate by the insertion of a heating element through the urethra tends to shrink the prostate. Treatments are carried out one or two times a week for several weeks to achieve desired results.

ACTIONS/INTERVENTIONS	RATIONALE

Collaborative

Balloon urethroplasty.

Inflation of a balloon-tipped catheter within the obstructed area displaces prostatic tissue, thus improving urinary flow.

NURSING DIAGNOSIS:	COMFORT, ALTERED: PAIN, ACUTE
May be related to:	Mucosal irritation: bladder distention, renal colic; urinary infection; radiation therapy
Possibly evidenced by:	Complaints of pain (bladder/rectal spasm)
	Narrowed focus; altered muscle tone, grimacing; distraction behaviors, restlessness
	Autonomic responses
PATIENT OUTCOMES/ EVALUATION CRITERIA:	Reports pain relieved/controlled. Appears relaxed, able to sleep/rest appropriately.

ACTIONS/INTERVENTIONS	RATIONALE

Independent

Assess pain, noting location, intensity (scale of 1–10), duration.

Provides information to aid in determining choice/effectiveness of interventions.

Tape drainage tube to thigh and catheter to the abdomen (if traction not required).

Prevents pull on the bladder and erosion of the penile–scrotal junction.

Maintain bedrest when indicated.

Bedrest may be needed initially during acute retention phase. However, early ambulation can help restore normal voiding patterns and relieve colicky pain.

Provide routine comfort measures, e.g., backrub; helping patient assume position of comfort; encouraging use of relaxation/deep breathing exercises; diversional activities.

Promotes relaxation, refocuses attention, and may enhance coping abilities.

Collaborative

Insert catheter and attach to straight drainage.

Draining bladder reduces bladder tension and irritability.

Do prostatic massage.

Aids in evacuation of ducts of gland to relieve congestion/inflammation. Contraindicated if infection is present.

Administer medications as indicated:

Narcotics, e.g., meperidine (Demerol);

Given to relieve severe pain, provide physical and mental relaxation.

Antibacterials, e.g., methenamine hippurate (Hiprex);

Reduces bacteria present in urinary tract as well as those introduced by drainage system.

Antispasmodics and bladder sedatives, e.g., flavoxate (Urispas), oxybutynin (Ditropan).

Relieves bladder irritability.

Provide sitz baths, warm soaks to perineum.

Promotes muscle relaxation.

599

NURSING DIAGNOSIS:	FLUID VOLUME DEFICIT, POTENTIAL
May be related to:	Postobstructive diuresis from rapid drainage of a chronically overdistended bladder
	Endocrine, electrolyte imbalances (renal dysfunction)
Possibly evidenced by:	[Not applicable; presence of signs and symptoms establishes an *actual* diagnosis.]
PATIENT OUTCOMES/ EVALUATION CRITERIA:	Maintains adequate hydration as evidenced by stable vital signs, palpable peripheral pulses, good capillary refill, and moist mucous membranes.

ACTIONS/INTERVENTIONS	RATIONALE

Independent

Monitor output carefully, hourly if indicated (100–200 ml/hr).	Too rapid diuresis causes the patient's total fluid volume to become depleted, because insufficient amounts of sodium are resorbed in renal tubules.
Encourage increased oral intake based on individual needs.	Patient may have restricted oral intake in an attempt to control urinary symptoms, reducing homeostatic reserves and increasing risk of dehydration/ hypovolemia in face of additional pathology.
Monitor BP, pulse frequently. Evaluate capillary refill and oral mucous membranes.	Enables early detection/intervention of systemic hypovolemia.
Promote bedrest with head elevated.	Decreases cardiac workload, facilitating circulatory homeostasis.

Collaborative

Monitor electrolytes, especially sodium.	As fluid is pulled from extracellular spaces, sodium may follow the shift, causing hyponatremia.
Administer IV fluids (hypertonic saline) as needed.	Replaces fluid and sodium losses to prevent/correct hypovolemia.

NURSING DIAGNOSIS:	FEAR/ANXIETY [SPECIFY LEVEL]
May be related to:	Change in health status: possibility of surgical procedure/malignancy
	Embarrassment/loss of dignity associated with genital exposure before, during, and after treatment; concern about sexual ability
Possibly evidenced by:	Increased tension, apprehension, worry
	Expressed concerns regarding perceived changes
	Fear of unspecific consequences
PATIENT OUTCOMES/ EVALUATION CRITERIA:	Appears relaxed and reports anxiety is reduced to a manageable level. Demonstrates calm attitude and verbalizes lessened fear.

ACTIONS/INTERVENTIONS

Independent

Be available to the patient. Establish trusting relationship with patient/SO.

Provide information about specific procedures and tests and what to expect afterward, e.g., catheter, bloody urine, bladder irritation. Be aware of how much information the patient wants.

Maintain matter-of-fact attitude in doing procedures/dealing with patient. Protect patient's privacy.

Encourage patient/SO to verbalize concerns/feelings.

Reinforce previous information patient has been given.

RATIONALE

Demonstrates concern and willingness to help. Helpful in discussing sensitive subjects.

Helps patient understand purpose of what is being done, and reduces concerns associated with the unknown, including fear of cancer. However, overload of information is not helpful and may increase anxiety.

Communicates acceptance and eases patient's embarrassment.

Defines the problem, providing opportunity to answer questions, clarify misconceptions, and problem-solve solutions.

Allows the patient to deal with reality and strengthens trust in care givers and information presented.

NURSING DIAGNOSIS:	KNOWLEDGE DEFICIT [LEARNING NEED] (SPECIFY)
May be related to:	**Lack of exposure/recall, information misinterpretation**
	Unfamiliarity with information resources
	Concern about sensitive area
Possibly evidenced by:	**Questions, request for information; verbalization of the problem/nonverbal indicators**
	Inaccurate follow-through of instructions, development of preventable complications.
PATIENT OUTCOMES/ EVALUATION CRITERIA:	**Verbalizes understanding of disease process/prognosis. Identifies relationship of signs/symptoms to the disease process. Initiates necessary lifestyle changes and participates in treatment regimen.**

ACTIONS/INTERVENTIONS

Independent

Review disease process, patient expectations.

Encourage verbalization of fears/feelings and concerns.

Give information that the causative agent is not venereal.

Recommend avoiding spicy foods, coffee and alcohol, long automobile rides, rapid intake of fluids (particularly alcohol).

Address sexual concerns, e.g., during acute episodes of prostatitis, intercourse is avoided, but may be helpful in treatment of chronic condition.

RATIONALE

Provides knowledge base on which patient can make informed therapy choices.

Helping patient work through feelings can be vital to rehabilitation.

May be an unspoken fear.

May cause prostatic irritation with resulting congestion. Sudden increase in urinary flow can cause bladder distention and loss of bladder tone, resulting in episodes of acute urinary retention.

Sexual activity can increase pain during acute episodes but may serve as massaging agent in chronic disease.

601

ACTIONS/INTERVENTIONS	RATIONALE
Independent	
Provide information about basic sexual anatomy. Encourage questions and promote a dialog about concerns.	Having information about anatomy involved helps patient understand the implications of proposed surgical procedure.
Review signs/symptoms requiring medical evaluation, e.g., cloudy, odorous urine; diminished urine output, inability to void; presence of fever/chills.	Prompt interventions may prevent more serious complications.
Discuss necessity of notifying other health care providers of diagnosis.	Reduces risk of inappropriate therapy; e.g., use of decongestants, anticholinergics and antidepressants increases urinary retention and may precipitate an acute episode.
Reinforce importance of medical follow-up for at least 6 months to a year, including rectal examination, urinalysis.	Recurrence of hypertrophy and/or infection (caused by same or different organisms) is not uncommon and will require changes in therapeutic regimen to prevent serious complications.

Prostatectomy

Transurethral Resection (TUR)
Obstructive prostatic tissue of the medial lobe surrounding the urethra is removed by means of a cystoscope/resectoscope introduced through the urethra.

Suprapubic Prostatectomy
Obstructing prostatic tissue is removed through a low midline incision made through the bladder. This approach is preferred if bladder stones are present.

Retropubic Prostatectomy
Hypertrophied prostatic tissue mass (located high in the pelvic region) is removed through a low abdominal incision without opening the bladder.

Perineal Prostatectomy
Prostatic tissue is removed through an incision between the scrotum and the rectum. A radical procedure is done for cancer. This procedure may result in impotence.

NURSING PRIORITIES

1. Maintain homeostasis.
2. Promote comfort.
3. Prevent complications.
4. Provide information about surgical procedure/prognosis, treatment, and rehabilitation needs.

DISCHARGE CRITERIA

1. Urinary flow restored/enhanced.
2. Pain relieved/controlled.
3. Complications prevented/minimized.
4. Procedure/prognosis, therapeutic regimen, and rehabilitation needs understood.

Refer to CPs: Surgical Intervention, p. 789; Cancer, p. 872, for additional nursing diagnoses and considerations.

NURSING DIAGNOSIS:	**URINARY ELIMINATION: ALTERED PATTERNS**
May be related to:	**Mechanical obstruction: blood clots, edema, trauma, surgical procedure** **Pressure and irritation of catheter/balloon** **Loss of bladder tone due to preoperative overdistention or continued decompression**
Possibly evidenced by:	**Frequency, urgency, hesitancy, dysuria, incontinence, retention** **Bladder fullness; suprapubic discomfort**
PATIENT OUTCOMES/ EVALUATION CRITERIA:	**Voiding normal amounts without retention. Demonstrates behaviors to regain bladder/urinary control.**

ACTIONS/INTERVENTIONS	RATIONALE
Independent	
Assess urine output and catheter/drainage system, especially when bladder irrigation is running.	Retention can occur because of surgical area edema, blood clots, and bladder spasms.

603

ACTIONS/INTERVENTIONS	RATIONALE

Independent

Assist patient to assume normal position to void, e.g., stand, walk to bathroom at frequent intervals after catheter is removed.

Encourages passage of urine and promotes sense of normality.

Note time, amount of voiding and size of stream after catheter is removed. Note complaints of bladder fullness; inability to void, urgency.

The catheter is usually removed 2–5 days after surgery, but voiding may continue to be a problem for some time because of urethral edema and loss of bladder tone.

Encourage patient to void when urge is noted but not more than every 2–4 hours per protocol.

Voiding with urge prevents urinary retention. Limiting voids to every 4 hours (if tolerated), increases bladder tone, and aids in bladder retraining.

Measure residual volumes if suprapubic catheter present.

Monitors effectiveness of bladder emptying. Residuals greater than 50 ml suggest need for continuation of catheter until bladder tone improves.

Encourage fluid intake of at least 2500 ml as tolerated, limiting fluids in evening.

Maintains adequate hydration and renal perfusion for urinary flow. Reduces need to void/interrupt sleep during the night.

Instruct patient in perineal exercises, e.g., tightening buttocks, stopping and starting urine stream.

Helps to regain bladder sphincter/urinary control, minimizing incontinence.

Advise patient that "dribbling" is to be expected after catheter is removed and should resolve as recuperation progresses.

Information helps patient to deal with the problem. Normal functioning may return in 2–3 weeks but can take up to 6 months following perineal approach.

NURSING DIAGNOSIS:	FLUID VOLUME DEFICIT, POTENTIAL
May be related to:	**Vascular nature of surgical area; difficulty controlling bleeding**
	Restricted intake preoperatively
Possibly evidenced by:	**[Not applicable; presence of signs and symptoms establishes an *actual* diagnosis.]**
PATIENT OUTCOMES/ EVALUATION CRITERIA:	**Maintains adequate hydration as evidenced by stable vital signs, palpable peripheral pulses, good capillary refill, moist mucous membranes, and appropriate urinary output. Bleeding minimized, controlled.**

ACTIONS/INTERVENTIONS	RATIONALE

Independent

Anchor catheter, avoid excessive manipulation.

Movement/pulling of catheter may cause bleeding or clot formation and plugging of the catheter, with bladder distention.

Monitor intake and output.

Indicator of fluid balance and replacement needs. With bladder irrigations, monitoring is essential for estimating blood loss and accurately assessing urine output.

Observe catheter drainage, noting excessive/con-

Bleeding is not unusual during first 24 hours for all but

ACTIONS/INTERVENTIONS	RATIONALE

Independent

tinued bleeding.

the perineal approach. Continued/heavy bleeding or recurrence of active bleeding requires medical evaluation/intervention.

Evaluate color, consistency of urine, e.g.:

Bright red with bright red clots;

Usually indicates arterial bleeding and requires aggressive therapy.

Increased viscosity, dark burgundy with dark clots;

Suggests venous source (the most common type of bleeding), which usually subsides on its own.

Note bleeding with absence of clots.

May indicate blood dyscrasias or hemolysis of blood.

Inspect dressings/wound drains. Weigh dressings if indicated. Note hematoma formation.

Bleeding may be evident or sequestered within tissues of the perineum.

Monitor vital signs, noting increased pulse and respiration, decreased BP, diaphoresis, pallor, delayed capillary refill, and dry mucous membranes.

Dehydration/hypovolemia requires prompt intervention to prevent impending shock.

Investigate restlessness, confusion, changes in behavior.

May reflect decreased cerebral perfusion (hypovolemia) or indicate cerebral edema from excessive solution absorbed into the venous sinusoids during TUR procedure.

Encourage fluid intake to 3000 ml/day unless contraindicated.

Flushes kidneys/bladder of bacteria and debris but may result in water intoxication/fluid overload if not monitored closely.

Avoid rectal temperatures and use of rectal tubes/enemas.

May result in referred irritation to prostatic bed and increased pressure on prostatic capsule with risk of bleeding.

Collaborative

Monitor laboratory studies as indicated, e.g.:

Hb/Hct, RBCs;

Useful in evaluating blood losses/replacement needs.

Coagulation studies, platelet count.

May indicate developing complications, e.g., depletion of clotting factors, disseminated intravascular coagulopathy (DIC).

Administer IV therapy/blood products as indicated.

May need additional fluids, if oral intake inadequate, or blood products, if losses are excessive.

Maintain traction on indwelling catheter, tape catheter to inner thigh.

Traction on the 30-ml balloon positioned in the prostatic uretheral fossa will create pressure on the arterial supply of the prostatic capsule to help prevent/control bleeding.

Release traction within 4–5 hours. Document period of application and release of traction, if used.

Prolonged traction may cause permanent trauma/problems with urinary control.

Administer stool softeners, laxatives as indicated.

Prevention of constipation/straining for stool reduces risk of rectal–perineal bleeding.

NURSING DIAGNOSIS: **INFECTION, POTENTIAL FOR**

    May be related to: **Invasive procedures: instrumentation during surgery, catheter, frequent bladder irrigation**

           Traumatized tissue, surgical incision (e.g., perineal)

ACTIONS/INTERVENTIONS	RATIONALE

Independent

Maintain sterile catheter system; provide routine catheter/meatal care with soap and water, applying antibiotic ointment around catheter site.	Prevents introduction of bacteria and resultant infection/sepsis.
Ambulate with drainage bag dependent.	Avoids backward reflux of urine, which may introduce bacteria into the bladder.
Monitor vital signs, noting low-grade fever, chills, rapid pulse and respiration, restlessness, irritability, disorientation.	Patient who has had cystoscopy and/or TURP are at increased risk for surgical shock related to manipulation/instrumentation.
Observe drainage from wounds, around suprapubic catheter.	Presence of drains, suprapubic incision increases risk of infection, as indicated by erythema, purulent drainage.
Change dressings frequently (supra/retropubic and perineal incisions), cleaning and drying skin thoroughly each time.	Wet dressings cause skin irritation and provide media for bacterial growth, increasing risk of wound infection.
Use ostomy-type skin barriers.	Provides protection for surrounding skin, preventing excoriation and reducing risk of infection.

Collaborative

Maintain continuous bladder irrigation (CBI).	Flushes bladder of debris and maintains patency of the catheter, minimizing risk of infection.
Administer antibiotics as indicated.	May be given prophylactically due to increased risk of infection with prostatectomy.

NURSING DIAGNOSIS:	**COMFORT, ALTERED: PAIN, ACUTE**
May be related to:	Irritation of the bladder mucosa; reflex muscle spasm associated with surgical procedure and/or pressure from bladder balloon (traction)
Possibly evidenced by:	Complaints of painful bladder spasms
	Facial grimacing, guarding, restlessness
	Autonomic responses
PATIENT OUTCOMES/ EVALUATION CRITERIA:	Reports pain is relieved/controlled. Demonstrates use of relaxation skills and diversional activities as indicated for individual situation. Appears relaxed.

ACTIONS/INTERVENTIONS	RATIONALE

Independent

Assess pain, noting location, intensity (1–10 scale).	Sharp, intermittent pain with urge to void/passage of

ACTIONS/INTERVENTIONS	RATIONALE
Independent	
	urine around catheter suggests bladder spasms, which tend to be more severe with suprapubic or TUR approaches (usually decrease by the end of 48 hours).
Maintain patency of catheter and drainage system. Keep tubings free of kinks and clots.	Maintaining a properly functioning catheter and drainage system decreases risk of bladder distention/spasm.
Promote intake of 2–3 liters of fluid.	Decreases irritation by maintaining a constant flow of fluid over the bladder mucosa.
Give patient accurate information about catheter, drainage, and bladder spasms.	Allays anxiety and promotes cooperation with necessary procedures.
Provide routine comfort measures (Therapeutic Touch, position changes, backrub) and diversional activities. Encourage use of relaxation techniques, including deep-breathing exercises, visualization, guided imagery.	Reduces muscle tension, refocuses attention and may enhance coping abilities.
Collaborative	
Administer antispasmodics, e.g.:	
Oxybutynin chloride (Ditropan), belladonna and opium (B&O) suppositories;	Relaxes smooth muscle, to provide relief of spasms and associated pain.
Propantheline bromide (Pro-Banthine).	Relieves bladder spasms by anticholinergic action. Usually discontinued 24–48 hours before anticipated removal of catheter to promote normal bladder contraction.
Provide sitz baths or heat lamp if indicated.	Promotes tissue perfusion, resolution of edema and enhances healing (perineal approach).

NURSING DIAGNOSIS:	**SEXUAL DYSFUNCTION [POTENTIAL]**
May be related to:	**Situational crisis (incontinence, leakage of urine after catheter removal, involvement of genital area)**
	Threat to self-concept/change in health status
Possibly evidenced by:	**[Not applicable; presence of signs and symptoms establishes an *actual* diagnosis.]**
PATIENT OUTCOMES/ EVALUATION CRITERIA:	**Appears relaxed and reports anxiety is reduced to a manageable level. Verbalizes understanding of individual situation. Demonstrates problem-solving skills.**

ACTIONS/INTERVENTIONS	RATIONALE
Independent	
Provide openings for patient/SO to talk about concerns of incontinence and sexual functioning.	May have anxieties about the effects of surgery and may be hesitant about asking necessary questions. Anxiety may have affected ability to access information given previously.

ACTIONS/INTERVENTIONS

Independent

Give accurate information about expectation of return of sexual function.

Discuss retrograde ejaculation if TUR/suprapubic approach is used.

Instruct in perineal and interruption/continuation of urinary stream exercises.

Collaborative

Refer to sexual counselor as indicated.

RATIONALE

Physiologic impotence occurs when the perineal nerves are cut during radical procedures; in other approaches, sexual activity can usually be resumed in 6–8 weeks. Note: Penile prosthesis may be recommended to facilitate erection and correct impotence following radical perineal procedure.

Seminal fluid goes into the bladder and is excreted with the urine. This does not interfere with sexual functioning but will cause infertility.

Promotes regaining muscular control of urinary continence and sexual function.

Persistent/unresolved problems may require professional intervention.

NURSING DIAGNOSIS:	KNOWLEDGE DEFICIT [LEARNING NEED] (SPECIFY)
May be related to:	Lack of exposure/recall; information misinterpretation
	Unfamiliarity with information resources
Possibly evidenced by:	Questions, request for information, statement of misconception
	Verbalization of the problem
	Inaccurate follow-through of instruction/development of preventable complications
PATIENT OUTCOMES/ EVALUATION CRITERIA:	Verbalizes understanding of surgical procedure and treatment. Correctly performs necessary procedures and explains reasons for actions. Initiates necessary lifestyle changes and participates in treatment regimen.

ACTIONS/INTERVENTIONS

Independent

Review implications of procedure and future expectations.

Discuss basic anatomy. Be honest in answers to patient's questions.

Stress necessity of good nutrition; encourage inclusion of fruits, increased fiber in diet.

Discuss initial activity restrictions, e.g., avoidance of

RATIONALE

Provides knowledge base on which patient can make informed choices.

The nerve plexus that controls erection runs posteriorly to the prostate through the capsule. In procedures that do not involve the prostatic capsule, impotence and sterility usually are not consequences. Surgical procedure may not provide a permanent cure, and hypertrophy may recur.

Promotes healing and prevents constipation, reducing risk of postoperative bleeding.

Increased abdominal pressure/straining places stress

ACTIONS/INTERVENTIONS	RATIONALE

Independent

heavy lifting, strenuous exercise, and prolonged sitting/long automobile trips.

on the bladder and prostate, potentiating risk of bleeding.

Encourage continuation of perineal exercises.

Facilitates urinary control and alleviation of incontinence.

Instruct in urinary catheter care if present. Identify source for supplies.

Promotes independence and competent self-care.

Instruct patient to avoid tub baths after discharge.

Decreases the possibility of infection, introduction of bacteria.

Review signs/symptoms requiring medical evaluation, e.g., erythema, purulent drainage from wound sites; changes in character/amount of urine, presence of urgency/frequency; heavy bleeding; fever/chills.

Prompt intervention may prevent serious complications. Note: Urine may appear cloudy for several weeks until postoperative healing occurs and will appear cloudy after intercourse because of retrograde ejaculation.

Urolithiasis

Kidney stones (calculi) are formed of mineral deposits, most commonly calcium oxalate and calcium phosphate; however, uric acid and other crystals are also calculus formers. Renal calculi can remain asymptomatic until passed into a ureter and/or urine flow is obstructed, when the potential for renal damage is acute.

PATIENT ASSESSMENT DATA BASE

ACTIVITY/REST

May report: Sedentary occupation, occupation in which patient is exposed to high environmental temperatures.

CIRCULATION

May exhibit: Elevated blood pressure/pulse (pain, anxiety, kidney failure).
Warm, flushed skin; pallor.

ELIMINATION

May report: History of recent/chronic urinary tract infection; previous obstruction (calculi).
Decreased urinary output, bladder fullness.
Burning, urgency with urination.
Diarrhea.

May exhibit: Oliguria, hematuria.
Alterations in voiding pattern.

FOOD/FLUID

May report: Nausea, abdominal tenderness.
Diet high in purines, calcium oxalate, and/or phosphates.
Insufficient fluid intake; does not drink fluids well.

May exhibit: Abdominal distention; decreased/absent bowel sounds.
Vomiting.

PAIN/COMFORT

May report: Acute episode of excruciating, colicky pain. Location is dependent on stone location, e.g., in the flank in the region of the costovertebral angle; may radiate to back, abdomen, and down to the groin/genitalia.
Pain may be described as acute, severe not relieved by positioning or any other measures.

May exhibit: Guarding; distraction behaviors.
Tenderness in renal areas on palpation.

SAFETY

May report: Use of alcohol.
Fever; chills.

TEACHING/LEARNING

May report: Family history of calculi, kidney disease, hypertension, gout, chronic UTI.
History of small bowel disease; previous abdominal surgery; bedrest/immobilization, e.g., debilitating disease, fractures.

Use of antibiotics, antihypertensives, sodium bicarbonate, allopurinal, phosphates, thiazides.

DIAGNOSTIC STUDIES

Urinalysis: color may be yellow, dark brown, bloody; commonly shows RBCs, WBCs, crystals (cystine, uric acid, calcium oxalate), casts, minerals, bacteria, pus; pH may be acid or alkaline.

Urine (24-hour): creatinine, uric acid, calcium, phosphorus, oxylate or cystine may be elevated.

Urine culture: may reveal UTI (Staphylococcus aureus, Proteus, Klebsiella, Pseudomonas).

Biochemical survey: elevated levels of magnesium, calcium, uric acid, phosphates, protein, electrolytes.

Serum and urine BUN/creatinine: abnormal (high in serum/low in urine) secondary to high obstructive stone in kidney causing ischemia/necrosis.

CBC: WBC: may be increased indicating infection/septicemia. *RBC:* usually normal. *Hb/Hct:* abnormal if patient is severely dehydrated or polycythemia is present (encourages precipitation of solids), or anemic (hemorrhage, kidney dysfunction/failure).

Parathyroid hormone: May be increased if kidney failure present. (PTH stimulates reabsorption of calcium from bones increasing circulating serum and urine calcium.)

KUB (kidney, ureter, bladder) x-ray: shows presence of calculi and/or anatomic changes in the area of the kidneys/ or along the course of the ureter.

IVP: provides rapid confirmation of urolithiasis as a cause of abdominal or flank pain. Shows abnormalities in anatomic structures (distended ureter) and outline of calculi.

Cystoureteroscopy: direct visualization of bladder and ureter may reveal stone and/or obstructive effects.

CT scan: identifies/delineates calculi and other masses; kidney, ureteral, and bladder distention.

NURSING PRIORITIES

1. Alleviate pain.
2. Maintain adequate renal functioning.
3. Prevent complications.
4. Provide information about disease process/prognosis and treatment needs.

DISCHARGE CRITERIA

1. Pain relieved/controlled.
2. Fluid/electrolyte balance maintained.
3. Complications prevented/minimized.
4. Disease process/prognosis and therapeutic regimen understood.

NURSING DIAGNOSIS:	COMFORT, ALTERED: PAIN, ACUTE
May be related to:	**Increased frequency/force of ureteral contractions**
	Tissue trauma, edema formation; cellular ischemia
Possibly evidenced by:	**Complaints of colicky pain**
	Guarding/distraction behaviors, restlessness, moaning, self-focusing, facial mask of pain, muscle tension
	Autonomic responses
PATIENT OUTCOMES/ EVALUATION CRITERIA:	**Reports pain is relieved with spasms controlled. Appears relaxed, able to sleep/rest appropriately.**

611

ACTIONS/INTERVENTIONS	RATIONALE
Independent	
Document location, duration, intensity (1–10 scale), and radiation. Note nonverbal signs, e.g., elevated BP and pulse, restlessness, moaning, thrashing about.	Helps evaluate progress of calculi movement. Flank pain often radiates to back, groin, genitalia due to proximity of nerve plexus and blood vessels supplying other areas. Sudden cessation of pain usually indicates stone passage.
Explain cause of pain and importance of notifying staff of pain occurrence/characteristics.	Provides opportunity for timely administration of analgesia (helpful in enhancing the patient's coping ability and may reduce anxiety) and alerts staff to possibility of passing of stone/developing complications. Note: Sudden severity of pain may precipitate fight–flight response manifested by apprehension, restlessness, severe anxiety.
Provide routine comfort measures, e.g., backrub, restful environment.	Promotes relaxation, reduces muscle tension, and enhances coping.
Assist with/encourage use of focused breathing, guided imagery, diversional activities.	Redirects attention and aids in muscle relaxation.
Encourage/assist with frequent ambulation as indicated and increased fluid intake of at least 3–4 l/day within cardiac tolerance.	Promotes passing of stone, prevents urinary stasis, and aids in prevention of further stone formation.
Note complaints of increased/persistent abdominal pain.	Complete obstruction of ureter, perforation, and extravasation of urine into perirenal space may occur due to increased ureteral pressure and represent an acute surgical emergency.
Collaborative	
Administer medications as indicated:	
Narcotics, e.g., meperedine (Demerol), morphine;	Usually given during acute episode to decrease ureteral colic and promote muscle/mental relaxation.
Antispasmotics, e.g., flavoxate (Urispas), oxybutynin (Ditropan);	Decreasing reflex spasm usually will decrease colic and pain.
Corticosteroids.	May be used to reduce tissue edema to facilitate movement of stone.
Apply warm compresses to back.	Relieves muscle tension and may reduce reflex spasms.
Maintain patency of catheters when used.	Prevents urinary stasis/retention, reduces risk of increased renal pressure and infection.

NURSING DIAGNOSIS:	URINARY ELIMINATION: ALTERED PATTERNS
May be related to:	Stimulation of the bladder by calculi, renal or ureteral irritation
	Mechanical obstruction, inflammation
Possibly evidenced by:	Urgency and frequency; oliguria (retention)
	Hematuria

PATIENT OUTCOMES/ EVALUATION CRITERIA:	Voiding in normal amounts and usual pattern, free of signs of obstruction.

ACTIONS/INTERVENTIONS

Independent

Monitor intake, output, and characteristics of urine.

Determine patient's normal voiding pattern, and note variations.

Encourage increased fluid intake.

Strain all urine. Document any stones expelled and send to laboratory for analysis.

Investigate complaints of bladder fullness; palpate for suprapubic distention. Note decreased urine output, presence of periorbital/dependent edema.

Observe for changes in mental status, behavior, or level of consciousness.

Collaborative

Monitor laboratory studies, e.g., electrolytes, BUN, creatinine.

Obtain urine for culture and sensitivities.

Administer medications as indicated, e.g.:

Acetazolamide (Diamox), sodium bicarbonate, allopurinol (Zyloprim);

Hydrochlorothiazide (Esidrix, HydroDIURIL), chlorthalidone (Hygroton);

Ammonium chloride; potassium or sodium phosphate (Sal-Hepatica);

Antibiotics.

Maintain patency of indwelling catheters (ureteral, urethral, or nephrostomy) when used.

Irrigate with acid or alkaline solutions as indicated.

Prepare patient for/assist with procedures, e.g.:

Basket procedure;

RATIONALE

Provides information about kidney function and presence of complications, e.g., infection and hemorrhage. Bleeding may indicate increased obstruction or irritation of ureter. Note: Hemorrhage due to ureteral ulceration is rare.

Calculi may cause nerve excitability, which causes sensations of urgent need to void. Usually frequency and urgency increase as calculus nears ureterovesical junction.

Increased hydration flushes bacteria, blood, and debris and may facilitate stone passage.

Retrieval of calculi allows for identification of type of stone and influences choice of therapy.

Urinary retention may develop, causing tissue distention (bladder/kidney) and potentiates risk of infection, renal failure. (Refer to CP: Renal Failure: Acute, p. 544.)

Accumulation of uremic wastes and electrolyte imbalances can be toxic to the CNS.

Elevated BUN, creatinine, and certain electrolytes indicate kidney dysfunction.

Determines presence of UTI, which may be causing/complicating symptoms.

Increases urine pH (alkalinity) to reduce formation of acid stones.

May be used to decrease calcium stone formation if not due to underlying disease process such as primary hyperthyroidism or vitamin D abnormalities.

Reduces phosphate stone formation.

Presence of UTI/alkaline urine potentiates stone formation.

May be required to facilitate urine flow/prevent retention and corresponding complications. Note: Tubes may be occluded by stone fragments.

Changing urine pH may help dissolve stones and prevent further stone formation.

Ureteral calculi may be removed by endoscopic cystoscope with capture of the stone in a basketing catheter.

613

ACTIONS/INTERVENTIONS	RATIONALE
Collaborative	
Ureteral stents;	Catheters are positioned above the stone to promote uretheral dilation/stone passage. Continuous or intermittent irrigation can be carried out to flush ureters and adjust pH of urine.
Ureterolithotomy;	Surgical removal of stone that is too large to pass through ureters.
Percutaneous ultrasonic lithotripsy (PUL);	Invasive shock wave treatment for stones in renal pelvis/calyx or upper ureters.
Extracorporeal shock-wave lithotripsy (ESWL).	Noninvasive procedure in which kidney stones are pulverized by shock waves delivered from outside the body.

NURSING DIAGNOSIS:	**FLUID VOLUME DEFICIT, POTENTIAL**
May be related to:	**Nausea, vomiting (generalized abdominal and pelvic nerve irritation from renal or ureteral colic)**
	Post obstructive diuresis
Possibly evidenced by:	**[Not applicable; presence of signs or symptoms establishes an *actual* diagnosis.]**
PATIENT OUTCOMES/ EVALUATION CRITERIA:	**Maintains adequate fluid balance as evidenced by vital signs and weight within patient's normal range, palpable peripheral pulses, moist mucous membranes, good skin turgor.**

ACTIONS/INTERVENTIONS	RATIONALE
Independent	
Monitor intake and output.	Comparing actual and anticipated output may aid in evaluating presence/degree of renal stasis/impairment. Note: Impaired kidney functioning and decreased urine output can result in higher circulating volumes with signs/symptoms of CHF.
Document incidence of vomiting, diarrhea. Note characteristics, frequency, as well as accompanying or precipitating events.	Celiac ganglion serves both kidneys and stomach; so nausea, vomiting, and diarrhea are commonly associated with renal colic. Documentation may help rule out other abdominal disturbances or pinpoint calculi and pain as causes of symptoms.
Increase fluid intake to 3–4 l/day within cardiac tolerance.	Dehydration and electrolyte imbalance may occur secondary to excessive fluid loss (vomiting and diarrhea). Maintains fluid balance for homeostasis as well as "washing" action that may flush the stone(s) out. Note: Concentrated urine potentiates stone formation.
Monitor vital signs. Evaluate pulses, capillary refill, skin turgor, and mucous membranes.	Indicators of hydration/circulating volume and need for intervention. Note: Decreased glomerular filtration rate stimulates production of renin, which acts to raise BP in an effort to increase renal blood flow.
Weigh daily.	Rapid weight gain may be related to water retention.

ACTIONS/INTERVENTIONS

Collaborative

Monitor Hct/Hb, electrolytes.

Administer IV fluids.

Administer appropriate diet, clear liquids, bland foods as tolerated.

Administer medications as indicated: antiemetics, e.g., prochlorperazine (Compazine).

RATIONALE

Assesses hydration and effectiveness of interventions.

Maintains circulating volume (if oral intake is insufficient) promoting renal function.

Easily digested foods decrease GI activity/irritation and helps maintain fluid and nutritional balance.

Reduces nausea and vomiting.

NURSING DIAGNOSIS:	KNOWLEDGE DEFICIT [LEARNING NEED] (SPECIFY)
May be related to:	Lack of exposure/recall; information misinterpretation Unfamiliarity with information resources
Possibly evidenced by:	Questions; request for information; statement of misconception Inaccurate follow-through of instructions, development of preventable complications
PATIENT OUTCOMES/ EVALUATION CRITERIA:	Verbalizes understanding of disease process. Correlates symptoms with causative factors. Initiates necessary lifestyle changes and participates in treatment regimen.

ACTIONS/INTERVENTIONS

Independent

Review disease process and future expectations.

Stress importance of increased fluid intake, e.g., 3–4 or as much as 6–8 l/day. Encourage patient to notice dry mouth, excessive diuresis/diaphoresis and to increase fluid intake whether feeling thirsty or not.

Review dietary regimen, as individually appropriate:

Low-purine diet, e.g., limited lean meat, turkey, legumes, whole grains, alcohol;

Low-calcium diet, e.g., limited milk, cheese, green leafy vegetables, yogurt;

Low-oxalate diet; e.g., restrict chocolate, caffeine-containing beverages, beets, spinach.

Shorr regimen: low calcium/phosphorus diet with aluminum carbonate gel 30–40 ml, 30 minutes pc/hs (watch for constipation).

Discuss medication regimen, avoidance of OTC drugs and reading of all product/food ingredient labels.

RATIONALE

Provides knowledge base on which patient can make informed choices.

Flushes renal system decreasing opportunity for urinary stasis and stone formation. Increased fluid losses/dehydration require additional intake beyond usual daily needs.

Diet depends on the type of stone. Knowledge of dietary alteration can be an important aspect of disease control.

Decreases oral intake of uric acid precursors.

Reduces risk of calcium stone formation.

Reduces calcium oxalate stone formation.

Prevents phosphatic calculi by forming an insoluble precipitate in the GI tract, reducing the load to the kidney nephron. Also effective against other forms of calcium calculi.

Drugs will be given to acidify or alkalize urine, dependent on underlying cause of stone formation. Ingestion

ACTIONS/INTERVENTIONS

Independent

Encourage regular activity/exercise program.

Active-listen concerns about therapeutic regimen/lifestyle changes.

Identify signs/symptoms requiring medical evaluation, e.g., recurrent pain, hematuria, oliguria.

Demonstrate proper care of incisions, catheters if present.

RATIONALE

of products containing individually contraindicated ingredients (e.g., calcium, phosphorus) potentiates recurrence of stones.

Inactivity contributes to stone formation through calcium shifts and urinary stasis.

Helps patient work through feelings and gain a sense of control over what is happening.

With increased probability of recurrence of stones, prompt interventions may prevent serious complications.

Promotes competent self-care and independence.

CHAPTER 11

ENDOCRINOLOGY

Addison's Disease (Adrenal Insufficiency/Crisis) _____

The primary form of the disease is caused by atrophy or destruction of the adrenal tissues, e.g., autoimmune response, tuberculosis, hemorrhagic infarction, malignancy, surgical removal.

The secondary form results from pituitary dysfunction/suppression, causing decreased levels of ACTH; but usually normal secretion of MSH remains.

PATIENT ASSESSMENT DATA BASE

ACTIVITY/REST

May report:	Exhaustion, muscle aches/weakness (progressively worse throughout the day). Inability to be active/work.
May exhibit:	Increased heart/pulse rate with minimal activity. Decreased strength, ROM. Depression, difficulty concentrating, decreased/lack of initiative. Lethargy.

CIRCULATION

May exhibit:	Hypotension, including postural. Tachycardia, dysrhythmias, diminished heart sounds. Weak peripheral pulses. Capillary refill may be delayed. Extremities cool; cyanosis, pallor. Mucous membranes bluish-black or slate gray (increased pigmentation).

EGO INTEGRITY

May report:	History of recent/multiple stress factors, including physical illness/surgery, change in lifestyle. Inability to cope with stress.
May exhibit:	Anxiety, irritability, depression, emotional instability.

ELIMINATION

May report: Diarrhea or constipation.
Abdominal cramps.
Changes in frequency, character of urine.

May exhibit: Diuresis, followed by oliguria.

FOOD/FLUID

May report: Marked anorexia (cardinal symptom); nausea/vomiting.
Craving salt.
Marked weight loss.

May exhibit: Skin turgor and moisture decreased, dry mucous membranes.

NEUROSENSORY

May report: Dizziness, syncope, trembling.
Headaches along with diaphoresis.
Muscle weakness.
Decreased tolerance to cold or stress.
Tingling/numbness/weakness.

May exhibit: Disorientation to time, place and person (low sodium level), lethargy, mental fatigue, irritability, apprehension/anxiety, coma (crisis).
Paresthesias, paralysis; asthenia (crisis).
Sense of taste/smell exaggerated; acuity of hearing increased.

PAIN/COMFORT

May report: Muscle aches, abdominal cramping, headache.
Severe back, abdominal, extremity pain (crisis).

RESPIRATION

May report: Dyspnea.

May exhibit: Increased respiratory rate, tachypnea.
Breath sounds: crackles, rhonchi (infection).

SAFETY

May exhibit: Hyperpigmentation of skin (brown, tan, or bronze), diffuse or patchy.
Temperature elevation; fever followed by hypothermia (crisis).
Muscle wasting.
Gait disturbances.

SEXUALITY

May report: History of premature menopause; amenorrhea.
Loss of secondary sex characteristics, e.g., decreased body hair (especially in females).
Loss of libido.

TEACHING/LEARNING

May report: Family history of diabetes, tuberculosis, cancer.
History of thyroiditis, diabetes mellitus, tuberculosis.

Discharge Plan Considerations: May need assistance with medication regimen, homemaker tasks.

DIAGNOSTIC STUDIES

Hormone levels:

Plasma cortisol: decreased with no response to IM (primary) or IV (secondary) ACTH administration.

ACTH: markedly increased (primary) or decreased (secondary).

ADH: increased.

Aldosterone: decreased.

Electrolytes: serum levels may be normal or sodium somewhat reduced and potassium slightly elevated. However, profound sodium and potassium abnormalities can occur in response to absence of aldosterone and cortisol deficiency (may precipitate/result from crisis).

Glucose: hypoglycemia.

BUN/creatinine: may be elevated (decreased renal perfusion).

ABGs: metabolic acidosis.

CBC: normocytic, normochromic anemia (may be masked by decreased fluid volume) and Hct elevated (hemoconcentration). Lymphocyte count may be low, eosinophils elevated.

Urine (24-hour): 17-ketosteroids, 17-hydroxycorticoids, and 17-ketogenic steroids decreased. Free cortisol level decreased. Note: Failure to achieve a rise in urine steroid levels after test administration of ACTH indicates primary Addison's disease (permanent adrenal gland atrophy), while increased levels suggest a secondary cause of hormone suppression. Urine sodium increased.

X-ray: small heart, adrenal calcifications, or tuberculosis (pulmonary, renal) may be noted.

NURSING PRIORITIES

1. Maintain fluid and electrolyte balance.
2. Improve nutritional status.
3. Prevent complications/crisis.
4. Support adjustment to condition.
5. Provide information about disease process/prognosis and lifelong therapy needs.

DISCHARGE CRITERIA

1. Homeostasis achieved.
2. Complications prevented/minimized.
3. Activities of daily living managed by self/with assistance.
4. Dealing realistically with current situation.
5. Disease process/prognosis and therapeutic regimen understood.

NURSING DIAGNOSIS:	FLUID VOLUME DEFICIT, ACTUAL 1 [REGULATORY FAILURE]
May be related to:	Aldosterone deficit promotes sodium and water losses (kidney, sweat glands, GI tract)
Possibly evidenced by:	Nausea, vomiting; weakness, thirst; weight loss
	Diarrhea; excessive urination, dilute urine
	Postural hypotension; tachycardia; weak, thready pulses
PATIENT OUTCOMES/	Demonstrates improved fluid balance, as evidenced by

ACTIONS/INTERVENTIONS	RATIONALE
Independent	
Obtain history from patient/SO related to the duration/intensity of present symptoms, e.g., vomiting, excessive urination.	Assists in estimation of total volume depletion.
Monitor vital signs, noting postural blood pressure changes, strength of peripheral pulses.	Postural hypotension is due in part to hypovolemia that results from aldosterone deficiency and from the reduced cardiac output that results from cortisol deficiency. Pulse may be weak, easily obliterated.
Measure intake and output. Weigh patient daily.	Provides ongoing estimate of volume replacement needs and effectiveness of therapy. Initial weight gain usually results from sodium and water retention related to steroid replacement therapy.
Assess patient for thirst; weak, rapid, thready pulse; delayed capillary refill; poor skin turgor; and dry mucous membranes. Note skin color and temperature.	Indicates extent of hypovolemia and influences replacement needs.
Investigate changes in mentation/sensorium.	Severe dehydration impairs cardiac output and tissue perfusion, especially in the brain.
Auscultate bowel sounds. Note complaints of nausea, presence of vomiting and diarrhea.	Impaired GI function can increase fluid/electrolyte losses and influences choice of routes for fluid and nutrient replacement.
Provide mouth care frequently.	Helps to reduce discomfort of dehydration and prevent mucous membrane breakdown.
Maintain comfortable environment. Cover patient with light blanket.	Avoids overheating which could promote further fluid loss.
Promote bedrest, assist with position changes and self-care activities.	Minimizes orthostatic hypotension, reducing risk of loss of consciousness and injury.
Encourage oral fluids up to 3000 ml/day as soon as patient can tolerate them.	Relief of GI symptoms and return of bowel function permits oral replacement of fluids/electrolytes.
Reposition frequently. Massage bony prominences.	Severe dehydration can greatly compromise circulation and skin breakdown can occur rapidly.
Observe for fatigue, rales, crackles, edema, increased heart rate.	Rapid replacement of fluids may lead to congestive heart failure in presence of cardiac strain.
Collaborative	
Administer fluids, e.g.:	
0.9% saline;	Patient may require up to 4–6 liters of fluid to replace losses. IV saline should be given rapidly in rates of up to 500–1000 ml/hr for a few hours to replace the sodium deficit.
Glucose solutions.	Added to help relieve hypoglycemia.
Administer medications as indicated:	
Cortisone (Cortone) or hydrocortisone (Cortef);	Drugs of choice to replace cortisol deficits and promote sodium resorption, which may reduce fluid losses and maintain cardiac output. Note: Patient may need salt restriction and potassium supplement if hy-

ACTIONS/INTERVENTIONS	RATIONALE
Collaborative	
	pertension occurs, if long-term cortisone therapy is needed and/or patient is taking a potassium-wasting diuretic.
Mineralocorticoids, e.g., fludrocortisone (Florinef), deoxycorticosterone (Cortate, DOCA-A);	Begun after completion of high-dose hydrocortisone therapy, the dosage of these potent salt-retaining steroids are adjusted according to their effect on BP, serum electrolyte levels, and alleviation of symptoms. Note: Not required in secondary adrenal insufficiency, because mineralocorticoid secretion is intact.
Insert/maintain indwelling urinary catheter.	Facilitates an accurate measurement of output.
Monitor laboratory studies, e.g.:	
Hct;	Elevated levels reflecting hemoconcentration should return to normal as rehydration occurs.
BUN/Cr;	Elevated values may reflect cellular breakdown from dehydration or signal the onset of renal failure.
Serum osmolality;	Elevated due to dehydration.
Sodium;	Hyponatremia reflects urinary loss due to impaired tubule reabsorption.
Potassium.	Decreased aldosterone levels allow sodium and water to be depleted while potassium is retained, resulting in hyperkalemia.

NURSING DIAGNOSIS:	**NUTRITION, ALTERED: LESS THAN BODY REQUIREMENTS**
May be related to:	**Glucocorticoid deficiency; abnormal fat, protein and carbohydrate metabolism**
	Nausea, vomiting, anorexia
Possibly evidenced by:	**Weight loss, muscle wasting, abdominal cramps and diarrhea**
	Severe hypoglycemia
PATIENT OUTCOMES/ EVALUATION CRITERIA:	**Reports relief of nausea and vomiting. Demonstrates stable weight or weight gain toward desired goal with absence of presenting signs and normalization of laboratory values.**

ACTIONS/INTERVENTIONS	RATIONALE
Independent	
Auscultate bowel sounds and assess for abdominal pain, nausea, vomiting.	Cortisol deficit can cause GI symptoms, affecting ingestion and absorption of nutrients.
Note presence of cool/clammy skin, changes in level of consciousness, rapid pulse, irritability, headache, shakiness.	Symptoms of hypoglycemia which signal the need for glucose, and may indicate a need for more glucocorticoids.

ACTIONS/INTERVENTIONS	RATIONALE
Independent	
Monitor dietary intake and weigh daily.	Aids in identifying nutritional needs and effectiveness of therapy. Note: Rapid weight gain may reflect fluid retention/effects of glucocorticoid replacement.
Record incidence, amount/other characteristics of vomiting.	This helps to determine degree of digestion/absorption of nutrients.
Provide/assist with mouth care.	A clean mouth can stimulate appetite.
Provide an environment conducive to eating, i.e., un-rushed atmosphere, absence of noxious odors, socialization.	May increase appetite, improve intake.
Obtain information about food preferences.	May stimulate appetite and facilitate intake when preferences are incorporated into meal plan.
Include SO in meal planning as indicated.	Understanding and involvement provides support and may enhance cooperation with diet.
Collaborative	
Maintain NPO status as indicated.	Promotes gastrointestinal rest, reduces discomfort and fluid/electrolyte loss associated with vomiting.
Perform fingerstick glucose testing, as indicated.	Serves as an ongoing assessment of serum glucose level/therapy needs. If decreased, dietary as well as glucocorticoid adjustments may need to be made.
Administer IV glucose and medications as indicated:	Corrects hypoglycemia, provides energy source for cellular function.
Glucocorticoids;	Stimulates gluconeogenesis, decreases utilization of glucose and promotes glucose storage as glycogen. Regular administration of drug is necessary for appropriate carbohydrate, protein, and fat metabolism.
Androgens, e.g., testosterone.	May be useful in debilitated/malnourished patients to improve appetite, foster a positive nitrogen balance, improve muscle tone/strength, and enhance sense of well-being.
Consult with dietician/nutritional support team.	Useful in determining individual nutritional/caloric needs and most appropriate route.
Provide liquids as tolerated; progress to small, frequent feedings of foods high in calories/protein when oral intake is resumed.	When nausea/vomiting and pain subside, beverages and small portions of solid foods can replace intravenous fluids. Increased caloric intake may be needed to foster weight gain and prevent hypoglycemia.
Increase sodium in diet, e.g., meats, fish, poultry, milk, eggs.	May help to prevent/correct hyponatremia.
Monitor Hb/Hct.	Presence of anemia can be due to nutritional deficits or may be attributed to a dilutional factor, which may occur from fluid retention associated with glucocorticoid administration.

NURSING DIAGNOSIS:	**FATIGUE**
May be related to:	**Decreased metabolic energy production**
	Altered body chemistry: fluid, electrolyte and glucose imbalance

Possibly evidenced by:	Unremitting/overwhelming lack of energy
	Inability to maintain usual routines, decreased performance
	Impaired ability to concentrate, lethargy, disinterest in surroundings
PATIENT OUTCOMES/ EVALUATION CRITERIA:	Reports feeling rested, increase in energy level, and decreased sense of fatigue. Verbalizes factors that contribute to fatigue. Displays improved ability to participate in desired activities.

ACTIONS/INTERVENTIONS	RATIONALE
Independent	
Discuss/review patient's fatigue level and identify activities that worsen fatigue.	Patient usually has decreased energy, muscle fatigue, which becomes progressively worse during the day due to disease process and sodium/potassium imbalance.
Monitor vital signs before and after activity. Observe for tachycardia, hypotension, pallor.	Circulatory collapse can occur as a result of activity stress if cardiac output is diminished.
Discuss the need for activity and plan the schedule with the patient. Identify activities that lead to fatigue.	Even though patient may initially feel too weak to engage in activity, gradual resumption of activity while receiving hormone replacement therapy improves muscle tone and strength, lessening fatigue. In addition, it provides hope that ability to perform desired activities will return.
Encourage patient to alternate periods of rest with activity.	Minimizes fatigue and prevents strain on the heart.
Discuss ways of conserving energy (e.g., sitting, rather than standing during activities), assist with/ provide self-care as necessary.	Patient will be able to accomplish more with a decreased expenditure of energy.
Have patient progressively do self-care.	Increases confidence level, and self-esteem as well as activity tolerance level.

NURSING DIAGNOSIS:	CARDIAC OUTPUT, ALTERED: DECREASED [POTENTIAL]
May be related to:	Decreased venous return/circulating volume
	Alterations in rate, rhythm, conduction (electrolyte imbalance)
	Inotropic changes in size/strength of cardiac muscle; abnormal metabolism with insufficient energy for cellular function (e.g., hypoglycemia)
Possibly evidenced by:	[Not applicable; presence of signs and symptoms establishes an *actual* diagnosis.]
PATIENT OUTCOMES/	Demonstrates adequate cardiac output, as evidenced by

ACTIONS/INTERVENTIONS	RATIONALE
Independent	
Monitor vital signs; heart rate/rhythm, documenting dysrhythmias.	Heart rate will elevate initially to compensate for hypovolemia and decreased cardiac output. Development of cardiac muscle failure/Addisonian crisis may cause sudden and profound hypotension. Irregular heart rate could result in decreased cardiac output or lead to MI. PVCs and depressed T waves may be present if patient is hypokalemic, or peaked T waves will occur with hyperkalemia.
Measure CVP if available.	CVP provides a more direct measurement of fluid volume and developing complications, e.g., cardiac failure.
Monitor temperature, noting sudden changes.	Sudden hyperpyrexia can occur, followed by hypothermia, as a result of hormonal, fluid, and electrolyte imbalance, affecting heart rate and cardiac output.
Assess skin color, temperature, capillary refill, peripheral pulses.	Pallor, cool/clammy skin, delayed capillary refill, weak/thready pulses may indicate impending shock.
Investigate changes in mentation and complaints of severe abdominal, back, or leg pain.	Mental changes (irritability, anxiety, apprehension) may be profound, reflecting decreased cardiac output/cerebral and peripheral perfusion, and/or severe hypoglycemia.
Measure urinary output.	Although polyuria is usual, falling output suggests reduced kidney perfusion, reflecting decreased cardiac output.
Place in quiet/cool room, avoiding loud noises and excessive activity. Avoid stressful topics and actions. Maintain bedrest; assist with or perform all care activities.	Patient's normal response to stressors is lacking, and stimuli that usually would not be of concern can negatively affect the patient.
Monitor for hypertension, dependent edema, crackles, weight gain, severe headache, irritability/confusion.	Excessive administration of corticosteroids and/or overzealous sodium and fluid replacement may potentiate fluid excess and cardiac failure.
Collaborative	
Administer IV fluids, blood, saline solutions and volume expanders as necessary. Avoid use of hypotonic or potassium-containing fluids.	Restoring circulating volume usually improves cardiac output. Because hyperkalemia is often present, exogenous potassium may cause severe dysrhythmias, cardiac arrest.
Administer medications as indicated:	
Hydrocortisone sodium succinate;	Rapid infusion of approximately 25–50 mg over 30–60 minutes, then 75–150 mg in next 4–8 hours, may prevent cardiovascular collapse.
Vasopressors, e.g., metaraminal bitartrate (Aramine);	Increases peripheral vascular resistance and venous return to improve cardiac output and BP.
Antipyretics, e.g., aspirin.	Fever greater than 40.6°C (105°F) occasionally occurs, contributing to stress situation and continuing sodium/water losses.
Provide supplemental oxygen.	Maximizes oxygenation; may help to reduce cardiac workload.

ACTIONS/INTERVENTIONS	RATIONALE
Collaborative	
Monitor serum potassium.	Patient is prone to hyperkalemia because as sodium levels decrease (secondary to an aldosterone deficit), potassium is retained by the kidneys.

NURSING DIAGNOSIS:	**THOUGHT PROCESSES, ALTERED [POTENTIAL]**
May be related to:	**Decreased sodium levels, hypoglycemia, dehydration, acid–base imbalance**
Possibly evidenced by:	**[Not applicable; presence of signs and symptoms establishes an *actual* diagnosis.]**
PATIENT OUTCOMES/ EVALUATION CRITERIA:	**Maintains usual level of mentation, free of injury.**

ACTIONS/INTERVENTIONS	RATIONALE
Independent	
Assign one nurse from each shift on a consistent basis if possible.	Provides best opportunity for early recognition of CNS changes and promotes a trusting relationship.
Monitor vital and neurologic signs.	Provides baseline for comparison/recognition of abnormal findings. Note: High temperature may affect mentation.
Address patient by name. Reorient to place, person, and time as needed. Give short explanations.	Helps to maintain orientation and decrease confusion.
Maintain consistent routine as possible. Schedule nursing time to provide for frequent rest periods.	Promotes orientation, prevents excessive fatigue.
Encourage patient to perform self-care to extent possible, with sufficient time to complete tasks.	Helps to keep the patient in touch with reality and maintain orientation to the environment.
Protect the patient from injury, e.g., bed in low position with siderails raised; assist with ambulation, changes in position; judicious use of restraints; provide padded bedrails/tongue blade (seizure precautions).	Disorientation increases risk of injury, especially at nighttime. Seizure precautions may be necessary to prevent physical injury, aspiration, etc.
Collaborative	
Monitor laboratory studies, e.g., blood glucose, serum osmolality, Hb/Hct.	As fluid, electrolyte and acid–base imbalances are corrected, thought processes should improve. Continued changes in mentation require further evaluation.

NURSING DIAGNOSIS:	**SELF-CONCEPT, DISTURBANCE IN: (SPECIFY) [POTENTIAL]**
May be related to:	**Presence of physical condition requiring lifelong therapy**
	Changes in skin pigmentation, weight, secondary sex characteristics, and role functioning

Possibly evidenced by:	[Not applicable; presence of signs and symptoms establishes an *actual* diagnosis.]
PATIENT OUTCOMES/ EVALUATION CRITERIA:	Verbalizes acceptance of self in situation. Demonstrates adaptation to changes/events that have occurred as evidenced by setting of realistic goals and active participation in work/play/personal relationships.

ACTIONS/INTERVENTIONS	RATIONALE

Independent

Arrange short periods of uninterrupted time and encourage patient to express feelings about effects of condition, e.g., change in appearance or roles, effect of illness on job. Demonstrate a caring, nonjudgmental manner.	Fosters rapport and promotes openness on the part of the patient. Helps in evaluating how much of a problem the various changes are to the patient.
Reduce excess stimuli in environment; provide private room if indicated. Encourage use of stress-management skills, e.g., relaxation techniques, visualization, guided imagery.	Minimizes feelings of stress, frustration; enhances coping abilities and promotes sense of control.
Encourage patient to enlist the aid of SO in dealing with stress.	Patient will not feel as alone if s/he confides in others and asks for assistance in problem solving. This also fosters understanding and a feeling of usefulness on the part of SO.
Encourage patient to make choices related to and participate in self-care.	May help to increase confidence level, improve self-esteem, decrease preoccupation with the changes and enhance sense of control.
Point out improvements that are occurring with treatment, e.g., decreasing skin pigmentation, weight gain, increasing hair growth (if male hormones have been given), resumption of the normal menstrual cycle.	These comments may lift patient's spirits and promote self-esteem.
Suggest visit with person whose disease is controlled and whose symptoms have subsided.	May be encouraging to the patient to see the results of treatment.

Collaborative

Refer to social services, counseling, support groups as needed.	A comprehensive approach may be needed for patient to maintain/regain coping behaviors.

NURSING DIAGNOSIS:	**KNOWLEDGE DEFICIT [LEARNING NEED] (SPECIFY)**
May be related to:	**Lack of exposure/recall; information misinterpretation**
	Cognitive limitation
Possibly evidenced by:	**Questions, request for information, verbalization of the problem**
	Inaccurate follow-through of instruction; development of preventable complications
PATIENT OUTCOMES/ EVALUATION CRITERIA:	**Verbalizes understanding of disease process and treatment. Identifies relationship of signs/symptoms to disease process and correlates symptoms with causative**

factors. Identifies stress situations and specific actions to deal with them. Initiates necessary lifestyle changes and participates in treatment regimen.

ACTIONS/INTERVENTIONS	RATIONALE
Independent	
Review disease process and future expectations.	Provides knowledge base on which patient can make informed choices.
Encourage patient to remain as active as possible, to maintain a regular schedule for eating, sleeping, and exercise.	Helps to promote feelings of well-being and good health and to understand that irregular physical activity may increase hormonal needs.
Explain reason for excessive fluid loss. Recommend that patient monitor intake/output and weight as applicable and to increase glucose, fluid, and salt intake during periods of stress, GI upset, excessive sweating (strenuous exercise, hot environment).	Knowledge may help prevent the problem in the future, and participation helps promote compliance with the therapy and provides opportunity for early recognition of changes.
Discuss dietary regimen, e.g., regular, nutritious diet with high carbohydrates and protein.	Prevents weight loss and reduces risk of hypoglycemia.
Review hormone replacement therapy and necessity of adherence to drug schedule;	Helps patient to understand reasons for treatment (daily medication enables patient to live normal, active life) which can enhance cooperation.
Take medications at mealtime/with snacks or with antacids;	Reduces GI upset and risk of peptic ulcer formation.
Take two thirds of cortisol dose in the am, one third in the late afternoon, or Florinef in the morning;	Mimics the body's natural secretion of corticoids.
Never omit a dose of the drug; take IM form of drug when ill (deep gluteal administration).	Failure to comply with replacement regimen places the patient at risk for crisis. Note: Subcutaneous injection potentiates risk of sterile abscess and tissue atrophy.
Stress need to wear an identification bracelet and to carry emergency drugs, e.g., IM or IV dexamethasone sodium (Decajet, Decadron Phosphate).	Assists with prompt/appropriate intervention in case of emergency.
Define and problem-solve ways to limit/control stressors, e.g., infection, dental work, trauma/accidents, personal or family crises, increased activity, prolonged exposure to hot temperatures.	The dosage of glucocortocoids may need to be adjusted (doubled or tripled) during periods of stress.
Discuss feelings related to taking drugs for the rest of the patient's life.	Discussing these factors may help patient to incorporate necessary changes into lifestyle.
Identify signs and symptoms requiring medical evaluation, e.g., nausea, vomiting, anorexia, weight loss, diarrhea, weakness, excess urination, irregular heartbeat; or weight gain and puffy face, neck, legs, or feet.	Prompt recognition of imbalance between hormone replacement and body needs (under/overdosing) may prevent development of life-threatening situation.
Stress importance of avoiding exposure to infection (crowds, persons with infectious processes; maintaining good handwashing/personal practices) and prompt reporting of signs of infection.	Suppression of the inflammatory response increases risk of infection and possibility of progression to a life-threatening situation.
Discuss necessity of regular medical follow-up.	Facilitates control of chronic condition and prevention of complications.

627

Hyperthyroidism (Thyrotoxicosis) _____

PATIENT ASSESSMENT DATA BASE

Data are dependent on the severity/duration of hormone imbalance and involvement of other organs.

ACTIVITY/REST

May report:	Nervousness, increased irritability, insomnia.
	Muscle weakness, incoordination.
	Extreme fatigue.
May exhibit:	Muscle atrophy.

CIRCULATION

May report:	Palpitations.
	Chest pain (angina).
May exhibit:	Dysrhythmias (atrial fibrillation); gallop rhythm, murmurs.
	Elevated BP with widened pulse pressure.
	Tachycardia at rest.
	Circulatory collapse, shock (thyrotoxic crisis).

ELIMINATION

May report:	Urinating in large amounts.
	Stool changes; diarrhea.

EGO INTEGRITY

May exhibit:	Emotional lability (mild euphoria to delerium); depression.

FOOD/FLUID

May report:	Recent/sudden weight loss.
	Increased appetite; large meals, frequent meals; thirst.
	Nausea, vomiting.
May exhibit:	Enlarged thyroid; goiter.
	Nonpitting fullness, especially in pretibial area.

NEUROSENSORY

May exhibit:	Rapid and hoarse speech.
	Mental status and behavior alterations, e.g., confusion, disorientation, nervousness, irritability, delirium, frank psychosis, stupor, coma.
	Fine tremor in hands; purposeless, quick, jerky movements of body parts.
	Hyperactive deep tendon reflexes.

PAIN/COMFORT

May report:	Orbital pain, photophobia (eye involvement).

RESPIRATION

May exhibit:	Increased respiratory rate, tachypnea.
	Dyspnea.
	Pulmonary edema (thyrotoxic crisis).

SAFETY

May report: Heat intolerance, excessive sweating.

Allergy to iodine (may be used in testing).

May exhibit: Elevated temperature (above 100°F), diaphoresis.

Skin smooth, warm and flushed; hair fine, silky, straight.

Exophthalmia; lid retraction; conjunctival irritation, tearing.

Pruritic, erythematous lesions (often in pretibial area) that become brawny.

SEXUALITY

May report: Decreased libido.

Hypomenorrhea, amenorrhea.

Impotence.

TEACHING/LEARNING

May report: Family history of thyroid problems.

History of hypothyroidism, thyroid hormone replacement therapy or antithyroid therapy, premature withdrawal of antithyroid drugs, recent partial thyroidectomy.

History of insulin-induced hypoglycemia, cardiac disorders or surgery, recent illness (pneumonia), trauma; x-ray contrast studies.

Recent stressful experience, e.g., emotional/physical.

Discharge Plan Considerations: May require assistance with treatment regimen.

DIAGNOSTIC STUDIES

Radioactive iodine uptake (RAIU) test: high in Grave's disease and toxic nodular goiter; low in thyroiditis.

Serum thyroxine (T_4) and triiodothyronine (T_3): increased.

Thyroid ^{131}I uptake: increased.

Protein-bound iodine (PBI): increased.

Blood sugar: elevated (related to adrenal involvement).

Plasma cortisol: low levels (less adrenal reserve).

Alkaline phosphatase and serum calcium: increased.

Liver function tests: abnormal.

Electrolytes: hyponatremia may reflect adrenal response or dilutional effect in fluid replacement therapy. Hypokalemia occurs owing to GI losses and diuresis.

Serum catecholamine: decreased.

Urine creatinine: increased.

ECG: atrial fibrillations; shorter systole time; cardiomegaly, heart enlarged with fibrosis and necrosis (late signs or in elderly with masked hyperthyroidism).

NURSING PRIORITIES

1. Reduce metabolic demands and support cardiovascular function.
2. Provide psychologic support.
3. Prevent complications.
4. Provide information about disease process/prognosis and therapy needs.

DISCHARGE CRITERIA

1. Achieves homeostasis.
2. Dealing with current situation.

629

3. Complications prevented/minimized.
4. Disease process/prognosis and therapeutic regimen understood.

NURSING DIAGNOSIS:	**CARDIAC OUTPUT, ALTERED: DECREASED [POTENTIAL]**
May be related to:	**Uncontrolled hyperthyroidism, hypermetabolic state increasing cardiac workload**
	Changes in venous return and systemic vascular resistance
	Alterations in rate, rhythm, conduction
Possibly evidenced by:	**[Not applicable; presence of signs and symptoms establishes an *actual* diagnosis.]**
PATIENT OUTCOMES/ EVALUATION CRITERIA:	**Maintains adequate cardiac output for tissue needs as evidenced by stable vital signs, palpable peripheral pulses, good capillary refill, usual mentation, and absence of dysrhythmias.**

ACTIONS/INTERVENTIONS	RATIONALE
Independent	
Monitor BP lying/sitting and standing, if able. Note widened pulse pressure.	General/orthostatic hypotension may occur as a result of excessive peripheral vasodilation and decreased circulating volume. Widened pulse pressure reflects compensatory increase in stroke volume and decreased systemic vascular resistance.
Monitor CVP if available.	Provides more direct measure of circulating volume and cardiac function.
Investigate complaints of chest pain/angina.	May reflect increased myocardial oxygen demands/ischemia.
Auscultate heart sounds, noting extra heart sounds, development of gallops and systolic murmurs.	Prominent S_1 and murmurs are associated with forceful cardiac output of hypermetabolic state; development of S_3 may warn of impending cardiac failure.
Monitor ECG, noting rate/rhythm. Document dysrhythmias.	Tachycardia (greater than normally expected with fever/increased circulatory demand) may reflect direct myocardial stimulation by thyroid hormone. Dysrhythmias often occur and may compromise cardiac function/output.
Auscultate breath sounds, noting adventitious sounds (e.g., crackles).	Early sign of pulmonary congestion, reflecting developing cardiac failure.
Monitor temperature; provide cool environment; limit bed linens/clothes; administer tepid sponge baths.	Fever (may exceed 104°F) may occur as a result of excessive thyroid levels and can aggravate diuresis and dehydration and cause increased peripheral vasodilation, venous pooling, and hypotension.
Observe signs/symptoms of severe thirst, dry mucous membranes, weak/thready pulse, poor capillary refill, decreased urine output, and hypotension.	Rapid dehydration can occur, which reduces circulating volume and compromises cardiac output.
Record intake/output. Note urine specific gravity.	Significant fluid losses (through vomiting, diarrhea, di-

ACTIONS/INTERVENTIONS	RATIONALE

Independent

Weigh daily.

uresis, diaphoresis) can lead to profound dehydration, concentrated urine, and weight loss.

Encourage chair/bed rest; limit nonessential activity.

Activity increases metabolic/circulatory demands, which may potentiate cardiac failure.

Note history of asthma/bronchoconstrictive disease, pregnancy, sinus bradycardia/heart blocks, advanced heart failure.

Presence of these conditions affect choice of therapy; e.g., use of beta-adrenergic blocking agents is contraindicated.

Observe for adverse side effects of adrenergic antagonists, e.g., severe decrease in pulse, BP; signs of vascular congestion/CHF; cardiac arrest.

Indicates need for reduction/discontinuation of therapy.

Collaborative

Administer intravenous fluids as indicated.

Rapid fluid replacement may be necessary to improve circulating volume but must be balanced against signs of cardiac failure/need for inotropic support.

Administer medications as indicated:

Beta-blockers, e.g., propranolol (Inderal), atenolol (Tenormin), nadolol (Corgard);

Given to control thyrotoxic effects of tachycardia, tremors, and nervousness and is first drug of choice for acute storm. Decreases heart rate/cardiac work by blocking beta-adrenergic receptor sites and blocking conversion of T_4 to T_3. Note: If severe bradycardia develops, atropine may be required.

Thyroid hormone antagonists, e.g., propylthiouracil (PTU), methimazole (Tapazole);

Blocks thyroid hormone synthesis and inhibits peripheral conversion of T_4 to T_3. May be definitive treatment or used to prepare patient for surgery; but effect is slow, and so may not relieve thyroid storm. Note: Once PTU therapy is begun, abrupt withdrawal may precipitate thyroid crisis.

Sodium iodine IV or supersaturated potassium iodide (SSKI) by mouth;

Temporarily acts to prevent release of thyroid hormone into circulation by increasing the amount of thyroid hormone stored within the gland. May interfere with radioactive iodine treatment and may exacerbate the disease in some people. May be used as surgical preparation to decrease size and vascularity of the gland or to treat thyroid storm. Note: Should be started 1–3 hours after initiation of antithyroid drug therapy to minimize hormone formation from the iodine.

Radioactive iodine;

Destroys functioning gland tissue. Peak results take 6–12 weeks (several treatments may be necessary).

Corticosteroids, e.g., dexamethazone (Decadron);

Provides glucocorticol support. Decreases hyperthermia, relieves relative adrenal insufficiency, inhibits calcium absorption, and reduces peripheral conversion of T_3 from T_4.

Digoxin (Lanoxin);

Digitalization may be required in congestive failure patients before beta-adrenergic blocking therapy can be considered/safely initiated.

Furosemide (Lasix);

Diuresis may be necessary if congestive failure occurs. Note: It also may be effective in reducing calcium level if neuromuscular function is impaired.

Acetaminophen (Tylenol);

Drug of choice to reduce temperature and associated

ACTIONS/INTERVENTIONS	RATIONALE
Collaborative	
	metabolic demands. Aspirin is contraindicated because it actually increases level of circulating thyroid hormones by blocking binding of T_3 and T_4 with thyroid-binding proteins.
Sedative, barbiturates;	Promotes rest, thereby reducing metabolic demands.
Muscle relaxants.	Reduces shivering associated with hyperthermia, which can further increase metabolic demands.
Monitor laboratory studies, as indicated, e.g.:	
Serum potassium (replace as indicated);	Hypokalemia resulting from intestinal losses, altered intake, or diuretic therapy may cause dysrhythmias and compromise cardiac function/output.
Serum calcium;	Elevation may alter cardiac contractility.
Sputum culture.	Pulmonary infection is most frequent precipitating factor of crisis.
Review serial ECGs;	May demonstrate effects of electrolyte imbalance or ischemic changes reflecting inadequate myocardial oxygen supply in presence of increased metabolic demands.
Chest x-rays.	Cardiac enlargement may occur in response to increased circulatory demands. Pulmonary congestion may be noted with cardiac decompensation.
Provide supplemental oxygen as indicated.	May be necessary to support increased metabolic demands/oxygen consumption.
Provide hypothermia blanket as indicated.	Occasionally used to lower uncontrolled hyperthermia (104°F and above) to reduce metabolic demands/ oxygen consumption, and cardiac workload.
Administer/assist with transfusions/plasmapheresis, hemoperfusion, dialysis.	May be done to achieve rapid depletion of extrathyroidal hormone pool in desperately ill/comatose patient.
Prepare for surgery.	Subtotal thyroidectomy (removal of five sixths of the gland) may be treatment of choice for hyperthyroidism once euthyroid state is achieved. (Refer to CP: Thyroidectomy, p. 639.)

NURSING DIAGNOSIS:	FATIGUE
May be related to:	**Hypermetabolic state with increased energy requirements; irritability of CNS; altered body chemistry**
Possibly evidenced by:	**Verbalization of overwhelming lack of energy to maintain usual routine, decreased performance**
	Emotional lability/irritability; nervousness, tension, jittery behavior
	Impaired ability to concentrate
PATIENT OUTCOMES/ EVALUATION CRITERIA:	**Verbalizes increase in level of energy. Displays improved ability to participate in desired activities.**

632

ACTIONS/INTERVENTIONS	RATIONALE
Independent	
Monitor vital signs, noting pulse rate at rest as well as when active.	Pulse is typically elevated and even at rest, tachycardia (up to 160) may be noted.
Note development of tachypnea, dyspnea, pallor, and cyanosis.	Oxygen demand and consumption is increased in hypermetabolic state, potentiating risk of hypoxia with activity.
Provide for quiet environment; cool room, decreased sensory stimuli, soothing colors, quiet music.	Reduces stimuli that may aggravate agitation, hyperactivity, and insomnia.
Encourage patient to restrict activity and rest in bed as much as possible.	Helps counteract effects of increased metabolism.
Provide routine comfort measures, e.g., judicious touch/massage, cool showers.	May decrease nervous energy, promoting relaxation.
Provide for diversional activities that are calming, e.g., reading, radio, televison.	Allows for use of nervous energy in a constructive manner and may reduce anxiety.
Avoid topics that irritate or upset the patient. Discuss ways to respond to these feelings.	Increased irritability of the CNS may cause patient to be easily excited, agitated, and prone to emotional outbursts.
Discuss with SO reasons for fatigue and emotional lability.	Understanding that the behavior is physically based may enhance coping with current situation and encourage SO to respond differently and provide support for the patient.
Collaborative	
Administer medications as indicated:	
Sedatives, e.g., phenobarbital (Luminal); tranquilizers, e.g., chlordiazepoxide (Librium).	Combats nervousness, hyperactivity, and insomnia.

NURSING DIAGNOSIS:	NUTRITION, ALTERED: LESS THAN BODY REQUIREMENTS [POTENTIAL]
May be related to:	Increased metabolism (increased appetite/intake with loss of weight)
	Nausea, vomiting, diarrhea
	Relative insulin insufficiency; hyperglycemia
Possibly evidenced by:	[Not applicable; presence of signs and symptoms establishes an *actual* diagnosis.]
PATIENT OUTCOMES/ EVALUATION CRITERIA:	Demonstrates stable weight with normal laboratory values and no signs of malnutrition.

ACTIONS/INTERVENTIONS	RATIONALE
Independent	
Auscultate bowel sounds.	Hyperactive bowel sounds reflect increased gastric motility, which can reduce/alter absorption.
Note complaints of anorexia, generalized weakness/aches, abdominal pain; presence of nausea/vomiting,	Increased adrenergic activity can cause impaired insulin secretion/resistance, resulting in hyperglycemia.

633

ACTIONS/INTERVENTIONS

Independent

polydipsia, polyuria; changes in respiratory rate/depth.

Monitor daily food intake. Weigh daily and report losses.

Encourage patient to eat and increase number of meals and snacks, using high-calorie foods that are easily digested.

Avoid foods that increase peristalsis (e.g., tea, coffee, fibrous and highly seasoned foods) and fluids that cause diarrhea (e.g., apple/prune).

Collaborative

Consult with dietician to provide diet high in calories, protein, carbohydrates, and vitamins.

Administer medications as indicated:

Glucose, vitamin B complex;

Insulin (small doses).

RATIONALE

Continued weight loss in face of adequate caloric intake may indicate failure of antithyroid therapy.

Aids in keeping caloric intake high enough to keep up with rapid expenditure of calories caused by hypermetabolic state.

Increased motility of GI tract may result in diarrhea and impair absorption of needed nutrients.

May need assistance to assure adequate intake of nutrients, identify appropriate supplements.

Given to meet energy requirements and prevent or correct hypoglycemia.

Aids in controlling serum glucose if elevated.

NURSING DIAGNOSIS:	TISSUE INTEGRITY, IMPAIRED [POTENTIAL]
May be related to:	**Alterations of protective mechanisms of eye: impaired closure of eyelid/exophthalmos**
Possibly evidenced by:	**[Not applicable; presence of signs and symptoms establishes an *actual* diagnosis.]**
PATIENT OUTCOMES/ EVALUATION CRITERIA:	**Maintains moist eye membranes, free of ulcerations. Identifies measures to provide protection for eyes and prevent complications.**

ACTIONS/INTERVENTIONS

Independent

Observe for periorbital edema, lid lag, and wide-eyed stare, excessive tearing; note complaints of photophobia, feeling of foreign object in eye; eye pain.

Evaluate visual acuity; note complaints of blurred or double vision.

Encourage use of dark glasses when awake and taping the eyelids shut during sleep if indicated.

Elevate the head of the bed and restrict salt intake if indicated.

RATIONALE

Common manifestations of excessive adrenergic stimulation related to thyrotoxicosis, requiring supportive interventions until therapeutic resolution of crisis state relieves symptomatology.

Infiltrative ophthalmopathy (Graves' disease) is result of increased retroorbital tissue, creating exophthalmos, and lymphocytic infiltration of extraocular muscles, causing weakness. Corresponding visual impairment may worsen or improve independent of therapy and clinical course of disease.

Protects exposed cornea if patient is unable to close eyelids completely due to edema/fibrosis of fat pads.

Decreases tissue edema when appropriate, e.g., CHF, which can aggravate existing exophthalmos.

ACTIONS/INTERVENTIONS

Independent

Instruct the patient in extraocular muscle exercises if appropriate.

Provide opportunity for patient to discuss feelings about altered appearance and measures to enhance self-image.

Collaborative

Administer medications as indicated:

    Methylcellulose drops;

    ACTH, prednisone;

    Antithyroid drugs;

    Diuretics.

Prepare for surgery as indicated.

RATIONALE

Improves circulation and maintains mobility of the eyelids.

Protruding eyes may be viewed as unattractive. Appearance can be enhanced with proper use of makeup, overall grooming, and use of shaded glasses.

Lubricates the eyes.

Given to decrease rapidly progressive and marked inflammation.

May decrease signs/symptoms or prevent worsening of the condition.

Can decrease edema in mild involvement.

Eyelids may need to be sutured shut temporarily to protect the corneas until edema resolves (rare); or increasing space within sinus cavity and adjusting musculature may return eye to a more normal position.

NURSING DIAGNOSIS:	ANXIETY [SPECIFY LEVEL]
May be related to:	**Physiologic factors: hypermetabolic state (CNS stimulation), pseudocatecholamine effect of thyroid hormones**
Possibly evidenced by:	**Increased feelings of apprehension, shakiness, loss of control, panic**
	Changes in cognition, distortion of environmental stimuli
	Extraneous movements, restlessness, tremors
PATIENT OUTCOMES/ EVALUATION CRITERIA:	**Appears relaxed. Reports anxiety reduced to a manageable level. Identifies healthy ways to deal with feelings.**

ACTIONS/INTERVENTIONS

Independent

Observe behavior indicative of level of anxiety.

Monitor physical responses, noting palpitations, repetitive movements, hyperventilation, insomnia.

RATIONALE

Mild anxiety may be displayed by irritability and insomnia. Severe anxiety progressing to panic state may produce feelings of impending doom, terror, inability to speak or move, shouting/swearing.

Increased number of beta-adrenergic receptor sites, coupled with effects of excess thyroid hormones, produces clinical manifestations of catecholamine excess even when normal levels of norepinephrine/ epinephrine exist.

635

ACTIONS/INTERVENTIONS	RATIONALE

Independent

Stay with patient, maintaining calm manner. Acknowledge fear and allow patient's behavior to belong to the patient.

Affirms to patient/SO that although patient feels out of control, environment is safe. Avoiding personal responses to inappropriate remarks or actions prevents conflicts/overreaction to stressful situation.

Describe/explain procedures, surrounding environment or sounds that may be heard by the patient.

Provides accurate information, which reduces distortions, misinterpretations, which can contribute to anxiety/fear reactions.

Speak in brief statements, using simple words.

Attention span may be shortened, concentration reduced, limiting ability to assimilate information.

Reduce external stimuli:

Place in quiet room; provide soft, soothing music; reduce bright lights; reduce number of persons contacting patient.

Creates a therapeutic environment; shows recognition that unit activity/personnel may increase patient's anxiety.

Discuss with patient/SO reasons for emotional lability/psychotic reaction. (Refer to ND: Thought Processes, Altered [Potential], below.)

Understanding that behavior is physically based can allow for different responses/approaches.

Reinforce expectation that emotional control should return as drug therapy progresses.

Provides information and reassures patient that the situation is temporary and will improve with treatment.

Collaborative

Administer antianxiety medications (tranquilizers, sedatives) and monitor effects.

May be used in conjunction with medical regimen to reduce effects of hyperthyroid secretion.

Refer to support systems as needed, e.g., counseling, social services, pastoral care.

Ongoing therapy support may be desired/required by patient/SO if crisis precipitates lifestyle alterations.

NURSING DIAGNOSIS:	THOUGHT PROCESSES, ALTERED [POTENTIAL]
May be related to:	**Physiologic changes: increased CNS stimulation/accelerated mental activity** **Altered sleep patterns**
Possibly evidenced by:	**[Not applicable; presence of signs and symptoms establishes an *actual* diagnosis.]**
PATIENT OUTCOMES/ EVALUATION CRITERIA:	**Maintains usual reality orientation. Recognizes changes in thinking/behavior and causative factors.**

ACTIONS/INTERVENTIONS	RATIONALE

Independent

Assess thinking processes, e.g., memory, attention span, orientation to person/place/time.

Determines extent of interference with sensory processing.

Note changes in behavior.

May be hypervigilant, restless, extremely sensitive, or crying or may develop frank psychosis.

Assess level of anxiety. (Refer to ND: Anxiety, p. 635.)

Anxiety may alter thought processes.

Provide quiet environment; decreased stimuli, cool

Reduction of external stimuli may decrease

ACTIONS/INTERVENTIONS

Independent

room, dim lights. Limit procedures/personnel.

Reorient to person/place/time.

Present reality concisely and briefly without challenging illogical thinking.

Provide clock, calendar, room with outside window; alter level of lighting to simulate day/night.

Provide safety measures, e.g., padded side rails, soft restraints, close supervision.

Encourage visits by family/SO. Provide support as needed.

Collaborative

Administer medications as indicated, e.g., sedatives/tranquilizers/antipsychotic drugs.

RATIONALE

hyperactivity/reflexia, CNS irritability, auditory/visual hallucinations.

Helps to establish and maintain awareness of reality/environment.

Limits defensive reaction.

Promotes continual orientation cues to assist patient in maintaining sense of normality.

Prevents injury to patient who may be hallucinating/disoriented.

Aids in maintaining socialization and orientation. Note: Patient's agitation/psychotic behavior may precipitate family quarrels/conflicts.

Promotes relaxation, reduces CNS hyperactivity/agitation.

NURSING DIAGNOSIS:	KNOWLEDGE DEFICIT [LEARNING NEED] (SPECIFY)
May be related to:	Lack of exposure/recall, information misinterpretation
	Unfamiliarity with information resources
Possibly evidenced by:	Questions; request for information; statement of misconception
	Inaccurate follow-through of instructions/development of preventable complications
PATIENT OUTCOMES/ EVALUATION CRITERIA:	Verbalizes understanding of disease process and treatment. Identifies relationship of signs/symptoms to the disease process and correlates symptoms with causative factors. Initiates necessary lifestyle changes and participates in treatment regimen.

ACTIONS/INTERVENTIONS

Independent

Review disease process and future expectations.

Provide information appropriate to individual situation.

Identify stressors, and discuss precipitators of thyroid crises, e.g., personal/social and job concerns, infection, pregnancy.

Provide information about signs/symptoms of hypothyroidism and the need for continuing follow-up care.

RATIONALE

Provides knowledge base on which patient can make informed choices.

Severity of condition, cause, age, and concurrent complications determines course of treatment.

Psychogenic factors are often of prime importance in the occurrence/exacerbation of this disease. (Refer to CP: Psychosocial Aspects of Acute Care, p. 773.)

The patient who has been treated for hyperthyroidism needs to be aware of possible development of hypo-

637

ACTIONS/INTERVENTIONS	RATIONALE
Independent	
	thyroidism, which can occur immediately after treatment or as long as 5 years later.
Discuss drug therapy, including need for adhering to regimen, and expected therapeutic and side effects.	Antithyroid medication (either as primary therapy or in preparation for thyroidectomy), requires adherence to a medical regimen over an extended period of time to inhibit hormone production. Agranulocytosis is the most serious side effect that can occur, and alternative drugs may be given when problems arise.
Identify signs/symptoms requiring medical evaluation, e.g., fever, sore throat, and skin eruptions.	Early identification of toxic reactions (thiourea therapy) and intervention are important in preventing development of agranulocytosis.
Explain need to check with physician/pharmacist before taking other prescribed or OTC drugs.	Antithyroid medications can affect or be affected by numerous other medications, requiring monitoring of medication levels, side effects, and interactions.
Emphasize importance of planned rest periods.	Prevents undue fatigue, reduces metabolic demands. As euthyroid state is achieved, stamina and activity level will increase.
Review need for nutritious diet and periodic review of nutrient needs; avoid caffeine, red/yellow food dyes, artificial preservatives.	Provides adequate nutrients to support hypermetabolic state. As hormonal imbalance is corrected, diet will need to be readjusted in order to prevent excessive weight gain. Irritants and stimulants should be limited to avoid cumulative systemic effects.
Stress necessity of continued medical follow-up.	Necessary for monitoring effectiveness of therapy and prevention of potentially fatal complications.

Thyroidectomy _____

Total thyroidectomy: The gland is removed completely. Usually done in the case of malignancy. Thyroid replacement therapy is necessary for life.

Subtotal thyroidectomy: Up to five sixths of the gland is removed when antithyroid drugs do not correct hyperthyroidism or radioactive iodine therapy is contraindicated.

PATIENT ASSESSMENT DATA BASE

Refer to CP: Hyperthyroidism, p. 628.

NURSING PRIORITIES

1. Reverse hyperthyroid state preoperatively.
2. Prevent complications.
3. Relieve pain.
4. Provide information about surgical procedure, prognosis and treatment needs.

DISCHARGE CRITERIA

1. Complications prevented/minimized.
2. Pain alleviated.
3. Surgical procedure/prognosis and therapeutic regimen understood.

PREOPERATIVE

NURSING DIAGNOSIS:	**CARDIAC OUTPUT, ALTERED: DECREASED [POTENTIAL]**
May be related to:	**Uncontrolled hyperthyroidism, hypermetabolic state, increasing cardiac workload**
	Changes in venous return and systemic vascular resistance
	Alterations in rate, rhythm, conduction
Possibly evidenced by:	**[Not applicable; presence of signs and symptoms establishes an *actual* diagnosis.]**
PATIENT OUTCOMES/ EVALUATION CRITERIA:	**Maintains adequate cardiac output for tissue needs as evidenced by stable vital signs, palpable peripheral pulses, good capillary refill, usual mentation, and absence of dysrhythmias. Achieves euthyroid state.**

ACTIONS/INTERVENTIONS	RATIONALE
Independent	
Promote restful environment, and reduce patient's exposure to anxiety-producing stimuli.	Limits external stimuli and reduces metabolic demands, cardiac workload.
Promote dietary intake, providing frequent full meals and snacks.	Because of increased metabolism, patient may need 4000–5000 calories/day to meet cellular energy

ACTIONS/INTERVENTIONS	RATIONALE

Independent

Restrict foods/fluids containing caffeine.

needs, prevent further depletion of glycogen stores, and maintain/regain lost weight as needed.

Stimulating effects of caffeine aggravate already existing hyperactive condition.

Note presence of rash; excessive tearing of the eyes, nasal discharge, salivation; and swelling of the buccal mucosa.

May indicate iodine toxicity requiring discontinuation of the drug. Usually given for 1–2 weeks preoperatively in combination with antithyroid drugs to achieve an euthyroid state and to reduce vascularity of the gland, decreasing risk of postoperative hemorrhage or thyroid storm.

Refer to CP: Hyperthyroidism, ND: Cardiac Output, Altered: Decreased [Potential], p. 630, for further concerns/interventions.

POSTOPERATIVE

NURSING DIAGNOSIS:	**AIRWAY CLEARANCE, INEFFECTIVE [POTENTIAL]**
May be related to:	**Tracheal obstruction: swelling, bleeding, laryngeal spasms**
Possibly evidenced by:	**[Not applicable; presence of signs and symptoms establishes an *actual* diagnosis.]**
PATIENT OUTCOMES/ EVALUATION CRITERIA:	**Maintains patent airway, with aspiration prevented.**

ACTIONS/INTERVENTIONS	RATIONALE

Independent

Monitor respiratory rate, depth and work of breathing.

Respirations may remain somewhat rapid, but development of respiratory distress is indicative of obstructive process.

Auscultate breath sounds, noting onset of rhonchi.

Rhonchi may indicate airway obstruction/accumulation of copious thick secretions.

Assess for dyspnea, stridor, "crowing," and cyanosis.

Indicators of tracheal obstruction/laryngeal spasm, requiring prompt evaluation and intervention.

Position with head of bed elevated 30–45 degrees.

Facilitates respirations, limits edema formation in surgical area and the accumulation of secretions in back of throat.

Assist with repositioning, deep breathing exercises and/or coughing as indicated.

Maintains clear airway and ventilation. Although coughing is not encouraged and may be painful, it may be needed to clear secretions.

Suction mouth and trachea, as indicated, noting color and characteristics of sputum.

Edema/pain may impair patient's ability to clear own airway.

Check dressing frequently, especially posterior portion.

If bleeding occurs, anterior dressing may appear dry as blood pools dependently.

Investigate complaints of difficulty swallowing, drooling of oral secretions.

May indicate edema/sequestered bleeding in tissues surrounding operative site.

ACTIONS/INTERVENTIONS	RATIONALE
Independent	
Keep tracheostomy tray at bedside.	Compromised airway may create a life-threatening situation requiring emergency procedure.
Collaborative	
Provide steam inhalation; humidify room air.	Reduces discomfort of sore throat and tissue edema and promotes expectoration of secretions.
Assist with/prepare for procedures, e.g., tracheostomy.	May be necessary to maintain airway if obstructed by edema of glottis or hemorrhage.
Return to surgery.	May require ligation of bleeding vessels.

NURSING DIAGNOSIS:	COMMUNICATION, IMPAIRED: VERBAL
May be related to:	Vocal cord injury/laryngeal nerve damage
	Tissue edema; pain
	Discomfort
Possibly evidenced by:	Impaired articulation, does not/cannot speak; use of nonverbal cues
PATIENT OUTCOMES/ EVALUATION CRITERIA:	Establishes method of communication in which needs can be expressed.

ACTIONS/INTERVENTIONS	RATIONALE
Independent	
Assess speech periodically; encourage voice rest.	Hoarseness and sore throat may occur secondary to tissue edema or surgical damage to recurrent laryngeal nerve and may last several days. Permanent nerve damage can occur (rare) that causes paralysis of vocal cords and/or compression of the trachea.
Keep communication simple, ask yes/no questions.	Reduces demand for response, promotes voice rest.
Provide alternate methods of communication as appropriate, e.g., slate board, letter/picture board. Place IV line to minimize interference with written communication.	Facilitates expression of needs.
Anticipate needs as possible. Visit patient frequently.	Reduces anxiety and patient's need to communicate.
Post notice of patient's voice limitations at central station and answer call bell promptly.	Prevents patient straining voice to make needs known/summon assistance.
Maintain quiet environment.	Enhances ability to hear whispered communication and reduces necessity for patient to raise/strain voice to be heard.

NURSING DIAGNOSIS:	INJURY, POTENTIAL FOR [TETANY]
May be related to:	Chemical imbalance: excessive CNS stimulation

641

ACTIONS/INTERVENTIONS	RATIONALE
Independent	
Monitor vital signs noting elevating temperature, tachycardia (140–200/min), dysrhythmias, respiratory distress, cyanosis (developing pulmonary edema/ CHF).	Manipulation of gland during surgery may result in increased hormone release, causing thyroid storm.
Evaluate reflexes periodically. Observe for neuromuscular irritability, e.g., twitching, numbness, paresthesias, positive Chvostek's and Trousseau's signs, seizures.	Hypocalcemia with tetany (usually transient) may occur 1–7 days postoperatively and indicates hypoparathyroidism, which can occur as a result of inadvertent trauma to/partial to total removal of parathyroid gland(s) during surgery.
Keep siderails raised/padded, bed in low position and airway at bedside. Avoid use of restraints.	Reduces potential for injury if seizures occur.
Collaborative	
Monitor serum calcium levels.	Levels below 7.5 mg/100 ml generally requires replacement therapy.
Administer medications as indicated:	
Calcium (gluconate, lactate);	Corrects deficiency which is usually temporary but may be permanent. Note: Use with caution in digitalized patient as calcium increases cardiac sensibility to digitalis, potentiating risk of toxicity.
Sedatives;	Promotes rest, reducing exogenous stimulation.
Anticonvulsants;	Controls seizures until corrective therapy is successful.
Phosphate-binding agents.	Helpful in lowering elevated phosphorus levels associated with hypocalcemia.

ACTIONS/INTERVENTIONS

Independent

Assess verbal/nonverbal complaints of pain, noting location, intensity (1–10 scale), and duration.

Place in semi-Fowler's position and support head/neck with sandbags or small pillows.

Maintain head/neck in neutral position and support during position changes. Instruct patient to use hands to support neck during movement and to avoid hyperextension of neck.

Keep call bell and frequently needed items within easy reach.

Give cool liquids by mouth or soft foods, such as ice cream or popsicles.

Encourage patient to use relaxation techniques, e.g., guided imagery, soft music, progressive relaxation.

Collaborative

Administer analgesics and/or analgesic throat sprays/lozenges as necessary.

Provide ice collar if indicated.

RATIONALE

Useful in evaluating pain, choice of interventions, effectiveness of therapy.

Prevents hyperextension of the neck and protects integrity of the suture line.

Prevents stress on the suture line and reduces muscle tension.

Limits stretching, muscle strain in operative area.

Soothing to sore throat but soft foods may be tolerated better if patient experiences difficulty swallowing.

Helps to refocus attention and assists patient to manage pain/discomfort more effectively.

Reduces pain and discomfort, enhances rest.

Reduces tissue edema and decreases perception of pain.

NURSING DIAGNOSIS:	KNOWLEDGE DEFICIT [LEARNING NEED] (SPECIFY)
May be related to:	Lack of exposure/recall, misinterpretation Unfamiliarity with information resources
Possibly evidenced by:	Questions; request for information; statement of misconception Inaccurate follow-through of instructions/development of preventable complications
PATIENT OUTCOMES/ EVALUATION CRITERIA:	Verbalizes understanding of surgical procedure and treatment. Initiates necessary lifestyle changes and participates in treatment regimen.

ACTIONS/INTERVENTIONS

Independent

Review surgical procedure and future expectations.

Discuss need for well-balanced, nutritious diet and inclusion of iodized salt.

Recommend avoidance of goitrogenic foods, e.g., excessive ingestion of seafood, soybeans, turnips.

RATIONALE

Provides knowledge base on which patient can make informed decisions.

Promotes healing and helps patient to regain/maintain appropriate weight. Use of iodized salt is often sufficient to meet iodine needs unless salt is restricted for other health care problems, e.g., CHF.

Contraindicated after partial thyroidectomy because these foods inhibit thyroid activity.

ACTIONS/INTERVENTIONS	RATIONALE
Independent	
Identify foods high in calcium (e.g., dairy products) and vitamin D (e.g., fortified dairy products, egg yolks, liver).	Maximizes supply and absorption of calcium if parathyroid function is impaired.
Encourage progressive general exercise program.	In patients with subtotal thyroidectomy, exercise can stimulate the thyroid gland and production of hormones, facilitating recovery of general well-being.
Review postoperative exercises, e.g., flexion, extension, rotation, and lateral movement of head and neck.	Regular ROM exercises strengthen neck muscles, enhance circulation and healing process.
Review importance of rest and relaxation, avoiding stressful situations and emotional outbursts.	Effects of hyperthyroidism usually subside completely, but it takes some time for the body to recover.
Instruct in incisional care, e.g., cleansing, dressing application.	Enables patient to provide competent self-care.
Give information about the use of loose fitting scarves to cover scar. Avoid the use of jewelry.	Covers the incision without aggravating healing or precipitating infections of suture line.
Apply cold cream after sutures have been removed.	Softens tissues and may help to minimize scarring.
Discuss possibility of change in voice.	Alteration in vocal cord function may cause changes in pitch and quality of voice, which may be temporary or permanent.
Review drug therapy, necessity of continuing even when feeling well.	If thyroid replacement is needed because of surgical removal of gland, patient needs to understand rationale for replacement therapy and consequences of failure to routinely take medication.
Identify signs/requiring medical evaluation, e.g., fever, chills, continued/purulent wound drainage, erythema, gaps in wound edges; sudden weight loss, intolerance to heat, nausea/vomiting, diarrhea, insomnia; weight gain, fatigue, intolerance to cold, constipation, drowsiness.	Early recognition of developing complications such as infection, hyperthyroidism, or hypothyroidism may prevent progression to life-threatening situation. Note: As many as 43% of patients with subtotal thyroidectomy will have hypothyroidism in time.
Stress necessity of continued medical follow-up.	Provides opportunity for evaluating effectiveness of therapy and prevention of complications.

Diabetes Mellitus/Diabetic Ketoacidosis _____

PATIENT ASSESSMENT DATA BASE

Data are dependent on the severity and duration of metabolic imbalance and effects on organ function.

ACTIVITY/REST

May report:
Weakness, exhaustion, difficulty walking/moving.
Muscle cramps, decreased muscle tone.
Sleep/rest disturbances.

May exhibit:
Tachycardia and tachypnea at rest or with activity.
Lethargy/disorientation, coma.
Decreased muscle strength.

CIRCULATION

May report:
History of hypertension; acute MI.
Claudication, numbness, tingling of extremities.
Leg ulcers, slow healing

May exhibit:
Tachycardia.
Postural BP changes; hypertension.
Decreased/absent pulses.
Dysrhythmias.
Crackles; jugular vein distention (CHF).
Hot, dry, flushed skin; sunken eyeballs.

EGO INTEGRITY

May report:
Stress; dependence on others.
Financial concerns related to condition.

May exhibit:
Anxiety, irritability.

ELIMINATION

May report:
Change in usual voiding pattern (polyuria), nocturia.
Pain/burning, difficulty voiding (infection), recent/recurrent urinary tract infection.
Abdominal tenderness.
Diarrhea.

May exhibit:
Pale, yellow, dilute urine; polyuria (may progress to oliguria/anuria if severe hypovolemia occurs).
Cloudy, odorous urine (infection).
Firm abdomen, bloating.
Bowel sounds diminished; hyperactive (diarrhea).

FOOD/FLUID

May report:
Nausea, vomiting.
Not following diet; increased intake of glucose/carbohydrates.
Weight loss over a period of days/weeks.
Use of diuretics (thiazides).

May exhibit:	Dry/cracked skin, poor skin turgor. Abdominal rigidity/distention, vomiting. Enlarged thyroid (increased metabolic needs with increased blood sugar). Halitosis/sweet, fruity odor (acetone breath).

NEUROSENSORY

May report:	Fainting spells/dizziness. Headaches. Tingling, numbness, weakness in muscles; paresthesias. Visual disturbances.
May exhibit:	Disorientation; drowsiness, lethargy, stupor/coma (later stages). Memory impairment (recent, remote); confusion. Deep tendon reflexes decreased (coma). Seizure activity (late stages of DKA).

PAIN/COMFORT

May report:	Abdominal bloating/pain (mild to severe).
May exhibit:	Facial grimacing with palpation; guarding.

RESPIRATION

May report:	Air hunger. Cough, with/without purulent sputum (infection).
May exhibit:	Increased respiratory rate, tachypnea; deep, rapid (Kussmaul's) respirations (metabolic acidosis). Rhonchi, wheezes. Yellow or green sputum (infection).

SAFETY

May report:	Dry, itching skin; skin ulcerations.
May exhibit:	Fever, diaphoresis. Skin breakdown, lesions/ulcerations. Decreased general strength/ROM. Paresthesia/paralysis of muscles including respiratory musculature (if potassium levels are markedly decreased).

SEXUALITY

May report:	Vaginal discharge (prone to infection). Problems with impotence; female orgasmic difficulty.

TEACHING/LEARNING

May report:	Familial risk factors: diabetes, heart disease, strokes, hypertension. Slow/delayed healing. Use of drugs, e.g., steroids, thiazide diuretics, Dilantin and phenobarbital (can increase glucose levels). May/may not be taking diabetic medications as ordered.
Discharge Plan Considerations:	May need assistance with dietary regimen, medication administration/supplies, self-care.

DIAGNOSTIC STUDIES

Serum glucose: increased 200–1000 mg/100 ml or more.

Plasma acetone (ketones): strongly positive.

Free fatty acids: lipids, and cholesterol elevated.

Serum osmolality: elevated but usually less than 330 mOsm/l.

Electrolytes:

    Sodium: may be normal, elevated or decreased.

    Potassium: normal or falsely elevated (cellular shifts), then decreased.

    Phosphorus:

*Glycosylated hen   reflect poor control of diabetes during past
4 months (life sp: g inadequate control versus incident-related
DKA (e.g., curren

ABGs: usually re   olic acidosis) with compensatory respiratory
alkalosis.

CBC: Hct may b   noconcentration, response to stress, or infection.

BUN: may be no   fusion).

Serum amylase: ause of DKA.

Serum insulin: m   pe II), indicating insulin insufficiency/improper
utilization (endog   secondary to formation of antibodies.

*Thyroid function   d glucose and insulin needs.

Urine: positive fo   ity may be elevated.

*Cultures and se   ions.

NURSING

1. Restore fluid/electrolyte, and acid–base balance.
2. Correct/reverse metabolic abnormalities.
3. Identify/assist with management of underlying cause/disease.
4. Prevent complications.
5. Provide information about disease process/prognosis, self-care, and treatment needs.

DISCHARGE CRITERIA

1. Homeostasis achieved.
2. Causative/precipitating factors corrected/controlled.
3. Complications prevented/minimized.
4. Disease process/prognosis, self-care needs, and therapeutic regimen understood.

NURSING DIAGNOSIS:	FLUID VOLUME DEFICIT, ACTUAL 1 [REGULATORY FAILURE]
May be related to:	**Osmotic diuresis (from hyperglycemia)**
	Excessive gastric losses: diarrhea, vomiting
	Restricted intake: nausea, confusion
Possibly evidenced by:	**Increased urine output, dilute urine**
	Weakness; thirst; sudden weight loss
	Dry skin/mucous membranes, poor skin turgor
	Hypotension, tachycardia, delayed capillary refill

Demonstrates adequate hydration as evidenced by stable vital signs, palpable peripheral pulses, good skin turgor and capillary refill, individually appropriate urinary output, and electrolyte levels within normal range.

ACTIONS/INTERVENTIONS	RATIONALE
Independent	
Obtain history from patient/SO related to duration/intensity of symptoms such as vomiting, excessive urination.	Assists in estimation of total volume depletion. Symptoms may have been present for varying amounts of time (hours to days). Presence of infectious process results in fever and hypermetabolic state, increasing insensible fluid losses.
Monitor vital signs; note orthostatic BP changes;	Hypovolemia may be manifested by hypotension and tachycardia. Estimates of severity of hypovolemia may be made when patient's systolic BP drops more than 10 mmHg from a recumbent to a sitting/standing position. Note: Cardiac neuropathy may block reflexes that normally increase heart rate.
Respiratory pattern, e.g., Kussmaul respirations, note acetone breath;	Lungs remove carbonic acid through respirations, producing a compensatory respiratory alkalosis for ketoacidosis. Acetone breath is due to breakdown of acetoacetic acid and should diminish as ketosis is corrected.
Respiratory rate and quality; use of accessory muscles, periods of apnea, and appearance of cyanosis;	Correction of hyperglycemia and acidosis will cause the respiratory rate and pattern to approach normal. However, increased work of breathing, shallow, rapid respirations and presence of cyanosis may indicate respiratory fatigue and/or that patient is losing ability to compensate for acidosis.
Temperature, skin color/moisture.	Although fever, chills, and diaphoresis are common with infectious process, fever with flushed, dry skin may reflect dehydration.
Assess peripheral pulses, capillary refill, skin turgor, and mucous membranes.	Indicators of level of hydration, adequacy of circulating volume.
Monitor intake and output; note urine specific gravity.	Provides ongoing estimate of volume replacement needs, kidney function, and effectiveness of therapy.
Weigh daily.	Provides the best assessment of current fluid status and adequacy of fluid replacement.
Maintain fluid intake of at least 2500 ml/day within cardiac tolerance when oral intake is resumed.	Maintains hydration/circulating volume.
Promote comfortable environment. Cover patient with light sheets.	Avoids overheating of patient, which could promote further fluid loss.
Investigate changes in mentation/sensorium.	Changes in mentation can be due to abnormally high or low glucose, electrolyte abnormalities, acidosis, decreased cerebral perfusion, or developing hypoxia. Regardless of the cause, impaired consciousness can predispose the patient to aspiration.
Note complaints of nausea, abdominal pain; presence of vomiting and gastric distention.	Fluid and electrolyte deficits alter gastric motility, frequently resulting in vomiting and potentiating the fluid/electrolyte losses.
Observe for increased fatigue, crackles, edema, increased weight, bounding pulse, vascular distention.	Rapid fluid replacement may potentiate overload and congestive heart failure.

ACTIONS/INTERVENTIONS	RATIONALE
Collaborative	
Administer fluids as indicated: normal or half-normal saline with/without dextrose;	Type and amount of fluid are dependent on degree of deficit and individual patient response.
Albumin, plasma, dextran.	Plasma expanders may occasionally be needed if the deficit is life-threatening/BP does not normalize with rehydration efforts.
Insert/maintain urinary catheter.	Provides for accurate/ongoing measurement of output, especially if autonomic neuropathies result in neurogenic bladder (urinary retention/overflow incontinence). May be removed when patient is stable to reduce risk of infection.
Monitor laboratory studies, e.g.:	
Hct;	Assesses level of hydration and is often elevated because of hemoconcentration that occurs after osmotic diuresis.
BUN/Cr;	Elevated values may reflect cellular breakdown from dehydration or signal the onset of renal failure.
Serum osmolality;	Elevated due to hyperglycemia and dehydration.
Sodium;	May be decreased reflecting shift of fluids from the intracellular compartment (osmotic diuresis). High sodium values reflect severe fluid loss/dehydration, or sodium reabsorption in response to aldosterone secretion.
Potassium.	Initially, intravascular hyperkalemia occurs in response to acidosis, but as this potassium is lost in the urine, the absolute potassium level in the body is depleted. As insulin is replaced and acidosis is corrected, serum potassium deficit becomes apparent.
Administer potassium and other electrolytes via IV and/or by oral route as indicated.	Potassium should be added to the IV (as soon as urinary flow is adequate) to prevent hypokalemia. Note: Potassium phosphate may be given if intravenous fluids contain sodium chloride, in order to prevent chloride overload.
Administer bicarbonate if pH is less than 7.0.	Given with caution to help correct acidosis in the presence of hypotension or shock.
Insert nasogastric tube and attach to suction as indicated.	Decompresses stomach and may relieve vomiting.

NURSING DIAGNOSIS:	**NUTRITION, ALTERED: LESS THAN BODY REQUIRE-MENTS**
May be related to:	**Insulin deficiency (decreased uptake and utilization of glucose by the tissues resulting in increased protein/fat metabolism)**
	Decreased oral intake; anorexia, nausea, gastric fullness, abdominal pain; altered consciousness
	Hypermetabolic state: release of stress hormones (e.g., epinephrine, cortisol, and growth hormone), infectious process

Possibly evidenced by:	Reported inadequate food intake, lack of interest in food
	Recent weight loss; weakness, fatigue, poor muscle tone
	Diarrhea
	Increased ketones (end products of fat metabolism)
PATIENT OUTCOMES/ EVALUATION CRITERIA:	Ingesting appropriate amounts of calories/nutrients. Displays usual energy level. Demonstrates stabilized weight or gain toward usual/desired range with normal laboratory values.

ACTIONS/INTERVENTIONS

Independent

Weigh daily or as indicated.

Ascertain patient's dietary program and usual pattern, compare with recent intake.

Auscultate bowel sounds. Note complaints of abdominal pain/bloating, nausea, vomiting of undigested food. Maintain NPO status as indicated.

Provide liquids containing nutrients and electrolytes as soon as patient can tolerate oral fluids; progress to more solid food as tolerated.

Identify food preferences, including ethnic/cultural needs.

Include SO in meal planning as indicated.

Observe for signs of hypoglycemia, e.g., changes in level of consciousness, cool/clammy skin, rapid pulse, hunger, irritability, anxiety, headache, lightheadedness, shakiness.

Collaborative

Perform fingerstick glucose testing.

RATIONALE

Assesses adequacy of nutritional intake (absorption and utilization).

Identifies deficits and deviations from therapeutic needs.

Hyperglycemia and fluid and electrolyte disturbances can decrease gastric motility/function (distention or ileus) affecting choice of interventions. Note: Long-term difficulties with decreased gastric emptying and poor intestinal motility suggest autonomic neuropathies affecting the GI tract and requiring symptomatic treatment.

Oral route is preferred when patient is alert and bowel function is restored.

If patient's food preferences can be incorporated into the meal plan, cooperation may be facilitated after discharge.

Promotes sense of involvement, provides information for SO to understand nutritional needs of the patient. Note: Various methods available for dietary planning include exchange list, point system, glycemic index, or preselected menus.

Once carbohydrate metabolism begins (blood glucose level reduced), and as insulin is being given, hypoglycemia can occur. If patient is comatose, hypoglycemia may occur without notable change in level of consciousness. This potentially life-threatening emergency should be assessed and treated quickly per protocol. Note: Type I diabetics of long-standing may not display usual signs of hypoglycemia because normal response to low blood sugar may be diminished.

Bedside analysis of serum glucose is more accurate (displays current levels) than monitoring urine sugar, which is not sensitive enough to detect fluctuations in serum levels and can be affected by patient's individual renal threshold or the presence of urinary

ACTIONS/INTERVENTIONS

Collaborative

RATIONALE

retention/renal failure. Note: Some studies have found that a urine glucose of 2% may be correlated to a blood glucose of 140–360 mg/dl.

Monitor laboratory studies, e.g., serum glucose, acetone, pH, HCO_3.

Blood sugar will decrease slowly with controlled fluid replacement and insulin therapy. With the administration of optimal insulin dosages, glucose can then enter the cells and be used for energy. When this happens, acetone levels decrease and acidosis is corrected.

Administer regular insulin by intermittent or continuous intravenous method, e.g., IV bolus followed by a continuous drip via pump of approximately 5–10 units per hour until glucose reaches 250 mg/100 ml.

Regular insulin has a rapid onset and thus will quickly help move glucose into cells. The intravenous route is the initial route of choice, because absorption from subcutaneous tissues may be erratic. Many believe the continuous method is the optimal way to facilitate transition to carbohydrate metabolism and reduce incidence of hypoglycemia.

Administer glucose solutions, e.g., dextrose and half-normal saline.

Glucose solutions are added after insulin and fluids have brought the blood glucose to approximately 250/100 ml. As carbohydrate metabolism approaches normal, care must be taken to avoid hypoglycemia.

Consult with dietician.

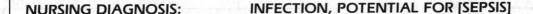

eful in calculating and adjusting diet to meet pant's needs; answers questions and can assist ient/SO in developing meal plans.

Provide di
20% prote
meals/snac

mplex carbohydrates (e.g., corn, peas, carrots, ccoli, dried beans, oats, apples) decrease glucose ls/insulin needs, reduce serum cholesterol, and mote satiation. Food intake will be scheduled acding to specific insulin characteristics (e.g., peak ct) and individual patient response. Note: HS k of complex carbohydrates is especially impor- if insulin is given in divided doses in order to pre- hypoglycemia during sleep and potential Somoesponse.

Administer m

be useful in treating symptoms related to auto- neuropathies affecting GI tract, thus enhancing ntake and absorption of nutrients.

NURSING DIAGNOSIS:	**INFECTION, POTENTIAL FOR [SEPSIS]**
May be related to:	**High glucose levels, decreased leukocyte function, alterations in circulation**
	Preexisting respiratory or urinary tract infection
Possibly evidenced by:	**[Not applicable; presence of signs and symptoms establishes an *actual* diagnosis.]**
PATIENT OUTCOMES/ EVALUATION CRITERIA:	**Identifies interventions to prevent/reduce risk of infection. Demonstrates techniques, lifestyle changes to prevent development of infection.**

ACTIONS/INTERVENTIONS	RATIONALE

Independent

Observe for signs of infection and inflammation, e.g., fever, flushed appearance, wound drainage, purulent sputum, cloudy urine.

Patient may be admitted with infection, which could have precipitated the ketoacidotic state, or may develop a nosocomial infection.

Promote good handwashing by staff and patient.

Reduces risk of cross-contamination.

Maintain aseptic technique for IV insertion procedure, administration of medications, and providing maintenance care. Rotate IV sites as indicated.

High glucose in the blood creates an excellent medium for bacterial growth.

Provide catheter/perineal care. Teach the female patient to clean from front to back after elimination.

Minimizes risk of UTI. Comatose patient may be at particular risk if urinary retention occurred prior to hospitalization. Note: Elderly female diabetic patients are especially prone to urinary/vaginal infections such as yeast.

Provide conscientious skin care; massage bony areas. Keep the skin dry, linens dry and wrinkle-free.

Peripheral circulation may be impaired which places the patient at increased risk for skin irritation/breakdown and infection.

Auscultate breath sounds.

Rhonchi indicates accumulation of secretions possibly related to pneumonia/bronchitis (may have precipitated the DKA). Pulmonary congestion/edema (crackles) may result from rapid fluid replacement/CHF.

Place in semi-Fowler's position.

Facilitates lung expansion, reduces risk of aspiration.

Reposition and encourage coughing/deep breathing if patient is alert and cooperative. Otherwise, suction airway, using sterile technique, as needed.

Aids in ventilating all lung areas and mobilization of secretions. Prevents stasis of secretions with increased risk of infection.

Provide tissues and trash bag in a convenient location for sputum and other secretions.

Minimizes spread of infection.

Assist with oral hygiene.

Reduces risk of oral/gum disease.

Encourage adequate dietary and fluid intake (approximately 3000 ml/day if not contraindicated).

Decreases susceptibility to infection. Increased urinary flow prevents stasis, aids in maintaining urine pH/acidity, reducing bacteria growth and flushing organisms out of system.

Collaborative

Obtain specimens for culture and sensitivities as indicated.

Identifies organism(s) so most appropriate drug therapy can be instituted.

Administer antibiotics as indicated.

Early treatment may help prevent sepsis.

NURSING DIAGNOSIS:	SENSORY-PERCEPTUAL ALTERATION: (SPECIFY) [POTENTIAL]
May be related to:	**Endogenous chemical alteration: glucose/insulin and/or electrolyte imbalance**
Possibly evidenced by:	**[Not applicable; presence of signs and symptoms establishes an *actual* diagnosis.]**
PATIENT OUTCOMES/ EVALUATION CRITERIA:	**Regains/maintains usual level of mentation. Recognizes and compensates for sensory impairments.**

ACTIONS/INTERVENTIONS	RATIONALE
Independent	
Monitor vital signs and mental status.	Baseline from which to compare abnormal findings; e.g., high temperature may affect mentation.
Address patient by name, reorient as needed, to place, person and time. Give short explanations, speaking slowly and enunciating clearly.	Decreases confusion and helps to maintain contact with reality.
Schedule nursing time to provide for uninterrupted rest periods.	Promotes restful sleep, reduces fatigue, and may improve cognition.
Keep patient's routine as consistent as possible. Encourage participation in activities of daily living as able.	Helps keep the patient in touch with reality and maintain orientation to the environment.
Protect patient from injury (e.g., restraints) when level of consciousness is impaired. Pad bedrails and provide padded tongue blade if patient is prone to seizures.	Disoriented patient is prone to injury, especially at night, and precautions need to be taken as indicated. Seizure precautions need to be taken to prevent physical injury, aspiration, etc.
Evaluate visual acuity as indicated.	Retinal edema/detachment, hemorrhage, presence of cataracts or temporary paralysis of extraocular muscles may impair vision requiring corrective therapy and/or supportive care.
Investigate complaints of hyperesthesia, pain, or sensory loss.	Peripheral neuropathies, especially involving feet/legs, may result in severe discomfort, lack of/distortion of tactile sensation potentiating risk of dermal injury and impaired balance. Note: Mononeuropathy affects a single nerve (most often femoral or cranial), causing sudden pain and loss of motor/sensory function along affected nerve path.
Provide bed cradle. Keep hands/feet warm, avoiding exposure to cool drafts/hot water or use of heating pad.	Reduces peripheral discomfort and potential for injury. Note: Sudden development of cold hands/feet may reflect hypoglycemia, suggesting need to evaluate serum glucose level.
Assist with ambulation/position changes.	Promotes patient safety, especially when balance is affected.
Collaborative	
Carry out prescribed regimen for correcting DKA as indicated.	Alteration in thought processes/potential for seizure activity is usually alleviated once hyperosmolar state is corrected.
Monitor laboratory values, e.g., blood glucose, serum osmolality, Hb/Hct, BUN/Cr.	With the correction of these values, mentation should improve. Note: If fluid is replaced too quickly, excess water may enter brain cells and cause alteration in the level of consciousness (water intoxication).
Assist with local nerve block, maintenance of TENs unit.	May provide relief of discomfort associated with neuropathies.

NURSING DIAGNOSIS:	**FATIGUE**
May be related to:	**Decreased metabolic energy production**
	Altered body chemistry: insufficient insulin
	Increased energy demands: hypermetabolic state/ infection

Possibly evidenced by:	Overwhelming lack of energy, inability to maintain usual routines, decreased performance, accident-prone
	Impaired ability to concentrate, listlessness, disinterest in surroundings
PATIENT OUTCOMES/ EVALUATION CRITERIA:	Verbalizes increase in level of energy. Displays improved ability to participate in desired activities.

ACTIONS/INTERVENTIONS	RATIONALE
Independent	
Discuss with patient the need for activity. Plan schedule with patient and identify activities that lead to fatigue.	Education may provide motivation to increase activity level even though patient may feel too weak initially.
Alternate activity with periods of rest/uninterrupted sleep.	Prevents excessive fatigue.
Monitor pulse, respiratory rate, and blood pressure before/after activity.	Indicates physiologic levels of tolerance.
Discuss ways of conserving energy while bathing, transferring, etc.	Patient will be able to accomplish more with a decreased expenditure of energy.
Increase patient participation in activities of daily living as tolerated.	Increases confidence level, self-esteem as well as tolerance level.

NURSING DIAGNOSIS:	**POWERLESSNESS**
May be related to:	Long-term/progressive illness that is not curable
	Dependence on others
Possibly evidenced by:	Reluctance to express true feelings; expressions of having no control/influence over situation
	Apathy, withdrawal, anger
	Does not monitor progress, nonparticipation in care/ decision making
	Depression over physical deterioration/complications despite patient cooperation with regimen
PATIENT OUTCOMES/ EVALUATION CRITERIA:	Acknowledges feelings of helplessness. Identifies healthy ways to deal with feelings. Assists in planning own care and independently takes responsibility for self-care activities.

ACTIONS/INTERVENTIONS	RATIONALE
Independent	
Encourage patient/SO to express feelings about hospitalization and disease in general.	Identifies concerns and facilitates problem solving.
Acknowledge normality of feelings.	Recognition that reactions are normal can help the pa-

ACTIONS/INTERVENTIONS	RATIONALE
Independent	
	tient to problem-solve and seek help as needed. Diabetic control is a full-time job that serves as a constant reminder of both presence of disease as well as threat to patient's health/life.
Assess how patient has handled problems in the past. Identify locus of control.	Knowledge of individual's style helps to determine needs for treatment goals. Patient whose locus of control is internal usually looks at ways to gain control over own treatment program. Patient who operates with an external locus of control wants to be cared for by others and may project blame for circumstances onto external factors.
Provide opportunity for SO to express concerns and discuss ways in which they can be helpful to the patient.	Enhances sense of being involved and gives SO a chance to problem-solve solutions to help patient prevent recurrence.
Ascertain expectations/goals of patient/SO.	Unrealistic expectations/pressure from others or self may result in feelings of frustration/loss of control and may impair coping abilities. Note: Even with rigid adherence to medical regimen, complications/setbacks may occur.
Determine whether a change in relationship with SO has occurred.	Constant energy and thought required for diabetic control often shifts the focus of a relationship. Development of psychologic concerns/visceral neuropathies affecting self-concept (especially sexual role function) may add further stress.
Encourage patient to make decisions related to care, e.g., ambulation, time for activities, etc.	Communicates to patient that some control can be exercised over care.
Support participation in self-care and give positive feedback for efforts.	Promotes feeling of control over situation.

NURSING DIAGNOSIS:	**KNOWLEDGE DEFICIT [LEARNING NEED] (SPECIFY)**
May be related to:	**Lack of exposure/recall, information misinterpretation**
	Unfamiliarity with information resources
Possibly evidenced by:	**Questions/request for information, verbalization of the problem**
	Inaccurate follow-through of instructions, development of preventable complications
PATIENT OUTCOMES/ EVALUATION CRITERIA:	**Verbalizes understanding of disease process. Identifies relationship of signs/symptoms to the disease process and correlates symptoms with causative factors. Correctly performs necessary procedures and explains reasons for the actions. Initiates necessary lifestyle changes and participates in treatment regimen.**

ACTIONS/INTERVENTIONS	RATIONALE

Independent

Create an environment of trust by listening to concerns, being available.

Rapport and respect need to be established before patient will be willing to take part in the learning process.

Work with patient in setting mutual goals for learning.

Participation in the planning promotes enthusiasm and cooperation with the principles learned.

Select a variety of teaching strategies, e.g., demonstrate needed skills and have patient do return demonstration, incorporate new skills into the hospital routine.

Use of different means of accessing information promotes learner retention.

Discuss essential elements, e.g.:

Normal glucose blood level and compare with patient's, type of diabetes mellitus patient has, relationship between insulin deficiency and a high glucose level;

Provides knowledge base on which patient can make informed lifestyle choices.

Reasons for the ketoacidotic episode;

Knowledge of the precipitating factors may help to avoid recurrences.

Acute and chronic complications of the disease, including visual disturbances, neurosensory and cardiovascular changes, renal impairment/hypertension.

Awareness helps patient to be more consistent with care and may prevent/delay onset of complications.

Demonstrate fingerstick testing in combination with testing urine ketones.

SMBG (self-monitoring of blood glucose) four or more times a day allows flexibility in self-care, promotes tighter control of serum levels (e.g., 60–150 mg/dl) and may prevent/delay development of long-term complications.

Discuss dietary plan, use of high-fiber foods and ways to deal with meals outside the home.

Awareness of importance of dietary control will aid patient in planning meals/sticking to regimen. Fiber can slow glucose absorption, decreasing fluctuations in serum levels, but may cause GI discomfort, increase flatus and affect vitamin/mineral absorption.

Review medication regimen, including onset, peak, and duration of prescribed insulin, as applicable with patient/SO.

Understanding all aspects of drug usage promotes proper use. Dose algorithms are created, taking into account drug dosages established during inpatient evaluation, usual amount and schedule of physical activity, and meal plan. Including SO provides additional support/resource for patient.

Review self-administration of insulin and care of equipment. Have patient demonstrate procedure (e.g., drawing up and injection or use of continuous pump).

Identifies understanding and correctness of procedure or potential problems (e.g., vision, memory, etc.) so that alternate solutions can be found for insulin administration.

Stress importance and necessity of maintaining diary of glucose testing, medication dose/time, dietary intake, activity, feelings/sensations, life events.

Aids in creating overall picture of patient situation to achieve better disease control and promotes self-care/independence.

Discuss factors that play a part in diabetic control, e.g., exercise (aerobic versus isometric), stress, surgery, and illness. Review Sick Day rules.

This information promotes diabetic control and can greatly reduce the occurrence of ketoacidosis. Note: Aerobic exercise (e.g., walking, swimming) promotes effective use of insulin, lowering glucose levels, and strengthens the cardiovascular system.

Review effects of smoking on insulin use. Encourage cessation of smoking.

Nicotine constricts the small blood vessels, and insulin absorption is delayed for as long as these vessels remain constricted. Note: It is estimated that insulin absorption can be reduced by as much as 30% below normal in the first half hour after smoking.

ACTIONS/INTERVENTIONS	RATIONALE
Independent	
Establish regular exercise/activity schedule and identify corresponding insulin concerns.	Exercise times should not coincide with the peak action of insulin. A snack should be ingested before or during exercise as needed, and rotation of injection sites should avoid the muscle group that will be used in the activity (e.g., abdominal site is preferred over thigh/arm before jogging or swimming) to prevent accelerated uptake of insulin.
Identify the symptoms of hypoglycemia (e.g., weakness, dizziness, lethargy, hunger, irritability, diaphoresis, pallor, tachycardia, tremors, headache, changes in mentation) and explain causes.	May promote early detection and treatment, preventing occurrence. Note: Early morning hyperglycemia may reflect "Dawn phenomenon" (indicating need for additional insulin) or a rebound response to hypoglycemia during sleep (Somogyi effect), requiring a decrease in insulin dosage/change in diet (e.g., HS snack). Testing serum levels at 3 AM aids in identifying the specific problem.
Instruct in importance of routine examination of the feet and proper foot care.	Prevents/delays complications associated with peripheral neuropathies and/or circulatory impairment.
Discuss sexual functioning and answer questions patient/SO may have.	Not infrequently, impotence occurs (may be first symptom of onset of diabetes mellitus). Note: Counseling and/or use of penile prosthesis may be of benefit.
Stress importance of use of identification bracelet.	Can promote quick entry into the health system with fewer resultant complications in the event of an emergency.
Recommend avoidance of OTC drugs without prior approval of health care provider.	These products may contain sugars/interact with prescribed medications.
Discuss importance of follow-up care.	Helps to maintain tighter control of disease process and may prevent exacerbations of diabetes mellitus, retarding development of systemic complications.
Review signs/symptoms requiring medical evaluation, e.g., fever; cold/flu symptoms; cloudy/odorous urine, painful urination; delayed healing of cuts/sores; sensory changes (pain/tingling) of lower extremities; changes in blood sugar level, presence of ketones in urine.	Prompt intervention may prevent development of more serious/life-threatening complications.
Demonstrate stress management techniques, e.g., deep-breathing exercises, guided imagery, visualization.	Promotes relaxation and control of stress response which may help to limit incidence of glucose/insulin imbalances.
Identify community resources, e.g., American Diabetic Association, VNA, weight loss/stop smoking clinic, contact person/diabetic instructor.	Continued support is usually necessary to sustain lifestyle changes and promote well-being.

Hyperglycemic Hyperosmotic Nonketotic Coma _____

Hyperglycemic hyperosmotic nonketotic coma (HHNC) is a coma/near coma state due to marked hyperglycemia, hyperosmolarity, hypernatremia, and dehydration. It is differentiated from DKA by the absence of ketosis and related acidosis. It usually occurs in non-insulin-dependent diabetics but may be precipitated in a nondiabetic person by a facilitating factor, e.g., use of TPN in patient with sepsis or pancreatitis. Mortality rates may range from 40% to 70% (usually due to circulatory collapse).

PATIENT ASSESSMENT DATA BASE

ACTIVITY/REST

May report:	Weakness and fatigue.
May exhibit:	ROM and muscle strength decreased.

CIRCULATION

May report:	History of concomitant cardiac disease; MI.
May exhibit:	Hypotension, including postural changes.
	Rapid, weak, easily obliterated pulses.
	Dysrhythmias.
	Pallor; cool, dry skin.
	Capillary refill delayed; sunken eyeballs.

ELIMINATION

May report:	History of kidney disease, e.g., pyelonephritis; peritoneal dialysis with hypertonic solution.
	Frequent urination of dilute, pale yellow urine.
May exhibit:	Profound diuresis; followed by oliguria/anuria.
	Abdominal tenderness.
	Bowel sounds decreased (decreased motility/ileus).

FOOD/FLUID

May report:	History of non-insulin-dependent diabetes (NIDD); use of oral hypoglycemia agents.
	History of pancreatitis; use of hyperalimentation.
	Anorexia; nausea/vomiting; thirst.
	Weight loss.
	Chronic use of diuretics.
May exhibit:	Skin: dry, turgor markedly decreased.
	Mucous membranes dry/cracked.
	Bowel sounds diminished (decreased motility/ileus).
	Urine positive for glucose, negative for ketones.

NEUROSENSORY

May report:	Dizziness (orthostatic hypotension).
	Headaches.
	Weakness in extremities.
	Visual changes.
May exhibit:	Drowsiness, lethargy, confusion, stupor.
	Pupil reaction may be absent (if cerebral edema present).

Hypo- or hyperreflexic deep tendon reflexes; positive Babinski's; general or focal seizures.

Aphasia; reversible hemiparesis.

PAIN/COMFORT

May report: Abdominal tenderness, pain; leg cramps.

RESPIRATION

May report: Dyspnea.

May exhibit: Increased respiratory rate, tachypnea without Kussmaul respirations and absence of acetone odor on breath.

Breath sounds: crackles, rhonchi (infection).

Restlessness.

SAFETY

May exhibit: History of use of glucocorticoids (aggravates insulin insufficiency).

History of current infection, sepsis.

Elevated temperature.

Skin integrity impaired; e.g., burns, infected skin ulcer.

TEACHING/LEARNING

May report: Family history of diabetes, heart/kidney disease.

Concurrent acute illness, surgery, dialysis.

Use of thiazide diuretics, corticosteroids.

Discharge Plan   May need assistance with medication administration, food preparation, self-care, and
Considerations: homemaker tasks.

DIAGNOSTIC STUDIES

Serum glucose: commonly greater than 900 mg/ml (higher levels than normally seen with DKA) sometimes approach 3000–4000 mg/100ml.

Serum osmolality: greater than 350 mOsm/kg (tends to be higher than with DKA).

Serum sodium: may be normal, or decreased but is more commonly elevated (reflecting severe dehydration related to hyperosmolality/hyperglycemia and effects of diuresis).

Serum potassium: may be low, normal or elevated, though elevation actually reflects intracellular depletion.

CBC: Hct elevated secondary to hemoconcentration. Leukocytosis may be marked (infection may be precipitator).

BUN/Cr: may be elevated with BUN disproportionately higher than creatinine, reflecting prerenal azotemia.

Phosphorus, calcium, magnesium: may be decreased.

ABGs: pH and bicarbonate low (metabolic acidosis) although lactic acidosis will also be present if shock is profound and prolonged.

Plasma and urine ketones: absent or mild (notable difference between DKA and HHNC).

Urine: sugar elevated, up to 5%; specific gravity is increased.

NURSING PRIORITIES

1. Restore/maintain circulating volume/perfusion.
2. Prevent complications.
3. Provide information about disease process/prognosis, and treatment needs.

DISCHARGE CRITERIA

1. Homeostasis achieved.
2. Complications prevented/minimized.
3. Disease process/prognosis and therapeutic regimen understood.

NURSING DIAGNOSIS:	FLUID VOLUME DEFICIT, ACTUAL 1 [REGULATORY FAILURE]
May be related to:	Osmotic diuresis: hyperglycemia/glycosuria Excessive gastric losses: vomiting Restricted intake: nausea, confusion/coma
Possibly evidenced by:	Increased urine output, dilute urine; profound diuresis Weakness, thirst; decreased skin moisture/turgor Hypotension, tachycardia
PATIENT OUTCOMES/ EVALUATION CRITERIA:	Demonstrates improved fluid balance as evidenced by stable vital signs; urine output within acceptable parameters; moist skin/mucous membranes, palpable pulses, good skin turgor and capillary refill.

ACTIONS/INTERVENTIONS	RATIONALE
Independent	
Obtain history concerning the duration/intensity of present symptoms, e.g., vomiting, excessive urination.	Assists in estimation of total volume depletion.
Monitor vital signs, noting:	
Decreased BP, including orthostatic hypotension;	Hypovolemia may cause severe hypotension. Estimates of severity of hypotension may be made when systolic blood pressure drops more than 10 mmHg when patient rises from a recumbent to a sitting/ standing position. Continued hypotension may be indicative of ineffective fluid replacement or cardiac complications.
Tachycardia, irregular rhythm;	Heart rate elevates initially to compensate for hypovolemia and decreased cardiac output/tissue perfusion. Electrolyte imbalances (especially hypokalemia) potentiate dysrhythmias, which also decrease cardiac output and may cause MI.
Fever.	May indicate infectious process or reflect severe dehydration. Hyperthermic patient is more likely to develop dysrhythmias, congestive heart failure, MI.
Measure CVP if available.	More direct indicator of circulating volume/replacement needs, developing complications, e.g., cardiac failure.
Assess for signs of thirst; weak, rapid, thready pulse; pallor, delayed capillary refill, poor skin turgor, and dry skin and mucous membranes.	Presence of symptoms indicates extent of hypovolemia and assists in determining effectiveness of fluid replacement therapy.

ACTIONS/INTERVENTIONS	RATIONALE

Independent

Measure/record intake and output, including GI and insensible fluid loss. Monitor urine specific gravity.

Provides ongoing estimate of volume replacement needs and renal function (ability to concentrate urine).

Weigh daily.

Provides the best assessment of current fluid status.

Auscultate bowel sounds. Note complaints of nausea, abdominal pain; presence of vomiting and gastric distention.

Fluid and electrolyte deficits alter gastric motility, frequently resulting in vomiting and potentiating fluid/electrolyte losses.

Encourage oral fluids when tolerated. Keep water at the bedside within easy reach of the patient. Provide mouth care frequently.

Relieves discomfort of dry mucous membranes. Improvement in orientation level and return of bowel sounds may indicate that patient can increase oral intake, facilitating rehydration and electrolyte replacement.

Maintain comfortable environment, use light covers; provide tepid sponge bath, apply ice bags under arms and in groin if indicated.

Avoids overheating/reduces fever which promotes further fluid loss.

Promote bedrest, assist with self-care needs, plan activities around patient's fatigue level.

Limits effects of orthostatic hypotension and reduces stress on heart.

Reposition frequently and massage bony prominences.

Severe dehydration can greatly compromise dermal circulation and skin breakdown can occur rapidly.

Evaluate mentation, neurologic status, reflexes.

Fluid/electrolyte imbalances and fever impair CNS function and may result in seizure activity.

Instruct patient to report symptoms such as chest pain, weakness, dizziness.

Myocardial ischemia may develop because of sustained tachycardia and reduced cardiac output/perfusion (hypovolemia).

Observe for fatigue, crackles, edema, increased heart rate when replacing fluids.

Rapid fluid replacement in presence of cardiac strain may cause heart failure.

Collaborative

Administer IV fluids as indicated, e.g.:

Saline 0.9% (isotonic); plasma expanders, e.g., albumin;

Fluid deficit may approach 20–25% total body water. Initial replacement is rapid (e.g., 1 l/hr to correct volume deficit. Normal saline is given to expand the intravascular volume if the patient is hypotensive/demonstrating symptoms of shock. Plasma expanders may occasionally be needed if the deficit is life-threatening/BP does not normalize with rehydration efforts.

Saline 0.45%;

One-half normal saline may be given if hypotension is not profound, because it will tend to restore intracellular volume and thus reverse the neurologic manifestations.

Dextrose 5% and saline 0.45%.

Dextrose fluids are added when the blood sugar has approached approximately 250 mg/100ml to prevent hypoglycemia because glucose levels can fall rapidly with rehydration.

Administer potassium and/or bicarbonate as needed.

Prevents/corrects hypokalemia and life-threatening acidosis (rarer in HHNC than in DKA). Note: Potassium phosphate may be given if chloride is included in the IV fluids to prevent chloride overload.

661

ACTIONS/INTERVENTIONS	RATIONALE
Collaborative	
Insert/maintain urinary catheter.	Provides method for accurate measurement of urinary output.
Monitor laboratory studies, e.g.:	
Hct;	Hematocrit is often elevated due to hemoconcentration that occurs with dehydration.
BUN/creatinine;	Elevated values may reflect cellular breakdown from dehydration or signal the onset of renal failure.
Serum osmolality;	Elevated due to hyperglycemia and dehydration.
Glucose (preferably by fingerstick method);	Frequent monitoring is necessary because glucose level may change quickly (patient is often very sensitive to exogenous insulin). Bedside analysis of serum levels is more accurate than monitoring urine sugars.
Sodium;	May be low, reflecting the urinary sodium loss that occurs with osmotic diuresis or dilution secondary to hyperglycemia. High sodium values reflect decreased glomerular filtration and sodium resorption in response to aldosterone secretion (response to dehydration).
Potassium;	Potassium may be depleted because of the osmotic diuresis if patient has been taking thiazides or loop diuretics and during insulin therapy. Patients with HHNC usually have enough insulin to prevent ketoacidosis; however, lactic acidosis may develop because of hypovolemic shock. If this occurs, potassium leaves the cell in exchange for hydrogen, and total available potassium is eventually depleted.
ABGs (pH).	Acidosis occurs only rarely, and ketoacidosis does not occur; however, baseline ABGs are useful in determining need for bicarbonate to correct metabolic acidosis.
Administer regular insulin by intermittent or continuous IV method.	Regular insulin has a rapid onset and thus will quickly help move glucose into the cells.
IV bolus of regular insulin or a continuous drip via pump of approximately 5 U/hr until glucose reaches 250 mg/100 ml.	Insulin should be given judiciously because most patients have some endogenous production and may be quite sensitive to exogenous administration. The total insulin dosage is much less in the patient with HHNC than in DKA. Subcutaneous administration is not recommended because tissue perfusion/absorption may be reduced. After rehydration, insulin therapy may not be necessary if patient has adequate endogenous insulin production and is not insulin-resistant.
Insert nasogastric tube and attach to suction as indicated.	May be needed to decompress stomach and relieve vomiting.
Administer antipyretic medications as indicated: acetaminophen (Tylenol).	Reduces fever.

NURSING DIAGNOSIS:	INJURY, POTENTIAL FOR: TRAUMA
May be related to:	**Weakness, balancing difficulties, reduced muscle coordination, uncontrolled muscle activity (seizures), cogni-**

tive impairment/decreased mentation.

Possibly evidenced by: [Not applicable; presence of signs and symptoms establishes an *actual* diagnosis.]

PATIENT OUTCOMES/ EVALUATION CRITERIA: Recognizes need for/seeks assistance to prevent accidents/injuries.

ACTIONS/INTERVENTIONS	RATIONALE
Independent	
Monitor vital/neurologic signs. Investigate changes in level of consciousness, responses to stimuli.	Intracellular dehydration and disturbance in electrolyte balance/oxygenation impair CNS function. In addition, rapid rehydration may cause life-threatening precipitous fall in serum osmolality with development of cerebral edema, and sudden hypoglycemia.
Address patient by name, reorient to place, person, and time. Give short explanations.	Helps to maintain orientation and decrease confusion.
Schedule nursing time to provide frequent/undisturbed rest periods.	When fatigue is lessened, patient is more likely to maintain orientation.
Keep the siderails raised and bed in low position. Provide assistance in ambulation, changing positions. Provide seizure precautions.	Precautionary measures can prevent injury.
Inform patient/SO about safety precautions and why they are needed.	Knowledge of potential problems can help to prevent injuries/accidents.
Collaborative	
Monitor fluid administration and laboratory studies, e.g., blood glucose, serum osmolality, Hb/Hct, electrolytes.	Cerebral edema may be avoided by attention to rate of fluid replacement as well as slow reduction of hyperglycemia and serum osmolality. If CNS function does not improve with correction of these values, further investigation and intervention is needed.
Assist with prescribed regimen for correcting HHNC.	Alteration in thought processes is usually alleviated once hyperosmolar state has been corrected.

NURSING DIAGNOSIS: KNOWLEDGE DEFICIT [LEARNING NEED] (SPECIFY)

May be related to: Lack of exposure/recall, information misinterpretation

Unfamiliarity with information resources

Possibly evidenced by: Questions, request for information

Statement of misconception

Inaccurate follow-through of instructions, development of preventable complications

PATIENT OUTCOMES/ EVALUATION CRITERIA: Verbalizes understanding of disease process and treatment. Identifies relationship of signs/symptoms to the disease process and correlates symptoms with causative factors. Participates in treatment regimen.

ACTIONS/INTERVENTIONS	RATIONALE

Independent

Assess knowledge and practices related to diabetic protocol. (Refer to CP: Diabetes Mellitus, ND: Knowledge Deficit, p. 655.)

Identifies areas of lack of knowledge that may have precipitated the crisis.

Review current episode and underlying pathology.

Provides knowledge base on which patient can make informed choices/take preventive measures, if appropriate.

Discuss general health measures, e.g., eating well-balanced diet, maintaining adequate fluids, exercise, and rest.

Optimal health aids in preventing recurrence of HHNC in the individual whose hyperosmolarity is preventable.

Provide written information regarding own situation and signs/symptoms which need to be reported to the health care provider.

Helps to prevent complications that may result if prompt medical care is not obtained.

Collaborative

Consult dietician/nutritional support team for assessment of present caloric needs and results of current therapy.

Patients with certain conditions (e.g., burns, severe infections, cancer, recent surgery) may already be on high-calorie diets or receiving hyperalimentation containing high levels of glucose/carbohydrates. These therapies may have to be adjusted and/or insulin given to prevent recurrence of HHNC.

CHAPTER 12

REPRODUCTIVE

Hysterectomy

Hysterectomy is surgical removal of the uterus, performed for malignancies and certain nonmalignant conditions (e.g., endometriosis/tumors) to control life-threatening bleeding/hermorrhage and in the event of intractable pelvic infection or irreparable rupture of the uterus.

Abdominal hysterectomy types include the following:

Subtotal (partial): body of the uterus is removed; cervical stump remains.

Total: removal of the uterus and cervix.

Total with bilateral salpingo-oophorectomy: removal of uterus, cervix, fallopian tubes, and ovaries is the treatment of choice for invasive cancer, fibroid tumors that are rapidly growing or produce severe abnormal bleeding, and endometriosis invading other pelvic organs.

The vaginal route may be used in certain conditions, such as uterine prolapse, cystocele/rectocele, carcinoma in situ, and extreme obesity. It is contraindicated if the diagnosis is obscure.

PATIENT ASSESSMENT DATA BASE

Data are dependent on the underlying disease process/need for surgical intervention (e.g., cancer, prolapse, dysfunctional uterine bleeding, severe endometriosis or pelvic infections unresponsive to medical management) and associated complications (e.g., anemia).

TEACHING/LEARNING

Discharge Plan Considerations: May need temporary help with transportation; homemaker tasks.

DIAGNOSTIC STUDIES

CBC: decreased Hb may reflect chronic anemia, while decreased Hct suggests active blood loss. WBC elevation may indicate inflammation/infectious process.

Pap smear: cellular dysplasia reflects possibility of/presence of cancer.

Schiller's test (staining of cervix with iodine): useful in identifying abnormal cells.

D & C with biopsy (endometrial/cervical): permits histopathologic study of cells to determine presence/location of cancer.

Ultrasound or CT scan: aids in identifying size/location of mass.

NURSING PRIORITIES

1. Support adaptation to change.
2. Prevent complications.
3. Provide information about procedure/prognosis and treatment needs.

DISCHARGE CRITERIA

1. Dealing realistically with situation.
2. Complications prevented/minimized.
3. Procedure/prognosis and therapeutic regimen understood.

Refer to CP: Surgical Intervention for general considerations and interventions, p. 789.

NURSING DIAGNOSIS:	SELF-CONCEPT, DISTURBANCE IN: (SPECIFY)
May be related to:	Concerns about inability to have children, changes in femininity, effect on sexual relationship Religious conflicts
Possibly evidenced by:	Expressions of specific concerns/vague comments about result of surgery; fear of rejection or of reaction of SO Withdrawal, depression
PATIENT OUTCOMES/ EVALUATION CRITERIA:	Verbalizes concerns and indicates healthy ways of dealing with them. Verbalizes acceptance of self in situation and adaptation to change in body/self image.

ACTIONS/INTERVENTIONS	RATIONALE
Independent	
Provide time to listen to concerns and fears of patient and SO. Discuss patient's perceptions of self related to change and how patient sees self as a woman in usual lifestyle functioning.	Conveys interest and concern, provides opportunity to correct misconceptions, e.g., may fear loss of femininity and sexuality, weight gain, menopausal body changes.
Assess emotional stress the patient is experiencing. Identify meaning of loss for patient/SO. Encourage patient to vent feelings appropriately.	Nurses need to be aware of what this operation means to the patient in order to avoid inadvertent casualness or oversolicitude. Depending on the reason for the surgery (e.g., cancer or long-term heavy bleeding) the woman can be frightened or relieved. She may fear inability to fulfill her reproductive role, may experience grief over loss.
Provide accurate information, reinforcing information previously given.	Provides opportunity for patient to question and assimilate information.
Ascertain individual strengths and identify previous positive coping behaviors.	Helpful to build on strengths already available for patient to use in coping with current situation.
Provide open environment for patient to discuss concerns about sexuality.	Promotes sharing of beliefs/values about sensitive subject and identifies misconceptions/myths that may interfere with adjustment to situation. (Refer to ND: Sexual Dysfunction [Potential], p. 669.)
Note withdrawn behavior, negative self-talk, use of denial or overconcern with actual/perceived changes.	Identifies stage of grief/need for interventions.

ACTIONS/INTERVENTIONS

Collaborative

Refer to professional counseling as necessary.

RATIONALE

May need additional help to resolve feelings about loss. (Refer to CP: Psychosocial Aspects of Acute Care, p. 773.)

NURSING DIAGNOSIS:	URINARY ELIMINATION, ALTERED PATTERNS/URINARY RETENTION [ACUTE]
May be related to:	Mechanical trauma, surgical manipulation, presence of local tissue edema, hematoma
	Sensory/motor impairment: nerve paralysis
Possibly evidenced by:	Sensation of bladder fullness, urgency
	Small frequent voiding or absence of urine output; overflow incontinence
	Bladder distention
PATIENT OUTCOMES/ EVALUATION CRITERIA:	Empties bladder regularly and completely.

ACTIONS/INTERVENTIONS

Independent

Note voiding pattern, and monitor urinary output.

Palpate bladder. Investigate complaints of discomfort, fullness, inability to void.

Provide routine voiding measures, e.g., privacy, normal position, running water in sink, pouring warm water over perineum.

Provide good perianal cleansing care, and catheter care (when present).

Assess urine characteristics, noting color, clarity, odor.

Collaborative

Catheterize when indicated/per protocol if patient is unable to void or is uncomfortable.

Decompress bladder slowly.

Maintain patency of indwelling catheter; keep drainage tubing free of kinks.

RATIONALE

May indicate urine retention if voiding frequently in small/insufficient amounts (<100 ml).

Perception of bladder fullness, distension of bladder above symphysis pubis indicates urinary retention.

Promotes relaxation of perineal muscles and may facilitate voiding efforts.

Promotes cleanliness reducing risk of ascending urinary infection.

Urinary retention, vaginal drainage, and possible presence of intermittent/retained catheter increase risk of infection, especially if patient has perineal sutures.

Edema or interference with nerve supply may cause bladder atony/urinary retention requiring decompression of the bladder. Note: Indwelling urethral or suprapubic catheter may be inserted intraoperatively if complications are anticipated.

When large amount of urine has accumulated, rapid bladder decompression releases pressure on pelvic vessels, which promotes venous pooling and decreases circulating blood volume, resulting in signs of shock.

Promotes free drainage of urine, reducing risk of urinary stasis/retention and infection.

ACTIONS/INTERVENTIONS

Collaborative

Check residual volume after voiding as indicated.

RATIONALE

May not be emptying bladder completely, and retention of urine increases possibility for infection and is uncomfortable/painful.

NURSING DIAGNOSIS:	BOWEL ELIMINATION, ALTERED (SPECIFY) [POTENTIAL]
May be related to:	**Physical factors: abdominal surgery, with manipulation of bowel, weakening of abdominal musculature**
	Pain/discomfort in abdomen or perineal area
	Changes in dietary intake
Possibly evidenced by:	**[Not applicable; presence of signs and symptoms establishes an *actual* diagnosis.]**
PATIENT OUTCOMES/ EVALUATION CRITERIA:	**Displays active bowel sounds/peristaltic activity and usual pattern of elimination.**

ACTIONS/INTERVENTIONS

Independent

Auscultate bowel sounds. Note abdominal distention, presence of nausea/vomiting.

Assist patient with sitting on edge of bed and walking.

Encourage adequate fluid intake, including fruit juices, when oral intake is resumed.

Collaborative

Restrict oral intake as indicated.

Maintain nasogastric tube, if present.

Provide clear/full liquids and advance to solid foods as tolerated.

Use rectal tube; apply heat to the abdomen, if appropriate.

Provide sitz baths.

Administer medications, e.g., stool softeners, mineral oil, laxatives as indicated.

RATIONALE

Indicators of presence/resolution of ileus, affecting choice of interventions.

Early ambulation helps stimulate intestinal function and return of peristalsis.

Promotes softer stool; may aid in stimulating peristalsis.

Prevents nausea/vomiting until peristalsis begins (1–2 days).

May be inserted in surgery to decompress stomach.

When peristalsis begins, food and fluid intake promote resumption of normal bowel elimination.

Promotes the passage of flatus.

Promotes muscle relaxation, minimizes discomfort.

Promotes formation/passage of softer stool.

NURSING DIAGNOSIS:	TISSUE PERFUSION, ALTERED: (SPECIFY) [POTENTIAL]
May be related to:	**Hypovolemia**
	Reduction/interruption of blood flow: pelvic congestion, postoperative tissue inflammation, venous stasis; in-

traoperative trauma or pressure on pelvic/calf vessels (lithotomy position during vaginal hysterectomy)

Possibly evidenced by:	[Not applicable; presence of signs and symptoms establishes an *actual* diagnosis.]
PATIENT OUTCOMES/ EVALUATION CRITERIA:	Demonstrates adequate perfusion, as evidenced by stable vital signs, palpable pulses, good capillary refill, usual mentation, individually adequate urinary output; and free of edema, signs of thrombus formation.

ACTIONS/INTERVENTIONS	RATIONALE
Independent	
Monitor vital signs; palpate peripheral pulses, and note capillary refill; assess urine output/characteristics. Evaluate changes in mentation.	Indicators of adequacy of systemic perfusion, fluid/ blood needs, and developing complications.
Inspect dressings and perineal pads, noting color, amount and odor of drainage. Weigh pads and compare with dry weight, if patient is bleeding heavily.	Proximity of large blood vessels to operative site and/ or potential for alteration of clotting mechanism (e.g., cancer) increase risk of postoperative hemorrhage.
Turn patient and encourage coughing and deep-breathing exercises frequently.	Prevents stasis of secretions and respiratory complications.
Avoid high Fowler's position and pressure under the knees or crossing of legs.	Creates vascular stasis by increasing pelvic congestion and pooling of blood in the extremities, potentiating risk of thrombus formation.
Assist with/instruct in foot and leg exercises and ambulate as soon as able.	Movement enhances circulation and prevents stasis complications.
Check for Homan's sign. Note erythema, swelling of extremity, or complaints of sudden chest pain with dyspnea.	May be indicative of development of thrombophlebitis/ pulmonary embolus. (Refer to CP: Thrombophlebitis: Deep Vein Thrombosis, p. 117.)
Collaborative	
Administer IV fluids, blood products as indicated.	Replacement of blood losses maintains circulating volume and tissue perfusion.
Apply antiembolus stockings.	Aids in venous return; reduces stasis and risk of thrombosis.
Assist with/encourage use of incentive spirometer.	Promotes lung expansion/minimizes atelectasis.

NURSING DIAGNOSIS:	**SEXUAL DYSFUNCTION [POTENTIAL]**
May be related to:	Altered body structure/function, e.g., shortening of vaginal canal; changes in hormone levels, decreased libido
	Possible change in sexual response pattern, e.g., absence of rhythmic uterine contractions during orgasm; vaginal discomfort/pain (dyspareunia)
Possibly evidenced by:	[Not applicable; presence of signs and symptoms establishes an *actual* diagnosis.]
PATIENT OUTCOMES/	Verbalizes understanding of changes in sexual

anatomy/function. Discusses concerns about body image, sex role, desirability as a sexual partner with SO. Identifies satisfying/acceptable sexual practices and some alternative ways of dealing with sexual expression.

ACTIONS/INTERVENTIONS	RATIONALE
Independent	
Listen to comments of patient/SO.	Sexual concerns are often disguised as humor and/or offhand remarks.
Assess patient/SO information regarding sexual anatomy/function and effects of surgical procedure.	May have misinformation/misconceptions which can affect adjustment. Negative expectations are associated with poor overall outcome. Changes in hormone levels can affect libido and/or decrease suppleness of the vagina. Although a shortened vagina can eventually stretch, initially intercourse may be uncomfortable/painful.
Identify cultural/value factors/conflicts present.	May affect return to satisfying sexual relationship.
Assist patient to be aware/deal with stage of grieving.	Acknowledging normal process of grieving for actual/perceived changes may enhance coping and facilitate resolution.
Encourage patient to share thoughts/concerns with partner.	Open communication can identify areas of agreement/problems and promote discussion and resolution.
Problem-solve solutions to potential problems, e.g., postponing sexual intercourse when fatigued, substituting alternate means of expression, positions that avoid pressure on abdominal incision, use of vaginal lubricant.	Assists patient to return to desired/satisfying sexual activity.
Discuss expected physical sensations/discomforts, changes in response as appropriate to the individual.	Vaginal pain may be marked following vaginal procedure or sensory loss may occur due to surgical trauma. Although sensory loss is usually temporary, it may take a period of weeks/months to resolve. In addition, changes in size of vagina, altered hormone levels, and loss of sensation of rhythmic contractions of the uterus during orgasm can impair sexual satisfaction. Note: Many patients experience few negative effects because fears of pregnancy are gone and relieved symptoms often improve enjoyment of intercourse.
Collaborative	
Refer to counselor, sex therapist as needed.	May need additional assistance to promote a satisfactory outcome.

NURSING DIAGNOSIS:	KNOWLEDGE DEFICIT [LEARNING NEED] (SPECIFY)
May be related to:	**Lack of exposure/recall; information misinterpretation**
	Unfamiliarity with information resources
Possibly evidenced by:	**Questions/request for information; statement of misconception**

	Inaccurate follow-through of instructions, development of preventable complications
PATIENT OUTCOMES/ EVALUATION CRITERIA:	**Verbalizes understanding of condition. Identifies relationship of signs/symptoms of surgical procedure and actions to deal with them.**

ACTIONS/INTERVENTIONS

Independent

Review effects of surgical procedure and future expectations; e.g., patient needs to know she will no longer menstruate or bear children, whether surgical menopause will occur, and the possible need for hormonal replacement.

Discuss complexity of problems anticipated during recovery, e.g., emotional lability and expectation of feelings of depression/sadness; excessive fatigue, sleep disturbances, urinary problems.

Discuss resumption of activity. Encourage light activities initially, with frequent rest periods and increased activities/exercise as tolerated. Stress importance of individual response in recuperation.

Identify individual restrictions, e.g., avoiding heavy lifting and strenuous activities (such as vacuuming, straining at stool); prolonged sitting/driving. Avoid tub baths/douching until physician allows.

Review recommendations for resumption of sexual intercourse. (Refer to ND: Sexual Dysfunction [Potential], p. 669.)

Identify dietary needs, e.g., high protein, additional iron.

Review replacement hormone therapy. Discuss possibility of "hot flashes" even though ovaries may remain.

Encourage taking prescribed drug(s) routinely (e.g., with meals).

Discuss potential side effects, e.g., weight gain, increased skin pigmentation or acne, breast ten-

RATIONALE

Provides knowledge base on which patient can make informed choices.

Physical, emotional, and social factors can have a cumulative effect, which may delay recovery, especially if hysterectomy was performed because of cancer. Providing an opportunity for problem solving may facilitate the process. Patient/SO may benefit from the knowledge that a period of emotional lability is normal and expected during recovery.

Patient can expect to feel tired when she goes home and needs to plan a gradual resumption of activities with return to work an individual matter. Prevents excessive fatigue, conserves energy for healing/tissue regeneration. Note: Some studies suggest that recovery from hysterectomy (especially when oophorectomy is done) may take four times as long as recovery from other major surgeries (12 months versus 3 months).

Strenuous activity intensifies fatigue and may delay healing. Activities that increase intraabdominal pressure can strain surgical repairs, and prolonged sitting potentiates risk of thrombus formation. Showers are permitted, but tub baths/douching may cause vaginal irritation or incisional infections as well as be a safety hazard.

When activity is cleared by the physician, it is best to resume sexual activity easily and gently, using alternate coital positions or expressing sexual feelings in other ways.

Facilitates healing/tissue regeneration and helpful in correcting anemia if present.

Total hysterectomy with bilateral salpingo-oophorectomy (surgically induced menopause) requires replacement hormones. In addition, hormone replacement may be needed in subtotal procedures because a portion of the blood supply to the ovaries is clamped during the procedure, possibly impairing long-term function.

Taking hormones with meals establishes routine for taking drug and reduces potential for initial nausea.

Development of some side effects is expected but may require problem-solving such as change in dos-

ACTIONS/INTERVENTIONS

Independent

derness, headaches, photosensitivity.

Recommend cessation of smoking when receiving estrogen therapy.

Review incisional care when appropriate.

Stress importance of follow-up care.

Identify signs/symptoms requiring medical evaluation, e.g., fever/chills, change in character of vaginal/wound drainage; bright bleeding.

RATIONALE

age or use of sun screen.

Some studies suggest an increased risk of thrombophlebitis, MI, CVA and pulmonary emboli.

Facilitates competent self-care, promoting independence.

Provides opportunity to ask questions and clear up misunderstandings as well as detect any beginning complications.

Early recognition and treatment of developing complications such as infection, hemorrhage may prevent life-threatening situations. Note: Hemorrhage may occur as late as 2 weeks postoperatively.

Mastectomy

The choice of treatment for breast cancer depends on tumor type, size, and location, as well as clinical characteristics (staging). Therapy may include surgical intervention with/without radiation, chemotherapy, and hormone therapy.

Types of surgery are generally grouped into three categories: radical mastectomy, total mastectomy, and more limited procedures (e.g., segmental, lumpectomy). Total (simple) mastectomy removes all breast tissue, but all or most axillary lymph nodes and chest muscles are left intact. Modified radical mastectomy removes the entire breast, some or most lymph nodes and sometimes the pectoralis minor chest muscles. Major chest muscles are left intact. Radical mastectomy (sometimes called Halsted mastectomy) is a procedure that requires removal of the entire breast, skin, major and minor pectoral muscles, axillary lymph nodes, and sometimes internal mammary or supraclavicular lymph nodes.

PATIENT ASSESSMENT DATA BASE

ACTIVITY/REST

May report: Work, activity involving arm movements.
Sleep style (e.g., sleeping on stomach).

CIRCULATION

May exhibit: Unilateral engorgement in affected arm (invaded lymph system).

FOOD/FLUID

May report: Loss of appetite.

EGO INTEGRITY

May report: Stress/fear.

PAIN/COMFORT

May report: Usually nontender lump and no complaints of pain (even with advanced metastatic destruction). Some experience discomfort or "funny feeling" in breast tissue.
Heavy, painful breasts premenstrually (fibrocystic disease).

SAFETY

May exhibit: Nodular axillary masses.
Edema, erythema of involved skin.

SEXUALITY

May report: History of early menarche (under age 12); late menopause (after age 50); late first pregnancy.
Concerns about sexuality/intimacy.

May exhibit: Change in breast contour/mass (visual/palpable nodule); may be fixed to chest wall (late).
Dimpling, puckering of skin; changes in skin color/texture, swelling, redness or heat in breast.
Retraction of nipple, discharge from nipple.

TEACHING/LEARNING

May report: Family history of breast cancer.

673

Discharge Plan Considerations: May need assistance with treatments/rehabilitation, decisions, homemaker tasks.

DIAGNOSTIC STUDIES

Mammography: visualizes internal structure of the breast; is capable of detecting nonpalpable cancers or tumors that are in early stages of development.

Ultrasound: may be helpful in distinguishing between solid masses and cysts and in women whose breast tissue is dense; complements findings of mammography.

Xeroradiography: reveals increased circulation around tumor site.

Thermography: identifies rapidly growing tumors as "hot spots," because of increased blood supply and corresponding higher skin temperature.

Diaphanography (transillumination): identifies tumor or mass by differentiating the way that tissues transmit and scatter light. Procedure remains experimental and is considered less accurate than mammography.

CT scan and MRI: scanning techniques that can detect breast disease, especially larger masses, or tumors in small, dense breasts that are difficult to examine by mammography. These techniques are not suitable for routine screening or substitute for mammography.

Breast biopsy (needle or excisional): provides definitive diagnosis of mass, and is useful for histologic classification (staging) and selection of appropriate therapies.

Hormone receptor assays: reveal whether cells of excised tumor or biopsy specimens contain hormone receptors (estrogen and progesterone). In malignant cells, the estrogen-plus receptor complex stimulates cell growth and division. About two-thirds of all women with breast cancer are estrogen-receptor (ER) positive and tend to respond favorably to hormone therapy following primary therapy to extend the disease-free period and survival.

Chest x-ray, liver function studies, CBC, and bone scan: done to assess for presence of metastasis.

NURSING PRIORITIES

1. Assist patient/SO in dealing with stress of situation/prognosis.
2. Prevent complications.
3. Establish individualized rehabilitation program.
4. Provide information about disease process, procedure, prognosis, and treatment needs.

DISCHARGE CRITERIA

1. Dealing realistically with situation.
2. Complications prevented/minimized.
3. Exercise regimen initiated.
4. Disease process, surgical procedure, prognosis, and therapeutic regimen understood.

Refer to CPs: Cancer, p. 870; Surgical Intervention, p. 789, for other considerations and interventions.

PREOPERATIVE

NURSING DIAGNOSIS:	**FEAR/ANXIETY [SPECIFY LEVEL]**
May be related to:	**Threat of death, e.g., extent of disease**
	Threat to self-concept: change of body image; scarring, loss of body part, sexual attractiveness
	Change in health status
Possibly evidenced by:	**Increased tension; apprehension; feelings of helplessness/inadequacy**
	Decreased self-assurance

Self-focus; restlessness; sympathetic stimulation

Expressed concerns regarding actual/anticipated changes in life

PATIENT OUTCOMES/ EVALUATION CRITERIA:	Acknowledges and discusses concerns. Demonstrates appropriate range of feelings. Reports lessened fear and anxiety reduced to a manageable level.

ACTIONS/INTERVENTIONS	RATIONALE
Independent	
Ascertain what information patient has about diagnosis, expected surgical intervention, and future therapies. Note presence of denial or extreme anxiety.	Provides knowledge base for the nurse to enable reinforcement of needed information and helps to identify patient with high anxiety, low capacity for information processing, and need for special attention. Note: Denial may be useful as a coping method for a period of time, but extreme anxiety needs to be dealt with immediately.
Explain purpose of preoperative tests and preparation.	Clear understanding of procedures and what is happening increases feelings of control and lessens anxiety.
Provide an atmosphere of concern, openness, and availability as well as privacy for the patient/SO. Suggest that SO be present as much as possible/desired.	Time and privacy are needed to provide support, discuss feelings of anticipated loss and other concerns. Therapeutic communication skills, open questions, listening, etc., facilitates this process.
Encourage questions and provide time for expression of fears.	Provides opportunity to identify and clarify misconceptions and offer emotional support.
Assess degree of support available to the patient. Give information about community resources, such as Reach to Recovery, Encore program of YWCA. Encourage/provide for visit with a woman who has recovered from a mastectomy.	Can be a helpful resource when patient is ready. A peer who has experienced the same process serves as a role model and can provide validity to the comments, hope for recovery/normal future.
Discuss/explain role of rehabilitation after surgery.	Rehabilitation is an essential component of therapy intended to meet physical, social, emotional, and vocational needs so that the patient can achieve the best possible level of physical and emotional functioning.

POSTOPERATIVE

NURSING DIAGNOSIS:	**SKIN/TISSUE INTEGRITY, IMPAIRED**
May be related to:	Surgical removal of skin/tissues; altered circulation, presence of edema, drainage; changes in skin elasticity, sensation; tissue destruction (radiation)
Possibly evidenced by:	Disruption of skin surface, destruction of skin layers/ subcutaneous tissues
PATIENT OUTCOMES/ EVALUATION CRITERIA:	Achieves timely wound healing, free of purulent drainage or erythema. Demonstrates behaviors/techniques to promote healing/prevent complications.

ACTIONS/INTERVENTIONS	RATIONALE

Independent

Assess dressings/wound for characteristics of drainage. Note edema, redness of the area. Monitor temperature.

Use of dressings depends on the extent of surgery and the type of wound closure. (Pressure dressings are usually applied initially and are reinforced, not changed). Drainage occurs because of the trauma of the procedure and manipulation of the numerous blood vessels and lymphatics in the area. Early recognition of developing infection can enable quickly instituted treatment.

Place in semi-Fowler's position on back, or unaffected side with arm elevated and supported by pillows.

Assists with drainage of fluid through use of gravity.

Do not take BP, insert IV, or give injections in affected arm.

Increases potential of constriction, infection, and lymphedema on affected side.

Inspect donor/graft site (if done) for color, blister formation; note drainage from donor site.

Color will be affected by availability of circulatory supply. Blister formation provides a site for bacterial growth/infection.

Empty wound drains periodically noting amount and characteristics of drainage.

Drainage of accumulated fluids (e.g., lymph, blood) enhances healing and reduces the susceptibility to infection. Suction devices (e.g., Hemovac, Jackson–Pratt) are often inserted during surgery to maintain negative pressure in wound. Tubes are usually removed between the third and fifth days or when drainage ceases.

Encourage wearing of loose-fitting/nonconstrictive clothing.

Prevents undue pressure on compromised tissues, which may impair circulation/healing.

Collaborative

Administer antibiotics as indicated.

May be given prophylactically or to treat specific infection and enhance healing.

NURSING DIAGNOSIS:	COMFORT, ALTERED: PAIN, ACUTE
May be related to:	**Surgical procedure; tissue trauma, interruption of nerves, dissection of muscles**
Possibly evidenced by:	**Complaints of stiffness, numbness in chest area, shoulder/arm pain; alteration of muscle tone**
	Self-focusing; distraction/guarding behavior
PATIENT/OUTCOMES/ EVALUATION CRITERIA:	**Expresses reduction in pain/discomfort. Appears relaxed, able to sleep/rest appropriately.**

ACTIONS/INTERVENTIONS	RATIONALE

Independent

Assess complaints of pain, noting location, duration, and intensity (1–10 scale). Note verbal and nonverbal clues.

Aids in identifying degree of discomfort and need for/ effectiveness of analgesia. The amount of tissue, muscle, and lymphatic system removed can affect the amount of pain experienced. Destruction of nerves in axillary region causes numbness in upper arm and scapular region, which may be more intolerable than

ACTIONS/INTERVENTIONS	RATIONALE

Independent

Discuss normality of phantom breast sensations.

Assist patient to find position of comfort.

Provide routine comfort measures (e.g., repositioning on back or unaffected side, backrub) and diversional activities. Encourage early ambulation and use of relaxation techniques, guided imagery, Therapeutic Touch.

Splint chest during coughing/deep-breathing exercises.

Medicate routinely before pain is severe/before activities are scheduled.

Collaborative

Administer narcotics/analgesics as indicated.

surgical pain. Note: Pain in chest wall can occur from muscle tension, be affected by extremes in heat and cold, and continue for several months.

Provides reassurance that sensations are not imaginary and that relief can be obtained.

Elevation of arm, size of dressings, presence of drains affects patient's ability to relax and rest/sleep effectively.

Promotes relaxation, helps to refocus attention, and may enhance coping abilities.

Facilitates participation in activity without undue discomfort.

Maintains comfort level and permits patient to exercise arm and to ambulate without pain hindering efforts.

Provides relief of discomfort/pain and facilitates rest, participation in postoperative therapy.

NURSING DIAGNOSIS:	SELF-CONCEPT, DISTURBANCE IN: (SPECIFY)
May be related to:	**Biophysical: disfiguring surgical procedure**
	Psychosocial: concern about sexual attractiveness
Possibly evidenced by:	**Actual change in structure/body contour**
	Verbalization of fear of rejection or of reaction by others, change in social involvement
	Negative feelings about body, preoccupation with change or loss, not looking at body, nonparticipation in therapy
PATIENT OUTCOMES/ EVALUATION CRITERIA:	**Demonstrates movement toward acceptance of self in situation. Recognizes and incorporates change into self-concept without negating self-esteem. Sets realistic goals and actively participates in therapy program.**

ACTIONS/INTERVENTIONS	RATIONALE

Independent

Encourage questions about current situation and future expectations. Provide emotional support when surgical dressings are removed.

Identify concerns about role as woman, wife, etc.

Loss of the breast causes many reactions, including feeling disfigured, fear of viewing scar by self/SO, and fear of partner's reaction to change in body.

May express hesitancy to resume/begin sexual rela-

Independent

tions for fear of rejection by partner or injury to surgical site.

Allow patient to express feelings, e.g., anger, hostility, and grief.

Loss of body part, disfigurement, and perceived loss of desirability engender grieving process that needs to be dealt with so patient can make plans for the future. Note: Grief may resurface when subsequent procedures are done (e.g., fitting for prosthesis, reconstructive procedure). (Refer to CP: Cancer, ND: Grieving, Anticipatory, p. 876.)

Discuss signs/symptoms of depression with patient/SO.

Common reaction to this type of procedure and needs to be recognized, acknowledged, and dealt with for prevention of exacerbation during extended recovery period.

Provide positive reinforcement for gains/improvement and participation in self-care/treatment program.

Encourages continuation of desired behaviors.

Review possibilities for reconstructive surgery and/or prosthetic augmentation.

If feasible, reconstruction provides less disfiguring/"near normal" cosmetic result. Variations in skin flap may be done for facilitation of future reconstructive process. Note: Although reconstruction is usually not done for 3–6 months, prolonged delay may result in increased tension in relationships and impair patient's incorporation of changes into self-concept.

Ascertain feelings/concerns of partner and provide information and support.

Negative responses directed at the patient may actually reflect concern for hurting patient, fear of cancer/death, difficulty in dealing with personality/behavior changes patient is experiencing, or simply "weak stomach" for viewing operative area.

Discuss and refer to support groups including "Men in Our Lives" for SO.

Provides a place to exchange concerns and feelings with others who have had a similar experience and identifies ways SO can facilitate patient's recovery.

Collaborative

Provide temporary soft prosthesis, if indicated.

Promotes social acceptance and allows patient to feel more comfortable about body image at the time of discharge. Prosthesis of nylon and Dacron fluff may be worn in bra until incision heals if reconstructive surgery is not performed at the time of mastectomy.

NURSING DIAGNOSIS:	MOBILITY, IMPAIRED PHYSICAL
May be related to:	Neuromuscular impairment; pain/discomfort; edema formation
Possibly evidenced by:	Reluctance to attempt movement
	Limited range of motion, decreased muscle mass, strength
PATIENT OUTCOMES/ EVALUATION CRITERIA:	Displays willingness to participate in therapy. Demonstrates techniques that enable resumption of activities. Increases strength of affected body parts.

ACTIONS/INTERVENTIONS	RATIONALE
Independent	
Elevate affected arm as indicated. Begin passive ROM (e.g., flexion/extension of elbow, pronation/supination of wrist, clenching/extending fingers) as soon as possible.	Promotes venous return lessening possibility of lymphedema. Early postoperative exercises are usually started in the first 24 hours to prevent joint stiffness which can further limit movement/mobility.
Have patient move fingers, noting sensations and color of hand on affected side.	Lack of movement may reflect problems with the intercostal brachial nerve, and discoloration can indicate impaired circulation.
Encourage patient to use affected arm for personal hygiene, e.g., feeding, combing hair, washing face.	Increases circulation, helps minimize edema, and maintains strength and function of the arm and hand. These activities use the arm without adduction, which can stress the suture line in the early postoperative period.
Help with self-care activities as necessary.	Conserves patient's energy; prevents undue fatigue.
Assist with ambulation, and encourage correct posture.	Patient will feel unbalanced and may need assistance until accustomed to change. Keeping back straight prevents shoulder from moving forward, avoiding permanent limitation in movement and posture.
Advance exercise as indicated, e.g., active extension of arm and rotation of shoulder while lying in bed, pendulum swings, rope turning, elevating arms to touch fingertips behind head.	Prevents joint stiffness, increases circulation, and maintains muscle tone of the shoulders and arm.
Progress to hand climbing (walking fingers up wall), clasping hands behind head, and full abduction exercises as soon as patient can manage.	Since this group of exercises can cause excessive tension on the incision, they are usually delayed until healing process is well established.
Evaluate presence/degree of exercise-related pain and changes in joint mobility. Measure upper and forearm if edema develops.	Monitors progression/resolution of complications. May need to postpone increasing exercises and wait until further healing occurs.
Discuss types of exercises to be done at home to reestablish strength and encourage circulation in the affected arm.	Exercise program needs to be continued to regain optimal function of the affected side.
Coordinate exercise program into self-care and homemaker activities, e.g., dressing self, washing, swimming, dusting, mopping.	Patient is usually more willing to participate or finds it easier to maintain an exercise program that fits into lifestyle and accomplishes tasks as well.
Assist patient to identify signs and symptoms of shoulder tension, e.g., inability to maintain posture, burning sensation in postscapular region. Instruct patient to avoid sitting or holding arm in dependent position for extended periods.	Altered weight and support puts tension on surrounding structures.
Collaborative	
Administer medications as indicated, e.g.:	
Analgesics;	Pain needs to be controlled prior to exercise or patient may not participate optimally, and incentive to exercise may be lost.
Diuretics.	May be useful in treating and preventing fluid accumulation/lymphedema.
Maintain integrity of elastic bandages or custom-fitted pressure-gradient elastic sleeve.	Promotes venous return and decreases risk/effects of edema formation.
Refer to physical/occupational therapist.	Provides individual exercise program. Assesses limitations/restrictions regarding employment requirements.

NURSING DIAGNOSIS:	KNOWLEDGE DEFICIT [LEARNING NEED] (SPECIFY)
May be related to:	Lack of exposure/recall
	Information misinterpretation
Possibly evidenced by:	Questions/request for information; statement of misconception
	Inaccurate follow-through of instructions/development of preventable complications
PATIENT OUTCOMES/ EVALUATION CRITERIA:	Verbalizes understanding of disease process and treatment. Performs necessary procedures correctly and explains reasons for actions. Initiates necessary lifestyle changes and participates in treatment regimen.

ACTIONS/INTERVENTIONS	RATIONALE
Independent	
Review disease process, surgical procedure, and future expectations.	Provides knowledge base on which patient can make informed choices including participation in radiation/chemotherapy programs. (Refer to CP: Cancer, p. 872.)
Discuss necessity for well-balanced, nutritious meals and adequate fluid intake.	Provides optimal nutrition and maintains circulating volume to enhance tissue regeneration/healing process.
Suggest alternating schedule of frequent rest and activity periods especially in situations where sitting is prolonged.	Prevents/limits fatigue, promotes healing, and enhances feelings of general well-being. Sitting with arms and head extended intensifies stress on affected structures, creating muscle tension/stiffness, and may interfere with healing.
Instruct patient to protect hands and arms when gardening; use thimble when sewing; use potholders when handling hot items; use plastic gloves when doing dishes; and so forth. Do not carry purse or wear jewelry/wristwatch on affected side.	Compromised lymphatic system causes tissues to be more susceptible to infection and/or injury.
Warn against having blood withdrawn or receiving IV fluids/medications or BP measurements on the affected side.	May restrict the circulation and increase risk of infection because the lymphatic system is compromised.
Recommend wearing of a Medic-Alert device.	Prevents unnecessary trauma (e.g., blood pressures, injections) to affected arm.
Demonstrate use of intermittent compression.	Pneumatic device aid is occasionally used in managing lymphedema by promoting circulation and venous return.
Suggest gentle massage of healed incision with emollients.	Stimulates circulation, promotes elasticity of skin, and reduces discomfort associated with phantom breast sensations.
Recommend use of different sexual positions that avoid pressure on chest wall or alternate forms of sexual expression during initial healing process/while operative area is still tender.	Promotes feelings of femininity and sense of ability to return to normal activities.

ACTIONS/INTERVENTIONS	RATIONALE

Independent

Encourage regular monthly self-examination of remaining breast. Determine recommended schedule for mammography.

Identifies changes in breast tissue indicative of recurrent/new tumor development.

Stress importance of regular medical follow-up.

Other treatment may be required as adjunctive therapy, such as radiation. Recurrence of malignant breast tumors can also be identified and managed by oncology. (Refer to CP: Cancer, p. 872.)

Identify signs/symptoms requiring medical evaluation, e.g., arm red, warm, swollen; erythema, edema, purulent wound drainage, fever/chills.

Lymphangitis can occur as result of infection causing lymphedema.

CHAPTER 13

ORTHOPEDIC AND CONNECTIVE TISSUE DISORDERS

Fractures _____

There are over 150 fracture classifications; 5 major ones are as follows:
1. *Incomplete:* fracture involves only a portion of the cross-section of the bone. One side breaks; the other usually just bends (green-stick).
2. *Complete:* fracture line involves entire cross-section of the bone, and bone fragments are usually displaced.
3. *Closed (simple):* the fracture does not extend through the skin.
4. *Open (compound):* bone fragments extend through the muscle and skin, potentially infected.
5. *Pathologic:* fracture occurs in diseased bone (such as cancer, osteoporosis), with no or only minimal trauma.

For discussion of cranial and spinal fractures, refer to CPs: Craniocerebral Trauma, p. 226; Spinal Cord Injury, p. 284.

PATIENT ASSESSMENT DATA BASE

Symptoms of fracture depend on site, severity, type of fracture, and amount of damage to other structures.

ACTIVITY/REST

May exhibit: Restricted/loss of function of affected part (may be immediate, owing to the fracture, or secondary, from tissue swelling, pain).

CIRCULATION

May exhibit: Hypertension (occasionally seen as a response to pain/anxiety or hypotension (blood loss).

Tachycardia (stress response, hypovolemia).

Pulse reduced/absent distal to local injury; delayed capillary refill, pallor of affected part.

Tissue swelling, or hematomo mass at site of injury.

NEUROSENSORY

May report: Loss of motion/sensation, muscle spasms.

Numbness/tingling (paresthesias).

May exhibit:	Local deformities; abnormal angulation, shortening, rotation, crepitation (grating sound), muscle spasms, visible weakness/loss of function.
	Agitation (may be related to pain/anxiety).

PAIN/COMFORT

May report:	Sudden severe pain at the time of injury (may be localized to the area of tissue/skeletal damage and be resolved upon immobilization); absence of pain suggests nerve damage.
	Muscle spasms/cramping (after immobilization).

SAFETY

May exhibit:	Skin lacerations, tissue avulsion, bleeding, color changes.
	Localized swelling (may increase gradually or suddenly).

TEACHING/LEARNING

May report:	Circumstances of injury.
Discharge Plan Considerations:	May require assistance with transportation, self-care and homemaker tasks.

DIAGNOSTIC STUDIES

X-ray examinations: determine location/extent of fractures/trauma.

Bone scans, tomograms, CT/MRI scans: visualize fractures; may also be used to identify soft-tissue damage.

Arteriograms: may be done if vascular damage is suspected.

CBC: Hct may be increased (hemoconcentration) or decreased (signifying hemorrhage at the fracture site or distant organs in multiple trauma). Increased WBC is a normal response after trauma.

Creatinine: muscle trauma increases load of creatinine for renal clearance.

Coagulation profile: alterations may occur owing to blood loss, multiple transfusions, or liver injury.

NURSING PRIORITIES

1. Prevent further bone/tissue injury.
2. Alleviate pain.
3. Prevent complications.
4. Provide information about condition/prognosis and treatment needs.

DISCHARGE CRITERIA

1. Fracture stabilized.
2. Pain controlled.
3. Complications prevented/minimized.
4. Condition, prognosis, and therapeutic regimen understood.

NURSING DIAGNOSIS:	**INJURY, POTENTIAL FOR: TRAUMA [ADDITIONAL]**
May be related to:	**Loss of skeletal integrity (fractures)**
Possibly evidenced by:	**[Not applicable; presence of signs and symptoms establishes an *actual* diagnosis.]**

ACTIONS/INTERVENTIONS	RATIONALE

Independent

Maintain bed/limb rest as indicated. Provide support of joints above and below fracture site when moving, turning.

Promotes stability, reduces possibility of disturbing alignment/healing.

Place a bed board under the mattress.

Soft or sagging mattress may deform a wet (green) cast, crack a dry cast, or interfere with pull of traction.

Casts/Splints

Support fracture site with pillows/folded blankets. Maintain neutral position of affected part with sandbags, splints, trochanter roll, footboard.

Prevents unnecessary movement and disruption of alignment. Proper placement of pillows can also prevent pressure deformities in the drying cast.

Use sufficient personnel for turning. Avoid using abduction bar for turning patient with spica cast.

Hip/body or multiple casts can be extremely heavy and cumbersome. Failure to properly support limbs in casts may cause the cast to break.

Evaluate splinted extremity for resolution of edema.

Coaptation splint (e.g., Jones–Sugar tong) may be used to provide immobilization of fracture while excessive tissue swelling is present. As edema subsides, readjustment of splint or application of plaster cast may be required for continued alignment of fracture.

Traction

Maintain position/integrity of traction (e.g., Buck's, Dunlop, Pearson, Russell):

Traction permits pull on the long axis of the fractured bone and overcomes muscle tension/shortening to facilitate alignment/union. Skeletal traction (pins, wires, tongs) permits use of greater weight for traction pull than can be applied to skin tissues.

Ascertain that all clamps are functional. Lubricate pulleys, and check ropes for fraying. Secure and wrap knots with adhesive tape.

Assures that traction setup is functioning properly to avoid interruption of fracture approximation.

Keep ropes unobstructed with weights hanging free, avoid lifting/releasing weights.

Optimal amount of traction weight is maintained. Note: Assuring free movement of weights during repositioning of patient avoids sudden excess pull on fracture with associated pain and muscle spasm.

Assist with placement of lifts under bed wheels if indicated.

Helps maintain proper patient position and function of traction by providing counterbalance.

Position the patient so that appropriate pull is maintained on the *long axis* of the bone.

Promotes bone alignment and reduced complications (e.g., delayed healing/nonunion).

Review restrictions imposed by therapy, e.g., not bending at waist/sitting up with Buck's traction, or not turning below the waist with Russell's traction.

Maintains integrity of pull of traction.

Assess integrity of external fixation device.

Hoffman traction provides stabilization and rigid support for fractured bone without use of ropes, pulleys, or weights, thus allowing for greater patient mobility/comfort and facilitating wound care. Loose or excessively tightened clamps/nuts can alter the compression of the frame, causing misalignment.

ACTIONS/INTERVENTIONS

Collaborative

Review follow-up/serial x-rays.

Maintain electrical stimulation if used.

RATIONALE

Provides visual evidence of beginning callus formation/healing process to determine level of activity and need for changes in/additional therapy.

May be indicated to promote bone growth in presence of delayed healing/nonunion.

NURSING DIAGNOSIS:	COMFORT, ALTERED: PAIN, ACUTE
May be related to:	Movement of bone fragments, edema, and injury to the soft tissue
	Traction/immobility device
	Stress, anxiety
Possibly evidenced by:	Complaints of pain
	Distraction; self-focusing/narrowed focus; facial mask of pain
	Guarding, protective behavior; alteration in muscle tone; autonomic responses
PATIENT OUTCOMES/ EVALUATION CRITERIA:	Verbalizes relief of pain. Displays relaxed manner; able to participate in activities, sleep/rest appropriately. Demonstrates use of relaxation skills and diversional activities as indicated for individual situation.

ACTIONS/INTERVENTIONS

Independent

Maintain immobilization of affected part by means of bedrest, cast, splint, traction. (Refer to ND: Injury, Potential for Trauma [Additional], p. 683.)

Elevate and support injured extremity.

Avoid use of plastic sheets/pillows under limbs in cast.

Provide bed cradle.

Evaluate complaints of pain/discomfort, noting location and characteristics, including intensity (1–10 scale). Note nonverbal pain cues (changes in vital signs and emotions/behavior).

Encourage patient to discuss problems related to injury.

Explain procedures before beginning them.

RATIONALE

Relieves pain and prevents bone displacement/ extension of tissue injury.

Promotes venous return, decreases edema, and may reduce pain.

Can increase discomfort by enhancing heat production in the drying cast.

Maintains body warmth without discomfort of pressure of bedclothes on affected parts.

Influences choice of/monitors effectiveness of interventions. Level of anxiety may affect perception of/ reaction to pain.

Helps to alleviate anxiety. Patient may feel need to relive the accident experience.

Allows patient to prepare mentally for activity as well as to participate in controlling level of discomfort.

ACTIONS/INTERVENTIONS	RATIONALE

Independent

Medicate before care activities.	Promotes muscle relaxation and enhances participation.
Perform and supervise active/passive range of motion exercises.	Maintains strength/mobility of unaffected muscles and facilitates resolution of inflammation in injured tissues.
Provide alternate comfort measures, e.g., massage, backrub, position changes.	Improves general circulation, reduces areas of local pressure and muscle fatigue.
Encourage use of stress management techniques, e.g., progressive relaxation, deep breathing exercises, visualization/guided imagery, Therapeutic Touch.	Refocuses attention, promotes sense of control and may enhance coping abilities in the management of pain, which is likely to persist for an extended period of time.
Identify diversional activities appropriate for patient age, physical abilities, and personal preferences.	Prevents boredom, reduces tension, can increase muscle strength, may enhance self-esteem and coping abilities.
Investigate any complaints of unusual/sudden pain or deep, progressive/poorly localized pain unrelieved by analgesics.	May signal a developing complication; e.g., infection, tissue ischemia, compartmental syndrome. (Refer to ND: Tissue Perfusion, Altered: Peripheral [Potential], following.)

Collaborative

Apply cold/ice pack first 24–48 hours and as necessary.	Reduces edema/hematoma formation, decreases pain sensation.
Administer medications as indicated: analgesics; muscle relaxants, e.g., diazepam (Valium), and hydroxyzine pamoate (Vistaril).	Given to reduce pain and/or muscle spasms. Note: Vistaril is often used to potentiate effects of narcotics to improve/prolong pain relief.
Instruct in/monitor PCA if indicated.	Patient controlled analgesia provides for timely drug administration, preventing fluctuations in pain with associated muscle tension/spasms.

NURSING DIAGNOSIS:	**TISSUE PERFUSION, ALTERED: PERIPHERAL [POTENTIAL]**
May be related to:	**Reduction/interruption of blood flow: direct vascular injury, tissue trauma, excessive edema, thrombus formation**
	Hypovolemia
Possibly evidenced by:	**[Not applicable; presence of signs and symptoms establishes an *actual* diagnosis.]**
PATIENT OUTCOMES/ EVALUATION CRITERIA:	**Maintains tissue perfusion as evidenced by palpable pulses, skin warm/dry, normal sensation, usual sensorium, stable vital signs and adequate urine output for individual situation.**

ACTIONS/INTERVENTIONS	RATIONALE

Independent

Remove jewelry from affected limb.	May restrict circulation when edema occurs.

ACTIONS/INTERVENTIONS	RATIONALE
Independent	
Evaluate presence/quality of peripheral pulse distal to injury via palpation/Doppler. Compare with normal limb.	Decreased/absent pulse may reflect vascular injury and necessitates immediate medical evaluation of circulatory status. Be aware that occasionally a pulse may be palpated even though circulation is blocked by a soft clot through which pulsations may be felt. In addition, perfusion through larger arteries may continue after increased compartment pressure has collapsed the arteriole/venule circulation in the muscle.
Assess capillary return, skin color, and warmth distal to the fracture.	Return of color should be rapid (3–5 seconds). White, cool skin indicates arterial impairment. Cyanosis suggests venous impairment. Note: Peripheral pulses, capillary refill, skin color, and sensation may be normal even in presence of compartmental syndrome, because superficial circulation is usually not compromised.
Perform neurovascular assessments, noting changes in motor/sensory function. Ask patient to localize pain/discomfort.	Impaired feeling, numbness, tingling, increased/diffuse pain occurs when there is inadequate circulation to nerves or nerve damage.
Test sensation of peroneal nerve by pinch/pinprick in the dorsal web between first and second toe and assess ability to dorsiflex toes if indicated.	Length and position of peroneal nerve increases risk of its injury in the presence of leg fracture, edema/compartmental syndrome, or malposition of traction apparatus.
Monitor position/location of supporting ring of splints/sling.	Traction apparatus can cause pressure on vessels/nerves, particularly in the axilla and groin, resulting in ischemia and possible permanent nerve damage.
Maintain elevation of injured extremity(ies) unless contraindicated.	Promotes venous drainage/decreases edema. Note: In presence of increased compartment pressure, elevation of extremity actually impedes arterial flow, decreasing perfusion.
Assess entire length of injured extremity for swelling/edema formation. Measure injured extremity and compare with uninjured extremity. Note appearance, spread of hematoma.	Increasing circumference of injured extremity may suggest general tissue swelling/edema, but may reflect hemorrhage. Note: A 1-inch increase in an adult thigh can equal approximately 1 unit of sequestered blood.
Note complaints of increasing pain on passive movement of extremity, development of paresthesia, muscle tension/tenderness with erythema.	Continued bleeding/edema formation within a muscle enclosed by tight fascia can result in impaired blood flow and ischemic myositis or compartmental syndrome, necessitating emergency interventions to relieve pressure/restore circulation.
Investigate sudden signs of limb ischemia; e.g., decreased skin temperature, pallor, increased pain.	Fracture dislocations of joints (especially the knee) may cause damage to adjacent arteries, with resulting loss of distal blood flow.
Encourage patient to routinely exercise digits/joints distal to injury. Ambulate as soon as possible.	Enhances circulation, reduces pooling of blood, especially in the lower extremities.
Investigate tenderness, swelling, pain on dorsiflexion of foot (positive Homans' sign).	There is an increased potential for thrombophlebitis and pulmonary emboli in patients immobile for 5 days or more.
Monitor vital signs. Note signs of general pallor/cyanosis, cool skin, changes in mentation.	Inadequate circulating volume will compromise systemic tissue perfusion.
Test stools/gastric aspirant for occult blood. Note continued bleeding at trauma/injection site(s), oozing from mucous membranes.	Increased incidence of gastric bleeding accompanies fractures/trauma and may be related to stress or occasionally reflects a clotting disorder requiring further evaluation.

ACTIONS/INTERVENTIONS	RATIONALE

Collaborative

Apply ice bags around fracture site as indicated.

Reduces edema/hematoma formation, which could impair circulation.

Split/bivalve cast as needed.

May be done on an emergency basis to relieve restriction of circulation resulting from edema formation in injured extremity.

Assist with/monitor intracompartmental pressures.

Elevation of pressure (usually to 30 mmHg or more) indicates need for prompt evaluation and intervention.

Prepare for surgical intervention (e.g., fibulectomy/fasciotomy) as indicated.

Failure to relieve pressure/correct compartmental syndrome within 4 to 6 hours of onset can result in severe contractures/loss of function and disfigurement of extremity distal to injury or even necessitate amputation.

Monitor Hb/Hct levels.

Assists in calculation of blood loss and needs/effectiveness of replacement therapy.

Administer IV fluids, blood products as needed.

Maintains circulating volume, enhancing tissue perfusion.

Apply antiembolic hose as indicated.

Decreases venous pooling and may enhance venous return, thereby reducing risk of thrombus formation.

NURSING DIAGNOSIS:	GAS EXCHANGE, IMPAIRED [POTENTIAL]
May be related to:	Altered blood flow; blood/fat emboli
	Alveolar-capillary membrane changes: interstitial, pulmonary edema, congestion
Possibly evidenced by:	[Not applicable; presence of signs and symptoms establishes an *actual* diagnosis.]
PATIENT OUTCOMES/ EVALUATION CRITERIA:	Maintains adequate respiratory function, as evidenced by absence of dyspnea/cyanosis; respiratory rate and ABGs within patient's normal limits.

ACTIONS/INTERVENTIONS	RATIONALE

Independent

Monitor respiratory rate and effort. Note stridor, use of accessory muscles, retractions, development of central cyanosis.

Tachypnea, dyspnea, and changes in mentation are early signs of respiratory insufficiency and may be the only indicator of developing pulmonary emboli in the early stage. Remaining signs/symptoms reflect advanced respiratory distress/impending failure.

Auscultate breath sounds noting development of unequal, hyperresonant sounds; presence of crackles, rhonchi, wheezes. Note inspiratory crowing/croupy sounds.

Changes in/presence of adventitious breath sounds reflects developing respiratory complications, e.g., atelectasis, pneumonia, emboli, ARDS. Inspiratory crowing reflects upper airway edema and is suggestive of fat emboli. (Refer to CPs: Bacterial Pneumonia, p. 138; Pulmonary Embolism, p. 148; Adult Respiratory Distress Syndrome (ARDS), p. 184.)

Handle injured tissues/bones gently, especially during first several days.

This may prevent the development of fat emboli (usually seen in first 12–72 hours), which are closely asso-

ACTIONS/INTERVENTIONS	RATIONALE
Independent	
	ciated with fractures, especially of long bone and pelvis.
Instruct and assist with deep breathing and coughing exercises. Reposition frequently.	Promotes alveolar ventilation and perfusion. Repositioning promotes drainage of secretions and decreases congestion in dependent lung areas.
Note increasing restlessness, confusion, lethargy, stupor.	Impaired gas exchange/presence of pulmonary emboli can cause deterioration in the patient's level of consciousness as hypoxemia/acidosis develops.
Observe sputum for signs of blood.	Hemoptysis may occur with pulmonary emboli.
Inspect skin for petechiae above nipple line; in axilla, spreading to abdomen/trunk; buccal mucosa, hard palate; conjunctival sacs and retina.	Most characteristic sign of fat emboli, which may appear within 2–3 days after injury.
Collaborative	
Assist with incentive spirometry.	Maximizes ventilation/oxygenation and minimizes atelectasis.
Administer supplemental oxygen if indicated.	Increases available oxygen for optimal tissue oxygenation.
Monitor laboratory studies, e.g.:	
Serial ABGs;	Decreased PaO_2 and increased $PaCO_2$ indicate impaired gas exchange/developing failure.
Hb, calcium, sedimentation rate (ESR), serum lipase, fat screen, platelets.	Anemia, hypocalcemia, elevated ESR and lipase levels, fat globules in blood/urine/sputum, and decreased platelet count (thrombocytopenia) are often associated with fat emboli.
Administer medications as indicated:	
Low-dose heparin;	Blocks the clotting cycle and prevents clot propagation in presence of thrombophlebitis.
Corticosteroids.	Steroids have been used with some success to prevent/treat fat embolus.

NURSING DIAGNOSIS:	**MOBILITY, IMPAIRED PHYSICAL**
May be related to:	**Neuromuscular skeletal impairment; pain/discomfort; restrictive therapies (limb immobilization)**
	Psychologic immobility
Possibly evidenced by:	**Inability to purposefully move within the physical environment, imposed restrictions**
	Reluctance to attempt movement; limited range of motion
	Decreased muscle strength/control
PATIENT OUTCOMES/ EVALUATION CRITERIA:	**Regains/maintains mobility at the highest possible level. Maintains position of function. Increases strength/**

689

function of affected and compensatory body parts. Demonstrates techniques that enable resumption of activities.

ACTIONS/INTERVENTIONS	RATIONALE
Independent	
Assess degree of immobility produced by injury/treatment and note patient's perception of immobility.	Patient may be restricted by self-view/self-perception out of proportion with actual physical limitations, requiring information/interventions to promote progress toward wellness.
Encourage participation in diversional/recreational activities. Maintain stimulating environment, e.g., radio, TV, newspapers, personal possessions/pictures, clock, calendar, visits from family/friends.	Provides opportunity for release of energy, refocuses attention, enhances patient's sense of self-control/self-worth, and aids in reducing social isolation.
Instruct/assist with active/passive ROM exercises of affected and unaffected extremities.	Increases blood flow to muscles and bone to improve muscle tone, maintain joint mobility; prevent contractures/atrophy, and bone resorption from disuse.
Encourage use of isometric exercises starting with the unaffected limb.	Isometrics contract muscles without bending joints or moving limbs and helps to maintain muscle strength and mass. Note: These exercises are contraindicated while acute bleeding/edema is present.
Provide footboard, wrist splints, trochanter/hand rolls as appropriate.	Useful in maintaining functional position of extremities, hands/feet and preventing complications (e.g., contractures/footdrop).
Place in supine position periodically, when traction used to stabilize lower limb fractures.	Reduces risk of flexion contracture of hip.
Instruct in/encourage use of trapeze and "post" position for lower limb fractures.	Facilitates movement during hygiene/skin care, linen changes, and reduces discomfort of remaining flat in bed. Post position involves placing the uninjured foot flat on the bed with the knee bent while grasping the trapeze and lifting the body off the bed.
Assist with/encourage self-care/hygiene (e.g., bathing, shaving).	Improves muscle strength and circulation, enhances patient control in situation, and promotes self-directed wellness.
Provide/assist with mobility by means of wheelchair, walker, crutches, canes as soon as possible. Instruct in safe use of mobility aids.	Early mobility reduces complications of bedrest (e.g., phlebitis), promotes healing and normalization of organ function. Learning the correct way to use aids is important to maintain optimal mobility and patient safety.
Monitor blood pressure with resumption of activity. Note complaints of dizziness.	Postural hypotension is a common problem following prolonged bedrest and may require specific interventions (e.g., tilt table with gradual elevation to upright position).
Reposition periodically and encourage coughing/deep-breathing exercises.	Prevents/reduces incidence of skin/respiratory complications (e.g., decubiti, atelectasis, pneumonia).
Auscultate bowel sounds. Monitor elimination habits and provide for regular bowel routine. Place on bedside commode, if feasible, or use fracture pan. Provide privacy.	Bedrest, use of analgesics, and changes in dietary habits can slow peristalsis and produce constipation. Nursing measures that facilitate elimination may prevent/limit complications. Fracture pan limits flexion of hips and lessens pressure on lumbar region/cast.
Encourage increased fluid intake to 2000–3000 ml/day, including acid/ash juices.	Keeps the body well hydrated, decreasing risk of urinary infection, stone formation, and constipation.

ACTIONS/INTERVENTIONS

Collaborative

Consult with physical/occupational therapist, rehabilitation specialist.

Provide diet high in proteins, carbohydrates, vitamins, and minerals via appropriate route.

Increase the amount of roughage in the diet. Avoid gas-forming foods.

Administer stool softeners, enemas, laxatives as indicated.

Refer to psychiatric nurse clinical specialist/therapist as indicated.

RATIONALE

Useful in creating individualized activity/exercise program. Patient may require long-term assistance with movement, strengthening, and weight-bearing activities, as well as use of adjuncts, e.g., walkers, crutches, canes; elevated toilet seats; pickup sticks, special eating utensils.

In the presence of musculoskeletal injuries, nutrients required for healing are rapidly depleted, often resulting in a weight loss of as much as 20–30 lb during skeletal traction. This can have a profound effect on muscle mass, tone, and strength.

Adding bulk to stool helps prevent constipation. Gas-forming foods may cause abdominal distention, especially in presence of decreased intestinal motility.

May be given to promote evacuation.

Patient/SO may require more intensive treatment to deal with reality of current condition/prognosis, prolonged immobility, perceived loss of control.

NURSING DIAGNOSIS:	SKIN/TISSUE INTEGRITY, IMPAIRED: ACTUAL/POTENTIAL
May be related to:	Puncture injury, compound fracture, surgical repair, insertion of traction pins, wires, screws
	Altered sensation, circulation; accumulation of excretions/secretions
	Physical immobilization
Possibly evidenced by:	Complaints of itching, pain, numbness, pressure of affected/surrounding area
	Disruption of skin surface; invasion of body structures; destruction of skin layers/tissues
PATIENT OUTCOMES/ EVALUATION CRITERIA:	Verbalizes relief of discomfort. Demonstrates behaviors/ techniques to prevent skin breakdown/facilitate healing as indicated. Achieves timely wound/lesion healing if present.

ACTIONS/INTERVENTIONS

Independent

Examine the skin for open wounds, foreign bodies, rashes, bleeding, discoloration, duskiness, blanching.

RATIONALE

Provides information regarding skin circulation and problems that may be caused by application and/or restriction of cast/splint or traction apparatus; or edema formation that may require further medical intervention.

ACTIONS/INTERVENTIONS	RATIONALE

Independent

Massage skin and bony prominences. Keep the bed dry and free of wrinkles. Provide elbow/heel pads as indicated.

Promotes circulation, reduces risk of abrasions/skin breakdown.

Reposition frequently. Encourage use of trapeze if possible.

Lessens constant pressure on same areas and minimizes risk of skin breakdown. Use of trapeze may reduce risk of abrasions to elbows/heels.

Assess position of splint ring of traction device.

Improper positioning may cause skin injury/breakdown.

Cast application and skin care:

Cleanse skin with soap and water. Rub gently with alcohol and/or dust with small amount of a borate or stearate of zinc powder;

Provides a dry, clean area for cast application. Too much powder may cake when it comes in contact with water/perspiration.

Cut a length of stockinette to cover the area and extend several inches beyond the cast;

Useful for padding bony prominences, finishing cast edges, and protecting the skin.

Use palm of hand to apply, hold or move cast, and support on pillows after application;

Prevents indentations/flattening over bony prominences and weight-bearing areas (e.g., back of heels), which would cause abrasions/tissue trauma. An improperly shaped or dried cast is irritating to the underlying skin and may lead to circulatory impairment.

Trim excess plaster from edges of cast as soon as casting is completed;

Uneven plaster is irritating to the skin and may result in abrasions.

Promote cast drying by removing bed linen, exposing to circulating air;

Prevents skin breakdown caused by prolonged moisture trapped under cast.

Observe for potential pressure areas, especially at the edges of and under the splint/cast;

Pressure can cause ulcerations, necrosis, and/or nerve palsies. These problems may be painless when nerve damage is present.

Pad (petal) the edges of the cast with waterproof tape;

Provides an effective barrier to cast flaking and moisture. Helps prevent breakdown of cast material at edges and reduces skin irritation/excoriation.

Cleanse excess plaster from skin while still wet, if possible;

Dry plaster may flake into completed cast and cause skin damage.

Protect cast and skin in perineal area. Provide frequent pericare;

Prevents tissue breakdown and infection by fecal contamination.

Instruct patient/SO to avoid inserting objects inside casts;

"Scratching an itch" may cause tissue injury.

Massage the skin around the cast edges with alcohol;

Has a drying effect, which toughens the skin. Creams and lotions are not recommended because excessive oils can seal cast perimeter, not allowing the cast to "breathe." Powders are not recommended because of potential for excessive accumulation inside the cast.

Turn frequently to include the uninvolved side and prone position with patient's feet over the end of the mattress.

Minimizes pressure on feet and around cast edges.

Skin traction application and skin care:

Cleanse the skin with warm soapy water;

Reduces level of contaminants on skin.

Apply tincture of benzoin;

"Toughens" the skin for application of skin traction.

Apply commercial skin traction tapes (or make some with strips of moleskin/adhesive tape) ~ngthwise on opposite sides of the affected limb;

Traction tapes encircling a limb may compromise circulation.

ACTIONS/INTERVENTIONS	RATIONALE
Independent	
Extend the tapes beyond the length of the limb;	Traction is inserted in line with the free ends of the tape.
Mark the line where the tapes extend beyond the extremity;	Allows for quick assessment of slippage.
Place protective padding under the leg and over bony prominences;	Minimizes pressure on these areas.
Wrap the limb circumference, including tapes and padding, with elastic bandages, being careful to wrap snugly but not too tightly;	Provides for appropriate traction pull without compromising circulation.
Palpate taped tissues daily and document any tenderness or pain;	If area under tapes is tender, suspect skin irritation, and prepare to remove the bandage system.
Remove skin traction every 24 hours, if allowed; inspect and give skin care.	Maintains skin integrity.
Skeletal traction application and skin care:	
Bend wire ends or cover ends of wires/pins with rubber or cork protectors or needle caps;	Prevents injury to other body parts.
Pad slings/frame with sheepskin, foam.	Prevents excessive pressure on skin and promotes moisture evaporation which reduces risk of excoriation.
Collaborative	
Use foam mattress, sheepskins, flotation pads, or air mattress as indicated.	Because of immobilization of body parts, bony prominences other than those affected by the casting may suffer from decreased circulation.
Monovalve, bivalve, or cut a window in the cast, per protocol.	Allows the release of pressure and provides access for wound/skin care.

NURSING DIAGNOSIS:	INFECTION, POTENTIAL FOR
May be related to:	**Inadequate primary defenses: broken skin, traumatized tissues; environmental exposure**
	Invasive procedures, skeletal traction
Possibly evidenced by:	**[Not applicable; presence of signs and symptoms establishes an *actual* diagnosis.]**
PATIENT OUTCOMES/ EVALUATION CRITERIA:	**Achieves timely wound healing, free of purulent drainage or erythema, and is afebrile.**

ACTIONS/INTERVENTIONS	RATIONALE
Independent	
Inspect the skin for preexisting irritation or breaks in continuity.	Pins or wires should not be inserted through skin infections, rashes, or abrasions (may lead to bone infection).
Assess pin sites/skin areas noting complaints of increased pain/burning sensation or presence of edema, erythema, foul odor/drainage.	May indicate onset of local infection/tissue necrosis, which can lead to osteomyelitis.

ACTIONS/INTERVENTIONS	RATIONALE

Independent

Provide sterile pin/wound care and meticulous hand-washing.

May prevent cross contamination and possibility of infection.

Instruct patient not to touch the insertion sites.

Minimizes opportunity for contamination.

Line perineal cast edges with plastic wrap.

Damp soiled casts can promote growth of bacteria.

Observe wounds for formation of bullae, crepitation, bronze discoloration of skin, forthy/fruity-smelling drainage.

Signs suggestive of gas gangrene infection.

Assess muscle tone, deep tendon reflexes, and ability to speak.

Muscle rigidity, tonic spasms of jaw muscles, dysphagia reflect development of tetanus.

Monitor vital signs. Note presence of chills, malaise, changes in mentation.

Hypotension, confusion may be seen with gas gangrene; tachycardia and chills/fever reflect developing sepsis.

Investigate abrupt onset of pain/limitation of movement with localized edema/erythema in injured extremity.

May indicate development of osteomyelitis.

Institute prescribed isolation procedures.

Presence of purulent drainage will require wound/linen precautions to prevent cross contamination.

Collaborative

Monitor laboratory studies, e.g.:

    CBC;

Anemia may be noted with osteomyelitis; leukocytosis is present with any infective process.

    ESR;

Elevated in osteomyelitis.

    Cultures and sensitivity of wound/serum/bone;

Identifies infective organism.

    Radioisotope scans.

Hot spots signify increased areas of vascularity, indicative of osteomyelitis.

Administer medications as indicated;

    IV/topical antibiotics;

Wide-spectrum antibiotics may be used prophylactically, or may be geared toward specific identified microorganism.

    Tetanus toxoid.

Given prophylactically because the possibility of tetanus exists with any open wound. Note: Risk increases when injury/wound(s) occur in outdoor/rural areas.

Provide wound/bone irrigations, application of warm/moist soaks as indicated.

Local debridement/cleansing of wounds reduces microorganisms and incidence of systemic infection. Continuous antimicrobial drip into bone may be necessary to treat osteomyelitis, especially if blood supply to bone is compromised.

Assist with procedures, e.g., incision/drainage, placement of drains, hyperbaric oxygen therapy.

Numerous procedures may be carried out in treatment of local infections, osteomyelitis, gas gangrene.

Prepare for surgery, as indicated.

Sequestrectomy (removal of necrotic bone) is necessary to facilitate healing and prevent extension of infectious process.

NURSING DIAGNOSIS: KNOWLEDGE DEFICIT [LEARNING NEED] (SPECIFY)

    May be related to: Lack of exposure/recall

	Information misinterpretation/unfamiliarity with information resources
Possibly evidenced by:	Questions/request for information, statement of misconception
	Inaccurate follow-through of instructions/development of preventable complications
PATIENT OUTCOMES/ EVALUATION CRITERIA:	Verbalizes understanding of condition, prognosis, and treatment. Correctly performs necessary procedures and explains reasons for actions.

ACTIONS/INTERVENTIONS	RATIONALE
Independent	
Review pathology, prognosis, and future expectations.	Provides knowledge base on which patient can make informed choices. Note: Internal fixation devices can ultimately compromise the bone's strength and intramedullary nails/rods or plates may be removed at a future date.
Instruct patient in methods of proper ambulation as indicated by individual situation.	Most fractures require casts, splints, or braces during the healing process. Further damage and delay in healing could occur secondary to improper use of ambulatory devices.
Suggest use of a backpack.	Provides place to carry necessary articles and leave hands free to manipulate crutches, or may prevent undue muscle fatigue when one arm is casted.
List activities the patient can perform independently and those that require assistance.	Organizes activities around need and who is available to provide help.
Identify available community services, VNA, homemaker service.	Provides assistance to facilitate self-care and support independence.
Encourage patient to continue active exercises for the joints above and below the fracture.	Prevents joint stiffness, contractures, and muscle wasting, promoting earlier return to activities of daily living.
Discuss importance of clinical follow-up appointments.	Fracture healing may take as long as a year for completion, and patient cooperation with the medical regimen is helpful for proper union of bone to take place.
Review proper pin/wound care.	Reduces risk of bone/tissue trauma and infection, which can progress to osteomyelitis.
Identify signs and symptoms requiring medical evaluation, e.g., severe pain, fever/chills, foul odors; changes in sensation, swelling, burning, numbness, tingling, skin discoloration, paralysis, white/cool toes, fingertips; warm spots, soft areas, cracks in cast.	Prompt intervention may reduce severity of complications such as infection/impaired circulation. Note: Some darkening of the skin may occur normally when walking on the casted extremity or using casted arm; however, this should resolve with rest and elevation.
Discuss care of "green" or wet cast.	Promotes proper curing to prevent cast deformities and associated misalignment/skin irritation. Note: Placing a "cooling" cast directly on rubber or plastic pillows traps heat and increases drying time.
Suggest the use of a blow-dryer to dry small areas of dampened casts.	Cautious use can hasten drying.
Demonstrate use of plastic bags to cover plaster cast during wet weather or while bathing. Clean soiled cast	Protects from moisture, which softens the plaster and weakens the cast. Note: Fiberglas casts are being

695

ACTIONS/INTERVENTIONS	RATIONALE

Independent

with a slightly dampened cloth and some scouring powder.

used more frequently because they are not affected by moisture. In addition, their light weight may enhance patient participation in desired activities.

Recommend use of adaptive clothing.

Facilitates dressing/grooming activities.

Suggest ways to cover toes, if appropriate, e.g. stockinette or soft socks.

Helps to maintain warmth.

Discuss post-cast removal instructions:

    Instruct the patient to continue exercises as permitted;

Reduces stiffness and improves strength and function of affected extremity.

    Inform the patient that the skin under the cast is commonly mottled and covered with scales or crusts of dead skin;

It will be several weeks before normal appearance returns.

    Wash the skin gently with soap, Betadine, or pHisoHex, and water. Lubricate with a protective emollient;

New skin is extremely tender because it has been protected beneath a cast.

    Inform the patient that muscles may appear flabby and atrophied (less muscle mass); recommend supporting the joint above and below the affected part and the use of mobility aids, e.g., elastic bandages, splints, braces, crutches, walkers, or canes;

Muscle strength will be reduced and new or different aches and pains may occur for awhile secondary to loss of support.

    Elevate the extremity.

Swelling and edema tend to occur after cast removal.

Amputation

Amputations are classified as upper- or lower-extremity. There are two types of amputations: (1) open, which requires strict aseptic techniques and later revisions; and (2) closed, or "flap."

PATIENT ASSESSMENT DATA BASE

Data are dependent on underlying reason/problem, need for surgical procedure, e.g., severe trauma, peripheral vascular/arterial occlusive disease, diabetic neuropathy, osteomyelitis, cancer.

ACTIVITY/REST

May report: Actual/anticipated limitations imposed by condition/amputation.

EGO INTEGRITY

May report: Concern about anticipated changes in lifestyle, financial situation, reaction of others. Feelings of helplessness, powerlessness.

May exhibit: Anxiety, apprehension, irritability, anger, fearfulness, withdrawal, false cheerfulness.

SEXUALITY

May report: Concerns about intimate relationships.

SOCIAL INTERACTION

May report: Problems related to illness/condition.
Concern about role function, reaction of others.

TEACHING/LEARNING

Discharge Plan Considerations: May require assistance with wound care/supplies, adaptation to prosthesis/ambulatory devices, transportation, homemaker tasks, possibly self-care activities and vocational retraining.

DIAGNOSTIC STUDIES

Studies are dependent on underlying condition necessitating amputation.
WBC/differential: elevation and "shift to left" suggests infectious process.
ESR: elevation indicates inflammatory response.
Wound cultures: identifies presence of infection and causative organism.
X-rays: identifies skeletal abnormalities.
CT scan: identifies neoplastic lesions, osteomyelitis, hematoma formation.
Angiography and Doppler flow studies: evaluates alteration in circulation/tissue perfusion.
Biopsy: confirms diagnosis of benign/malignant mass.

NURSING PRIORITIES

1. Support psychologic and physiologic adjustment.
2. Alleviate pain.
3. Prevent complications.
4. Promote mobility.
5. Provide information about surgical procedure/prognosis and treatment needs.

DISCHARGE CRITERIA

1. Dealing with current situation realistically.
2. Pain relieved/controlled.
3. Complications prevented/minimized.
4. Optimal mobility facilitated.
5. Surgical procedure, prognosis and therapeutic regimen understood.

Refer to CP: Surgical Intervention, p. 789, for general considerations and interventions.

NURSING DIAGNOSIS:	**SELF-CONCEPT, DISTURBANCE IN: BODY IMAGE, ROLE PERFORMANCE**
May be related to:	**Biophysical factor: loss of body part**
Possibly evidenced by:	**Anticipated changes in lifestyle; fear of rejection/reaction by others**
	Negative feelings about body
	Focus on past strength, function or appearance
	Feelings of helplessness, powerlessness
	Preoccupation with missing body part, not looking at/or touching body part
	Perceived change in usual patterns of responsibility/physical capacity to resume role
PATIENT OUTCOMES/ EVALUATION CRITERIA:	**Begins to show adaptation and verbalize acceptance of self in situation (amputee). Recognizes and incorporates changes into self-concept in accurate manner without negating self-esteem. Developing realistic plans for adapting to new role/role modifications.**

ACTIONS/INTERVENTIONS

Independent

Encourage expression of fears, negative feelings, and grief over loss of body part.

Reinforce preoperative information including type/location of amputation, type of prosthetic fitting if appropriate (immediate, delayed), expected postoperative course, including pain control and rehabilitation.

Assess degree of support available to the patient.

Encourage/provide for visit by another amputee.

Discuss patient's perceptions of self related to change, and how patient sees self in usual lifestyle role functioning.

RATIONALE

Venting emotions helps patient begin to deal with the fact and reality of life without a limb.

Provides opportunity for patient to question and assimilate information, begin to deal with changes in body image and function, which can facilitate postoperative recovery.

Sufficient support by SO and friends can facilitate rehabilitation process.

A peer who has been through a similar experience serves as a role model and can provide validity to comments, hope for recovery and a normal future. (Refer to CP: Psychosocial Aspects of Acute Care, p. 773.)

Aids in defining concerns in relation to previous lifestyle and facilitates problem solving. For example, may fear loss of independence, ability to work, etc.

ACTIONS/INTERVENTIONS

Independent

Ascertain individual strengths and identify previous positive coping behaviors.

Encourage participation in ADLs. Provide opportunities to view/care for stump using the moment to point out positive signs of healing.

Provide open environment for patient to discuss concerns about sexuality.

Note withdrawn behavior, negative self-talk, use of denial or overconcern with actual/perceived changes.

Collaborative

Discuss availability of various resources, e.g., psychiatric/sexual counseling, occupational therapist.

RATIONALE

Helpful to build on strengths which are already available for patient to use in coping with current situation.

Promotes independence and enhances feelings of self-worth. Although integrating of stump into body image can take months or even years, looking at the stump and hearing positive comments (made in a normal, matter-of-fact manner) can help patient with this acceptance.

Promotes sharing of beliefs/values about sensitive subject and identifies misconceptions/myths that may interfere with adjustment to situation.

Identifies stage of grief/need for interventions.

May need assistance for these concerns to facilitate optimal adaptation and rehabilitation.

NURSING DIAGNOSIS:	COMFORT, ALTERED: PAIN, ACUTE
May be related to:	Physical injury/tissue and nerve trauma
	Psychologic impact of loss of body part
Possibly evidenced by:	Complaints of pain
	Narrowed self-focus
	Autonomic responses, guarding/protective behavior
PATIENT OUTCOMES/ EVALUATION CRITERIA:	Reports pain is relieved/controlled. Appears relaxed and able to rest/sleep appropriately. Verbalizes understanding of phantom pain and methods to provide relief.

ACTIONS/INTERVENTIONS

Independent

Document location and intensity of pain (1–10 scale). Investigate changes in pain characteristics, e.g., numbness, tingling.

Elevate affected part by raising foot of bed slightly or use of pillow/sling for upper limb amputation.

Acknowledge reality of phantom limb sensations and that this is usually self-limiting.

Provide routine comfort measures (e.g., frequent turning, backrub) and diversional activities. Encourage use of stress management techniques (e.g., deep-

RATIONALE

Aids in evaluating need for and effectiveness of interventions. Changes may indicate developing complications, e.g., necrosis/infection.

Lessens edema formation by enhancing venous return, reduces muscle fatigue and skin/tissue pressure.

Knowing about these sensations allows the patient to understand this is a normal phenomenon that may develop several weeks postoperatively. Although the sensations usually resolve on their own, some individuals continue to experience the discomfort for several months/years.

Refocuses attention, promotes relaxation, may enhance coping abilities and may decrease occurrence of phantom limb pain.

ACTIONS/INTERVENTIONS

Independent

breathing exercises, visualization, guided imagery) and Therapeutic Touch.

Provide gentle massage to stump as tolerated once dressings are discontinued.

Investigate complaints of progressive/poorly localized pain unrelieved by analgesics.

Collaborative

Administer medications, as indicated, e.g.: analgesics, muscle relaxants. Instruct in PCA.

Maintain TENS device if used.

Provide topical heat as indicated.

RATIONALE

Enhances circulation, reduces muscle tension.

May indicate developing compartmental syndrome, especially following traumatic injury. (Refer to CP: Fractures, ND: Tissue Perfusion, Altered: Peripheral [Potential], p. 686.)

Reduces pain/muscle spasms. Note: Patient-controlled analgesia provides for timely drug administration preventing fluctuations in pain with associated muscle tension/spasms.

Provides continuous low level nerve stimulation, blocking transmission of pain sensation.

May be used to promote muscle relaxation, enhance circulation, and facilitate resolution of edema.

NURSING DIAGNOSIS:	TISSUE PERFUSION, ALTERED: PERIPHERAL [POTENTIAL]
May be related to:	**Reduced arterial/venous blood flow; tissue edema, hematoma formation**
	Hypovolemia
Possibly evidenced by:	**[Not applicable; presence of signs and symptoms establishes an *actual* diagnosis.]**
PATIENT OUTCOMES/ EVALUATION CRITERIA:	**Maintains adequate tissue perfusion as evidenced by palpable peripheral pulses, skin warm/dry, timely wound healing.**

ACTIONS/INTERVENTIONS

Independent

Monitor vital signs. Palpate peripheral pulses, noting strength and equality.

Perform periodic neurovascular assessments, e.g., sensation, movement, pulse, skin color and temperature.

Inspect dressings/drainage device, noting amount and characteristics of drainage.

Keep tourniquet at bedside.

Evaluate lower limb(s) for inflammation, positive Homans' sign.

RATIONALE

General indicators of circulatory status and adequacy of perfusion.

Postoperative tissue edema, hematoma formation, restrictive dressings may impair circulation to stump/ resulting in tissue necrosis.

Continued blood loss may indicate need for additional fluid replacement and evaluation for coagulation defect or surgical intervention to ligate bleeder.

Immediately available if hemorrhage occurs.

Increased incidence of thrombus formation in patients with preexisting peripheral vascular disease/diabetic changes.

ACTIONS/INTERVENTIONS	RATIONALE
Collaborative	
Administer IV fluids, blood products as indicated.	Maintains circulating volume to maximize tissue perfusion.
Apply antiembolic hose.	Effectiveness is controversial but may enhance venous return reducing venous pooling and risk of thrombophlebitis.
Administer low-dose anticoagulant as indicated.	May be useful in preventing thrombus formation without increasing risk of postoperative bleed/hematoma formation.
Monitor laboratory studies, e.g.:	
Hb/Hct;	Indicators of hypovolemia/dehydration which can impair tissue perfusion.
PT/APTT.	Evaluates need for/effectiveness of anticoagulant therapy and identifies developing complication, e.g., post-traumatic DIC.

NURSING DIAGNOSIS:	INFECTION, POTENTIAL FOR
May be related to:	**Inadequate primary defenses (broken skin, traumatized tissue)**
	Invasive procedures; environmental exposure
	Chronic disease, altered nutritional status
Possibly evidenced by:	**[Not applicable; presence of signs and symptoms establishes an *actual* diagnosis.]**
PATIENT OUTCOMES/ EVALUATION CRITERIA:	**Achieves timely wound healing; free of purulent drainage or erythema; and is afebrile.**

ACTIONS/INTERVENTIONS	RATIONALE
Independent	
Maintain aseptic technique when changing dressings/caring for wound.	Minimizes opportunity for introduction of bacteria.
Inspect dressings and wound, note characteristics of drainage.	Early detection of developing infection provides opportunity for timely intervention and prevention of more serious complications (e.g., osteomyelitis).
Maintain patency and routinely empty drainage device.	Hemovac, Jackson/Pratt drains facilitate removal of drainage, promoting wound healing and reducing risk of infection.
Cover dressing with plastic when using the bedpan, or if incontinent.	Prevents contamination in lower limb amputation.
Expose stump to air; wash with mild soap and water after dressings are discontinued.	Maintains cleanliness, minimizes skin contaminants and promotes healing of tender/fragile skin.
Monitor vital signs.	Temperature elevation, tachycardia may reflect developing sepsis.

701

ACTIONS/INTERVENTIONS

Collaborative

Obtain wound/drainage cultures as appropriate.

Administer antibiotics as indicated.

RATIONALE

Identifies presence of infection/specific organisms.

Wide-spectrum antibiotics may be used prophylactically, or antibiotic therapy may be geared toward specific identified organisms.

NURSING DIAGNOSIS:	MOBILITY, IMPAIRED PHYSICAL
May be related to:	Loss of a limb (particularly a lower extremity); pain/discomfort; perceptual impairment (altered sense of balance)
Possibly evidenced by:	Reluctance to attempt movement
	Impaired coordination; decreased muscle strength, control, and mass
PATIENT OUTCOMES/ EVALUATION CRITERIA:	Verbalizes understanding of individual situation, treatment regimen, and safety measures. Displays willingness to participate in activities. Maintains position of function as evidenced by absence of contractures. Demonstrates techniques/behaviors that enable resumption of activities.

ACTIONS/INTERVENTIONS

Independent

Provide routine stump care, e.g., inspect area, cleanse and dry thoroughly, and rewrap stump with elastic bandage or air splint, or apply a stump shrinker (heavy stockinette sock), for "delayed" prosthesis. Measure circumference periodically.

Rewrap stump immediately with an elastic bandage, elevate if "immediate/early" cast is accidentally dislodged. Prepare for reapplication of cast.

Assist with specified ROM exercises for the affected as well as unaffected limbs beginning early in postoperative stage.

Encourage active/isometric exercises for upper torso and arms.

Provide trochanter rolls as indicated.

Instruct patient to lie in prone position as tolerated at least twice a day with pillow under abdomen and lower extremity stump.

RATIONALE

Provides opportunity to evaluate healing and note complications (unless covered by immediate prosthesis). Wrapping stump controls edema and helps form stump into conical shape to facilitate fitting of prosthesis. Note: Air splint may be preferred, because it permits visual inspection of the wound. Measurement is done to estimate shrinkage to assure proper fit of sock and prosthesis.

Edema will occur rapidly, and rehabilitation can be delayed.

Prevents contracture deformities, which can develop rapidly and could delay prosthesis usage.

Increases muscle strength to facilitate transfers/ambulation.

Prevents external rotation of lower limb stump.

Strengthens extensor muscles and prevents flexion contracture of the hip.

702

ACTIONS/INTERVENTIONS	RATIONALE

Independent

Caution against keeping pillows under lower extremity stump or allowing BKA (below-the-knee amputation) limb to hang dependently over side of bed or chair.

Use of pillows can cause permanent flexion contracture of hip, and a dependent position of stump impairs venous return and may increase edema formation.

Demonstrate/assist with transfer techniques and use of mobility aids, e.g., trapeze, crutches or walker.

Facilitates self-care and patient's independence. Proper transfer techniques prevent shearing abrasions/dermal injury related to "scooting."

Assist with ambulation.

Reduces potential for injury. Ambulation after lower limb amputation is dependent upon timing of prosthesis placement. *Immediate postoperative fitting:* A rigid plaster of Paris dressing is applied to the stump and a pylon and artificial foot is attached. Weight-bearing begins within 24–48 hours. *Early postoperative fitting:* Weight-bearing does not occur until 10–30 days postoperatively. *Delayed fitting:* More common in areas that do not have facilities available for immediate/early application of prosthesis or when the condition of the stump and/or the patient precludes these choices.

Help patient continue preoperative muscle exercises as able/when allowed out of bed; e.g., patient should (while holding on to chair for balance) perform abdominal tightening exercises, knee bends, hop on foot, stand on toes.

Contributes to gaining improved sense of balance and strengthens compensatory body parts.

Instruct patient in stump-conditioning exercises, e.g., pushing the stump against a pillow initially, then progressing to harder surface.

Hardens the stump by toughening the skin and altering feedback of resected nerves to facilitate use of prosthesis.

Collaborative

Refer to rehabilitation team, e.g., physical and occupational therapy.

Provides for creation of exercise/activity program to meet individual needs and strengths, and identifies mobility aids to promote independence. Note: Vocational counseling/retraining may be indicated.

Provide foam/flotation mattress.

Reduces pressure on skin/tissues that can impair circulation, potentiating risk of tissue ischemia/breakdown.

NURSING DIAGNOSIS:	KNOWLEDGE DEFICIT [LEARNING NEED] (SPECIFY)
May be related to:	Lack of exposure/recall
	Information misinterpretation
Possibly evidenced by:	Questions/request for information, verbalization of the problem
	Inaccurate follow-through of instructions/development of preventable complications
PATIENT OUTCOMES/ EVALUATION CRITERIA:	Verbalizes understanding of condition/disease process and treatment. Correctly performs necessary procedures and explains reasons for the actions. Initiates necessary lifestyle changes and participates in treatment regimen.

ACTIONS/INTERVENTIONS	RATIONALE
Independent	
Review disease process/surgical procedure and future expectation.	Provides knowledge base on which patient can make informed choices.
Instruct in dressing/wound care, inspection of stump using mirror to visualize all areas, skin massage, and appropriate wrapping of the stump.	Promotes competent self-care; facilitates healing and fitting of prosthesis and reduces potential for complications.
Discuss general stump care, e.g.:	
Massage the stump after dressings are discontinued and suture line is healed;	Massage softens scar and prevents adherence to the bone, decreases tenderness and stimulates circulation.
Avoid use of lotions/powders;	Although small amount of lotion may be indicated if skin is dry, emollients/creams soften skin and may cause maceration when a prosthesis is worn. Powder may cake, potentiating skin irritation.
Wear only properly fitted, clean, wrinkle-free limb sock;	Stump may continue to shrink for up to 2 years, and improperly fitting sock or one that is mended or dirty can cause skin irritation/breakdown.
Use of clean cotton T-shirt under harness for upper limb prosthesis.	Absorbs perspiration, prevents skin irritation from harness.
Demonstrate care of prosthetic device. Stress importance of routine maintenance/periodic refitting.	Assures proper fit, reduces risk of complications and prolongs life of prosthesis.
Encourage continuation of postoperative exercise program.	Enhances circulation/healing and function of affected part, facilitating adaptation to prosthetic device.
Identify techniques to manage phantom pain, e.g., gentle massage/pressure, intermittent pressure, use of dry/moist heat, or to visualize exercising of lost limb.	Reduces muscle tension and provides alternative nerve stimulation, enhancing control of situation and coping abilities.
Stress importance of well-balanced diet and adequate fluid intake.	Provides needed nutrients for tissue regeneration/healing, aids in maintaining circulating volume and normal organ function, and aids in maintenance of proper weight (weight changes affect fit of prosthesis).
Recommend cessation of smoking.	Smoking potentiates peripheral vasoconstriction, impairing circulation as well as oxygenation.
Identify signs/symptoms requiring medical evaluation, e.g., edema, erythema, increased/odorous drainage from incision; changes in sensation, movement, skin color; persistent phantom pain.	Prompt intervention may prevent serious complication and/or loss of function. Note: Chronic phantom limb pain may indicate neuroma, requiring surgical resection.
Identify community support groups, VNA, homemaker services as needed.	Facilitates transfer to home, supports independence, and enhances coping.

Total Joint Replacement

Joint replacement is indicated for irreversibly damaged joints and unremitting pain (e.g., degenerative and rheumatoid arthritis); selected fractures (e.g., femoral neck); joint instability; congenital hip disease. The surgery can be performed on any joint except the spine, hip and knee replacement being the most common. The prosthesis may be metallic or polyethylene (or a combination) and implanted with an acrylic cement, or it may be a porous, coated implant that encourages bone growth into the joint area.

PATIENT ASSESSMENT DATA BASE

ACTIVITY/REST

May report: Difficulty with ambulation; stiffness in joints (worse in the morning or after period of inactivity).
History of occupation that wears on particular joint.
Inability to participate in occupational/recreational activities at desired level.

CIRCULATION

May exhibit: Presence of edema; diminished pulses in affected joint, limb/digits.

NEUROSENSORY

May exhibit: Impaired range of motion of affected joints.

PAIN/COMFORT

May report: Pain (dull, aching, persistent) in affected joint(s), worsened by movement.

TEACHING/LEARNING

May report: History of inflammatory, debilitating arthritis (rheumatoid or osteoarthritis); aseptic necrosis of the joint head.
Severe accident destroying the joint, e.g., sports, auto accident.
Current medication use, e.g., antiinflammatory, analgesics/narcotics; steroids.

Discharge Plan Considerations: May need assistance with resumption of activities; self-care, homemaker tasks, transportation; placement in extended care facility for rehabilitation if needed.

DIAGNOSTIC STUDIES

X-rays and scans of bones/joints: determines extent of degeneration and rules out malignancy.

NURSING PRIORITIES

1. Prevent complications.
2. Promote optimal mobility.
3. Alleviate pain.
4. Provide information about diagnosis, prognosis, and treatment needs.

DISCHARGE CRITERIA

1. Complications prevented/minimized.
2. Mobility increased.
3. Pain relieved/controlled.
4. Diagnosis, prognosis and therapeutic regimen understood.

Refer to CP: Surgical Intervention, p. 789, for general considerations and interventions.

NURSING DIAGNOSIS:	INFECTION, POTENTIAL FOR
May be related to:	Inadequate primary defenses (broken skin, exposure of joint)
	Inadequate secondary defenses/immunosuppression (long-term corticosteroid use, cancer)
	Invasive procedures; surgical manipulation; implantation of foreign body
	Decreased mobility
Possibly evidenced by:	[Not applicable; presence of signs and symptoms establishes an *actual* diagnosis.]
PATIENT OUTCOMES/ EVALUATION CRITERIA:	Achieves timely wound healing, free of purulent drainage or erythema; and is afebrile.

ACTIONS/INTERVENTIONS	RATIONALE
Independent	
Promote good handwashing by staff and patient.	Reduces risk of cross-contamination.
Use strict aseptic or clean techniques as indicated to reinforce/change dressings and when handling drains.	Contamination can lead to wound infection.
Maintain patency of drainage devices (e.g., Hemovac/Jackson–Pratt). Note characteristics of wound drainage.	Reduces risk of infection by preventing accumulation of blood and secretions in the joint space (medium for bacterial growth). Purulent, nonserous, odorous drainage is indicative of infection, and continuous drainage from incision may reflect developing skin tract, which can potentiate infectious process.
Assess skin/incision color, temperature and integrity; note presence of erythema/inflammation, loss of wound approximation.	Provides information about status of healing process and alerts staff to early signs of infection. Note: Infection is devastating because joint cannot be saved once infection and prosthetic loss occurs.
Monitor temperature. Note presence of chills.	Although temperature elevations are common in early postoperative phase, elevations occurring 5 or more days postoperatively and/or presence of chills usually indicate developing infection requiring intervention to prevent more serious complications, e.g., sepsis, osteomyelitis, tissue necrosis, and prosthetic failure.
Encourage fluid intake, high-protein diet with roughage.	Maintains fluid and nutritional balance to support tissue perfusion and provide nutrients necessary for cellular regeneration and tissue healing.
Collaborative	
Maintain reverse isolation, if appropriate.	May be done initially to reduce contact with sources of possible infection, especially in elderly, immunosuppressed, or diabetic patient.
Administer antibiotics as indicated.	May be used prophylactically to prevent infection.
Culture drainage routinely/as needed.	Verifies presence of infection, identifies causative organism. Anaerobic or aerobic bacteria may be present, which affect choice of antibiotic and therapy.

NURSING DIAGNOSIS:	MOBILITY, IMPAIRED PHYSICAL
May be related to:	Pain and discomfort, musculoskeletal impairment Surgery/restrictive therapies
Possibly evidenced by:	Reluctance to attempt movement, difficulty purposefully moving within the physical environment Complaints of pain/discomfort on movement Limited range of motion; decreased muscle strength/control
PATIENT OUTCOMES/ EVALUATION CRITERIA:	Maintains position of function, as evidenced by absence of contracture. Displays increased strength and function of affected joint and limb. Verbalizes understanding of individual treatment regimen and participates in rehabilitation program.

ACTIONS/INTERVENTIONS	RATIONALE
Independent	
Maintain initial bedrest with affected joint in prescribed position and body in alignment.	Provides time for stabilization of prosthesis and recovery from effects of anesthesia, reducing risk of injury. Length of bedrest depends on joint replaced (e.g., usually 24–72 hours for hip).
Limit use of semi/high Fowler's position, if indicated.	Prolonged hip flexion may strain/dislocate new prosthesis.
Elevate extremity by raising foot of bed, not knee gatch. Limit movement as indicated; e.g., keep operative leg slightly abducted after total hip or knee to prevent crossing of legs/inward rotation of joint.	Enhances venous return to prevent excessive edema formation; may prevent dislocation of prosthesis. Use of knee gatch or pillow under knee can compromise circulation.
Medicate prior to procedures/activities.	Muscle relaxants, narcotics/analgesics decrease pain, reduce muscle tension/spasm, and facilitate participation in therapy.
Turn on unoperated side using adequate number of personnel and maintaining operated extremity in neutral alignment. Support position with pillows/wedges.	Prevents dislocation of prosthesis and prolonged skin/tissue pressure reducing risk of tissue ischemia/breakdown.
Demonstrate/assist with transfer techniques and use of mobility aids, e.g., trapeze, walker.	Facilitates self-care and patient's independence. Proper transfer techniques prevent shearing abrasions of skin and falls.
Inspect skin, observe for reddened areas. Keep linens dry and wrinkle-free. Massage skin/bony prominences routinely.	Prevents skin irritation/breakdown.
Perform/assist with ROM to unaffected joints.	Patient with degenerative joint disease can quickly lose joint function during periods of restricted activity.
Promote participation in routine exercise program, e.g.:	
Total hip: quadriceps and gluteal muscle setting, hip-hiking, isometrics, leg lifts, dorsiflexion, plantar flexion of the foot. *Total knee:* quadriceps setting,	Strengthens muscle groups, increasing muscle tone and mass; stimulates circulation; prevents decubiti. Active use of the joint may be painful but will not injure

ACTIONS/INTERVENTIONS

Independent

gluteal contraction, flexion/extension exercises, isometrics, and straight leg lifts.

Other joints: exercises are individually designed, e.g., toes and knee movements (for ankle joint replacement); arm and unaffected fingers (for finger joint replacement).

Observe appropriate limitations based on specific joint; e.g., avoid marked flexion/rotation of hip, flexion or hyperextension of leg; adhere to weight-bearing restrictions; wear knee immobilizer as indicated.

Investigate sudden increased pain and shortening of limb, changes in skin color, temperature, and sensation.

Encourage participation in ADL.

Provide positive reinforcement for efforts.

Collaborative

Consult with physical/occupational therapists and rehabilitation specialist.

Provide foam/flotation mattress.

RATIONALE

the joint. In fact, continuous passive exercise is usually mechanically performed on the knee joint in the first 48–72 hours.

Meets individual needs of the joint that is replaced.

Joint stress is to be avoided at all times during stabilization period to prevent dislocation of new prosthesis.

Indicative of slippage of prosthesis, requiring medical evaluation/intervention.

Enhances self-esteem, promotes sense of control and independence.

Promotes a positive attitude and encourages involvement in therapy.

Useful in creating individualized activity/exercise program. Patient may require ongoing assistance with movement, strengthening, and weight-bearing activities as well as use of adjuncts, e.g., walkers, crutches, canes; elevated toilet seat, pickup sticks, etc.

Reduces skin/tissue pressure; limits feelings of fatigue and general discomfort.

NURSING DIAGNOSIS:	TISSUE PERFUSION, ALTERED: PERIPHERAL [POTENTIAL]
May be related to:	Reduced arterial/venous blood flow: trauma to blood vessels; tissue edema, improper location/dislocation of prosthesis Hypovolemia
Possibly evidenced by:	[Not applicable; presence of signs and symptoms establishes an *actual* diagnosis.]
PATIENT OUTCOMES/ EVALUATION CRITERIA:	Demonstrates adequate tissue perfusion as evidenced by palpable pulses, skin warm/dry, stable vital signs.

ACTIONS/INTERVENTIONS

Independent

Palpate pulses. Evaluate capillary refill, skin color and temperature. Compare with nonoperated limb.

RATIONALE

Diminished/absent pulses, delayed capillary refill time, pallor, blanching, cyanosis, coldness of skin reflect diminished circulation/perfusion. Comparison with un-

ACTIONS/INTERVENTIONS	RATIONALE
Independent	operated limb provides clues as to whether problem is localized or generalized.
Assess motion, sensation of operated extremity.	Increasing pain, numbness/tingling, inability to perform expected movements (e.g., flex foot) suggest nerve injury, compromised circulation, or dislocation of prosthesis, requiring immediate intervention.
Test sensation of peroneal nerve by pinch/pinprick in the dorsal web between first and second toe and assess ability to dorsiflex toes after hip/knee replacement.	Position and length of peroneal nerve increases risk of direct injury or compression by tissue edema/hematoma.
Monitor vital signs.	Tachycardia and decreasing BP may reflect response to hypovolemia/blood loss or suggest anaphylaxis related to absorption of methyl-methacrylate into systemic circulation. Note: This occurs less often because of the advent of prosthetics with a porous layer that fosters ingrowth of bone instead of total reliance on adhesives to internally fix the device.
Monitor amount and characteristics of drainage on dressings/from suction device.	May indicate excessive bleeding/hematoma formation, which can potentiate neurovascular compromise.
Ensure that stabilizing devices (e.g., trochanter rolls, sling on splint device, traction apparatus) are in correct position and are not exerting undue pressure on skin and underlying tissue. Avoid use of pillow or knee gatch under knees.	Reduces risk of pressure on underlying nerves or compromised circulation to extremity on which operation was performed.
Evaluate for calf tenderness, positive Homans' sign, inflammation.	Early identification of thrombus development and intervention may prevent embolus formation.
Observe for signs of continued bleeding, oozing from puncture sites/mucous membranes, or ecchymosis following minimal trauma.	Depression of clotting mechanisms/sensitivity to anticoagulants may result in bleeding episodes that can affect RBC level/circulating volume.
Observe for restlessness, confusion, sudden chest pain, dyspnea, tachycardia, fever, development of petechiae.	Fat emboli can occur (usually in first 72 hours postoperatively) because of traumatic manipulation of bone marrow during implantation of hip prosthesis.
Collaborative	
Administer IV fluids, blood/plasma expanders as needed.	Restores circulating volume to maintain perfusion.
Monitor laboratory studies, e.g.:	
Hct;	Usually done 24–48 hours postoperatively for evaluation of blood loss, which can be quite large because of high vascularity of surgical site.
Coagulation studies.	Evaluates presence/degree of alteration in clotting mechanisms and effects of anticoagulant/antiplatelet agents when used.
Administer medications as indicated, e.g.: warfarin (Coumadin), heparin, aspirin, low molecular weight dextran.	Anticoagulants/antiplatelet agents may be used to reduce risk of thrombophlebitis and fat emboli.
Apply cold/heat as indicated.	Ice packs are used initially to limit edema/hematoma formation. Heat may then be used to enhance circulation, facilitating resolution of tissue edema.
Apply elastic leg wraps or antiembolic stockings.	Promotes venous return and prevents venous stasis, reducing risk of thrombus formation.

ACTIONS/INTERVENTIONS

Collaborative

Prepare for surgical procedure as indicated.

RATIONALE

Evacuation of hematoma or relocation of prosthesis may be required to correct compromised circulation.

NURSING DIAGNOSIS:	COMFORT, ALTERED: PAIN, ACUTE
May be related to:	Injuring agents: biologic, physical/psychologic (e.g., surgical procedure, preexisting chronic joint diseases, elderly age, anxiety)
Possibly evidenced by:	Complaints of pain; distraction/guarding behaviors Narrowed focus/self-focusing Alteration in muscle tone; autonomic responses
PATIENT OUTCOMES/ EVALUATION CRITERIA:	Reports pain relieved/controlled. Demonstrates use of relaxation skills and diversional activities as indicated by individual situation. Appears relaxed, able to rest/ sleep appropriately.

ACTIONS/INTERVENTIONS

Independent

Assess complaints of pain, noting intensity (scale of 1–10), duration, and location.

Maintain proper position of operated extremity.

Provide routine comfort measures (e.g., frequent repositioning, backrub) and diversional activities. Encourage stress management techniques (e.g., progressive relaxation, guided imagery, visualization) and use of Therapeutic Touch.

Medicate prior to activities/procedures.

Investigate complaints of sudden, severe joint pain with muscle spasms and changes in joint mobility; sudden, severe chest pain with dyspnea and restlessness.

Collaborative

Administer narcotics, analgesics, and muscle relaxants as needed.

Apply ice packs as indicated.

Maintain TENS unit if used.

RATIONALE

Provides information on which to base and monitor effectiveness of interventions.

Reduces muscle spasm and undue tension on new prosthesis and surrounding tissues.

Reduces muscle tension, refocuses attention, promotes sense of control, and may enhance coping abilities in the management of discomfort/pain, which can persist for an extended period of time.

Reduces muscle tension, facilitates participation.

Early recognition of developing problems, such as dislocation of prosthesis or pulmonary emboli (blood/fat), provides opportunity for prompt intervention and prevention of more serious complications.

Relieves surgical pain and reduces muscle tension/ spasm, which contributes to overall discomfort.

Promotes vasoconstriction to reduce bleeding/tissue edema in surgical area and lessens perception of discomfort.

Provides constant low level nerve stimulation to block transmission of sensations of pain.

710

NURSING DIAGNOSIS:	KNOWLEDGE DEFICIT [LEARNING NEED] (SPECIFY)
May be related to:	Lack of exposure/recall
	Information misinterpretation
Possibly evidenced by:	Questions/request for information, statement of misconception
	Inaccurate follow-through of instructions/development of preventable complications
PATIENT OUTCOMES/ EVALUATION CRITERIA:	Verbalizes understanding of surgical procedure and prognosis. Correctly performs necessary procedures and explains reasons for the actions.

ACTIONS/INTERVENTIONS	RATIONALE
Independent	
Review disease process, surgical procedure, and future expectations.	Provides knowledge base on which patient can make informed choices.
Encourage alternating rest periods with activity.	Conserves energy for healing, prevents undue fatigue, which can increase risk of injury/fall.
Stress importance of continuing prescribed exercise/rehabilitation program within patient's tolerance: crutch/cane walking, weight-bearing exercises, stationary bicycling, or swimming.	Increases muscle strength and joint mobility. Some patients may be involved in formal rehabilitation programs or be followed by physical therapists in extended-care facilities. Muscle aching indicates too much weight-bearing or activity, signaling a need to cut back.
Review long-term activity limitations, dependent on joint replaced, e.g., sitting for long periods or in low chair/toilet seat, jogging, jumping, excessive bending, lifting, twisting or crossing legs.	Prevents undue stress on implant.
Discuss need for safe environment in home (e.g., removing scatter rugs and unnecessary furniture) and use of assistive devices (e.g., handrails in tub/toilet, raised toilet seat, cane for long walks).	Reduces risk of falls, excessive stress on joints.
Review incisional/wound care.	Promotes independence in self-care, reducing risk of complications.
Stress importance of continuing to wear antiembolic stockings.	Prevents venous pooling, enhances venous return to reduce risk of thrombophlebitis.
Identify signs/symptoms requiring medical evaluation, e.g., fever/chills, incisional inflammation, unusual wound drainage, pain in calf or upper thigh, or development of "strep" throat, dental infections.	Bacterial infections require prompt treatment to prevent progression to osteomyelitis in the operative area and prosthesis failure, which could occur at any time, even years later.
Review drug regimen, e.g., anticoagulants or antibiotics for invasive procedures (e.g., tooth extraction).	Prophylactic therapy may be necessary for a prolonged period after discharge to limit risk of thromboemboli/infection. Procedures known to cause bacteremia can result in osteomyelitis and prosthesis failure.
Identify bleeding precautions, e.g., use of soft toothbrush, electric razor, avoidance of trauma/forceful blowing of nose, and routine laboratory follow-up.	Reduces risk of therapy-induced bleeding/hemorrhage.

711

CHAPTER 14

INTEGUMENTARY DISORDERS

Burns: Thermal/Chemical/Electrical (Acute and Convalescent Phase) _____

Thermal burns: Injuring agent can be flame, hot liquid, or contact with hot object. Flame burns are associated with smoke/inhalation injury.

Chemical burns: Occur from type/content of injuring agent, as well as concentration and temperature of agent.

Electrical burns: Occur from type/voltage of current which generates heat in proportion to resistance offered, and travels the pathway of least resistance (i.e., nerves offer the least resistance and bones the greatest resistance). Underlying injury will be more severe than visible injury.

Superficial partial-thickness burns (first degree): Involve only the epidermis. Wounds appear bright pink to red with minimal edema and no blisters. The skin is often warm/dry.

Moderate partial-thickness burns (second degree): Involve the epidermis and dermis. Wounds appear red to pink with moderate edema and moist, weeping blisters.

Deep partial-thickness burns (second degree): Involve the deep dermis. Wounds appear pink to pale ivory with moderate edema and blisters. These wounds are dryer than the moderate partial thickness burns.

Full-thickness burns (third degree): Involve all layers of skin, subcutaneous fat and may involve the muscle, nerves, and blood supply. Wound appearance varies from white, cherry red, to brown or black, with blistering uncommon. These wounds have a dry, leathery texture.

Full-thickness burns (fourth degree): Involve all skin layers plus muscle, organ tissue, and bone. Charring occurs.

PATIENT ASSESSMENT DATA BASE

Data are dependent on type, severity, and body surface area involved.

ACTIVITY/REST

May exhibit:	Decreased strength, endurance.
	Limited range of motion of involved areas.
	Impaired muscle mass, altered tone.

CIRCULATION

May exhibit (with burn injury involving more than 20% TBSA):	Hypotension (shock).
	Peripheral pulses diminished distal to extremity injury.
	Tachycardia (shock/anxiety/pain).

Dysrhythmias (electrical shock).

Tissue edema formation (all burns).

EGO INTEGRITY

May report: Concerns about family, job, finances.

ELIMINATION

May exhibit: Urine output decreased/absent during emergent phase. Color may be reddish black if myoglobin present, indicating deep muscle damage.

Diuresis (after capillary leak sealed and fluids mobilized back into circulation).

Bowel sounds decreased/absent, especially in cutaneous burns of greater than 20% as stress reduces gastric motility/peristalsis.

FOOD/FLUID

May exhibit: Generalized tissue edema.

Anorexia, nausea, vomiting.

NEUROSENSORY

May report: Mixed areas of numbness, tingling.

May exhibit: Changes in orientation, affect, behavior.

Decreased deep tendon reflexes in injured extremities.

PAIN/COMFORT

May report: Complaints of pain vary, e.g., first-degree burns are extremely sensitive to touch, pressure, air movement and temperature changes; second-degree moderate-thickness burns are very painful, while pain response in second-degree deep-thickness burns is dependent upon intactness of nerve endings; third-degree burns are painless.

RESPIRATION

May exhibit: Hoarseness, wheezy cough, carbonaceous particles in sputum, drooling/inability to swallow oral secretions, and cyanosis, indicative of inhalation injury.

Thoracic excursion may be limited in presence of circumferential chest burns.

Upper airway stridor/wheezes (obstruction due to laryngospasm, laryngeal edema).

Breath sounds: crackles (pulmonary edema), stridor (laryngeal edema), profuse airway secretions (rhonchi).

SAFETY

May exhibit: Skin: General: Exact depth of tissue destruction may not be evident for 3–5 days due to the process of microvascular thromboses in some wounds. Unburned skin areas may be cool/clammy, pale, with slow capillary refill in the presence of decreased cardiac output due to fluid loss/shock state.

Flame injury: There may be areas of mixed depth of injury due to varied intensity of heat produced by burning clothing. Singed nasal hairs; dry, red mucosa of nose and mouth; blisters on posterior pharynx; circumoral and/or circumnasal edema.

Chemical injury: Appearance of wound varies according to causative agent. Skin may be yellowish brown with soft leatherlike texture; blisters, ulcers, necrosis, or thick eschar. Injuries are generally deeper than they appear cutaneously and tissue destruction can continue for up to 72 hours after injury.

Electrical injury: The external cutaneous injury is usually much less than the underlying necrosis. Appearance of wounds varies and may include entry/exit wounds of current, arc burns from current moving in close proximity to body, and thermal burns due to ignition of clothing.

713

TEACHING/LEARNING

May report: History of trauma, e.g., fractures, soft tissue/internal organ damage from falls, explosions, motor vehicular accidents, or following contact with electrical current, which causes strong tetanic muscle contractions.

Discharge Plan Considerations: May require assistance with treatments, wound care/supplies, self-care/homemaker tasks, transportation, finances, vocational counseling; changes in physical layout of home or living facility other than home during prolonged rehabilitation.

DIAGNOSTIC STUDIES

CBC: initial increased Hct suggests hemoconcentration due to fluid shift/loss. Later decreased Hct and RBCs may occur due to heat damage to vascular endothelium.

WBCs: leukocytosis can occur due to loss of cells at wound site and inflammatory response to injury.

ABGs: baseline especially important with suspicion of inhalation injury. Reduced PaO_2/increased $PaCO_2$ may be seen with carbon monoxide retention. Acidosis may occur due to reduced renal function and loss of compensatory respiratory mechanisms.

COHbg (carboxyhemoglobin): elevation of greater than 15% indicates carbon monoxide poisoning/inhalation injury.

Serum electrolytes: potassium may be initially elevated due to injured tissues/red blood cell destruction and decreased renal function, hypokalemia can occur when diuresis starts; magnesium may be decreased. Sodium initially may be decreased with body water losses; hypernatremia can occur later as renal conservation occurs.

Alkaline phosphatase: elevated due to interstitial fluid shifts/impairment of sodium pump.

Serum glucose: elevation reflects stress response.

Serum albumin: albumin/globulin ratio may be reversed due to loss of protein in edema fluid.

BUN/creatinine: elevation reflects decreased renal perfusion/function; however, creatinine can elevate because of tissue injury.

Urine: presence of albumin, hemoglobin, and myoglobin indicates deep tissue damage and protein loss (especially seen with serious electrical burns). Reddish black color of urine is due to presence of myoglobin.

Wound cultures: may be obtained for baseline data and repeated periodically.

Chest x-ray: may appear normal in early postburn period even with inhalation injury; however, a true inhalation injury will present as a progressive whiteout on x-ray (ARDS).

Fiberoptic bronchoscopy: useful in diagnosing extent of inhalation injury; findings can include edema, hemorrhage, and/or ulceration of upper respiratory tract.

Flow volume loop: provides noninvasive assessment of effects/extent of inhalation injury.

Lung scan: may be done to determine extent of inhalation injury.

ECG: signs of myocardial ischemia/dysrhythmias may occur with electrical burns.

Photographs of burns: provides documentation for later burn wound healing.

NURSING PRIORITIES

1. Maintain patent airway/respiratory function.
2. Restore hemodynamic stability/circulating volume.
3. Alleviate pain.
4. Prevent complications.
5. Provide emotional support for patient/SO.
6. Provide information about condition, prognosis, and treatment needs.

DISCHARGE CRITERIA

1. Homeostasis achieved.
2. Pain controlled/reduced.
3. Complications prevented/minimized.
4. Dealing with current situation realistically.
5. Condition/prognosis and therapeutic regimen understood.

NURSING DIAGNOSIS:	AIRWAY CLEARANCE, INEFFECTIVE [POTENTIAL]
May be related to:	Tracheobronchial obstruction: mucosal edema and loss of ciliary action (smoke inhalation); circumferential full-thickness burns of the neck, thorax and chest with compression of the airway or limited chest excursion
	Trauma: direct upper airway injury by flame, steam, hot air, and chemicals/gases
	Fluid shifts, pulmonary edema, decreased lung compliance
Possibly evidenced by:	[Not applicable; presence of signs and symptoms establishes an *actual* diagnosis.]
PATIENT OUTCOMES/ EVALUATION CRITERIA:	Demonstrates clear breath sounds, respiratory rate within normal range, free of dyspnea/cyanosis.

ACTIONS/INTERVENTIONS	RATIONALE

Independent

Assess gag/swallow reflexes; note drooling, inability to swallow, hoarseness, wheezy cough.	Suggestive of inhalation injury.
Monitor respiratory rate, rhythm, depth; note presence of pallor/cyanosis and carbonaceous or pink-tinged sputum.	Tachypnea, use of accessory muscles, presence of cyanosis, and changes in sputum suggest developing respiratory distress/pulmonary edema, and need for medical intervention.
Auscultate lungs, noting stridor, wheezing/crackles, diminished breath sounds, brassy cough.	Airway obstruction/respiratory distress can occur very quickly or may be delayed, e.g., up to 48 hours after burn.
Note presence of pallor or cherry red color of uninjured skin.	Suggests presence of hypoxemia or carbon monoxide.
Elevate head of bed.	Promotes optimal lung expansion/respiratory function.
Encourage coughing/deep breathing exercises and frequent position changes.	Promotes lung expansion, mobilization and drainage of secretions.
Suction (if necessary) with extreme care, maintaining sterile technique.	Helps to maintain clear airway, but should be done cautiously because of mucosal edema and inflammation. Sterile technique reduces risk of infection.
Promote voice rest but assess ability to speak and/or swallow oral secretions periodically.	Increasing hoarseness/decreased ability to swallow suggests increasing tracheal edema and may indicate need for prompt intubation.
Investigate changes in behavior/mentation, e.g., restlessness, agitation, confusion.	Although often related to pain, changes in consciousness may reflect developing/worsening hypoxia.
Monitor 24-hour fluid balance, noting variations/changes.	Fluid shifts or excess fluid replacement increases risk of pulmonary edema. Note: Inhalation injury increases fluid demands as much as 35% or more because of obligatory edema.

Collaborative

Administer humidified oxygen via appropriate mode, e.g., face mask.	Oxygen corrects hypoxemia/acidosis. Humidity decreases drying of respiratory tract and reduces viscosity of sputum.

715

ACTIONS/INTERVENTIONS

Collaborative

Monitor/graph serial ABGs.

Review serial x-rays.

Provide/assist with chest physiotherapy/incentive spirometry.

Prepare for/assist with intubation or tracheostomy as indicated.

RATIONALE

Baseline is essential for further assessment of respiratory status and as a guide to treatment. PaO_2 less than 50, $PaCO_2$ greater than 50, and decreasing pH reflect smoke inhalation and developing pneumonia/ARDS.

Changes reflecting atelectasis, pulmonary edema may not occur for 2–3 days after burn.

Chest physiotherapy drains dependent areas of the lung, while incentive spirometry may be done to improve lung expansion, thereby promoting respiratory function and reducing atelectasis.

Intubation/mechanical support is required when airway edema or circumferential burn injury interferes with respiratory function/oxygenation.

NURSING DIAGNOSIS:	FLUID VOLUME DEFICIT, POTENTIAL
May be related to:	**Loss of fluid through abnormal routes, e.g., wounds**
	Increased need: hypermetabolic state, insufficient intake
	Hemorrhagic losses
Possibly evidenced by:	**[Not applicable; presence of signs and symptoms establishes an *actual* diagnosis.]**
PATIENT OUTCOMES/ EVALUATION CRITERIA:	**Demonstrates improved fluid balance as evidenced by individually adequate urinary output with normal specific gravity, stable vital signs, moist mucous membranes.**

ACTIONS/INTERVENTIONS

Independent

Monitor vital signs, CVP. Note capillary refill and strength of peripheral pulses.

Monitor urine output and specific gravity. Observe urine color and hematest as indicated.

Estimate wound drainage and insensible losses.

RATIONALE

Serves as a guide to fluid replacement needs and assess cardiovascular response. Note: Invasive monitoring is indicated for patients with major burns, smoke inhalation or patients with preexisting cardiac disease.

Generally, fluid replacement should be titrated to ensure urinary output of 50 ml/hr (in the adult). Urine can appear red to black, with massive muscle destruction due to presence of blood and release of myoglobin. If gross myoglobinuria is present, minimum urine output should be 75–100 ml/hr to prevent tubular damage/ necrosis.

Increased capillary permeability, protein shifts, inflammatory process and evaporative losses greatly affect circulating volume and urinary output, especially during initial 24–72 hours after burn.

ACTIONS/INTERVENTIONS	RATIONALE

Independent

Maintain cumulative record of amount and type of fluid intake.

Massive/rapid replacement with different types of fluids and fluctuations in rate of administration requires close tabulation to prevent constituent imbalances or fluid overload.

Weigh daily.

Fluid replacement formulas partly depend on admission weight and subsequent changes. A 15–20% weight gain in the first 72 hours during fluid replacement can be anticipated with return to preburn weight approximately 10 days after burn.

Measure circumference of burned extremities daily as indicated.

May be helpful in estimating extent of edema/fluid shifts affecting circulating volume and urine output.

Investigate changes in mentation.

Deterioration in the level of consciousness may indicate inadequate circulating volume/reduced cerebral perfusion.

Observe for gastric distention, hematemesis, tarry stools. Hematest NG drainage and stools periodically.

Stress (Curling's) ulcer occurs in up to half of all severely burned patients (can occur as early as first week). (Refer to CP: Upper Gastrointestinal/Esophageal Bleeding, p. 397.)

Collaborative

Insert/maintain indwelling urinary catheter.

Allows for close observation of renal function and prevents stasis or reflux of urine. Retention of urine with its byproducts of tissue cell destruction can lead to renal dysfunction and infection.

Insert/maintain large bore IV catheter(s).

To accommodate rapid infusion of fluids.

Administer calculated IV replacement of fluids, electrolytes, plasma, albumin.

Fluid resuscitation replaces lost fluids/electrolytes and helps to prevent complications, e.g., shock, acute tubular necrosis. Replacement formulas vary (e.g., Brooke, Evans, Parkland) but are based on extent of injury, amount of urine output, and weight.

Monitor laboratory studies, e.g., Hgb/Hct, electrolytes.

Identifies blood loss/red cell destruction, and fluid and electrolyte replacement needs.

Administer medications as indicated:

Diuretics, e.g., mannitol (Osmitrol);

May be indicated to enhance urine output, and clear tubules of debris/prevent necrosis.

Potassium;

Although hyperkalemia often occurs during first 24–48 hours (tissue destruction), subsequent replacement may be necessary because of large urinary losses.

Antacids, e.g., calcium carbonate (Titralac), magaldrate (Riopan); Histamine inhibitors, e.g., cimetidine (Tagamet)/ranitidine (Zantac).

Antacids may reduce gastric acidity, while histamine inhibitors decrease production of hydrochloric acid to reduce risk of gastric irritation/bleeding.

Add electrolytes to water used for wound debridement.

Washing solution that approximates tissue fluids may minimize osmotic fluid shifts.

NURSING DIAGNOSIS:	INFECTION, POTENTIAL FOR
May be related to:	**Inadequate primary defenses: destruction of skin barrier, traumatized tissues**
	Inadequate secondary defenses: decreased hemoglobin, suppressed inflammatory response

	Environmental exposure, invasive procedures
Possibly evidenced by:	[Not applicable; presence of signs and symptoms establishes an *actual* diagnosis.]
PATIENT OUTCOMES/ EVALUATION CRITERIA:	Achieves timely wound healing free of purulent exudate; and is afebrile.

ACTIONS/INTERVENTIONS

Independent

Implement appropriate isolation techniques as indicated.

Use gowns, gloves, masks and strict aseptic technique during direct wound care, and provide sterile or freshly laundered bed linens/gowns.

Monitor/limit visitors, if necessary. Explain isolation procedure to visitors if utilized.

Shave/clip all hair from around burned areas to include a one inch border (excluding eyebrows).

Provide special care for eyes; e.g., use eye covers and tear formulas as appropriate.

Prevent skin to skin surface contact (e.g., wrap each burned finger/toe separately; do not allow burned ear to touch scalp).

Remove dressings and cleanse burned areas in a hydrotherapy/whirlpool tub or in a shower stall with hand-held shower head. Maintain temperature of water at 100°F (37.8°C). Wash areas with a mild cleansing agent or surgical soap, such as betadine.

Debride necrotic/loose tissue with scissors and forceps. Do not disturb intact blisters if they are smaller than 2–3 cm, do not interfere with joint function and do not appear infected.

Examine wounds daily, note/document changes in appearance, odor or quantity of drainage.

Monitor vital signs for fever and increased respiratory rate/depth in association with changes in sensorium, decreased platelet count, and hyperglycemia with glycosuria.

Collaborative

Obtain routine cultures and sensitivities of wounds/drainage.

RATIONALE

Dependent on type/extent of wounds, and the choice of wound treatment (e.g., open versus closed), isolation may range from simple wound/skin to complete/reverse to reduce risk of cross-contamination/exposure to multiple bacterial flora.

Prevents exposure to infectious organisms.

Prevents cross-contamination from visitors.

Hair is a good medium for bacterial growth; however, eyebrows act as a protective barrier for the eyes.

Eyes may be swollen shut and/or become infected by drainage from surrounding burns. If lids are burned, eye covers may be needed to prevent corneal damage.

Prevents adherence to surface it may be touching and encourages proper healing. Note: Ear cartilage has limited circulation and is prone to pressure necrosis.

Water softens and aids in removal of dressings and eschar (slough layer of dead skin or tissue). Sources vary as to whether bath or shower is best. Bath has advantage of water providing support for exercising extremities but may promote cross-contamination of wounds. Showering enhances wound inspection and prevents contamination from floating debris.

Promotes healing. Prevents autocontamination. Small, intact blisters help to protect skin unless the burn injury is the result of chemicals (in which case fluid contained in blisters may continue to cause tissue destruction).

Identifies presence of healing (granulation tissue) and provides for early detection of burn wound infection.

Indicators of sepsis (often occurs with full thickness burn) requiring prompt evaluation and intervention.

Allows early recognition and specific treatment of wound infection.

ACTIONS/INTERVENTIONS	RATIONALE

Collaborative

Assist with excisional biopsies when infection is suspected.

Bacteria can colonize the wound surface without invading the underlying tissue; therefore, biopsies may be obtained for diagnosing infection.

Photograph wound initially and at periodic intervals.

Provides baseline and documentation of healing process.

Administer medications as indicated:

Topical agents, e.g.:

The following agents help to prevent/control wound infections and prevent drying of wound, which can cause further tissue destruction.

Silver sulfadiazine (Silvadene),

Wide-spectrum antimicrobial that is relatively painless but has less eschar penetration than Sulfamylon and may cause rash or depression of WBCs.

Mafenide acetate (Sulfamylon),

Antibiotic of choice with confirmed invasive burn wound infection. Useful against gram-negative/positive organisms. Causes burning/pain on application and for 30 minutes following. Can cause rash, metabolic acidosis, and decreased $PaCO_2$.

Silver nitrate,

Effective against staphylococcus aureus, Escherichia coli, and Pseudomonas aeruginosa, but has poor eschar penetration, is painful, and may cause electrolyte imbalance. Dressings must be constantly saturated. Product stains skin/surfaces black.

Providone-iodine (Betadine);

Broad spectrum antimicrobial but is painful on application and may cause metabolic acidosis/increased iodine absorption.

Subeschar clysis/systemic antibiotics;

Local and systemic antibiotics are given to control pathogens identified by culture/sensitivity. Subeschar clysis has been found effective against pathogens to prevent sepsis in granulated tissues at the line of demarcation between viable/nonviable tissue.

Tetanus toxoid or clostridial antitioxin as appropriate.

Tissue destruction/altered defense mechanisms increases risk of developing tetanus or gas gangrene, especially in deep burns such as those caused by electricity.

NURSING DIAGNOSIS:	COMFORT, ALTERED: PAIN, ACUTE
May be related to:	Destruction of skin/tissues; edema formation
	Manipulation of injured tissues, e.g., wound debridement
Possibly evidenced by:	Complaints of pain
	Narrowed focus, facial mask of pain
	Alteration in muscle tone; autonomic responses
	Distraction guarding behaviors; anxiety/fear

ACTIONS/INTERVENTIONS	RATIONALE

Independent

Cover wounds as soon as possible unless open air exposure burn care method required.

Temperature changes and air movement can cause great pain to exposed nerve endings.

Elevate burned extremities periodically.

Elevation may be required initially to reduce edema formation; thereafter changes in position and elevation reduce discomfort as well as risk of joint contractures.

Provide bed cradle as indicated.

Elevation of linens off wounds may help to reduce pain.

Wrap digits/extremities in position of function (avoiding flexed position of affected joints) using splints and footboards as necessary.

Position of function reduces deformities/contractures and promotes comfort. Although flexed position of injured joints may feel more comfortable, it can lead to flexion contractures.

Change position frequently and assist with active and passive range of motion as indicated.

Movement and exercise reduces joint stiffness and muscle fatigue but type of exercise is dependent on location and extent of injury.

Maintain comfortable environmental temperature.

Temperature regulation may be lost with major burns. External heat sources may be necessary to prevent chilling.

Assess complaints of pain, noting location/character and intensity (1–10 scale).

Pain is nearly always present to some degree because of varying severity of tissue involvement/destruction, but is usually most severe during dressing changes and debridement. Changes in location/character/intensity of pain may indicate developing complications (e.g., limb ischemia) or herald improvement/return of nerve function/sensation.

Perform dressing changes and debridement after patient is medicated and/or in hydrotherapy.

Reduces severe physical and emotional distress associated with dressing changes and debridement.

Encourage expression of feelings about pain.

Verbalization allows outlet for emotions and may enhance coping mechanisms.

Explain procedures/provide frequent information as appropriate, especially during wound debridement.

Empathic support can help to alleviate pain/promote relaxation. Knowing what to expect provides opportunity for patient to prepare self and enhances sense of control.

Provide routine comfort measures, e.g., massage of uninjured areas, frequent position changes.

Promotes relaxation, reduces muscle tension and general fatigue.

Encourage use of stress management techniques, e.g., progressive relaxation, breathing exercises, guided imagery, and visualization.

Refocuses attention, promotes relaxation, and enhances sense of control, which may reduce pharmacologic dependency.

Provide diversional activities appropriate for age/condition.

Helps to lessen concentration on pain experience and refocus attention.

Promote uninterrupted sleep periods.

Sleep deprivation can increase perception of pain/reduce coping abilities.

Collaborative

Administer analgesics (narcotic and nonnarcotic) as indicated.

IV method is often used initially to maximize drug effect. Concerns of patient addiction or doubts regard-

ACTIONS/INTERVENTIONS

Collaborative

Provide/instruct in use of PCA.

RATIONALE

ing degree of pain experienced are not valid during emergent/acute phase of care, but narcotics should be decreased as soon as feasible and alternate methods for pain relief initiated.

Patient-controlled analgesia provides for timely drug administration, preventing fluctuations in intensity of pain, often at lower total dosage than would be given by conventional methods.

NURSING DIAGNOSIS:	**TISSUE PERFUSION, ALTERED [POTENTIAL]**
May be related to:	**Reduction/interruption of arterial/venous blood flow, e.g., circumferential burns of extremities with resultant edema**
	Hypovolemia
Possibly evidenced by:	**[Not applicable; presence of signs and symptoms establishes an *actual* diagnosis.]**
PATIENT OUTCOMES/ EVALUATION CRITERIA:	**Maintains palpable peripheral pulses of equal quality/ strength; good capillary refill and skin color normal in uninjured areas.**

ACTIONS/INTERVENTIONS

Independent

Assess color, sensation, movement, peripheral pulses (via Doppler), and capillary refill on extremities with circumferential burns. Compare with findings of unaffected limb.

Elevate affected extremities, as appropriate. Remove jewelry/arm band. Avoid taping around a burned extremity/digit.

Remove BP cuff after each reading.

Investigate complaints of deep/throbbing ache, numbness.

Encourage active range of motion exercises of unaffected body parts.

Investigate irregular pulses.

RATIONALE

Edema formation can readily compress blood vessels, thereby impeding circulation and increasing venous stasis/edema. Comparisons with unaffected limbs aid in differentiating localized versus systemic problems (e.g., hypovolemia/decreased cardiac output).

Promotes systemic circulation/venous return and may reduce edema or other deleterious effects of constriction of edematous tissues. Prolonged elevation can impair arterial perfusion if BP falls or tissue pressures rise excessively.

If BP readings must be obtained on an injured extremity, leaving the cuff in place may increase edema formation/reduce perfusion, and convert partial-thickness burn to a more serious injury.

Indicators of decreased perfusion, and/or increased pressure within enclosed space, such as may occur with a circumferential burn of an extremity (compartment syndrome).

Promotes local and systemic circulation.

Cardiac dysrhythmias can occur as a result of electrolyte shifts, electrical injury, or release of myocardial depressant factor, compromising cardiac output/tissue perfusion.

721

ACTIONS/INTERVENTIONS	RATIONALE

Collaborative

Maintain fluid replacement per protocol. (Refer to ND: Fluid Volume Deficit, Potential, p. 716.)

Maximizes circulating volume, and tissue perfusion.

Monitor electrolytes, especially sodium, potassium, calcium. Administer replacement therapy as indicated.

Losses/shifts of these electrolytes, affect cellular membrane potential/excitability, thereby altering myocardial conductivity and potentiating risk of dysrhythmias, reducing cardiac output/tissue perfusion.

Measure intracompartmental pressures as indicated. (Refer to CP: Fractures, ND: Tissue Perfusion, Altered, p. 721.)

Ischemic myositis may develop due to decreased perfusion.

Assist with/prepare for escharotomy/fasciotomy, as indicated.

Enhances circulation by relieving constriction caused by rigid nonviable tissue (eschar) or edema formation.

NURSING DIAGNOSIS:	NUTRITION, ALTERED: LESS THAN BODY REQUIREMENTS
May be related to:	**Hypermetabolic state (can be as much as 50–60% greater than normal proportional to the severity of injury)**
	Protein catabolism
Possibly evidenced by:	**Decrease in total body weight, loss of muscle mass and subcutaneous fat, and development of negative nitrogen balance**
PATIENT OUTCOMES/ EVALUATION CRITERIA:	**Demonstrates nutritional intake adequate to meet metabolic needs as evidenced by stable weight/muscle mass measurements, positive nitrogen balance, and tissue regeneration.**

ACTIONS/INTERVENTIONS	RATIONALE

Independent

Auscultate bowel sounds, noting hypoactive/absent sounds.

Ileus is often associated with postburn period but usually subsides within 36–48 hours, at which time oral feedings can be initiated.

Maintain strict caloric count. Weigh daily. Reassess percent of open body surface area/wounds weekly.

Appropriate guides to proper caloric intake. As burn wound heals, percentage of burned areas is reevaluated to calculate prescribed dietary formulas, and appropriate adjustments are made.

Monitor triceps skinfold/arm muscle circumference as indicated.

May be useful in estimating muscle mass/subcutaneous fat reserves if upper extremity not burned.

Provide small, frequent meals and snacks.

Helps to prevent gastric distention/discomfort and may enhance intake.

Encourage patient to view diet as a treatment and to make food/beverage choices high in calories/protein.

Calories and proteins are needed to maintain weight, meet metabolic needs, and promote wound healing.

Ascertain food likes/dislikes. Encourage SO to bring food from home, as appropriate.

Provides patient/SO sense of control, enhances participation in care and may improve intake.

ACTIONS/INTERVENTIONS	RATIONALE
Independent	
Encourage patient to sit up for meals, and visit with others.	Sitting helps to prevent aspiration and aids in proper digestion of food. Socialization promotes relaxation and may enhance intake.
Provide oral hygiene before meals.	Clean mouth/clear palate enhances taste and helps promote a good appetite.
Perform clinitest/acetest as indicated.	Monitors for development of hyperglycemia related to hormonal changes/demands, or use of hyperalimentation to meet caloric needs.
Collaborative	
Refer to dietician/nutritional support team.	Useful in establishing individual nutritional needs based on weight, and body surface area of injury and identifying appropriate routes.
Provide diet high in calories/protein with vitamin supplements.	Calories (as many as 5000/day), proteins and vitamins are needed to meet metabolic needs, maintain weight, and encourage tissue regeneration. Note: Oral route is most preferable once gastrointestinal function returns.
Insert/maintain small feeding tube for enteric feedings/supplements if needed.	Provides continuous/or supplemental feedings when patient is unable to consume total daily calorie requirements orally.
Administer parenteral hyperalimentation as indicated. (Refer to CP: Total Nutritional Support, p. 894.)	Hyperalimentation will maintain nutritional intake/meet metabolic needs in presence of severe complications or sustained esophageal/gastric injuries that do not permit enteral feedings.
Monitor laboratory studies e.g., serum albumin, creatinine, transferrin; urine urea nitrogen.	Indicators of nutritional needs and adequacy of diet/therapy.
Administer insulin as indicated.	Elevated serum glucose levels may develop due to stress response to injury, high caloric intake, pancreatic fatigue.

NURSING DIAGNOSIS:	**MOBILITY, IMPAIRED PHYSICAL**
May be related to:	**Neuromuscular impairment, pain/discomfort, decreased strength and endurance**
	Restrictive therapies, limb immobilization; contractures
Possibly evidenced by:	**Reluctance to move/inability to purposefully move**
	Limited range of motion, decreased muscle strength control and/or mass
PATIENT OUTCOMES/ EVALUATION CRITERIA:	**Verbalizes and demonstrates willingness to participate in activities. Maintains position of function as evidenced by absence of contractures. Maintains or increases strength and function of affected and/or compensatory body part. Demonstrates techniques/behaviors that enable resumption of activities.**

ACTIONS/INTERVENTIONS	RATIONALE

Independent

Maintain proper body alignment with supports or splints (including use of footboard) especially for burns over joints.

Promotes functional positioning of extremities and prevents contractures, which are more likely over joints.

Note circulation, motion, sensation of digits frequently.

Edema may compromise circulation to extremities potentiating tissue necrosis/development of contractures.

Initiate the rehabilitative phase on admission.

It is easier to enlist participation when the patient is aware of the possibilities for recovery that exist.

Perform range of motion exercises consistently, initially passive, then active.

Prevents progressively tightening scar tissue and contractures, enhances maintenance of muscle/joint functioning and reduces loss of calcium from the bone.

Medicate for pain before activity/exercises.

Reduces muscle/tissue stiffness and tension enabling patient to be more active and facilitating participation.

Schedule treatments and care activities to provide periods of uninterrupted rest.

Increases patient's strength and tolerance for activity.

Instruct and assist with mobility aids, e.g., cane, walker, crutches as appropriate.

Promotes safe ambulation.

Encourage family/SO support and assistance with ROM exercises.

Enables family/SO to be active in patient care and provides more constant/consistent therapy.

Incorporate activities of daily living with physical therapy, hydrotherapy, and nursing care.

Combining activities produces improved results by enhancing effects of each.

Encourage patient participation in all activities as individually able.

Promotes independence, enhances self-esteem, and facilitates recovery process.

Collaborative

Provide foam, water/air mattress or kinetic therapy/CircOlectric bed as indicated.

Prevents prolonged pressure on tissues, reducing potential for tissue ischemia/necrosis and decubitus formation.

Excise and cover burn wounds quickly.

Early excision is known to reduce scarring as well as risk of infection, thereby facilitating healing.

Maintain pressure garment when used.

Hypertrophic scarring can develop around grafted areas or at the site of deep, partial-thickness wounds. Pressure dressings minimize scar tissue by keeping it flat, soft, and pliable.

Consult with rehabilitation, physical and occupational therapists.

Provides integrated activity/exercise program and specific assistive devices based on individual needs and facilitates intensive long-term management of potential deficits.

NURSING DIAGNOSIS:	**SKIN INTEGRITY, IMPAIRED: ACTUAL [GRAFTS]**
May be related to:	**Trauma: disruption of skin surface with destruction of skin layers (partial/full-thickness burn)**
Possibly evidenced by:	**Absence of viable tissue**
PATIENT OUTCOMES/ EVALUATION CRITERIA:	**Demonstrates tissue regeneration. Achieves timely healing of burned areas.**

ACTIONS/INTERVENTIONS	RATIONALE
Independent	
Preoperative	
Assess/document size, color, depth of wound, noting necrotic tissue and condition of surrounding skin.	Provides baseline information about need for skin grafting and possible clues about circulation in area to support graft.
Provide appropriate burn care and infection control measures. (Refer to ND: Infection, Potential for, p. 717.)	Prepares tissues for grafting and reduces risk of infection/graft failure.
Postoperative	
Maintain wound covering as indicated:	
Biosynthetic dressing, e.g., Biobrane;	Nylon fabric/silicon membrane containing collagenous porcine peptides which adheres to wound surface until removed or sloughed off by spontaneous skin reepithelialization. Useful for wounds awaiting autografts because it can remain in place 2 weeks or longer and is permeable to topical antimicrobial agents.
Synthetic dressings, e.g., DuoDerm,	Hydroactive dressing that adheres to the skin to cover small partial-thickness burns and interacts with wound exudate to form a soft gel which facilitates debridement.
Op-Site.	Thin, transparent, elastic, waterproof, occlusive dressing (permeable to moisture and air) that is used to cover clean partial-thickness wounds and clean donor sites.
Elevate grafted area if possible/appropriate.	Reduces swelling; limits risk of graft separation.
Maintain desired position and immobility of area when indicated.	Movement of tissue under graft can dislodge it, interfering with optimal healing.
Maintain dressings over newly grafted area and/or donor site as indicated, e.g., mesh, petroleum, nonadhesive.	Areas may be covered by translucent, nonreactive surface material (between graft and outer dressing) in order to eliminate shearing of new epithelium/protect healing tissue.
Keep skin free from pressure.	Promotes circulation and prevents ischemia/necrosis and graft failure.
Evaluate color of grafted and donor sites, note presence/absence of healing.	Evaluates effectiveness of circulation and identifies developing complications.
Wash sites with mild soap, rinse, and lubricate with cream (e.g., Nivea) several times daily, after dressings are removed and healing is accomplished.	Newly grafted skin and healed donor sites require special care to maintain flexibility.
Collaborative	
Prepare for/assist with surgical procedure/biologic dressings, e.g.:	
Homograft (allograft);	Skin grafts obtained from living persons or cadavers used as a temporary covering for extensive burns until person's own skin is ready for grafting (test graft), to cover excised wounds immediately after escharotomy, or to protect granulation tissue.
Heterograft (xenograft, porcine);	Skin grafts obtained from synthetic or animal skin with use same as for homograft as well as to cover meshed autografts and/or partial-thickness burns that are eschar-free and clean.

ACTIONS/INTERVENTIONS

Collaborative

Autograft.

RATIONALE

Skin graft obtained from uninjured part of patient's own skin; may be full-thickness or partial-thickness.

NURSING DIAGNOSIS:	FEAR/ANXIETY
May be related to:	Situational crises: hospitalization/isolation procedures, interpersonal transmission and contagion, memory of the trauma experience, threat of death and/or disfigurement
Possibly evidenced by:	Expressed concern regarding changes in life, fear of unspecific consequences
	Apprehension; increased tension
	Feelings of helplessness, uncertainty, decreased self-assurance
	Sympathetic stimulation, extraneous movements, restlessness, insomnia
PATIENT OUTCOMES/ EVALUATION CRITERIA:	Verbalizes awareness of feelings and healthy ways to deal with them. Reports anxiety/fear reduced to manageable level. Demonstrates problem-solving skills, effective use of resources.

ACTIONS/INTERVENTIONS

Independent

Provide frequent explanations and information about care procedures.

Demonstrate willingness to listen and talk to patient when free of painful procedures.

Assess mental status, including mood/affect, comprehension of events, and content of thoughts, e.g., illusions or manifestations of terror/panic.

Investigate changes in mentation and presence of hyper/hypovigilance, hallucinations, sleep disturbances (e.g., nightmares), agitation/apathy, disorientation, labile affect, all of which may vary from moment to moment.

Provide constant and consistent orientation.

Encourage the patient to talk about the burn circumstances when ready.

RATIONALE

Knowing what to expect usually reduces fear and anxiety, clarifies misconceptions and promotes cooperation.

Helps patient/SO to know that support is available, and that care giver is interested in the person, not just care of the burn.

Initially the patient may use denial and repression to reduce and filter information which might be overwhelming. Some patients display calm manner and alert mental status, representing a dissociation from reality, which is also a protective mechanism.

Indicators of extreme anxiety/delirium state in which the patient is literally fighting for life. Although cause can be psychologically based, pathologic life-threatening causes (e.g., shock, sepsis, hypoxia) must be ruled out.

Helps the patient stay in touch with surroundings and reality.

Patient may need to tell the story of what happened over and over in order to make some sense out of what is a terrifying situation.

ACTIONS/INTERVENTIONS

Independent

Explain to patient what happened. Provide opportunity for questions and give open/honest answers.

Identify previous methods of coping/handling of stressful situations.

Assist the family to express their feelings of grief and guilt.

Be nonjudgmental in dealing with the patient and family.

Encourage family/SO to visit and discuss family happenings. Remind patient of past and future events.

Collaborative

Involve entire burn team in care from admission to discharge, including psychiatric resources.

Administer mild sedation/tranquilizers as indicated, e.g., haloperidol (Haldol) or lorazepam (Ativan).

RATIONALE

Compassionate statements reflecting the reality of the situation can help the patient/SO acknowledge that reality and begin to deal with what has happened.

Past successful behavior can be used to assist in dealing with the present situation.

The family may initially be most concerned about the patient dying and/or feel guilty, believing that in some way they could have prevented the incident.

Family relationships are disrupted; financial, lifestyle/role changes make this a difficult time for those involved with the patient, and they may react in many different ways.

Maintains contact with a familiar reality, creating a sense of attachment and continuity of life.

Provides a wider support system and promotes continuity of care and coordination of activities.

Antianxiety medications may be necessary for brief period of time until patient is more physically stable and internal locus of control is regained.

NURSING DIAGNOSIS:	SELF-CONCEPT, DISTURBANCE IN: BODY IMAGE; ROLE PERFORMANCE
May be related to:	**Situational crisis: traumatic event, dependent patient role; disfigurement, pain**
Possibly evidenced by:	**Negative feelings about body/self, fear of rejection/reaction by others**
	Focus on past appearance, abilities; preoccupation with change/loss
	Change in physical capacity to resume role; change in social involvement
PATIENT OUTCOMES/ EVALUATION CRITERIA:	**Verbalizes acceptance of self in situation. Talking with family/SO about situation, changes that have occurred. Develops realistic goals/plans for the future. Incorporates changes into self-concept without negating self-esteem.**

ACTIONS/INTERVENTIONS

Independent

Assess meaning of loss/change to patient/SO.

RATIONALE

Traumatic episode results in sudden, unanticipated changes, creating feelings of grief over actual/perceived losses. This necessitates support to work through to optimal resolution.

ACTIONS/INTERVENTIONS	RATIONALE

Independent

Acknowledge and accept expression of feelings of frustration, dependency, anger, grief and hostility. Note withdrawn behavior and use of denial.

Acceptance of these feelings as a normal response to what has occurred facilitates resolution. It is not helpful or possible to push patient before ready to deal with situation. Denial may be prolonged and be an adaptive mechanism, because patient is not ready to cope with personal problems.

Set limits on maladaptive behavior (e.g., manipulative/aggressive). Maintain nonjudgmental attitude while giving care, and help patient to identify positive behaviors that will aid in recovery.

Patient and SO tend to deal with this crisis in the same way in which they have dealt with problems in the past. Staff may find it difficult and frustrating to handle behavior that is disrupting/not helpful to recuperation but should realize that the behavior is usually directed toward situation and not the care giver.

Be realistic and positive during treatments, in health teaching, and in setting goals within limitations.

Enhances trust and rapport between patient and nurse.

Provide hope within parameters of individual situation; do not give false reassurance.

Promotes positive attitude and provides opportunity to set goals and plan for future based on reality.

Give positive reinforcement of progress and encourage endeavors toward attainment of rehabilitation goals.

Words of encouragement can support development of positive coping behaviors.

Show slides or pictures of burn care/other patient outcomes, being selective in what is shown as appropriate to the individual situation. Encourage discussion of feelings about what they have seen.

Allows patient/SO to be realistic in expectations. Also assists in demonstration of importance of/necessity for certain devices and procedures.

Encourage family interaction with each other and in rehabilitation team.

Maintains/opens lines of communication and provides ongoing support for patient and family.

Provide support group for SO, giving them information about how they can be helpful to the patient.

Promotes ventilation of feelings and allows for more helpful responses to the patient.

Collaborative

Refer to physical/occupational therapy, vocational counselor, and psychiatric counseling, e.g., clinical specialist psychiatric nurse, social services, psychologist as needed.

Helpful in identifying ways/devices to maintain independence. Patient may need further assistance to resolve emotional problems if they persist (e.g., post-trauma response).

NURSING DIAGNOSIS:	**KNOWLEDGE DEFICIT [LEARNING NEED] (SPECIFY)**
May be related to:	**Lack of exposure/recall, information misinterpretation**
	Unfamiliarity with resources
Possibly evidenced by:	**Questions/request for information, statement of misconception**
	Inaccurate follow-through of instructions/development of preventable complications
PATIENT OUTCOMES/ EVALUATION CRITERIA:	**Verbalizes understanding of condition, prognosis and treatment. Correctly performs necessary procedures and explains reasons for actions. Initiates necessary lifestyle changes and participates in treatment regimen.**

ACTIONS/INTERVENTIONS	RATIONALE
Independent	
Review condition, prognosis, and future expectations.	Provides knowledge base on which patient can make informed choices.
Discuss patient's expectations of returning home, to work, and to normal activities.	Patient frequently has a difficult adjustment to discharge. Problems often occur (e.g., sleep disturbances, nightmares, reliving the accident, difficulty with resumption of intimacy/sexual activity, emotional lability) that interfere with successful adjustment to resuming normal life.
Review proper burn, skin graft and wound care techniques. Identify appropriate sources for outpatient care and supplies.	Promotes competent self-care after discharge and enhances independence.
Discuss skin care, e.g., use of moisturizers and sunscreens.	Itching, blistering, and sensitivity of healing wounds/graft sites can be expected for an extended period of time.
Explain scarring process and necessity for/proper use of pressure garments when used.	Promotes optimal regrowth of skin, preventing development of contractures and facilitating healing process. Note: Consistent use of the pressure garment over a long period of time can reduce the need for reconstructive surgery to release contractures and remove scars.
Encourage continuation of prescribed exercise program and scheduled rest periods.	Maintains mobility, reduces complications, and prevents fatigue, facilitating recovery process.
Identify specific limitations of activity as individually appropriate.	Imposed restrictions are dependent on severity/location of injury and stage of healing.
Stress importance of sustained intake of high protein/calorie diet.	Optimal nutrition enhances tissue regeneration and general feeling of well-being.
Review medications, including purpose, dosage, route, and expected/reportable side effects.	Reiteration allows opportunity for patient to ask questions and be sure understanding is accurate.
Advise patient/SO of potential for exhaustion, boredom, emotional lability, adjustment problems. Provide information about possibility of discussion/interaction with appropriate professional counselors.	Provides perspective to some of the problems patient/SO may encounter and helps them to be aware that help/assistance is available when necessary.
Identify signs/symptoms requiring medical evaluation, e.g., inflammation, increased or changes in wound drainage, fever/chills; changes in pain characteristics or loss of mobility/function.	Early detection of developing complications (e.g., infection, delayed healing) may prevent progression to more serious/life-threatening situations.
Stress necessity/importance of follow-up care/rehabilitation.	Long-term support with continual reevaluation and changes in therapy are required to achieve optimal recovery.
Provide phone number for contact person.	Provides easy access to treatment team to reinforce teaching, clarify misconceptions, and reduce potential for complications.
Identify community resources, e.g., crisis centers, recovery groups, mental health, Red Cross, VNA, Ambli-Cab, homemaker service.	Facilitates transition to home, provides assistance with meeting individual needs, and supports independence.

CHAPTER 15
IMMUNOLOGIC DISORDERS

The HIV-Positive Patient

The individual who has tested positive for the human immunodeficiency virus (HIV) may live for many years before meeting the Centers for Disease Control (CDC) criteria for a diagnosis of acquired immune deficiency syndrome (AIDS). While imminent death is not a realistic concern, these patients need to make major behavioral and lifestyle changes to prolong their life expectancy and may have significant problems that require information and assistance. The person who is well supported medically may survive opportunistic infection episodes over a longer period of time.

NURSING DIAGNOSIS: **KNOWLEDGE DEFICIT [LEARNING NEED] (SPECIFY)**

    May be related to: **Lack of exposure/recall; information misinterpretation**

             Unfamiliarity with information resources

             Cognitive limitation

    Possibly evidenced by: **Statement of misconception/request for information**

             Inaccurate follow-through of instructions/development of preventable complications

    PATIENT OUTCOMES/
    EVALUATION CRITERIA: **Verbalizes understanding of condition/disease process and treatment. Identifies relationship of signs/symptoms to the disease process and correlates symptoms with causative factors. Initiates necessary lifestyle changes and participates in treatment regimen.**

ACTIONS/INTERVENTIONS	RATIONALE
Independent	
Determine current understanding and perception of diagnosis. Discuss difference between HIV-positivity and AIDS.	Provides opportunity to clarify misconceptions/myths, make informed choices and allows for development of individualized plan of care.

ACTIONS/INTERVENTIONS	RATIONALE

Independent

Assess emotional ability to assimilate information and understand instructions. Respect patient's need to use "denial" coping techniques initially.

Initial shock and anxiety can block intake of information. Self-esteem, lifestyle, guilt, and denial of own responsibility in acquiring disease become issues; denial may serve as a protective mechanism promoting more effective self-care.

Encourage safe expression of feelings, denial, shock, and other coping strategies.

Promotes awareness of feelings and establishes base on which resolution of own situation can occur.

Provide information about normal immune system/response and how the HIV affects it, transmission of the virus, behaviors/factors believed to increase probability of progression. Encourage questions.

Patient needs to be aware of own personal risk as well as risk to others in order to make immediate and long-range decisions and establish a basis for goal-setting. Also, establishes rapport and provides opportunity to identify concerns and assimilate information.

Provide realistic, optimistic information on first visit.

Necessary to provide realistic hope to reduce risk of suicide. Many patients have been exposed to media information about AIDS, or have friends/lovers who have died of the disease. These persons may feel suicidal upon being diagnosed. Persons with HIV-positive testing may also believe untimely death is imminent.

Plan short sessions for additional information.

Patient will need time and repeated contacts to absorb information.

Review signs/symptoms that may be a consequence of HIV positivity, e.g., mild persistent fever, anorexia, weight loss, fatigue, night sweats, diarrhea, dry cough, rashes, headaches, and sleep disturbances.

Patient may experience an acute illness 2–6 weeks after infection; however, it is more common for infection to be subclinical, with the individual feeling unwell and experiencing one or more of these signs/symptoms.

Discuss signs/symptoms that require medical evaluation, e.g., persistent cough or swollen lymph glands; profound fatigue that is unrelieved by rest; weight loss of 10 pounds in less than 2 months; severe, persistent diarrhea; fever; blurred vision; skin discoloration or rash that persists or spreads; open sores anywhere.

Early recognition of progression of disease/development of complications provides for timely intervention and may prevent more serious situations.

Provide information about necessary lifestyle changes and health maintenance factors.

Evidence suggests that specific dietary and lifestyle factors may affect the progression of HIV to ARC/AIDS. Prevention and/or early detection and treatment of infection is crucial to prevention of further impairment of the immune system and development of opportunistic diseases.

Avoid crowds and people with infections; Get adequate sleep and rest; alternate rest periods with activity;

Exercise to limit of ability, avoiding undue fatigue;

Eat regularly, even if appetite is reduced. Try small, frequent meals and snacks;

Practice good oral hygiene and examine mouth regularly for sores, and have regular dental checkups;

Examine skin for rashes, bruises, breaks in skin integrity;

Practice safe sex at all times;

Avoid use of IV drugs; however, if using, do not share needles, and clean "works" with bleach solution.

ACTIONS/INTERVENTIONS	RATIONALE
Independent	
Stress importance of follow-up care. Review procedures and tests that will be necessary for continuous assessment of status.	Even though patient may be asymptomatic, periodic evaluation may prevent development of complications/progression of the disease. Knowledge about what to expect promotes sense of control over situation.
Assess potential for inappropriate/high-risk behavior: continued IV drug abuse, unsafe sexual practices.	High denial/anger, drug addiction may result in behaviors that are high-risk for spread of the virus. A person's sexuality and identity are threatened by the discovery of the diagnosis.
Discuss active changes in sexual behaviors that the patient can make that will satisfy sexual needs and are designed to prevent transmission.	Promotes a sense of responsibility and control and may reduce sexual tensions.
Provide written information.	Patient may feel overwhelmed, and written materials allow for later review and reinforcement when patient has had an opportunity to calm down.
Encourage daily contact with SO as needed.	Initiates sense of support and concern for SO, promoting involvement and understanding of patient and situation.
Collaborative	
Refer to support groups, peer counselors, and mental health professionals.	Patient will experience a variety of emotional and psychologic responses to the diagnosis and may need additional assistance to promote optimal adjustment.

Acquired Immunodeficiency Syndrome (AIDS) _____

Current literature recommends that the diagnosis of AIDS be reserved for a person who has a life-threatening, opportunistic infection, progressive dementia, wasting syndrome, or Kaposi's sarcoma (under 60 years), certain other cancers, or dissemination of generally localized diseases (e.g., tuberculosis), while having an underlying immunodeficiency with no known cause and/or being antibody-positive for HIV.

Persons with AIDS have currently been found to fall into six risk groups:
1. Homosexual men
2. Bisexual men
3. Intravenous drug users
4. Recipients of infected blood or blood products
5. Heterosexual partners of a person with HIV infection
6. Children born to an infected mother

PATIENT ASSESSMENT DATA BASE

Data are dependent on the organs/body tissues involved and the specific opportunistic infection or cancer.

ACTIVITY/REST

May report: Tires easily, reduced tolerance for usual activities, progressing to profound fatigue/malaise.

Altered sleep patterns.

May exhibit: Muscle weakness, wasting of muscle mass.

Physiologic response to activity, e.g., changes in blood pressure, heart rate, respiration.

CIRCULATION

May report: Slow healing; bleed longer with injury.

May exhibit: Tachycardia, postural blood pressure changes.

Decreased pulse volume.

Pallor or cyanosis; delayed capillary refill.

EGO INTEGRITY

May report: Stress factors related to relationship status, financial, spiritual, lifestyle concerns.

Concern about appearance; alopecia, disfiguring lesions.

Denial of diagnosis, feelings of powerlessness, hopelessness, helplessness, worthlessness, guilt, loss of control, depression.

May exhibit: Denial, anxiety, depression, fear, withdrawal.

Angry behaviors, dejected body posture, crying, poor eye contact.

Failure to keep appointments.

ELIMINATION

May report: Intermittent, persistent to frequent diarrhea with or without abdominal cramping.

Flank pain, burning on urination.

May exhibit: Loose-formed to watery stools with or without mucus or blood.

Frequent, copious diarrhea.

Abdominal tenderness.

Rectal, perianal lesions or abscesses.

Changes in urine output, color, character.

FOOD/FLUID

May report: Anorexia, food intolerance, nausea, vomiting.
Rapid/progressive weight loss.
Dysphagia, retrosternal pain with swallowing.

May exhibit: Vomiting.
Weight loss; thin frame; decreased subcutaneous fat/muscle mass.
Poor skin turgor.
Lesions of the oral cavity, white patches, discoloration.
Poor dental/gum health.
Edema (generalized, dependent).

HYGIENE

May report: Unable to complete activities of daily living.

May exhibit: Disheveled appearance.
Deficits in many or all personal care, self-care activities.

NEUROSENSORY

May report: Fainting spells/dizziness; headache.
Changes in mental status, loss of mental acuity/ability to solve problems, forgetfulness, poor concentration.
Impaired sensation, or sense of position and vibration.
Muscle weakness, tremors, changes in visual acuity.

May exhibit: Mental status changes ranging from confusion to dementia, forgetfulness, poor concentration, decreased alertness, apathy, psychomotor retardation/slowed responses.
Paranoid ideation, free floating anxiety, unrealistic expectations.
Abnormal reflexes and decreased muscle strength.
Fine/gross motor tremors, focal motor deficits; seizures.
Retinal hemorrhages and exudates (cytomegalovirus [CMV] retinitis).

PAIN/COMFORT

May report: Generalized/localized pain, aching.
Headache (CNS involvement).
Pleuritic chest pain.

May exhibit: Swelling of joints, painful nodules, tenderness.
Decreased ROM, gait changes/limp.
Muscle guarding.

RESPIRATION

May report: Frequent, persistent upper respiratory infections.
Progressive shortness of breath.
Cough (ranging from mild to severe); nonproductive/productive of sputum (Pneumocystis carinii pneumonia [PCP] has a nonproductive cough).
Congestion or tightness in chest.

May exhibit: Tachypnea, respiratory distress.
Changes in breath sounds/adventitious breath sounds.
Sputum (yellow in sputum-producing pneumonia).

SAFETY

May report:　　History of frequent or multiple blood transfusions (e.g., hemophiliac, major vascular surgery, traumatic incident).

History of immune deficiency diseases, e.g., advanced cancer; ARC.

History of/current infection with sexually transmitted diseases (STDs).

Recurrent fevers, low grade, intermittent temperature elevations/spikes; night sweats.

Slow-healing wounds.

May exhibit:　　Changes in skin integrity; eczema, exanthemas, psoriasis, discolorations; changes in size, color of nevi; tattoos; unexplained, easy bruising.

Rectal, perianal lesions or abscesses.

Nodules, enlarged lymph nodes in two or more areas of body (e.g., neck, armpits, groin).

Alterations in general strength, muscle tone, gait.

SEXUALITY

May report:　　History of high-risk behavior, e.g., homosexual, bisexual partner who is HIV antibody-positive (Ab+)/has AIDS, multiple sexual partners, unprotected sexual activity, and anal sex.

Loss of libido.

Inconsistent use of birth control measures/condoms.

Use of birth control pills (enhanced susceptibility to virus).

May exhibit:　　Pregnant or at risk for pregnancy.

Genitalia: mucocutaneous manifestations (e.g., herpes, warts); discharge.

SOCIAL INTERACTION

May report:　　Problems imposed by diagnosis, e.g., loss of family/SO, friends, support.

Fear of telling others; fear of rejection/loss of income.

Isolation, loneliness, close friends or sexual partners who have died of AIDS.

Questioning of ability to remain independent, unable to plan.

May exhibit:　　Changes in family/SO interaction pattern.

Disorganized activities, poor goal-setting.

TEACHING/LEARNING

May report:　　Failure to comply with treatment, continued high-risk behavior (sexual or IV drug use).

IV drug use/abuse, current smoking, alcohol abuse.

Evidence of failure to improve from last hospitalization.

Discharge Plan Considerations:　　May require assistance with finances, medications/treatments, wound care/supplies, transportation, food shopping and preparation, self-care, homemaker tasks, provision for child care; changes in living facilities.

DIAGNOSTIC STUDIES

CBC: anemia and thrombocytopenia.

WBC: lymphopenia may be present, differential shift to the left suggests infectious process (PCP); shift to the right may be noted. With certain infections, low T-cell count or T-cell tumor, no shift may occur.

Anergy panel: cutaneous anergy (lack of reactivity to antigens patient has been exposed to previously) is a common indicator of depressed cell-mediated immunity.

Serologic:

　　Serum antibody test: HIV screen by enzyme-linked immunosorbent assay (ELISA). A positive test result may be indicative of exposure to HIV but is not diagnostic, and indicates the need for other testing. (Sensitivity varies with the incidence of false-positive results as high as 25%.)

735

Western blot test: identifies antibodies to specific viral proteins and is used as a confirming test.

T-lymphocyte cells: total count reduced.

T4 helper cells (immune system indicator which mediates several immune system processes and signals B cells to produce antibodies to foreign germs): numbers below normal (often less than 400, may be less than 200) indicate immune deficiency response.

TB (cytopathic suppressor cells): Reversed ratio (2:1 or greater) of suppressor cells to helper cells (T8 to T4) indicates immune suppression.

P24 (primary protein of HIV): increased quantitative values of this core protein can be indicative of progression of infection. (May not be detectable during very early stages of HIV infection.)

Immunoglobin (Ig) levels: usually elevated, especially IgG and IgA, with normal to near normal IgM (indicator of the ability of the body to show whether infectious processing is intact, but is not used frequently because other factors can alter it, such as a change in environmental pollutants).

PCR (polymerase chain reaction): Detects viral DNA in small number of infected peripheral mononuclear cells.

STD testing: Hepatitis B envelope and core antibodies, syphillis, CMV may be positive.

Cultures: histologic, cytologic studies of urine, blood, stool, spinal fluid, lesions, sputum and secretions may be done to identify the opportunistic infection. Some of the most commonly identified are the following:

Protozoa and helminthic infections: PCP, cryptosporidiosis, toxoplasmosis.

Fungal infections: Candida albicans (candidiasis), cryptococcus neoformans (cryptococcosis); Histoplasma capsulatum (histoplasmosis).

Bacterial infections: Mycobacterium avium-intercellulare, Shigella (shigellosis), Salmonella (salmonellosis).

Viral infections: CMV infection, herpes simplex, herpes zoster.

Radiologic studies:

MRI: detects progressive multifocal leukoencephalopathy.

Chest x-ray: may initially be normal, or may reveal progressive interstitial infiltrates from advanced PCP (most common opportunistic disease) or other pulmonary complications.

Gallium scan: diffuse pulmonary uptake occurs in PCP and other forms of pneumonia.

Biopsies: may be done for differential diagnosis of Kaposi's sarcoma or other neoplastic lesions.

Bronchoscopy/tracheobronchial washings: may be done with biopsy when PCP or lung malignancies are suspected (diagnostic confirming test for PCP).

Endoscopy: Disseminated Candida may be present, especially in esophagus. Kaposi's sarcoma may be present in gastrointestinal system.

NURSING PRIORITIES

1. Prevent infections.
2. Maintain homeostasis.
3. Promote comfort.
4. Support psychosocial adjustment.
5. Provide information about disease process/prognosis and treatment needs.

DISCHARGE CRITERIA

1. Infection prevented.
2. Complications prevented/minimized.
3. Pain/discomfort alleviated.
4. Dealing with current situation realistically.
5. Diagnosis, prognosis, and therapeutic regimen understood.

NURSING DIAGNOSIS:	INFECTION, POTENTIAL FOR [PROGRESSION TO SEPSIS/ONSET OF NEW OPPORTUNISTIC INFECTION]
May be related to:	**Inadequate primary defenses: broken skin, traumatized tissue, stasis of body fluids**

Depression of the immune system; use of antimicrobial agents

Environmental exposure, invasive techniques

Chronic disease; malnutrition

Possibly evidenced by: [Not applicable; presence of signs and symptoms establishes an *actual* diagnosis.]

PATIENT OUTCOMES/ EVALUATION CRITERIA: Identifies/participates in behaviors to reduce risk of infection. Achieves timely healing of wounds/lesions; is afebrile and free of purulent drainage/secretions.

ACTIONS/INTERVENTIONS	RATIONALE
Independent	
Wash hands before and after all care contacts. Instruct patient/SO to wash hands as indicated.	Reduces risk of cross contamination.
Provide a clean, well-ventilated environment. Screen visitors/staff for signs of infection and maintain isolation precautions as indicated.	Reduces possibility of patient contracting an iatrogenic infection.
Clean up spills of body fluids/blood with bleach solution (1:10).	Controls microorganisms on hard surfaces.
Discuss extent and rationale for isolation precautions and maintenance of personal hygiene.	Promotes cooperation with regimen and may lessen feelings of isolation.
Monitor vital signs, including temperature.	Provides information for baseline data; frequent temperature elevations or new fever onset indicates that body is responding to new infectious process.
Assess respiratory rate/depth; note dry cough, changes in characteristics of sputum and presence of wheezes, rhonchi. (Refer to ND: Breathing Pattern, Ineffective, p. 739.)	Respiratory congestion/distress may indicate developing pneumocystic carinii pneumoniae (PCP), the most common opportunistic disease. However, other fungal, viral, and bacterial infections may occur that compromise the respiratory system.
Investigate complaints of headache, stiff neck, alterations in vision. Note changes in mentation and behavior. Monitor for nuchal rigidity/seizure activity.	Neurologic abnormalities are common and may be related to the HIV or secondary infections. Symptoms may vary from subtle changes in mood/sensorium (personality changes or depression) to hallucinations, memory loss, severe dementias, seizures, and loss of vision. Central nervous system infections (encephalitis is the most common) may be caused by protozoa and helminthic organisms, or fungus.
Examine skin/oral mucous membranes for white patches/lesions. (Refer to ND: Skin Integrity, Impaired: Potential/Actual, p. 744.)	Oral candidiasis, Kaposi's sarcoma (KS), and herpes are common opportunistic diseases affecting the cutaneous membranes.
Monitor complaints of heartburn, dysphagia, retrosternal pain on swallowing, increased abdominal cramping, profuse diarrhea.	Esophagitis may occur secondary to oral candidiasis or herpes. Cryptosporidiosis is a parasitic infection responsible for watery diarrhea (often > 15 liters/day). (Refer to ND: Fluid Volume Deficit, Potential, p. 738.)
Inspect wounds/site of invasive devices, noting signs of local inflammation/infection.	Early identification/treatment of secondary infection may prevent sepsis. (Refer to CP: Sepsis/Septicemia, p. 763.)
Wear gloves and gowns during direct contact with secretions/excretions or anytime there is a break in	Depending on protocol, gloves may be worn when direct contact with patient fluids is anticipated. Use of

ACTIONS/INTERVENTIONS	RATIONALE

Independent

skin of care givers hands. Wear mask and protective eyewear to protect nose, mouth, and eyes from secretions during procedures (e.g., suctioning) or when splattering may occur (e.g., dialysis, angiogram).

masks, gowns, and gloves is required for direct contact with body fluids, e.g., blood/blood products, semen, vaginal secretions. Note: Although other fluids have not been shown to transmit infection, all body fluids and tissues should be regarded as potentially infectious.

Dispose of needles/sharps in rigid, puncture-resistant containers.

Prevents accidental innoculation of care givers. Use of needle cutters and recapping is not to be practiced. Note: Accidental inoculations/punctures should be reported immediately and follow-up evaluations done per protocol. Encourage bleeding of the site of puncture and washing immediately with hot soapy water.

Label blood bags, body fluid containers, soiled dressings/linens and package appropriately for disposal per isolation protocol.

Alerts appropriate personnel/departments to exercise their own isolation procedures.

Collaborative

Monitor laboratory studies, e.g.:

 CBC/differential;

Shifts in the differential and changes in WBC indicates infectious process.

 Culture/sensitivity studies of lesions, blood, urine and sputum.

May be done to identify cause of fever, diagnose infecting organisms/appropriate course of treatment.

Administer antibiotic antifungal/antimicrobial agents, e.g., trimethroprim (Bactrim, Septra), nystatin (Mycostatin), pentamidine; or experimental drugs such as AZT and DHPG.

Combats infectious process. Some drugs are targeted for specific organisms/affected system. Other drugs are targeted to improve immune function. Although no cure is currently available, experimental agents such as AZT are aimed at blocking the enzyme that enables the virus to begin reproducing, thereby retarding the progression of the disease. DHPG is used when CMV is present to prevent blindness/life threatening dissemination. Note: AZT may potentiate acute CMV, and usage may be limited.

NURSING DIAGNOSIS:	FLUID VOLUME DEFICIT, POTENTIAL
May be related to:	Excessive losses: copious diarrhea, profuse sweating, vomiting
	Hypermetabolic state, fever
	Restricted intake: nausea, anorexia; lethargy
Possibly evidenced by:	[Not applicable; presence of signs/symptoms establishes an *actual* diagnosis.]
PATIENT OUTCOMES/ EVALUATION CRITERIA:	Maintains hydration as evidenced by moist mucous membranes, good skin turgor, stable vital signs, individually adequate urine output.

ACTIONS/INTERVENTIONS	RATIONALE
Independent	
Monitor vital signs, including CVP if available. Note hypotension, including postural changes.	Indicators of circulating fluid volume.
Note temperature elevation, duration of febrile episode. Administer tepid sponge baths as indicated. Keep clothing and linens dry. Maintain comfortable environmental temperature.	Increased metabolic demands and excessive diaphoresis associated with fever result in increased insensible fluid losses.
Assess skin turgor, mucous membranes, and thirst.	Indirect indicators of fluid status.
Measure urine output and specific gravity. Measure/estimate amount of diarrheal loss. Note insensible losses. Weigh as indicated.	Increased specific gravity/decreasing output reflects altered renal perfusion/circulating volume. Note: Monitoring fluid balance is difficult because of excessive gastrointestinal/insensible losses. In addition, weight loss may reflect muscle wasting as well as state of hydration.
Monitor oral intake and encouarge fluids of up to 2500 ml/day. Make fluids easily accessible to patient; use fluids which are tolerable to the patient and which replace needed electrolytes, e.g., Gatorade, broth.	Restores fluid balance, reduces thirst, and moisturizes mucous membranes. If nausea prevents oral intake, fluids may be replaced by feeding tube or parenteral route. Certain fluids may be too painful to consume (e.g., acidic juices) because of mouth lesions.
Eliminate foods potentiating diarrhea, e.g., spicy/high-fat foods, nuts, cabbage, milk products. Adjust rate/concentration of tube feedings if indicated.	May help reduce diarrhea.
Collaborative	
Administer IV fluids/electrolytes.	May be necessary to support/augment circulating volume, especially if oral intake is inadequate.
Monitor laboratory studies as indicated, e.g.:	
Hb/Hct;	Useful in estimating fluid needs.
Serum/urine electrolytes;	Alerts to possible electrolyte disturbances and determines replacement needs.
BUN/creatinine.	Evaluates renal perfusion/function.
Administer medications as indicated:	
Antiemetics, e.g., prochlorperazine maleate (Compazine), trimethobenzamide hydrochloride (Tigan), metoclopramide hydrochloride (Reglan);	Reduces incidence of vomiting to reduce further loss of fluids/electrolytes.
Antidiarrheals, e.g., diphenoxylate (Lomotil), Imodium, Paregoric, or antispasmotics, e.g., mepenzolate bromide (Cantil);	Decreases the amount and fluidity of stool; may reduce intestinal spasm and peristalsis. Note: Antibiotics may also be used to treat diarrhea if caused by infection.
Antipyretics, e.g., acetominophen (Tylenol). Maintain hypothermia blanket if used.	Helps to reduce fever and hypermetabolic response decreasing insensible losses. Note: Acetominophen is contraindicated when patient is receiving AZT (Retrovir).

NURSING DIAGNOSIS:	**BREATHING PATTERN, INEFFECTIVE [POTENTIAL]**
May be related to:	**Muscular impairment (wasting of respiratory musculature), decreased energy/fatigue, decreased lung expansion, retained secretions (tracheobronchial obstruction)**
	Inflammatory process, pain

Possibly evidenced by:	[Not applicable; presence of signs and symptoms establishes an *actual* diagnosis.]
PATIENT OUTCOMES/ EVALUATION CRITERIA:	Maintain effective respiratory pattern; free of dyspnea/cyanosis with breath sounds and chest x-ray clear/improving and ABGs within patient's normal range.

ACTIONS/INTERVENTIONS	RATIONALE
Independent	
Auscultate breath sounds, noting areas of decreased/absent ventilation and presence of adventitious sounds, e.g., crackles, wheezes, rhonchi.	Suggests developing pulmonary complications/infection, e.g., atelectasis/pneumonia. Note: PCP is often advanced before changes in breath sounds occur.
Note rate/depth of respiration, cyanosis, use of accessory muscles/increased work of breathing and presence of dyspnea, anxiety.	Tachypnea, cyanosis, restlessness and increased work of breathing reflect respiratory distress and need for increased surveillance/medical intervention.
Elevate head of bed. Turn, cough, deep breathe as indicated.	Promotes optimal pulmonary function, and reduces incidence of aspiration or infection due to atelectasis.
Suction airway as indicated, using sterile technique and observing safety precautions, e.g., mask, protective eyewear.	Assists in clearing the ventilatory passages, thereby facilitating gas exchange.
Assess changes in level of consciousness.	Hypoxemia can result in changes ranging from anxiety and confusion to unresponsiveness.
Investigate complaints of chest pain.	Pleuritic chest pain may reflect nonspecific pneumonitis or pleural effusions associated with malignancies.
Allow adequate rest periods between care activities. Maintain a quiet environment.	Reduces oxygen consumption.
Collaborative	
Monitor/graph serial ABGs.	Reflects the oxygenation and ventilation status of the patient.
Review serial chest x-rays.	Presence of diffuse infiltrates may suggest pneumonia, PCP, while areas of congestion/consolidation may reflect other pulmonary complications, e.g., atelectasis or KS lesions.
Instruct in use of incentive spirometer. Provide chest physiotherapy, e.g., percussion, vibration, and postural drainage.	Encourages proper breathing technique and improves lung expansion. Loosens secretions, dislodges mucus plugs to promote airway clearance. Note: In the event of multiple skin lesions, chest physiotherapy may be discontinued.
Provide humidified supplemental oxygen via appropriate means, e.g., cannula, mask, intubation/mechanical ventilation.	Maintains effective ventilation/oxygenation to prevent/correct respiratory crisis. (Refer to CP: Ventilatory Assistance (Mechanical), p. 191.)
Administer medications as indicated:	
Antimicrobials, e.g.: trimethoprim (Bactrim, Septra); pentamidine isoethionate (Pentam);	These drugs are useful in treating PCP; however, choice of therapy is dependent on individual situation/infecting organism(s).
Bronchodilators, expectorants, depressants.	May be needed to improve/maintain airway patency or help clear secretions.

NURSING DIAGNOSIS:	INJURY, POTENTIAL FOR: ALTERED CLOTTING FACTORS
May be related to:	Decreased vitamin K absorption, alteration in hepatic function, presence of autoimmune antiplatelet antibodies, malignancies (Kaposi's sarcoma); and/or circulating endotoxins (sepsis).
Possibly evidenced by:	[Not applicable; presence of signs/symptoms establishes an *actual* diagnosis.]
PATIENT OUTCOMES/ EVALUATION CRITERIA:	Displays homeostasis as evidenced by absence of mucosal bleeding and free of ecchymosis.

ACTIONS/INTERVENTIONS	RATIONALE

Independent

Hematest body fluids for occult blood, e.g., urine, stool, vomitus.	Prompt detection of bleeding/initiation of therapy may prevent critical hemorrhage. (Refer to CP: Upper Gastrointestinal/Esophageal Bleeding, p. 397.)
Observe for/report epistaxis, hemoptysis, hematuria, nonmenstrual vaginal bleeding, or oozing from lesions/body orifices, IV insertion sites.	Spontaneous bleeding may indicate development of disseminated intravascular coagulation (DIC) or immune thrombocytopenia.
Monitor for changes in vital signs and skin color, e.g., BP, pulse, respirations, skin pallor/discoloration.	Presence of bleeding/hemorrhage may lead to circulatory failure/shock.
Monitor for change in level of consciousness and visual disturbances.	Change may reflect cerebral bleeding.
Avoid IM injections, rectal temperatures/suppositories, rectal tubes.	Protects patient from procedure-related causes of bleeding; e.g., insertion of thermometers, rectal tubes can damage or tear rectal mucosa.
Maintain a safe environment; e.g., keep all necessary objects and call bell within patient's reach and keep bed in low position.	Reduces accidental injury, which could result in bleeding.
Maintain bed/chair rest when platelets are below 10,000 or as individually appropriate. Assess medication regimen.	Reduces possibility of injury, although activity needs to be maintained. May need to discontinue or reduce drug, e.g., AZT.

Collaborative

Review laboratory studies, e.g., PT, PTT, clotting time, platelets, Hb/Hct.	Detects alterations in clotting capability, identifies therapy needs.
Administer blood products as indicated.	Transfusions may be required in the event of persistent/massive spontaneous bleeding.
Avoid use of aspirin products.	Reduces platelet aggregation, impairing/prolonging the coagulation process.

NURSING DIAGNOSIS:	NUTRITION, ALTERED: LESS THAN BODY REQUIREMENTS
May be related to:	Inability to ingest, digest and/or absorb nutrients: nausea/vomiting, hyperactive gag reflex, intestinal disturbances

	Increased metabolic activity/nutritional needs (fever/infection)
Possibly evidenced by:	**Weight loss, decreased subcutaneous fat/muscle mass**
	Lack of interest in food, aversion to eating, altered taste sensation
	Abdominal cramping, hyperactive bowel sounds, diarrhea
	Sore, inflamed buccal cavity
PATIENT OUTCOMES/ EVALUATION CRITERIA:	**Displays weight gain toward desired goal, free of signs of malnutrition. Demonstrates positive nitrogen balance and improved energy level.**

ACTIONS/INTERVENTIONS

Independent

Assess ability to chew, taste, and swallow.

Auscultate bowel sounds.

Remove existing noxious environmental stimuli or conditions that aggravate gag reflex.

Provide frequent mouth care, observing secretion precautions. Avoid alcohol-containing mouth washes.

Weigh as indicated.

Plan diet with patient/SO; suggest "foods from home" if appropriate. Provide small, frequent meals/snacks of nonacidic foods and beverages, with choice of foods palatable to patient. Encourage high-calorie/nutrition foods, some of which may be considered appetite stimulants. Note time of day when appetite is best, and try to serve larger meal at that time.

Limit food(s) that induce nausea/vomiting or are poorly tolerated by the patient because of mouth sores/dysphagia. Avoid serving very hot liquids/foods. Serve foods easy to swallow, e.g., eggs, ice cream, cooked vegetables.

Schedule medications between meals (if tolerated) and limit fluid intake with meals, unless fluid has nutritional value.

Encourage as much physical activity as possible.

Provide rest period before meals. Avoid stressful procedures close to mealtime.

Encourage patient to sit up for meals.

Record caloric intake.

RATIONALE

Lesions of the mouth, throat, and esophagus may cause dysphagia, limiting patient's ability to ingest food and reducing desire to eat.

Hypermotility of intestinal tract is common and is associated with vomiting and diarrhea, which may affect choice of diet/route.

Reduces stimulus of the vomiting center in the medulla.

Promotes comfort by reducing discomfort associated with nausea/vomiting, oral lesions, mucosal dryness, and halitosis. Clean mouth may enhance appetite.

Indicator of nutritional needs/adequacy of intake.

Including patient in planning gives sense of control of environment and may enhance intake. Fulfilling cravings for noninstitutional food may also improve intake.

Prevents interference with intake, enhancing nutrition.

Gastric fullness diminishes appetite and food intake.

May improve appetite and general feelings of well-being.

Minimizes fatigue, increases energy available for work of eating.

Facilitates swallowing and reduces risk of aspiration.

Identifies need for supplements or alternate feeding methods.

ACTIONS/INTERVENTIONS

Collaborative

Review laboratory studies, e.g., BUN, glucose, liver function studies, electrolytes, protein, and albumin.

Maintain NPO status when appropriate.

Insert/maintain nasogastric tube if indicated.

Consult with dietician/nutritional support team.

Administer TPN (hyperalimentation/intralipids) as indicated.

Administer medications as indicated:

Antiemetics, e.g., metoclopramide hydrochloride (Reglan);

Parenteral vitamin supplements.

RATIONALE

Indicates nutritional status and organ function, and identifies replacement needs.

May be needed to reduce vomiting.

May be needed to reduce nausea/vomiting, or to administer tube feedings. Note: Esophageal irritation from existing infection (Candida/herpes or KS) may provide site for secondary infections/trauma, therefore, tube should be used with caution.

Provides for diet based on individual needs/appropriate route.

Occasionally parenteral nutrients may be required if oral/enteral feedings are not tolerated. (Refer to CP: Total Nutritional Support, p. 894.)

Reduces incidence of vomiting, promotes gastric function.

Vitamin deficiencies result from decreased food intake and/or disorders of digestion and absorption in the GI system. When oral intake resumed/tolerated, vitamins may be administered orally.

NURSING DIAGNOSIS:	**COMFORT, ALTERED: PAIN, ACUTE/CHRONIC**
May be related to:	**Tissue inflammation/destruction: infections, internal/external cutaneous lesions, rectal excoriation, malignancies, necrosis**
	Myalgias and arthralgias
	Abdominal cramping
Possibly evidenced by:	**Complaints of pain**
	Self-focusing; narrowed focus
	Alteration in muscle tone; guarding behaviors
	Autonomic responses; restlessness
PATIENT OUTCOMES/ EVALUATION CRITERIA:	**Reports pain relieved/controlled. Demonstrates relaxed posture/facial expression and is able to sleep/rest appropriately.**

ACTIONS/INTERVENTIONS

Independent

Assess pain, noting location, intensity (1–10 scale), frequency and time of onset. Note nonverbal cues, e.g., restlessness, tachycardia, grimacing.

Encourage verbalization of feelings.

RATIONALE

Indicates need for/effectiveness of interventions and may signal development/resolution of complications.

Can reduce anxiety and fear and thereby reduce perception of intensity of pain.

ACTIONS/INTERVENTIONS

Independent

Provide diversional activities, e.g., reading, visiting, television.

Perform palliative measures e.g., repositioning, massage, ROM of affected joints.

Apply warm/moist packs to pentamidine injection/IV sites for 20 minutes after administration.

Instruct patient in/encourage use of visualization/guided imagery, progressive relaxation, deep breathing techniques.

Provide oral care. (Refer to ND: Oral Mucous Membranes, altered, p. 745.)

Collaborative

Administer analgesics/antipyretics; narcotic analgesics.

RATIONALE

Refocuses attention, may enhance coping abilities.

Promotes relaxation/decreases muscle tension.

These injections are known to cause sterile abscesses and pain.

May decrease the need for narcotic analgesics (CNS depressants) where there is already a neuro/motor degenerative process involved. May not be useful when secondary dementia is present, even though minor.

Oral ulcerations/lesions may cause severe discomfort.

Provides relief of pain/discomfort, reduces fever. Note: Acetaminophen is contraindicated if patient is receiving AZT (Retrovir) as metabolism of AZT may be impaired, potentiating risk of toxicity.

NURSING DIAGNOSIS:	SKIN INTEGRITY, IMPAIRED: POTENTIAL/ACTUAL
May be related to:	**Immunologic deficit: AIDS-related dermatitis; bacterial and fungal infections (e.g., herpes, Candida); opportunistic disease processes (e.g., Kaposi's sarcoma)**
	Decreased level of activity, altered sensation, skeletal prominence, changes in skin turgor
	Malnutrition, altered metabolic state
Possibly evidenced by:	**Skin lesions; ulcerations; decubitus ulcer formation**
PATIENT OUTCOMES/ EVALUATION CRITERIA:	**Demonstrates behaviors/techniques to prevent skin breakdown/promote healing. Displays improvement in wound/lesion healing.**

ACTIONS/INTERVENTIONS

Independent

Assess skin daily. Note color, turgor, circulation and sensation. Describe lesions and observed changes.

Maintain/instruct in good skin hygiene, e.g., wash thoroughly, pat dry carefully, and massage with lotion or appropriate cream.

RATIONALE

Establishes baseline with which changes in status can be compared, and appropriate interventions instituted.

Maintaining clean, dry skin provides a barrier to infection. Patting skin dry instead of rubbing reduces risk of dermal trauma to dry/fragile skin. Massaging increases circulation to the skin and promotes comfort. Note: Isolation precautions, e.g., gloves, linen, diapers, are required, especially if extensive mucocutaneous herpes lesions are present.

ACTIONS/INTERVENTIONS	RATIONALE

Independent

Reposition frequently. Protect bony prominences with pillows, heel/elbow pads, sheepskin.

Reduces stress on pressure points and possibility of ulceration/decubiti.

Maintain clean, dry, wrinkle-free linen.

Skin friction caused by wet or wrinkled sheets leads to irritation and potentiates infection.

Encourage ambulation/out of bed as tolerated.

Decreases pressure on skin from prolonged bedrest.

Cleanse perianal area. Remove stool with water and mineral oil. Avoid use of toilet paper if vesicles present. Apply protective creams, e.g., zinc oxide, A&D ointment.

Prevents maceration caused by diarrhea and keeps perianal lesions dry. Note: Use of toilet paper may abrade lesions.

Cover open pressure ulcers with sterile dressings or protective barrier, e.g., DuoDerm, as indicated.

May reduce bacterial contamination, promote healing.

Collaborative

Provide foam/flotation mattress/or bed.

Decreases potential for tissue ischemia, reducing pressure on skin/tissue.

Obtain cultures of open skin lesions.

Identifies infectious pathogens and appropriate treatment choices.

Apply/administer systemic/topical drugs as indicated, e.g., acyclovir sodium (Zovirax).

Used in treatment of herpes infectious processes. In the event of multidose ointments, care must be taken to avoid cross-contamination.

Cover ulcerated KS lesions with wet-to-wet dressings or antibiotic ointment and Telfa as indicated.

Protects ulcerated areas from contamination and promotes healing.

NURSING DIAGNOSIS:	ORAL MUCOUS MEMBRANES, ALTERED [POTENTIAL]
May be related to:	Immunologic deficit: presence of Candida, herpes, Kaposi's sarcoma
	Dehydration, malnutrition
	Ineffective oral hygiene
	Side effects of drugs, chemotherapy
Possibly evidenced by:	[Not applicable; presence of signs and symptoms establishes an *actual* diagnosis.]
PATIENT OUTCOMES/ EVALUATION CRITERIA:	Displays intact mucous membranes, which are pink and moist and free of inflammation/ulcerations.

ACTIONS/INTERVENTIONS	RATIONALE

Independent

Note ability to swallow, handle secretions.

Edema, open lesions, and crusting on oral mucous membranes and throat may cause difficulty with swallowing and increase risk of aspiration.

Provide oral care using soft toothbrush, nonabrasive toothpaste, nonalcohol mouthwash and lip moisturizer. Use gloves when in direct contact with lesions, secretions, mucous membranes.

Reduces risk of further infection, alleviates discomfort and promotes feeling of well-being. Use of gloves reduces risk to care giver.

ACTIONS/INTERVENTIONS

Independent

Rinse oral mucosal lesions with saline/hydrogen peroxide solutions. Apply lip balm.

Plan diet to avoid salty, spicy, abrasive, and acidic foods or beverages. Check for temperature tolerance of foods.

Encourage oral intake of at least 2500 ml/day.

Collaborative

Obtain culture specimens as indicated.

Administer medications, as indicated, e.g., nystatin (Mycostatin), solution/troches.

Refer for dental consultation, if appropriate.

RATIONALE

Reduces spread of lesions and encrustations from candidiasis and promotes comfort.

Abrasive foods may open healing lesions. Open lesions will be painful and aggravated by salt, spice, acidic foods/beverages. Extreme cold or heat can cause pain to sensitive mucous membranes.

Maintains hydration, prevents drying of oral cavity.

Reveals causative agents and identifies appropriate therapies.

Specific drug choice is dependent on individual situation/infecting organism(s), e.g., Candida.

Gingivitis may require additional therapy to prevent dental losses.

NURSING DIAGNOSIS:	FATIGUE
May be related to:	**Decreased metabolic energy production, increased energy requirements (hypermetabolic state)**
	Overwhelming psychologic/emotional demands
	Altered body chemistry: side effects of medication, chemotherapy
Possibly evidenced by:	**Unremitting/overwhelming lack of energy, inability to maintain usual routines, decreased performance**
	Impaired ability to concentrate, lethargy/listlessness
	Disinterest in surroundings
PATIENT OUTCOMES/ EVALUATION CRITERIA:	**Reports improved sense of energy. Performs activities of daily living and participates in desired activities at level of ability.**

ACTIONS/INTERVENTIONS

Independent

Plan care to allow for rest periods. Schedule activities for periods when patient has most energy. Involve patient/SO in schedule planning.

Establish realistic activity goals with patient.

Assist with self-care needs; keep bed in low position, travelways clear of furniture, assist with ambulation.

RATIONALE

Frequent rest periods are needed to restore/conserve energy. Planning will allow patient to be active during times when energy level is higher, which may restore a feeling of well-being and a sense of control.

Provides for a sense of control and feelings of accomplishment.

Weakness may make ADLs almost impossible for the patient to complete. Protects patient from injury during activities.

ACTIONS/INTERVENTIONS	RATIONALE

Independent

Encourage patient to do whatever possible, e.g., self-care, up in chair, walking. Increase activity level as indicated.

May increase strength, stamina and enable patient to become more active without undue fatigue.

Monitor physiologic response to activity, e.g., changes in blood pressure, or heart/respiratory rate.

Tolerance varies greatly depending on the stage of the disease process, nutrition state, fluid balance, and number/type of opportunistic diseases that the patient has been subject to.

Encourage nutritional intake. (Refer to ND: Nutrition, Altered: Less Than Body Requirements, p. 741.)

Adequate intake/utilization of nutrients is necessary to meet energy needs for activity.

Collaborative

Provide supplemental oxygen as indicated.

Presence of anemia/hypoxemia reduces oxygen available for cellular uptake and contributes to fatigue.

Refer to physical/occupational therapy.

Programmed daily exercises and activities help patient to maintain/increase strength and muscle tone, enhance sense of well-being.

NURSING DIAGNOSIS:	THOUGHT PROCESSES, ALTERED
May be related to:	**Hypoxemia, CNS infection by HIV, brain malignancies, and/or disseminated systemic opportunistic infection**
	Alteration of drug metabolism/excretion, accumulation of toxic elements: renal failure, severe electrolyte imbalance, hepatic insufficiency
Possibly evidenced by:	**Altered attention span; distractibility**
	Memory deficit
	Disorientation; cognitive dissonance; delusional thinking
	Sleep disturbances
	Impaired ability to make decisions/problem-solve; inability to follow complex commands/mental tasks, loss of impulse control
PATIENT OUTCOMES/ EVALUATION CRITERIA:	**Maintains usual reality orientation and optimal cognitive functioning.**

ACTIONS/INTERVENTIONS	RATIONALE

Independent

Assess mental/neurologic status, noting changes in orientation, level of response to stimuli, ability to problem-solve, altered sleep patterns, hallucinations, paranoid ideation, general anxiety.

Establishes functional neurologic level at time of admission and alerts the nurse to changes in status which may be asssociated with exacerbation of CNS infection/opportunistic disease, environmental stressors, psychologic stress, or side effects of drug therapy.

ACTIONS/INTERVENTIONS	RATIONALE

Independent

Consider effects of emotional distress, e.g., grieving and/or effects of medications.

May contribute to reduced alertness, confusion, withdrawal, hypoactivity and require further evaluation and intervention.

Review drug regimen.

Prolonged drug half-life/altered excretion results in cumulative effects, potentiating risk of toxic reactions, while some drugs may simply have adverse side effects; e.g., Haldol can seriously impair motor function in patients with AIDS dementia complex (ADC).

Monitor for signs of CNS infection, e.g., headache, nuchal rigidity, vomiting, fever.

CNS symptoms associated with disseminated meningitis/encephalitis may range from subtle personality changes to confusion, irritability, drowsiness, stupor, seizures, and dementia.

Maintain a pleasant environment with appropriate auditory, visual and cognitive stimuli. Provide cues for reorientation, e.g., radio, television, calendars, clocks, room with an outside view. Use patient's name; identify yourself. Maintain structured schedules as appropriate.

Providing normal environmental stimuli can help in maintaining some sense of reality orientation. Frequent reorientation to place and time may be necessary, especially during periods of fever/acute CNS involvement. Sense of continuity may reduce associated anxiety.

Reduce provocative/noxious stimuli. Maintain bedrest in quiet, darkened room if indicated.

If the patient is prone to seizures or increased intracranial pressure, reducing external stimuli may become necessary.

Encourage family/SO to provide reorientation with current news, family events.

Familiar contacts are often helpful in maintaining reality orientation, especially if patient is hallucinating.

Maintain safe environment: e.g., excess furniture out of the way, call bell within patient's reach, bed in low position/rails up; restriction of smoking (unless monitored by care giver/SO); seizure precautions; soft restraints if indicated.

Decreases the possibility of patient injury.

Set limits on maladaptive/abusive behavior; avoid open-ended choices.

Provides sense of security/stability in an otherwise confusing situation.

Provide support for SO. Encourage discussion of concerns/fears.

Bizarre behavior, deterioration of abilities may be very frightening for SO and makes management of care/dealing with situation difficult. They may feel a loss of control as stress, anxiety, burnout, and anticipatory grieving impairs usual coping abilities.

Provide information about care on an ongoing basis. Answer questions simply and honestly. Repeat explanations as needed. Discuss causes/future expectations of dementia.

Can reduce anxiety and fear of unknown, enhance patient's understanding and involvement/cooperation in treatment when possible.

Collaborative

Assist with diagnostic studies, e.g., spinal tap, and monitor laboratory studies as indicated, e.g., BUN/creatinine, electrolytes, ABGs.

Choice of tests/studies are dependent on clinical manifestations and index of suspicion, as changes in mental status may reflect a wide variety of causative factors, e.g., CMV meningitis/encephalitis, drug toxicity, electrolyte imbalances, and altered organ function.

Administer medications as indicated:

    Amphotericin B (Fungizone);

Antifungal useful in treatment of cryptococcosis meningitis.

    Zidovudine/AZT (Retrovis);

May reverse neurologic effects of the virus and enhance mental functioning.

ACTIONS/INTERVENTIONS	RATIONALE
Collaborative	
Antipsychotics, e.g., haloperidol (Haldol), and/or antianxiety agents, e.g., lorazepam (Ativan).	Cautious use may improve sleeplessness, emotional lability; decrease hallucinations, suspiciousness and agitation. Note: Combined use of Ativan and Haldol may allow lower drug dosage, reducing adverse effects.
Provide controlled environment/behavioral management.	May be required to protect patient when mental impairment (e.g., delusions) threaten patient safety.
Refer to psychiatric counseling as indicated.	May help patient gain control in presence of psychotic symptomatology.

NURSING DIAGNOSIS:	ANXIETY/FEAR [SPECIFY]
May be related to:	**Threat to self-concept, threat of death, change in health/socioeconomic status, role functioning**
	Interpersonal transmission and contagion
	Separation from support system
	Fear of transmission of the disease to family/loved ones
Possibly evidenced by:	**Increased tension, apprehension, feelings of helplessness/hopelessness**
	Expressed concern regarding changes in life
	Fear of unspecific consequences
	Somatic complaints, insomnia; sympathetic stimulation, restlessness
PATIENT OUTCOMES/ EVALUATION CRITERIA:	**Verbalizes awareness of feelings and healthy ways to deal with them. Displays appropriate range of feelings and lessened fear/anxiety. Demonstrates problem-solving skills. Uses resources effectively.**

ACTIONS/INTERVENTIONS	RATIONALE
Independent	
Assure patient of strict confidentiality.	Provides reassurance and opportunity for patient to problem-solve solutions to anticipated situations.
Maintain frequent contact with patient. Talk with and touch the patient. Limit use of isolation clothing and masks.	Provides assurance that the patient is not alone or rejected, conveys respect for and acceptance of the person, fostering trust.
Provide accurate, consistent information regarding prognosis. Avoid arguing about patient's perceptions of the situation.	Can reduce anxiety and enable patient to make decisions/choices based on realities.
Be alert to signs of denial/depression, e.g., withdrawal, angry inappropriate remarks. Determine presence of suicidal ideation and assess potential on a scale of 1–10.	Patient may use defense mechanism of denial and express hope that diagnosis is inaccurate. Feelings of guilt and spiritual distress may cause the patient to become withdrawn and believe that suicide is a viable alternative.

749

ACTIONS/INTERVENTIONS	RATIONALE

Independent

Provide open environment in which patient feels safe to discuss feelings or to refrain from talking.

Helps patient to feel accepted in present condition without feeling judged and promotes sense of dignity and control.

Permit expressions of anger, fear, despair without confrontation. Give information that feelings are normal and are to be appropriately expressed.

Acceptance of feelings allows patient to begin to deal with situation.

Recognize and support level patient/family are at in the grieving process. (Refer to CP: Cancer, ND: Grieving, Anticipatory, p. 876.)

Choice of interventions is dictated by stage of grief, coping behaviors, e.g., anger/withdrawal, denial.

Explain procedures, providing opportunity for questions and honest answers. Stay with patient during anxiety-producing procedures and consultations.

Accurate information allows the patient to deal more effectively with the reality of the situation, thereby reducing anxiety and fear of the unknown.

Identify and encourage patient interaction with support systems. Encourage verbalization/interaction with family/SO.

Reduces feeling of isolation. If family support systems are not available, outside sources may be needed immediately, e.g., local AIDS Task Force.

Provide reliable and consistent information and support for SO.

Allows for better interpersonal interaction and reduction of anxiety and fear.

Include SO as indicated when major decisions are to be made.

Ensures a support system for the patient, and allows the SO the chance to participate in patient's life.

Collaborative

Refer to psychiatric counseling.

May require further assistance in dealing with diagnosis/prognosis especially when suicidal thoughts are present.

NURSING DIAGNOSIS:	SOCIAL ISOLATION
May be related to:	Major alterations in established social/professional/sexual patterns (altered state of wellness, changes in body image, probable loss of job, finances, home, and insurance)
	Physical isolation
Possibly evidenced by:	Expressed feeling of aloneness imposed by others, feelings of rejection.
	Absence of supportive SO: partners, family, acquaintances/friends
PATIENT OUTCOMES/ EVALUATION CRITERIA:	Expresses increased sense of self-worth. Participates in activities/programs at level of ability/desire.

ACTIONS/INTERVENTIONS	RATIONALE

Independent

Ascertain patient's perception of situation.

Isolation may be partly self-imposed as patient fears rejection/reaction of others.

ACTIONS/INTERVENTIONS	RATIONALE
Independent	
Spend time talking with patient during and between care activities. Be supportive, allowing for verbalization. Treat with dignity and regard for patient's feelings.	Patient may experience physical isolation due to current medical status and some degree of social isolation secondary to diagnosis of AIDS.
Limit/avoid use of mask when possible, e.g., when talking to patient.	Reduces patient's sense of physical isolation and provides positive social contact, which may enhance self-esteem.
Identify support systems available to patient, including presence of/relationship with immediate and extended family.	When patient has assistance from SO, feelings of loneliness and rejection will be diminished. Note: Patient may not receive "usual"/needed support for coping with life-threatening illness and associated grief because of fear and lack of understanding (AIDS hysteria).
Explain isolation precautions/procedures to patient/SO.	Gloves, gowns, mask are not routinely required with a diagnosis of AIDS. Misuse of these barriers enhances feelings of emotional as well as physical isolation. When precautions are necessary, explanations help patient understand reasons for procedures and provide feeling of inclusion in what is happening.
Encourage open visitation (as able), telephone contacts, and social activities within tolerated level.	Participation with others can foster a feeling of belonging.
Encourage active role of contact with SO.	Helps to reestablish a feeling of participation in a social relationship. May lessen likelihood of suicide attempts.
Develop a plan of action with patient: look at available resources; support healthy risk-taking behaviors. Help patient problem-solve solutions to short-term/imposed isolation.	Having a plan promotes a sense of control over own life and gives patient something to look forward to/ actions to accomplish.
Be alert to verbal/nonverbal cues, e.g., withdrawal, statements of despair, sense of aloneness. Ask the patient if thoughts of suicide are being entertained.	Indicators of despair and suicidal ideation are often present; and when these cues are acknowledged by the care giver, the patient is usually willing to talk about thoughts of suicide, sense of isolation and hopelessness.
Collaborative	
Refer to resources, e.g., social services, counselors, and AIDS Task Force (local/national).	Establishes support systems, may reduce feelings of isolation.
Provide for placement in sheltered community when necessary.	May need more specific care when unable to be maintained at home or when SO cannot manage care.

NURSING DIAGNOSIS:	POWERLESSNESS
May be related to:	**Confirmed diagnosis of a terminal disease, incomplete grieving process**
	Social ramifications of AIDS; alteration in body image, desired lifestyle; advancing CNS involvement
Possibly evidenced by:	**Feelings of loss of control over own life**
	Depression over physical deterioration that occurs despite patient compliance with regimen

Anger, apathy, withdrawal, passivity

Dependence on others for care/decision-making resulting in resentment, anger, guilt

PATIENT OUTCOMES/ EVALUATION CRITERIA:	**Acknowledges feelings and healthy ways to deal with them. Verbalizes some sense of control over present situation. Makes choices related to and is involved in care.**

ACTIONS/INTERVENTIONS	RATIONALE

Independent

Identify factors that contribute to the patient's feelings of powerlessness, e.g., diagnosis of a terminal illness, lack of support systems, lack of knowledge about present situation.

Patients with AIDS are usually aware of the current literature and prognosis. Fear of AIDS (by the general population as well as the patient's family/SO) is the most profound cause of the patient's isolation. For some patients, this may be the first time that the family has been made aware that the patient has chosen an alternative lifestyle.

Assess degree of feelings of helplessness, e.g., verbal/nonverbal expressions indicating lack of control ("It won't make any difference"), flat affect, lack of communication.

Determines the status of the individual patient and allows for appropriate intervention when the patient is immobilized by depressed feelings.

Encourage active role in planning activities, establishing realistic/attainable daily goals. Encourage patient control and responsibility as much as possible. Identify things that the patient can and cannot control.

May enhance feelings of control and self-worth and sense of personal responsibility. Note: Many factors associated with the treatments used in this debilitating, and often fatal disease process, place the patient at the mercy of medical personnel and other unknown people who may be making decisions for and about the patient without regard for the patient's loss of independence.

NURSING DIAGNOSIS:	**KNOWLEDGE DEFICIT [LEARNING NEED] (SPECIFY)**
May be related to:	**Lack of exposure/recall; information misinterpretation**
	Cognitive limitation
	Unfamiliarity with information resources
Possibly evidenced by:	**Questions/request for information; statement of misconception**
	Inaccurate follow-through of instructions/development of preventable complications
PATIENT OUTCOMES/ EVALUATION CRITERIA:	**Verbalizes understanding of condition/disease process and treatment. Identifies relationship of signs/ symptoms to the disease process and correlates symptoms with causative factors. Correctly performs necessary procedures and explains reasons for actions. Initiates necessary lifestyle changes and participates in treatment regimen.**

ACTIONS/INTERVENTIONS	RATIONALE

Independent

Review disease process and future expectations.	Provides knowledge base on which patient can make informed choices.
Identify person's level of dependence and physical condition.	Helps to plan amount of care and symptom management required.
Assess extent of care and support available from family/SO and need for other care givers.	Identifies resources to help carry out treatment plan.
Review modes of transmission of disease.	Corrects myths and misconceptions; promotes safety for patient/others.
Instruct patient and care givers concerning infection control, e.g.: good handwashing for everyone (patient, family, care givers); use of gloves when handling bedpans, dressings/soiled linens; wearing mask if patient has productive cough; placing soiled/wet linens in plastic bag and separating from family laundry; washing with detergent and hot water; cleaning surfaces with solution of 1 part bleach to 10 parts water; disinfecting toilet bowl/bedpan with full-strength bleach; preparing patient's food in clean area; washing dishes, utensils in hot soapy water (can be washed with the family dishes).	Reduces transmission of diseases.
Review dietary needs (high-protein and -calorie) and ways to improve intake when anorexia, diarrhea, weakness, depression interfere with intake.	Promotes adequate nutrition necessary for healing and support of immune system, enhances feeling of well-being.
Discuss medication regimen, interactions and side effects.	Enhances cooperation with/increases probability of success with therapeutic regimen.
Stress importance of adequate rest.	Prevents/reduces fatigue, enhances abilities.
Encourage activity/exercise to patient tolerance.	Stimulates release of endorphins in the brain, enhancing sense of well-being.
Stress necessity of continued health care and follow-up.	Provides opportunity for altering regimen to meet individual/changing needs.
Recommend cessation of smoking.	Smoking increases risk of respiratory infections and can impair immune system (decrease oxygen-combining power with RBCs).
Identify signs/symptoms requiring medical evaluation, e.g., persistent fever/night sweats, swollen glands, continued weight loss, diarrhea, skin blotches/lesions, headache, chest pain, dyspnea.	Early recognition of developing complications and timely interventions may prevent progression to life-threatening situation.
Identify community resources, e.g., hospice/residential care centers, VNA, homecare services, Meals-on-Wheels, peer group.	Facilitates transfer from acute care setting; supports recovery and independence.

Rheumatoid Arthritis _____

Rheumatoid arthritis (RA) is a chronic inflammatory systemic disease of unknown cause, characterized by destruction and proliferation of the synovial membrane, resulting in joint destruction, ankylosis, and deformity. Immunologic mechanisms appear to play an important role in the initiation and perpetuation of the disease.

PATIENT ASSESSMENT DATA BASE

Data are dependent on severity and involvement of other organs (e.g., eyes, heart, lungs), stage (i.e., acute exacerbation or remission), and coexistence of other forms of arthritis.

ACTIVITY/REST

May report: Joint pain with motion, or tenderness, worsened by stress placed on joint; morning stiffness.

Functional disability (ADLs, job performance, sexual activity).

May exhibit: Malaise.

Limited ROM; atrophy of muscle, skin; joint and muscle contractures.

EGO INTEGRITY

May report: Acute/chronic stress factors; e.g., financial, employment, disability, relationship factors.

Hopelessness and powerlessness (incapacitating situation).

Threat to self-concept, body image, personal identity (dependent on others).

FOOD/FLUID

May report: Inability to obtain/consume adequate food/fluids, nausea.

May exhibit: Weight loss.

Dryness of mucous membranes.

HYGIENE

May report: Difficulty performing the simplest self-care activities.

NEUROSENSORY

May report: Paresthesia of hands and feet.

May exhibit: Symmetric joint swelling.

PAIN/COMFORT

May report: Acute episodes of pain (may/may not be accompanied by soft tissue swelling in joints).

Chronic aching pain and stiffness (mornings are most difficult).

SAFETY

May report: Shiny, taut skin; subcutaneous nodules.

Skin/periarticular local warmth, erythema.

Compromised skin/tissue integrity.

Difficulty managing homemaker/maintenance tasks.

Low-grade fever.

Dryness of eyes, mucous membranes.

SOCIAL INTERACTION

May report: Impaired interactions with family/others; change in roles; isolation.

TEACHING/LEARNING

May report: Familial history of RA (in juvenile onset).

Use of health foods, vitamins, untested arthritis "cures".

Discharge Plan Considerations: May require assistance with transportation, self-care, and homemaker tasks; changes in physical layout of home.

DIAGNOSTIC STUDIES

Latex fixation: positive in 75% of typical cases.

Agglutination reactions: positive in over 50% of typical cases

Sedimentation rate (ESR): usually greatly increased (80–100 in 1 hour). May return to normal as symptoms improve.

WBC: elevated when inflammatory processes are present.

Immunoglobins (IgM and IgG): elevation strongly suggests autoimmune process as cause for RA.

X-rays of involved joints: reveals soft tissue swelling, erosion of joints, and osteoporosis of adjacent bone (early changes) progressing to bone cyst formation, narrowing of joint space, and subluxation. Concurrent osteoarthritic changes.

Radionuclide scans: identify inflamed synovium.

Direct arthroscopy: visualization of area reveals bone irregularities/degeneration of joint.

Synovial fluid aspirate: may reveal volume greater than normal; opaque, cloudy, yellow appearance (inflammatory response, bleeding, degenerative waste products); elevated WBCs and leukocytes.

NURSING PRIORITIES

1. Alleviate pain.
2. Increase mobility.
3. Promote positive self-concept.
4. Support independence.
5. Provide information about disease process/prognosis and treatment needs.

DISCHARGE CRITERIA

1. Pain relieved/controlled.
2. Dealing realistically with current situation.
3. Managing ADLs by self/with assistance as needed.
4. Disease process/prognosis and therapeutic regimen understood.

NURSING DIAGNOSIS:	COMFORT, ALTERED: PAIN, ACUTE/CHRONIC
May be related to:	**Injuring agents: distention of tissues by accumulation of fluid/inflammatory process**
Possibly evidenced by:	**Complaints of pain/discomfort, fatigue**
	Self/narrowed focus
	Distraction behaviors/autonomic responses
	Guarding/protective behavior

755

PATIENT OUTCOMES/ EVALUATION CRITERIA:	Reports pain is relieved/controlled. Appears relaxed, able to sleep/rest and participate in activities appropriately. Follows prescribed pharmacologic regimen. Incorporates relaxation skills and diversional activities into pain control program.

ACTIONS/INTERVENTIONS	RATIONALE
Independent	
Investigate complaints of pain, noting location, and intensity (scale of 1–10). Note precipitating factors and nonverbal pain cues.	Helpful in determining pain management needs and effectiveness of program.
Provide firm mattress, bedboards. Use bed cradle as needed.	Soft/sagging mattress prevents maintenance of proper body alignment, placing stress on affected joints. Elevation of bed linens reduces pressure on inflamed/painful joints.
Have patient assume position of comfort while in bed or sitting in chair. Promote bedrest as indicated.	In severe disease/acute exacerbation, total bedrest may be necessary (until objective and subjective improvements are seen) to limit pain/injury to joint.
Maintain neutral position of affected joints with pillows, sandbags, trochanter rolls, splints, braces.	Rests painful joints.
Encourage frequent changes of position. Assist patient to move in bed, supporting affected joints above and below, avoiding jerky movements.	Prevents general fatigue and joint stiffness. Stabilizes joint, decreasing joint movement/pain.
Recommend patient take warm bath or shower on arising. Apply warm moist compresses to affected joints several times a day.	Heat promotes muscle relaxation and mobility, decreases pain and relieves morning stiffness.
Monitor water temperature of compress.	Sensitivity to heat may be diminished and dermal injury may occur.
Provide gentle massage.	Promotes relaxation/reduces muscle tension.
Encourage use of stress management techniques, e.g., progressive relaxation, Therapeutic Touch, biofeedback, visualization, guided imagery, self-hypnosis, and controlled breathing.	Promotes relaxation, provides sense of control and may enhance coping abilities.
Involve in diversional activities appropriate for individual situation.	Refocuses attention, provides stimulation, and enhances self-esteem and feelings of general well-being.
Medicate prior to planned activities/exercises as indicated.	Promotes relaxation, reduces muscle tension/spasms, facilitating participation in therapy.
Collaborative	
Administer medications as indicated, e.g.:	
Acetylsalicylates (aspirin);	ASA exerts an antiinflammatory and mild analgesic effect decreasing stiffness and increasing mobility. Must be taken regularly in order to sustain a blood level between 18–25 mg. Exact mechanism is unknown but may be due to salicylate-induced reduction of capillary permeability, inhibition of mucopolysaccharide syntheses, and oxidative phosphorylation.
Other nonsteroid antiinflammatory drugs (NSAIDs), e.g., ibuprofen (Motrin), naproxen (Naprosyn);	May be used when patient does not respond to aspirin or to enhance effects of aspirin.

ACTIONS/INTERVENTIONS	RATIONALE
Collaborative	
D-penicillamine (Cuprimine);	May control systemic effects of RA if other therapies have not been successful. High rate of side effects (e.g., thrombocytopenia, leukopenia, aplastic anemia) necessitates close monitoring. Note: Drug should be given between meals because drug absorption is impaired by food as well as antacids and iron products.
Antacids;	Given with NSAID agents to minimize gastric irritation/discomfort.
Codeine products.	Although narcotics are generally contraindicated because of chronic nature of condition, short-term use may be required during periods of acute exacerbation to control severe pain.
Assist with physical therapy, e.g., paraffin glove, whirlpool baths.	Provides sustained heat to affected joints.
Apply ice or cold packs when indicated.	Cold relieves pain and swelling. Heat may be contraindicated in the presence of hot, swollen joints.
Maintain TENS unit if used.	Constant low-level electrical stimulus blocks transmission of pain sensations.
Prepare for surgical interventions, e.g., synovectomy.	Removal of inflamed synovium can alleviate pain and limit progression of degenerative changes.

NURSING DIAGNOSIS:	MOBILITY, IMPAIRED PHYSICAL
May be related to:	**Skeletal deformity**
	Pain, discomfort
	Intolerance to activity; decreased muscle strength
Possibly evidenced by:	**Reluctance to attempt movement/inability to purposefully move within the physical environment**
	Limited range of motion, impaired coordination, decreased muscle strength/control and mass (late)
PATIENT OUTCOMES/ EVALUATION CRITERIA:	**Maintains position of function and absence of contractures. Maintains or increases strength and function of affected and/or compensatory body part. Demonstrates techniques/behaviors that enable resumption/continuation of activities.**

ACTIONS/INTERVENTIONS	RATIONALE
Independent	
Evaluate/continuously monitor degree of joint inflammation/ pain.	Level of activity/exercise is dependent on progression/resolution of inflammatory process.
Maintain bed/chair rest when indicated and encourage frequent rest periods.	Systemic rest is mandatory during acute exacerbations and important throughout all phases of disease.

ACTIONS/INTERVENTIONS	RATIONALE

Independent

Assist with active/passive ROM as well as resistive exercises and isometrics when able.

Maintains/improves joint function, muscle strength and general stamina. Note: Inadequate exercise leads to joint stiffening, whereas excessive activity can damage joints.

Reposition frequently with adequate personnel. Demonstrate/assist with transfer techniques and use of mobility aids, e.g., trapeze.

Relives pressure on tissues and promotes circulation. Facilitates self-care and patient's independence. Proper transfer techniques prevent shearing abrasions of skin.

Position with pillows, sandbags, trochanter rolls, splints, braces.

Promotes joint stability (reducing risk of injury) and maintains proper joint position and body alignment, minimizing contractures.

Use small/thin pillow under neck.

Prevents flexion of neck.

Provide safe environment, e.g., raised chairs/toilet seat, use of handrails in tub/shower and toilet, proper use of mobility aids/wheelchair safety.

Avoids accidental injuries/falls.

Collaborative

Consult with physical/occupational therapists and vocational specialist.

Useful in formulating exercise/activity program based on individual needs and in identifying mobility devices/adjuncts.

Provide foam/alternating pressure mattress.

Decreases pressure on fragile tissues to reduce risks of immobility.

Administer medications as indicated:

Antirheumatic agents, e.g., gold, sodium thiomaleate (Myochrysine) or auranofin (Ridaura);

Chrysotherapy (gold salts) may produce dramatic/sustained remission but may result in rebound inflammation if discontinued or serious side effects occur, e.g., nitritoid crisis with dizziness, blurred vision, flushing, progressing to anaphylactic shock.

Steroids.

May be necessary to suppress acute systemic inflammation.

Prepare for surgical interventions, e.g.:

Arthroplasty;

Correction of periarticular weakness and subluxation promotes joint stability.

Tunnel release procedures, tendon repair, ganglionectomy;

Corrects associated connective tissue defects, enhances function and mobility.

Joint implant.

Replacement may be needed to restore optimal functioning and mobility. (Refer to CP: Total Joint Replacement, p. 705.)

NURSING DIAGNOSIS:	SELF-CONCEPT, DISTURBANCE IN: (SPECIFY)
May be related to:	**Changes in ability to perform usual tasks**
	Increased energy expenditure; impaired mobility
Possibly evidenced by:	**Change in structure/function of affected parts**
	Negative self-talk, focus on past strength/function, appearance

Change in lifestyle/physical ability to resume roles, loss of employment, dependence on SO for assistance

Change in social involvement; sense of isolation

Feelings of helplessness, hopelessness

PATIENT OUTCOMES/ EVALUATION CRITERIA: Verbalizes increased confidence in ability to deal with illness, changes in lifestyle, and possible limitations, and makes realistic goals/plans for future.

ACTIONS/INTERVENTIONS	RATIONALE
Independent	
Encourage verbalization about concerns of disease process, future expectations.	Provides opportunity to identify fears/misconceptions and deal with directly.
Discuss meaning of loss/change to patient/SO. Ascertain how patient views self as a man/woman in usual lifestyle functioning, including sexual aspects. Discuss patient's perception of how SO perceives limitations.	Identifying how illness affects perception of self and interactions with others will determine need for further intervention/counseling. Verbal/nonverbal cues from SO may have a major impact on how patient views self.
Acknowledge and accept feelings of grief, hostility, dependency.	Constant pain is wearing, and feelings of anger and hostility are common. Acceptance provides feedback that feelings are normal.
Note withdrawn behavior, use of denial or overconcern with body/changes.	May suggest emotional exhaustion or maladaptive coping methods, requiring more in-depth intervention/ psychologic support.
Set limits on maladaptive behavior. Assist patient to identify positive behaviors that will aid in coping.	Helps patient to maintain self-control, which enhances self-esteem.
Involve patient in planning care and scheduling activities.	Enhances feelings of competency/self-worth, encourages independence, and participation in therapy.
Assist with grooming needs as necessary.	Maintaining appearance enhances self-image.
Give positive reinforcement for accomplishments.	Allows patient to feel good about self. Reinforces positive behavior. Enhances self-confidence.

(Refer to CP: Psychosocial Aspects of Acute Care, p. 773.)

Collaborative	
Refer to psychiatric counseling, e.g., clinical specialist psychiatric nurse, psychiatrist/psychologist, social worker.	Patient/SO may require ongoing support to deal with long-term/debilitating process.
Administer medications as indicated, e.g.:	
Tranquilizers and mood-elevating drugs.	May be needed in presence of severe depression until patient develops more effective coping skills.

NURSING DIAGNOSIS: SELF-CARE DEFICIT: (SPECIFY)

May be related to: Musculoskeletal impairment; decreased strength, endurance, pain on movement

Depression

Possibly evidenced by:	Inability to manage ADLs (feeding, bathing, dressing, and toileting)
PATIENT OUTCOMES/ EVALUATION CRITERIA:	Performs self-care activities at a level consistent with individual capabilities. Demonstrates techniques/ lifestyle changes to meet self-care needs. Identifies personal/community resources that can provide needed assistance.

ACTIONS/INTERVENTIONS

Independent

Discuss usual level of functioning (0–4) prior to onset/ exacerbation of illness and potential changes now anticipated.

Maintain mobility, pain control, and exercise program.

Assess barriers to participation in self-care. Identify/ plan for environmental modifications.

Allow patient sufficient time to complete tasks to fullest extent of ability. Capitalize on individual strengths.

Collaborative

Arrange VNA home evaluation prior to discharge with follow-up afterward.

Arrange for consult with other agencies, e.g., Meals-on-Wheels, home care service, nutritionist.

RATIONALE

May be able to continue usual activities with necessary adaptations to current limitations.

Supports physical/emotional independence.

Prepares for increased independence, which enhances self-esteem.

May need more time to complete tasks by self but provides an opportunity for greater sense of self-confidence and self-worth.

Identifies problems that may be encountered because of current level of disability. Provides for more successful team efforts with others who are involved in care, e.g., occupational therapy team.

May need additional kinds of assistance to continue in home setting.

NURSING DIAGNOSIS:	HOME MAINTENANCE MANAGEMENT, IMPAIRED [POTENTIAL]
May be related to:	Long-term degenerative disease process
	Inadequate support systems
Possibly evidenced by:	[Not applicable; presence of signs and symptoms establishes an *actual* diagnosis.]
PATIENT OUTCOMES/ EVALUATION CRITERIA:	Maintains safe, growth-promoting environment. Demonstrates appropriate, effective use of resources.

ACTIONS/INTERVENTIONS

Independent

Assess level of physical functioning.

Evaluate environment to assess ability to care for self.

RATIONALE

Identifies degree of assistance/support required.

Determines feasibility of remaining in/changing home layout to meet individual needs.

ACTIONS/INTERVENTIONS

Independent

Determine financial resources to meet needs of individual situation. Identify support systems available to patient, e.g., extended family, friends/neighbors.

Develop plan for maintaining a clean, healthful environment, e.g., sharing of household repair/tasks between family members or by contract services.

Identify sources for necessary equipment, e.g., lifts, elevated toilet seat, wheelchair.

Collaborative

Refer to community resources, e.g., VNA, homemaker service, social services, senior citizens groups.

RATIONALE

Availability of personal resources/community supports will affect ability to problem-solve solutions.

Assures that needs will be met on an ongoing basis.

Provides opportunity to acquire equipment before discharge.

Can facilitate transfer to/support continuation in home setting.

NURSING DIAGNOSIS:	KNOWLEDGE DEFICIT [LEARNING NEED] (SPECIFY)
May be related to:	**Lack of exposure/recall**
	Information misinterpretation
Possibly evidenced by:	**Questions/request for information, statement of misconception**
	Inaccurate follow-through of instruction/development of preventable complications
PATIENT OUTCOMES/ EVALUATION CRITERIA:	**Verbalizes understanding of condition/prognosis, treatment. Develops a plan for self-care, including lifestyle modifications consistent with mobility and/or activity restrictions.**

ACTIONS/INTERVENTIONS

Independent

Review disease process, prognosis, and future expectations.

Discuss patient's role in management of disease process through diet, medication, and balanced program of exercise and rest.

Assist in planning a realistic and integrated schedule of activity, rest, personal care, drug administration, physical therapy, and stress management.

Stress importance of continued pharmacotherapeutic management.

Recommend use of enteric coated/buffered aspirin or nonacetylated salicylates, e.g., choline salicylate (Arthropan) or choline magnesium trisalicylate (Trilisate).

RATIONALE

Provides knowledge base on which patient can make informed choices.

Goal of disease control is to suppress inflammation in joints/other tissues to maintain joint function and prevent deformities.

Provides structure and defuses anxiety when managing a complex chronic disease process.

Benefits of drug therapy are dependent on correct dosage; e.g., aspirin must be taken regularly in order to sustain therapeutic blood levels of 18–25 mg.

Coated/buffered preparations ingested with food, etc., minimize gastric irritation, reducing risk of bleeding/hemorrhage. Note: Nonacetylated products have a longer half-life, requiring less frequent administration in addition to producing less gastric irritation.

ACTIONS/INTERVENTIONS	RATIONALE

Independent

Suggest ingestion of medications with meals, milk products or antacids and at bedtime.	Limits gastric irritation. Reduction of pain at HS enhances sleep and increased blood level decreases early morning stiffness.
Identify adverse drug effects, e.g., tinnitus, gastric intolerance, GI bleeding, purpuric rash.	Prolonged, maximal doses of aspirin may result in overdose. Tinnitus usually indicates high therapeutic blood levels. If tinnitus occurs, the dosage is usually decreased by one tablet every 2–3 days until it stops.
Stress importance of reading product labels and refraining from OTC drug usage without prior medical approval.	Many products contain hidden salicylates (e.g., cold remedies, antidiarrheals) that increase risk of drug overdose/harmful side effects.
Review importance of balanced diet with foods high in vitamins, protein, and iron.	Promotes general well-being and tissue repair/regeneration.
Encourage obese patient to lose weight and supply with weight reduction information as appropriate.	Weight loss will reduce stress on joints, especially hips, knees, ankles, feet.
Provide information about assistive devices, e.g., wheeled dolly/wagon for moving items, pickup sticks, light-weight dishes and pans, raised toilet seats, safety handle bars.	Reduces force exerted on joints and enables individual to participate more comfortably in needed/desired activities.
Discuss energy-saving techniques, e.g., sitting instead of standing to prepare meals, shower.	Prevents fatigue, facilitates self-care and independence.
Encourage maintenance of correct body position and posture both at rest and during activity, e.g., keeping joints extended, not flexed, wearing splints for prescribed time periods, avoidance of remaining in one position for extended periods of time.	Good body mechanics must become a part of the patient's lifestyle to lessen joint stress and pain.
Review necessity of frequent inspection of skin and meticulous skin care under splints, casts, supporting devices. Demonstrate proper padding.	Reduces risk of skin irritation/breakdown.
Discuss necessity of medical follow-up/laboratory studies, e.g., ESR, salicylate levels, prothrombin time.	Drug therapy requires frequent assessment/refinement to assure optimal effect and to prevent overdose/dangerous side effects, e.g., aspirin prolongs prothrombin time, increasing risk of bleeding. Chrysotherapy depresses platelets, potentiating risk of thrombocytopenia.
Provide for sexual counseling as necessary.	Information about different positions and techniques and/or other options for sexual fulfillment may enhance personal relationships and feelings of self-worth/self-esteem.
Identify community resources, e.g., Arthritis Foundation.	Assistance/support from others promotes maximal recovery.

CHAPTER 16

SYSTEMIC INFECTIONS

Sepsis/Septicemia _____

Sepsis is a syndrome characterized by clinical signs and symptoms of severe infection which may progress to septicemia and septic shock.

Septicemia implies the presence of a systemic infection of the blood caused by rapidly multiplying microorganisms or their toxins which can result in profound physiologic changes. The pathogens can be bacteria, fungi, viruses, or rickettsiae. The most common causes of septicemia are gram-negative organisms. If the defense system of the body is not effective in controlling the invading microorganisms, septic shock may result, characterized by altered hemodynamics, impaired cellular function, and multiple system failure.

PATIENT ASSESSMENT DATA BASE

Data are dependent on the type, location, duration of the infective process and organ involvement. (Refer to specific CPs as appropriate, e.g., Bacterial Pneumonia, p. 138; Pulmonary Tuberculosis, p. 202; Inflammatory Cardiac Conditions, p. 109; Intracranial Infections, p. 258; Peritonitis, p. 444; AIDS, p. 733.)

ACTIVITY/REST

May report: Malaise.

CIRCULATION

May exhibit: Blood pressure normal/slightly low normal range (as long as cardiac output remains elevated).

Peripheral pulses bounding, rapid (hyperdynamic phase); weak/thready/easily obliterated, extreme tachycardia (shock).

Heart sounds: dysrhythmias and development of S_3 suggest myocardial dysfunction, effects of acidosis/electrolyte imbalance.

Skin warm, dry, flushed (vasodilation), pale, cold, clammy, mottled (vasoconstriction).

ELIMINATION

May report: Diarrhea.

FOOD/FLUID

May report: Anorexia; nausea/vomiting.

May exhibit:	Weight loss, decreased subcutaneous fat/muscle mass (malnutrition).
	Urine output decreased, concentrated; progressing to oliguria, anuria.

NEUROSENSORY

May report:	Headache; dizziness, fainting.
May exhibit:	Restlessness, apprehension, confusion, disorientation, delirium/coma.

PAIN/COMFORT

May report:	Abdominal tenderness, localized pain/discomfort.
	Generalized urticaria/pruritus.

RESPIRATION

May exhibit:	Tachypnea with decreased respiratory depth, dyspnea.
	Basilar crackles, rhonchi, wheezes (developing pulmonary complications/onset of cardiac decompensation).

SAFETY

May report:	Immunosuppression: cancer therapies, corticosteroid use.
May exhibit:	Temperature: usually elevated (101°F or greater) but may be normal in elderly or compromised patient; occasionally subnormal (under 98.6°F).
	Fever, shaking chills.
	Poor/delayed wound healing, purulent drainage, localized erythema.
	Macular erythematous rash.

SEXUALITY

May report:	Perineal pruritus.
	Recent childbirth/abortion.
May exhibit:	Maceration of vulva, purulent vaginal drainage.

TEACHING/LEARNING

May report:	Chronic/debilitating health problems, e.g., liver, renal, cardiac disease; cancer; alcoholism.
	History of splenectomy.
	Recent surgery/invasive procedures, traumatic wounds.
	Antibiotic use (recent or long-term).
Discharge Plan Considerations:	May require assistance with wound care/supplies, treatments, self-care, and homemaker tasks.

DIAGNOSTIC STUDIES

Cultures (wound, sputum, urine, blood): may identify organism(s) causing the sepsis. Sensitivity determines most effective drug choices. Catheter/intravascular line tips may need to be removed and cultured if the portal of entry is unknown.

CBC: Hct may be elevated in hypovolemic states due to hemoconcentration. Leukopenia (decreased WBCs) occurs early, followed by a rebound leukocytosis with increased bands (shift to the left) indicating rapid production of immature WBCs.

Serum electrolytes: various imbalances may occur due to acidosis, fluid shifts, and altered renal function.

Clotting studies:

　Platelets: decreased levels (thrombocytopenia) can occur due to platelet aggregation.

PT/PTT: may be prolonged indicating coagulopathy associated with liver ischemia/circulating toxins/shock state.

Serum lactate: elevated in metabolic acidosis, liver dysfunction, shock.

Serum glucose: hyperglycemia occurs reflecting gluconeogenesis and glycogenolysis in the liver in response to cellular starvation/alteration in metabolism.

BUN/creatinine: increased levels are associated with dehydration, renal impairment/failure, and liver dysfunction/failure.

ABGs: respiratory alkalosis and hypoxemia may occur early. In later stages, respiratory and metabolic acidosis occur due to failure of compensatory mechanisms.

Urinalysis: presence of WBCs/bacteria suggests infection.

X-rays: abdominal and lower chest films indicating free air in the abdomen may suggest infection due to perforated abdominal/pelvic organ.

NURSING PRIORITIES

1. Eliminate infection.
2. Support tissue perfusion/circulatory volume.
3. Prevent complications.
4. Provide information about disease process, prognosis, and treatment needs.

DISCHARGE CRITERIA

1. Infection eliminated/controlled.
2. Homeostasis maintained.
3. Complications prevented/minimized.
4. Disease process, prognosis, and therapeutic regimen understood.

NURSING DIAGNOSIS:	INFECTION, POTENTIAL FOR [PROGRESSION OF SEPSIS TO SEPTIC SHOCK/DEVELOPMENT OF OPPORTUNISTIC INFECTIONS]
May be related to:	Compromised immune system
	Failure to recognize/treat infection, and/or exercise proper preventive measures
	Environmental exposure (nosocomial)
Possibly evidenced by:	[Not applicable; presence of signs and symptoms establishes an *actual* diagnosis.]
PATIENT OUTCOMES/ EVALUATION CRITERIA:	Achieves timely healing, free of purulent secretions/drainage or erythema, and is afebrile.

ACTIONS/INTERVENTIONS	RATIONALE
Independent	
Provide isolation/monitor visitors as indicated.	Wound/linen isolation may be all that is required for draining wounds while reverse isolation/restriction of visitors may be needed to protect the immunosuppressed patient. Reduces risk of opportunistic infections.
Wash hands before/after each care activity even if sterile gloves are used.	Reduces risk of cross contamination.

ACTIONS/INTERVENTIONS	RATIONALE

Independent

Encourage frequent change of position, deep breathing/coughing.

Good pulmonary toilet may prevent pneumonia.

Encourage patient to cover mouth and nose with tissue during coughs/sneezes.

Prevents spread of infection via airborne droplets.

Limit use of invasive devices/procedures when possible.

Reduces number of sites for entry of opportunistic organisms.

Inspect wounds/site of invasive devices daily, paying particular attention to hyperalimentation lines. Note signs of local inflammation/infection, changes in character of wound drainage or sputum, urine.

May provide clue to portal of entry, type of infecting organism(s), as well as early identification of secondary infections. Note: High nutrient content of TPN provides excellent media for bacterial growth.

Use sterile technique when changing dressings/suctioning/providing site care, e.g., invasive line, urinary catheter.

Prevents introduction of bacteria, reducing risk of nosocomial infection.

Wear gloves/gowns when caring for open wounds/anticipating direct contact with secretions or excretions.

Prevents spread of infection/cross-contamination.

Dispose of soiled dressings/materials in double bag.

Reduces contamination/soilage of area, limits spread of airborne organisms.

Monitor temperature trends.

Fever (101–105°F/38.5–40°C) is caused by the effect of endotoxins on the hypothalamus and pyrogen-released endorphins. Hypothermia (<96°F/36°C) is a grave sign reflecting advancing shock state/decreased tissue perfusion.

Observe for shaking chills and profuse diaphoresis.

Chills often precede temperature spikes in presence of generalized infection.

Monitor for signs of deterioration of condition/failure to improve during therapy.

May reflect inappropriate/inadequate antibiotic therapy or overgrowth of resistant/opportunistic organisms.

Inspect oral cavity. Investigate complaints of vaginal/perineal itching or burning.

Depression of immune system and use of antibiotics increases risk of secondary infections, particularly yeast.

Collaborative

Obtain specimens of urine, blood, sputum, wound, invasive lines/tubes as indicated for Gram stain, culture and sensitivity.

Identification of portal of entry and organism causing the septicemia is crucial to effective treatment.

Administer medications as indicated:

Broad-spectrum antibiotics, e.g., ampicillin (Omnipen); gram-negative, e.g., Ticarcillin disodium (Ticar); gram-positive, e.g., nafcillin (Nafcil), vancomycin (Vancocin); aminoglycosides, e.g., tobramycin (Nebcin), gentamicin (Garamycin); cephalosporins, e.g., cefotaxime (Claforan);

Specific antibiotics are determined by culture results, but therapy is usually initiated prior to obtaining results, using broad-spectrum antibiotics and/or based on most likely infecting organisms. Concomitant use of antimicrobials is often beneficial, but dosage must be balanced against renal function/clearance.

Immune globulins as appropriate.

May boost/provide temporary immunity to general infection or specific illness, e.g., varicella zoster, rabies.

Assist with/prepare for incision and drainage of wound, irrigation, application of warm/moist soaks as indicated.

Facilitates removal of purulent material/necrotic tissue and promotes healing.

NURSING DIAGNOSIS:	HYPERTHERMIA
May be related to:	Increased metabolic rate, illness
	Dehydration
	Direct effect of circulating endotoxins on the hypothalmus, altering temperature regulation
Possibly evidenced by:	Increase in body temperature above normal range
	Flushed skin, warm to touch
	Increased respiratory rate, tachycardia
PATIENT OUTCOMES/ EVALUATION CRITERIA:	Demonstrates temperature within normal range, free of chills and associated complications.

ACTIONS/INTERVENTIONS

Independent

Monitor patient temperature (degree and pattern), note shaking chills/profuse diaphoresis.

Monitor environmental temperature; limit/add bed linens as indicated.

Provide tepid sponge baths; avoid use of alcohol.

Collaborative

Administer antipyretics, e.g., acetylsalicylic acid (aspirin), acetaminophen (Tylenol).

Provide cooling blanket.

RATIONALE

Temperature of 102–106°F (38.9–41.1°C) suggests acute infectious disease process. Fever pattern may aid in diagnosis; e.g., sustained or continuous fever curves lasting more than 24 hours suggest pneumococcal pneumonia, scarlet or typhoid fever; remittent fever (varying only a few degrees in either direction) reflects pulmonary infections; intermittent curves or fever that returns to normal once in 24-hour period suggest septic episode, septic endocarditis, or tuberculosis. Chills often precede temperature spikes. Note: Use of antipyretics alters fever patterns.

Room temperature/number of blankets should be altered to maintain near normal temperature.

May help reduce fever. Note: Use of ice water/alcohol may cause chills, actually elevating temperature. In addition, alcohol is very drying to skin.

Used to reduce fever by its central action on the hypothalamus, although fever may be beneficial in limiting growth of organisms and enhancing autodestruction of infected cells.

Used to reduce fever usually greater than 104–105°F (39.5–40°C), when brain damage/seizures can occur.

NURSING DIAGNOSIS:	TISSUE PERFUSION, ALTERED: DECREASED [POTENTIAL]
May be related to:	Relative/actual hypovolemia
	Reduction of arterial/venous blood flow: selective vasoconstriction, vascular occlusion (intimal damage/ microemboli)

767

Possibly evidenced by:	[Not applicable; presence of signs and symptoms establishes an *actual* diagnosis.]
PATIENT OUTCOMES/ EVALUATION CRITERIA:	Displays adequate perfusion as evidenced by stable vital signs, palpable peripheral pulses, skin warm and dry, usual level of consciousness, individually appropriate urine output, and active bowel sounds.

ACTIONS/INTERVENTIONS	RATIONALE
Independent	
Maintain bedrest; assist with ADLs.	Decreases myocardial workload and oxygen consumption, maximizing effectiveness of tissue perfusion.
Monitor trends in blood pressure, noting progressive hypotension and changes in pulse pressure.	Hypotension develops as microorganisms invade the bloodstream, stimulating release or activation of chemical and hormonal substances, which initially results in peripheral vasodilation, decreased systemic vascular resistance, and relative hypovolemia. As shock progresses, cardiac output becomes severely depressed because of major alterations in contractility and preload/afterload, producing profound hypotension.
Monitor heart rate, rhythm. Note dysrhythmias.	Tachycardia occurs, due to sympathetic nervous system stimulation secondary to stress response and to compensate for the relative hypovolemia and hypotension. Cardiac dysrhythmias can occur as a result of hypoxia, acid-base/electrolyte imbalance, and/or low-flow perfusion state.
Note quality/strength of peripheral pulses.	Initially the pulse is strong/bounding because of increased cardiac output. Pulse may become weak/thready because of sustained hypotension, decreased cardiac output, and peripheral vasoconstriction if the shock state progresses.
Assess respiratory rate, depth and quality. Note onset of severe dyspnea.	Increased respirations occur in response to direct effects of endotoxins on the respiratory center in the brain, as well as developing hypoxia, stress and fever. Respiration can become shallow as respiratory insufficiency develops, creating risk of acute respiratory failure. (Refer to ND: Gas Exchange, Impaired, p. 770.)
Investigate changes in sensorium, e.g., mental cloudiness, agitation, restlessness, personality changes, delirium, stupor, coma.	Changes reflect alterations in cerebral perfusion, hypoxemia, and/or acidosis.
Assess skin for changes in color, temperature, moisture.	Compensatory mechanism of vasodilitation results in warm, dry, pink skin, which is characteristic of hyperperfusion in hyperdynamic phase of early septic shock. If shock state progresses, compensatory vasoconstriction occurs, shunting blood to vital organs, reducing peripheral blood flow, and creating cool, clammy, pale/dusky skin.
Record hourly urine output and specific gravity.	Decreasing urinary output with increased specific gravity indicates diminished renal perfusion related to fluid shifts and selective vasoconstriction. There may be transient polyuria during hyperdynamic phase (while cardiac output is elevated) but may progress to oliguria. (Refer to CP: Renal Failure; Acute, p. 544.)

ACTIONS/INTERVENTIONS	RATIONALE
Independent	
Auscultate bowel sounds.	Reduced blood flow to the mesentery (splanchnic vasoconstriction) decreases peristalsis and may lead to paralytic ileus.
Monitor gastric pH as indicated. Hematest gastric secretions, stools for occult blood.	Stress of illness and use of steroids increase risk of gastric mucosal erosion/bleeding.
Evaluate lower extremities for local tissue swelling, erythema, positive Homans' sign.	Venous stasis and infectious process may result in the development of thrombosis.
Monitor for signs of bleeding, e.g., oozing from puncture sites/suture lines, petechiae, ecchymoses, hematuria, epistaxis, hemoptysis, hematemesis.	Coagulapathy/DIC may occur related to accelerated clotting in the microcirculation (activation of chemical mediators, vascular insufficiency and cell destruction), creating a life-threatening hemorrhagic situation/multiple emboli.
Note drug effects, and monitor for signs of toxicity.	Massive doses of antibiotics are often ordered which have potentially toxic effects when hepatic/renal perfusion is compromised.
Collaborative	
Administer parenteral fluids. (Refer to ND: Fluid Volume Deficit, Potential, following.)	In order to maintain tissue perfusion, large amounts of fluid may be required to support circulating volume.
Administer drugs as indicated:	
Steroids;	Although controversial, steroids' potential advantages include decreased capillary permeability, increased renal perfusion, and inhibition of microemboli formation.
Sodium bicarbonate;	Impaired tissue perfusion and production of lactate results in metabolic acidosis, requiring base replacement therapy.
Antacids: e.g., aluminum hydroxide (Amphojel).	Decreases potential for gastric bleeding related to stress response/altered perfusion.
Monitor laboratory studies, e.g., ABGs, lactate levels.	Development of respiratory/metabolic acidosis reflects loss of compensatory mechanisms, e.g., decreased renal perfusion/hydrogen excretion; and accumulation of lactic acid due to circulatory shunting/stagnation.
Administer supplemental oxygen.	Maximizes oxygen available for cellular uptake.
Maintain body temperature, using adjunctive aids as necessary. (Refer to ND: Hyperthermia, p. 767.)	Temperature elevations increase metabolic/oxygen demands beyond cellular resources, hastening tissue ischemia/cellular destruction.
Transfer to critical care setting as indicated.	Progression of shock state will require more aggressive therapy (e.g., hemodynamic monitoring and vasoactive drugs).

NURSING DIAGNOSIS:	**FLUID VOLUME DEFICIT, POTENTIAL**
May be related to:	**Marked increase in vascular compartment/massive vasodilatation**
	Capillary permeability/fluid leaks into the interstitial space (third-spacing)

ACTIONS/INTERVENTIONS	RATIONALE
Independent	
Measure/record urine output and specific gravity. Note cumulative I&O imbalances (including all/insensible losses), and correlate with daily weight. Encourage oral fluids to tolerance.	Decreasing urine output with a high specific gravity suggests hypovolemia. Continued positive fluid balance with corresponding weight gain may indicate third spacing and tissue edema, suggesting need to alter fluid therapy/replacement components.
Monitor blood pressure, heart rate. Measure CVP.	Reduction in the circulating fluid volume reduces blood pressure/CVP, initiating compensatory mechanisms of tachycardia in order to improve cardiac output and increase systemic blood pressure.
Palpate peripheral pulses.	Weak, easily obliterated pulses suggest hypovolemia.
Assess for dry mucous membranes, poor skin turgor and thirst.	Hypovolemia/third spacing of fluid gives rise to signs of dehydration.
Observe for dependent/peripheral edema in sacrum, scrotum, back, legs.	Fluid losses from the vascular compartment into the interstitial space create tissue edema.
Collaborative	
Administer IV fluids, e.g., crystalloids (D5W, NS) and colloids (albumin, fresh frozen plasma) as indicated.	Large volumes of fluid may be required to overcome relative hypovolemia (peripheral vasodilation); replace losses from increased capillary permeability (e.g., sequestration of fluid in the peritoneal cavity) and increased insensible sources (e.g., fever/diaphoresis).
Monitor laboratory values, e.g.:	
Hct/RBC count;	Evaluates changes in hydration/blood viscosity.
BUN/creatinine.	Moderate elevations of BUN reflect dehydration, high values of BUN/creatinine may indicate renal dysfunction/failure.

NURSING DIAGNOSIS:	GAS EXCHANGE, IMPAIRED [POTENTIAL]
May be related to:	**Altered oxygen supply: effects of endotoxins on the respiratory center in the medulla (resulting in hyperventilation/respiratory alkalosis); hypoventilation**
	Altered blood flow (changes in vascular resistance), alveolar-capillary membrane changes (increased capillary permeability leading to pulmonary congestion)
	Interference with oxygen delivery/utilization in the tissues (endotoxin-induced damage to the cells/capillaries)
Possibly evidenced by:	**[Not applicable; presence of signs and symptoms establishes an *actual* diagnosis.]**

PATIENT OUTCOMES/ EVALUATION CRITERIA:	Displays ABGs and respiratory rate within patient's normal range; absence of dyspnea/cyanosis; breath sounds clear, and chest x-ray clear/improving.

ACTIONS/INTERVENTIONS	RATIONALE

Independent

Maintain patent airway. Place patient in position of comfort with head of bed elevated.	Enhances lung expansion, respiratory effort.
Monitor respiratory rate and depth. Note use of accessory muscles/work of breathing.	Rapid/shallow respirations occur because of hypoxemia, stress, and circulating endotoxins. Hypoventilation and dyspnea reflect ineffective compensatory mechanisms and are an indication that ventilatory support is needed.
Auscultate breath sounds. Note crackles, wheezes, areas of decreased/absent ventilation.	Respiratory distress and the presence of adventitious sounds are indicators of pulmonary congestion/interstitial edema, atelectasis. Note: Respiratory complications, including pneumonia and ARDS are a prime cause of death. (Refer to CP: Adult Respiratory Distress Syndrome (ARDS), p. 184.)
Note presence of circumoral cyanosis.	Reflects inadequate systemic oxygenation/hypoxemia.
Investigate alterations in sensorium: agitation, confusion, personality changes, delirium, stupor, coma.	Cerebral function is very sensitive to decreases in oxygenation (e.g., hypoxemia/reduced perfusion).
Note cough and purulent sputum production.	Pneumonia is a common nosocomial infection, which can occur by aspiration of oropharyngeal organisms or spread from other sites.
Reposition frequently. Encourage cough and deep breathing exercises. Suction with lavage, as indicated.	Good pulmonary toilet is necessary for reducing ventilation/perfusion imbalance, mobilizing and facilitating removal of secretions, to maximize gas exchange.

Collaborative

Monitor ABGs.	Hypoxemia is related to decreased ventilation/pulmonary changes (e.g., interstitial edema, atelectasis, and pulmonary shunting) and increased demands (e.g., fever). Respiratory acidosis (pH below 7.35 and $PaCO_2$ greater than 40 mmHg) occurs because of hypoventilation and ventilation-perfusion imbalance. As septic condition worsens, metabolic acidosis (pH below 7.35 and bicarbonate less than 22–24 mEq/l) arises due to buildup of lactic acid from anaerobic metabolism.
Administer supplemental oxygen via appropriate route, e.g., nasal cannula, mask, high-flow rebreathing mask.	Necessary for correction of hypoxemia with failing respiratory effort/progressing acidosis. Note: Intubation/mechanical ventilation may be required if respiratory failure develops.
Review chest x-rays.	Changes reflect progression/resolution of pulmonary complications, e.g., infiltrates/edema.

NURSING DIAGNOSIS:	KNOWLEDGE DEFICIT [LEARNING NEED] (SPECIFY)
May be related to:	Lack of exposure/recall; information misinterpretation
	Cognitive limitation

Possibly evidenced by:	Questions/request for information, statement of misconception
	Inaccurate follow-through of instructions/development of preventable complications
PATIENT OUTCOMES/ EVALUATION CRITERIA:	Verbalizes understanding of disease process and prognosis. Correctly performs necessary procedures and explains reasons for the actions. Initiates necessary lifestyle changes and participates in treatment regimen.

ACTIONS/INTERVENTIONS

Independent

Review disease process and future expectations.

Review individual risk factors and mode of transmission/portal of entry of infections.

Identify signs/symptoms requiring medical evaluation, e.g., persistent temperature elevation(s), tachycardia, syncope, rashes of unknown origin, unexplained fatigue, anorexia, increased thirst, and changes in bladder function.

Provide information about drug therapy, interactions, side effects, and importance of adherence to regimen.

Discuss need for good nutritional intake/balanced diet.

Encourage adequate rest periods with scheduled activities.

Review necessity of personal hygiene and environmental cleanliness.

Discuss proper use or avoidance of tampons as indicated.

Stress importance of prophylactic immunization as needed.

RATIONALE

Provides knowledge base on which patient can make informed choices.

Glucocorticoid therapy, kidney/liver dysfunction, neoplastic disease, rheumatic heart disease, valve dysfunction, and diabetes may predispose to septicemia. Being aware of how infection is transmitted provides opportunity to plan for/institute protective measures.

Early recognition of developing/recurring infection allows for timely intervention and reduces risk for progression to life-threatening situation.

Promotes understanding of and enhances cooperation in treatment/prophylaxis and reduces risk of recurrence and complications.

Necessary for optimal healing and general well-being.

Prevents fatigue, conserves energy and promotes healing.

Helps to control environmental exposure by diminishing the number of pathogens present.

Superabsorbent tampons/infrequent changing potentiates risk of staphylococcus aureus infection (toxic shock syndrome).

Used for prevention of infection.

Psychosocial Aspects of Acute Care _____

The emotional response of the patient in the acute care setting is of extreme importance. The mind–body connection is well established; for example, when a physiologic response occurs, there is a corresponding psychologic response. Also, there are physiologic conditions that have a psychologic component, for example, the emotional instability of Cushing's syndrome/steroid therapy and the irritability of hypoglycemia. It is not necessarily the event, but rather the patient's perception of the event, that creates problems: unmet psychologic needs drain energy resources needed for healing. Although the stress of illness is well recognized, the effect on the individual is unpredictable.

ASSESSMENT FACTORS TO BE CONSIDERED

INDIVIDUAL

Age and sex.

Religious affiliation: church attendance, importance of religion in patient's life, belief in life after death.

Level of knowledge/education. How does the individual access information (auditory, visual, kinesthetic)?

How does patient define and perceive illness?

Behavior when anxious, afraid, impatient, or angry.

How is patient experiencing illness versus what illness actually is?

Emotional response to current treatment and hospitalization? Past experience with illness and hospitalization?

Describe emotional reaction in feeling (sensory) terms: e.g., "States 'I feel scared.' "

Patterns of communication with significant others, with health care givers? Style of speech?

Perception of body and its functions. When well? In illness? This illness?

What is past experience with health care systems?

SIGNIFICANT OTHERS

Marital status. Who are significant others? Nuclear family? Extended family? Recurring or patterned relationships?

Family developmental cycle: Just married? Children? Young? Adolescent? Children leaving home? Retired?

Patient's role in family tasks and functions.

How are SOs affected by the illness and prognosis?

What are the interaction processes within the family?

Lifestyle differences which need to be considered. Dietary? Spiritual? Sexual preference? Other community?

SOCIOECONOMIC

Employment; finances.

Environmental factors: home, work, and recreation.

Out of usual environment (on vacation, visiting).

Social class; value system.

Social acceptability of disease.

CULTURAL

Ethnic background.

Health-seeking behaviors; illness referral system.

Values related to health and treatment.

Cultural factors in pain response.

Beliefs regarding caring and curing.

DISEASE (ILLNESS)

Kind of illness. How has it been treated? Will it be treated? Should it be treated? Anticipated response to treatment?

Cause of the illness.

What is the threat to others?

Is this an acute/chronic illness? Is it inherited?

If terminal illness, what do the patient and SO know and anticipate?

Is the condition "appropriate" to the afflicted individual?

Is the illness related to personality factors, such as type A (may be myth or valid)?

NURSE-RELATED

Basic knowledge of human beings and the current situation related to response of the individual.

Basic knowledge of biologic, psychologic, social, and cultural issues, as well as therapeutic communication skills.

Knowledge of own value and belief systems.

Willingness to look at own behavior in relation to interaction with others and make changes as necessary.

Respect of patient's privacy; confidentiality.

NURSING PRIORITIES

1. Reduce anxiety/fear.
2. Support grieving process.
3. Facilitate integration of self-concept and body-image changes.
4. Encourage effective coping skills of patient/SO.
5. Promote safe environment/patient well-being.

NURSING DIAGNOSIS:	ANXIETY [SPECIFY LEVEL]/FEAR
May be related to:	**Unconscious conflict about essential values**
	Situational and/or maturational crises
	Interpersonal transmission and contagion
	Threat to self-concept; threat of death; change in health status; unmet needs
	Separation from support system; knowledge deficit
	Sensory impairment; environmental stimuli

Possibly evidenced by:	Reports of increased tension; feelings of helplessness, inadequacy; apprehension, uncertainty; being scared; overexcitedness
	Expressed concern regarding changes in life events; dread of an identifiable problem recognized by the patient; fear of unspecific consequences
	Focus on self; fight/flight behavior
	Facial tension; sympathetic stimulation; extraneous movements
PATIENT OUTCOMES/ EVALUATION CRITERIA:	**Acknowledges and discusses fears. Appears relaxed and reports anxiety is reduced to a manageable level. Verbalizes awareness of feelings of anxiety and healthy ways to deal with them. Demonstrates problem-solving and uses resources effectively.**

ACTIONS/INTERVENTIONS	RATIONALE
Independent	
Note palpitations, elevated pulse/respiratory rate.	Changes in vital signs may suggest the degree of anxiety being experienced by the patient or reflect the impact of physiologic factors, e.g., endocrine imbalances.
Acknowledge fear/anxieties. Validate observations with patient, e.g., "You seem to be afraid?"	Feelings are real, and it is helpful to bring them out in the open so they can be discussed and dealt with.
Assess degree/reality of threat to patient and level of anxiety (e.g., mild, moderate, severe) by observing behavior such as clenched hands, wide eyes, startle response, furrowed brow, clinging to family/staff, or physical/verbal lashing out.	Individual responses can vary according to culturally learned patterns. Distorted perceptions of the situation may magnify feelings.
Note narrowed focus of attention (e.g., patient concentrates on one thing at a time).	Narrowed focus usually reflects extreme fear/panic.
Observe speech content and patterns: rapidity, words, repetition, laughter.	Provides clues about such factors as the level of anxiety, ability to comprehend, brain damage, or possible language differences.
Assess level of severity of pain if present. Delay gathering of information until later if pain is too severe.	Severe pain and anxiety leave little energy for thinking and other activities.
Identify patient's/SO perception(s) of the situation.	Regardless of the reality of the situation, perception affects how each individual deals with the illness/ stress.
Acknowledge reality of the situation as the patient sees it without challenging the belief.	Patient may need to deny reality until ready to deal with it. It is not helpful to force the patient to face facts.
Evaluate coping/defense mechanisms being used to deal with the perceived or real threat.	May be dealing well with the situation at the moment; e.g., denial and regression may be helpful coping mechanisms for a time. However, they use energy the patient needs for healing and need to be dealt with at some point in time.
Review coping mechanisms used in the past if possible, e.g., problem-solving skills, recognizing/asking for help.	Provides opportunity to build on resources the patient/ SO may have available.

ACTIONS/INTERVENTIONS	RATIONALE

Independent

Maintain frequent contacts with the patient/SO. Be available for listening and talking as needed.

Establishes rapport, promotes expression of feelings, and helps patient and SO look at realities of the illness/treatment without confronting issues they are not ready to deal with.

Acknowledge feelings as they are expressed. If actions are unacceptable, take necessary steps to control/deal with behavior. (Refer to ND: Violence, Potential for, p. 785.)

Often acknowledging feelings will enable patient to deal more appropriately with situation. May need chemical/physical control for brief periods of time.

Identify ways in which patient can get help when needed.

Provides assurance that staff is available for assistance/support.

Stay with or arrange to have someone stay with patient as indicated.

Continuous support may help patient regain internal locus of control and reduce anxiety/fear to a manageable level.

Provide accurate information as appropriate and requested by the patient/SO. Answer questions freely and honestly and in language that is understandable by all. Repeat information as necessary; correct misconceptions.

Complex and/or anxiety-provoking information can be given in manageable amounts over an extended period of time. As opportunities arise and facts are given, individuals will accept what they are ready for. Note: Words/phrases may have different meanings for each individual; therefore, clarification is necessary to ensure understanding.

Avoid empty reassurances, e.g., statements of "everything will be all right." Instead, provide specific information: e.g., "Your heart rate is regular, your pain is being easily controlled, and that is what we want."

It is not possible for the nurse to know how the specific situation will be resolved, and false reassurances may be interpreted as lack of understanding/honesty, further isolating the patient. Sharing observations used in assessing condition/prognosis provides opportunity for patient/SO to feel reassured.

Note expressions of concern/anger about treatment/staff.

Anxiety about self and outcome may be masked by comments/angry outbursts directed at therapy/care givers.

Ask the patient/SO to identify what they can/cannot do about what is happening.

Assists in identifying areas in which control is available as well as those in which control is not possible.

Provide as much order and predictability as possible in scheduling care/activities, visitors.

Helps patient anticipate and prepare for difficult treatments/movements, as well as look forward to pleasant occurrences.

Instruct in ways to use positive self-talk, e.g., "I know I can manage this pain for now."

Internal dialog is often negative. When this is shared out loud, the patient becomes aware and can be directed in the use of positive self-talk, which can help reduce anxiety.

Encourage/instruct in mental imagery/relaxation methods; e.g., imaging a pleasant place, use of music/tapes, slow breathing, and meditation.

Promotes release of endorphins and aids in developing internal locus of control, reducing anxiety. May enhance coping skills, allowing body to go about its work of healing.

Use touch, Therapeutic Touch, and other adjunctive therapies as indicated.

Aids in meeting basic human need, decreasing sense of isolation and assisting the patient to feel less anxious. Note: Therapeutic Touch is a method of using the hands to direct human energies to help or to heal.

Collaborative

Administer medications as needed: diazepam (Valium), clorazepate dipotassium (Tranxene), chlordiazepoxide hydrochloride (Librium).

Antianxiety agents may be useful for brief periods of time to assist the patient/SO to reduce anxiety to manageable levels, providing opportunity for initiation of coping skills.

NURSING DIAGNOSIS:	GRIEVING [SPECIFY]
May be related to:	Actual or perceived loss; chronic and/or fatal illness
	Thwarted grieving response to a loss; lack of resolution of previous grieving response/absence of anticipatory grieving
Possibly evidenced by:	Verbal expression of distress/unresolved issues
	Denial of loss
	Altered eating habits, sleep and dream patterns, activity levels, libido
	Crying; labile affect; feelings of sorrow, guilt, anger
	Difficulty in expressing loss; alterations in concentration and/or pursuit of tasks
PATIENT OUTCOMES/ EVALUATION CRITERIA:	Verbalizes a sense of progress toward resolution of the grief and hope for the future. Functioning at an adequate level, participating in work and ADLs.

ACTIONS/INTERVENTIONS	RATIONALE
Independent	
Provide open environment in which the patient feels free to discuss feelings and concerns realistically.	Therapeutic communication skills of Active-listening, silence, being available, and acceptance can allow the patient the opportunity to talk freely and deal with the perceived/actual loss.
Identify stage of grieving/dysfunction:	Awareness allows for appropriate choice of interventions as individuals handle grief in many different ways.
Denial: Be aware of avoidance behaviors; anger, withdrawal, etc. Allow patient to talk about what he/she chooses, and do not try to force patient to "face the facts."	Denying the reality of diagnosis and/or prognosis is an important phase in which the patient protects self from the pain and reality of the threat of loss. Each person does this in an individual manner based on previous experiences with loss and cultural/religious factors.
Anger: Note behaviors of withdrawal, lack of cooperation, and direct expression of anger. Allow verbalization of anger with acknowledgment of feelings and setting of limits regarding destructive behavior.	Denial gives way to feelings of anger, rage, guilt, and resentment. Patient may find it difficult to express anger directly and may feel guilty about feeling angry. Although staff may have difficulty dealing with angry behaviors, acceptance of it allows patient to work through the anger and move on to more effective coping behaviors.
Bargaining: Allow verbalization without confrontation about realities.	Helpful in beginning resolution and acceptance. May be working through feelings of guilt about things done or undone.
Depression: Give permission to be where he/she is. Provide comfort and availability as well as caring for physical needs.	When patient can no longer deny the reality of the loss, feelings of helplessness and hopelessness replace feelings of anger. The patient needs information that this is a normal progression of feelings.
Acceptance: Respect the patient's needs and wishes for quiet, privacy, and/or talking.	Having worked through the denial, anger and depression, patient often prefers to be alone and does not

ACTIONS/INTERVENTIONS

Independent

Active-listen patient's concerns and be available for help as necessary.

Identify and problem-solve existing physical responses, e.g., eating, sleeping, activity levels and sexual desire.

Assess needs of SO and assist as indicated.

Collaborative

Refer to other resources, e.g., counseling, psychotherapy as indicated.

RATIONALE

want to talk much at this point. Patient may still cling to hope, which can be sustaining through whatever is happening at this point.

The process of grieving does not proceed in an orderly fashion, but fluctuates with various aspects of all stages present at one time or another. If process is being dysfunctional, or prolonged, more aggressive interventions may be required to facilitate the process.

May need additional assistance to deal with the physical aspects of grieving.

Identification of dysfunctional grieving allows for individual interventions.

May need additional help to resolve grief, make plans, and look toward the future.

NURSING DIAGNOSIS:	SELF-CONCEPT, DISTURBANCE IN: (SPECIFY)
May be related to:	Biophysical, psychosocial, cognitive perceptual, cultural, or spiritual factors, e.g., changes in body image, self-esteem, role performance, personal identity
	Failure at life events
	Situational, developmental, health/illness crisis
	Organic brain syndrome; biochemical body change; poor ego differentiation; panic/dissociative state
Possibly evidenced by:	Fear of rejection/reaction by others
	Negative feelings about body/self; focus on past abilities, strengths, function or appearance; preoccupation with change/loss
	Feelings of helplessness, hopelessness, or powerlessness
	Change in lifestyle, social involvement, usual role patterns/responsibility
	Self-negating verbalization
	Denial of problems obvious to others
	Projection of blame/responsibility for problems
PATIENT OUTCOMES/ EVALUATION CRITERIA:	Verbalizes realistic view and acceptance of self in situation. Identifies remaining strengths and views self as capable person. Recognizes and incorporates change into self concept in accurate manner without negating self-esteem. Demonstrates adaptation to changes/events that have occurred as evidenced by setting of realistic

goals and active participation in work/play/personal relationships.

ACTIONS/INTERVENTIONS	RATIONALE
Independent	
Use the patient's name. Ask what the patient would like to be called.	Shows courtesy, respect and acknowledges person.
Identify SO from whom the patient derives comfort and who should be notified in case of emergency.	Allows provisions to be made for this person(s) to visit or remain close and provide needed support for patient. Note: May or may not be legal next of kin.
Active-listen patient concerns and fears.	Conveys sense of caring and can more effectively identify the needs and problems as well as patient's coping strategies and how effective they are. Provides opportunity to identify problems and begin a problem-solving process.
Encourage verbalization of feelings, accepting what is said.	Helps patient/SO begin to adapt to change and reduces anxiety about altered function/lifestyle.
Discuss stages of grief and the importance of grief work. (Refer to ND: Grieving [Specify], p. 777.)	Grieving is a necessary step for integration of change/loss into self-concept.
Provide nonthreatening environment.	Promotes feelings of safety, encouraging verbalization.
Observe nonverbal communication, e.g., body posture and movements, eye contact, gestures, use of touch.	Contains large percentage of communication and therefore is extremely important. How the person uses touch provides information about how it is used for communication and how comfortable the individual is with being touched.
Reflect back to the patient what has been said, for clarification and verification.	Information must be validated by the patient as assumptions may be inaccurate.
Observe and describe behavior in objective terms.	All behavior has meaning, some of which is obvious and some of which needs to be identified. This is a process of educated guesswork and needs to be validated by the patient.
Identify developmental level.	More important than age and may be useful in anticipating and identifying some needs. Some degree of regression occurs during illness, dependent on many factors such as the normal coping skills of the individual and severity of the illness.
Discuss patient's view of body image and how this illness might affect it.	The patient's perception of a change in body image may occur over a period of time or suddenly (e.g., actual loss of a body part through injury/surgery or a perceived loss, as in a heart attack) or be a continuous subtle process, as in chronic illness, eating disorders, or aging. Awareness can alert the nurse to the need for appropriate interventions tailored to the individual need.
Encourage discussion of physical changes in simple, direct and factual manner. Give realistic feedback and discuss options, e.g., rehabilitation services.	Provides opportunity to begin incorporating actual changes in an accepting and hopeful atmosphere.
Acknowledge efforts at problem-solving, resolution of current situation, and future planning.	Provides encouragement and reinforces continuation of desired behaviors.
Introduce tasks at patient's level of functioning, progressing to more complex activities as tolerated.	Provides for success experiences, reaffirming capabilities and enhancing self-esteem.

779

ACTIONS/INTERVENTIONS	RATIONALE

Independent

Ascertain how the patient sees own role within the family system, e.g., breadwinner, homemaker, husband/wife.

Illness may create a temporary or permanent problem in role expectations. Sexual role and how the patient views self in relation to the current illness also play important parts in recovery.

Assist patient/SO with clarifying expected roles and those that may need to be relinquished or altered.

Provides opportunity to identify misconceptions, begin to look at options and promotes reality orientation.

Assess impact of illness/surgery on sexuality.

Sexuality encompasses the whole person in the total environment. Many times problems of illness are superimposed on already existing problems of sexuality. Some problems are more obvious than others, such as illness involving the reproductive parts of the body. Others are less obvious, such as sexual values, role in family, e.g., mother, wage-earner, single parent, etc.

Be alert to comments and innuendos which may mean the patient has a concern in this area.

People are often reluctant and/or embarrassed to ask direct questions about sexual/sexuality concerns.

Be aware of nurse's feelings about dealing with this subject.

Nurses/care givers are often as reluctant and embarrassed in dealing with sexuality issues as most patients.

Provide information, and referral to hospital and community resources.

Enables patient/SO to be in contact with interested groups with access to assistive and supportive devices, services and counseling.

Collaborative

Refer to psychiatric support/therapy group, social services, as indicated.

May be needed to assist patient/SO to achieve optimal recovery.

Refer to appropriate resources, for sex therapy as need indicates.

May be someone with comfort level and knowledge who is available or may be necessary to refer to professional resources for additional help and support.

NURSING DIAGNOSIS:	COPING, INEFFECTIVE INDIVIDUAL/DECISIONAL CONFLICT
May be related to:	Situational crises/personal vulnerability; multiple life changes/maturational crises; inadequate coping methods
	Inadequate support systems
	No vacations/inadequate relaxation
	Impairment of nervous system; memory loss
	Impaired adaptive behaviors and problem-solving skills
	Severe pain/overwhelming threat to self
	Unclear personal values/beliefs; perceived threat to value system; lack of experience/interference with decision-making; lack of information
Possibly evidenced by:	Verbalization of inability to cope/asking for help
	Muscular tension, frequent headaches/neck aches

Chronic worry, fatigue, insomnia, anxiety/depression

Poor self-esteem; inappropriate use of defense mechanisms; inability to meet role expectations, basic needs, problem-solve

Alteration in social participation; change in usual communication patterns

High illness/accident rate; overeating; excessive smoking/drinking

Destructive behavior toward self or others

Uncertainty about choices; vacillation between alternative actions; delayed decision-making

PATIENT OUTCOMES/ EVALUATION CRITERIA: Identifies ineffective coping behaviors and consequences. Verbalizes awareness of own coping/problem-solving abilities. Meets psychologic needs as evidenced by appropriate expression of feelings, identification of options, and use of resources. Makes decisions and expresses satisfaction with choices.

ACTIONS/INTERVENTIONS

Independent

Review pathophysiology affecting the patient and extent of feelings of hopelessness/helplessness/loss of control over life, level of anxiety.

Establish therapeutic nurse–patient relationship.

Note expressions of indecision, dependence on others, and inability to manage own ADLs.

Assess presence of positive coping skills, e.g., use of relaxation techniques, willingness to express feelings.

Encourage patient to talk about what is happening at this time and what has occurred to precipitate feelings of helplessness and anxiety.

Correct misperceptions patient may have. Provide factual information.

Provide quiet, nonstimulating environment. Determine what patient needs, and provide if possible. Give simple, factual information about what patient can expect, and repeat as necessary.

Allow patient to be dependent in the beginning with gradual resumption of independence in ADLs, self-care, and other activities. Make opportunities for patient to make decisions about care when possible, accepting choice not to do so.

RATIONALE

Indicators of degree of disequilibrium and need for intervention to prevent or resolve the crisis.

Patient may feel freer to verbalize feelings of helplessness, powerlessness, and to discuss changes that may be necessary in the patient's life.

May indicate need to lean on others for a period of time. Early recognition and intervention can help patient regain equilibrium.

When the individual has coping skills that have been successful in the past, they may be used in the current situation to relieve tension and preserve the individual's sense of control.

Provides clues to assist patient to develop coping skills to regain equilibrium.

Assists in identification and correction of perception of reality and enables problem solving to begin.

Decreases anxiety and provides control for the patient during crisis situation.

Promotes feelings of security (patient will know nurse will provide safety). As control is regained, patient has the opportunity to develop adaptive coping/problem-solving skills.

781

ACTIONS/INTERVENTIONS	RATIONALE

Independent

Accept verbal expressions of anger, setting limits on maladaptive behavior.

Verbalizing angry feelings is an important process for resolution of grief and loss. However, preventing destructive actions (such as striking out at others) preserves patient's self esteem.

Discuss feelings of self-blame/projection of blame on others.

While these mechanisms may be protective at the moment of crisis, they are counterproductive and intensify feelings of helplessness and hopelessness.

Note expressions of inability to find meaning in life/reason for living, feelings of futility or alienation from God.

Crisis situation may evoke questioning of spiritual beliefs affecting ability to cope with current situation and plan for the future.

Problem-solve solutions for current situation. Provide information, support and reinforce reality as patient begins to ask questions, look at what is happening.

Helping patient/SO to brainstorm possible solutions (giving consideration to the pros and cons of each) promotes feelings of self-control/esteem.

Identify new coping behaviors patient is displaying and reinforce positive adaptation.

During crisis, patient develops new ways of dealing with problems, which can assist with resolution of current situation as well as future crises.

NURSING DIAGNOSIS: COPING, INEFFECTIVE FAMILY, COMPROMISED/DISABLING

May be related to: Inadequate or incorrect information or understanding by a primary person

Temporary preoccupation by a significant person who is trying to manage emotional conflicts and personal suffering and is unable to perceive or to act effectively with regard to patient's needs

Temporary family disorganization and role changes

Patient providing little support in turn for the primary person

Prolonged disease/disability progression that exhausts the supportive capacity of significant persons

Significant person with chronically unexpressed feelings of guilt, anxiety, hostility, despair

Highly ambivalent family relationships

Possibly evidenced by: Patient expresses/confirms a concern or complains about SO's response to patient's health problem, despair about family reactions/lack of involvement

Neglectful relationships with other family members

SO describes preoccupation about personal reactions; displays intolerance, abandonment, rejection

SO attempts assistive/supportive behaviors with less than satisfactory results; withdraws or enters into limited or temporary personal communication with patient; displays protective behavior disproportionate (too little or too much) to patient's abilities or need for autonomy

FAMILY OUTCOMES/ EVALUATION CRITERIA:	Identifies resources within themselves to deal with situation. Provides opportunity for patient to deal with situation in own way. Expressing more realistic understanding and expectations of the patient; visiting regularly and participating positively in care of patient, within limits of abilities.

ACTIONS/INTERVENTIONS	RATIONALE
Independent	
Assess level of anxiety present in family/SO.	Anxiety level needs to be dealt with before problem solving can begin. Individuals may be so preoccupied with own reactions to situation that they are unable to respond to another's needs.
Establish rapport and acknowledge difficulty of the situation for the family.	May assist SO to accept what is happening and be willing to share problems with staff.
Assess preillness/current behaviors that are interfering with the care/recovery of the patient.	Information about family problems (e.g., divorce/ separation, alcoholism, drug abuse, abusive situation) will be helpful in developing an appropriate plan of care.
Determine current knowledge of the situation.	Provides information on which to begin planning care and make informed decisions.
Assess current actions of SO and how they are received by patient.	May be trying to be helpful but are not perceived as helpful by the patient. May be withdrawn or may be too protective.
Involve SO in information giving, problem solving, and care of patient as feasible.	Information can reduce feelings of helplessness and uselessness. Involvement in care enhances feelings of control and self-worth.
Encourage seeking help appropriately. Give information about persons and agencies available to them.	Permission to seek help as needed allows them to choose to take advantage of what is available.

NURSING DIAGNOSIS:	COPING, FAMILY: POTENTIAL FOR GROWTH
May be related to:	Basic needs are sufficiently gratified and adaptive tasks effectively addressed to enable goals of self-actualization to surface
	Willingness to deal with one's own needs and to begin to problem-solve with the patient
Possibly evidenced by:	[Not applicable; presence of signs and symptoms establishes an *actual* diagnosis.]
FAMILY OUTCOMES/ EVALUATION CRITERIA:	Expresses willingness to look at own role in family's growth; desire to undertake tasks leading to change; feelings of self-confidence and satisfaction with progress being made.

ACTIONS/INTERVENTIONS	RATIONALE
Independent	
Provide opportunities for SO to talk with patient and/or staff.	Reduces anxiety and allows expression of what has been learned and how they are managing, as well as opportunity to make plans for the future and share support.
Listen to family's expressions of hope, planning, effect on relationships/life.	Provides clues to avenues to explore for assistance with growth.
Provide opportunities for and instruction in how SO can care for patient. Discuss ways in which they can support patient in meeting own needs.	Enhances feelings of control and involvement in situation where SO cannot do many things. Also provides opportunity to learn how to be most helpful when patient is discharged.
Provide a role model with which family may identify.	Having a positive example can help with adoption of new behaviors to promote growth.
Assist family to develop effective communication skills of Active-listening, "I-messages," and problem solving.	Helps individuals to express needs and wants in ways that will develop family cohesiveness.
Collaborative	
Refer to support group(s) and other resources as indicated.	Provides opportunities for sharing experiences; provides mutual support and practical problem solving; and can aid in decreasing alienation and helplessness.

NURSING DIAGNOSIS:	NONCOMPLIANCE [COMPLIANCE, ALTERED] (SPECIFY)
May be related to:	Patient value system: health beliefs, spiritual values, cultural influences
	Patient and provider relationships
	Fear/anxiety; side effects of therapy
Possibly evidenced by:	Statements of unwillingness to follow treatment regimen
	Behavior indicative of failure to adhere to treatment regimen, e.g., not keeping appointments
	Evidence of development of complications; failure to progress
PATIENT OUTCOMES/ EVALUATION CRITERIA:	Participates in the development of goals and treatment plan. Verbalizes accurate knowledge of disease and understanding of treatment regimen. Makes choices at level of readiness based on accurate information.

ACTIONS/INTERVENTIONS	RATIONALE
Independent	
Determine reason(s) for behavior/problems which are interfering with treatment. Assess level of anxiety, locus of control, sense of powerlessness, etc.	Many factors may be involved in behavior that is disruptive to the treatment regimen (e.g., fear, pain, anxiety, hypoxemia, chemical imbalance).

ACTIONS/INTERVENTIONS	RATIONALE
Independent	
Discuss patient's/SO's view of illness/treatment. Determine cultural/spiritual/health beliefs, as possible.	Provides insight into thoughts/factors related to individual situation.
Note length of illness.	Patients tend to become passive and dependent in long-term, debilitating illness.
Assess support systems available to the patient.	Access to helpful resources may assist patient in meeting treatment goals/provide purpose for living.
Review patient's knowledge and understanding of the need for treatment/medication as well as consequences of actions/choices.	Provides opportunities to clarify viewpoints/misconceptions. Verifies that patient has accurate/factual information with which to make informed choices.
Review treatment plan with patient/SO. Establish graduated goals or modified regimen as necessary; work out alternate solutions.	Provides opportunities to exchange accurate information and to clarify viewpoints/misconceptions. Promotes patient involvement/independence, provides opportunity for compromise, and may enhance cooperation with regimen.
Contract with the patient for participation in care.	Patient who agrees to own responsibility is more apt to cooperate.
Accept the patient's choice/point of view, even it if appears to be self-destructive, e.g., decision to continue smoking.	Confrontation is not beneficial and may actually be detrimental to future cooperation and goal achievement.
Develop a system for self-monitoring. Share data pertinent to patient's condition, e.g., laboratory results, blood pressure.	Provides a sense of control and enables patient to follow own progress and to assist with making choices.
Have some personnel care for patient as much as possible.	Enables relationship to develop in which the patient can begin to trust/participate in care.
Be aware of own (care giver's) response to patient's treatment choices (e.g., refusal of blood or chemotherapy, Living Will).	Negative feelings regarding these choices may be expressed in judgmental behaviors that block or interfere with patient's wishes, comfort, and/or care.

NURSING DIAGNOSIS:	**VIOLENCE, POTENTIAL FOR: DIRECTED AT SELF/OTHERS**
May be related to:	**Attempt to deal with the threat to self-concept that illness can represent**
	Antisocial character; catatonic/manic excitement; panic states; rage reactions
	Suicidal ideation/behavior, depression
	Hormonal imbalance; temporal lobe epilepsy; toxic reactions to medication
	Negative role modeling; developmental crisis
Possible indicators:	**Suspicion of others, paranoid ideation, delusions, hallucinations**
	Expressed intent or desire to harm self/others (directly or indirectly); hostile verbalizations
	Body language: rigid posture, clenched fists, facial expressions

Increased motor activity, excitement, irritability, agitation

Overt and aggressive acts; self-destructive behavior

Substance abuse/withdrawal

PATIENT OUTCOMES/ EVALUATION CRITERIA:	Acknowledges realities of the situation. Verbalizes understanding of reason(s) for behavior/precipitating factors. Expresses increased self-concept/esteem. Demonstrates self-control, as evidenced by relaxed posture, nonviolent behavior.

ACTIONS/INTERVENTIONS

Independent

Observe for early signs of distress.

Help patient identify more adequate solutions. Give as much autonomy as is possible in the situation.

Provide protection within the environment, e.g., constant observation, removal of objects that might be used to harm self/others.

Give permission to express angry feelings in acceptable ways. Make time to listen to verbalization of these feelings.

Accept patient's anger without reacting on an emotional basis.

Remain calm and state limits on behavior in a firm manner. Be truthful.

Assume that the patient has control and is responsible for own behavior.

Identify conditions that may interfere with ability to control own behavior.

Tell patient to "stop."

Hold patient; place in restraints or seclusion. Do so in a calm, positive, nonstimulating/nonpunitive manner.

Monitor for suicidal intent, e.g., morbid or anxious feelings while with the patient; warning from the patient, "It doesn't matter," "I'd be better off dead"; mood swings, putting affairs in order, suicide attempt.

Assess suicidal intent (1–10 scale) by asking directly if patient is thinking of killing self.

RATIONALE

Irritability, lack of cooperation and demanding behavior may all be signs of increasing anxiety.

Enhances feelings of power and control in a situation where many things are not within individual's control.

May need more structure to maintain control until own internal locus of control is regained.

Encouraging acceptable expression can be helpful in defusing feelings of helplessness and anger, as well as decreasing guilt.

Responding with anger is not helpful in resolving the situation and may result in escalating patient's behavior.

Understanding that helplessness and fear underlie this behavior can be helpful.

Often enables the individual to exercise control. Note: When violent behavior is the result of drugs, patient may not be able to respond appropriately.

Acute or chronic brain syndrome, drug-induced or post-surgical confusion may precipitate violent behavior.

May be sufficient to help patient control own actions if exhibiting hostile actions. Note: Patient is often afraid of own actions.

As a last resort, physical restraint may be necessary while the patient regains control. Note: These measures are meant to *protect* patient, not punish the behavior.

Indicators of need for further assessment, evaluation, and intervention/psychiatric care.

Provides guidelines for necessity/urgency of interventions. Direct quesiton is most helpful when done in a caring, concerned manner.

ACTIONS/INTERVENTIONS

Collaborative

Refer to psychiatric resource(s), e.g., clinical specialist psychiatric nurse, psychiatrist, psychologist, social worker.

Administer medications, e.g., tranquilizers, sedatives, narcotics.

RATIONALE

More in-depth assistance may be needed to deal with patient and defuse situation.

May be indicated to quiet/control behavior. Note: May need to be withheld if they are suspected to be the cause of/contribute to the behavior.

NURSING DIAGNOSIS:	POST-TRAUMA RESPONSE
May be related to:	**Disasters (e.g., floods, earthquakes, tornadoes, airplane crashes, combat); wars, epidemics, rape, incest, assault, torture, catastrophic illness or accident, being held hostage**
Possibly evidenced by:	**Reexperiencing traumatic event (may be identified in cognitive, affective, and/or sensory motor activities, e.g., flashbacks, intrusive thoughts, repetitive dreams or nightmares, excessive verbalization of the traumatic event, verbalization of survival guilt or guilt about behavior required for survival)**
	Altered lifestyle (self-destructiveness); loss of interest in usual activities; loss of feeling of intimacy/sexuality; development of phobia; poor impulse control/irritability and explosiveness
	Disturbance of mood, e.g., depression, anxiety, embarrassment, fear, self-blame, low self-esteem
	Cognitive disruption: confusion, loss of memory/concentration, indecisiveness
PATIENT OUTCOMES/ EVALUATION CRITERIA:	**Verbalizes reduced anxiety/fear. Demonstrates ability to deal with emotional reactions in an individually appropriate manner. Expresses own feelings/reactions; avoids projection. Demonstrates appropriate changes in lifestyle/getting support from SO as needed. Participates in plans for follow-up care/counseling.**

ACTIONS/INTERVENTIONS

Independent

Determine when incident occurred: present or past.

Assess physical trauma if present and individual reaction to occurrence, e.g., physical symptoms such as numbness, headache, tightness in chest, and psychologic responses of anger, shock, acute anxiety, confusion, denial.

RATIONALE

Manifestations of acute and chronic post-trauma responses may require different interventions.

Provides information on which to develop plan of care, make informed choices.

ACTIONS/INTERVENTIONS

Independent

Evaluate behavior (e.g., calm/agitated, excited/hysterical; inappropriate laughter, crying), expressions of disbelief and/or self-blame.

Note ethnic background/cultural perceptions and beliefs about the incident.

Assess signs/stage of grieving.

Tell patient that painful emotional reactions are normal. Phrase this information in neutral terms: "You may or may not experience. . . ."

Discuss things patient can do to feel better, e.g., physical exercise alternated with relaxation; keeping busy with normal activities; talking to others; acknowledging that it is all right to feel upset; writing about the experience in a journal; being kind to yourself.

Identify supportive persons for patient.

Note signs of severe/prolonged depression, presence of flashbacks, nightmares, chronic pain, somatic complaints.

Collaborative

Refer to counselors/therapists for further therapy, e..g, psychotherapy (in conjunction with medications); implosive therapy, flooding, hypnosis, Rolfing, memory work or cognitive restructuring as indicated.

RATIONALE

Indicators of extent of individual response to traumatic incident and degree of disorganization.

May influence patient's response to what has happened, e.g., may believe it is retribution from God.

Patient may be suffering from sense of loss of self and/or others.

Understanding that experiencing these uncomfortable feelings is not unusual following a traumatic event may reduce patient's anxiety/fear of "going crazy" and enhance coping.

Enhances sense of control and helps patient achieve resolution of uncomfortable feelings. Often when the patient begins these activities within the first 24 hours of the event, further therapy may not be required.

Having positive support systems can help patient reach optimal recovery.

If patient did not deal with trauma when it occurred, behavioral manifestations may reveal extent of problem in the present.

When post-trauma response has become chronic, patient may need more in-depth assistance from sensitive, trained individuals who are skilled in dealing with these problems.

Surgical Intervention _____

Surgery may be needed to diagnose or cure a specific disease process, correct a structural deformity, or restore a functional process and may be performed in the acute care center or an ambulatory surgical setting.

PATIENT ASSESSMENT DATA BASE

Data are dependent on the duration, severity of underlying problem, and involvement of other body systems. Refer to specific CP (e.g., Cardiac surgery, Laminectomy, Thyroidectomy, Mastectomy, Amputation, Cholecystectomy, Prostatectomy) for data and diagnostic studies relevant to the procedure and additional nursing diagnoses.

CIRCULATORY

May report:	History of cardiac problems, CHF, pulmonary edema, peripheral vascular disease, or vascular stasis (increases risk of thrombus formation).

EGO INTEGRITY

May report:	Feelings of anxiety, fear, anger, apathy.
	Multiple stress factors, e.g., financial, relationship, lifestyle.
May exhibit:	Restlessness, increased tension/irritability.
	Sympathetic stimulation.

FOOD/FLUID

May report:	Pancreatic insufficiency (predisposing to hypoglycemia/ketoacidosis).
May exhibit:	Malnutrition (including obesity).
	Dry mucous membranes (limited intake/NPO period preoperatively).

RESPIRATION

May report:	Infections, chronic conditions/cough, smoking.

SAFETY

May report:	Immune deficiencies (increases risk of systemic infections and delayed healing).
	Allergies or sensitivities to medications, food, tape, and solution(s).
	Family history of malignant hyperthermia/reaction to anesthesia.
	History of hepatic disease (affects drug detoxification and may alter coagulation).
	History of blood transfusion(s)/transfusion reaction.
May exhibit:	Presence of existing infectious process; fever.

TEACHING/LEARNING

May report:	Use of anticoagulants, steroids, antibiotics, antihypertensives, cardiotonic glycosides, antidysrhythmics, bronchodilators, diuretics, decongestants, analgesics, antiinflammatories, anticonvulsants, or tranquilizers as well as OTC, street, or recreational drugs.
	Use of alcohol (risk of liver damage affecting coagulation and choice of anesthesia as well as potential for postoperative withdrawal).
Discharge Plan Considerations:	May require assistance with transportation, dressing(s)/supplies, self-care, and homemaker tasks.

DIAGNOSTIC STUDIES

General preoperative requirements: urinalysis, CBC, prothrombin, PTT, chest x-ray.

Other studies: dependent on type of operative procedure, current medications, systemic processes, age, and weight, e.g., BUN, creatinine, glucose, ABGs, electrolytes, thyroid studies. Deviations from normal should be corrected if possible prior to safe administration of anesthetic agents.

Urinalysis: presence of WBCs or bacteria indicates infection.

Pregnancy test: positive results affect timing of procedure and choice of pharmacologic agents.

CBC: WBC elevation is indicative of inflammatory process (may be diagnostic, e.g., appendicitis); decreased WBC count suggests viral processes (requiring evaluation because immune system may be dysfunctional). Hg decrease suggests anemia/blood loss (impairs tissue oxygenation and reduces the Hg available to bind with inhalation anesthetics); may suggest need for cross-match/blood transfusion. Hct elevation may indicate dehydration; decreased Hct suggests fluid overload.

Electrolytes: imbalances impair organ function, e.g., decreased potassium affects cardiac muscle contractility, leading to decreased cardiac output.

ABGs: evaluates current respiratory status.

Coagulation times: may be prolonged, interfering with intra/postoperative homeostasis.

Chest x-ray: should be free of infiltrates, pneumonia; used for identification of masses and COPD.

ECG: abnormal findings require attention prior to administering anesthetics.

NURSING PRIORITIES

1. Reduce anxiety and emotional trauma.
2. Provide for physical safety.
3. Prevent complications.
4. Alleviate pain.
5. Facilitate recovery process.
6. Provide information about disease process/surgical procedure, prognosis, and treatment needs.

DISCHARGE CRITERIA

1. Dealing realistically with current situation.
2. Injury prevented.
3. Complications prevented/minimized.
4. Pain relieved/controlled.
5. Wound healing/organ function progressing toward normal.
6. Disease process/surgical procedure, prognosis, and therapeutic regimen understood.

PREOPERATIVE

NURSING DIAGNOSIS:	**KNOWLEDGE DEFICIT [LEARNING NEED] (SPECIFY)**
May be related to:	**Lack of exposure/recall, information misinterpretation**
	Unfamiliarity with information resources
Possibly evidenced by:	**Statement of the problem/concerns, misconceptions**
	Request for information
	Inappropriate, exaggerated behaviors (e.g., agitated, apathetic, hostile)
	Inaccurate follow-through of instructions/development of preventable complications
PATIENT OUTCOMES/ EVALUATION CRITERIA:	**Verbalizes understanding of disease process/peri-operative process. Correctly performs necessary proce-**

dures and explains reasons for the actions. Initiates necessary lifestyle changes and participates in treatment regimen.

ACTIONS/INTERVENTIONS	RATIONALE
Independent	
Assess patient's level of understanding.	Facilitates planning of preoperative teaching program.
Review specific pathology and anticipated surgical procedure.	Provides knowledge base on which patient can make informed therapy choices and consent for procedure, and presents opportunity to clarify misconceptions.
Use resource teaching materials, audiovisuals as available.	Specifically designed materials can facilitate the patient's learning.
Implement individualized preoperative teaching program: Pre/postoperative procedures and restrictions, e.g., urinary and bowel changes; dietary considerations; activity levels/transfers; respiratory and cardiovascular exercises; pain control.	Enhances patient's understanding/control and enables participation in postoperative care. Explanation of anticipated IV lines and tubes (e.g., nasogastric tubes, drains, and catheters) can relieve stress related to the unknown/unexpected. Increased understanding of the importance of performing activities and cooperating with restrictions reduces the possibility of postoperative complications and promotes a rapid return to normal body function.
Provide opportunity to practice coughing, deep breathing, and muscular exercises.	Enhances learning and continuation of activity postoperatively.
Inform patient/SO about itinerary, physician/SO communications.	Logistical information on schedule and places (e.g., recovery room, postoperative room assignment) as well as where and when the surgeon will communicate with SO relieves stress and miscommunications, preventing confusion and doubt over patient's well-being.

NURSING DIAGNOSIS:	FEAR/ANXIETY
May be related to:	**Situational crisis; unfamiliarity with environment**
	Threat of death; change in health status
	Separation from usual support systems
Possibly evidenced by:	**Increased tension, apprehension, decreased self-assurance**
	Expressed concern regarding changes, fear of consequences
	Facial tension, restlessness, focus on self
	Sympathetic stimulation
PATIENT OUTCOMES/ EVALUATION CRITERIA:	**Acknowledges feelings and identifies healthy ways to deal with them. Appears relaxed, able to rest/sleep appropriately. Reports decreased fear, and anxiety reduced to a manageable level.**

ACTIONS/INTERVENTIONS	RATIONALE

Independent

Provide for visit with OR personnel before surgery when possible. Discuss anticipated things that may frighten/concern patient, e.g., masks, lights, IVs, BP cuff, electrodes, bovie pad, autoclave noises, child crying.

Can provide reassurance and alleviate patient's anxiety, as well as provide information for formulating intraoperative care. Acknowledges that foreign environment may be frightening, alleviates associated fears.

Inform patient/SO of nurse's intraoperative advocate role.

Develops trust/rapport, decreasing fear of loss of control in a foreign environment.

Identify fear levels that may necessitate postponement of surgical procedure.

Overwhelming or persistent fears result in excessive stress reaction, potentiating risk of adverse reaction to procedure/anesthetic agents.

Validate source of fear. Provide accurate, factual information. Active-listen concerns.

Identification of specific fear helps patient to deal realistically with it, e.g., misidentification/wrong operation, dismemberment, disfigurement, loss of dignity/control, or being awake/aware with local anesthesia. Patient may have misinterpreted preoperative information or have misinformation regarding surgery/disease process. Previous experiences, family/acquaintances' fears may be unresolved.

Note expressions of distress/feelings of helplessness, preoccupation with anticipated change/loss, choked feelings.

Patient may already be grieving the loss represented by the anticipated surgical procedure/diagnosis/prognosis of illness.

Tell patient anticipating local/spinal anesthesia that drowsiness/sleep occurs, that more sedation may be requested and will be given if needed, and that surgical drapes will block view of the operative field.

Reduces anxiety/fear that patient may "see" the procedure.

Introduce staff at time of transfer.

Establishes rapport and psychologic comfort.

Compare surgery schedule, chart, patient identification band, and signed operative consent.

Provides for positive identification, reducing fear that wrong procedure may be done.

Prevent unnecessary body exposure during transfer and in OR suite.

Patients are concerned about loss of dignity and inability to exercise control.

Give simple, concise directions/explanations to sedated patient. Review environmental concerns as needed.

Impairment of thought processes makes it difficult for patient to understand lengthy instructions.

Control external stimuli.

Extraneous noises and commotion may accelerate anxiety.

Collaborative

Refer to pastor/spiritual care, psychiatric nurse clinical specialist, psychiatric counseling if indicated.

Professional counseling may be required for patient to resolve fear.

Discuss postponement/cancellation of surgery with physician, anesthesiologist, patient and family.

May be necessary if overwhelming fears are not reduced/resolved.

Administer medications as indicated, e.g.:

Sedatives, hypnotics;

Used to promote sleep the evening before surgery, may enhance coping abilities.

IV tranquilizers.

May be needed in the holding area to reduce nervousness and provide comfort.

(Refer to CP: Psychosocial Aspects of Acute Care, p. 773.)

INTRAOPERATIVE

NURSING DIAGNOSIS:	INJURY, POTENTIAL FOR
May be related to:	Interactive conditions between individual and environment
	External environment, e.g., physical design, structure of environment, exposure to electrical machines, use of pharmaceutical agents
	Internal environment, e.g., tissue hypoxia, abnormal blood profile/altered clotting factors, broken skin
Possibly evidenced by:	[Not applicable; presence of signs and symptoms establishes an *actual* diagnosis.]
CARE GIVER OUTCOMES/ EVALUATION CRITERIA:	Identifies individual risk factors. Modifies environment as indicated to enhance safety and uses resources appropriately.

ACTIONS/INTERVENTIONS	RATIONALE
Independent	
Remove partial plates or bridges preoperatively. Inform anesthesiologist of loose teeth.	Foreign bodies may be aspirated at intubation.
Remove artificial devices preoperatively or after induction, dependent on sensory/perceptual alterations and mobility impairment.	Contact lenses may cause corneal abrasions while under anesthesia; eyeglasses and hearing aids are obstructive and may break; however, patients may feel more in control of environment if hearing and visual aids are left on as long as possible. Artificial limbs may be damaged and skin integrity impaired if left on.
Remove jewelry preoperatively.	Metals conduct electrical current and provide an electrocautery hazard. In addition, loss or damage to patient's personal property can easily occur in the foreign environment.
Verify patient identity and scheduled operative procedure by comparing patient chart, arm band, and surgical schedule. Verbally ascertain correct name, procedure, and physician.	Assures correct patient and procedure.
Give simple and concise directions to the sedated patient.	Impairment of thought process makes it difficult for patient to understand lengthy directions.
Stabilize both patient cart and OR table when transferring patient to and from OR table, using adequate numbers of personnel for transfer and support of extremities.	Unstabilized cart/table can separate, causing patient to fall. Both side rails must be in the down position for care giver(s) to assist patient transfer and prevent loss of balance.
Anticipate movement of extraneous lines and tubes during the transfer and secure or guide them into position.	Prevents undue tension and dislocation of IV lines, NG tubes, catheters, and chest tubes, and maintains gravity drainage when appropriate.
Secure patient on OR table with safety belt over thighs, explaining necessity.	OR tables and arm boards are narrow, and patient or extremity may fall off, causing injury, especially during vesiculation. Sedated or emerging patient may be-

793

ACTIONS/INTERVENTIONS

Independent

Prepare equipment and padding for required position, according to operative procedure and patient's specific needs.

Position extremities so they may be periodically checked for safety, circulation, nerve pressure, and alignment. Periodically check peripheral pulses.

Ascertain electrical safety of equipment used in surgical procedure, e.g., intact cords, grounds, medical engineering verification labels.

Place electrocautery pad over greatest available muscle mass, ensuring its contact.

Prevent pooling of prep solutions under and around patient.

Assist with induction as needed; e.g., stand by to apply cricoid pressure during intubation or stabilize position during lumbar puncture for spinal block.

Monitor intake and output during procedure.

Confirm and document correct sponge, instrument, needle, and blade counts.

Handle, label, and document specimens appropriately, ensuring proper medium and transport for test desired.

Collaborative

Limit/avoid use of epinephrine to Fluothane-anesthetized patient.

RATIONALE

come resistive or combative, furthering potential for injury.

Depending on individual patient's size, weight, and preexisting conditions, extra padding materials may be required to protect bony prominences, prevent circulatory compromise, nerve pressure and allow for optimum chest expansion for ventilation.

Prevents accidental trauma, e.g., hands, fingers, and toes may be inadvertently scraped, pinched, or amputated by moving table attachments; positional pressure to brachial plexus, peroneal and ulnar nerves can cause damage; prolonged plantar flexion may result in footdrop.

Malfunction of equipment can occur during the operative procedure, causing not only delays and unnecessary anesthesia but also injury and death, e.g., short circuits, faulty grounds, laser misalignment. Periodic electrical safety checks are imperative for all OR equipment.

Provides a ground for maximal conductivity to prevent electrical burns.

Antiseptic solutions may chemically burn skin as well as conduct electricity.

Facilitates safe administration of anesthesia.

Potential for fluid volume deficit exists, affecting safety of anesthesia, organ function, and patient well-being.

Foreign bodies remaining in body cavities at closure not only cause inflammation, infection, perforation, abscess formation, but also may result in disastrous complications, leading to death.

Proper identification of specimens to patient is imperative. Frozen sections, preserved or fresh examination, and cultures all have different requirements. OR nurse advocate must be knowledgeable of specific hospital laboratory requirements for validity of examination.

Fluothane sensitizes the myocardium to catecholamines and may produce dysrhythmias.

NURSING DIAGNOSIS:	**INFECTION, POTENTIAL FOR**
May be related to:	**Broken skin, traumatized tissues, stasis of body fluids**
	Presence of pathogens/contaminants, environmental exposure, invasive procedures
Possibly evidenced by:	**[Not applicable; presence of signs and symptoms establishes an *actual* diagnosis.]**

| CARE GIVER OUTCOMES/ EVALUATION CRITERIA: | Identifies individual risk factors and interventions to reduce potential for infection. Maintains safe aseptic environment. |

ACTIONS/INTERVENTIONS

Independent

Adhere to hospital infection control, sterilization, and aseptic policies/procedures.

Verify sterility of all manufacturers' items.

Review laboratory studies for possibility of systemic infections.

Verify that preoperative skin, vaginal and bowel cleansing procedures have been done as needed.

Prepare operative site according to specific procedures.

Examine skin for breaks or ongoing infection.

Maintain dependent gravity drainage of indwelling catheters, tubes, and/or positive pressure of parenteral or irrigation lines.

Identify breaks in aseptic technique and resolve immediately upon occurrence.

Contain contaminated fluids/materials in specific site in operating room suite, and dispose of according to hospital protocol.

Provide sterile dressing.

Collaborative

Do copious wound irrigation, e.g., saline, water, antibiotic or antiseptic.

Obtain cultures/Gram stain.

RATIONALE

Established mechanisms designed to prevent infection.

Prepackaged items may appear to be sterile, however, each item must be scrutinized for manufacturers' statement of sterility, breaks in packaging, environmental effect on package, and delivery techniques. Package sterilization/expiration dates, lot/serial numbers must be documented on implant items for further follow-up if necessary.

Increased WBC may indicate ongoing infection, which the operative procedure will alleviate (e.g., appendicitis, abscess, inflammation from trauma); or presence of systemic/organ infection, which may contraindicate surgical procedure and/or anesthesia (e.g., pneumonia, kidney).

Cleansing reduces bacterial counts on the skin, vaginal mucosa, and alimentary tract.

Minimizes bacterial counts at operative site.

Disruptions of skin integrity at or near the operative site are sources of contamination to the wound. Careful shaving is imperative to prevent abrasions and nicks in the skin.

Prevents stasis and reflux of body fluids.

Contamination by environmental/personnel contact renders the sterile field unsterile thereby increasing the risk of infection.

Containment of blood and body fluids and items in contact with an infected wound and patient will prevent spread of infection to environment/other patients/personnel.

Prevents environmental contamination of fresh wound.

May be used intraoperatively to reduce bacterial counts at the site and cleanse the wound of debris, e.g., bone, ischemic tissue, bowel contaminants, toxins.

Immediate identification of type of infective organism by Gram stain allows prompt treatment while more specific identification by cultures can be obtained over a period of hours/days.

ACTIONS/INTERVENTIONS

Collaborative

Administer antibiotics as indicated.

RATIONALE

May be given parenterally for suspected infection or contamination.

NURSING DIAGNOSIS:	BODY TEMPERATURE, ALTERED, POTENTIAL
May be related to:	**Exposure to cool environment**
	Use of medications, anesthetic agents
	Extremes of age, weight
	Dehydration
Possibly evidenced by:	[Not applicable; presence of signs and symptoms establishes an *actual* diagnosis.]
PATIENT OUTCOMES/ EVALUATION CRITERIA:	**Maintains body temperature within normal range.**

ACTIONS/INTERVENTIONS

Independent

Note preoperative temperature.

Monitor temperature throughout intraoperative phase.

Assess environmental temperature and modify as needed, e.g., providing infant warmers, warming and cooling blankets, increasing room temperature.

Cover skin areas outside of operative field.

Provide cooling measures for patient with preoperative temperature elevations.

Note rapid temperature elevation and treat promptly per protocol.

Apply warm blankets at emergence.

Collaborative

Use temperature-controlled humidifier.

RATIONALE

Used as baseline for monitoring intraoperative temperature. Preoperative temperature elevations are indicative of disease process, e.g., appendicitis, abscess, or systemic disease requiring treatment preoperatively and possibly postoperatively.

Temperature elevation may indicate adverse response to anesthesia. Temperature decreases may require warming.

May assist in maintaining/stabilizing patient's temperature.

Heat losses will occur as skin (e.g., legs, arms, head) is exposed to cool environment.

Cool irrigations and exposure of skin surfaces to air may be required to decrease temperature. Note: Use of atropine or scopolamine may further increase temperature.

Anaphylaxis (malignant hyperthermia) must be recognized and treated promptly to avoid serious complications.

Inhalation anesthetics depress the hypothalamus, resulting in poor body temperature regulation.

Continuous warm/cool humidified inhalation anesthetics are used to maintain humidity and temperature balance within the tracheobronchial tree.

ACTIONS/INTERVENTIONS

Collaborative

Place warming/cooling blanket under patient. Provide iced saline as indicated.

Obtain dantrolene (Dantrium) for IV administration.

RATIONALE

Maintains appropriate body temperature in cool environment. Note: Lavage of body cavity with iced saline may help reduce hyperthermic responses.

Immediate action to control temperature is necessary to prevent death from malignant hyperthermia.

POSTOPERATIVE

NURSING DIAGNOSIS:	**BREATHING PATTERN, INEFFECTIVE**
May be related to:	**Neuromuscular, perceptual/cognitive impairment**
	Decreased lung expansion, energy
	Tracheobronchial obstruction
Possibly evidenced by:	**Changes in respiratory rate and depth**
	Reduced vital capacity, apnea, cyanosis, noisy respirations
PATIENT OUTCOMES/ EVALUATION CRITERIA:	**Establishes a normal/effective respiratory pattern free of cyanosis or other signs of hypoxia.**

ACTIONS/INTERVENTIONS

Independent

Maintain patent airway by head tilt, jaw hyperextention, oral pharyngeal airway.

Auscultate breath sounds. Listen for gurgling, wheezing, crowing, and/or silence after extubation.

Observe respiratory rate, depth, use of accessory muscles, chest expansion, retraction or flaring of nostrils, skin color and airflow.

Monitor vital signs continuously.

Position patient appropriately dependent on respiratory effort and type of surgery.

Observe for return of muscle function, especially respiratory.

RATIONALE

Airway obstruction may still occur with oral airway in place.

Indicative of obstruction by mucus or tongue corrected by suctioning/positioning. Diminished breath sounds suggest atelectasis. Wheezing indicates bronchospasm, whereas crowing or silence reflects partial to total laryngospasm.

Ascertains effectiveness of respirations immediately so corrective measures can be initiated.

Increased respirations, tachycardia, and/or bradycardia suggest hypoxia.

Head elevation and left lateral Sims' position prevent aspiration of vomitus, enhances ventilation to lower lobes, and relieves pressure on diaphragm.

After administration of intraoperative muscle relaxants, return of muscle function occurs first to the diaphragm, intercostals, and larynx; followed by large muscle groups, neck, shoulders, and abdominal muscles; then by midsize muscles, tongue, pharynx, extensors, and flexors; and finally by eyes, mouth, face, and fingers.

ACTIONS/INTERVENTIONS	RATIONALE
Independent	
Initiate *stir-up* regimen as soon as patient is reactive and continue into the postoperative period.	Active deep ventilation inflates alveoli, breaks up secretions, increases oxygen transfer, and removes anesthetic gases; coughing enhances removal of secretions from the pulmonary system.
Observe for excessive somnolence.	Narcotic-induced respiratory depression or presence of muscle relaxants in the system may be cyclical in recurrence, creating sine-wave pattern of depression and reemergence. In addition, pentothal is absorbed in the fatty tissues; and as circulation improves, it may be redistributed throughout the bloodstream.
Suction as necessary.	Airway obstruction can occur because of blood or mucus in throat or trachea.
Collaborative	
Administer supplemental oxygen as indicated.	Maximizes oxygen for uptake to bind with Hb in place of anesthetic gases to enhance removal of inhalation agents.
Administer IV medications, e.g., naloxone (Narcan) or doxapram (Dopram).	Narcan reverses narcotic-induced CNS depression, and Dopram stimulates respiratory muscles. Both drugs are cyclical in nature, and respiratory depression may return.
Provide/maintain ventilator assistance.	Dependent on cause of respiratory depression or type of surgery (e.g., pulmonary, extensive abdominal, cardiac), endotracheal tube may be left in place and connected to ventilator.
Assist with use of respiratory aids, e.g., incentive spirometer, blow bottles.	Maximal respiratory efforts reduce potential for atelectasis and infection.

NURSING DIAGNOSIS:	**SENSORY-PERCEPTUAL ALTERATION: (SPECIFY)/ THOUGHT PROCESSES, ALTERED**
May be related to:	**Chemical alteration: use of pharmaceutical agents, hypoxia**
	Therapeutically restricted environments; excessive sensory stimuli
	Physiologic stress
Possibly evidenced by:	**Disorientation to person, place, time; change in usual response to stimuli**
	Impaired ability to concentrate, reason, make decisions
	Motor incoordination
PATIENT OUTCOMES/ EVALUATION CRITERIA:	**Regains usual level of consciousness/mentation. Recognizes limitations and seeks assistance as necessary.**

ACTIONS/INTERVENTIONS	RATIONALE

Independent

Continuously reorient patient to time and place; confirm that surgery is completed.

As patient regains consciousness, support and assurance will help to alleviate anxiety.

Speak in normal, clear voice without shouting, being aware of what you are saying. Minimize discussion of negatives (e.g., patient/personnel problems) within patient's hearing. Explain procedures even if patient does not seem aware.

Cannot tell when patient is aware, but sense of hearing returns first; so it is important not to say things that may be misinterpreted. Providing information helps patient to preserve dignity and to prepare for activity.

Evaluate sensation/movement of extremities and trunk as appropriate.

Return of function following local or spinal nerve blocks is dependent on type/amount of agent used and duration of procedure.

Use bed rail padding, restraints as necessary.

Provides for patient safety during emergence stage. Prevents injury to head and extremities if patient becomes combative while disoriented.

Secure parenteral lines, endotracheal tube, catheters, if present, and check for patency.

Disoriented patient may pull on lines and drainage systems, disconnecting or kinking them.

Maintain quiet, calm environment.

External stimuli, e.g., noise, lights, touch may cause psychic aberrations when dissociative anesthetics (e.g., ketamine) have been administered.

Observe for hallucinations, delusions, depression, or an excited state.

May develop following trauma and indicate delirium. In patient who has used alcohol to excess, may suggest impending delirium tremens. (Refer to CP: Alcoholism, p. 825.)

Reassess return of sensory abilities and thought processes thoroughly prior to discharge, as indicated.

Ambulatory surgical patient must be able to fend for self with the help of SO to prevent personal injury after discharge.

Collaborative

Maintain extended stay in postoperative recovery area prior to discharge.

Disorientation may persist, and SO may not be able to protect the patient at home.

NURSING DIAGNOSIS:	FLUID VOLUME DEFICIT, POTENTIAL
May be related to:	**Restriction of oral intake (medical/presence of nausea)**
	Loss of fluid through abnormal routes, e.g., indwelling tubes, drains; normal routes, e.g., vomiting
	Loss of vascular integrity, changes in clotting ability
	Extremes of age and weight
Possibly evidenced by:	**[Not applicable; presence of signs and symptoms establishes an *actual* diagnosis.]**
PATIENT OUTCOMES/ EVALUATION CRITERIA:	**Demonstrates adequate fluid balance, as evidenced by stable vital signs, palpable pulses of good quality, normal skin turgor, moist mucous membranes, and individually appropriate urinary output.**

ACTIONS/INTERVENTIONS	RATIONALE

Independent

Measure and record intake and output (including GI losses). Review intraoperative record.

Accurate documentation helps identify fluid losses/replacement needs and influences choice of interventions.

Assess urinary output specifically for type of operative procedure done.

May be decreased or absent after procedures on the genitourinary system and/or adjacent structures (e.g., ureteroplasty, ureterolithotomy, abdominal or vaginal hysterectomy), indicating malfunction or obstruction of the urinary system.

Provide routine voiding measures as needed, e.g., privacy, sitting position, running water in sink, pouring warm water over perineum.

Promotes relaxation of perineal muscles and may facilitate voiding efforts.

Monitor vital signs.

Hypotension, tachycardia, increased respirations may indicate fluid deficit, e.g., dehydration/hypovolemia.

Inspect dressings, drainage devices at regular intervals. Assess wound for swelling.

Excessive bleeding can lead to hypovolemia/circulatory collapse. Note: Local swelling may indicate hematoma formation/hemorrhage.

Monitor skin temperature, palpate peripheral pulses.

Cool/clammy skin, weak pulses indicate decreased peripheral circulation and need for additional fluid replacement.

Collaborative

Administer parenteral fluids, blood products, and/or plasma expanders as indicated. Increase IV rate if needed.

Replaces documented fluid loss. Timely replacement of circulating volume decreases potential for complications of deficit, e.g., electrolyte imbalance, dehydration, cardiovascular collapse. Note: Increased volume may be required initially to support circulating volume/prevent hypotension because of decreased vasomotor tone following fluothane administration.

Insert urinary catheter with or without urimeter as necessary.

Provides mechanism for accurate monitoring of urinary output.

Resume oral intake gradually as indicated.

Oral intake is dependent on return of gastrointestinal function.

Administer antiemetics as appropriate.

Relieves nausea/vomiting, which may impair intake/add to fluid losses.

Monitor laboratory studies, e.g., Hg/Hct. Compare preoperative and postoperative blood studies.

Indicators of hydration/circulating volume. Anemia and/or low Hct preoperatively combined with unreplaced fluid losses intraoperatively will further potentiate deficit.

NURSING DIAGNOSIS:	**COMFORT, ALTERED: PAIN, ACUTE**
May be related to:	**Disruption of skin, tissue, and muscle integrity, musculoskeletal/bone trauma**
	Presence of tubes and drains
Possibly evidenced by:	**Complaints of pain**
	Alteration in muscle tone; facial mask of pain; distraction/guarding/protective behaviors

	Self-focusing; narrowed focus
	Autonomic responses
PATIENT OUTCOMES/ EVALUATION CRITERIA:	**Reports pain relieved/controlled. Appears relaxed, able to rest/sleep and participate in activities appropriately.**

ACTIONS/INTERVENTIONS	RATIONALE

Independent

Review intraoperative/recovery room record for medications previously administered.	Presence of narcotics and droperidol in system will potentiate narcotic analgesia, whereas patients anesthetized with Fluothane and Ethrane have no residual analgesic effects. In addition, intraoperative local/regional blocks have varying duration, e.g., 1–2 hours for regionals or up to 2–6 hours for locals.
Evaluate pain noting characteristics, location, and intensity (1–10 scale).	Provides information about need for/effectiveness of interventions.
Assess vital signs, noting tachycardia, hypertension, and increased respiration.	May indicate pain and discomfort.
Assess causes of possible discomfort other than operative procedure.	Discomfort can be caused/aggravated by presence of nonpatent indwelling catheters, nasogastric tube, parenteral lines (e.g., bladder pain, gastric fluid and gas accumulation, and infiltration pressure of IV fluids/medications).
Provide information about transitory nature of discomfort, as appropriate.	Understanding the cause of the discomfort (e.g., sore muscles from administration of succinylcholine may persist up to 48 hours postoperatively, whereas sore throat due to intubation is transitory) provides emotional reassurance.
Reposition as indicated, e.g., semi-Fowler's; lateral Sims'.	May relieve pain and enhance circulation. Semi-Fowler's position will relieve abdominal muscle tension and arthritic back muscle tension, whereas lateral Sims' will relieve dorsal pressures.
Encourage use of relaxation techniques, e.g., deep-breathing exercises, guided imagery, visualization.	Relieves muscle and emotional tension, enhances sense of control and may improve coping abilities.
Provide routine oral care, occasional ice chips/sips of fluids as tolerated.	Reduces discomfort associated with dry mucous membranes due to anesthetic agents, oral restrictions.
Observe effects of analgesia.	Respirations may decrease upon administration of narcotic, and synergistic effects with anesthetic agents may occur.

Collaborative

Administer medications as indicated:	
Analgesics IV (after reviewing anesthesia record for contraindications and/or presence of agents that may potentiate analgesia);	Analgesics given IV reach the pain centers immediately, providing more effective relief with small doses of medication. IM administration takes longer, and its effectiveness is dependent on absorption rates and circulation. Note: Narcotic dosage should be reduced one fourth to one third after use of Innovar or doperidol to prevent profound tranquilization during first 10 hours postoperatively.

ACTIONS/INTERVENTIONS	RATIONALE

Collaborative

PCA;

Patient-controlled analgesia (PCA) needs detailed instruction in its use and must be monitored closely but is considered very effective in managing acute postoperative pain with smaller amounts of narcotic.

Local anesthetics, e.g., epidural block.

Analgesics may be injected into the operative site or nerves to the site may be kept blocked in the immediate postoperative phase to prevent pain.

NURSING DIAGNOSIS:	SKIN/TISSUE INTEGRITY, IMPAIRED
May be related to:	**Mechanical interruption of skin/tissues**
	Altered circulation, effects of medication; accumulation of drainage; altered metabolic state
Possibly evidenced by:	**Disruption of skin surface/layers and tissues**
PATIENT OUTCOMES/ EVALUATION CRITERIA:	**Achieves timely wound healing. Demonstrates behaviors/techniques to promote healing and to prevent complications.**

ACTIONS/INTERVENTIONS	RATIONALE

Independent

Reinforce initial dressing/change as indicated. Use strict aseptic techniques.

Protects wound from mechanical injury and contamination. Prevents accumulation of fluids that may cause excoriation.

Gently remove tape and dressings when changing.

Reduces risk of skin trauma and disruption of wound.

Apply skin sealants/barriers before tape if needed. Use paper/silk (hypoallergenic) tape or Montgomery straps/elastic netting for dressings requiring frequent changing.

Reduces potential for skin trauma/abrasions and provides additional protection for delicate skin/tissues.

Check tension of dressings. Avoid wrapping tape around extremity.

Can impair/occlude circulation to wound as well as distal portion of extremity.

Inspect wound routinely, noting characteristics and integrity.

Early recognition of delayed healing/developing complications may prevent a more serious situation.

Assess amount and characteristics of drainage.

Decreasing drainage suggests evolution of healing process, while continued drainage or presence of bloody/odoriferous exudate suggests complications (e.g., fistula formation, hemorrhage, infection).

Maintain patency of drainage tubes; apply collection bag over drains/incisions in presence of copious or caustic drainage.

Facilitates approximation of wound edges; reduces risk of infection and chemical injury to skin/tissues.

Elevate operative area if feasible.

Promotes venous return and limits edema formation.

Splint incisional area with pillow or pad during coughing/movement.

Equalizes pressure on the wound, minimizing risk of dehiscence/rupture.

Caution patient not to touch wound if avoidable.

Prevents contamination of wound.

ACTIONS/INTERVENTIONS	RATIONALE

Independent

Leave wound open to air as soon as possible, or cover with small gauze/Telfa pad as needed.

Aids in drying wound and facilitates healing processes. Light covering may be necessary to prevent irritation if sutures/wound edges rub against linens.

Cleanse skin surface with diluted hydrogen peroxide, or running water and mild soap after incision is sealed.

Reduces skin contaminants, aids in removal of exudate.

Collaborative

Apply ice if appropriate.

Reduces edema formation that may cause undue pressure on incision during initial postoperative period.

Use abdominal binder if indicated.

Provides additional support for high risk incisions (e.g., obese patient).

Irrigate wound; assist with debridement as needed.

Removes infectious exudate/necrotic tissue to promote healing.

NURSING DIAGNOSIS:	TISSUE PERFUSION, ALTERED [POTENTIAL]
May be related to:	**Interruption of flow: arterial, venous**
	Hypovolemia
Possibly evidenced by:	**[Not applicable; presence of signs and symptoms establishes an *actual* diagnosis.]**
PATIENT OUTCOMES/ EVALUATION CRITERIA:	**Demonstrates adequate perfusion evidenced by stable vital signs, peripheral pulses present and strong; skin warm/dry; usual mentation and individually appropriate urinary output.**

ACTIONS/INTERVENTIONS	RATIONALE

Independent

Change position slowly in bed and at transfer (especially Fluothane-anesthetized patient).

Vasoconstrictor mechanisms are depressed and quick movement may lead to hypotension.

Assist with ROM exercises, including active ankle/leg exercises.

Stimulates peripheral circulation, aids in preventing venous stasis to reduce risk of thrombus formation.

Encourage/assist with early ambulation.

Enhances circulation and return of normal organ function.

Avoid use of knee Gatch/pillow under knees. Caution patient against crossing legs or sitting with legs dependent for prolonged period of time.

Prevents stasis of venous circulation and reduces risk of thrombophlebitis.

Assess lower extremities for erythema, positive Homans' sign.

Circulation may be restricted by some positions used during surgery, while anesthetics and decreased activity alter vasomotor tone, potentiating vascular pooling and increasing risks of thrombus formation. (Refer to CP: Thrombophlebitis: Deep Vein Thrombosis, p. 117.)

ACTIONS/INTERVENTIONS

Independent

Monitor vital signs; palpate peripheral pulses; note skin temperature/color and capillary refill. Evaluate urine output/time of voiding.

Collaborative

Administer IV fluids/blood products as needed.

Apply antiembolic hose as indicated.

RATIONALE

Indicators of adequacy of circulating volume and tissue perfusion/organ function.

Maintains circulating volume, supports perfusion. (Refer to ND: Fluid Volume Deficit, Potential, p. 799.)

Promotes venous return and prevents venous stasis of legs to reduce risk of thrombosis.

NURSING DIAGNOSIS:	KNOWLEDGE DEFICIT [LEARNING NEED] (SPECIFY)
May be related to:	Lack of exposure/lack of recall, information misinterpretation
	Unfamiliarity with information resources
	Cognitive limitation
Possibly evidenced by:	Questions/request for information
	Statement of misconception
	Inaccurate follow-through of instructions/development of preventable complications
PATIENT OUTCOMES/ EVALUATION CRITERIA:	Verbalizes understanding of condition, effects of procedure and treatment. Correctly performs necessary procedures and explains reasons for actions. Initiates necessary lifestyle changes and participates in treatment regimen.

ACTIONS/INTERVENTIONS

Independent

Review condition, specific procedure done, and future expectations.

Demonstrate dressing/wound care. Identify source for supplies.

Review avoidance of environmental risk factors, e.g., exposure to crowds/persons with infections.

Discuss drug therapy, including use of prescribed and OTC analgesics.

Identify specific activity limitations.

Recommend planned/progressive exercise.

Schedule adequate rest periods.

RATIONALE

Provides knowledge base on which patient can make informed choices.

Promotes competent self-care and enhances independence.

Reduces potential for acquired infections.

Enhances cooperation with regimen, reduces risk of adverse reactions/untoward effects.

Prevents undue strain on operative site.

Promotes return of normal function and enhances feelings of general well-being.

Prevents fatigue and conserves energy for healing.

ACTIONS/INTERVENTIONS	RATIONALE
Independent	
Review importance of nutritious diet and adequate fluid intake.	Provides elements necessary for tissue regeneration/ healing and support of tissue perfusion and organ function.
Encourage cessation of smoking.	Increases risk of pulmonary infections. Causes vaso-constriction and reduces oxygen-binding capacity of blood, affecting cellular perfusion and potentially impairing healing.
Identify signs/symptoms requiring medical evaluation, e.g., nausea/vomiting; difficulty voiding; fever, continued/odiferous wound drainage; incisional swelling, erythema or separation of edges; unresolved, or changes in characteristics of, pain.	Early recognition and treatment of developing complications (e.g., ileus, urinary retention, infection, delayed healing) may prevent progression to more serious or life-threatening situation.
Stress necessity of follow-up visits.	Monitors progress of healing and evaluates effectiveness of regimen.
Include SO in teaching program. Provide written instructions/teaching materials.	Provides additional resource for reference after discharge.

Long-Term Care

Patients in the acute care setting may be discharged to an extended care facility. Patients requiring relatively short-term rehabilitation as well as those needing long-term care/permanent nursing care are included in this group. Coordination and knowledge are essential in providing continuity and quality care for these patients. The needs of the patient (e.g., physical, occupational, and rehabilitation therapy) are frequently the deciding factors in the choice of placement.

Refer to appropriate CPs (e.g., Spinal Cord Injury; Cerebrovascular Accident/Stroke; Multiple Sclerosis; Craniocerebral Trauma; Fractures) for additional interventions and considerations.

PATIENT ASSESSMENT DATA BASE

Data are dependent on underlying physical/psychosocial conditions necessitating continuation of structured care.

TEACHING/LEARNING

Discharge Plan Considerations: May require assistance with treatments, self-care/homemaker tasks or alternate living arrangements (e.g., group home).

DIAGNOSTIC STUDIES

ECG: provides baseline data; detects abnormalities.

Chest x-ray: reveals size of heart, lung abnormalities, changes of the large blood vessels and bony structure of the chest.

Tonometer test: measures intraocular pressure.

Visual acuity testing: identifies cataracts/other vision problems.

Pap smear: checks for cancer of the cervix, vagina.

CBC: reveals problems such as infection, anemia, other abnormalities.

Urinalysis: provides information about kidney function; determines presence of UTI or diabetes.

Electrolytes: identifies imbalances.

Drug screen: as indicated by usage to identify therapeutic or toxic levels.

NURSING PRIORITIES

1. Promote physiologic and psychologic well-being.
2. Provide for security and safety.
3. Prevent complications of disease and/or aging process.
4. Promote effective coping skills and independence.
5. Encourage continuation of "healthy" habits, participation in plan of care to meet individual needs and wishes.

DISCHARGE CRITERIA

1. Dealing realistically with current situation.
2. Homeostasis maintained.
3. Injury prevented.
4. Complications prevented/minimized.
5. Meeting ADLs by self/with assistance as necessary.

NURSING DIAGNOSIS:	ANXIETY [SPECIFY LEVEL]/FEAR
May be related to:	**Change in health status, role functioning, interaction patterns, socioeconomic status, environment**
	Unmet needs; recent life changes, loss of friends/SO

Possibly evidenced by:	Apprehension; restlessness; repetitive questioning; pacing, purposeless activity
	Various behaviors (appears overexcited, withdrawn, worried, fearful); presence of facial tension, trembling, hand tremors
	Expressed concern regarding changes in life events
	Insomnia
	Focus on self; lack of interest in activity
PATIENT OUTCOMES/ EVALUATION CRITERIA:	Appears relaxed. Reports anxiety is reduced to a manageable level. Demonstrates problem-solving skills and uses resources effectively.

ACTIONS/INTERVENTIONS	RATIONALE

Independent

Provide patient/SO with copy of "Patients' Bill of Rights" and review it with them. Discuss facility's rules, e.g., visiting, off-grounds visits.	Provides information that can foster confidence that individual rights do continue in this setting and the patient is still "his own person" and has some control over what happens.
Determine patient/SO attitude toward admission to facility.	When patient is giving up own home and way of life, feelings of helplessness, loss, and grieving are to be expected.
Assess level of anxiety and discuss reasons when possible.	Identifying specific problems will enable individual to deal more realistically with them.
Make time to listen to patient about concerns, and encourage free expression of feelings; e.g., anger, hostility, fear and loneliness.	Being available in this way allows patient to feel accepted, begin to acknowledge and deal with feelings related to circumstances of admission.
Acknowledge reality of situation and feelings of patient. Accept expressions of anger while limiting aggressive, acting-out behavior.	Permission to express feelings allows for beginning resolution. Acceptance promotes sense of self-worth.
Develop nurse/patient relationship.	Trusting relationships among patient/SO/staff promotes optimal care and support.
Orient to physical aspects of facility, schedules and activities. Introduce to roommate(s) and staff. Give explanation of roles.	Getting acquainted is an important part of admission. Knowledge of where things are and who patient can expect assistance from can be helpful in reducing anxiety.
Provide above information in written or taped form as well.	Overload of information is difficult to remember. Patient can refer to written or taped material as needed to refresh memory, learn new information.
Give careful thought to room placement. Provide help and encouragement in placing own belongings around room. Do not transfer from one room to another without patient approval/documentable need.	Location, roommate compatibility, and place for personal belongings are important considerations for helping the patient feel "at home." Changes are often met with resistance and can result in emotional upset and decline in physical condition.

Collaborative

Refer to social service or other appropriate agency for assistance. Have social worker discuss ramifications	Often patient is not aware of the resources available, and providing current information about individual

807

ACTIONS/INTERVENTIONS

Collaborative

of Medicare/Medicaid if patient is eligible for these resources.

RATIONALE

coverage and other possible sources of support will assist with adjustment to new situation.

NURSING DIAGNOSIS:	GRIEVING, ANTICIPATORY
May be related to:	Perceived, actual or potential loss of physiopsychosocial well-being, personal possessions, or SO; cultural beliefs about aging
Possibly evidenced by:	Denial of feelings, depression, sorrow, guilt
	Alterations in activity level, sleep patterns, eating habits, libido
PATIENT OUTCOMES/ EVALUATION CRITERIA:	Identifies and expresses feelings appropriately; progressing through the grieving process. Enjoying the present and planning for the future, one day at a time.

ACTIONS/INTERVENTIONS

Independent

Assess emotional state.

Make time to listen to the patient. Encourage free expression of hopeless feelings and desire to die.

Assess suicidal potential.

Involve SO in discussions and activities to the level of their willingness.

Provide liberal touching/hugs as individually accepted.

Collaborative

Refer to other resources as indicated, e.g., clinical specialist, social worker.

Assist with/plan for specifics as necessary (e.g., making of will, funeral arrangements).

RATIONALE

Anxiety and depression are common reactions to changes/losses associated with long-term illness or debilitating condition.

More helpful to allow these feelings to be expressed and dealt with than to deny them.

May be related to physical disease, social isolation, and grief and is more common in men. (Refer to CP: Psychosocial Aspects of Acute Care, p. 773.)

When SO are involved, there is more potential for successful problem solving. Note: SO may not be available or may not choose to be involved.

Conveys sense of concern/closeness to reduce feelings of isolation and enhance sense of self-worth. Note: Touch may be viewed as a threat by some patients and escalate feelings of anger.

May need further assistance to resolve some problems.

Having these issues resolved can help patient/SO deal with the grieving process and may provide peace of mind.

NURSING DIAGNOSIS:	THOUGHT PROCESSES, ALTERED
May be related to:	Physiologic changes of aging; loss of cells and brain atrophy; decreased blood supply; altered sensory input

Pain; effects of medications

Psychologic conflicts: disrupted life pattern

Possibly evidenced by: Slower reaction times, gradual memory loss, altered attention span; disorientation; inability to follow

Altered sleep patterns

Personality changes

PATIENT OUTCOMES/ EVALUATION CRITERIA: Maintains usual reality orientation. Recognizes changes in thinking and behavior. Identifies interventions to deal effectively with situation/deficits.

ACTIONS/INTERVENTIONS	RATIONALE
Independent	
Allow adequate time for patient to respond to questions/comments and to make decisions.	Reaction time may be slowed with aging or with brain injuries and some neuromuscular conditions.
Discuss happenings of the past. Place familiar objects in room. Encourage the display of SO/friends photographs/photo-albums; frequent visits.	Events of the past may be more readily available to the patient, because long-term memory often remains intact. Reminiscence/life review and companionship have been shown to be beneficial to the elderly patient.
Note patient's problem of short-term memory loss, and provide with aids (e.g., calendars, clocks, room signs, pictures) to assist in continual reorientation.	Short-term memory loss presents a challenge for nursing care, especially if the patient cannot remember such things as how to use the call bell or how to get to the bathroom. This problem is not in patient's control but may be less frustrating if simple reminders are used. It may be helpful for older person to know that short-term memory loss is common and is not necessarily a sign of "senility."
Evaluate individual stress level, and deal with it appropriately.	Stress level may be greatly increased because of recent losses, e.g., health, death of SO, loss of home. In addition, some conflicts that occur with age come from previously unresolved problems that may need to be dealt with now.
Assess physical status/psychiatric symptoms. Institute interventions appropriate to findings.	Not all mental changes are the result of aging and it is important to rule out physical causes before accepting these as unchangeable. May be the result of metabolic, toxic, drug-induced, infectious or cardiac and respiratory disorders. (Refer to CP: Alzheimer's Disease, p. 313.)

NURSING DIAGNOSIS: COPING, INEFFECTIVE FAMILY: COMPROMISED

May be related to: Placement of family member in long-term care facility

Temporary family disorganization and role changes

Situational crises SO may be facing

Patient providing little support for SO

Prolonged disease or disability progression that ex-

Possibly evidenced by:	SO describes significant preoccupation with personal reactions, e.g., fear, anticipatory grief, guilt, anxiety
	SO attempts assistive/supportive behaviors with unsatisfactory results
	SO withdraws from patient
	SO displays protective behavior disproportionate (too little or too much) to patient's abilities/need for autonomy
FAMILY OUTCOMES/ EVALUATION CRITERIA:	Identifies/verbalizes resources within themselves to deal with the situation. Interacts appropriately with the patient and staff, providing support and assistance as indicated. Verbalizes knowledge and understanding of situation.

ACTIONS/INTERVENTIONS

Independent

Introduce staff and provide SO with information about facility and care. Be available for questions. Provide tour of facility.

Encourage SO participation in care at level of desire and capability and within limits of safety. Include in social events/celebrations.

Accept choices of SO regarding level of involvement in care.

Identify staff's own feelings of anger and frustration about patient/SO choices and goals that differ from staff, and deal with appropriately.

Collaborative

Inform SO of services available to them (meal tickets, family cooking time, group care conference, VNA, caseworker, social services).

RATIONALE

Helpful to establish beginning relationships. Offers opportunities for enhancing feelings of involvement.

Helps family to feel at ease and allows them to feel supportive and a part of the patient's life.

May choose to ignore patient or project feelings of guilt in criticism of staff. Note: Feelings of dissatisfaction with the staff may be transferred to the patient.

Group care conferences or individual counseling may be helpful in problem solving.

Promotes feeling of involvement, eases transition in adjustment to patient's admission.

NURSING DIAGNOSIS:	**INJURY, POTENTIAL FOR [DRUG TOXICITY]**
May be related to:	Reduced metabolism; impaired circulation; precarious physiologic balance, presence of multiple diseases/organ involvement
	Use of multiple prescribed/OTC drugs
Possibly evidenced by:	[Not applicable; presence of signs and symptoms establishes an *actual* diagnosis.]
PATIENT OUTCOMES/	Maintains prescribed drug regimen free of untoward

810

EVALUATION CRITERIA: side effects.

ACTIONS/INTERVENTIONS	RATIONALE
Independent	
Determine allergies and other past drug history.	Avoids repetition/creation of problems.
Use resources (e.g., drug manuals, pharmacist) for information about toxic symptoms and side effects. List drug interactions and medications that are given with or without foods, as well as those that should not be crushed.	Provides information about drugs being taken and identifies possible interactions. Toxicity can be increased in the debilitated and older patient with symptoms not as apparent.
Discuss self-administration of OTC products.	Limits interference with prescribed regimen/desired drug action and organ function. May prevent inadvertent overdosing/toxic reactions.
Identify interferences with swallowing or reluctance to take tablets or capsules.	May not be able to or want to take medication.
Give pills in a spoonful of soft foods, e.g., applesauce, ice cream; or use liquid form of medication if available.	Enables proper dosage if patient is unable to swallow pills normally.
Open capsules or crush tablets only when appropriate.	Should not be done unless absolutely necessary as this may alter absorption of medications, e.g., enteric-coated tablets may be absorbed in stomach when crushed, instead of the intestines.
Make sure medication has been swallowed.	Ensures effective therapeutic use of medication and prevents hoarding.
Observe for changes in condition/behavior.	Behavior may be only indication of drug toxicity and early identification of problems provides for appropriate intervention.
Use discretion in the administration of sedatives.	A quiet place where the patient can pace or seclusion may be more helpful. If patient is destructive or excessively disruptive, pharmacologic or mechanical control measures may be required. Convenience of the staff is never a reason for sedating patients, but rights of other patients need to be taken into consideration.
Collaborative	
Review drug regimen routinely with physician, pharmacist.	Provides opportunity to alter therapy (e.g., reduce dosage, discontinue medications) as patient's needs and organ functions change.
Obtain serum drug levels as indicated.	Determines therapeutic/toxicity levels.

NURSING DIAGNOSIS:	COMMUNICATION, IMPAIRED VERBAL
May be related to:	**Degenerative changes (e.g., reduced cerebral circulation, hearing loss); progressive neurologic disease (e.g., Parkinson's disease, Alzheimer's)**
	Laryngectomy; stroke
Possibly evidenced by:	**Impaired articulation, difficulty with phonation, inability to modulate speech, find words, name or identify objects**

	Diminished hearing ability
	Aphasia, dysarthria
PATIENT OUTCOMES/ EVALUATION CRITERIA:	**Establishes method of communication by which needs can be expressed. Demonstrates congruent verbal and nonverbal communication.**

ACTIONS/INTERVENTIONS	RATIONALE
Independent	
Investigate how SO communicates with the patient.	Provides opportunity to develop/continue effective communication patterns, which have already been established.
Assess reason for lack of communicaton, including CNS and neuromuscular functioning, gag/swallow reflexes, and hearing.	Identification of the problem is essential to appropriate intervention. Sometimes patients do not want to talk, may think they talk when they do not, may expect others to know what they want, may not be able to comprehend or be understood.
Determine whether patient is bilingual or whether English is primary language.	With declining cerebral function/diminished thought processes, increased level of stress, patient may mix languages/revert to original language.
Check for excess cerumen.	Hardened earwax may decrease hearing acuity and causes tinnitus.
Assess patient knowledge base and level of comprehension. Treat the patient as an adult, avoiding pity and impatience.	Knowing how much to expect of the patient can help to avoid frustration and unreasonable demands for performance. However, having an expectation that the patient will understand may help to raise level of performance.
Establish therapeutic nurse-patient relationship through Active-listening, being available for problem solving.	Aids in dealing with communication problems.
Be aware that behavioral problems may indicate hearing loss.	Anger, explosive temper outbursts, frustration, embarrassment, depression, withdrawal, and paranoia may be attempts to deal with communication problems.
Make patient aware of presence when entering the room by turning a light off and on, touching patient or mattress as appropriate.	Getting attention is the first step in communication.
Make eye contact, lower self to patient's level, and speak face to face.	Conveys interest and promotes contact.
Speak slowly and distinctly, using simple sentences, yes or no questions. Avoid speaking loudly or shouting. Supplement with written communication when possible/needed. Allow sufficient time for reply; remain relaxed with patient.	Assists in comprehension and overall communication. Patient may respond poorly to high-pitched sounds; shouting also obscures consonants and amplifies vowels.
Use other creative measures to assist in communication, e.g., picture chart, alphabet board, sign language when appropriate.	Many options are available, depending on individual situation. Note: Sign language also may be used effectively with other than hearing-impaired individuals.
Collaborative	
Refer to speech therapists, or for audiometry as needed to determine extent of hearing loss and whether a hearing aid is appropriate.	May be helpful to patient and staff in improving communication. Testing may ascertain precise nature of the hearing deficit. Some sources believe 90% of the

ACTIONS/INTERVENTIONS	RATIONALE
Collaborative	

patients in long-term care facilities have some degree of loss. Presbycusis is a common age change. Hearing aids are most effective with conductive losses and may help with sensorineural losses.

NURSING DIAGNOSIS:	SLEEP PATTERN DISTURBANCE
May be related to:	Internal factors: illness, psychologic stress, inactivity
	External factors: environmental changes, facility routines
Possibly evidenced by:	Complaints of difficulty in falling asleep/not feeling well rested
	Interrupted sleep, awakening earlier than desired
	Change in behavior/performance
	Increasing irritability, listlessness
PATIENT OUTCOMES/ EVALUATION CRITERIA:	Reports improvement in sleep/rest pattern. Verbalizes increased sense of well-being and feeling rested.

ACTIONS/INTERVENTIONS	RATIONALE
Independent	
Determine normal sleep habits and changes that are occurring.	Assesses need for and identifies appropriate interventions.
Obtain comfortable bedding. Provide some of own possessions, e.g., pillow, afghan.	Increases comfort for sleep as well as physiologic/psychologic support.
Establish sleep routine suitable to old pattern and new environment.	When new routine contains as many aspects of old habits as possible, stress and related anxiety may be reduced.
Encourage some light physical activity during the day. Make sure patient stops activity several hours before bedtime.	Daytime activity can help patient expend energy and be ready for nighttime sleep. However, continuation of activity close to bedtime may act as a stimulant, delaying sleep.
Provide warm bath and massage, warm milk, wine, or brandy at bedtime.	Promotes a relaxing soothing effect. Note: Milk has soporific qualities, enhancing synthesis of serotonin, a neurotransmitter that helps patient fall asleep faster and sleep longer.
Instruct in relaxation measures.	Helps to induce sleep.
Reduce noise and light.	Provides atmosphere conducive to sleep.
Encourage position of comfort, assist in turning.	Repositioning alters areas of pressure and promotes rest.
Use side rails as indicated; lower bed when possible.	May have fear of falling because of change in size and height of bed. Side rails provide safety and may be used to assist with turning.

813

ACTIONS/INTERVENTIONS

Independent

Avoid interruptions (e.g., drug and therapy schedule).

Collaborative

Administer sedatives, hypnotics, as indicated.

RATIONALE

Uninterrupted sleep is more restful, and patient may be unable to return to sleep when wakened.

May be given to help patient sleep/rest during transition period from home to new setting. Note: Avoid habitual use, because these drugs decrease REM sleep time.

NURSING DIAGNOSIS:	**NUTRITION, ALTERED: LESS/MORE THAN BODY REQUIREMENTS**
May be related to:	**Impaired dentition; dulling of senses of smell and taste**
	Cognitive limitations, depression
	Sedentary activity level
Possibly evidenced by:	**Reported/observed dysfunctional eating patterns**
	Weight under/over ideal for height and frame
	Poor muscle tone, pale conjunctiva/mucous membranes
PATIENT OUTCOMES/ EVALUATION CRITERIA:	**Maintains normal weight or progresses toward weight goal with normalization of laboratory values and free of signs of malnutrition/obesity. Demonstrates eating patterns/behaviors to maintain appropriate weight.**

ACTIONS/INTERVENTIONS

Independent

Assess causes of weight loss/gain, e.g., dysphagia caused by neuro/psychogenic disturbances, tumors, muscular dysfunction or dysfunctional eating patterns related to depression.

Weigh on admission and on a regular basis.

Evaluate activity pattern.

Observe condition of skin; note muscle-wasting, brittle nails, dry, lifeless hair, and signs of poor healing.

Check state of patient's dental health, including fit and condition of dentures, if present.

Incorporate favorite foods and maintain as near normal food consistency as possible, e.g., soft or finely ground food with gravy or liquid added. Avoid baby food whenever possible.

Encourage the use of spices (other than sodium) to

RATIONALE

Aids in creating plan of care/choice of interventions.

Monitors nutritional state and effectiveness of interventions.

Extremes of exercise (e.g., sedentary life, continuous pacing) affect caloric needs.

Reflects lack of adequate nutrition.

Oral infections/dental problems, shrinking gums, with resultant loose denture fit, decrease patient's ability to chew.

Aids in maintaining intake, especially when mouth and dental problems exist. Baby food is often unpalatable and can decrease appetite and lower self-esteem.

Reduction in number of taste buds results in food tast-

ACTIONS/INTERVENTIONS

Independent

patient's personal taste.

Provide small, frequent feedings as indicated.

Promote a pleasant environment for eating, with company if possible.

Encourage exercise and activity program within individual ability.

Collaborative

Consult with dietician.

Provide high-protein diet with individually appropriate complex carbohydrates and calories. Include supplements between meals as indicated.

Refer for dental care routinely and as needed.

RATIONALE

ing bland and decreases enjoyment of food and desire to eat.

Decreased gastric motility causes patient to feel full and reduces intake.

Eating is in part a social event, and appetite can improve with increased socialization.

Promotes sense of well-being and may improve appetite.

Aids in establishing specific nutritional program to meet individual patient needs.

Adjustments may be needed to deal with the body's decreased ability to process protein, as well as decreased metabolic rate and levels of activity.

Maintenance of oral/dental health and good dentition can enhance intake.

NURSING DIAGNOSIS:	SELF-CARE DEFICIT: (SPECIFY)
May be related to:	**Depression, discouragement, loss of mobility, general debilitation; perceptual/cognitive impairment**
Possibly evidenced by:	**Inability to manage ADLs; unkempt appearance**
PATIENT OUTCOMES/ EVALUATION CRITERIA:	**Performs self-care activities within level of own ability. Demonstrates techniques/lifestyle changes to meet own needs. Uses resources effectively.**

ACTIONS/INTERVENTIONS

Independent

Determine current capabilities (0–4 scale) and barriers to participation in care.

Involve patient in formulation of care plan at level of ability.

Encourage self care. Work with present abilities; do not pressure patient beyond capabilities. Have expectation of improvement and assist as needed.

Provide and promote privacy.

Utilize specialized equipment as needed, e.g., tub transfer seat, grab bars, raised toilet seat.

Give tub bath, using a two-person lift if necessary. Use shower chair and spray attachment. Avoid chilling.

RATIONALE

Identifies need for/level of interventions required.

Enhances sense of control and aids in cooperation and development of independence.

Doing for oneself enhances feeling of self-worth. Failure can produce discouragement and depression.

Modesty may lead to reluctance to participate in care or perform activities in the presence of others.

Enhances ability to move/perform activities safely.

Provides safety for those who cannot get into the tub alone. Shower may be more feasible for some patients. Elderly/debilitated patients are more prone to chilling.

Independent

Shampoo hair as needed.

Aids in maintaining appearance.

Acquire clothing with modified fasteners as needed.

Use of velcro instead of buttons/shoe laces can facilitate process of dressing/undressing.

Encourage/assist with routine mouth/teeth care daily.

Reduces risk of gum disease/tooth loss, promotes proper fitting of dentures.

Collaborative

Consult with physical/occupational therapist and rehabilitation specialist.

Useful in establishing exercise/activity program and in identifying assistive devices to meet individual needs/facilitate independence.

Encourage use of barber/beauty salon regularly.

Enhances self-image and self-esteem, preserving dignity of the patient.

NURSING DIAGNOSIS:	SKIN INTEGRITY, IMPAIRED: POTENTIAL
May be related to:	General debilitation; reduced mobility; changes in skin and muscle mass associated with aging, sensory/motor deficits
	Altered circulation; edema; poor nutrition
	Excretions/secretions (bladder and bowel incontinence)
	Problems with self-care
Possibly evidenced by:	[Not applicable; presence of signs and symptoms establishes an *actual* diagnosis.]
PATIENT OUTCOMES/ EVALUATION CRITERIA:	Maintains intact skin. Identifies individual risk factors. Demonstrates behaviors/techniques to prevent skin breakdown/facilitate healing.

Independent

Anticipate and use preventive measures in patients who are at risk, such as anyone who is thin, obese, aging, or debilitated.

Decubitus ulcers are difficult to heal and prevention is the best treatment.

Assess nutritional status and initiate corrective measures as indicated. Provide balanced diet, e.g., adequate protein, vitamins A and E.

A positive nitrogen balance and improved nutritional state can help prevent skin breakdown and promote ulcer healing. Note: May need additional calories and protein if draining ulcer present.

Maintain strict skin hygiene, using mild, nondetergent soap (if any), drying gently and thoroughly, and lubricating with lotion or emollient.

A daily bath is usually not necessary because there is less waste excretion on skin surface (atrophy of sebaceous and sweat glands), and bathing may create dry-skin problems. However, as epidermis thins with age, cleansing skin and use of lubricants keep it soft/pliable and protect skin susceptible to breakdown.

Change position frequently, in bed and chair. Recommend 10 minutes of exercise each hour and/or per-

Improves circulation, muscle tone, and joint motion and promotes activity.

ACTIONS/INTERVENTIONS	RATIONALE

Independent

form passive range of motion.

Use a rotation schedule in turning patient on all four sides unless contraindicated.

Allows for longer periods free of pressure. Note: Use of prone position is dependent on patient tolerance.

Massage bony prominences gently with lotion or cream.

Enhances circulation to tissues, increases vascular tone, and reduces tissue edema.

Keep sheets and bedclothes clean, dry, and free from wrinkles, crumbs, and other irritating material.

Avoids friction/abrasions of skin.

Use elbow/heel protectors; foam pads, sheepskin for positioning in bed and when up in chair.

Reduces risk of tissue abrasions, and decreases pressure that can impair cellular blood flow. Promotes circulation of air along skin surface to dissipate heat/moisture.

Provide for safety during ambulation.

Loss of muscle control and debilitation may result in impaired coordination.

Limit exposure to temperature extremes/use of heating pad or ice pack.

Decreased sensation of pain/heat/cold increases risk of tissue trauma.

Examine feet and nails routinely and provide foot and nail care as indicated.

Foot problems are common among patients who are bedfast/debilitated.

Keep nails cut short and smooth;

Jagged, rough nails can cause tissue infection by scratching adjacent skin areas.

Use lotion, softening cream on feet;

Prevents drying/cracking of skin; promotes maintenance of healthy skin.

Check for fissures between toes. Swab with hydrogen peroxide or dust with antiseptic powder and place a wisp of cotton between the toes;

Prevents spread of infection and/or tissue injury.

Rub feet with witch hazel or a mentholated preparation and have patient wear lightweight cotton stockings.

Even though rash may not be present, burning and itching may be a problem. Witch hazel may be contraindicated if skin is dry.

Inspect skin surface/folds and bony prominences routinely. Increase preventive measures when reddened areas are noticed.

Skin breakdown can occur quickly with potential for infection and necrosis, possibly involving muscle and bone.

Continue regimen for redness and irritation when break in skin occurs.

Aggressive measures are important because decubitus can develop in a matter of a few hours.

Observe for decubitus ulcer development, and treat immediately.

Timely intervention may prevent extensive damage.

Cleanse ulcer daily.

Removes dead tissue and allows new epidermis to form.

Change dressings daily or as indicated. Employ sterile dressing technique, using light dressings.

Wet or soiled dressings potentiate skin breakdown and bacterial growth/infections. Dry dressings allow for air circulation and skin respiration.

Expose ulcer to air and sunlight/heat lamp.

Helps dry wound/inhibit growth of bacteria and promotes healing.

Collaborative

Provide waterbed, alternating pressure/eggcrate mattress, padded chair.

Provides protection and improves circulation by decreasing amount of pressure on tissues.

Monitor Hb/Hct and blood sugar.

Anemia and elevated blood sugar levels are factors in skin breakdown and can impair healing.

817

ACTIONS/INTERVENTIONS

Collaborative

Refer to podiatrist as indicated.

Provide whirlpool treatments.

Assist with topical applications; skin barrier dressings; collagenase therapy; absorbable gelatin sponges (Gelfoam); aerosol sprays.

Administer iron and vitamin C supplements.

Prepare for/assist with skin grafting. (Refer to CP: Burns, ND: Skin Integrity, Impaired: Actual, p. 724.)

RATIONALE

May need professional care for such problems as ingrown toenails, corns, bony changes, skin/tissue ulceration.

Increases circulation and has a debriding action.

Although there are differing opinions about the efficacy of these agents, individual or combination use may enhance healing.

Aids in healing/cellular regeneration.

May be needed to close large ulcers.

NURSING DIAGNOSIS:	URINARY ELIMINATION: ALTERED PATTERNS [POTENTIAL]
May be related to:	Changes in fluid/nutritional pattern Neuromuscular changes Perceptual/cognitive impairment
Possibly evidenced by:	[Not applicable; presence of signs and symptoms establishes an *actual* diagnosis.]
PATIENT OUTCOMES/ EVALUATION CRITERIA:	Maintains/regains effective pattern of elimination. Initiates necessary lifestyle changes and participates in treatment regimen to correct/control situation, e.g., bladder training program or use of indwelling catheter.

ACTIONS/INTERVENTIONS

Independent

Monitor voiding pattern. Identify possible reasons for changes, e.g., disorientation, neuromuscular impairment, psychotropic medications.

Palpate bladder. Observe for "overflow" voiding; determine frequency and timing of dribbling/voiding.

Promote fluid intake of 2000–3000 ml/day within cardiac tolerance; include fruit juices, especially cranberry juice. Schedule fluid intake times appropriately.

Institute bladder program (including scheduled voiding times, Kegel exercise) involving patient and staff in a positive manner.

Assist patient to sit upright on bedpan/commode.

RATIONALE

Essential to plan for care, and influences choice of individual interventions.

Bladder distention indicates urinary retention, which may cause incontinence and infection.

Maintains adequate hydration and promotes kidney function. Acid-ash juices act as an internal pH acidifier, retarding bacterial growth. Note: Patient may decrease fluid intake in an attempt to control incontinence and become dehydrated. Instead, fluids may be scheduled to decrease frequency of incontinence (e.g., limit fluids after 6 PM to reduce need to void during the night).

Regular toileting times may help to control incontinence. Program is more apt to be successful when positive attitudes and cooperation are present.

Provides functional position for voiding.

ACTIONS/INTERVENTIONS

Independent

Provide/encourage perineal care daily and PRN.

Use adult diapers if needed. Keep patient clean and dry. Provide frequent skin care.

Avoid verbal or nonverbal signs of rejection, disgust or disapproval over failures.

Provide routine catheter care and maintain patency if indwelling catheter is present.

Collaborative

Administer medications as indicated, e.g.:

Oxybutynin chloride (Ditropan);

Vitamin C, methenamine hippurate (Hiprex), methenamine mandelate (Mandelamine).

Insert/maintain indwelling catheter.

Irrigate catheter with acetic acid, if indicated.

RATIONALE

Reduces risk of contamination/ascending infection.

When training is unsuccessful, this is the preferred method of management.

Expressions of disapproval lower self-esteem and are not helpful to a successful program.

Prevents infection and/or minimizes reflux.

Promotes sphincter control.

Bladder pH acidifiers that retard bacterial growth.

May be used if continence cannot be maintained, in order to prevent skin breakdown and resultant problems.

May be done to maintain acid pH and retard bacterial growth.

NURSING DIAGNOSIS:	BOWEL ELIMINATION, ALTERED: (SPECIFY) [POTENTIAL]
May be related to:	Changes in/inadequate nutritional/fluid intake; poor muscle tone; change in level of activity
	Medication side effects
	Perceptual/cognitive impairment, depression
	Lack of privacy
Possibly evidenced by:	[Not applicable; presence of signs and symptoms establishes an *actual* diagnosis.]
PATIENT OUTCOMES/ EVALUATION CRITERIA:	Establishes/maintains normal patterns of bowel functioning. Demonstrates changes in lifestyle as necessitated by risk or contributing factors. Participates in bowel program, as indicated.

ACTIONS/INTERVENTIONS

Independent

Ascertain usual bowel pattern and aids used (e.g., previous long-term laxative use). Compare with current routine.

Assess reasons for problems; rule out medical causes, e.g., cancer, hemorrhoids, drugs, impaction.

RATIONALE

Determines extent of problem and indicates need for/ type of interventions appropriate. Many patients may already be laxative-dependent, and it is important to reestablish as near normal functioning as possible.

Identification/treatment of underlying medical condition is necessary to achieve optimal bowel function.

ACTIONS/INTERVENTIONS	RATIONALE
Independent	
Determine presence of food/drug sensitivities.	May contribute to diarrhea.
Institute individualized program of exercise, rest, diet, and bowel-retraining.	Depends on the needs of the patient. Loss of muscular tone reduces peristalsis or may impair control of rectal sphincter.
Provide diet high in bulk in the form of whole grain cereals, breads, fresh fruits (especially prunes, plums).	Improves stool consistency.
Decrease or eliminate foods such as dairy products.	These foods are known to be constipating.
Encourage increased fluid intake.	Promotes normal stool consistency.
Use adult diapers, if needed. Keep patient clean and dry. Provide frequent skin care. Apply baby oil to anal area.	Prevents skin breakdown.
Keep air freshener in room/at bedside or in bathroom.	Limits noxious odors and may help reduce patient embarrassment/concern.
Give emotional support to patient.	Decreases feelings of frustration and embarrassment.
Collaborative	
Administer medications as indicated:	
Bulk-providers/stool softeners, e.g., Metamucil;	Promotes regularity by increasing bulk and/or improving stool consistency.
Camphorated tincture of opium (Paregoric), diphenoxylate with atropine (Lomotil).	May be needed on a short-term basis when diarrhea persists.

NURSING DIAGNOSIS:	MOBILITIY, IMPAIRED PHYSICAL
May be related to:	**Decreased strength and endurance, neuromuscular impairment**
	Pain/discomfort
	Perceptual/cognitive impairment
Possibly evidenced by:	**Impaired coordination, limited range of motion; decreased muscle mass, strength, control**
	Reluctance to attempt movement; inability to purposefully move
PATIENT OUTCOMES/ EVALUATION CRITERIA:	**Verbalizes willingness to/and participates in activities. Demonstrates techniques/behaviors that enable continuation or resumption of activities. Maintains/increases strength and function of affected body parts.**

ACTIONS/INTERVENTIONS	RATIONALE
Independent	
Determine functional ability (0–4 scale) and reasons for impairment.	Identifies need for/degree of intervention required. (Refer to specific CPs as indicated, e.g., Cerebrovascular Accident/Stroke, p. 243; Multiple Sclerosis, p.

ACTIONS/INTERVENTIONS	RATIONALE
Independent	339; Fractures, p. 82.)
Note emotional/behavioral responses to altered ability.	Physical changes and loss of independence often create feelings of anger, frustration, and depression that may be manifested as reluctance to engage in activity.
Plan activities/visits with adequate rest periods as necessary.	Prevents fatigue, conserves energy for continued participation.
Encourage participation in self-care, occupational/recreational activities.	Promotes independence and self-esteem, may enhance willingness to participate.
Assist with transfers and ambulation if indicated; show patient/SO ways to move safely.	Prevents accidental falls/injury.
Obtain supportive shoes and well-fitting, nonskid slippers.	Assists patient to walk with a firm step, maintain sense of balance and prevents slipping.
Remove extraneous furniture from pathways.	Prevents patient from bumping into furniture and reduces risk of falling/injuring self.
Encourage use of handrails in hallway, stairwells, and bathrooms.	Promotes independence in mobility; reduces risk of falls.
Review safe use of mobility aids/adjunctive devices, e.g., walkers, braces, prosthetics.	Facilitates activity; reduces risk of injury.
Provide chairs with firm, high seats and lifting chairs when indicated.	Facilitates rising from seated position.
Provide for environmental changes to meet visual deficiencies.	Prevents accidents and sensory deprivation. If patient is blind, will need assistance and ongoing orientation to surroundings.
Speak to patient when entering the room, and let patient know when leaving.	Special actions help patient who cannot see to know when someone is there.
Encourage the patient with glasses/contacts to wear them. Be sure glasses are kept clean.	Optimal visual acuity facilitates participation in activities and reduces risk of falls/injury.
Determine reason if glasses are not being worn.	Patient may not be wearing glasses because they need adjustment or change in correction.
Collaborative	
Consult with physical/occupational therapist, rehabilitation specialist.	Useful in creating individual exercise/activity program and identifying adjunctive aids.
Arrange for eye examination as necessary.	Identifies specific vision problem, e.g., myopia, hyperopia, presbyopia, astigmatism, cataract and glaucoma development, tunnel vision, and blindness.

NURSING DIAGNOSIS:	**DIVERSIONAL ACTIVITY DEFICIT**
May be related to:	**Environmental lack of diversional activity; long-term care**
	Physical limitations; psychologic condition, e.g., depression
Possibly evidenced by:	**Statements of boredom, depression, lack of energy**
	Disinterest, lethargy, withdrawn behavior, hostility

PATIENT OUTCOMES/ EVALUATION CRITERIA:	Recognizes own response and initiates appropriate coping actions. Engages in satisfying activities within personal limitations.

ACTIONS/INTERVENTIONS

Independent

Determine avocation/hobbies patient previously pursued. Incorporate activities, if appropriate, into present program.

Encourage participation in mix of activities/stimuli, e.g., music, news program, educational presentations, crafts as appropriate.

Provide change of scenery when possible, alter personal environment, encourage trips to shop/participate in local/family events.

Collaborative

Refer to occupational therapist, activity director.

RATIONALE

Encourages involvement and helps to stimulate patient mentally/physically to improve overall condition.

Offering different activities helps patient to try out new ideas and develop new interests. Activities need to be personally meaningful for the patient to derive the most enjoyment from them (e.g., talking or braille books for the blind, closed-captioned TV broadcasts for the deaf/hard of hearing).

Stimulates energy and provides new outlook for patient.

Can introduce and design new programs to provide positive stimuli for the patient.

NURSING DIAGNOSIS:	SEXUALITY PATTERNS, ALTERED [POTENTIAL]
May be related to:	**Biopsychosocial alteration of sexuality**
	Interference in psychologic/physical well-being; self-image
	Lack of privacy/SO
Possibly evidenced by:	**[Not applicable; presence of signs and symptoms establishes an *actual* diagnosis.]**
PATIENT OUTCOMES/ EVALUATION CRITERIA:	**Verbalizes knowledge and understanding of sexual limitations, difficulties or changes that have occurred. Demonstrates improved communication and relationship skills.**

ACTIONS/INTERVENTIONS

Independent

Note patient/SO cues regarding sexuality.

Evaluate cultural and religious/value factors and conflicts that may be present.

Assess developmental and lifestyle issues.

RATIONALE

May be concerned that condition/environmental restrictions may interfere with sexual function or ability, but be afraid to ask directly.

Affects patient's perception of existing problems.

Factors such as menopause and aging, adolescence and young adulthood need to be taken into consideration with regard to sexual concerns about illness and

ACTIONS/INTERVENTIONS

Independent

Provide atmosphere in which discussion of sexuality is encouraged/permitted.

Provide privacy for patient/SO.

Collaborative

Refer to sex counselor/therapist, family therapy when needed.

RATIONALE

long-term care.

When concerns are identifed and discussed, problem solving can occur.

Demonstrates acceptance of need for intimacy and provides opportunity to continue previous patterns of interaction as much as possible.

May require additional assistance for resolution of problems.

NURSING DIAGNOSIS:	HEALTH MAINTENANCE, ALTERED
May be related to:	Lack of, or significant alteration in, communication skills
	Complete or partial lack of gross and/or fine motor skills
	Perceptual/cognitive impairment, lack of ability to make deliberate/thoughtful judgments
	Lack of material resources
Possibly evidenced by:	Demonstrated lack of knowledge regarding basic health practices
	Reported/observed inability to take responsibility for meeting basic health needs; impairment of personal support system
	Demonstrated lack of behaviors adaptive to internal or external environmental changes
PATIENT OUTCOMES/ EVALUATION CRITERIA:	Verbalizes understanding of factors contributing to current situation. Adopts lifestyle changes supporting individual health care goals. Assumes responsibility for own health care needs when possible.

ACTIONS/INTERVENTIONS

Independent

Assess level of adaptive behavior; knowledge and skills about health maintenance, environment, and safety.

Provide information about individual health care needs.

Note patient's previous use of professional services, and continue as appropriate. Include in choice of new health care providers as able.

RATIONALE

Identifies areas of concern/need and aids in choice of interventions.

Provides knowledge base as encourages participation in decision-making.

Preserves continuity and promotes independence in meeting own health care needs.

ACTIONS/INTERVENTIONS	RATIONALE
Independent	
Maintain adequate hydration; and balanced diet with sufficient protein intake.	Promotes general well-being and aids in disease prevention.
Schedule adequate rest with progressive activity program.	Prevents fatigue and enhances general well-being.
Promote good handwashing and personal hygiene. Use aseptic techniques as necessary.	Prevents contamination/cross-contamination, reducing risk of illness/infection.
Protect from exposure to infections; avoid extremes of temperature and require the wearing of masks/other interventions as indicated.	Staff and/or visitors may have colds/other infections and may expose patient to these illnesses.
Encourage cessation of smoking.	Smokers are prone to bronchitis and ineffective clearing of secretions.
Encourage reporting of signs/symptoms as they occur.	Provides opportunity for early recognition of developing complications and timely intervention to prevent serious illness.
Observe for/monitor changes in vital signs, e.g., temperature elevation.	Early identification of onset of illness allows for timely intervention and may prevent serious complications. Note: Elderly persons often display subnormal temperatures; so presence of a low-grade fever may be of serious concern.
Collaborative	
Administer medications as indicated:	
Immunizations, e.g., Haemophilus influenzae;	Reduces risk of acquiring contagious/potentially life-threatening diseases.
Antibiotics.	May be used prophylactically and to treat infections.
Schedule preventive/routine health care appointments based on individual needs, e.g., with cardiologist, podiatrist, ophthalmologist, dentist.	Promotes optimal recovery/maintenance of health.

Alcoholism (Acute): Intoxication/Overdose _____

Although patients are not generally admitted to the acute care setting with this diagnosis, withdrawal from alcohol may occur secondarily during hospitalization.

PATIENT ASSESSMENT DATA BASE

Data are dependent on the duration/extent of use of alcohol, concurrent use of other drugs, and degree of organ involvement.

ACTIVITY/REST

May report: Difficulty sleeping.

CIRCULATION

May exhibit: Generalized tissue edema (due to protein deficiencies).

Peripheral pulses weak, irregular, or rapid.

Hypertension common in early withdrawal stage but may become labile/progress to hypotension.

Tachycardia common during acute withdrawal; numerous dysrhythmias may be identified. (Other abnormalities depend on underlying heart disease.)

ELIMINATION

May report: Diarrhea.

Constant upper abdominal pain and tenderness radiating to the back (pancreatic inflammation).

FOOD/FLUID

May report: Nausea/vomiting; food intolerance.

May exhibit: Gastric distention; ascites, liver enlargement (seen with cirrhosis).

Muscle wasting, dry/dull hair, swollen salivary glands, inflamed buccal cavity, capillary fragility (malnutrition).

Bowel sounds varied, related to gastric complications, such as gastric hemorrhage or distention.

NEUROSENSORY

May report: "Internal shakes."

Headache, dizziness, blurred vision.

May exhibit: Psychopathology, e.g., paranoid schizophrenia, major depression (may indicate dual diagnosis).

Level of consciousness/orientation: confusion, stupor, hyperactivity, distorted thought processes, slurred/incoherent speech.

Memory loss/confabulation.

Affect/mood/behavior: may be fearful, anxious, easily startled, inappropriate, silly, euphoric, irritable, physically/verbally abusive, depressed, and/or paranoid.

Hallucinations—visual, tactile, olfactory and auditory, e.g., patient may be picking items out of air or responding verbally to unseen person/voices.

Nystagmus (associated with cranial nerve palsy).

Pupil constriction (may indicate CNS depression).

Arcus senilis (ringlike opacity of the cornea): although normal in aging populations, suggests alcohol-related changes in younger patients.

Fine motor tremors of face, tongue, and hands; seizures (commonly grand mal).

Gait unsteady (ataxia)—may be due to thiamine deficiency, or cerebellar degeneration (Wernicke's encephalopathy).

RESPIRATION

May exhibit: Tachypnea (hyperactive state of alcohol withdrawal).

Cheyne–Stokes respirations or respiratory depression.

Breath sounds diminished/adventitious sounds (suggests pulmonary complications, e.g., respiratory depression, pneumonia).

SAFETY

May report: History of recurrent accidents, such as falls, fractures, lacerations, burns, blackouts, or automobile.

May exhibit: Skin: flushed face/palms of hand, scars, ecchymotic areas, cigarette burns on fingers, spider nevis (impaired portal circulation); fissures at corners of mouth (vitamin deficiency).

Fractures—healed or new (signs of recent/recurrent trauma).

Temperature elevation (dehydration and sympathetic stimulation); flushing/diaphoresis (suggests presence of infection).

Suicidal ideation/suicide attempts (some research suggests alcoholic suicide attempts are 30% higher than national average for general population).

SOCIAL INTERACTION

May report: Frequent sick days off work/school; fighting with others, arrests (disorderly conduct, motor vehicle violations/DUIs).

Mood changes.

That alcohol intake does not have any significant effect on present condition (denial).

Dysfunctional family system of origin.

TEACHING/LEARNING

May report: History of alcohol and/or drug use/abuse.

Ignorance and/or denial of addiction to alcohol, or inability to cut down or stop drinking despite repeated efforts.

Large amount of alcohol consumed in last 24–48 hours, previous periods of abstinence/withdrawal.

Previous hospitalizations for alcoholism/alcohol-related diseases, e.g., cirrhosis, esophageal varices.

Family history of alcoholism.

Discharge Plan Considerations: May require assistance to maintain abstinence and begin to participate in rehabilitation program.

DIAGNOSTIC STUDIES

Blood alcohol/drug levels: alcohol level may/may not be severely elevated, depending on amount consumed and length of time between consumption and testing. In addition to alcohol, numerous controlled substances may be identified in a poly-drug screen, e.g., morphine, Percodan, Quaalude.

CBC: decreased Hg/Hct may reflect such problems as iron-deficiency anemia or acute/chronic GI bleeding. WBC count may be increased with infection or decreased if immunosuppressed.

Glucose: hyperglycemia/hypoglycemia may be present, related to pancreatitis, malnutrition, or depletion of liver glycogen stores.

Electrolytes: hypokalemia and hypomagnesemia are common.

Liver function tests: SGOT/AST, SGPT/ALT, and amylase may be elevated, reflecting liver or pancreatic damage.

Nutritional tests: albumin may be low and total protein decreased. Vitamin deficiencies are usually present, reflecting malnutrition/malabsorption.

Urinalysis: infection may be identified; ketones may be present, related to breakdown of fatty acids in malnutrition (pseudodiabetic condition).

Chest x-ray: may reveal right lower lobe pneumonia (malnutrition, depressed immune system, aspiration) or chronic lung disorders associated with tobacco use.

ECG: dysrhythmias, cardiomyopathies, and/or ischemia may be present owing to direct effect of alcohol on the cardiac muscle and/or conduction system, as well as effects of electrolyte imbalance.

Addiction severity index (ASI): an assessment tool that produces a "problem severity profile" of the patient, including chemical, medical, psychologic, legal, family/social, and employment/support aspects, indicating areas of treatment needs.

NURSING PRIORITIES

1. Maintain physiologic stability during acute withdrawal phase.
2. Promote patient safety.
3. Provide appropriate referral and follow-up.
4. Encourage/support SO involvement in "Intervention" (confrontation) process.
5. Provide information about condition/prognosis and treatment needs.

DISCHARGE CRITERIA

1. Homeostasis achieved.
2. Sobriety being maintained on a day-to-day basis.
3. Transferred to rehabilitation program/attending group therapy, e.g., Alcoholics Anonymous.
4. Condition, prognosis, and therapeutic regimen understood.

NURSING DIAGNOSIS:	BREATHING PATTERN, INEFFECTIVE [POTENTIAL]
May be related to:	**Direct effect of alcohol toxicity on respiratory center, and/or sedative drugs given to decrease alcohol withdrawal symptoms** **Tracheobronchial obstruction** **Presence of chronic respiratory problems, inflammatory process** **Decreased energy/fatigue**
Possibly evidenced by:	**[Not applicable; presence of signs and symptoms establishes an *actual* diagnosis.]**
PATIENT OUTCOMES/ EVALUATION CRITERIA:	**Maintains effective breathing pattern with respiratory rate within normal range; lungs clear, free of cyanosis and other signs/symptoms of hypoxia.**

ACTIONS/INTERVENTIONS	RATIONALE
Independent	
Monitor respiratory rate/depth and pattern as indicated. Note periods of apnea, Cheyne–Stokes respirations.	Frequent assessment is important because toxicity levels may change rapidly. Hyperventilation is common during acute withdrawal phase. Kussmaul respirations are sometimes present due to acidotic state as-

ACTIONS/INTERVENTIONS

Independent

Elevate head of bed.

Encourage cough/deep breathing exercises and frequent position changes.

Auscultate breath sounds. Note presence of adventitious sounds, e.g., rhonchi, wheezes.

Have suction equipment, airway adjuncts available.

Collaborative

Administer supplemental oxygen if necessary.

Review chest x-rays, ABGs as indicated.

RATIONALE

sociated with vomiting and malnutrition. However, marked respiratory depression can occur due to CNS depressant effects from alcohol. This may be compounded by drugs used to control alcohol withdrawal symptoms.

Decreases possibility of aspiration, lowers diaphragm to enhance lung inflation.

Facilitates lung expansion and mobilization of secretions to reduce risk of atelectasis/pneumonia.

Patient is at risk for atelectasis related to hypoventilation and pneumonia. Right lower lobe pneumonia is common in alcohol debilitated patients and is often due to aspiration. Chronic lung diseases are also common, e.g., emphysema, chronic bronchitis.

Sedative effects of alcohol/drugs potentiates risk of aspiration, relaxation of oropharyngeal muscles, and respiratory depression, requiring intervention to prevent respiratory arrest.

Hypoxia may occur with CNS/respiratory depression.

Monitors presence of secondary complications such as atelectasis/pneumonia; evaluates effectiveness of respiratory effort.

NURSING DIAGNOSIS:	CARDIAC OUTPUT, ALTERED: DECREASED [POTENTIAL]
May be related to:	Direct effect of alcohol on the heart muscle
	Altered systemic vascular resistance
	Electrical alterations in rate; rhythm; conduction
Possibly evidenced by:	[Not applicable; presence of signs and symptoms establishes an *actual* diagnosis.]
PATIENT OUTCOMES/ EVALUATION CRITERIA:	Displays vital signs within patient's normal range; absence of/reduced frequency of dysrhythmias. Demonstrates an increase in activity tolerance. Verbalizes understanding of the effect of alcohol on the heart.

ACTIONS/INTERVENTIONS

Independent

Monitor vital signs frequently during acute withdrawal.

RATIONALE

Hypertension frequently occurs in acute withdrawal phase. Extreme hyperexcitability, accompanied by catecholamine release and increased peripheral vascular resistance, raises blood pressure (and heart rate), but blood pressure may become labile/progress

ACTIONS/INTERVENTIONS	RATIONALE

Independent

	to hypotension. Note: May have underlying cardiovascular disease, which is compounded by alcohol withdrawal.
Monitor cardiac rate/rhythm. Document irregularities/dysrhythmias.	Long-term alcohol abuse may result in cardiomyopathy/congestive heart failure. Tachycardia is common due to sympathetic response to increased circulating catecholamines. Irregularities/dysrhythmias may develop with electrolyte shifts/imbalance. All of these may have an adverse effect on cardiac function/output.
Monitor body temperature.	Elevation may occur due to sympathetic stimulation, dehydration, and/or infections, increasing the vascular bed (vasodilation) and compromising venous return/cardiac output.
Monitor intake/output. Note 24-hour fluid balance.	Preexisting dehydration, vomiting, fever, and diaphoresis may result in decreased circulating volume which can compromise cardiovascular function. Note: Hydration is difficult to assess in the alcoholic because the usual indicators are not reliable, and overhydration is a risk in the presence of compromised cardiac function.
Be prepared for/assist in cardiopulmonary resuscitation.	Causes of death during acute withdrawal stages include cardiac dysrhythmias, respiratory depression/arrest, oversedation, excessive psychomotor activity, severe dehydration or overhydration, and massive infections. Mortality for unrecognized/untreated delirium tremens (DTs) may be as high as 15–25%.

Collaborative

Monitor laboratory studies, e.g., serum electrolyte levels.	Electrolyte imbalance, e.g., potassium/magnesium, potentiate risk of cardiac dysrhythmias and CNS excitability.
Administer medications as indicated, e.g.:	
Clonidine (Catapres);	Provides for greater mean reductions in heart rate and systolic blood pressure with less nausea and vomiting.
Potassium.	Corrects deficits which can result in life-threatening dysrhythmias.

NURSING DIAGNOSIS:	INJURY, POTENTIAL FOR: (SPECIFY)
May be related to:	Cessation of alcohol intake with varied autonomic nervous system responses to the system's suddenly altered state
	Involuntary clonic/tonic muscle activity (seizures)
	Equilibrium/balancing difficulties, reduced muscle and hand/eye coordination
Possibly evidenced by:	[Not applicable; presence of signs and symptoms establishes an *actual* diagnosis.]

829

Demonstrates absence of untoward effects of withdrawal, and physical injury is prevented.

ACTIONS/INTERVENTIONS	RATIONALE

Independent

Identify stage of alcohol withdrawal symptoms, i.e., stage I is associated with signs/symptoms of hyperactivity (e.g., tremors, sleeplessness, nausea/vomiting, diaphoresis, tachycardia, hypertension). Stage II is manifested by increased hyperactivity plus hallucinations and/or seizure activity. Stage III symptoms include DTs and extreme autonomic hyperactivity with profound confusion, anxiety, insomnia, fever.

Prompt recognition and intervention may halt progression of symptoms and enhance recovery/improve prognosis. In addition, recurrence/progression of symptoms indicates need for changes in drug therapy/more intense treatment to prevent death.

Monitor/document seizure activity. Maintain patent airway. Provide environmental safety, e.g., padded side rails, bed in low position.

Grand mal seizures are most common and may be related to decreased magnesium levels, hypoglycemia, elevated blood alcohol, or previous history of seizures. Note: In absence of previous history of seizures, they usually stop spontaneously, requiring only symptomatic treatment.

Check deep tendon reflexes. Assess gait, if possible.

Reflexes may be depressed, absent, or hyperactive. Peripheral neuropathies are common, especially in malnourished patient. Ataxia (gait disturbance) is associated with Wernicke's syndrome (thiamine deficiency) and cerebellar degeneration.

Assist with ambulation and self-care activities as needed.

Prevents falls with resultant injury.

Provide for environmental safety when indicated. (Refer to ND: Sensory-Perceptual Alteration, following.)

May be required when equilibrium, hand/eye coordination problems exist.

Collaborative

Administer IV/po fluids with caution, as indicated.

Cautious replacement corrects dehydration and promotes renal clearance of toxins while reducing risk of overhydration.

Administer medications as indicated:

Benzodiazepines, e.g., chlordiazepoxide (Librium), diazepam (Valium);

Commonly used to control neuronal hyperactivity that occurs as alcohol is detoxified. IV/oral administration is perferred route, because intramuscular absorption is unpredictable. Muscle-relaxant qualities are particularly helpful to patient in controlling "the shakes," trembling, and ataxic quality of movements. Patient may initially require large doses to achieve desired effect, and then drugs may be tapered and discontinued, usually within 96 hours. Note: These agents must be used cautiously in patient with hepatic disease, because they are metabolized by the liver.

Oxazepam (Serax);

Although less dramatic for control of withdrawal symptoms, may be drug of choice in patient with liver disease because of its shorter half-life.

Phenobarbital;

Useful in suppressing withdrawal symptoms as well as an effective anticonvulsant. Use must be monitored so that exacerbation of respiratory depression is prevented.

ACTIONS/INTERVENTIONS

Collaborative

Magnesium sulfate.

RATIONALE

Reduces tremors and seizure activity by decreasing neuromuscular excitability.

NURSING DIAGNOSIS:	SENSORY-PERCEPTUAL ALTERATION: (SPECIFY)
May be related to:	**Chemical alteration: exogenous (e.g., alcohol consumption/sudden cessation) and endogenous (e.g., electrolyte imbalance, elevated ammonia and BUN)**
	Sleep deprivation
	Psychologic stress (anxiety/fear)
Possibly evidenced by:	**Disorientation to time/place or person**
	Changes in usual response to stimuli; exaggerated emotional responses, change in behavior
	Bizarre thinking
	Fear/anxiety
PATIENT OUTCOMES/ EVALUATION CRITERIA:	**Regains/maintains usual level of consciousness. Reports absence of/reduced hallucinations. Identifies external factors that affect sensory-perceptual abilities.**

ACTIONS/INTERVENTIONS

Independent

Assess level of consciousness; ability to speak, response to stimuli/commands.

Observe behavioral responses, e.g., hyperactivity, disorientation, confusion, sleeplessness, irritability.

Note onset of hallucinations. Document as auditory, visual, and/or tactile.

Provide quiet environment. Speak in calm, quiet voice. Regulate lighting as indicated. Turn off radio/TV during sleep.

Provide care by same personnel whenever possible.

RATIONALE

Speech may be garbled, confused, or slurred. Response to commands may reveal inability to concentrate, impaired judgment, or muscle coordination deficits.

Hyperactivity related to CNS disturbances may escalate rapidly. Sleeplessness is common due to loss of sedative effect gained from alcohol usually consumed prior to bedtime. Sleep deprivation may aggravate disorientation/confusion. Progression of symptoms may indicate impending hallucinations (stage II) or DTs (stage III).

Auditory hallucinations are reported to be more frightening/threatening to patient. Visual hallucinations occur more at night and often include insects, animals, or faces of friends/enemies. Patients are frequently observed "picking the air." Yelling may occur if patient is calling for help from perceived threat (usually seen in stage III).

Reduces external stimuli during hyperactive stage. P tient may become more delirious when surroundir cannot be seen, but some respond better to c darkened room.

Promotes recognition of care givers and a consistency, which may reduce fear.

ACTIONS/INTERVENTIONS	RATIONALE

Independent

Encourage SO to stay with patient whenever possible.

May have a calming effect, and may provide a reorienting influence.

Reorient frequently to person, place, time, and surrounding environment as indicated.

May reduce confusion/misinterpretation of external stimuli.

Avoid bedside discussion about patient or topics unrelated to the patient that do not include the patient.

Patient may hear and misinterpret conversation, which can aggravate hallucinations.

Provide environmental safety, e.g., place bed in low position, leave doors in full open or closed position, observe frequently, place call light/bell within reach, remove articles that can harm patient.

Patient may have distorted sense of reality, be fearful, or be suicidal, requiring protection from self.

Collaborative

Provide seclusion, restraints as necessary.

Patients with excessive psychomotor activity, severe hallucinations, violent behavior, and/or suicidal gestures may respond better to seclusion. Restraints are usually ineffective and add to patient's agitation, but occasionally may be required to prevent self-harm.

Monitor laboratory studies, e.g., electrolytes, liver function studies, ammonia, BUN, glucose, ABGs, magnesium levels.

Changes in organ function may precipitate or potentiate sensory-perceptual deficits. Electrolyte imbalance is common. Liver function is often impaired in the chronic alcoholic. Ammonia intoxication can occur if the liver is unable to convert ammonia to urea. Ketoacidosis is sometimes present without glycosuria; however, hyperglycemia or hypoglycemia may occur, suggesting pancreatitis or impaired gluconeogenesis in the liver. Hypoxemia and hypercarbia are common manifestations in chronic alcoholics who are also heavy smokers.

Administer medications as indicated: e.g.:

Minor tranquilizers as indicated. (Refer to ND: Anxiety [Specify Level]/Fear), p. 834.)

Reduces hyperactivity, promoting relaxation/sleep. This group of drugs has little effect on dreaming and allows dream recovery (REM rebound) to occur, which has been suppressed by alcohol use.

Thiamine, C and B complex, multi-vitamins, Stresstabs.

Vitamin deficiency (especially thiamine) is associated with ataxia, loss of eye movement and pupillary response, palpitations, postural hypotension, and exertional dyspnea.

NURSING DIAGNOSIS:	NUTRITION, ALTERED: LESS THAN BODY REQUIREMENTS
May be related to:	Poor dietary intake (replaced by alcohol consumption)
	Effects of alcohol on organs involved in digestion, e.g., stomach, pancreas, liver; interference with absorption and metabolism of nutrients and amino acids; and increased loss of vitamins in the urine
Possibly evidenced by:	Reports of inadequate food intake, altered taste sensation, abdominal pain, lack of interest in food

Body weight 20% or more under ideal

Pale conjunctiva and mucous membranes; sore inflammed buccal cavity/cheilosis

Poor muscle tone, skin turgor

Hyperactive bowel sounds, diarrhea

Third spacing of circulating blood volume (e.g., edema of extremities, ascites)

Presence of neuropathies

Laboratory evidence of decreased red cell count (anemias), vitamin deficiencies, reduced serum albumin, or electrolyte imbalance

PATIENT OUTCOMES/ EVALUATION CRITERIA: Demonstrates stable weight or progressive weight gain toward goal with normalization of laboratory values and absence of signs of malnutrition. Verbalizes understanding of effects of alcohol ingestion and reduced dietary intake on nutritional status. Demonstrates behaviors, lifestyle changes to regain/maintain appropriate weight.

ACTIONS/INTERVENTIONS	RATIONALE
Independent	
Evaluate presence/quality of bowel sounds. Note abdominal distention, tenderness.	Irritation of gastric mucosa is common and may result in epigastric pain, nausea, and hyperactive bowel sounds. More serious effects on GI system may occur secondary to cirrhosis and hepatitis.
Note presence of nausea/vomiting, diarrhea.	Nausea and vomiting are often among first signs of alcohol withdrawal and may interfere with achieving adequate nutritional intake.
Assess ability to feed self.	Tremors, altered mentation or hallucinations may interfere with ingestion of nutrients and indicate need for assistance.
Provide frequent, small, easily digested feedings/ snacks and advance as tolerated.	May limit distress, enhance intake and tolerance of nutrients. As appetite and ability to tolerate food increases, diet should be adjusted to provide the necessary calories and nutrition for cellular repair and restoration of energy.
Collaborative	
Review laboratory studies, e.g., SGOT/AST, SGPT/ ALT, LDH, serum albumin, transferrin.	Assesses liver function, adequacy of nutritional intake; influences choice of diet and need for/effectiveness of supplemental therapy.
Refer to dietician/nutritional support team.	Useful in establishing individual nutritional program.
Provide diet high in protein with at least half of calories obtained from carbohydrates.	Stabilizes blood sugar, thereby reducing risk of hypoglycemia while providing for energy needs and cellular regeneration.
Administer medications as indicated, e.g.:	
Antacids, antiemetics, antidiarrheals;	Reduces gastric irritation and effects of sympathetic

833

ACTIONS/INTERVENTIONS

Collaborative

Vitamins, thiamine.

Institute/maintain NPO status as indicated.

RATIONALE

stimulation.

Replace losses. Note: All patients should receive thiamine, because vitamin deficiencies (either clinical or sub-clinical) exist in most, if not all, chronic alcoholics.

Provides GI rest to reduce harmful effects of gastric/pancreatic stimulation in presence of GI bleeding or excessive vomiting.

NURSING DIAGNOSIS:	**ANXIETY [SPECIFY LEVEL]/FEAR**
May be related to:	**Cessation of alcohol intake/physiologic withdrawal**
	Situational crisis (hospitalization)
	Threat to self-concept, perceived threat of death
Possibly evidenced by:	**Feelings of inadequacy, shame, self-disgust, and remorse**
	Increased helplessness/hopelessness with loss of control of own life
	Increased tension, apprehension
	Fear of unspecified consequences
PATIENT OUTCOMES/ EVALUATION CRITERIA:	**Verbalizes reduction of fear and anxiety to an acceptable and manageable level. Expresses sense of regaining some control of situation/life. Demonstrates problem-solving skills and uses resources effectively.**

ACTIONS/INTERVENTIONS

Independent

Identify cause of anxiety, involving patient in the process. Explain that alcohol withdrawal increases anxiety and uneasiness. Reassess level of anxiety on an ongoing basis.

Develop a trusting relationship through frequent contact. Project an accepting attitude about alcoholism.

Inform patient about what you plan to do and why. Include patient in planning process and provide choices when possible.

Reorient frequently. (Refer to ND: Sensory-Perceptual Alteration, p. 831.)

RATIONALE

Person in acute phase of withdrawal may be unable to identify and/or accept what is happening. Anxiety may be physiologically or environmentally caused. Continued alcohol toxicity will be manifested by increased anxiety and agitation as effects of tranquilizers wear off.

Provides patient with a sense of humanness, helping to decrease paranoia and distrust. Patient will be able to detect biased or condescending attitude of care givers.

Enhances sense of trust, and may increase cooperation or reduce anxiety. Provides sense of control over self in circumstance where loss of control is a significant factor.

Patient may experience periods of confusion resulting in increased anxiety.

834

ACTIONS/INTERVENTIONS	RATIONALE

Collaborative

Administer medications as indicated:

Benzodiazepines, e.g., chlordiazepoxide (Librium), diazepam (Valium).

This group of drugs has little effect on dreaming and allows dream recovery (REM rebound) to occur, which has been suppressed by alcohol use. Minor tranquilizers are given during acute withdrawal to help patient relax, be less hyperactive, and feel more in control.

Barbiturates, e.g., phenobarbital, or secobarbital, (Seconal) pentobarbital (Nembutal).

These drugs for suppression of alcohol withdrawal symptoms need to be used with caution because they are respiratory depressants and REM inhibitors.

Arrange "Intervention" (confrontation) to assist patient to accept that substance use is creating a problem.

Process of Intervention, wherein SOs, supported by staff, provide information about how patient's drinking and behavior has affected each one of them, helps patient acknowledge that drinking is a problem and has resulted in current situational crisis.

Provide consultation for referral to detoxification/crisis center for ongoing treatment program as soon as medically stable (e.g., oriented to reality).

Patient is more likely to contract for treatment while still "hurting" and experiencing fear and anxiety from last drinking episode. Motivation decreases as well-being increases and person again feels able to control the problem. Direct contact with available treatment resources provides realistic picture of help. Decreases time for patient to "think about it"/change mind or restructure and strengthen denial systems.

(Refer to CP: Substance Dependence/Abuse Rehabilitation, p. 861, for postacute interventions/considerations and learning needs.)

Hallucinogens (LSD, PCP, Cannabis): Intoxication/Overdose

Of the drugs that produce mood changes and perceptual changes varying from sensory illusion to hallucinations, the most popular and well-known are LSD and other LSD-like hallucinogenic drugs, e.g, MDA, MDMA (Ecstasy), Mescaline, synthetic THC, DOM (STP), Morning Glory Seeds, Nutmeg; phencyclidine (PCP); and cannabis (marijuana, hashish, THC).

PATIENT ASSESSMENT DATA BASE

Factors that can affect the kind of reaction (positive or negative) experienced by the hallucinogen user include individual circadian rhythms (fatigue), previous drug-taking experience, personality, mood, expectations, and concurrent use of alcohol/other drugs can compound symptoms/reactions. The educational level can also cause different perceptions.

ACTIVITY/REST

May report:	Insomnia
May exhibit:	Disturbances of sleep/wakefulness.
	Hyperactivity (LSD, mescaline, PCP).

CIRCULATORY

May report:	Palpitations.
May exhibit:	Increased vital signs (LSD).
	Decreased diastolic BP (cannabis, high-dose PCP); hypertension, hypertensive crisis (low to moderate dose PCP).
	Tachycardia; possible dysrhythmias (high-dose PCP).

EGO INTEGRITY

May exhibit:	Highly dependent nature, with characteristics of poor impulse control, low frustration tolerance, low self-esteem; depersonalization.
	Weak superego possibly resulting in absence of guilt feelings for behavior or self-reproach, excessive guilt, fearfulness.
	Moods reflecting depression or anxiety.
	Preoccupation with the idea that brain is destroyed and/or will not return to a normal state.

FOOD/FLUID

May report:	Nausea/vomiting, increased salivation.

NEUROSENSORY

May report:	Blurred vision, altered depth perception.
	Dizziness, headache (LSD).
	Flashback (spontaneous transitory recurrence of a drug-induced experience [LSD] in a drug-free state).
	"Bad trips" (self-limiting and confined to period of intoxication [hallucinogenic drugs]):
	LSD: Three kinds: (1) bad body trip, e.g., "my body is purple"; (2) bad environment trip, visual distortions so real the person thinks s/he is going crazy; (3) bad mind trip, e.g., unexpected subconscious material bursts forth into consciousness, as in, "I'm responsible for my mother's death."
	PCP: Aggravates any underlying psychopathology.

Cannabis: Rare; however, when they do occur, panic attacks are usually seen.

May exhibit: Eyes: pupil constriction, vertical and horizontal nystagmus (PCP); pupillary dilation, catatonic staring (LSD, mescaline).

Muscle incoordination/tremors, seizures; increased muscle strength may be noted with PCP, due to the anesthetic effect that deadens pain perception; deep tendon reflexes increased (low to moderate dose PCP) or depressed (high-dose PCP); opisthotonos.

Level of consciousness: usually responsive, coma may be noted (especially if intracranial hemorrhage occurs with PCP); slurred speech, mutism often present.

Mental status: sensation of slowed time, perceptual changes, perceptions enhanced (colors richer, music more profound, smells and tastes heightened), synesthesia (merging of senses, colors are "heard" or sounds are "seen"), changes in body image, depersonalization.

Delirium with clouded state of consciousness (sensory misperception, difficulty in sustaining attention, disordered stream of thought, psychomotor activity), including misinterpretations, illusions, hallucinations (rare with cannabis intoxication), disorientation, and memory impairment. May occur within 24 hours after use or after recovery, days after PCP has been taken.

Mood: euphoria/dysphoria, anxiety, emotional lability, apathy, grandiosity.

Behavioral findings: may include assaultiveness, bizarre behavior, impulsivity, unpredictability, belligerence, impaired judgment, paranoid ideation, panic attacks.

Delusions occurring in a normal state of consciousness may persist beyond 24 hours after cessation of hallucinogen use; persecutory delusions can follow cannabis use immediately or may occur during the course of cannabis intoxication.

PAIN/COMFORT

May report: Decreased awareness of pain.

RESPIRATION

May exhibit: Decreased rate/depth of respiration (PCP, heavy cannabis use).
Rhonchi, gurgling sounds.

SAFETY

May exhibit: Skin: diaphoretic.

SOCIAL INTERACTION

May report: Dysfunctional family system; one parent who is absent or who is an overpowering tyrant and/or one who is weak and ineffectual.
Substance abuse as the primary coping method.
Overwhelming peer pressure leading to involvement with drugs.
Impaired social or occupational functioning (fights, loss of friends, absence from work, loss of job, or legal difficulties).

TEACHING/LEARNING

May report: Family history of substance abuse.

Discharge Plan Considerations: May need assistance with abstinence and/or transfer to rehabilitation program.

DIAGNOSTIC STUDIES

Drug screen/urinalysis: to identify drug(s) being used.

ASI: to assess substance abuse and determine treatment needs.

NURSING PRIORITIES

1. Protect patient/others from injury.
2. Promote physiologic/psychologic stability.
3. Provide appropriate referral and follow-up.
4. Support patient/family in "Intervention" (confrontation) process for decision to stop using drugs.
5. Provide information about dependency/prognosis and treatment needs.

DISCHARGE CRITERIA

1. Homeostasis achieved.
2. Abstinence from drug(s) maintained.
3. Dependency condition, prognosis, and therapeutic regimen understood.
4. Enrolled in/transferred to drug rehabilitation program.

NURSING DIAGNOSIS:	**VIOLENCE, POTENTIAL FOR: DIRECTED AT SELF/OTHERS**
May be related to:	**Chemical alteration, exogenous (CNS stimulants/mind-altering drug); toxic reaction to drug(s)**
	Organic brain syndrome (drug anesthetizes mind and body)
	Psychologic state (narrowed perceptual field)
Possible indicators:	**Synesthesias, hallucinations, illusions, visual/auditory distortions; panic state; suspiciousness of others, paranoid ideation, delusions**
	Hostile threatening verbalizations; unpredictable behavior
	Change in behavior pattern; exaggerated emotional response
	Increased motor activity, pacing, excitement, irritability, agitation
	Overt and aggressive acts; self-destructive behavior
	Increasing anxiety, fear and feelings of loss of control
	Decreased response to pain
PATIENT OUTCOMES/ EVALUATION CRITERIA:	**Demonstrates self-control, as evidenced by relaxed posture, nonviolent behavior. Acknowledges reality of situation and understanding of relationship of behavior to drug use. Participates in treatment program.**

ACTIONS/INTERVENTIONS	RATIONALE
Independent	
Place in darkened, quiet, nonthreatening environment with a nonintrusive observer.	Lowered stimulation decreases the likelihood of confusion and fear, thus reducing chance of violent response. Use of an observer promotes safety. Note:

ACTIONS/INTERVENTIONS

Independent

Speak in a soft, nonthreatening voice. Use "Talk-downs" when LSD has been taken. If technique is tried with other drugs (PCP), and agitation increases, stop immediately.

Observe for increasing anxiety, fear, irritability, and agitation.

Accept patient's anger, without reacting on an emotional basis.

Provide protection within the environment via constant observation and removal of objects that may be used to hurt self or others.

Observe behavior before administering drugs.

Collaborative

Administer medications as necessary, e.g.:

　　Diazepam (Valium);

　　Haloperidol (Haldol).

Avoid use of phenothiazine neuroleptics.

Apply restraints, if needed and document reason(s) for use.

RATIONALE

PCP users often seek help only after the situation has gotten out of hand, and it is therefore important to take safe action immediately.

Nonthreatening communication may have a calming effect. However, "Talk-downs" (the use of orientation, support and reassuring words/touch) may be deleterious resulting in an increase in the user's agitation level in the presence of PCP intoxication.

May indicate potential for change to violent behavior. Note: Patient is not in complete control because of drug use.

Responding emotionally on a personal level, is not constructive and may escalate reactions.

Reduces risk of injury to patient and/or staff. Patient may not feel pain and may not be able to follow directions because of the drug.

A period of drug-free observation should precede any decision to administer medications (e.g., tranquilizers), so that a clear clinical picture can develop. In addition, because it is not known what other drugs may also have been ingested, it is not generally advisable to add another drug.

Used to reduce muscle spasms and/or restlessness in PCP user.

Preferred to control psychosis and assaultive behavior.

Durgs such as thorazine should probably be avoided because of the possibility of potentiating PCP anticholinergic effects.

Restraints should be avoided in a frightened, hallucinating patient but may be necessary because of potential injury to self or others, or where other dangerous drugs have been taken. PCP users are unpredictable; so it is best to err on the side of safety (using restraints with sufficient documentation), rather than risking injury.

NURSING DIAGNOSIS:	INJURY, POTENTIAL FOR: (SPECIFY)
May be related to:	**Muscle incoordination; reduced hand/eye coordination**
	Decreased response to/perception of pain, reduced temperature/tactile sensation
	Clouded sensorium and impaired judgment; unfamiliar environment; fear
	Clonic movements, muscle rigidity (may precede/occur

839

with generalized seizure activity)

Internal factors, host: psychologic perception (hallucinations)

Interactive conditions between individual and environment that impose a risk to the defensive and adaptive resources of the individual, e.g., placing hand in open flame, "flying out of window"

Possibly evidenced by: [Not applicable; presence of signs and symptoms establishes an *actual* diagnosis.]

PATIENT OUTCOMES/ EVALUATION CRITERIA: Verbalizes understanding of factors (e.g., drug use) that contribute to possibility of injury and takes steps to correct situation. Demonstrates behaviors and lifestyle changes necessary to minimize and/or prevent injury. Maintains/achieves physiologic stability, as evidenced by patent airway and adequate respiratory/cardiac function.

ACTIONS/INTERVENTIONS	RATIONALE
Independent	
Ascertain what drugs have been taken when possible.	Necessary for appropriate intervention/anticipation of needs. Lethal overdoses of hallucinogenic drugs (except for PCP) are rare; however, caution must be taken because adulterants such as sedative-hypnotics, anticholinergics, and PCP are often added. Note: Two reasons one might not know what drug was taken are (1) that the patient lies because of legal concerns or feels embarrassed and (2) that the person who sold the drugs to the patient either did not know what it was or lied to the patient. In either case, the nurse should listen to the patient but be aware that the information the patient gives may not be accurate.
Anticipate some form of unpredictability and be prepared for the unexpected, including physiologic as well as psychologic emergencies.	These drugs can be dangerous because they can lead to bizarre thinking/harmful behavior. Also, because drugs are often mixed or "cut" with other drugs, it is difficult to know what drugs may actually be involved.
Maintain patient under close observation. Note precursors that might indicate increasing agitation, e.g., body tension, rising voice tone, quickening movements.	PCP alters thinking and is an anesthetic, and patient may hurt self because of bizarre thinking, e.g., attempt to jump out window or escape from restraints.
Remove objects that may be used to hurt self or others.	Provides protection within the environment.
Provide a hockey/bicycle helmet as indicated.	If patient is banging head against hard objects, a helmet can decrease the potential for/severity of injury.
Monitor vital signs, respiratory rate/depth and rhythm.	Decreased diastolic blood pressure (cannabis) or hypertensive crisis (PCP) may develop. Bradypnea/respiratory arrest can occur, especially with PCP or heavy cannabis use.
Assess gag/swallow response and character of respi-	Hypersalivation and vomiting, especially in the pres-

ACTIONS/INTERVENTIONS	RATIONALE

Independent

rations.

ence of ineffective cough and/or loss of muscle tone may result in occlusion of airway, crowing/gurgling/choked respirations and respiratory arrest.

Position patient on side.

Facilitates drainage of vomitus and buildup of saliva, and prevent choking in sedated/comatose patient.

Encourage taking fluids frequently, if patient is able to swallow safely.

Adequate hydration keeps secretions loose and easier to expectorate and enhances renal clearance of drugs.

Have emergency equipment (including airway adjunct/suction) and medications available.

Toxic effects of PCP on the heart and respiratory system may result in cardiac/respiratory arrest requiring prompt intervention to prevent death.

Collaborative

Administer IV fluids and ammonium chloride or ascorbic acid, as indicated.

Forced diuresis and acidifying urine enhance renal clearance of PCP. (Effects are dose-related: > 5 mg = low dose; > 10 mg = high dose; > 20 mg can lead to hypertensive crisis, coma/death due to respiratory/cardiac failure).

Administer medications as indicated, e.g.:

　　Diazepam (Valium);

May be useful to reduce agitation and hyperactivity after drug use is clear.

Apply restraints with caution when used.

May prevent injury to self or others. However, restraints should be avoided, if possible, in a frightened, hallucinating patient.

NURSING DIAGNOSIS:	TISSUE PERFUSION, ALTERED: CEREBRAL [POTENTIAL]
May be related to:	**Alterations in blood flow (hypertensive crisis)**
Possibly evidenced by:	**[Not applicable; presence of signs and symptoms establishes an *actual* diagnosis.]**
PATIENT OUTCOMES/ EVALUATION CRITERIA:	**Regains/maintains usual level of consciousness free of adverse neurologic symptoms/complications.**

ACTIONS/INTERVENTIONS	RATIONALE

Independent

Elevate head of the bed; keep head in midline position.

Enhances venous drainage, thereby reducing risk of vascular congestion, increasing intracranial pressure, and possibility of hemorrhage in PCP intoxication.

Observe for pupillary or vital sign changes, decreased level of consciousness and/or motor function.

Provides for early detection and intervention to minimize intracranial pressure/injury.

Encourage rest and quiet. Reduce environmental stimuli.

Promotes relaxation and may assist with lowering of blood pressure.

Collaborative

Administer antihypertensive medications, e.g., diazox-

Effective in lowering blood pressure to prevent hyper-

ACTIONS/INTERVENTIONS

Collaborative

ide (Hyperstat) and hydralazine (Apresoline).

RATIONALE

tensive crisis, which can be associated with PCP intoxication.

NURSING DIAGNOSIS:	**THOUGHT PROCESSES, ALTERED**
May be related to:	**Physiologic changes (use of hallucinogenic substance)**
	Impaired judgment with loss of memory
Possibly evidenced by:	**Inaccurate interpretation of environment, memory impairment, bizarre thinking, disorientation**
	Inability to make decisions; unpredictable behavior
	Cognitive dissonance; distractibility
	Inappropriate/nonreality based thinking
	Sleep deprivation
	Inability to communicate needs/desires effectively (mutism or confusion)
PATIENT OUTCOMES/ EVALUATION CRITERIA:	**Observed return of memory and ability to function. Communicating effectively. Reports absence of visual/ auditory distortions. Verbalizes understanding that the drug is the cause of/contributes to alteration in perception.**

ACTIONS/INTERVENTIONS

Independent

Observe closely, do not leave unattended, make sure restraints are secure when used. Remove objects from the environment that patient could use to harm self and others. (Refer to ND: Violence, Potential for: Directed at Self/Others, p. 838.)

Anticipate some form of unpredictable behavior and be prepared for the unexpected.

Tell patient that current thoughts and feelings are a result of the PCP, if indicated.

Allow patient to sleep whenever possible.

Observe for psychotic indicators, e.g., paranoia, delusions, hallucinations.

Note altered speech ability/patterns. Refer to loss of speech as temporary.

RATIONALE

PCP alters thinking, is an anesthetic, and patient may hurt self via attempt to jump out window, jump in front of cars, escape from restraints, and so forth. Removal of potentially harmful objects provides for protection and safety.

Use of hallucinogens can lead to bizarre thinking/ harmful responses.

This information may be helpful to the patient who can accept it; however, it may cause agitation.

Sleep cycle is disturbed by PCP; patient will need sleep after being agitated and expending excessive amounts of energy; sleeping also provides time for drug(s) to clear system.

Overdose may precipitate psychotic episode, which will clear within hours to days. When psychosis remains, preexisting condition, e.g., schizophrenia, may have been precipitated.

Mutism and confusion may occur, and information may reassure patient that problem is drug-induced and that it will improve with time. Note: "Talk-down"

Independent

approach may agitate the patient and should be used with caution.

Anticipate patient's needs and allow more time for patient to respond to any necessary questions and/or comments.

May reduce need to communicate in presence of confusion/interference with memory. Adequate time allows full expression. Note: Be aware that touching and/or physical closeness may increase anxiety and agitation.

Collaborative

Administer medications as indicated, e.g.: diazepam (Valium) or chlordiazepoxide (Librium).

Chronic PCP users in whom psychiatric complications develop may require further treatment for the thought disorder or depressive illness. The response may be very slow because of the persistence of PCP in the body tissues, sometimes for a period of several months.

NURSING DIAGNOSIS:	ANXIETY [SPECIFY LEVEL]/FEAR
May be related to:	Situational crisis; threat to/change in health status
	Perceived threat of death
	Inexperience or unfamiliarity with the effect of drug(s), (e.g., PCP, LSD)
	Impaired thought processes; sensory impairment
Possibly evidenced by:	Assumptions of "losing my mind, losing control"; verbalized concern about unknown consequences/outcomes
	Sympathetic stimulation, e.g., cardiovascular excitation, superficial vasoconstriction, pupil dilation, vomiting/diarrhea, restlessness, trembling
	Preoccupation with feelings of impending doom; apprehension
	Attack behavior
PATIENT OUTCOMES/ EVALUATION CRITERIA:	Verbalizes/demonstrates lessened anxiety. Identifies the fear and verbalizes feelings of control of self and situation. Reports anxiety reduced to a manageable level.

INTERVENTIONS

RATIONALE

Independent

Assess level of anxiety on an ongoing basis.

Increased anxiety may lead to agitation and violent behavior because patient is not in complete control of actions/responses.

Place in darkened, quiet, nonthreatening environment with a nonintrusive observer.

Lowered stimulation decreases the likelihood of confusion and fear.

843

ACTIONS/INTERVENTIONS	RATIONALE

Independent

Orient person to surroundings, time, and who is with the patient. Speak in soft voice, in a nonthreatening manner.

Use "Talk-downs" with caution, telling the patient that the ingested drug is the cause of feelings of anxiety, the effects are only temporary, and permanent damage should not occur.

Encourage verbal expression of changes in perception that are occurring.

Collaborative

Administer sedatives if necessary, e.g., diazepam (Valium) or chlordiazepoxide (Librium).

Knowing where one is can increase the feeling of security when experiencing a "bad trip."

Reassurance can be the single most important therapeutic intervention. "Talk-downs" are effective with persons who have taken LSD or similar substances. If the patient can realize that the perceptions are drug related, then an increase in control can take place. However, in some situations (e.g., PCP) "Talk-downs" can result in an increase in fear and agitation.

Can be used for assessment and provides guidance on direction for support.

Drugs of choice to be used in extreme cases in order to calm patient. Note: Medications are often discouraged because "bad trips" are usually self-limiting and time is the best remedy for treating negative effects.

NURSING DIAGNOSIS:	**SELF-CARE DEFICIT: (SPECIFY)**
May be related to:	**Perceptual/cognitive impairment**
	Therapeutic management (restraints)
Possibly evidenced by:	**Inability to meet own physical needs**
PATIENT OUTCOMES/ EVALUATION CRITERIA:	**Resumes/performs self care activities within level of own ability. Verbalizes commitment to lifestyle changes to meet self-care needs.**

ACTIONS/INTERVENTIONS	RATIONALE

Independent

Provide care as needed/permitted.

Involve patient in formulation of care plan, as possible.

Work with patient's present abilities. Do not pressure to perform beyond capabilities.

Provide and promote privacy within limits of safety needs.

Collaborative

Problem-solve with patient, using input from other team members as indicated.

Patient may be agitated and care will need to be postponed until control is regained.

Enables patient to participate at level of ability and enhances sense of control. Note: PCP user is often unable to interact without becoming agitated.

Failure can produce discouragement, depression, and agitation.

Important to enhance self-esteem.

Multidisciplinary approach with involvement of everyone who is caring for the patient, along with the patient, increases probability of plan being effective/successful.

ACTIONS/INTERVENTIONS

Collaborative

(Refer to CP: Substance Dependence/Abuse Rehabilitation, p. 861, for postacute interventions, considerations, and learning needs.)

RATIONALE

Stimulants (Amphetamines, Cocaine, Caffeine, Tobacco): Intoxication/Overdose

PATIENT ASSESSMENT DATA BASE

Data are dependent on stage of withdrawal, concurrent use of alcohol/other drugs or contaminants in drug "cut."

ACTIVITY/REST

May report: Insomnia; hypersomnia.

May exhibit: Hyperactivity, wide awake, or falling asleep during activities.

Inability to tolerate or to correct chronic fatigue (depression and/or loneliness may be a factor).

CIRCULATION

May exhibit: Elevated blood pressure, tachycardia.

Diaphoresis.

EGO INTEGRITY

May exhibit: Underdeveloped ego; highly dependent nature, with characteristics of poor impulse control, low frustration tolerance, and low self-esteem; weak superego.

Absence of guilt feelings for behavior.

May be seen or view self as susceptible to influence by others, having an inability to say "no." Need to feel elated, sociable, happy with self; desire to prove self-worth, improve self-esteem.

FOOD/FLUID

May report: Nausea/vomiting, anorexia.

May exhibit: Weight loss; thin, cachectic appearance.

NEUROSENSORY

May report: Emotional/psychologic symptoms: e.g., elation, grandiosity, loquacity, hypervigilance.

May exhibit: Pupillary dilation.

Delirium with tactile and olfactory hallucinations as well as hallucinations of insects or vermin crawling in/under the skin (formication); labile affect, violent or aggressive behavior, symptoms of a paranoid delusional disorder (amphetamine or similarly acting substances).

Fixed delusional system of a persecutory nature, lasting weeks to a year or more.

Psychosis can occur with a one-time high dose of amphetamine (especially with intravenous administration) or with long-term use at moderate or high doses.

Ideas of reference.

Aggressiveness, hostility, violence, quick response to anger; psychomotor agitation.

Stereotyped compulsive motor behavior, e.g., sorting, taking things apart and putting them back together, moving mouth from side to side in a stereotypic grimacing pattern.

Anxiety; impaired judgment and perception.

Compulsion regarding stimulant use, or may use denial of powerlessness over the stimulant (use of drug for celebration or crisis; believing drug can be used in small quantities, often resulting in binge use).

May think of recovery process as notion of willpower, subject to impulse control.

SAFETY

May exhibit: Fever/chills.

SEXUALITY

May report: Diminished/enhanced sexual desire.

SOCIAL INTERACTION

May report: Dysfunctional system (family of origin).

Impairment in social or occupational functioning.

TEACHING/LEARNING

May report: Pattern of habitual use of the particular drug/patholologic abuse, with inability to reduce or to stop use, occurring for at least 1 month duration.

Intoxication throughout the day, sometimes with daily involvement.

Episodes of overdose wherein hallucinations and delusions occur (cocaine).

Previous hospitalization or having been in residential treatment program.

Health beliefs about use of drugs.

Attendance at recovery groups, e.g., Narcotics/Alcoholics Anonymous, or other drug-specific recovery groups.

Discharge Plan Considerations: May need assistance to maintain abstinence and begin to participate in rehabilitation program

DIAGNOSTIC STUDIES

Urine: screen for presence of drug(s).

ASI: produces a "problem severity profile," which indicates areas of treatment needs.

NURSING PRIORITIES

1. Maintain physiologic stability.
2. Promote safety and security.
3. Prevent complications.
4. Support patient's acceptance of reality of situation.
5. Promote family involvement in "Intervention"/treatment process.
6. Provide information about dependency, prognosis, and treatment needs.

DISCHARGE CRITERIA

1. Homeostasis maintained.
2. Complications prevented/minimized.
3. Dealing with situation realistically/planning for the future.
4. Abstinence from drug(s) maintained.
5. Dependence condition, prognosis, and therapeutic regimen understood.
6. Transferred to rehabilitation program/attending group.

NURSING DIAGNOSIS:	CARDIAC OUTPUT, ALTERED: DECREASED [POTENTIAL]
May be related to:	Drug (cocaine) effect on myocardium (dependent on purity/quantity ingested)
	Pre-existing myocardiopathy (with or without previous

prolonged drug abuse)

Alterations in electrical rate/rhythm/conduction

Possibly evidenced by:	[Not applicable; presence of signs and symptoms establishes an *actual* diagnosis.]
PATIENT OUTCOMES/ EVALUATION CRITERIA:	Reports absence of chest pain. Demonstrates adequate cardiac output free of signs of shock, dysrhythmias.

ACTIONS/INTERVENTIONS

Independent

Monitor cardiac rate and rhythm. Document dysrhythmias.

Investigate complaints of chest pain, indigestion/heartburn.

Have emergency equipment/medications available.

Review physical assessment periodically.

Obtain information specific to pattern of drug use over past month, immunizaiton history, allergies, medications used for other purposes.

Collaborative

Administer medications as indicated, e.g.:

    Propranolol (Inderal);

    Lidocaine.

RATIONALE

Ventricular dysrhythmias/cardiac arrest may occur at any time, especially with toxic levels of cocaine.

Increased incidence of myocardial infarction in cocaine users.

Prompt treatment of dysrhythmias may prevent cardiac arrest.

Can reveal daily changes and problem areas and identifies opportunities for providing information for health promotion and problem prevention.

Initial factual history can reveal information essential to physical treatment; where person obtained drug could assist in investigating possible "cut" with other drugs.

Beta-adrenergic blocker that reduces cardiac oxygen demand by blocking catecholamine-induced increases in heart rate, blood pressure, and force of myocardial contraction.

Used in emergency situation to control/prevent ventricular dysrhythmias.

NURSING DIAGNOSIS:	**VIOLENCE, POTENTIAL FOR: DIRECTED AT SELF/OTHERS**
May be related to:	Toxic reaction to drug, panic state, profound depression/suicidal behavior
	Organic brain syndrome
Possible indicators:	Overt and aggressive acts
	Increased motor activity
	Possession of destructive means
	Suspicion of others, paranoid ideation, delusions, and hallucinations
	Expressed intent directly/indirectly
PATIENT OUTCOMES/	Acknowledges fearfulness and realities of situation.

Verbalizes understanding of behavior and precipitating factors. Demonstrates self-control.

ACTIONS/INTERVENTIONS	RATIONALE
Independent	
Decrease stimuli, provide quiet in own room or place in stimulus-reduction room with supervision.	Reduces reactivity, enhances calm feelings.
Allow SO to remain in room during procedures when appropriate.	Can provide a calming effect to see someone that patient knows/cares about.
Remove potentially harmful objects from environment.	Reduces opportunity for patient to carry out suicidal ideas. Patient may be suicidal when/if rebound CNS depression occurs secondary to stimulant withdrawal.
Explain consistent rules of unit, e.g., no violence, no threats.	Secure environment enhances sense of safety which can decrease perceived threat. Enhances opportunity for patient to learn ways to cope with aggressive feelings before reacting.
Maintain high staff profile in situations where potential violence can occur.	May prevent onset of violence.
Allow chance for verbal expression of aggressive feelings.	Encouragement of new avenue of expression helps patient learn new coping skills.
Assist patient in identifying what provokes anger.	Awareness of reaction is the first step in learning change.
Provide outlets for expression that involve physical activity, e.g., stationary bicycle, racquetball/basketball/volleyball.	Gross motor activity in protected environment can lessen aggressive drive.
Discuss consequences of aggressive behavior.	Learning choices assists patient to gain control of situation and self.
Be alert to violence potential, e.g., increased pacing, verbalization of delusional persecutory content, hypervigilance regarding specific persons in the milieu, gesturing aggressively, threatening others verbally or physically.	Recognizing potential and assisting patient to gain control can be more effective prior to violent outbreak.
Isolate immediately if patient becomes violent, using adequate staff trained in assaultive management. Maintain calm, nonpunitive attitude.	Patient will feel safer if others take control until internal locus of control can be regained. An attitude of acceptance is important while refusing to tolerate the violent behavior.
Negotiate conditions for coming out of isolation when the patient is calm, based on agreement of social appropriateness.	Clear expectations aid patient in feeling secure about own control.
Build trust: follow through on commitments/agreements, maintain consistent staff and frequent brief contact with patient.	Trust is essential to working with all patients. Brief contacts can prevent overstimulation.
Collaborative	
Administer medications as indicated, e.g.:	
Chlorpromazine (Thorazine); haloperidol (Haldol);	Short-term use of major tranquilizers during acute intoxication/psychosis assists patient in gaining self-control; promotes sedation/rest when agitated, assaultive, overstimulated. Note: Thorazine may cause postural hypotension, and Haldol may provoke acute extrapyramidal reaction, requiring additional

ACTIONS/INTERVENTIONS

Collaborative

Diazepam (Valium), chlordiazepoxide (Librium);

L-tryptophan.

Avoid the use of restraints/seclusion.

RATIONALE

evaluation/medication.

Occasionally useful for treatment of acute cocaine intoxication. Either drug is useful for preventing DTs when substance use is combined with alcohol.

Useful in agitation and irritability, decreases anxiety.

In stimulated state, may exacerbate hyperactivity.

NURSING DIAGNOSIS:	**SENSORY-PERCEPTUAL ALTERATION: (SPECIFY)**
May be related to:	**Chemical alteration: exogenous (CNS stimulants or depressants, mind-altering drugs)/decreased pain perception**
	Altered sensory reception, transmission and/or integration: altered status of sense organs
Possibly evidenced by:	**Preoccupation with/appears to be responding to internal stimuli from hallucinatory experiences, e.g., "listening pose," laughing and talking to self, stopping in mid-sentence and listening, "picking" at self and clothing**
PATIENT OUTCOMES/ EVALUATION CRITERIA:	**Distinguishes reality from altered perceptions. States awareness that hallucinations may result from stimulant use.**

ACTIONS/INTERVENTIONS

Independent

Notice patient's preoccupation, responses, gesturing, social skill.

Assist patient in checking perceptions verbally; provide reality information.

Acknowledge patient's emotional state; reassure regarding safety.

Explore ways of calming and relaxing patient.

Be aware that altered sensation and perception may cause injury, e.g., be alert for patient burning self with cigarette, excessive scratching at skin to rid self of insects or drug (which may feel as though it is in the skin), accidentally harming self through poor judgment or misperceptions. (Refer to ND: Violence, Potential for: Directed at Self/Others, p. 848.)

Inform patient, if calm enough, of temporary nature of hallucinations that have resulted from stimulant use.

RATIONALE

Helps to assess whether or not patient is hallucinating without overstimulating verbally.

Can calm the patient and provide reassurance of safety and that formication (illusion of insects crawling on the body) or other misperceptions are not occurring.

Empathetic response can diminish intensity of fear.

Relaxation can promote positive outlook, distracting from negativity and enhancing clarity of perceptions.

Amphetamine use causes impaired judgment, increasing risk of injury/self-harm.

Learning cause, effect and possible temporary nature of misperceptions may reduce fear, anxiety, and negativity. May inject hope and positive attitude.

NURSING DIAGNOSIS:	FEAR/ANXIETY [SPECIFY LEVEL]
May be related to:	Paranoid delusions associated with stimulant use
Possibly evidenced by:	Feelings/beliefs that others are conspiring against or are about to kill patient
PATIENT OUTCOMES/ EVALUATION CRITERIA:	Recognizes frightening feelings before preoccupying self or becoming violent. Discusses reality base of persecutory fears with staff. Reports fear/anxiety reduced to manageable level. Demonstrates appropriate range of feelings and appears relaxed.

ACTIONS/INTERVENTIONS	RATIONALE
Independent	
Establish consistent staff. Build trust by being reliable, honest, genuine, prompt.	Trust and rapport are necessary for overcoming fear.
Acknowledge awareness of patient's feelings, e.g., fear, terror, overwhelmed, panic, anxiety, confusion.	Empathy can assist patient to tolerate/deal with own feelings.
Be concrete, clear in communication. Assess patient's readiness for humor and/or touch.	Fear negatively influences one's ability to laugh. Fear is serious to the perceiver and must be respected. Touch can be misinterpreted/increase anxiety.
Encourage verbalization of fears/anxieties.	Venting feelings to trusted staff can lessen intensity of fearfulness. Provides opportunity to clarify misunderstandings and comfort patient.
Assist patient in reality-checking fears. Use gentle confrontation.	Patient can reduce fear if s/he understands difference between reality and delusions. Should be used cautiously because reality-checking a delusional system puts trust at risk.

NURSING DIAGNOSIS:	NUTRITION, ALTERED: LESS THAN BODY REQUIREMENTS
May be related to:	Anorexia (stimulant use)
	Insufficient/inappropriate use of financial resources
Possibly evidenced by:	Reported inadequate intake
	Lack of interest in food; weight loss
	Poor muscle tone
	Signs/laboratory evidence of vitamin deficiencies
PATIENT OUTCOMES/ EVALUATION CRITERIA:	Demonstrates progressive weight gain toward goal. Verbalizes understanding of causative factors and individual needs. Identifies appropriate dietary choices, lifestyle changes to regain/maintain desired weight.

851

ACTIONS/INTERVENTIONS	RATIONALE

Independent

Ascertain dietary intake pattern over past several weeks.	Stimulants cause decreased appetite and impaired judgment regarding nutritional needs.
Discuss needs/likes/dislikes about food choices.	Will be more likely to maintain desired intake if individual preferences are considered.
Anticipate hyperphagia and weigh every other day.	Often a consequence of stimulant withdrawal and may result in sudden/inappropriate weight gain.
Provide meals in a relaxed, nonstimulating environment.	Stimulus reduction aids relaxation and ability to focus on eating.
Encourage frequent nutritional snacks, small nutritious meals.	Small amounts of food frequently can prevent/reduce GI distress.

Collaborative

Obtain/review routine laboratory work, e.g., CBC, serum protein, albumin, UA.	Assessment of nutritional state is necessary to treat preexisting deficiencies, rule out anemia, dehydration, or ketosis.
Consult with dietitian.	Useful in establishing individual nutritional needs/dietary program.

NURSING DIAGNOSIS:	INFECTION, POTENTIAL FOR
May be related to:	IV drug use techniques; impurities in drugs injected
	Localized trauma; nasal septum damage (snorting cocaine)
	Malnutrition; altered immune state
Possibly evidenced by:	[Not applicable; presence of signs and symptoms establishes an *actual* diagnosis.]
PATIENT OUTCOMES/ EVALUATION CRITERIA:	Verbalizes understanding of individual risk factors. Identifies interventions to prevent/reduce risk factors. Demonstrates lifestyle changes to promote safe environment. Achieves timely healing of infectious process if present/develops and is afebrile.

ACTIONS/INTERVENTIONS	RATIONALE

Independent

Assess skin integrity and character. Assist as needed with body and oral hygiene; provide clean clothes, properly fitting shoes.	Skin integrity requires cleanliness. Sores may need care for prevention of infection.
Use blood/body fluid precautions per hospital policy, when appropriate.	Protects care giver from possible contamination by infectious disease viruses, e.g., hepatitis, AIDS.
Monitor vital signs. Assess level of consciousness.	Abnormal signs, including fever, can indicate presence of infection. Cerebral complications, e.g., meningitis, brain abscess, may occur, affecting mentation.

ACTIONS/INTERVENTIONS	RATIONALE

Independent

Observe for nasal stuffiness, pain, bleeding, abnormal mucus production.

Cocaine snorting can cause erosion of the nasal septum, requiring additional therapy/interventions.

Investigate complaints of acute/chronic bone pain, tenderness, guarding with movement, regional muscle spasm.

Symptoms of osteomyelitis usually due to hematogenous spread of bacteria, most often affecting lumbar vertebrae.

Ascertain health status of family members/SO currently in contact with patient.

May expose patient to diseases such as colds, hepatitis, AIDS.

Collaborative

Review laboratory studies, e.g., UA, CBC, SMA, RPR, ESR, ELISA/Western Blot test.

May identify complications of IV cocaine and amphetamine use such as hepatitis, nephritis, tetanus, vasculitis, septicemia, subacute bacterial endocarditis, embolic phenomena, malaria. Toxic allergic reactions may result from other substances in the "cut" and immunologic abnormalities may occur due to repeated antigenic stimulation. Note: IV needle drug users are at high risk for contamination with AIDS and hepatitis viruses.

NURSING DIAGNOSIS:	SLEEP PATTERN DISTURBANCE
May be related to:	**CNS sensory alterations: External factor (stimulant use), internal factors (psychologic stress)**
Possibly evidenced by:	**Altered sleep cycle; initial signs of insomnia and then hypersomnia**
	Constant alertness; racing thoughts that prevent rest
	Denial of need to sleep or reports of inability to stay awake
PATIENT OUTCOMES/ EVALUATION CRITERIA:	**Sleeping 6–8 hours at night. Resting minimally, appropriately, during the day. Verbalizes feeling rested when awakens.**

ACTIONS/INTERVENTIONS	RATIONALE

Independent

Establish sleep cycle where patient sleeps at night, is awake during day with brief rest periods as needed.

Adequate rest and sleep can improve emotional state. Restoration of regular pattern is a priority in a sleep-deprived stimulant user.

Decrease external stimuli and enhance relaxation prior to bedtime; encourage use of presleep routines, e.g., hot bath, warm milk, stretching.

Patient may need calming in order to attempt rest.

Provide opportunities for fresh air, mild exercise, non-caffeinated beverages, quiet environment as patient can tolerate.

Promotes drowsiness/desire for sleep.

ACTIONS/INTERVENTIONS

Collaborative

Administer medications as indicated, e.g., L-tryptophan.

(Refer to CP: Substance Dependence/Abuse Rehabilitation, p. 861, for continuation of care and learning needs.)

RATIONALE

Patient may initially require chemical assistance to attain appropriate sleep cycle.

Depressants (Benzodiazepines, Barbiturates, Opioids): Intoxication/Overdose

CNS depressants prescribed for symptoms of anxiety, depression, and sleep disturbances are among the most widely used and abused drugs. These drugs are very likely to be abused when the underlying conditions remain untreated.

PATIENT ASSESSMENT DATA BASE

Data are dependent on stage of withdrawal and concurrent use of alcohol/other drugs.

ACTIVITY/REST

May report:
Interference with sleep pattern.
General malaise.

May exhibit:
Lethargy.

CIRCULATION

May exhibit:
Tachycardia (suggests withdrawal syndrome); atrial fibrillation, ventricular dysrhythmias.
Hypotension.

EGO INTEGRITY

May report:
Substance use for stress management.
Feelings of helplessness, hopelessness, powerlessness.

May exhibit:
Underdeveloped ego; highly dependent nature, with characteristics of poor impulse control, low frustration tolerance, and low self-esteem.
Weak superego, with absence of guilt feelings.
Psychostructural factors (e.g., personality) are seen as significant with substance use/abuse (maladaptive coping mechanisms).

FOOD/FLUID

May report:
Nausea.

May exhibit:
Vomiting.

NEUROSENSORY

May report:
Muscle aches; twitching.

May exhibit:
Mental status: impaired judgment with some affective change; alterations in consciousness, from extreme agitation to coma.
Behavior: mood swings, aggression, combativeness (related to general "disinhibiting" effect of the drug, loss of impulse control).
Temporary psychosis with acute onset of auditory hallucinations and paranoid delusions (unexplained neuropsychiatric presentation may be indicative of drug use).
Psychomotor activity increased.
Hypersensitivity, e.g., anxiety, tremors, hypotension, irritability, restlessness, and seizures.
Pupils small/pinpoint constriction (opiates), dilated (barbiturates).
Gait unsteady/staggering, loss of coordination; positive Romberg sign.
Speech slurred.

855

PAIN/COMFORT

May report: Headache, abdominal pain/severe cramping.

Deep muscle/bone pain (methadone abusers).

RESPIRATION

May report: Continued rhinorrhea, excessive lacrimation, sneezing.

May exhibit: Respiratory depression (noted in overdose).

Increased rate (withdrawal syndrome).

SAFETY

May report: Hot/cold flashes.

May exhibit: Thermoregulation instability with hyperpyrexia, hypothermia.

Skin: piloerection ("gooseflesh"); puncture wounds on arms, hands, legs, under tongue, indicating IV drug use.

SOCIAL INTERACTION

May report: Dysfunctional family of origin system.

History from family member/significant other(s) may reveal dysfunctional patterns of interaction.

TEACHING/LEARNING

May report: Preexisting physical/psychologic conditions.

Family history of substance use/abuse.

Discharge Plan Considerations: May need assistance to maintain abstinence and begin to participate in rehabilitation program.

DIAGNOSTIC STUDIES

Drug screen: identifies drug(s) being used.

ASI: produces a "problem severity profile," which indicates areas of treatment needs.

NURSING PRIORITIES

1. Promote physiologic stability.
2. Protect patient from injury.
3. Provide appropriate referral and follow-up.
4. Promote family involvement in the withdrawal/rehabilitation process.
5. Provide information about dependency/prognosis and treatment needs.

DISCHARGE CRITERIA

1. Homeostasis achieved.
2. Abstinence from drug(s) maintained.
3. Transferred to rehabilitation program/attending group therapy, e.g., Narcotics Anonymous.
4. Dependency condition, prognosis, and therapeutic regimen understood.

NURSING DIAGNOSIS:	INJURY, POTENTIAL FOR: (SPECIFY)
May be related to:	**CNS depression (effect of overdose)**

CNS agitation (effect of abrupt withdrawal)

Hypersensitivity to the drug(s)

Psychologic stress (narrowed perceptual fields seen with anxiety)

Possibly evidenced by:	**[Not applicable; presence of signs and symptoms establishes an *actual* diagnosis.]**
PATIENT OUTCOMES/ EVALUATION CRITERIA:	**Verbalizes understanding of risk factors of taking drugs. Refrains from acting on hallucinations/impaired judgment. Completes withdrawal without injury to self/ development of complications.**

ACTIONS/INTERVENTIONS	RATIONALE

Independent

Determine degree of impairment by talking to patient/ SO, noting when person was last seen well; sleep patterns and duration of problems.	Information provides an approximate time frame for impairment, with sleep disruption often the first observable sign of a problem. Prescription information provides clues to identity of drug(s) and amount taken.
Identify drug(s) taken, when taken, and route used if possible.	Helpful to identify interventions for specific drug. Determining drug(s) taken may be difficult outside of blood/urine testing because the patient may not feel free to tell because of embarrassment or for legal reasons or may not know what has been ingested.
Assess level of consciousness, e.g., agitated, stuporous, lethargic, confused, or unconscious. Note pinpoint pupils.	May be indicator of degree of intoxication and level of intervention required. Constricted pupils are a classic sign of opioid (heroin) ingestion.
Evaluate for evidence of head trauma.	Important for differential diagnosis to prevent permanent damage/death.
Determine when food was last eaten. Note complaints of nausea.	May slow absorption of drug(s) into the bloodstream; however, may present risk of vomiting and aspiration if level of consciousness is depressed.
Monitor temperature as indicated. Observe for signs of dehydration.	Hypothermia may be seen in intoxication, while hyperpyrexia may occur with withdrawal or indicate infectious process. Note: Dehydration often accompanies hyperpyrexia, requiring additional intervention/fluid replacement.
Monitor vital signs (BP, pulse, respirations).	Changes depend on drug taken, e.g., diazepam (Valium) may be evidenced by hypotension, tachycardia.
Provide quiet, lighted room. An isolation room with simple furniture may be needed.	Reduces stimuli, internal or external, that may lead to injury as the patient responds.
Observe patient at all times; use staff or family member as available.	Patient with varying level of consciousness should not be left alone because of the danger of accidental injury.
Provide orientation as needed.	Maintaining contact provides reassurance, reduces anxiety when consciousness returns.
Note presence of tremors.	Involuntary movements of one or more parts of the body may result from abrupt removal of drug.

857

ACTIONS/INTERVENTIONS	RATIONALE

Independent

Provide seizure precautions, e.g., padded side rails, bed in low position, airway adjunct/suction at bedside.

Precautions can prevent injury if seizures occur during withdrawal.

Note changes in behavior indicative of psychosis, e.g., distorted reality, altered mood, impaired language and memory.

Drug intoxication can precipitate an alteration in perceptions/psychotic behavior.

Assess emotional state, noting psychiatric history and suicide gestures/attempts. Note use/abuse of other substances.

Patterns of drug use will indicate likelihood of intentional or accidental overdose. Substance abuse/suicide attempts may be symptom of or response to underlying psychiatric illness or to hallucinations caused by sensitivity to drug.

Determine history of hallucinations.

May be auditory, visual, tactile, and very frightening. May also trigger suicidal/homicidal behavior.

Institute suicide precautions, as indicated.

May need environmental restraints to protect patient until own coping abilities improve and internal locus of control is regained.

Collaborative

Start/maintain IV line.

Provides an open line for emergency treatment.

Administer 50% glucose IV with thiamine added.

Acute thiamine deficiency and hypoglycemia may mimic drug intoxication if patient is comatose.

Assist with gastric lavage if indicated.

May be done when drug has been recently ingested, consciousness is depressed, making vomiting hazardous, or when induced emesis has failed.

Administer medication per current treatment/protocol:

    Emetics, e.g., apomorphine, syrup of ipecac;

Induced vomiting is an efficient and effective way to empty the stomach when the patient is fully conscious. It is of questionable value unless performed within a few hours of drug ingestion because of rapid gastrointestinal absorption.

    Activated charcoal;

Binds with many substances in the GI tract, reducing absorption of ingested drug(s).

    Phenobarbital;

Prolonged effect provides smoother sedation without "high" of more rapidly acting drugs, and has an anticonvulsant effect.

    Methadone.

Replaces heroin or other narcotic analgesics in detoxification program, reducing/minimizing withdrawal symptoms.

Assist with barbiturate detoxification program.

Reintoxication should be done before drug withdrawal is attempted. This establishes an independent estimate of prior drug use and provides a baseline to begin the detoxification schedule. Reintoxication should begin as soon as there are signs of intoxication, e.g., nystagmus, slurred speech, ataxia on backward and frontward tandem gait.

Prepare for/assist with dialysis if indicated.

Occasionally effective for clearance of toxic/lethal levels of phenobarbital.

Refer to rehabilitation program, involve in "Intervention" (confrontation) and/or therapy as indicated.

Patient will need ongoing assistance to acknowledge and maintain drug-free existence.

NURSING DIAGNOSIS:	BREATHING PATTERN, INEFFECTIVE/GAS EXCHANGE, IMPAIRED [POTENTIAL]
May be related to:	Neuromuscular impairment
	Decreased energy/fatigue
	Inflammatory process
	Decreased lung expansion
Possiby evidenced by:	[Not applicable; presence of signs and symptoms establishes an *actual* diagnosis.]
PATIENT OUTCOMES/ EVALUATION CRITERIA:	Establishes normal/effective breathing pattern with absence of cyanosis/symptoms of respiratory distress.

ACTIONS/INTERVENTIONS	RATIONALE

Independent

Monitor respiratory rate, depth, rhythm, and breath sounds.	Sedative/depressant effects on CNS may result in loss of airway patency and/or respiratory depression. Prompt treatment is necessary to prevent respiratory arrest. Note: Acute pulmonary edema is a common complication in heroin overdose/intoxication.
Have suction equipment, airway adjuncts available.	Sedative effects of drugs, increased salivation, vomiting potentiate risk of aspiration. Relaxation of oropharyngeal muscles and respiratory depression require prompt intervention to prevent respiratory arrest.

Collaborative

Administer medications as indicated, e.g., naloxone (Narcan).	Narcotic antagonist that may reverse effects of respiratory depression in opioid intoxication. Note: May trigger acute withdrawal syndrome.
Provide supplemental oxygen.	May be necessary to improve oxygen intake in presence of respiratory depression.
Review chest x-ray.	Common complications of depressant (opiate) abuse include pneumonia, aspiration pneumonitis, lung abscess, atelectasis, which will require specific treatment.
Monitor ABGs, pulmonary function studies when indicated.	Chronic addiction may result in decreased vital capacity and pulmonary diffusion, affecting gas exchange. Presence of septic pulmonary emboli or pulmonary fibrosis (from talc granulomatosis) may further compromise respiratory function.

NURSING DIAGNOSIS:	INFECTION, POTENTIAL FOR
May be related to:	IV drug use techniques; impurities in injected drugs
	Localized trauma
	Malnutrition; altered immune state

859

Possibly evidenced by:	[Not applicable; presence of signs and symptoms establishes an *actual* diagnosis.]
PATIENT OUTCOMES/ EVALUATION CRITERIA:	Verbalizes understanding of and demonstrates lifestyle changes to reduce risk factor(s). Achieves timely healing of infectious process if present or develops and is afebrile.

ACTIONS/INTERVENTIONS	RATIONALE

Independent

Refer to CP: Stimulants, ND: Infection, Potential for, p. 852, for interventions specific to this nursing diagnosis. (Refer to CP: Substance Dependence/Abuse Rehabilitation, p. 861, for continuation of care and learning needs.)

Substance Dependence/Abuse Rehabilitation _____

Alcohol; amphetamines or similarly acting sympathomimetics; cannabis, cocaine, hallucinogens, barbiturates, opioids; sedatives/hypnotics/anxiolytics.

PATIENT ASSESSMENT DATA BASE

Refer to appropriate acute CP: Alcoholism, p. 825; Stimulants, p. 846; Hallucinogens, p. 836; Depressants, p. 855.

TEACHING/LEARNING

Discharge Plan Considerations: May need assistance with long-range plan for recovery.

DIAGNOSTIC STUDIES

ASI: an assessment tool that produces a "problem severity profile" of the patient, including chemical, medical, psychologic, legal, family/social and employment/support aspects, indicating areas of treatment needs.

NURSING PRIORITIES

1. Provide support for decision to stop substance use.
2. Strengthen individual coping skills and facilitate learning of new ways to reduce anxiety.
3. Promote family involvement in rehabilitation program.
4. Facilitate family growth/development.
5. Provide information about condition, prognosis, and treatment needs.

DISCHARGE CRITERIA

1. Responsibility for own life and behavior assumed.
2. Plan to maintain substance-free life formulated.
3. Family relationships/co-dependency issues being addressed.
4. Treatment program successfully completed.
5. Condition, prognosis, and therapeutic regimen understood.

NURSING DIAGNOSIS:	COPING, INEFFECTIVE INDIVIDUAL
May be related to:	**Personal vulnerability; difficulty handling new situations**
	Previous ineffective/inadequate coping skills with substitution of drug(s)
	Anxiety/fear
Possibly evidenced by:	**Denial (one of the strongest and most resistant symptoms of substance abuse); lack of acceptance that drug use is causing the present situation**
	Altered social patterns/participation
	Impaired adaptive behavior and problem-solving skills
	Decreased ability to handle stress of illness/hospitalization
	Financial affairs in disarray; employment difficulties

	(usually the last area to be affected), e.g., losing time on job/not maintaining steady employment
PATIENT OUTCOMES/ EVALUATION CRITERIA:	Verbalizes awareness of relationship of substance abuse to current situation. Identifies ineffective coping behaviors/consequences. Uses effective coping skills/ problem solving. Initiates necessary lifestyle changes. Attends support group (e.g., Cocaine/Narcotics/ Alcoholics Anonymous) regularly.

ACTIONS/INTERVENTIONS

Independent

Ascertain what name patient would like to be addressed by.

Determine understanding of current situation and previous/other methods of coping with life's problems.

Confront and examine denial in peer group.

Remain nonjudgmental. Be alert to changes in behavior, e.g., restlessness, increased tension.

Provide positive feedback for expressing awareness of denial in self/others.

Maintain firm expectation that patient attend recovery support/therapy groups regularly.

Structure diversional activity that relates to recovery (e.g., social activity within support group) wherein issues of being chemically free are examined.

Use peer support to examine ways of coping with drug hunger.

Provide information about addictive use versus experimental, occasional; biochemical/genetic disorder theory (genetic predisposition); use activated by environment; pharmacology of stimulant; compulsive desire as a lifelong occurrence.

Encourage and support patient's taking responsibility for own recovery (e.g., development of alternative behaviors to drug urge). Assist patient to learn own responsibility for recovering.

Assist patient to learn/encourage use of relaxation skills, guided imagery, visualizations.

Be aware of staff enabling behaviors and feelings.

Collaborative

Administer medications as indicated, e.g.:

RATIONALE

Shows courtesy and respect. Gives sense of orientation and control.

Provides information about degree of denial, identifies coping skills that may be used in present plan of care.

Because denial is the major defense mechanism in addictive disease, confrontation by peers can help the patient accept the reality that drug use is a major problem.

Confrontation can lead to an increase in agitation, which may compromise safety of patient/staff.

Positive feedback is necessary to enhance self-esteem and to reinforce desired behavior.

Attending is related to admitting need for help, to working with denial and for maintenance of a long-term drug-free existence.

Discovery of alternative methods for coping with drug hunger can remind patient that addiction is a lifelong process and opportunity for changing patterns is available.

Addictive self-help groups are valuable for learning and promoting abstinence in each member as well as in using peer pressure.

Progression of use in the addict is from recreational to addictive use. Comprehending this process is important in combating denial. Education may relieve patient of blame, may help awareness of recurring addictive characteristics.

Denial can be replaced with responsible action when patient accepts the reality of own responsibility.

Helps patient to relax, develop new ways to deal with stress, problem-solve.

Lack of understanding of enabling and codependence can result in nontherapeutic approaches to addicts.

ACTIONS/INTERVENTIONS	RATIONALE
Collaborative	
Disulfiram (Antabuse);	This drug can be helpful in maintaining abstinence from alcohol while other therapy is undertaken. By inhibiting alcohol oxidation, the drug leads to an accumulation of acetaldehyde with a highly unpleasant reaction if alcohol is consumed.
Methadone.	This drug is thought to blunt the craving for/diminish the effects of heroin and is used to assist in withdrawal and long-term maintenance programs. It has fewer side effects and allows the individual to maintain daily activities and ultimately withdraw from drug use.
Encourage involvement with self-help associations, e.g., Alcoholics/Narcotics Anonymous.	Puts patient in direct contact with support systems necessary for continued sobriety/drug-free life.

NURSING DIAGNOSIS: POWERLESSNESS

May be related to:

Substance addiction with/without periods of abstinence

Episodic compulsive indulgence; attempts at recovery

Lifestyle of helplessness

Possibly evidenced by:

Ineffective recovery attempts; statements of inability to stop behavior/requests for help

Continuous/constant thinking about drug and/or obtaining drug

Alteration in personal, occupational and social life.

PATIENT OUTCOMES/ EVALUATION CRITERIA:

Admits inability to control drug habit, surrenders to powerlessness. Verbalizes acceptance of need for treatment and awareness that willpower alone cannot control abstinence. Engages in peer support. Demonstrates active participation in program. Regains and maintains healthful status with a drug-free lifestyle.

ACTIONS/INTERVENTIONS	RATIONALE
Independent	
Use crisis intervention techniques:	Patient is more amenable to acceptance of need for treatment at this time.
Assist patient to recognize problem exists;	While patient is hurting, it is easier to admit drug(s) is a problem.
Identify goals for change;	Helpful in planning direction for care, promoting belief that change can occur.
Discuss alternative solutions;	Brainstorming helps creatively identify possibilities and provides sense of control.
Assist in selecting most appropriate alternative;	As possibilities are discussed, the most useful solution becomes clear.
Support in decision and implementation of selected alternative(s).	Helps the patient to persevere in process of change.

ACTIONS/INTERVENTIONS	RATIONALE

Independent

Discuss need for help in a caring, nonjudgmental way.	A caring confrontive manner is more therapeutic because the patient may respond defensively to a moralistic attitude, blocking recovery.
Discuss ways in which drug has interfered with life, occupation, personal/interpersonal relationships.	Awareness of how the drug has controlled life is important in combatting denial.
Explore support in peer group. Encourage sharing of drug hunger, situations that increase the desire to indulge, ways that substance has influenced life.	May need assistance in expressing self, speaking about powerlessness, admitting need for help in order to face up to problem and begin resolution.
Assist patient to learn ways to enhance health and structure healthy diversion from drug use, e.g., a balanced diet, adequate rest, acupuncture, biofeedback, deep meditative techniques, exercise (e.g., walking, slow/long distance running).	Learning to empower self in constructive areas can strengthen ability to continue recovery. These activities help restore natural biochemical balance, aid detoxification, and manage stress, anxiety, use of free time. These diversions can increase self-confidence, thereby improving self-esteem. Note: Release of endorphins from lengthy exercise can create a feeling of well-being.
Assist patient in self-examination of spirituality, faith.	Surrendering to and faith in a power greater than oneself has been found effective in substance recovery; may decrease sense of powerlessness.
Assist patient to learn assertive communication.	Effective in assisting in ability to refuse use, to stop relationships with users and dealers, to build healthy relationships, regain control of own life.
Provide treatment information on an ongoing basis.	Helps patient know what to expect. Creates opportunity for patient to be a part of what is happening and make informed choices about participation/outcomes.

Collaborative

Refer to/assist with making appointment to treatment program for continuation after discharge, e.g., partial hospitalization drug treatment programs, Narcotics/Alcoholics Anonymous.	Follow-through on appointments may be easier than making the initial contact, and continuing treatment is essential to positive outcome.

NURSING DIAGNOSIS:	**NUTRITION, ALTERED: LESS THAN BODY REQUIREMENTS**
May be related to:	**Insufficient dietary intake to meet metabolic needs for psychologic, physiologic or economic reasons**
Possibly evidenced by:	**Weight loss; weight below norm for height/body build; decreased subcutaneous fat/muscle mass**
	Reported altered taste sensation; lack of interest in food
	Poor muscle tone
	Sore, inflamed buccal cavity
	Laboratory evidence of protein/vitamin deficiencies
PATIENT OUTCOMES/ EVALUATION CRITERIA:	**Demonstrates progressive weight gain toward goal with normalization of laboratory values and absence of**

signs of malnutrition. Verbalizes understanding of effects of substance abuse, reduced dietary intake on nutritional status. Demonstrates behaviors, lifestyle changes to regain and maintain appropriate weight.

ACTIONS/INTERVENTIONS	RATIONALE

Independent

Assess height/weight, age, body build, strength, activity/rest level. Note condition of oral cavity.

Provides information about individual on which to base dietary plan. Type of diet/foods may be affected by condition of mucous membranes and teeth.

Take triceps skinfold measurements.

Calculates subcutaneous fat and muscle mass to aid in determining dietary needs.

Note total daily calorie intake; maintain a diary of intake, times and patterns of eating.

Information about patient's dietary pattern will identify nutritional needs/deficiencies.

Evaluate energy expenditure (e.g., pacing or sedentary), and establish an individualized exercise program.

Activity level affects nutritional needs. Exercise enhances muscle tone, may stimulate appetite.

Provide opportunity to choose foods/snacks to meet dietary plan.

Enhances participation/sense of control and may promote resolution of nutritional deficiencies.

Weigh weekly and record.

Provides information regarding effectiveness of dietary plan.

Collaborative

Consult with dietician.

Useful in establishing individual dietary needs/plan. Provides additional resource for learning.

Review lab work as indicated, e.g., glucose, serum albumin, electrolytes.

Identifies anemias, electrolyte imbalances, other abnormalities that may be present, requiring specific therapy.

Refer for dental consultation as necessary.

Teeth are essential to good nutritional intake and dental hygiene/care is often a neglected area in this population.

NURSING DIAGNOSIS:	SELF-CONCEPT, DISTURBANCE IN: SELF-ESTEEM; PERSONAL IDENTITY; ROLE PERFORMANCE
May be related to:	Social stigma attached to substance abuse
	Social expectation that one control behavior
	Biochemical body change (e.g., withdrawal from alcohol/drugs)
	Situational crisis with loss of control over life events
Possibly evidenced by:	Not taking responsibility for self/self-care; lack of follow-through
	Self-destructive behavior
	Change in usual role patterns or responsibility (family, job, legal)
	Confusion about self, purpose or direction in life

865

Denial that substance use is a problem

PATIENT OUTCOMES/ EVALUATION CRITERIA:	Identifies feelings and methods for coping with negative perception of self. Verbalizes acceptance of self as is and an increased sense of self-esteem. Sets goals and participates in realistic planning for lifestyle changes necessary to live without drugs.

ACTIONS/INTERVENTIONS	RATIONALE
Independent	
Provide opportunity for and encourage verbalization/ discussion of individual situation.	Patient often has difficulty expressing self, even more difficulty accepting the degree of importance substance has assumed in life and its relationship to present situation.
Assess mental status. Note presence of other psychiatric disorders (dual diagnosis).	Many patients use substances (alcohol and other drugs) to seek relief from depression or anxiety. Note: Approximately 60% of substance-dependent patients also have mental illness problems, and there is an increasing awareness that treatment for both is imperative.
Spend time with patient. Discuss patient's behavior/ use of substance in a nonjudgmental way.	Presence of the nurse conveys acceptance of the individual as a worthwhile person. Discussion provides opportunity for insight into the problems abuse has created for the patient.
Provide positive reinforcement for positive actions and encourage the patient to accept this input.	Failure and lack of self-esteem have been problems for this patient, who needs to learn to accept self as an individual with positive attributes.
Observe SO dynamics/support.	Substance abuse is a family disease, and how the members act and react to the patient's behavior affects the course of the disease and how patient sees self. Many unconsciously become "enablers," helping the individual to cover up the consequences of the abuse. (Refer to ND: Coping, Ineffective Family: Compromised/Disabling, p. 867.)
Encourage expression of feelings of guilt, shame, and anger.	The patient often has lost respect for self and believes that the situation is hopeless. Expression of these feelings helps the patient to begin to accept responsibility for self and take steps to make changes.
Help the patient to acknowledge that substance use is the problem and that problems can be dealt with without the use of drugs. Confront the use of defenses, e.g., denial, projection, rationalization.	When drugs can no longer be blamed for the problems that exist, the patient can begin to plan a life without substance use. Confrontation helps the patient accept the reality of the problems as they exist.
Ask the patient to list past accomplishments and positive happenings.	There are things in everyone's life that have been successful. Often when self-esteem is low, it is difficult to remember these successes.
Use techniques of role rehearsal.	Assists patient to practice the development of skills to cope with new role as a person who no longer uses or needs drugs to handle life's problems.
Collaborative	
Involve in group therapy.	Group sharing helps encourage verbalization as other members of group are in various stages of abstinence from drugs and can address the patient's concerns/

ACTIONS/INTERVENTIONS

Collaborative

Refer to other resources, such as Narcotics/Alcoholics Anonymous.

Formulate plan to treat other mental illness problems.

Administer antipsychotic medications as necessary.

RATIONALE

denial. The patient can gain new skills, hope, and a sense of family/community from group participation.

One of the oldest and most popular forms of group treatment, which uses a basic strategy known as the Twelve Steps. The patient admits powerlessness over drug and seeks help from a "higher power." Members help one another, and meetings are available at many different times and places in most communities. The philosophy of "one day at a time" helps attain the goal of abstinence.

Patients who seek relief for other mental health problems through drugs will continue to do so once discharged. Both the substance use and the mental health problems need to be treated together to maximize abstinence potential.

Prolonged psychosis following LSD or PCP use can be treated with these drugs as it is probably the result of an underlying functional psychosis that has now emerged. Note: Avoid the use of phenothiazines because they may decrease seizure threshold and cause hypotension in the presence of LSD/PCP.

NURSING DIAGNOSIS:	COPING, INEFFECTIVE FAMILY: COMPROMISED/DISABLING
May be related to:	Personal vulnerability of individual family members; codependency issues
	Situational crises
	Compromised social systems; family disorganization/role changes
	Prolonged disease progression that exhausts supportive capability of family members
	Significant person(s) with chronically unexpressed feelings of guilt, anger, hostility, despair
Possibly evidenced by:	Denial (one of the strongest and most resistant symptoms); lack of acceptance that drinking/drug use is causing the present situation, or belief that *all* problems are due to substance use
	Severely dysfunctional family, e.g., family violence, spouse/child abuse, separation/divorce, children displaying acting-out behaviors
	Financial affairs in disarray; employment difficulties
	Altered social patterns/participation
	SO demonstrating enabling or codependent behaviors, e.g., avoiding and shielding, attempting to control, tak-

867

	ing over responsibilities, rationalizing and accepting, co-operating and collaborating, rescuing and subserving
FAMILY OUTCOMES/ EVALUATION CRITERIA:	**Verbalizes understanding of dynamics of co-dependence and participates in individual and family programs. Identifies ineffective coping behaviors/ consequences. Demonstrates/plans for necessary life-style changes. Takes action to change self-destructive behaviors/alters behavior that contributes to partner's addiction.**

ACTIONS/INTERVENTIONS	RATIONALE
Independent	
Assess family history; explore roles of family members, circumstances involving drug use, strengths, areas for growth.	Determines areas for focus, potential for change.
Explore how the SO has coped with the addict's habit, e.g., denial, repression, rationalization, hurt, loneliness, projection.	Co-dependent also suffers from the same feelings as the patient (e.g., anxiety, self-hatred, helplessness, low self-worth, guilt) and needs help in learning new/ effective coping skills.
Determine understanding of current situation and previous methods of coping with life's problems.	Provides information on which to base present plan of care.
Assess current level of functioning of family members.	Affects individual's ability to cope with situation.
Determine extent of "enabling" behaviors being evidenced by family members, explore with individual/ patient.	"Enabling" is doing for the patient what s/he needs to do for self. People want to be helpful and do not want to feel powerless to help their loved one to stop drinking and change the behavior that is so destructive. However, the substance abuser relies on others to cover up own inability to cope with daily responsibilities.
Provide information about enabling behavior, addictive disease characteristics for both user and non-user co-dependent.	Awareness and knowledge provide opportunity for individuals to begin the process of change.
Provide factual information to patient and family about the effects of addictive behaviors on the family and what to expect after discharge.	Many patients/SO are not aware of the nature of addiction. If patient is using legally obtained drugs, may believe this does not constitute abuse.
Encourage SOs to be aware of their own feelings, look at the situation with perspective and objectivity. They can ask themselves: "Am I being conned? Am I acting out of fear, shame, guilt, or anger? Do I have a need to control?"	When the co-dependent family members become aware of their own actions that perpetuate the addict's problems, they need to decide to change themselves. If they change, the patient can then face the consequences of the patient's own actions and may choose to get well.
Provide support for co-dependent partner(s). Encourage group work.	Families/SOs need support as much as addicts in order to produce change.
Assist the co-dependent partner to become aware that patient's abstinence and drug use is not the partner's responsibility.	Partners need to learn that user's habit may or may not change despite partner's involvement in treatment.
Help the recovering (former user) co-dependent to distinguish between destructive aspects of enabling behavior and genuine motivation to aid the user.	Enabling behavior can be partner's attempts at personal survival.
Note how the co-dependent partner relates to the	Determines enabling style. A parallel exists between

ACTIONS/INTERVENTIONS	RATIONALE

Independent

treatment team/staff.

how partner relates to user and to staff, based on partner's feelings about self and situation.

Assess co-dependent's conflicting feelings about treatment, e.g., may have feelings similar to those of abuser (blend of anger, guilt, fear, exhaustion, embarrassment, loneliness, distrust, grief, and possibly relief).

Useful in establishing co-dependent's need for therapy. Own identity may have been lost, may fear self-disclosure to staff, and may have difficulty giving up the dependent relationship.

Involve SO in discharge referral plans.

Drug abuse is a family illness. Because the family has been so involved in dealing with the substance abuse behavior, they need help adjusting to the new behavior of sobriety/abstinence. Incidence of recovery is almost doubled when the family is treated along with the patient.

Be aware of staff enabling behaviors and feelings about patient and co-dependent partners.

Lack of understanding of enabling and co-dependence can result in nontherapeutic approaches to addicts and their families.

Collaborative

Encourage involvement with self-help associations, Alcoholics/Narcotics Anonymous, Al-Anon, Al-Ateen, and professional family therapy.

Puts patient/family in direct contact with support systems necessary for continued sobriety and to assist with problem resolution.

NURSING DIAGNOSIS:	SEXUAL DYSFUNCTION
May be related to:	**Altered body function: neurologic damage and debilitating effects of drug use (particularly alcohol and opiates)**
Possibly evidenced by:	**Progressive interference with sexual functioning in men and women** **In men: a significant degree of testicular atrophy is noted (testes are smaller and softer than normal); gynecomastia (breast enlargement); impotence/decreased sperm counts** **In women: loss of body hair, thin soft skin, and spider angioma (elevated estrogen); amenorrhea/increase in miscarriages**
PATIENT OUTCOMES/ EVALUATION CRITERIA:	**Verbally acknowledges effects of drug use on sexual functioning/reproduction. Identifies interventions to correct/overcome individual situation.**

ACTIONS/INTERVENTIONS	RATIONALE

Independent

Assess patient's current information and have patient describe problem in own words.

Determines level of knowledge, what patient needs are.

Encourage and accept individual expressions of concern.

Most people find it difficult to talk about this sensitive subject and may not ask directly for information.

ACTIONS/INTERVENTIONS

Independent

Provide education opportunity (e.g., pamphlets, consultation from appropriate persons) for patient to learn effects of drug on sexual functioning.

Provide information about individual's condition.

Provide information about effects of drugs on the reproductive system/fetus (e.g., increased risk of premature birth, brain damage and fetal malformation). Assess drinking/drug history of pregnant patient.

Discuss prognosis for sexual dysfunction, e.g., impotence.

Collaborative

Refer for sexual counseling, if indicated.

Review results of sonogram if pregnant.

RATIONALE

Much of denial and hesitancy to seek treatment may be decreased with sufficient and appropriate information.

Sexual functioning may have been affected by drug (alcohol) intake, physiologic and/or psychologic factors (such as stress). Information will assist patient to understand own situation and identify actions to be taken.

Awareness of the negative effects of alcohol/other drugs on reproduction may motivate patient to stop using drug(s). When patient is pregnant, identification of potential problems aids in planning for future fetal needs/concerns.

In about 50% of cases, impotence is reversed with abstinence from drug(s), in 25% the return to normal functioning is delayed, and approximately 25% remain impotent.

Patient may need additional assistance to resolve more severe problems/situations. Patient may have difficulty adjusting if drug has improved sexual experience (e.g., heroin decreases dyspareunia in women/premature ejaculation in men). Further, the patient may have engaged enjoyably in bizarre erotic and sexual behavior under influence of the stimulant; patient may have found no substitute for the drug, may have driven a partner away, and may have no motivation to adjust to sexual experience without drugs.

Assesses fetal growth and development to identify possibility of fetal alcohol syndrome (FAS) and future needs.

NURSING DIAGNOSIS:	KNOWLEDGE DEFICIT [LEARNING NEED] (SPECIFY)
May be related to:	Lack of information; information misinterpretation
	Cognitive limitations/interference with learning (other mental illness problems/organic brain syndrome); lack of recall
Possibly evidenced by:	Statements of concern; questions/misconceptions
	Inaccurate follow-through of instructions/development of preventable complications
	Continued use in spite of complications/bad trips
PATIENT OUTCOMES/ EVALUATION CRITERIA:	Verbalizes understanding of own condition/disease process, prognosis, and treatment plan. Identifies/initiates necessary lifestyle changes to remain drug-free. Participates in treatment program.

ACTIONS/INTERVENTIONS	RATIONALE

Independent

Be aware of and deal with anxiety of patient and family members.

Anxiety can interfere with ability to hear and assimilate information.

Provide an active role for the patient/SO in the learning process, e.g., discussions, group participation, role-playing.

Learning is enhanced when persons are actively involved.

Provide written and verbal information as indicated. Include list of articles and books related to patient/family needs and encourage reading and discussing what they learn.

Helps patient/SO to make informed choices about future. Bibliotherapy can be a useful addition to other therapy approaches.

Assess patient's knowledge of own situation, e.g., disease, complications, and needed changes in lifestyle.

Assists in planning for long-range changes necessary for maintaining sobriety/drug-free status. Patient may have street knowledge of the drug but be ignorant of medical facts.

Review condition and prognosis/future expectations.

Provides knowledge base on which patient can make informed choices.

Time activities to individual needs.

Facilitates learning as information is more readily assimilated when pacing is considered.

Discuss relationship of drug use to current situation.

Often patient has misperception (denial) of real reason for admission to the medical (psychiatric) setting.

Discuss effects of drug(s) used, e.g., PCP is deposited in body fat and may reactivate (flashbacks) even after long interval of abstinence; alcohol use may result in mental deterioration/liver involvement/damage; cocaine can damage postcapillary vessels, increase platelet aggregation, promoting thomboses and infarction of skin/internal organs, causing localized atrophie blanche or sclerodermatous lesions.

Information will help patient understand possible long-term effects of drug use.

Discuss potential for reemergence of withdrawal symptoms in stimulant abuse as early as 3 months or as late as 9–12 months.

While symptoms of intoxication may have passed, patient may manifest denial, drug hunger, periods of "flare up" wherein there is a delayed reoccurrence of withdrawal symptoms, e.g., anxiety, depression, irritability, sleep disturbance, compulsiveness with food (especially sugars).

Inform patient of effects of Antabuse with alcohol intake and importance of avoiding use of alcohol containing products, e.g., cough syrups or foods/candy.

Interaction of alcohol and Antabuse results in nausea and hypotension, which may produce fatal shock. Individuals on Antabuse are sensitive to alcohol on a continuum with some being able to drink on the drug, and others can have a reaction with only slight exposure, e.g., alcohol-containing foods or products such as aftershave. Reactions appear to be dose-related as well.

Review specific post-care needs; e.g., PCP user should drink cranberry juice and continue use of ascorbic acid; alcohol abuser with liver damage should refrain from drugs/anesthetics/household cleaning products detoxified in the liver.

Promotes individualized care related to specific situation. Cranberry juice and ascorbic acid enhance clearance of PCP from the system. Substances that have the potential for liver damage are more dangerous in the presence of already damaged liver.

Discuss variety of helpful organizations and programs that are available for assistance/referral.

Long-term support is necessary to maintain optimal recovery. Psychosocial needs may require addressing as well as other issues.

Cancer

Cancer is a general term used to describe a disturbance of cellular growth and refers to a group of diseases and not a single disease entity. There are currently over 150 different known types of cancer. Because cancer is a cellular disease, it can arise from any body tissue, with manifestations that are the result of failure to control the proliferation and maturation of cells.

There are four main classifications of cancer according to tissue type: (1) lymphomas (cancers originating in infection-fighting organs); (2) leukemias (cancers originating in blood forming organs); (3) sarcomas (cancers originating in bones, muscle, or connective tissue); and (4) carcinomas (cancers originating in epithelial cells). Within these broad categories, a cancer is classified by histology, stage, and grade.

Through years of observation and documentation, it has been noted that the metastatic behavior of cancers varied according to the primary site of diagnosis. This behavior pattern is known as the "natural history." An example is the metastatic pattern for primary breast cancer: breast–bone–lung–liver–brain. Knowledge of the etiology and natural history of a cancer type is important in planning the patient's care and in evaluation of the patient's progress, prognosis, and physical complaints.

PATIENT ASSESSMENT DATA BASE

Refer to CPs: Radical Neck Surgery: Laryngectomy (Postoperative Care), p. 171; Mastectomy, p. 673; Leukemias, p. 530; and Lymphomas, p. 538 for specific signs and symptoms.

ACTIVITY/REST

May report:

Weakness and/or fatigue.

Changes in rest pattern and usual hours of sleep per night; presence of factors affecting sleep, e.g., pain, anxiety, night sweats.

Limitations of participation in hobbies, exercise.

Occupation or profession with environmental carcinogen exposure, high stress level.

CIRCULATION

May report: Palpitations, chest pain on exertion.

May exhibit: Changes in blood pressure.

EGO INTEGRITY

May report:

Stress factors (financial, job, role changes) and ways of handling stress (e.g., smoking, drinking, delay in seeking treatment, religious/spiritual belief).

Concern about appearance; alopecia, disfiguring lesions, surgery.

Denial of diagnosis, feelings of powerlessness, hopelessness, helplessness, worthlessness, guilt, loss of control, depression.

May exhibit: Denial, withdrawal, anger.

ELIMINATION

May report:

Changes in bowel pattern, e.g., blood in stools, pain with defecation.

Changes in urinary elimination, e.g., pain or burning on urination, hematuria, frequent micturition.

May exhibit: Changes in bowel sounds, abdominal distention.

FOOD/FLUID

May report:

Poor dietary habits (e.g., low-fiber, high-fat, additives, preservatives).

Anorexia, nausea, vomiting.

Food intolerances.

Changes in weight; severe weight loss.

| **May exhibit:** | Changes in skin moisture/turgor; edema. |

NEUROSENSORY

| **May report:** | Dizziness; syncope. |

PAIN/COMFORT

| **May report:** | No pain, or varying degrees, e.g., mild discomfort to severe pain (associated with disease process). |

RESPIRATION

| **May report:** | Smoking (tobacco, marijuana, living with someone who smokes).
Asbestos exposure. |

SAFETY

| **May report:** | Exposure to toxic chemicals, carcinogens.
Excessive/prolonged sun exposure. |
| **May exhibit:** | Fever.
Skin rashes, ulcerations. |

SEXUALITY

| **May report:** | Sexual concerns, e.g., impact on relationship, change in level of satisfaction.
Nulligravida greater than 30 years of age.
Multigravida, multiple sex partners, early sexual activity.
Genital herpes. |

SOCIAL INTERACTION

| **May report:** | Inadequate/weak support system.
Marital history (regarding in-home satisfaction, support or help).
Concerns about role function/responsibility. |

TEACHING/LEARNING

| **May report:** | Family history of cancer, e.g., mother or aunt with breast cancer.
Primary site: of primary disease, date discovered/diagnosed.
Metastatic disease: additional sites involved; if none, natural history of primary will provide important information for looking for metastasis.
Treatment history: previous treatment for cancer—place and treatments given. |
| **Discharge Plan Considerations:** | May require assistance with finances, medications/treatments, wound care/supplies, transportation, food shopping and preparation, self-care, homemaker tasks, provision for child care; changes in living facilities. |

DIAGNOSTIC STUDIES

Test selection depends on history, clinical manifestations, and index of suspicion for a particular cancer.

Scans (e.g., MRI, CT, gallium) and ultrasound: may be done for identification of metastasis, diagnostic purposes, and evaluation of response to treatment.

Biopsy (aspiration, excision, needle, punch): done to differentiate diagnosis and delineate treatment and may be taken from bone marrow, skin, organ, etc. Examples: Bone marrow is done in myeloproliferative diseases for diagnosis; in solid tumors for staging.

Tumor markers: Carcinogenic embryonic antigen (CEA), prostate specific antigen (PSA), alpha-fetoprotein (AFP), human chorionic gonadotropin (HCG), prostatic acid phosphatase (PAP), lactic dehydrogenose (LDH), human lymphocytic surface markers can help in diagnosing cancer but are more useful as prognostic indices and/or therapeutic monitors.

Tissue studies (estrogen and progesterone receptors): done on breast tissue to provide information about whether or not hormonal manipulation would be therapeutic in metastatic disease control.

Screening chemistry tests: e.g., electrolytes (sodium, potassium, calcium); renal tests (BUN/creatinine); liver tests (bilirubin, SGOT/AST, alkaline phosphatase, LDH); bone tests (alkaline phosphatase, calcium).

CBC with differential and platelets: may reveal anemia, changes in red and white blood cells; reduced or increased platelets.

Chest x-ray: screens for primary or metastatic disease of lungs.

NURSING PRIORITIES

1. Support adaptation and independence.
2. Promote comfort.
3. Maintain optimal physiologic functioning.
4. Prevent complications.
5. Provide information about disease process/condition, prognosis, and treatment needs.

DISCHARGE CRITERIA

1. Dealing with current situation realistically.
2. Pain alleviated/controlled.
3. Homeostasis achieved.
4. Complications prevented/minimized.
5. Disease process/condition, prognosis, and therapeutic choices and regimen understood.

NURSING DIAGNOSIS:	**FEAR/ANXIETY (SPECIFY LEVEL)**
May be related to:	**Situational crisis (cancer)**
	Threat to/change in health/socioeconomic status, role functioning, interaction patterns
	Threat of death
	Separation from family (hospitalization, treatments)
	Interpersonal transmission/contagion of feelings
Possibly evidenced by:	**Increased tension, shakiness, apprehension, restlessness**
	Expressed concerns regarding changes in life events
	Feelings of helplessness, hopelessness, inadequacy
	Sympathetic stimulation, somatic complaints
PATIENT OUTCOMES/ EVALUATION CRITERIA:	**Displays appropriate range of feelings and lessened fear. Appears relaxed and reports anxiety is reduced to a manageable level. Demonstrates use of effective coping mechanisms and active participation in treatment regimen.**

ACTIONS/INTERVENTIONS	RATIONALE

Independent

Review patient's/SO's previous experience with cancer. Determine what the doctor has told patient and what conclusion patient has reached.

Assists in identification of fear(s) and misconceptions based on past experience with cancer.

Encourage patient to share thoughts and feelings.

Provides opportunity to examine realistic fears as well as misconceptions about diagnosis.

Provide open environment in which patient feels safe to discuss feelings or to refrain from talking.

Helps patient to feel accepted in present condition without feeling judged and promotes sense of dignity and control.

Maintain frequent contact with patient. Talk with and touch patient as appropriate.

Provides assurance that the patient is not alone or rejected; conveys respect for and acceptance of the person, fostering trust.

Be aware of effects of isolation on patient when required for immunosuppression or radiation implant. Limit use of isolation clothing/masks as possible.

Sensory deprivation may result when sufficient stimulation is not available and may intensify feelings of anxiety/fear.

Assist patient/SO in recognizing and clarifying fears to begin developing coping strategies for dealing with these fears.

Coping skills are often impaired after diagnosis and during early phase of treatment. Support and counseling are often necessary to enable individual to recognize and begin to deal with fear and to realize control/coping strategies available.

Provide accurate, consistent information regarding prognosis. Avoid arguing about patient's perceptions of situation.

Can reduce anxiety and enable patient to make decisions/choices based on realities.

Permit expressions of anger, fear, despair without confrontation. Give information that feelings are normal and are to be appropriately expressed.

Acceptance of feelings allows patient to begin to deal with situation.

Explain the recommended treatment, its purpose and potential side effects. Help patient prepare for treatments.

The goal of cancer treatment is to destroy malignant cells while minimizing damage to normal ones. Treatment may include surgery (curative, preventive, palliative) as well as chemotherapy, radiation (internal, external) or newer/organ specific treatments such as whole-body hyperthermia or immunotherapy.

Explain procedures, providing opportunity for questions and honest answers. Stay with patient during anxiety-producing procedures and consultations.

Accurate information allows patient to deal more effectively with reality of situation, thereby reducing anxiety and fear of the unknown.

Provide primary or consistent care givers whenever possible.

May help reduce anxiety by fostering therapeutic relationship and facilitating continuity of care.

Promote calm, quiet environment.

Facilitates rest, conserves energy and may enhance coping abilities.

Identify stage/degree of grieving patient and SO are currently experiencing. (Refer to ND: Grieving, Anticipatory, following.)

Choice of interventions are dictated by stage of grief, coping behaviors, e.g., anger/withdrawal, denial.

Note ineffective coping, e.g., poor social interactions, helplessness, giving up everyday functions and usual sources of gratification.

Identifies individual problems and provides support for patient/SO in using effective coping skills.

Be alert to signs of denial/depression, e.g., withdrawal, anger, inappropriate remarks. Determine presence of suicidal ideation and assess potential on a scale of 1–10.

Patient may use defense mechanism of denial and express hope that diagnosis is inaccurate. Feelings of guilt, spiritual distress, or physical symptoms, lack of cure may cause the patient to become withdrawn and believe that suicide is a viable alternative.

ACTIONS/INTERVENTIONS

Independent

Encourage and foster patient interaction with support systems.

Provide reliable and consistent information and support for SO.

Include SO as indicated when major decisions are to be made.

RATIONALE

Reduces feelings of isolation. If family support systems are not available, outside sources may be needed immediately, e.g., local cancer support groups.

Allows for better interpersonal interaction and reduction of anxiety and fear.

Ensures a support system for the patient and allows the SO to be involved appropriately.

NURSING DIAGNOSIS:	GRIEVING, ANTICIPATORY
May be related to:	**Anticipated loss of physiologic well-being (e.g., loss of body part; change in body function); change in lifestyle**
	Perceived potential death of patient
Possibly evidenced by:	**Changes in eating habits, alterations in sleep patterns, activity levels, libido, and communication patterns**
	Denial of potential loss, choked feelings, anger
PATIENT OUTCOMES/ EVALUATION CRITERIA:	**Identifies and expresses feelings appropriately continuing normal life activities, looking toward/planning for the future, one day at a time. Verbalizes understanding of the dying process and feelings of being supported in grief work.**

ACTIONS/INTERVENTIONS

Independent

Expect initial shock and disbelief following diagnosis of cancer and/or traumatizing procedures (e.g., disfiguring surgery, colostomy, amputation).

Assess patient/SO for stage of grieving currently being experienced. Explain process as appropriate.

Provide open, nonjudgmental environment. Use therapeutic communication skills of Active-Listening, acknowledgement, etc.

Encourage verbalization of thoughts/concerns and accept expressions of sadness, anger, rejection. Acknowledge normality of these feelings.

Be aware of mood swings, hostility, and other acting-out behavior. Set limits on inappropriate behavior.

Visit frequently and provide physical contact as appropriate/desired. Move patient closer to nurses station if frightened; leave door open if comfortable for patient.

RATIONALE

Few patients are fully prepared for reality of the changes that can occur.

Identification of stages of grieving provides information about the normality of feelings/reactions and can help patient deal more effectively with them.

Promotes and encourages realistic dialogue about feelings and concerns.

Patient may feel supported in expression of feelings by the understanding that deep and often conflicting emotions are normal and experienced by others in this difficult situation.

Indicators of ineffective coping and need for additional interventions. Preventing destructive actions enables patient to maintain control and sense of self-esteem.

Helps reduce feelings of isolation and abandonment.

ACTIONS/INTERVENTIONS	RATIONALE

Independent

Reinforce teaching regarding disease process and treatments and provide information as requested/appropriate about dying. Be honest; do not give false hope while providing emotional support.

Review past life experiences, role changes, and coping skills.

Identify positive aspects of the situation.

Discuss ways patient/SO can plan together for the future. Encourage setting of realistic goals.

Assist patient/SO to identify strengths in self/situation and support systems.

Encourage participation in care and treatment decisions.

Note evidence of conflict, expressions of anger and statements of despair, guilt, hopelessness, "nothing to live for."

Assess way that patient/SO understand and respond to death, e.g., cultural expectations, learned behaviors, past experience with death (close family members/friends), beliefs about life after death, faith in higher being (God).

Provide open environment for discussion with patient/SO (when appropriate) about desires/plans pertaining to death; e.g., making will, burial arrangements, tissue donation, death benefits, insurance, time for family gatherings.

Be aware of own feelings about cancer, impending death. Accept whatever methods patient/SO have chosen to help each other through process.

Collaborative

Refer to appropriate counselor as needed (e.g., psychiatric clinical nurse specialist, social worker, clergyman).

Refer to community hospice program, if appropriate, or VNA, home health agency service as needed.

RATIONALE

Patient/SO benefit from factual information. Individuals may ask direct questions about death, and honest answers promote trust and provide reassurance that correct information will be given.

Opportunity to identify skills that may help individuals cope with grief of current situation more effectively.

Possibility of remission and slow progression of disease and/or new therapies can offer hope for the future.

Having a part in problem-solving/planning can provide a sense of control over anticipated events.

Recognizing these resources provides opportunity to work through feelings of grief.

Allows patient to retain some control over life.

Interpersonal conflicts/angry behavior may be patient's ways of expressing/dealing with feelings of despair/spiritual distress and could be indicative of suicidal ideation.

These factors affect how each individual deals with the possibility of death and influences how they may respond and interact.

If the patient/SO are mutually aware of impending death, they may more easily deal with unfinished business or desired activities.

Care giver's anxiety and unwillingness to accept reality of possibility of own death may block ability to be helpful to the patient/SO, necessitating enlisting the aid of others to provide needed support.

Can help to alleviate distress or palliate feelings of grief to facilitate coping and foster growth.

Provides support in meeting physical and emotional needs of patient/SO, and can supplement the care family and friends are able to give.

NURSING DIAGNOSIS:	SELF-CONCEPT, DISTURBANCE IN: (SPECIFY)
May be related to:	**Biophysical: disfiguring surgery, chemotherapy or radiotherapy side effects, e.g., loss of hair, nausea and vomiting, weight loss, anorexia, impotence, sterility, overwhelming fatigue, uncontrolled pain**

	Psychosocial: threat of death; feelings of lack of control and doubt regarding acceptance by others; fear and anxiety
Possibly evidenced by:	**Verbalization of change in lifestyle; fear of rejection/reaction of others; negative feelings about body; feelings of helplessness, hopelessness, powerlessness**
	Preoccupation with change or loss
	Not taking responsibility for self-care, lack of follow-through
	Change in self/other's perception of role
PATIENT OUTCOMES/ EVALUATION CRITERIA:	**Verbalizes understanding of body changes, acceptance of self in situation. Begins to develop coping mechanisms to deal effectively with problems. Demonstrates adaptation to changes/events that have occurred as evidenced by setting of realistic goals and active participation in work/play/personal relationships as appropriate.**

ACTIONS/INTERVENTIONS	RATIONALE
Independent	
Discuss with patient/SO how the diagnosis and treatment are affecting the patient's personal life, home and work activities.	Aids in defining concerns to begin problem-solving process.
Review anticipated side effects associated with a particular treatment, including possible effects on sexual activity and sense of attractiveness/desirability, e.g., alopecia, disfiguring surgery. Tell patient that not all side effects occur.	Anticipatory guidance can help patient/SO begin the process of adaptation to new state and to prepare for some side effects, e.g., buy a wig before radiation, schedule time off from work as indicated. (Refer to ND: Sexuality Patterns, Altered [Potential], p. 889.)
Encourage discussion of/problem-solve concerns about effects of cancer/treatments on role as homemaker, wage earner, parent, and so forth.	May help reduce problems which interfere with acceptance of treatment or stimulate progression of disease.
Acknowledge difficulties patient may be experiencing. Give information that counseling is often necessary and important in the adaptation process.	Validates reality of patient's feelings and gives permission to take whatever measures are necessary to cope with what is happening.
Evaluate support structures available to and used by patient/SO.	Helps with planning for care while hospitalized as well as after discharge.
Provide emotional support for patient/SO during diagnostic tests and treatment phase.	Although some patients adapt/adjust to cancer effects or side effects of therapy, many need additional support during this period.
Use touch during interactions, if acceptable to patient, and maintain eye contact.	Affirmation of individuality and acceptance are important in reducing patient's feelings of insecurity and self-doubt.
Collaborative	
Refer patient/SO to supportive group programs (e.g., CanSurmount, I Can Cope, Reach to Recovery, Encore).	Group support is usually very beneficial for both patient/SO, providing contact with other patients with cancer at various levels of treatment and/or recovery.
Refer to professional counseling if indicated.	May be necessary to regain and maintain a positive psychosocial structure if patient/SO suport systems are deteriorating.

878

NURSING DIAGNOSIS:	COMFORT, ALTERED: PAIN, ACUTE
May be related to:	The disease process (compression of nerve tissue, infiltration of nerves or their vascular supply, obstruction of a nerve pathway, inflammation)
Possibly evidenced by:	Complaints of pain
	Self-focusing/narrowed focus
	Alteration in muscle tone; facial mask of pain
	Distraction/guarding behaviors
	Autonomic responses, restlessness
PATIENT OUTCOMES/ EVALUATION CRITERIA:	Reports maximal pain relief/control with minimal interference with ADLs. Follows prescribed pharmacologic regimen. Demonstrates use of relaxation skills and diversional activities as indicated for individual situation.

ACTIONS/INTERVENTIONS	RATIONALE

Independent

Determine pain history, e.g., location of pain, frequency, duration and intensity (1–10 scale), and relief measures used.	Information provides baseline data to evaluate need for/effectiveness of interventions. Note: The pain experience is an individualized one composed of both neurologic and emotional responses.
Provide routine comfort measures (e.g., repositioning, backrub) and diversional activities (e.g., music, television).	Promotes relaxation and helps refocus attention.
Encourage use of stress management skills (e.g., relaxation techniques, visualization, guided imagery), laughter, music, and Therapeutic Touch.	Enables patient to participate actively and enhances sense of control.
Evaluate pain relief/control. Adjust medication regimen as necessary.	Goal is maximum pain control with minimum interference with ADL.

Collaborative

Develop pain management plan with the patient and physician.	An organized plan improves chance for pain control. Particularly with chronic pain, patient/SO must be active participants in home management.
Administer analgesics as indicated, e.g.: Brompton's cocktail, morphine, methadone, or specific IV narcotic mixtures.	Pain is a frequent complication of cancer, although individual responses differ. As changes in the disease/treatment occur, adjustments in dosage and delivery will be needed. Note: Addiction to or dependency on drug is not a concern.
Provide/instruct in use of PCA as appropriate.	Patient-controlled analgesia provides for timely drug administration, preventing fluctuations in intensity of pain, often at lower total dosage than would be given by conventional methods.
Prepare for/assist with procedures, e.g., nerve block, cordotomy, commissural myelotomy.	May be used in severe/intractable pain unresponsive to other measures.

879

NURSING DIAGNOSIS:	NUTRITION, ALTERED: LESS THAN BODY REQUIRE-MENTS
May be related to:	Hypermetabolic state associated with cancer
	Consequences of chemotherapy, radiation, surgery, e.g., anorexia, gastric irritation, taste distortions, nausea
	Emotional distress, fatigue, poorly controlled pain
Possibly evidenced by:	Reported inadequate food intake, altered taste sensation, loss of interest in food, perceived/actual inability to ingest food
	Body weight 20% or more under ideal for height and frame, decreased subcutaneous fat/muscle mass
	Sore, inflamed buccal cavity
	Diarrhea and/or constipation, abdominal cramping
PATIENT OUTCOMES/ EVALUATION CRITERIA:	Demonstrates stable weight (or progressive weight gain toward goal) with normalization of laboratory values and free of signs of malnutrition. Verbalizes understanding of individual interferences to adequate intake. Participates in specific interventions to stimulate appetite/increase dietary intake.

ACTIONS/INTERVENTIONS

Independent

Monitor daily food intake; keep food diary as indicated.

Measure height, weight and tricep skinfold thickness. Ascertain amount of recent weight loss. Weigh daily or as indicated.

Assess for pallor, delayed wound healing, enlarged parotid glands.

Encourage patient to eat high-calorie nutrient-rich diet, with adequate fluid intake. Encourage use of supplements and frequent/smaller meals spaced throughout the day.

Adjust diet prior to and immediately after treatment, e.g., clear, cool liquids, light/bland foods, dry crackers, toast, carbonated drinks. Give liquids 1 hour before or 1 hour after meals.

Control environmental factors (e.g., strong/noxious odors or noise). Avoid overly sweet, fatty, or spicy foods.

RATIONALE

Identifies nutritional needs.

If these measurements fall below minimum standards, patient's chief source of stored energy (fat tissue) is depleted.

Helps in identification of protein-calorie malnutrition, especially when weight and tricep skinfold measurement are below normal.

Metabolic tissue needs are increased as well as fluids (to eliminate waste products). Supplements can play an important role in maintaining adequate caloric and protein intake.

The effectiveness of diet adjustment is very individualized in relief of posttherapy nausea. Patients must experiment to find best solution/combination.

Can trigger nausea and vomiting response.

ACTIONS/INTERVENTIONS	RATIONALE

Independent

Create pleasant dining atmosphere; share meals with family/friends.

Encourage use of relaxation techniques, visualization, guided imagery, moderate exercise before meals.

Identify the patient with anticipatory nausea and vomiting.

Encourage open communication regarding anorexia problem.

Administer antiemetic on a regular schedule before/during and after administration of antineoplastic agent as appropriate.

Evaluate effectiveness of antiemetic.

Hematest stools, gastric secretions.

Collaborative

Review laboratory studies as indicated, e.g., total lymphocyte count, serum transferrin, and albumin.

Administer medications as indicated:

Phenothiazines, e.g., prochlorperazine (Compazine), thiethylperazine (Torecan); antihistamines, e.g., diphenhydramine (Benadryl); corticosteroids, e.g., dexamethasone (Decadron); cannabinoids, e.g., 9-tetrahydrocannabinol; benzodiazepines, e.g., diazepam (Valium);

Vitamins, especially A, D, E, and B_6;

Antacids.

Refer to dietician/nutritional support team.

Insert/maintain NG/feeding tube for enteric feedings, or central line for parenteral hyperalimentation if indicated.

Makes mealtime more enjoyable which may enhance intake.

May prevent onset or reduce severity of nausea, decrease anorexia and enable patient to increase oral intake.

Psychogenic nausea/vomiting occurring before chemotherapy begins generally does not respond to antiemetic drugs. Change of treatment environment or patient routine on treatment day may be effective.

Often a source of emotional distress, especially for SO who wants to feed patient frequently. When patient refuses, SO may feel rejected/frustrated.

Nausea/vomiting are frequently the most disabling and psychologically stressful side effects of chemotherapy.

Individuals respond differently to all medications. First-line antiemetics may not work, requiring alteration in or combination drug therapy.

Certain therapies (e.g., antimetabolites) inhibit renewal of epitheleal cells lining the gastrointestinal tract, which may cause changes ranging from mild erythema to severe ulceration with bleeding.

Helps identify the degree of biochemical imbalance/malnutrition and influences choice of dietary interventions.

Most antiemetics act to interfere with stimulation of true vomiting center (TVC) and chemoreceptor trigger zone (CTZ) agents also act peripherally to inhibit reverse peristalsis. Note: Combination therapy (e.g., Torecan with Decadron or Valium) is often more effective than single agents.

Prevents deficit related to decreased absorption of fat-soluble vitamins. Deficiency of B_6 can contribute to/exacerbate depression, irritability.

Minimizes gastric irritation and reduces risk of mucosal ulceration.

Provides for specific dietary plan to meet individual needs and reduce problems associated with protein-calorie malnutrition and micronutrient deficiencies.

When oral feeding is not sufficient to correct patient's dietary deficits, tube feeding or TPN may be needed. In the presence of severe malnutrition (e.g., loss of 7% body weight in two months, or patient has been NPO for 5 days and is unlikely to be able to eat for another week), aggressive therapy is necessary to meet nutritional needs. (Refer to CP: Total Nutritional Support, p. 894.)

```
┌──────────────────────────────────────────────────────────────────────────┐
│  NURSING DIAGNOSIS:              FLUID VOLUME DEFICIT, POTENTIAL           │
│                                                                            │
│     May be related to:           Excessive losses through normal (e.g.,    │
│                                  vomiting, diar- rhea) and/or abnormal      │
│                                  routes (e.g., indwelling tubes, wounds)    │
│                                                                            │
│                                  Hypermetabolic state                      │
│                                                                            │
│                                  Impaired intake of fluids                 │
│                                                                            │
│     Possibly evidenced by:       [Not applicable; presence of signs        │
│                                  and/or symptoms es- tablishes an actual    │
│                                  diagnosis.]                               │
│                                                                            │
│  PATIENT OUTCOMES/              Displays adequate fluid balance as         │
│  EVALUATION CRITERIA:           evidenced by stable vital signs, moist     │
│                                  mucous membranes, good skin turgor,        │
│                                  prompt capillary refill, and individually  │
│                                  adequate uri- nary output.                │
└──────────────────────────────────────────────────────────────────────────┘
```

ACTIONS/INTERVENTIONS

Independent

Monitor intake/output and specific gravity; include all output sources, e.g., emesis, diarrhea, draining wounds. Calculate 24-hour balance.

Weigh as indicated.

Monitor vital signs. Evaluate peripheral pulses, capillary refill.

Assess skin turgor and moisture of mucous membranes. Note complaints of thirst.

Encourage increased fluid intake to 3000 ml/day as individually appropriate/tolerated.

Observe for bleeding tendencies, e.g., oozing from mucous membranes, puncture sites; presence of ecchymosis or petechiae.

Minimize venipunctures (e.g., combine IV starts with blood draws).

Avoid trauma and apply pressure to puncture sites.

Collaborative

Provide IV fluids as indicated.

Administer antiemetic therapy. (Refer to ND: Nutrition, Altered: Less Than Body Requirements, p. 880.)

Monitor laboratory studies, e.g., CBC, electrolytes, serum albumin.

RATIONALE

Continued negative fluid balance, decreasing renal output/concentration of urine suggests developing dehydration and need for increased fluid replacement.

Sensitive measurement of fluctuations in fluid balance.

Reflects adequacy of circulating volume.

Indirect indicators of hydration status/degree of deficit.

Assists in maintenance of fluid requirements and reduces risk of harmful side effects, e.g., hemorrhagic cystitis in patient receiving Cytoxan.

Early identification of problems (which may occur as a result of cancer, and/or therapies) allows for prompt intervention.

Eliminates potential route of infection and hemorrhage.

Reduces potential for bleeding/hematoma formation.

Given for general hydration as well as to dilute antineoplastic drugs and reduce adverse side effects, e.g., nausea, vomiting, or nephrotoxicity.

Alleviation of nausea/vomiting decreases gastric losses and allows for increased oral intake.

Provides information about level of hydration and corresponding deficits. Note: Malnutrition and effects of decreased albumin levels potentiates fluid shifts/edema formation.

ACTIONS/INTERVENTIONS

Collaborative

Administer transfusions as indicated, e.g.:

RBCs;

Platelets.

Avoid use of aspirin, gastric irritants or platelet inhibitors.

RATIONALE

May be needed to restore blood count and prevent manifestations of anemia often present in cancer patients, e.g., tachycardia, tachypnea, dizziness, and weakness.

Thrombocytopenia (which may occur as a side effect of chemotherapy, radiation, or cancer process) increases the risk of bleeding from mucous membranes and other body sites. Spontaneous bleeding generally occurs with platelets below 20,000.

Potentiates risk of bleeding.

NURSING DIAGNOSIS:	FATIGUE
May be related to:	Decreased metabolic energy production, increased energy requirements (hypermetabolic state)
	Overwhelming psychologic/emotional demands
	Altered body chemistry: side effects of medications, chemotherapy
Possibly evidenced by:	Unremitting/overwhelming lack of energy, inability to maintain usual routines, decreased performance
	Impaired ability to concentrate, lethargy/listlessness
	Disinterest in surroundings
PATIENT OUTCOMES/ EVALUATION CRITERIA:	Reports improved sense of energy. Performs ADLs and participates in desired activities at level of ability.

ACTIONS/INTERVENTIONS

Independent

Plan care to allow for rest periods. Schedule activities for periods when patient has most energy. Involve patient/SO in schedule planning.

Establish realistic activity goals with patient.

Assist with self-care needs when indicated; keep bed in low position, pathways clear of furniture; assist with ambulation.

Encourage patient to do whatever possible, e.g., self-bath, sitting up in chair, walking. Increase activity level as able.

RATIONALE

Frequent rest periods are needed to restore/conserve energy. Planning will allow patient to be active during times when energy level is higher, which may restore a feeling of well-being and a sense of control.

Provides for a sense of control and feelings of accomplishment.

Weakness may make activities of daily living difficult to complete or place the patient at risk for injury during activities.

Enhances strength/stamina and enables patient to become more active without undue fatigue.

ACTIONS/INTERVENTIONS

Independent

Monitor physiologic response to activity, e.g., changes in blood pressure, or heart/respiratory rate.

Encourage nutritional intake. (Refer to ND: Nutrition, Altered: Less Than Body Requirements, p. 880.)

Collaborative

Provide supplemental oxygen as indicated.

Refer to physical/occupational therapy.

RATIONALE

Tolerance varies greatly depending on the stage of the disease process, nutrition state, fluid balance, and reaction to therapeutic regimen.

Adequate intake/utilization of nutrients is necessary to meet energy needs for activity.

Presence of anemia/hypoxemia reduces oxygen available for cellular uptake and contributes to fatigue.

Programmed daily exercises and activities help patient to maintain/increase strength and muscle tone, enhance sense of well-being. Use of adaptive devices may help conserve energy.

NURSING DIAGNOSIS:	INFECTION, POTENTIAL FOR
May be related to:	**Inadequate secondary defenses and immunosuppression, e.g., bone marrow suppression (dose-limiting side effect of both chemotherapy and radiation)**
	Malnutrition, chronic disease process
	Invasive procedures
Possibly evidenced by:	**[Not applicable; presence of signs and symptoms establishes an *actual* diagnosis.]**
PATIENT OUTCOMES/ EVALUATION CRITERIA:	**Identifies and participates in interventions to prevent/ reduce risk of infection. Remains afebrile and achieves timely healing as appropriate.**

ACTIONS/INTERVENTIONS

Independent

Promote good handwashing procedures by staff and visitors. Screen/limit visitors who may have infections. Place in reverse isolation as indicated.

Emphasize personal hygiene.

Monitor temperature.

Assess all systems (e.g., skin, respiratory, genitourinary) for signs/symptoms of infection on a continual basis.

RATIONALE

Protects patient from sources of infection, such as visitors and staff who may have URI.

Limits potential sources of infection and/or secondary overgrowth.

Temperature elevation may occur (if not masked by corticosteroids or antiinflammatory drugs) because of various factors, e.g., chemotherapy side effects, response of disease process as well as infection. Early identification of infectious process enables appropriate therapy to be started promptly.

Early recognition and intervention may prevent progression to more serious situation/sepsis.

ACTIONS/INTERVENTIONS	RATIONALE

Independent

Reposition frequently; keep linens dry and wrinkle-free.

Reduces pressure and irritation to tissues and may prevent skin breakdown (potential site for bacterial growth).

Promote adequate rest/exercise periods.

Limits fatigue, yet encourages sufficient movement to prevent stasis complications, e.g., pneumonia, decubitus, and thrombus formation.

Collaborative

Monitor CBC with differential WBC and granulocyte count and platelets as indicated.

Bone marrow activity may be inhibited by effects of chemotherapy, the disease state, or radiation therapy. Monitoring status of myelosuppression is important, for preventing further complications (e.g., infection, anemia or hemorrhage) and scheduling drug delivery. Note: The nadir (point of lowest drop in blood count) is usually seen 7–10 days after administration of chemotherapy.

Obtain cultures as indicated.

Identifies causative organism(s) and appropriate therapy.

Administer medications as indicated, e.g.:

    Antibiotics;

May be used to treat identified infection or given prophylactically in immunocompromised patient.

    Steroids.

May improve clinical picture.

Transfuse granulocytes as indicated.

May be given when WBC remains suppressed. Severe or sustained granulocytopenia may be determinant in home care versus hospital care and enhances risk of sepsis, which could be life-threatening.

NURSING DIAGNOSIS:	ORAL MUCOUS MEMBRANE, ALTERED [POTENTIAL]
May be related to:	**Side effect of some chemotherapeutic agents (e.g., antimetabolites) and head/neck radiation**
Possibly evidenced by:	**[Not applicable; presence of signs and symptoms establishes an *actual* diagnosis.]**
PATIENT OUTCOMES/ EVALUATION CRITERIA:	**Displays intact mucous membranes, which are pink, moist, and free of inflammation/ulcerations. Verbalizes understanding of causative factors. Demonstrates techniques to maintain/restore integrity of oral mucosa.**

ACTIONS/INTERVENTIONS	RATIONALE

Independent

Assess dental health and oral hygiene on admission.

Identifies prophylactic treatment that may be needed prior to initiation of chemotherapy or radiation and provides baseline data in current oral hygiene care.

Discuss with patient areas needing improvement and demonstrate methods for good oral care.

Good care is critical during treatment to control stomatitis complications.

ACTIONS/INTERVENTIONS	RATIONALE
Independent	
Initiate oral hygiene program to include:	
Avoidance of commercial mouthwashes, lemon-glycerine swabs;	Products containing alcohol or phenol may exacerbate mucous membrane dryness/irritation.
Use of mouthwash made from warm saline, dilute solution of hydrogen pyroxide or baking soda and water;	May be soothing to the membranes.
Brush with soft toothbrush or toothette;	Prevents trauma to delicate/fragile tissues.
Floss gently or use WaterPik cautiously;	Removes food particles that can promote bacterial growth.
Keep lips moist with Vaseline, K-Y Jelly, Chapstick, etc.;	Promotes comfort and prevents drying/cracking of tissues.
Encourage use of mints/hard candy or artificial saliva (Ora-lub, Salivert) if indicated.	Stimulates/provides moisture to maintain integrity of mucous membranes, especially in presence of dehydration/reduced saliva production.
Assess oral cavity daily, noting changes in mucous membrane integrity (e.g., dry, reddened). Ascertain whether patient notices changes in voice quality, ability to swallow, development of thick/viscous saliva.	The range of response extends from mild erythema to severe ulceration, which can be very painful, inhibit oral intake, and be potentially life-threatening. Early identification enables prompt treatment.
Instruct regarding dietary changes: e.g., avoid hot or spicy foods, acidic juices; suggest use of straw; ingestion of soft or blenderized foods, Popsicles, and ice cream as tolerated.	Severe stomatitis may interfere with nutritional and fluid intake leading to negative nitrogen balance or dehydration. Dietary modifications may make foods easier to swallow and feel soothing.
Encourage fluid intake as individually tolerated.	Adequate hydration helps keep mucous membranes moist, preventing drying/cracking.
Discuss limitation of smoking and alcohol intake.	May cause further irritation and dryness of mucous membranes. Note: May need to compromise if these activities are important to emotional status.
Monitor for and explain to patient signs of oral superinfection (e.g., thrush).	Early recognition ensures prompt initiation of treatment.
Collaborative	
Refer to dentist before initiating chemotherapy or head/neck radiation.	Prophylactic examination and repair work prior to therapy reduces risk of infection.
Administer medications as indicated, e.g.:	
Analgesics, topical xylocaine jelly;	Aggressive analgesia program may be required to relieve intense pain.
Antimicrobial mouthwash preparation, e.g., nystatin (Mycostatin).	May be needed to treat/prevent secondary oral infections.

NURSING DIAGNOSIS:	**SKIN/TISSUE INTEGRITY, IMPAIRED: POTENTIAL**
May be related to:	**Effects of radiation and chemotherapy**
	Immunologic deficit
	Altered nutritional state, anemia

Possibly evidenced by:	**[Not applicable; presence of signs and symptoms establishes an *actual* diagnosis.]**
PATIENT OUTCOMES/ EVALUATION CRITERIA:	**Identifies interventions appropriate for specific condition. Participates in techniques to prevent complications/promote healing as appropriate.**

ACTIONS/INTERVENTIONS	RATIONALE
Independent	
Assess skin frequently for side effects of cancer therapy; note breakdown/delayed wound healing. Stress importance of reporting open areas to care giver.	A reddening and/or tanning effect (radiation reaction) may develop within the field of radiation. Dry desquamation (dryness and pruritis), moist desquamation (blistering), ulceration, hair loss, loss of dermis, and sweat glands may also be noted. In addition, skin reactions (e.g., allergic rashes, hyperpigmentation, pruritis, and alopecia) may occur with some chemotherapy agents.
Bathe with lukewarm water and mild soap.	Maintains cleanliness without irritating the skin.
Encourage patient to avoid scratching and to pat skin dry instead of rubbing.	Helps prevent skin friction/trauma.
Turn/reposition frequently.	Promotes circulation and prevents undue pressure on skin/tissues.
Advise patient to avoid any skin creams, ointments, and powders unless physician approves.	May actually increase irritation/reaction.
Review skin care protocol for patient receiving radiation therapy:	Designed to minimize trauma to area of radiation therapy.
Avoid rubbing or use of soap, lotions, or deodorants on area; avoid applying heat or attempting to wash off marks/tattoos placed on skin to identify area of irradiation;	Can potentiate or otherwise interfere with radiation delivery.
Recommend wearing soft, loose clothing next to area; have patient avoid wearing bra if it creates pressure;	Skin is very sensitive during treatment, and all irritation should be avoided to prevent dermal injury.
Apply cornstarch to area as needed, and Eucerin (or other recommended cream) to area twice daily after radiation is completed;	Helps to control dampness or pruritis. Maintenance care is required until skin tissues have regenerated and are back to normal.
Review use of sunscreen/block.	Protects skin from ultraviolet rays and reduces risk of recall reactions.
Review skin care protocol for patient receiving chemotherapy, e.g.:	
Ascertain that IV is infusing well, dilute anticancer drug per protocol.	Reduces risk of tissue irritation/injury.
Instruct patient to notify care giver promptly of discomfort at IV insertion site.	Development of irritation indicates need for alteration of rate/dilution of chemotherapy and/or change of IV site to prevent more serious reaction.
Assess skin/IV site and vein for erythema, edema, tenderness; weltlike patches, itching/burning; or swelling, burning, soreness, blisters progressing to ulceration/tissue necrosis.	Presence of phlebitis, vein flare (localized allergic reaction) or extravasation requires immediate discontinuation of antineoplastic agent and medical intervention.

887

ACTIONS/INTERVENTIONS	RATIONALE

Independent

Wash skin immediately with soap and water if anti-neoplastic agents are spilled on unprotected skin (patient or care giver).

Dilutes drug to reduce risk of skin irritation/burn.

Advise patients receiving 5FU and methotrexate to avoid sun exposure. Withhold methotrexate if sunburn present.

Sun can cause exacerbation of burn spotting (a side effect of 5FU) or can cause a red "flash" area with methotrexate, which can exacerbate drug's effect.

Review expected dermatologic side effects seen with chemotherapy, e.g., rash, hyperpigmentation, and peeling of palms with 5FU.

Anticipatory guidance helps decrease concern if side effects do occur.

Inform patient that if alopecia occurs, hair could grow back after completion of chemotherapy, but may not grow back after radiation therapy.

Anticipatory guidance may help adjustment to/preparation for baldness. Men are often as sensitive to hair loss as women. Radiation's effect on hair follicles may be permanent, depending on rad dosage.

Collaborative

Administer appropriate antidote if extravasation should occur, e.g.:

Reduces local tissue damage.

Topical DMSO;

May be useful for mitomycin, doxorubicin (Adriamycin)/daunorubicin. Note: Injection of Benadryl may relieve symptoms of vein flare.

Hyaluronidase (Wydase);

Injected subcutaneously for vincristine.

Sodium bicarbonate;

Injected IV and/or into surrounding tissues for Bisantrene.

Thiosulfate.

Injected subcutaneously for nitrogen mustard.

Apply topical ointment, e.g., silver sulfadiazine (Silvadene) as appropriate.

May be used to prevent infection/facilitate healing if chemical burn (extravasation) occurs.

Apply ice pack/warm compresses per protocol.

Controversial intervention is dependent on type of agent used to restrict blood flow, keeping drug localized, or to enhance dispersion of antidote.

NURSING DIAGNOSIS:	**BOWEL ELIMINATION, ALTERED: (SPECIFY) [POTENTIAL]**
May be related to:	**Irritation of the gastrointestinal mucosa from either chemotherapy or radiation therapy; malabsorption of fat**
	Hormone-secreting tumor, carcinoma of colon
	Poor fluid intake, low bulk diet, lack of exercise, use of opiates/narcotics
Possibly evidenced by:	**[Not applicable; presence of signs and symptoms establishes an *actual* diagnosis.]**
PATIENT OUTCOMES/ EVALUATION CRITERIA:	**Maintains usual bowel consistency/pattern. Verbalizes understanding of factors and appropriate interventions/ solutions related to individual situation.**

ACTIONS/INTERVENTIONS	RATIONALE

Independent

Ascertain usual elimination habits.

Data required as baseline for future evaluation.

Assess bowel sounds and monitor/record bowel movements including frequency, consistency (particularly during first 3–5 days of Vinca alkaloid therapy).

Defines problem, i.e., diarrhea, constipation. Note: Constipation is one of the earliest manifestations of neurotoxicity.

Monitor I & O and weight.

Dehydration, weight loss, and electrolyte imbalance are complications of diarrhea. Inadequate fluid intake may potentiate constipation.

Encourage adequate fluid intake (e.g., 2 qt/24 hr), increased fiber in diet; exercise.

May reduce potential for constipation by improving stool consistency and stimulating peristalsis; can prevent dehydration (diarrhea).

Provide small, frequent meals of foods low in residue (if not contraindicated), maintaining needed protein and carbohydrates (e.g., eggs, cooked cereal, bland cooked vegetables).

Reduces gastric irritation. Use of low-fiber foods can decrease irritability and provide bowel rest when diarrhea present.

Adjust diet as appropriate: avoid foods high in fat (e.g., butter, fried foods, nuts); foods with high-fiber content; those known to cause diarrhea or gas (e.g., cabbage, baked beans, chili); food/fluids high in caffeine; or extremely hot/cold food/fluids.

GI stimulants which may increase gastric motility/frequency of stools.

Check for impaction if patient has not had BM in 3 days or abdominal distention, cramping, headache are present.

Further interventions/alternative bowel care may be needed.

Collaborative

Monitor laboratory studies as indicated, e.g., electrolytes.

Electrolyte imbalances may be the result of/contribute to altered GI function.

Administer IV fluids;

Prevents dehydration, dilutes chemotherapy agents to diminish side effects.

Antidiarrheal agents;

May be indicated in severe diarrhea.

Stool softeners, laxatives, enemas as indicated.

Prophylactic use may prevent further complications in some patients (e.g., those who will receive Vinca alkaloid, have poor bowel pattern prior to treatment, or have decreased motility).

NURSING DIAGNOSIS:	SEXUALITY PATTERNS, ALTERED [POTENTIAL]
May be related to:	**Knowledge/skill deficit about alternative responses to health-related transitions, altered body function/structure, illness and medical treatment**
	Overwhelming fatigue
	Fear and anxiety
	Lack of privacy/SO
Possibly evidenced by:	**[Not applicable; presence of signs and symptoms establishes an *actual* diagnosis.]**

ACTIONS/INTERVENTIONS	RATIONALE

Independent

Discuss with patient/SO the nature of sexuality and re- actions when it is altered or threatened. Provide infor- mation about normality of these problems and that many people find it helpful to seek assistance with adaptation process.	Provides legitimacy to the problem. Sexuality encom- passes the way men and women view themselves as individuals and how they relate between and among themselves in every area of life.
Advise patient of side effects of prescribed cancer treatment that are known to affect sexuality.	Anticipatory guidance can help patient and SO begin the process of adaptation to new state.
Provide private time for hospitalized patient. Knock on door and receive permission from patient/SO before entering.	Sexuality needs do not end because the patient is hos- pitalized. Intimacy needs continue and an open and accepting attitude for the expression of those needs is essential.

NURSING DIAGNOSIS:	FAMILY PROCESS, ALTERED [POTENTIAL]
May be related to:	Situational/transitional crises; long-term illness, change in roles/economic status
	Developmental: anticipated loss of a family member
Possibly evidenced by:	[Not applicable; presence of signs and symptoms estab- lishes an *actual* diagnosis.]
FAMILY OUTCOMES/ EVALUATION CRITERIA:	Expresses feelings freely. Demonstrates individual in- volvement in problem-solving process directed at appro- priate solutions for the situation. Encourages and al- lows member who is ill to handle situation in own way.

ACTIONS/INTERVENTIONS	RATIONALE

Independent

Note components of family, presence of extended family and others, e.g., friends/neighbors.	Helps to know who is available to assist with care/ provide respite, provide support, and be available as needed.
Identify patterns of communication in family and pat- terns of interaction between family members.	Provides information about effectiveness of communi- cation and identifies problems that may interfere with family's ability to assist patient and adjust positively to diagnosis/treatment of cancer.
Assess role expectations of family members and en- courage discussion about them.	Each person may see the situation in own individual manner, and clear identification and sharing of these expectations promotes understanding.
Assess energy direction, e.g., are efforts at resolution/ problem-solving purposeful or scattered?	Provides clues about interventions that may be appro- priate to assist patient and family in directing energies in a more effective manner.

890

ACTIONS/INTERVENTIONS	RATIONALE
Independent	
Note cultural/religious beliefs.	Affects patient/SO reaction and adjustment to diagnosis, treatment, and outcome of cancer.
Listen for expressions of helplessness.	Helpless feelings may contribute to difficulty adjusting to diagnosis of cancer and cooperating with treatment regimen.
Deal with family members in a warm, caring, respectful way. Provide information (verbal/written), and reinforce as necessary.	Provides feeling of empathy and promotes individual's sense of worth and competence in ability to handle current situation.
Encourage appropriate expressions of anger without reaction.	Feelings of anger are to be expected when individuals are dealing with the difficult/potentially fatal illness of cancer. Appropriate expression enables progress toward resolution of the stages of the grieving process.
Acknowledge difficulties of the situation, e.g., diagnosis and treatment of cancer, possibility of death.	Communicates acceptance of the reality the patient/family are facing.
Identify and encourage use of previous successful coping behaviors.	Most people have developed effective coping skills which can be useful in dealing with current situation.
Stress importance of continuous open dialogue between family members.	Promotes understanding and assists family members to maintain clear communication and resolve problems effectively.
Collaborative	
Refer to support groups, clergy, family therapy as indicated.	May need additional assistance to resolve problems of disorganization which may accompany diagnosis of potentially terminal illness (cancer).

NURSING DIAGNOSIS:	**KNOWLEDGE DEFICIT [LEARNING NEED] (SPECIFY)**
May be related to:	**Lack of exposure/recall; information misinterpretation, myths**
	Unfamiliarity with information resources
	Cognitive limitation
Possibly evidenced by:	**Questions/request for information, verbalization of problem**
	Statement of misconception
	Inaccurate follow-through of instructions/development of preventable complications
PATIENT OUTCOMES/ EVALUATION CRITERIA:	**Verbalizes accurate information about diagnosis and treatment regimen at own level of readiness. Correctly performs necessary procedures and explains reasons for the actions. Initiates necessary lifestyle changes and participates in treatment regimen.**

891

ACTIONS/INTERVENTIONS	RATIONALE

Independent

Review with patient/SO understanding of specific diagnosis, treatment alternatives, and future expectations.	Validates current level of understanding, identifies learning needs, and provides knowledge base on which patient can make informed decisions.
Determine patient's perception of cancer and cancer treatment(s); ask about patient's own/previous experience or experience with other people who have (or had) cancer.	Aids in identification of ideas, attitudes, fears, misconceptions, and gaps in knowledge about cancer.
Provide clear, accurate information in a factual but sensitive manner. Answer questions specifically, but do not bombard with unessential details.	Helps with adjustment to the diagnosis of cancer, by providing needed information along with time to absorb it. Note: Rate and method of giving information may need to be altered in order to decrease patient's anxiety and enhance ability to assimilate information.
Provide anticipatory guidance with patient/SO regarding treatment protocol, length of therapy, expected results, possible side effects. Be honest with patient.	Patient has the ''right to know'' (be informed) and participate in decision tree. Accurate and concise information helps to dispel fears and anxiety, helps clarify the expected routine, and enables patient to maintain some degree of control.
Ask patient for verbal feedback, and correct misconception about individual's type of cancer and treatment.	Misconceptions about cancer may be more disturbing than facts and can interfere with treatments/reduce healing.
Outline normally expected limitations (if any) on ADLs (e.g., limit sun exposure, alcohol intake; loss of work time because of in hospital treatments).	If limitations are required, enables patient/SO to begin to put them into perspective and begin adaptation as indicated.
Provide written materials about cancer, treatment, and available support systems.	Anxiety and preoccupation with thoughts about life and death often interfere with patient's ability to assimilate adequate information. Written, take-home materials provide reinforcement and clarification about information as patient needs it.
Review specific medication regimen and use of OTC drugs.	Enhances ability to manage self care and avoid potential complications, drug reactions/interactions.
Address specific home care needs, e.g., ability to live alone, perform necessary treatments/procedures, and acquire supplies.	Provides information regarding changes that may be needed in current plan of care to meet therapeutic needs.
Do predischarge home evaluation as indicated.	Aids in transition to home setting by providing information about needed changes in physical layout, acquisition of needed supplies.
Refer to community resources as indicated: e.g., social services, VNA, Meals-on-Wheels, local American Cancer Society chapter.	Promotes competent self-care and optimal independence.
Review with patient/SO the importance of maintaining optimal nutritional status.	Promotes well-being, facilitates recovery, and is critical in enabling the patient to tolerate treatments.
Encourage diet variations and experimentation in meal planning and food preparation, e.g., cooking with sweet juices, wine; serving foods cold or at room temperature as appropriate (egg salad, ice cream).	Creativity may enhance flavor and intake, especially when protein foods taste bitter.
Provide cookbooks that are designed for cancer patients.	Helpful in providing specific menu/recipe ideas.
Recommend increased fluid intake and fiber in diet as well as routine exercise.	Improves consistency of stool and stimulates peristalsis.

ACTIONS/INTERVENTIONS	RATIONALE

Independent

Instruct patient to assess oral mucous membranes routinely, noting erythema, ulceration.

May impair oral intake and provides avenue for infection.

Advise patient concerning skin and hair care: e.g., avoid harsh shampoos, hair dyes, permanents, salt water, chlorinated water; avoid exposure to strong wind and extreme heat or cold; avoid sun exposure to target area for 1 year after end of radiation treatments and apply sunblock (SPF 15 or greater).

Prevents additional hair damage, and skin irritation and may prevent recall reactions.

Review signs and symptoms, requiring medical evaluation, e.g., infection, delayed healing, drug reactions, increased pain (dependent on individual situation).

Early identification and treatment may limit severity of complications.

Stress importance of continuing medical follow-up.

Provides ongoing monitoring of progression/resolution of disease process and opportunity for timely diagnosis and treatment of complications. Note: Some complications can develop long after therapy is completed, e.g., pathologic fractures, radiation cystitis/nephritis.

Total Nutritional Support: Parenteral/Enteral Feeding ___

Specifically designed nutritional therapy can be administered by the parenteral or enteral route when the use of standard diets via the oral route is inadequate or not possible, to prevent/correct protein-calorie malnutrition.

Enteral nutrition is preferred for the patient who has a functional GI tract but is unable to consume an adequate nutritional intake, or oral intake is contraindicated/impossible. Feeding may be done via nasogastric or orogastric tube, esophagostomy, gastrostomy, duodenostomy, or jejunostomy.

Parenteral nutrition may be chosen because of altered metabolic states or when mechanical or functional abnormalities of the GI tract prevent enteral feeding. Amino acids, fat, carbohydrates, trace elements, vitamins, and electrolytes may be infused via a central or peripheral vein.

PATIENT ASSESSMENT DATA BASE

Clinical signs listed below are dependent on degree and duration of malnutrition and include observations indicative of vitamin and mineral as well as protein/calorie deficiency.

ACTIVITY/REST

May exhibit: Muscle wasting (temporal, intercostal, gastrocnemius, dorsum of hand); thin extremities, flaccid muscles, decreased activity tolerance.

CIRCULATION

May exhibit: Mucous membranes dry, pale, red, swollen.

Diaphoresis, cyanosis.

Tachycardia, bradycardia.

ELIMINATION

May report: Diarrhea or constipation; flatulence associated with food intake.

May exhibit: Abdominal distention/increased girth, ascites; tenderness on palpation.

Stools may be loose, hard-formed, fatty, or clay-colored.

FOOD/FLUID

May report: Weight loss of 10% of body weight within previous 6 months.

Problems with chewing, swallowing, choking, or saliva production.

Changes in the taste of food; anorexia, nausea/vomiting; inadequate oral intake (NPO) status for 7–10 days, long-term use of 5% dextrose intravenously.

May exhibit: Actual weight (measured) as compared with usual or preillness weight is less than 90% of ideal body weight for height, sex, and age or equal to or greater than 120% of ideal body weight (patient risk in obesity is a tendency to overlook protein and calorie requirements). A distorted actual weight may occur due to the presence of edema, ascites, organomegaly, tumor bulk, anasarca, amputation.

Edentulous or with ill-fitting dentures.

Bowel sounds diminished, hyperactive, or absent.

Thyroid, parotid enlargement.

Lips dry, cracked, red, swollen; angular stomatitis.

Tongue may be smooth, pale, slick, coated. Color often magenta, beefy red. Lingual papillae atrophy/swelling.

Gums swollen/bleeding, multiple caries.

NEUROSENSORY

May exhibit: Lethargy, apathy, listlessness, irritability, disorientation, coma.

Gag/swallow reflex may be decreased/absent, e.g., CVA, head trauma, nerve injury.

RESPIRATION

May exhibit: Increased respiratory rate; respiratory distress.

Dyspnea, increased sputum production.

Breath sounds: crackles (protein deficiency-related fluid shifts).

SAFETY

May exhibit: Hair may be fragile, coarse, lackluster. Alopecia, decreased pigmentation may be present.

Skin dry, scaly, tented; "flaky paint" dermatosis; edema; draining or unhealed wounds, pressure sores; ecchymoses, perifollicular petechiae, subcutaneous fat loss.

Eyes sunken, dull, dry, with pale conjunctiva; Bitot's spots (triangular, shiny, gray spots on the conjunctiva seen in vitamin A deficiency), or scleral icterus.

Nails may be brittle, thin, flattened, ridged, spoon-shaped.

SEXUALITY

May report: Loss of libido.

Amenenorrhea.

TEACHING/LEARNING

May report: History of conditions causing protracted protein losses, e.g., malabsorption or short-gut syndrome with increased diarrhea, renal dialysis, fistulas, draining wounds, thermal injuries.

Presence of factors known to alter nutritional requirements/increase energy demands, e.g., single or multiorgan failure; sepsis; fever; trauma; extensive burns; use of steroids, antitumor agents, immunosuppressants.

Use of medications that cause untoward drug/nutrient interactions, e.g., laxatives, anticonvulsants, diuretics, antacids, narcotics, immunosuppressants, chemotherapy.

Illness of psychiatric origin, e.g., anorexia nervosa/bulimia.

Educational/social factors, e.g., lack of nutrition knowledge, kitchen facilities, reduced/limited financial resources.

Discharge Plan Considerations: May require assistance with solution preparation, therapy supplies, and maintenance of feeding device for home nutritional care.

DIAGNOSTIC STUDIES

Anthropometrics:

Weight for height less than 90% or equal to or greater than 120% ideal body weight per hospital formula.

Tricep skinfold measurement: estimates subcutaneous fat stores; fat reserves less than 10th precentile suggest advanced depletion; levels less than the 30th percentile suggest mild to moderate depletion.

Midarm muscle circumference: measures somatic muscle mass and is used in combination with tricep skinfold measurement; a decrease of 15–20 percentiles from the expected value suggests a significant reduction.

Visceral proteins:

Serum albumin (the classic marker measured): values of 2.7–3.4 g/dl indicate mild depletion; 2.1–2.7 g/dl, moderate depletion; and less than 2.1 g/dl, severe depletion. (Decreased levels are due to poor protein intake, nephrotic syndrome, sepsis, burns, congestive heart failure, cirrhosis, eclampsia, protein-losing enteropathy. Above normal values [>4.5 g/dl] are seen in dehydration.)

Serum transferrin: more sensitive to changes in visceral protein stores than albumin; levels of 150–200 mg/dl reflect mild depletion; 100–150 mg/dl, moderate depletion; and 100 mg/dl, severe depletion. (Elevated values are seen with iron deficiency, pregnancy, hypoxia, and chronic blood loss. Decreased values are seen with pernicious anemia, chronic infection, liver disease, iron overload, and protein-losing enteropathy.)

Thyroxine-binding prealbumin: reflects rapid changes in hepatic protein synthesis and thus is a more sensitive indicator of visceral protein depletion. (Decreased levels less than 200 μg/ml are noted with cirrhosis, inflammation, and surgical trauma.)

Amino acid profile: alterations reflect an imbalance of plasma proteins with depressed levels of branch chain amino acids (common with hepatic encephalopathy or sepsis).

Tests of immune system:

Total lymphocyte count: less than 1500 cells/mm indicates leukopenia and results from decreased generation of T cells, which are very sensitive to malnutrition. (Levels are also altered by infection and administration of immunosuppressants.)

Electrolytes/minerals/trace elements:

Potassium: deficiency occurs with inadequate intake and with loss of potassium-containing fluids (e.g., urine, diarrhea, vomiting, fistula drainage, continuous nasogastric suctioning). Potassium is also lost from cells during muscle wasting and is excreted by the kidneys.

Sodium: levels are dependent on state of hydration/presence of active loss as may exist in excessive diuresis, GI suctioning, burns.

Phosphorus: may be decreased reflecting inadequate intake or may be elevated in renal failure.

Magnesium: deficiency is common in alcoholics, vomiting, diarrhea; may be elevated in renal failure.

Calcium; levels will be decreased with conditions associated with hypoalbuminemia, e.g., renal failure (majority of calcium is bound to albumin). Absorption is decreased by fat malabsorption and low protein diet.

Zinc: deficiency is seen in alcoholic cirrhosis; or may be secondary to hypoalbuminemia and GI losses (diarrhea).

Tests reflecting protein (nitrogen) loss:

Nitrogen balance studies: nitrogen (protein) excretion via urine, stool and insensible losses often exceeds nitrogen intake in the acutely ill, reflecting catabolic response to stress and use of endogenous protein stores for energy production (gluconeogenesis). *BUN* may be severely decreased as a result of chronic malnutrition and depletion of skeletal protein stores.

24-hour creatinine excretion: because creatinine is concentrated in muscle mass, there is a good correlation between lean body mass and 24-hour creatinine excretion. Actual values are compared with ideal values (based on height and weight) times 100, known as the *Creatinine height index (CHI):* CHI of 60–80% indicates moderate depletion; less than 60%, severe depletion.

Tests of gastrointestinal function:

Tests of malabsorption include Schilling test, D-xylose test, 72-hour stool fat, GI series.

Chest x-ray: may be normal or show evidence of pleural effusion; small heart silhouette.

ECG: may be normal or demonstrate low voltage, dysrhythmias/patterns reflective of electrolyte imbalances.

NURSING PRIORITIES

1. Promote consistent intake of estimated calorie and protein requirements.
2. Prevent complications.
3. Minimize energy losses/needs.
4. Provide information about condition, prognosis and treatment needs.

DISCHARGE CRITERIA

1. Nutritional intake adequate for individual needs.
2. Complications prevented/minimized.
3. Fatigue alleviated.
4. Condition, prognosis, and therapeutic regimen understood.

NURSING DIAGNOSIS:	NUTRITION, ALTERED: LESS THAN BODY REQUIREMENTS
May be related to:	Conditions that interfere with nutrient intake or increase nutrient need/metabolic demand, e.g., cancer and associated treatments, anorexia, surgical procedures, dysphagia/difficulty swallowing, depressed mental status/level of consciousness.
Possibly evidenced by:	Body weight 10% or more under ideal
	Decreased subcutaneous fat/muscle mass, poor muscle tone
	Changes in gastric motility and stool characteristics
PATIENT OUTCOMES/ EVALUATION CRITERIA:	Demonstrates stable weight or progressive weight gain toward goal with normalization of laboratory values and free of signs of malnutrition.

ACTIONS/INTERVENTIONS	RATIONALE
Independent	
General	
Document oral intake by use of 24-hour recall, food history, calorie counts as appropriate.	Identifies imbalance between estimated nutritional requirements and actual intake.
Assure accurate collections of specimens (urine, stool, drainage) for nitrogen balance studies.	Inaccurate collections can alter test results, leading to improper interpretation of patient's current status and needs.
Administer nutritional solutions at prescribed rate via infusion control device as needed. Adjust rate to prescribed hourly rate but never "catch up."	Nutrition support prescriptions are based on estimated caloric and protein requirements. A consistent rate of nutrient administration will assure proper utilization with fewer side effects, such as hyperglycemia or dumping syndrome. Note: Continuous infusion of enteral formulas is better tolerated than bolus feedings and results in improved absorption.
Be familiar with electrolyte content of nutritional solutions.	Metabolic complications of nutritional support often result from a lack of appreciation of changes that can occur as a result of refeeding, e.g., HHNC, electrolyte imbalances.
Schedule activities with adequate rest periods. Promote relaxation techniques.	Conserves energy/reduces calorie needs. (Refer to ND: Fatigue, p. 904.)
Assess nutritional status continually, during daily nursing care, noting energy level; condition of skin, nails, hair, oral cavity, desire to eat/anorexia.	Provides the opportunity to observe deviations from normals/patient baseline and influences choices of interventions.
Weigh daily and compare with admission weight.	Establishes baseline, aids in monitoring effectiveness of therapeutic regimen, and alerts nurse to inappropriate trends in weight loss/gain.
Parenteral	
Observe appropriate "hang" time of parenteral solutions per protocol.	Effectiveness of intravenous vitamins diminishes after 24 hours.

897

ACTIONS/INTERVENTIONS	RATIONALE

Independent

Monitor urine sugar/acetone or fingerstick glucose per protocol.

High glucose content of solutions may lead to pancreatic fatigue, requiring use of supplemental insulin to prevent HHNC. Note: Fingerstick determination of glucose level is more accurate/may be preferred over urine testing because of variations in renal glucose threshold.

Enteral

Assess gastrointestinal function and tolerance to enteral feedings: note bowel sounds; complaints of nausea/vomiting, abdominal discomfort; presence of diarrhea/constipation; development of weakness, lightheadedness, diaphoresis, tachycardia, abdominal cramping.

Because protein turnover of the gastrointestinal mucosa occurs approximately every 3 days, the GI tract is at great risk for early dysfunction and atrophy from disease and malnutrition. Intolerance of formula/presence of dumping syndrome may require alteration of rate of administration/concentration of formula or change to parenteral administration.

Check gastric residuals if bolus feedings are done; hold feeding/return aspirate per protocol for type/rate of feeding used if residual is greater than predetermined level.

Delayed gastric emptying can be caused by a specific disease process, e.g., paralytic ileus/surgery, shock; by drug therapy (especially narcotics); or the protein/fat content of the individual formula. Note: Replacement of gastric aspirate reduces loss of gastric acid/electrolytes.

Maintain patency of enteral feeding tubes by flushing with warm water, cranberry juice, etc., as indicated.

Enteral formulas contain protein that can clog small-bore feeding tubes, necessitating removal/replacement of tube.

Transitional

Stress importance of transition to oral feedings.

Although patient may have little interest or desire to eat, transition to oral feedings is preferred in view of potential side effects/complications of nutritional support therapy.

Assess gag reflex, ability to chew/swallow, and motor skills when progressing to transitional feedings.

May require additional interventions, e.g., retraining by dysphagia expert (speech therapist) or long-term nutritional support.

Provide self-help utensils as indicated, e.g., plate guard, utensils with built-up handles, lidded cups.

Patients with neuromuscular deficits, e.g., post-CVA, brain injury, may require use of special aids developed for feeding.

Create optimal environment, e.g., remove noxious stimuli, bedpans, soiled linens. Provide cheerful, attractive tray/table, soft music, companionship.

Encourages patient's attempts to eat, reduces anorexia, and introduces some of the social pleasures usually associated with mealtime.

Allow adequate time for chewing, swallowing, savoring food; provide socialization and feeding assistance as indicated.

Patients need extra encouragement/assistance to overcome underlying problems such as anorexia, fatigue, muscular weakness.

Offer small, frequent feedings; incorporate patient likes/dislikes in meal planning as much as possible, and include "home foods" as appropriate.

May enhance patient's desire for food and amount of intake.

Collaborative

Refer to nutritional team/registered dietitian.

Aids in identification of nutrient deficits and need for parenteral/enteral nutritional intervention.

Calculate basal energy expenditure (BEE) using formula based on sex, height, weight, age and estimated energy requirements.

Provides an estimation of calorie and protein needs.

ACTIONS/INTERVENTIONS	RATIONALE
Collaborative	
Review results of indirect calorimetry test if available.	Measures oxygen consumption at basal or resting metabolic rate, to aid in estimating calorie/protein requirements.
Assist with insertion and confirm proper placement of infusion line (e.g., chest x-ray for central venous catheter or aspiration of gastric contents from feeding tube) prior to administration of solutions.	Reduces risk of feeding-induced complications, including pneumo/hemothorax, hydrothorax, air embolus, arterial puncture (central venous line), or aspiration (nasogastric tube).
Administer intralipid fat emulsions as indicated.	Useful in meeting excessive calorie requirements (e.g., burns) or as a source of essential fatty acids during long-term hyperalimentation. Note: May be contraindicated in patients with alterations in fat metabolism or in the presence of pancreatitis, liver damge, anemia, coagulation disorders, pulmonary disease.
Administer medications, as indicated, e.g.:	
Insulin;	High glucose content of solutions may require exogenous insulin for metabolism especially in presence of pancreatic insufficiency or disease.
Diphenoxylate with atropine (Lomotil), camphorated tincture of opium (Paregoric), and metoclopramide (Reglan).	Gastrointestinal side effects of enteral feeding may need to be controlled with antidiarrheal agents (Lomotil/paregoric) or peristaltic stimulants (Reglan) if more conservative measures such as alteration of rate/strength or type of formula are not successful.
Monitor laboratory studies, e.g., serum glucose, electrolytes, transferrin, albumin, total protein, PO_4, BUN/Cr, liver enzymes, CBC, ABGs.	Untoward metabolic effects of TPN include: hypokalemia, hyponatremia and fluid retention, hyperglycemia, hypophosphatemia, increased carbon dioxide production resulting in respiratory compromise, elevation of liver function tests, renal dysfunction.
Provide calorie containing beverages, when oral intake is possible, e.g., juices/Jello water, dietary supplements (Sustacal, Ensure) or add Polycase to beverages/water.	Maximizes calorie intake when oral intake is limited/restricted.

NURSING DIAGNOSIS:	**INFECTION, POTENTIAL FOR**
May be related to:	**Invasive procedures: insertion of venous catheter, surgically placed gastrostomy, jejunostomy feeding tube**
	Malnutrition; chronic disease
	Environmental exposure: access devices in place for extended periods of time, improper preparation/handling/contamination of the feeding solution
Possibly evidenced by:	**[Not applicable; presence of signs and symptoms establishes an *actual* diagnosis.]**
PATIENT OUTCOMES/ EVALUATION CRITERIA:	**Displays absence of fever or chills; with catheter/feeding tube insertion sites clean, free of drainage and no erythema/edema present.**

ACTIONS/INTERVENTIONS	RATIONALE

Independent

Parenteral

Maintain an optimal aseptic environment during bedside insertion of central venous catheters and during changes of TPN bottles and administration tubing.

Catheter related sepsis may result from entry of pathogenic microorganisms through skin insertion tract, or from touch contamination during manipulations of TPN system.

Secure external portion of catheter/administration tubing to dressing with tape. Note intactness of skin suture.

Manipulation of catheter in/out of insertion site can result in tissue trauma (coring) and potentiate entry of skin organisms into catheter tract.

Maintain a sterile occlusive dressing over catheter insertion site. Perform central/peripheral venous catheter dressing care per protocol.

Protects catheter insertion sites from potential sources of contamination. Note: Central venous catheter sites can easily become contaminated from tracheostomy or endotracheal secretions or from wounds of the head, neck, and chest.

Inspect insertion site of catheter for erythema, induration, drainage, tenderness.

The catheter is a potential irritant to the surrounding skin and subcutaneous skin tract, and extended use may result in insertion site irritation and infection.

Refrigerate premixed amino acid/dextrose solutions prior to use; observe a 24-hour hang time for amino acid solutions and a 12-hour hang time for intravenous fat emulsions.

TPN solutions and fat emulsions have been shown to support the growth of a wide variety of pathogenic organisms once contaminated.

Monitor temperature and glucose.

A rise in temperature or loss of glucose tolerance (glycosuria, hyperglycemia) are early indications of possible catheter-related sepsis.

Enteral

Keep manipulations of enteral feeding system to a minimum and wash hands before opening system.

Touch contamination by care giver during enteral formula administration has been shown to cause contamination of formula.

Alternate nares for tube placement in long-term NG feedings.

Reduces risk of trauma/infection of paranasal tissue (especially important in facial trauma/burns).

Provide daily/prn site care to abdominally placed feeding tubes.

Gastrointestinal secretions leaking through or around gastrostomy/jejunostomy tube tracts can cause skin breakdown severe enough to require removal of the feeding tube.

Refrigerate reconstituted enteral formulas before use; observe a 4–8-hour hang time; discard unused formula after 24 hours.

Enteral formulas easily support bacterial growth and can be contaminated during formula preparation. For example, bacterial growth has been shown to occur within 4 hours after contamination.

Collaborative

Aseptically prepare parenteral solutions/enteral formulas for administration.

TPN solutions should be prepared under a laminar flow hood in the department of pharmacy. Enteral formulas should be mixed in a clean environment in the dietary or pharmacy department, although with the advent of canned/modular formulas, this may not be necessary. Note: Additives to TPN solutions, as a rule, should not be made on the unit because of the potential for contamination and drug incompatibilities.

Notify physician if signs of infection present. Follow protocol for obtaining appropriate culture specimens, e.g., blood, solutions. Change bottle/tubing as indicated.

Necessary to identify source of infection and initiate appropriate therapy. May require removal of TPN line and culture of catheter tip.

ACTIONS/INTERVENTIONS	RATIONALE

Collaborative

Administer antibiotics as indicated.

May be given prophylactically or for specifically identified organism.

NURSING DIAGNOSIS:	INJURY, POTENTIAL FOR [MULTIFACTOR]
May be related to:	External environment: catheter-related complications (air emboli and septic thrombophlebitis)
	Internal factors: aspiration; effects of therapy/drug interactions
Possibly evidenced by:	[Not applicable; presence of signs and symptoms establishes an *actual* diagnosis.]
PATIENT OUTCOMES/ EVALUATION CRITERIA:	Free of complications associated with nutritional support. Modifies environment/corrects hazards to enhance safety.

ACTIONS/INTERVENTIONS	RATIONALE

Independent

Parenteral

Maintain a closed central intravenous system using Luer-Lok connections/taping of all connections.

Inadvertent disconnection of central intravenous system can result in lethal air emboli.

Administer appropriate TPN solution via peripheral or central venous route.

Solutions containing high concentrations of dextrose (greater than 10%) must be delivered via a central vein, because they will result in chemical phlebitis when delivered through small peripheral veins.

Monitor patient for potential drug/nutrient interactions.

For example, digoxin, in conjunction with diuretic therapy, can cause hypomagnesemia; hypokalemia may result from chronic use of laxatives, mineralocorticosteroids, diuretics, or amphotericin.

Assess catheter for signs of displacement out of central venous position, i.e., extended length of catheter on skin surface; leaking of IV solution onto dressing; patient complaints of neck pain, tenderness at catheter site, or swelling of extremity on side of catheter insertion.

Central venous catheter tip may slip out of superior vena cava and position itself into smaller innominate and jugular veins, causing a chemical thrombophlebitis. Incidence of subclavian or superior vena cava thrombosis is increased with extended use of central venous catheters.

Inspect peripheral TPN catheter site routinely and change sites at least every 3 days or per protocol.

Peripheral TPN solutions (although less hyperosmolar), can still irritate small veins and cause phlebitis. Peripheral venous access is often limited in malnourished patients, but site should still be changed if signs of irritation develop.

Investigate complaints of severe chest pain/coughing. Turn patient to left side in Trendelenburg position if indicated and notify physician.

Suggests presence of air embolus requiring immediate intervention to displace air into apex of heart away from the pulmonary artery.

Maintain an occlusive dressing on catheter insertion sites for 24 hours after subclavian catheter removed.

Extended catheter use may result in development of catheter skin tract. Once the catheter is removed, air embolus is still a potential risk until skin tract has sealed.

901

ACTIONS/INTERVENTIONS	RATIONALE

Independent

Enteral

Assess gastrostomy or jejunostomy tube sites for evidence of malposition.

Indwelling and mushroom catheters are still frequently used for feeding tubes inserted via the abdomen. Migration of the catheter balloon can result in duodenal or jejunal obstruction. Improperly sutured gastrostomy tubes may easily fall out.

Collaborative

Review chest x-ray as indicated.

Central parenteral line placement is routinely confirmed by x-ray.

Consult with pharmacist in regard to site/time of delivery of drugs whose action might be adversely affected by enteral formula.

Absorption of vitamin D is impaired by administration of mineral oil (inhibits micelle formation of bile salts) and by neomycin (inactivates bile salts). Aluminum-containing antacids bind with the phosphorus in the feeding solution, potentiating hypophosphatemia.

NURSING DIAGNOSIS:	ASPIRATION, POTENTIAL FOR
May be related to:	**Presence of the gastrointestinal tubes, bolus tube feedings, medication administration**
	Increased intragastric pressure, delayed gastric emptying
Possibly evidenced by:	**[Not applicable: presence of signs and symptoms establishes an *actual* diagnosis.]**
PATIENT OUTCOMES/ EVALUATION CRITERIA:	**Maintains clear airway, free of signs of aspiration.**

ACTIONS/INTERVENTIONS	RATIONALE

Independent

Confirm placement of nasoenteral feeding tubes. Determine feeding tube position in stomach by x-ray, confirmation of pH of 2 or 3 of the gastric fluid withdrawn through tube, or auscultation of injected air prior to intermittent feedings. Observe for ability to speak/cough.

Malplacement of nasoenteral feeding tubes may result in aspiration of enteral formula. Patients at particular risk include those who are intubated or obtunded; following CVA or surgery of the head/neck, upper gastrointestinal system.

Maintain aspiration precautions during enteral feedings:

Aspiration of enteral formulas is irritating to the lung parenchyma and may result in pneumonia and respiratory compromise.

Keep head of bed elevated at 30–45 degrees during feeding and at least 1 hour after feeding;

Inflate tracheostomy cuff during and for 1 hour after intermittent feeding;

Interrupt feeding when patient is in prone position;

ACTIONS/INTERVENTIONS

Independent

Add blue food coloring to enteral formula as indicated.

Monitor gastric residuals after bolus feedings (as previously noted in ND: Nutrition, Altered: Less Than Body Requirements, p. 897).

Note characteristics of sputum/tracheal aspirate. Investigate development of dyspnea, cough, tachypnea, cyanosis. Auscultate breath sounds.

Note indicators of nasogastric tube intolerance, e.g., absence of gag reflex, high risk of aspiration, frequent removal of nasogastric feeding tubes.

Collaborative

Review abdominal x-ray if done.

RATIONALE

Helps identify aspiration of enteral formula and/or tracheal esophageal fistula, if discovered in sputum/lung secretions. Note: Avoid use of methylene blue dye, which may cause false-positive guaiac test when assessing for GI bleeding.

Presence of large gastric residuals may potentiate an incompetent esophageal sphincter, leading to vomiting and aspiration.

Presence of formula in tracheal secretions or signs/symptoms reflecting respiratory distress suggests aspiration.

May require consideration of surgically placed feeding tubes (e.g., gastrostomy, jejunostomy) for patient safety and consistency of enteral formula delivery.

Confirmation of gastric feeding tube may be obtained by x-ray.

NURSING DIAGNOSIS:	FLUID VOLUME, ALTERED: [FLUCTUATION]
May be related to:	Active loss and/or failure of regulatory mechanisms (specific to underlying disease process/trauma); complications of nutrition therapy, e.g., high-glucose solutions, hyperglycemia (hyperosmolar nonketotic coma and severe dehydration) Inability to obtain/ingest fluids
Possibly evidenced by:	[Not applicable; presence of signs and symptoms establishes an *actual* diagnosis.]
PATIENT OUTCOMES/ EVALUATION CRITERIA:	Displays moist skin/mucous membranes, stable vital signs, individually adequate urinary output; free of edema and excessive weight loss/inappropriate gain.

ACTIONS/INTERVENTIONS

Independent

Assess for clinical signs of dehydration (e.g., thirst, dry skin/mucous membranes, hypotension); or fluid excess (e.g., peripheral edema, tachycardia, adventitious breath sounds).

Incorporate knowledge of caloric density of enteral formulas into assessment of fluid balance.

Provide additional water/flush tubing as indicated.

RATIONALE

Early detection and intervention may prevent occurrence/excessive fluctuation in fluid balance. Note: Severely malnourished patients have an increased risk of developing refeeding syndrome, e.g., life-threatening fluid overload, intracellular electrolyte shifts, and cardiac strain occurring during initial 3–5 days of therapy.

Enteric solutions are usually concentrated and do not meet free water needs.

With higher calorie formula, additional water is needed to prevent dehydration/HHNC.

ACTIONS/INTERVENTIONS

Independent

Record intake and output; calculate fluid balance. Measure urine specific gravity.

Weigh daily or as indicated; evaluate changes.

Collaborative

Monitor laboratory studies, e.g.:

    Serum potassium/phosphorus;

    Hct;

    Serum albumin.

Dilute formula or change from hypertonic to isotonic formula as indicated.

RATIONALE

Excessive urinary losses may reflect developing HHNC. Specific gravity is an indicator of hydration and renal function.

Rapid weight gain (reflecting fluid retention) can predispose/potentiate congestive heart failure or pulmonary edema. Gain of greater than 0.5 lb/day indicates fluid retention and not deposition of lean body mass.

Hypokalemia/phosphatemia can occur due to intracellular shifts during initial refeeding and may compromise cardiac function if not corrected.

Reflects hydration/circulating volume.

Hypoalbuminemia/decreased colloidal osmotic pressure leads to third spacing of fluid (edema).

May decrease gastric intolerance reducing occurrence of diarrhea and associated fluid losses.

NURSING DIAGNOSIS:	FATIGUE
May be related to:	Decreased metabolic energy production; increased energy requirements (hypermetabolic states, healing process) Altered body chemistry: medications, chemotherapy
Possibly evidenced by:	Overwhelming lack of energy, inability to maintain usual routines/accomplish routine tasks Lethargy, impaired ability to concentrate
PATIENT OUTCOMES/ EVALUATION CRITERIA:	Reports increased sense of well-being/energy level. Demonstrates measurable increase in physical activity.

ACTIONS/INTERVENTIONS

Independent

Monitor physiologic response to activity, e.g., changes in blood pressure, or heart/respiratory rate.

Establish realistic activity goals with patient.

Plan care to allow for rest periods. Schedule activities for periods when patient has most energy. Involve patient/SO in schedule planning.

RATIONALE

Tolerance varies greatly, depending on the stage of the disease process, nutritional state and fluid balance.

Provides for a sense of control and feelings of accomplishment.

Frequent rest periods are needed to restore/conserve energy. Planning will allow patient to be active during times when energy level is higher, which may restore a feeling of well-being and a sense of control.

ACTIONS/INTERVENTIONS	RATIONALE

Independent

Encourage patient to do whatever possible, e.g., self-care, sitting up in chair, walking. Increase activity level as indicated.

Increases strength, stamina and enables patient to become more active without undue fatigue.

Provide passive/active range of motion exercises to bedridden patients.

The deposition of lean body mass is dependent on the provision of both isotonic and isometric exercises.

Keep bed in low position, pathways clear of furniture; assist with ambulation.

Protects patient from injury during activities.

Assist with self-care needs as necessary.

Weakness may make activities of daily living almost impossible for the patient to complete.

Collaborative

Provide supplemental oxygen as indicated.

Presence of anemia/hypoxemia reduces oxygen available for cellular uptake and contributes to fatigue.

Refer to physical/occupational therapy.

Programmed daily exercises and activities help patient to maintain/increase strength and muscle tone and enhance sense of well-being.

NURSING DIAGNOSIS:	KNOWLEDGE DEFICIT [LEARNING NEED] (SPECIFY)
May be related to:	**Lack of exposure/recall, information misinterpretation**
	Cognitive limitation
Possibly evidenced by:	**Request for information, questions/statement of misconception**
	Inaccurate follow-through of instructions/development of preventable complications
PATIENT OUTCOMES/ EVALUATION CRITERIA:	**Verbalizes understanding of condition/disease process and individual nutritional needs. Correctly performs necessary procedures and explains reasons for the actions.**

ACTIONS/INTERVENTIONS	RATIONALE

Independent

Assess patient's/SO knowledge of nutritional state. Review individual situation, signs/symptoms of malnutrition, future expectations, transitional feeding needs.

Provides information on which the patient/SO can base informed choices. Knowledge of the interaction between malnutrition and illness is helpful to understanding need for special therapy.

Discuss reasons for use of parenteral/enteral nutrition support.

May experience anxiety regarding inability to eat and may not comprehend the nutritional value of the prescribed TPN/tube feedings.

Provide adequate time for patient/SO teaching when patient is going home on enteral/parenteral feedings. Document patient/SO understanding and ability/competence to deliver safe home therapy.

Generally 3–4 days is sufficient for patient/SO to become proficient with tube feedings. Parenteral therapy is more complex and may require a week or longer for patient/SO to feel ready for home management and requires follow-up in the home.

ACTIONS/INTERVENTIONS	RATIONALE

Independent

Discuss proper handling, storage, preparation of nutritional solutions, or blenderized feedings; aseptic or clean techniques for care of insertion sites, use of dressings.

Reduces risk of metabolic complications and infection.

Review use/care of nutritional support devices.

Patient understanding and cooperation is key to the safe insertion and maintenance of nutritional support access devices as well as prevention of complications.

Review specific precautions dependent on type of feeding, e.g., checking placement of tube, sitting upright for enteral feeding, maintaining patency of tube, anchoring of tubing.

Promotes safe self-care and reduces risk of complications.

Demonstrate reinsertion of gastric feeding tube if appropriate.

Tube may be changed routinely or only inserted for feedings. Intermittent feedings enhance patient mobility and aid in transition to regular feeding pattern.

Identify signs/symptoms requiring medical evaluation, e.g., nausea/vomiting, abdominal cramping/bloating, diarrhea, rapid weight changes; erythema, drainage, foul odor at tube insertion site, fever/chills; coughing/choking or difficulty breathing during enteral feeding.

Early evaluation and treatment of problems (e.g., feeding intolerance, infection, aspiration) may prevent progression to more serious complications.

Instruct patient/SO in urine/serum glucose monitoring if indicated.

Timely recognition of changes in blood sugar levels, reduces risk of hypoglycemic reactions in patient on hyperalimentation.

Discuss signs/symptoms and treatment of hyper/hypoglycemia.

Hyperglycemia is more common for patient receiving parenteral feedings and those who have pancreas or liver disease, or are on large doses of corticosteroids. Rebound hypoglycemia can occur when feedings are intentionally/accidentally discontinued.

Encourage use of diary for recording test results, physical feelings/reactions, activity level, etc.

Provides resource for review by health care providers for optimal management of individual situation.

Recommend daily exercise/activity to tolerance, scheduling of adequate rest periods.

Enhances gastric motility for enteral/transition feedings, promotes feelings of general well-being, and prevents undue fatigue.

Ascertain that all supplies are in place in the home prior to discharge; make arrangements as needed with suppliers, e.g., hospital, pharmacy, medical equipment suppliers.

Provides for successful and competent home therapy.

Refer to nutritional support nurses, home health care agency, VNA, etc. Provide with immediate access phone numbers.

Patient/SO need ready support persons to assist with home therapy, equipment problems, and emotional adjustments in long-term therapy.

Fluid and Electrolyte Imbalances _____

The body's fluid balance depends on the net gain or loss of two components, water and its dominant electrolyte, sodium (Na^+). Note: Because these problems usually occur in conjunction with other medical conditions, the following files are offered as a reference. The interventions are presented in a general format for inclusion in the primary care plan.

HYPERVOLEMIA (EXTRACELLULAR FLUID VOLUME EXCESS)

PREDISPOSING/CONTRIBUTING FACTORS

Excess sodium intake/hypertonic fluid replacement.

Excessive, rapid administration of parenteral fluids.

Increased release of ADH; excessive ACTH production, hyperaldosteronism.

Decreased plasma proteins as may occur with chronic liver disease with ascites, major abdominal surgery, malnutrition/protein depletion.

Chronic kidney disease/acute renal failure.

Congestive heart failure.

PATIENT ASSESSMENT DATA BASE

ACTIVITY/REST

May report: Fatigue.

CIRCULATION

May exhibit: Hypertension, elevated CVP.

Pulse full/bounding; tachycardia usually present; bradycardia (late sign of cardiac decompensation).

Extra heart sounds (S_3).

Edema: dependent, pitting, facial, periorbital, anasarca.

Neck vein distention.

ELIMINATION

May report: Decreased urinary output.

FOOD/FLUID

May report: Anorexia, nausea/vomiting, thirst.

May exhibit: Abdominal girth increased with visible fluid wave on palpation.

Acute weight gain, often in excess of 5% of total body weight.

NEUROSENSORY

May exhibit: Changes in level of consciousness, from confusion to coma.

Aphasia.

Seizures.

RESPIRATION

May exhibit: Tachypnea with/without dyspnea, orthopnea; productive cough.

Crackles.

SAFETY

May exhibit: Fever.

Skin changes in color, temperature, turgor, e.g., taut and cool where edematous.

TEACHING/LEARNING

Refer to predisposing/contributing factors.

Discharge Plan Considerations: May require assistance with changes in therapeutic regimen, dietary management.

DIAGNOSTIC STUDIES

CBC: Hct, Hb, and RBC usually decreased (hemodilution).

Serum sodium: may be high, low, or normal.

Urine sodium: may be low because of sodium retention.

Total protein: albumin may be decreased.

Serum osmolality: usually unchanged, although hypoosmolality may occur.

Serum potassium and BUN: normal or decreased, unless renal damage present.

Urine specific gravity: decreased.

Chest X-ray: may reveal signs of congestion.

ACTIONS/INTERVENTIONS	RATIONALE
Independent	
Monitor vital signs and CVP.	Tachycardia and hypertension are common manifestations. Tachypnea usually present with/without dyspnea. Elevated CVP may be noted before dyspnea and adventitious breath sounds occur.
Auscultate lungs and heart sounds.	Adventitious sounds (crackles) and extra heart sounds (S_3) are indicative of fluid excess. Pulmonary edema may develop rapidly.
Assess for presence/location of edema formation.	Edema may be generalized or localized in dependent areas. Elderly patients may develop dependent edema with relatively little excess fluid. Note: Patients in a supine position can have an increase of 4–8 liters of fluid before edema is readily detected.
Note presence of neck vein distention, along with pitting edema, dyspnea.	Signs of cardiac decompensation/congestive heart failure.
Maintain accurate I&O. Note decreased urine output, positive fluid balance on 24-hour calculations.	Decreased renal perfusion, cardiac insufficiency, and fluid shifts may cause decreased urine output and edema formation.
Weigh as indicated.	One liter of fluid retention equals a weight gain of 2.2 lb.
Give oral fluids with caution. If fluids are restricted, set up a 24-hour schedule for fluid intake.	Fluid restrictions, as well as extracellular shifts, can cause drying of mucous membranes, and patient may desire more fluids than are prudent.
Monitor infusion rate of parenteral fluids closely; administer via control device/pump as necessary.	Sudden fluid bolus/prolonged excessive administration potentiates volume overload/risk of cardiac decompensation.
Encourage coughing/deep breathing exercises.	Pulmonary fluid shifts potentiate respiratory complications.
Maintain semi-Fowler's position if dyspnea or ascites is present.	Gravity improves lung expansion by lowering diaphragm, and shifting fluid to lower abdominal cavity.

908

ACTIONS/INTERVENTIONS	RATIONALE
Independent	
Turn, reposition, and provide skin care at regular intervals.	Reduces pressure and friction on edematous tissue, which is more prone to breakdown than normal tissue.
Promote bedrest. Schedule care to provide frequent rest periods.	Limited cardiac reserves result in fatigue/activity intolerances.
Provide safety precautions as indicated, e.g., use of side rails, bed in low position, frequent observation, soft restraints (if required).	Fluid shifts may cause cerebral edema/changes in mentation, especially in the geriatric population.
Collaborative	
Assist with identification/treatment of underlying cause.	Refer to listing of predisposing/contributing factors.
Monitor laboratory studies as indicated, e.g., electrolytes, BUN, ABGs.	Extracellular fluid shifts, sodium/water restriction and renal function all affect serum sodium levels. Potassium deficit may occur with diuretic therapy. BUN may be increased as a result of renal dysfunction/failure. ABGs may reflect metabolic acidosis.
Provide high-protein, low-sodium diet. Restrict fluids as indicated.	Increased serum proteins can enhance colloidal osmotic gradients and promote return of fluid to the vascular space. Restriction of sodium/water decreases extracellular fluid retention.
Administer diuretics, e.g., furosemide (Lasix).	Decreases total body water.
Replace potassium losses as indicated.	Potassium deficit (which may occur if patient is receiving potassium-wasting diuretic) can cause lethal cardiac dysrhythmias if untreated.
Prepare for/assist with dialysis/ultrafiltration, if indicated.	May be done to rapidly reduce fluid overload, especially in the presence of severe cardiac/renal failure.

HYPOVOLEMIA (EXTRACELLULAR FLUID VOLUME DEFICIT)

PREDISPOSING/CONTRIBUTING FACTORS

Excessive losses: vomiting, gastric suctioning, diarrhea, diaphoresis, wounds or burns, intraoperative fluid loss, hemorrhage.

Insufficient/decreased fluid intake, e.g., pre/postoperative NPO status.

Systemic infections, fever.

Intestinal obstruction or fistulas.

Pancreatitis, peritonitis, cirrhosis/ascites.

Kidney disease, diabetic ketoacidosis, HHNC, diabetes insipidus.

PATIENT ASSESSMENT DATA BASE

ACTIVITY/REST

May report: Fatigue, generalized weakness.

CIRCULATION

May exhibit: Hypotension, including postural changes.
Pulse weak/thready; tachycardia.
Neck veins flattened; CVP decreased.

909

ELIMINATION

May report:	Constipation or occasionally diarrhea, abdominal cramps.
May exhibit:	Urine volume decreased, dark/concentrated color; oliguria (severe fluid depletion).

FOOD/FLUID

May report:	Thirst, anorexia, nausea/vomiting.
May exhibit:	Weight loss often exceeding 5% of total body weight.
	Abdominal distention.
	Mucous membranes dry, furrows on tongue; decreased tearing and salivation.
	Skin dry with poor turgor; or pale, moist, clammy (shock).

NEUROSENSORY

May report:	Tingling of the extremities, vertigo, syncope.
	Behavior change, apathy, restlessness, confusion.

RESPIRATIONS

May exhibit:	Tachypnea, rapid/shallow breathing.

SAFETY

May exhibit:	Temperature usually subnormal, although fever may occur.

TEACHING/LEARNING

Refer to predisposing/contributing factors.

Discharge Plan Considerations:	May require assistance with changes in therapeutic regimen, dietary management.

DIAGNOSTIC STUDIES

Serum sodium: may be normal, high, or low.

Urine sodium: usually decreased (less than 10 mEq/l when losses are from external causes; usually above 20 mEq/l if the cause is renal or adrenal).

CBC: Hct, Hb, and RBC usually increased (hemoconcentration); decrease suggests hemorrhage.

Serum glucose: normal or elevated.

Serum protein: increased.

BUN and creatinine: increased, with BUN out of proportion to creatinine.

Urine specific gravity: increased.

ACTIONS/INTERVENTIONS	RATIONALE
Independent	
Monitor vital signs and CVP.	Tachycardia is present as well as varying degrees of hypotension, depending on degree of fluid deficit. CVP measurements are useful in determining degree of fluid deficit and response to replacement therapy.
Palpate peripheral pulses; note capillary refill, skin color/temperature; assess mentation.	Conditions that contribute to extracellular fluid deficit can result in inadequate organ perfusion to all areas and may cause circulatory collapse/shock.

910

ACTIONS/INTERVENTIONS	RATIONALE

Independent

Monitor urine output. Measure/estimate all sources, e.g., gastric losses, wound drainage, diaphoresis.

A decreased urine output may indicate insufficient renal perfusion/hypovolemia. Fluid replacement needs are based on correction of current deficits and ongoing losses. Note: A diaphoretic episode requiring a full linen change may represent a fluid loss of as much as 1 liter.

Weigh daily and compare with 24-hour fluid balance. Mark/measure edematous areas, e.g., abdomen, limbs.

Changes in weight may not accurately reflect intravascular volume, e.g., third spaced fluid accumulation cannot be used by the body for tissue perfusion.

Ascertain patient's beverage preferences, and set up a 24-hour schedule for fluid intake. Encourage foods with high fluid content.

Relieves thirst and discomfort of dry mucous membranes and augments parenteral replacement.

Turn frequently, massage skin and protect bony prominences.

Tissues are susceptible to breakdown because of vasoconstriction, and increased cellular fragility.

Provide skin and mouth care. Bathe every other day using mild soap.

Skin and mucous membranes are dry, with decreased elasticity, because of vasoconstriction and reduced intracellular water.

Provide safety precautions as indicated, e.g., use of side rails, bed in low position, frequent observation, soft restraints (if required).

Decreased cerebral perfusion frequently results in changes in mentation/altered thought processes, requiring protective measures to prevent patient injury.

Investigate complaints of sudden/sharp chest pain, dyspnea, cyanosis, increased anxiety, restlessness.

Hemoconcentration (sludging) and increased platelet aggregation may result in systemic emboli formation.

Monitor for sudden/marked elevation of blood pressure, restlessness, moist cough, dyspnea, basalar crackles, frothy sputum.

Too rapid a correction of fluid deficit may compromise the cardiopulmonary system, especially if colloids are used in general fluid replacement (increased osmotic pressure potentiates fluid shifts).

Collaborative

Assist with identification/treatment of underlying cause.

Refer to listing of predisposing/contributing factors.

Monitor laboratory studies as indicated, e.g., electrolytes, glucose, pH/PCO_2, coagulation studies.

Depending on the avenue of fluid loss, differing electrolyte/metabolic imbalances may be present/require correction; e.g., use of glucose solutions in patients with underlying glucose intolerance may result in serum glucose elevation and increased urinary water losses.

Administer IV solutions as indicated:

Isotonic solutions, e.g., normal saline, 5% dextrose/water, lactated Ringer's;

Crystalloids provide prompt circulatory improvement, although the benefit may be transient (increased renal clearance). Note: Use of buffered crystalloids (LR) may potentiate the risk of metabolic acidosis.

Colloids, e.g., dextran, Plasmanate/albumin, Hetastarh (Hespan);

Corrects plasma protein concentration deficits, thereby increasing intravascular osmotic pressure and facilitating return of fluid into vascular compartment.

Whole blood/packed red blood cell transfusion.

Indicated when hypovolemia is related to active blood loss.

Administer sodium bicarbonate ($NaHCO_3$), if indicated.

May be given to correct severe acidosis while correcting fluid balance.

SODIUM

Sodium is the major cation of extracellular fluid (ECF) and is primarily responsible for osmotic pressure in that compartment. Sodium enhances neuromuscular conduction/transmission of impulses and is essential for maintaining acid–base balance. Normal serum range is 135–145 mEq/l; intracellular, 10 mEq/l. Note: Chloride is carried by sodium and will display the same imbalances. Normal serum range is 95–105 mEq/l.

HYPONATREMIA (SODIUM DEFICIT)

PREDISPOSING/CONTRIBUTING FACTORS

Primary hyponatremia: lack of sufficient dietary sodium, severe malnutrition, infusion of sodium free solutions. Excessive sodium loss through sweating (e.g., heat exhaustion), wounds/trauma (hemorrhage), gastric suctioning, vomiting, diarrhea, small bowel obstruction, peritonitis, salt-wasting renal dysfunction, adrenal insufficiency (Addison's disease).

Dilutional hyponatremia: excessive water intake, electrolyte-free IV infusion, water intoxication (IV therapy, tap water enemas), gastric irrigations with electrolyte-free solutions; SIADH (syndrome of inappropriate ADH), CHF, renal failure/nephrotic syndrome, hepatic cirrhosis, diabetes mellitus (hyperglycemia), freshwater near-drowning; use of hypoglycemia medications, barbiturates, aminophylline or morphine (may stimulate pituitary gland to secrete excessive amounts of ADH).

Note: A pseudohyponatremia may occur in presence of multiple myeloma, hyperlipidemia, or hypoproteinemia but does not reflect an actual abnormality of water metabolism.

PATIENT ASSESSMENT DATA BASE

General

ACTIVITY/REST

May report: Generalized weakness, faintness, muscle cramps.

FOOD/FLUID

May report: Nausea, anorexia, thirst.

NEUROSENSORY

May report: Headache, blurred vision, vertigo.

May exhibit: Loss of coordination.

TEACHING/LEARNING

Refer to predisposing/contributing factors.

**Discharge Plan
Considerations:**   May require assistance with changes in therapeutic regimen, dietary management.

Sodium/Water Deficit

CIRCULATION

May exhibit: Hypotension, tachycardia.
                   Peripheral pulses diminished.

ELIMINATION

May report:	Abdominal cramping, diarrhea.
May exhibit:	Urine output decreased.

FOOD/FLUID

May report:	Vomiting.
May exhibit:	Poor skin turgor; soft/sunken eyeballs.
	Mucous membranes dry, decreased saliva/perspiration.

NEUROSENSORY

May exhibit:	Muscle twitching.
	Lethargy, restlessness, confusion, stupor.

RESPIRATION

May exhibit:	Tachypnea.

SAFETY

May exhibit:	Skin flushed, dry, hot.
	Fever.

Sodium Deficit/Water Excess

CIRCULATION

May exhibit:	Hypertension.
	Generalized edema.

ELIMINATION

May exhibit:	Urinary output increased.

Severe Sodium Deficit

CIRCULATION

May exhibit:	Hypotension with vasomotor collapse.
	Rapid thready pulse.
	Cold/clammy skin, fingerprinting on sternum; cyanosis.

NEUROSENSORY

May exhibit:	Hyperreflexia.
	Convulsions/coma.

DIAGNOSTIC STUDIES

Serum sodium: decreased, <135 mEq/l.
Urine sodium: <20 mEq/l unless sodium wasting nephropathy present.
Serum potassium: may be decreased as the kidneys attempt to conserve sodium at the expense of potassium.
Serum chloride/bicarbonate: levels are decreased, depending on which ion is lost with the sodium.

Osmolality: commonly low, but may be normal (pseudohyponatremia), or high (HHNC).
Urine osmolality: usually <100 mOsmol/l unless SIADH present in which case it will exceed serum osmolality.
Urine specific gravity: may be decreased (<1.010) or increased (>1.020) if SIADH is present.
Hct: is dependent on fluid balance, e.g., fluid excess versus dehydration.
BUN: may be elevated in presence of fluid excess.

ACTIONS/INTERVENTIONS	RATIONALE
Independent	
Monitor intake and output. Calculate fluid balance. Weigh daily.	Indicators of fluid balance are important, because either fluid excess or deficit may occur with hyponatremia.
Assess level of consciousness/neuromuscular response.	Sodium deficit may result in decreased mentation (to point of coma), as well as generalized muscle weakness/cramps/convulsions.
Maintain quiet environment; provide safety/seizure precautions.	Reduces CNS stimulation and risk of injury from neurologic complications, e.g., seizures.
Note respiratory rate and depth.	Co-occurring hypochloremia may produce slow/shallow respirations as the body compensates for metabolic alkalosis.
Encourage foods and fluids high in sodium, e.g., milk, meat, eggs, carrots, beets, and celery. Use fruit juices and bouillion instead of plain water.	Unless sodium deficit causes serious symptoms requiring immediate IV replacement, the patient may benefit from slower replacement by oral method or removal of previous salt restriction.
Irrigate nasogastric tube (when used) with normal saline instead of water.	Isotonic irrigation will minimize loss of GI electrolytes.
Collaborative	
Assist with identification/treatment of underlying cause.	Refer to listing of predisposing/contributing factors.
Monitor serum electrolytes, osmolality.	Evaluates therapy needs/effectiveness.
Administer/restrict fluids dependent on fluid volume status.	In presence of hypovolemia, volume losses are replaced with isotonic saline (e.g., normal saline), or, on occasion, hypertonic solution (3% NaCl) in life-threatening situations. In the presence of normal/hypervolemia (SIADH), fluid restriction is indicated.
Administer medications as indicated, e.g.:	
Furosemide (Lasix);	Effective in reducing fluid excess to correct sodium/water balance.
Sodium chloride (NaCl);	Used to replace deficits/prevent recurrence in the presence of chronic/ongoing losses.
Potassium chloride (KCl);	Corrects potassium deficit, especially when diuretic is used.
Demeclocycline (Declomycin).	Useful in treating SIADH, especially when severe water restriction may not be tolerated, e.g., COPD. Note: May be contraindicated in patients with liver disease because nephrotoxicity may occur.

HYPERNATREMIA (SODIUM EXCESS)

PREDISPOSING/CONTRIBUTING FACTORS

Excessive water losses: polyuria (as may occur with diabetes mellitus or insipidus); use of osmotic diuretics (such as mannitol); presence of fever, vomiting, diarrhea, or disease processes that increase extracellular fluid volume (e.g., renal disease, primary aldosteronism, excessive steroids/Cushing's disease).

Insufficient water intake: administration of tube feedings/high protein diets with minimal fluid intake, ulcer diets primarily using half and half.

Excessive ingestion of sodium chloride; salt water near-drowning.

PATIENT ASSESSMENT DATA BASE

Sodium Excess/Water Deficit

ACTIVITY/REST

May exhibit: Muscle rigidity/tremors, generalized weakness.

CIRCULATION

May exhibit: Postural hypotension.
Tachycardia.

ELIMINATION

May exhibit: Urinary output decreased.

FOOD/FLUID

May report: Thirst.

May exhibit: Mucous membranes dry, sticky.

NEUROSENSORY

May exhibit: Irritability, lethargy/coma, seizures.

SAFETY

May exhibit: Hot, dry flushed skin.
Fever.

Sodium/Water Excess

CIRCULATION

May exhibit: Elevated blood pressure, hypertension.

ELIMINATION

May exhibit: Polyuria.

FOOD/FLUID

May exhibit: Skin pale, moist, taut with pitting edema.
Weight gain.

NEUROSENSORY

May exhibit: Confusion, lethargy.

RESPIRATION

May exhibit: Dyspnea.

TEACHING/LEARNING

Refer to predisposing/contributing factors.

Discharge Plan Considerations: May require assistance with changes in therapeutic regimen, dietary management.

DIAGNOSTIC STUDIES

Serum sodium: increased, >145 mEq/l. Serum levels greater than 160 mEq/l may be accompanied by severe neurologic signs.

Serum chloride: increased, >106 mEq/l.

Serum potassium: decreased.

Serum osmolality: >295 mOsm/l when dehydrated; lower in presence of extracellular fluid excess.

Hct: may be normal or elevated.

Urine sodium: <50 mEq/l.

Urine chloride: <50 mEq/l.

Urine osmolality: >800 mOsm/l.

Urine specific gravity: increased, >1.030, if water deficit present except when hypernatremia is due to polyuria.

ACTIONS/INTERVENTIONS	RATIONALE
Independent	
Monitor blood pressure.	Either hypertension or hypotension may be present, depending on the fluid status. Presence of postural hypotension may affect activity tolerance.
Note respiratory rate, depth.	Deep labored respirations with air hunger suggest metabolic acidosis (hyperchloremia), which can lead to cardiopulmonary arrest if not corrected.
Monitor intake/output, urine specific gravity. Weigh daily. Assess presence/location of edema.	These parameters are variable depending on fluid status and are indicators of therapy needs/effectiveness.
Assess level of consciousness and muscular strength, tone, movement.	Sodium imbalance may cause changes, which vary from confusion and irritability to seizures and coma. In presence of water deficit, rapid rehydration may cause cerebral edema.
Maintain seizure precautions, if indicated.	Sodium excess/cerebral edema increases risk of convulsions.
Assess skin turgor, color, temperature, and mucous membrane moisture.	Water deficit will be manifested by signs of dehydration.
Provide meticulous skin care and frequent repositioning.	Maintains skin integrity.
Provide frequent oral care. Avoid use of mouthwash/rinse that contains alcohol.	Promotes comfort and prevents further drying of mucous membranes.
Recommend avoidance of foods high in sodium, e.g., canned soups/vegetables, processed foods, snack foods, and condiments.	Reduces risk of sodium-associated complications.

ACTIONS/INTERVENTIONS	RATIONALE
Collaborative	
Assist with identification/treatment of underlying cause.	Refer to listing of predisposing/contributing factors.
Monitor serum electrolytes, osmolality, and ABGs as indicated.	Evaluates therapy needs/effectiveness. Note: Co-occurring hyperchloremia may cause metabolic acidosis, requiring buffering, e.g., sodium bicarbonate.
Increase oral/IV fluid intake, e.g., 5% dextrose (in water in presence of dehydration); 0.9% NaCl (if extracellular deficit is present).	Replacement of total body water deficit will gradually restore sodium/water balance. Note: Rapid reduction of serum sodium level with corresponding decrease in serum osmolality can cause cerebral edema/convulsions.
Restrict sodium intake and administer diuretics as indicated.	Restriction of sodium intake while promoting renal clearance lowers serum sodium levels in the presence of extracellular fluid excess.

POTASSIUM

Potassium is the major cation of the intracellular fluid and is responsible for maintaining intracellular osmotic pressure. Potassium also regulates neuromuscular excitability, aids in maintenance of acid–base balance, synthesis of protein, and metabolism of carbohydrates. Normal serum range 3.5 to 5.0 mEq/l (body total of 42 mEq/l).

HYPOKALEMIA (POTASSIUM DEFICIT)

PREDISPOSING/CONTRIBUTING FACTORS

Renal loss: use of potassium wasting diuretics, diuretic phase of ATN, healing phase of burns; diabetic acidosis; Cushing's syndrome; nephritis, hypomagnesemia, steroid administration.

Gastrointestinal loss: profuse vomiting, excessive diarrhea, frequent use of laxatives, GI suction, inflammatory bowel disease, fistulas.

Liver disease.

Inadequate dietary intake: starvation, high sodium diet; use of hyperalimentation, or conditions resulting in hypersecretion of insulin.

Severe alkalosis or use of IV glucose/insulin solutions to reverse acidosis; mechanical hyperventilation, e.g., correction of increased intracranial pressure.

PATIENT ASSESSMENT DATA BASE

ACTIVITY/REST

May report: Generalized weakness, lethargy, fatigue.

CIRCULATION

May exhibit: Hypotension.
Pulses weak/diminished, irregular.
Heart sounds distant.
Dysrhythmias: PVCs, ventricular tachycardia/fibrillation.

ELIMINATION

May exhibit: Nocturia, polyuria if factors contributing to hypokalemia include CHF or diabetes mellitus.

917

Bowel sounds diminished, decreased bowel motility, paralytic ileus. Abdominal distention.

FOOD/FLUID

May report: Anorexia, nausea/vomiting.

NEUROSENSORY

May report: Paresthesias.

May exhibit: Depressed mental state/confusion, apathy, drowsiness, irritability, coma. Hyporeflexia, tetany, paralysis.

PAIN/COMFORT

May report: Muscle pain/cramps.

RESPIRATION

May exhibit: Hypoventilation/decreased respiratory depth due to muscle weakness/paralysis of diaphragm; apnea, cyanosis.

TEACHING/LEARNING

Refer to predisposing/contributing factors.

Discharge Plan Considerations: May require assistance with changes in therapeutic regimen, dietary management.

DIAGNOSTIC STUDIES

Serum potassium: decreased, <3.5 mEq/l.

Serum chloride: often decreased, <98 mEq/l.

Plasma bicarbonate: increased, >29 mEq/l.

Urine osmolality: decreased.

ECG: low voltage; flat or inverted T wave, appearance of U wave, depressed S–T segment, peaked P waves; prolonged Q–T interval, ventricular dysrhythmias.

ACTIONS/INTERVENTIONS	RATIONALE
Independent	
Monitor heart rate/rhythm.	Tachycardia may develop, and potentially life-threatening dysrhythmias, e.g., PVCs, sinus bradycardia, AV blocks, AV dissociation, ventricular tachycardia.
Monitor respiratory rate, depth, effort. Encourage cough/deep breathing exercises; reposition frequently.	Respiratory muscle weakness may proceed to paralysis and eventual respiratory arrest.
Assess level of consciousness and neuromuscular function, e.g., strength, sensation, movement.	Apathy, drowsiness, irritability, tetany, parathesias, and coma may occur.
Auscultate bowel sounds, noting decrease/absence/change.	Paralytic ileus commonly follows gastric losses through vomiting/gastric suction.
Maintain accurate record of urinary, gastric, and wound losses.	Guide for calculating fluid/potassium replacement needs.

ACTIONS/INTERVENTIONS	**RATIONALE**

Independent

Monitor rate of IV potassium administration using micro/minidrop infusion devices. Check for side effects. Provide ice pack as indicated.

Assures controlled delivery of medication to prevent bolus effect and reduce associated discomfort, e.g., burning sensation at IV site. When solution cannot be administered via central vein, and slowing rate is not possible/effective, ice pack to infusion site may help relieve discomfort.

Encourage intake of foods and fluids high in potassium, e.g., bananas, oranges, dried fruits, red meat, turkey, salmon, coffee, colas, tea, leafy vegetables, peas, baked potatoes, tomatoes, winter squash. Discuss use of potassium chloride salt substitutes for patient receiving long-term diuretics.

Potassium may be replaced/level maintained through the diet when the patient is allowed oral food and fluids.

Review drug regimen for potassium wasting drugs, e.g., furosemide (Lasix), hydrochlorothiazide (Diamox), IV catecholamines, gentamicin (Garamycin), carbenicillin (Geocillin), amphotericin (Fungizone).

If alternate agents (e.g., potassium-sparing diuretics such as Aldactone, Dyrenium, Midamar) cannot be administered, continued use will require close monitoring of potassium level.

Dilute oral potassium supplements (SSKI) with 4 oz water/juice and give after meals.

May prevent/reduce GI irritation. Tablet forms of potassium may be used when gastric irritation is a recurrent problem, e.g., Micro-K.

Watch for signs of digitalis intoxication when used (e.g., complaints of nausea/vomiting, blurred vision, increasing atrial dysrhythmias, and heart block).

Low potassium enhances effect of digitalis, slowing cardiac conduction. Note: Combined effects of digitalis, diuretics, and hypokalemia may produce lethal dysrhythmias.

Observe for signs of metabolic alkalosis, e.g., hypoventilation, tachycardia, dysrhythmias, tetany, changes in mentation. (Refer to CP: Metabolic Alkalosis, p. 933.)

Frequently preceeds/follows hypokalemia.

Collaborative

Assist with identification/treatment of underlying cause.

Refer to listing of predisposing/contributing factors.

Monitor laboratory studies, e.g.:

    Serum potassium;

Levels should be checked frequently during replacement therapy, especially in the presence of insufficient renal function. Sudden excess/elevation may cause cardiac dysrhythmias.

    ABGs;

Correction of alkalosis will increase serum potassium level and reduce replacement needs. Correction of acidosis will drive potassium back into cells, resulting in decreased serum levels and increased replacement needs.

    Serum magnesium;

Hypomagnesemia impairs potassium retention.

    Serum chloride.

Use of diuretics, e.g., Lasix, HydroDiuril may also cause chloride as well as potassium depletion.

Administer oral (e.g., KCl elixir, S–lor, Slow–K) and/or IV potassium.

Parenteral replacement should not exceed 40 mEq/2-hour period. Dietary supplementation may also be used to produce a gradual equilibration if patient is able to take oral food and fluids.

HYPERKALEMIA (POTASSIUM EXCESS)

PREDISPOSING/CONTRIBUTING FACTORS

Potassium retention: decreased renal excretion (e.g., renal disease/acute failure), hypovolemia, use of potassium-sparing diuretics.

Excessive potassium intake: salt substitutes, drugs containing potassium (e.g., penicillin), too rapid IV administration of potassium.

Release of potassium into serum by destruction of tissue/cells, e.g., severe catabolism, burns, crush injuries, myocardial infarction, severe hemolysis, rhabdomyolysis, massive transfusion of banked blood, chemotherapy with cytotoxic drugs.

Adrenocortical insufficiency (inadequate amounts of glucocorticoid and mineralocorticoid hormones).

Shifts of potassium out of the cell due to metabolic acidosis, anoxia, insulin deficiency.

PATIENT ASSESSMENT DATA BASE

Data are dependent on degree of elevation as well as length of time condition has existed.

ACTIVITY/REST

May exhibit: Generalized weakness.

CIRCULATION

May exhibit: Irregular pulse, bradycardia.

ELIMINATION

May report: Abdominal cramps, diarrhea.

May exhibit: Urine volume decreased.
Hyperactive bowel sounds.

FOOD/FLUID

May report: Nausea, vomiting.

NEUROSENSORY

May report: Paresthesias (often of face, tongue, hands, feet).

May exhibit: Decreased deep tendon reflexes; progressive, ascending flaccid paralysis; twitching, seizures.
Apathy, confusion.

TEACHING/LEARNING

Refer to predisposing/contributing factors.

Discharge Plan Considerations: May require assistance with changes in therapeutic regimen, dietary management.

DIAGNOSTIC STUDIES

Serum potassium: increased, >5.5 mEq/l.

Renal function studies: may be altered indicating failure.

Leukocyte or thrombocyte count: elevation may cause a pseudohyperkalemia affecting choice of interventions.

ECG changes: T waves tall and peaked/tented, prolonged P–R interval, loss of P waves, widening of QRS complex, shortened Q–T interval, and S–T segment depression; atrial/ventricular dysrhythmias, e.g., bradycardia, atrial arrest, complete heart block, ventricular fibrillation, cardiac arrest.

ACTIONS/INTERVENTIONS	RATIONALE
Independent	
Monitor respiratory rate and depth. Elevate head of bed. Encourage cough/deep breathing exercises.	Patients may hypoventilate and retain carbon dioxide, leading to respiratory acidosis. Muscular weakness can affect respiratory muscles and lead to respiratory complications of infection/respiratory failure.
Monitor heart rate/rhythm. Be aware that cardiac arrest can occur.	Excess potassium depresses myocardial conduction. Bradycardia can progress to cardiac fibrillation/arrest.
Monitor urine output.	In kidney failure, potassium is retained because of improper excretion. Potassium should not be given if oliguria or anuria is present.
Assess level of consciousness, neuromuscular function, e.g., movement, strength, sensation.	Patient is usually awake and alert, while muscular paresthesia, weakness, and flaccid paralysis may occur.
Assist with active/passive range of motion exercises.	Improves muscular tone and reduces muscle cramps and pain.
Encourage frequent rest periods; assist with care activities, as indicated.	General muscle weakness decreases activity tolerance.
Review drug regimen for medications containing/affecting potassium excretion, e.g., penicillin G, Aldactone, Midamar, Dyazide, Maxzide.	May require alternate drug choices or changes in dosage/frequency.
Identify/discontinue dietary sources of potassium, e.g., tomatoes, broccoli, orange juice, bananas, bran, chocolate, dairy products, dried fruits.	Facilitates reduction of potassium level and may prevent recurrence of hyperkalemia.
Stress importance of patient notifying future care givers when chronic condition potentiates development of hyperkalemia.	May help prevent recurrence.
Collaborative	
Assist with identification/treatment of underlying cause.	Refer to listing of predisposing/contributing factors.
Monitor laboratory results, e.g., serum potassium, ABGs, BUN/creatinine, glucose as indicated.	Evaluates therapy needs/effectiveness. Note: Hypoventilation may result in respiratory acidosis, thereby increasing serum potassium levels.
Administer medications as indicated:	
Diuretics, e.g., furosemide (Lasix);	Promotes renal clearance and excretion of potassium.
IV glucose with insulin, $NaHCO_3$;	Short term emergency measure to move potassium into the cell, thus reducing toxic serum level. Note: Use with caution in presence of CHF or hypernatremia.
Calcium gluconate/chloride;	Temporary measure that antagonizes toxic potassium depressant effects on heart and stimulates cardiac contractility. Note: Calcium is contraindicated in patients on digitalis because it increases the cardiotonic effects of the drug and may cause dysrhythmias.
Sodium chloride;	Enhances renal excretion of potassium.
Kayexalate, with sorbitol per nasogastric tube/enema.	Resin that exchanges potassium for sodium or calcium in the GI tract. Sorbitol enhances evacuation. Note: Use cautiously in patients with CHF, edema, and

ACTIONS/INTERVENTIONS	RATIONALE
Collaborative	
	the elderly because it contains sodium. In addition, Kayexalate may cause hyperchloremia.
Restrict potassium-containing fluids and salt substitutes. Increase carbohydrates/fats and foods low in potassium, e.g., canned fruits, refined cereals, apple/cranberry juice.	Reduces exogenous sources of potassium and prevents catabolic tissue breakdown with release of cellular potassium.
Infuse potassium-based medication/solutions slowly.	Prevents administration of concentrated bolus, allows time for kidneys to clear excess free potassium.
Provide fresh blood or washed RBCs (when possible) if transfusions required.	Fresh blood has less potassium than banked blood, because breakdown of older red cells releases potassium.
Prepare for/assist with dialysis (peritoneal or hemodialysis).	May be required when more conservative methods fail or are contraindicated, e.g., severe CHF. (Refer to CP: Renal Dialysis, p. 567.)

CALCIUM

Calcium is involved in bone formation/reabsorption, neural transmission/muscle contraction, regulation of enzyme systems and is a coenzyme in blood coagulation. Normal serum level is 4.5–5.3 mEq/l, or 8.5 to 10.5 mg/dl.

HYPOCALCEMIA (CALCIUM DEFICIT)

PREDISPOSING/CONTRIBUTING FACTORS

Excessive gastrointestinal losses: draining fistula, diarrhea, fat malabsorption, chronic laxative use (particularly phosphate-containing laxatives/enemas).

Massive subcutaneous tissue infections, burns, peritonitis, acute pancreatitis, malignancies.

Extreme stress situations with mobilization and excretion of calcium.

Diuretic and terminal phase of renal failure.

Inadequate dietary intake, lack of milk/vitamin D, excessive protein diet.

Use of anticonvulsants, antibiotics, corticosteroids, multiple infusion of citrated blood, calcium-free infusions; rapid infusion of Plasmanate.

Primary hypoparathyroidism: hyperphosphatemia, hypomagnesemia.

Malignant neoplasms with bone metastases.

Alkalosis.

PATIENT ASSESSMENT DATA BASE

CIRCULATION

May exhibit:	Hypotension.
	Pulses weak/decreased, irregular (weak cardiac contraction/premature dysrhythmias).

ELIMINATION

May report:	Diarrhea, abdominal pain.
May exhibit:	Abdominal distention (paralytic ileus).

FOOD/FLUID

May report: Nausea/vomiting.

NEUROSENSORY

May report: Circumoral paresthesia, numbness of fingers, muscle cramps.

May exhibit: Anxiety, depression, psychoses.

Muscle spasms (carpopedal and laryngeal), increased deep tendon reflexes; tetany, tonic/clonic seizures, positive Trousseau and Chvostek signs.

RESPIRATION

May exhibit: Labored shallow breathing.

SAFETY

May exhibit: Bleeding with no or minimal trauma.

TEACHING/LEARNING

Refer to predisposing/contributing factors.

Discharge Plan Considerations: May require assistance with changes in therapeutic regimen, dietary management.

DIAGNOSTIC STUDIES

Calcium: decreased, <4.5 mEq/l, or 8.5 mg/dl.

Urine Sulkowitch test: shows no precipitate.

ECG: prolonged Q–T interval (characteristic). In severe deficiency, T waves may flatten or invert giving appearance of hypokalemia or myocardial ischemia; ventricular tachycardia may develop.

ACTIONS/INTERVENTIONS	RATIONALE
Independent	
Monitor heart rate/rhythm.	Calcium deficit weakens cardiac muscle/contractility.
Assess respiratory rate, rhythm, effort. Have tracheostomy equipment available.	Laryngeal stridor may develop and result in respiratory emergency/arrest.
Observe for neuromuscular irritability, e.g., tetany, seizures. Assess for presence of Chvostek/Trousseau signs.	Calcium deficit causes repetitive and uncontrolled nerve transmission leading to muscle spasms and hyperirritability.
Provide quiet environment, and seizure precautions.	Reduces CNS stimulation and protects patient from potential injury.
Promote relaxation/stress reduction techniques, e.g., deep-breathing exercises, guided imagery, visualization.	Tetany can be potentiated by hyperventilation and stress. Note: Direct pressure on the nerves (e.g., tightening blood pressure cuff) may also cause tetany.
Check for bleeding from any source (mucous membranes, puncture sites, wounds/incisions, etc.). Note presence of ecchymosis, petechiae.	Alterations in coagulation can occur as a result of calcium deficiency.
Review patient's drug regimen, e.g., use of insulin, mithramycin, parathyroid injection, digitalis.	Some drugs can lower magnesium levels. Digitalis is enhanced by calcium, and, in patient receiving calcium, digitalis intoxication may develop.
Discuss use of laxatives/antacids.	Those containing phosphate may negatively affect calcium metabolism.

ACTIONS/INTERVENTIONS	RATIONALE

Independent

Review dietary intake of vitamins and fat.

Insufficient ingestion of vitamin D and fat impairs absorption of calcium.

Identify sources to increase calcium and vitamin D in diet, e.g., dairy products, beans, cauliflower, eggs, oranges, pineapples, sardines, shellfish. Restrict intake of phosphorus, e.g., barley, bran, whole wheat, rye, liver, nuts, chocolate.

Vitamin D aids in absorption of calcium from intestinal tract. Phosphorus competes with calcium for intestinal absorption.

Encourage use of calcium-containing antacids if needed (e.g., Titralac, Dicarbosil, Tums).

Possible sources for oral replacement to help maintain calcium levels.

Stress importance of meeting calcium needs.

Adverse effects of long-term deficiency include tooth decay, eczema, cataracts, and osteoporosis.

Collaborative

Assist with identification/treatment of underlying cause.

Refer to listing of predisposing/contributing factors.

Monitor laboratory studies, e.g.:

Serum calcium and magnesium; serum albumin, ABGs;

Evaluates therapy needs/effectiveness. Note: Low serum albumin levels or serum pH affects calcium levels, e.g., a low albumin level causes a deceptively low calcium level; alkalosis causes surplus bicarbonate to bind with free calcium, impairing function; acidosis frees calcium, potentiating hypercalcemia.

PT, platelets.

Calcium is an essential part of the clotting mechanism and deficit may lead to excessive bleeding.

Administer calcium gluconate/chloride/gluceptate IV;

Provides rapid treatment in acute calcium deficit (especially in presence of tetany/convulsions).

Oral preparations, e.g., calcium lactate/carbonate;

Oral preparations are useful in correcting subacute deficiencies.

Magnesium sulfate IV/PO if indicated.

Hypomagnesemia is a precipitating factor in calcium deficit.

HYPERCALCEMIA (CALCIUM EXCESS)

PREDISPOSING/CONTRIBUTING FACTORS

Hyperparathyroidism, hyperthyroidism, multiple myeloma/other malignancies, renal disease, skeletal muscle paralysis, parathyroid tumor, sarcoidosis, adrenal insufficiency, tuberculosis.

Excessive administration of vitamin D/A and calcium-containing antacids; prolonged use of thiazides/diuretics, lithium.

Multiple fractures, bone tumors, osteoporosis, osteomalacia, prolonged immobilization causing release of calcium stores.

Milk-alkali syndrome as a side effect of milk/antacid ulcer therapy.

Hypophosphatasia, hyperproteinemia.

PATIENT ASSESSMENT DATA BASE

ACTIVITY/REST

May report:	General malaise, fatigue/weakness.
	Incoordination, ataxia, joint pain.

CIRCULATION

May exhibit: Hypertension.

Irregular pulse, dysrhythmias, bradycardia.

ELIMINATION

May report: Constipation or diarrhea.

May exhibit: Polyuria, nocturia.

Kidney stones/calculi.

FOOD/FLUID

May report: Anorexia, nausea/vomiting, thirst.

Abdominal pain.

NEUROSENSORY

May report: Headache.

May exhibit: Hypotonicity/muscular relaxation, flaccid paralysis, depressed/absent deep tendon reflexes.

Drowsiness, lethargy, apathy, paranoia, personality changes, memory loss, depression, psychosis, stupor/coma (with high calcium levels).

Slurred speech.

PAIN/COMFORT

May report: Epigastric, deep flank, or bone pain.

TEACHING/LEARNING

Refer to predisposing/contributing factors.

Discharge Plan Considerations: May require assistance with changes in therapeutic regimen, dietary management.

DIAGNOSTIC STUDIES

Serum calcium: increased, >5.8 mEq/l, or 10.5 mg/dl.

BUN: increased (calculi can damage kidney).

Serum phosphorus: decreased levels may be noted.

Urine Sulkowitch test: shows heavy precipitate.

Urine calcium: increased.

Urine osmolality: decreased.

Urine specific gravity: decreased.

X-ray: may reveal evidence of bone cavitation, pathologic fracture, osteoporosis, urinary calculi.

ECG changes: shortened S–T segment and Q–T interval, inverted T waves. In severe deficit, QRS may widen, P–R interval lengthen, and ventricular prematurities develop.

ACTIONS/INTERVENTIONS	RATIONALE

Independent

Monitor cardiac rate/rhythm. Be aware that cardiac arrest can occur in hypercalcemic crisis.

Overstimulation of cardiac muscle occurs with resultant dysrhythmias and ineffective cardiac contraction. Sinus bradycardia, sinus dysrhythmias, wandering pacemaker, and AV block may be noted. Hypercalcemia creates a predisposition to cardiac arrest.

925

ACTIONS/INTERVENTIONS	RATIONALE

Independent

Assess level of consciousness and neuromuscular status, e.g., muscle movement, strength, tone.	Nerve and muscle activity is depressed. Lethargy and fatigue can progress to convulsion/coma.
Monitor intake/output; calculate fluid balance.	Efforts to reduce dehydration and encourage urinary clearance of calcium potentiate the risk of fluid imbalance.
Strain urine if flank pain occurs.	Large amount of calcium present in kidney parenchyma may lead to stone formation.
Encourage increased fluid intake (2000–3000 ml/day) and use of acid-ash juices, e.g., cranberry and prune.	Maintains urine flow and acidity, reduces risk of stone formation.
Auscultate bowel sounds.	Hypotonicity leads to constipation when the smooth muscle tone is inadequate to produce peristalsis.
Maintain bulk in diet.	Constipation may be a problem because of decreased gastrointestinal tone.
Turn frequently, and do range-of-motion and/or muscle-setting exercises with caution. Encourage ambulation if able.	Muscle activity may reduce calcium shifting from the bones that occurs during immobilization. Note: Increased risk for pathologic fractures exists due to calcium shifts out of the bones.
Provide safety measures, e.g., gentle handling when moving/transferring patient.	Reduces risk of pathologic fractures.
Review drug regimen, noting use of heparin, tetracyclines, methicillin, phenytoin.	These drugs can elevate calcium level.
Identify/restrict sources of calcium intake, e.g., dairy products, eggs, and spinach; calcium-containing antacids (Titralac, Dicarbosil, Tums).	Foods or drugs containing calcium may need to be limited in chronic conditions causing hypercalcemia.

Collaborative

Assist with identification/treatment of underlying cause.	Refer to listing of predisposing/contributing factors.
Monitor laboratory studies, e.g., calcium, magnesium, phosphate.	Monitors therapy needs/effectiveness. Note: Phosphate levels may be low when parathyroid hormone inversely promotes calcium uptake and calcium competes with phosphate for absorption/transport with vitamin D.
Administer isotonic saline and sodium sulfate IV/orally.	Dilutes extracellular calcium concentration and inhibits tubular reabsorption of calcium, increasing urinary excretion.
Administer medications as indicated:	
Diuretics, e.g., furosemide (Lasix);	Diuresis promotes renal excretion of calcium and reduces risks of fluid excess from isotonic saline infusion.
Sodium bicarbonate (NaHCO$_3$);	Induces alkalosis, thereby reducing the ionized calcium fraction.
Phosphate;	Rapid acting agent which induces calcium excretion, inhibits resorption of bone.
Steroid therapy;	Inhibits intestinal absorption of calcium and reduces inflammation and associated stress response that mobilizes calcium from the bone.
Mithramycin (Mithracin);	Antibiotic which lowers serum calcium by inhibiting bone resorption.

ACTIONS/INTERVENTIONS	RATIONALE
Collaborative	
Ethylenediaminetetraacetic acid (EDTA);	Chelating action lowers serum calcium level.
Calcitonin;	Promotes movement of serum calcium into bones temporarily reducing serum calcium levels especially in the presence of increased parathyroid hormone.
Neutra-Phos, Fleet Phospho-Soda.	These drugs bind calcium in the GI tract promoting excretion.
Prepare for/assist with hemodialysis.	Rapid reduction of serum calcium may be necessary to correct life-threatening situation.

MAGNESIUM

Magnesium influences carbohydrate metabolism, secretion of parathyroid hormone, sodium/potassium transport across the cell membrane, and synthesis of protein and nucleic acid; activates ATP; and mediates neural transmission within the CNS. Normal serum range, 1.5–2.5 mEq/l or 1.8–3.0 mg/dl.

HYPOMAGNESEMIA (MAGNESIUM DEFICIT)

PREDISPOSING/CONTRIBUTING FACTORS

Gastrointestinal losses: biliary/intestinal fistula; surgery (bowel resection, small bowel bypass), impaired GI absorption/malabsorption syndrome, gastric cancer, prolonged GI suction.

Starvation or severe protein malnutrition.

Prolonged intravenous infusion of magnesium-free solutions.

Chronic alcoholism.

Toxemia of pregnancy.

Severe renal disease/diuretic phase of ARF; vigorous and/or prolonged diuresis with mercurial thiazides or loop diuretics, gentamycin toxicity, or use of chemotherapeutic drugs.

Diabetic ketoacidosis, malignancies.

Acute pancreatitis, hypoparathyroidism, SIADH, multiple transfusions of citrated blood.

Primary hyperaldosteronism, hypercalcemia, hyperthyroidism, vitamin D intoxication.

PATIENT ASSESSMENT DATA BASE

ACTIVITY/REST

May report:	Generalized weakness, insomnia.
	Ataxia, vertigo.

CIRCULATION

May exhibit:	Tachycardia, dysrhythmias.
	Hypotension (vasodilation); occasional hypertension.

FOOD/FLUID

May report:	Anorexia, nausea, vomiting, diarrhea.

NEUROSENSORY

May report:	Paresthesia (legs, feet).
	Vertigo.

927

May exhibit:	Nystagmus.
	Musculoskeletal fasciculations/tremors, neuromuscular irritability/spasticity, spontaneous carpopedal spasms, hyperactive deep tendon reflexes, clonus.
	Tetany, convulsions; positive Babinski, Chvostek, and Trousseau signs.
	Disorientation, apathy, depression, irritability, agitation, hallucinations/psychoses, coma.

TEACHING/LEARNING

Refer to predisposing/contributing factors.

| **Discharge Plan Considerations:** | May require assistance with changes in therapeutic regimen, dietary management. |

DIAGNOSTIC STUDIES

Serum magnesium: decreased, <1.6 mEq/l.
Calcium: may be decreased.
ECG: prolonged P–R and Q–T interval, broadened or flat T waves, occasional shortened S–T segment.

ACTIONS/INTERVENTIONS	RATIONALE
Independent	
Monitor cardiac rate/rhythm.	Magnesium influences sodium/potassium transport across the cell membrane and affects excitability of cardiac tissue.
Monitor for signs of digitalis intoxication when used (e.g., complaints of nausea/vomiting, blurred vision; increasing atrial dysrhythmias and heart block).	Magnesium deficit may precipitate digitalis toxicity.
Assess level of consciousness, and neuromuscular status, e.g., movement, strength, reflexes/tone; note presence of Chvostek/Trousseau signs.	Confusion, irritability and psychosis may occur. However, more common manifestations are muscular, e.g., muscle tremors, spasticity, generalized tetany.
Take seizure/safety precautions, e.g., side rails, bed in low position, frequent observation.	Changes in mentation or the development of seizures increases the risk of patient injury.
Provide quiet environment and subdued lighting.	Reduces extraneous stimuli, promotes rest.
Provide range of motion exercises as tolerated.	Reduces deleterious effects of muscle weakness/spasticity.
Place footboard/cradle on bed.	Elevation of linens may prevent spasms.
Auscultate bowel sounds.	Muscle weakness/spasticity may reduce peristalsis and bowel function.
Encourage intake of dairy products, whole grains, green leafy vegetables, meat and fish.	Provides oral replacement of mild magnesium deficits; may prevent recurrence.
Observe for signs of magnesium toxicity, e.g., thirst, feeling hot and flushed, diaphoresis, anxiety, drowsiness, hypotension, increased muscular and nervous system irritability, loss of patellar reflex.	Rapid, excessive IV replacement may lead to toxicity and life-threatening complications.
Collaborative	
Assist with identification/treatment of underlying cause.	Refer to list of predisposing/contributing factors.
Monitor laboratory studies, e.g., serum magnesium and calcium levels.	Evaluates therapy needs/effectiveness.

ACTIONS/INTERVENTIONS	RATIONALE

Collaborative

Administer medications as indicated:

Magnesium sulfate (MgSO₄) or magnesium chloride (MgCl) IV:	IV replacement is preferred in severe deficit because absorption of magnesium from intestinal tract varies inversely with calcium absorption. Note: Calcium gluconate is the antidote should hypermagnesemia occur as evidenced by respiratory depression and hypotension.
MgSO₄ IM, or Mg hydroxide PO;	May be given prophylactically or in nonemergent situations. Injections should be deep IM because they may be painful.
Magnesium-based antacids, e.g., Mylanta, Maalox, Gelusil, Riopan.	Can supplement dietary replacement. Note: Use of these products may cause diarrhea, which can be alleviated by concurrent use of aluminum-containing products, e.g., Amphojel, Basaljel.

HYPERMAGNESEMIA (MAGNESIUM EXCESS)

PREDISPOSING/CONTRIBUTING FACTORS

Excessive intake/absorption: e.g., too rapid replacement of magnesium; excessive use of magnesium-containing drugs/products, e.g., Maalox, Milk of Magnesia, Epsom salts.

Chronic renal disease/failure or untreated diabetic acidosis.

Hyperparathyroidism, aldosterone deficiency, adrenal insufficiency.

Saltwater near-drowning, hypothermia, shock.

Chronic diarrhea; diseases that interfere with gastric absorption.

PATIENT ASSESSMENT DATA BASE

ACTIVITY/REST

May report:	Generalized weakness, lethargy.

CIRCULATION

May exhibit:	Hypotension.
	Pulses weak/irregular, bradycardia.

FOOD/FLUID

May report:	Nausea/vomiting.

NEUROSENSORY

May exhibit:	Decreased level of consciousness, lethargy progressing to coma.
	Depressed deep tendon reflexes progressing to flaccid paralysis.
	Slurred speech.
	Skin flushing, sweating.

RESPIRATION

May exhibit:	Hypoventilation progressing to apnea.

929

TEACHING/LEARNING

Refer to predisposing/contributing factors.

Discharge Plan Considerations: May require assistance with changes in therapeutic regimen, dietary management.

DIAGNOSTIC STUDIES

Serum magnesium: symptomatic levels >3 mEq/l (increase to 12–15 mEq/l results in death).
ECG: prolonged P–R interval, wide QRS, elevated T waves, development of heart block, cardiac arrest.

ACTIONS/INTERVENTIONS	RATIONALE
Independent	
Monitor cardiac rate/rhythm.	Dysrhythmias may develop progressing to cardiac arrest as a direct result of hypermagnesemia on cardiac muscle.
Monitor vital signs.	Hypotension is an early sign of toxicity.
Assess level of consciousness and neuromuscular status, e.g., reflexes/tone, movement, strength.	CNS and neuromuscular depression can cause decreasing level of alertness, progressing to coma, and depressed muscular responses, progressing to flaccid paralysis.
Monitor respiratory rate/depth/rhythm. Encourage cough/deep breathing exercises. Elevate head of bed as indicated.	Neuromuscular transmissions are blocked by magnesium excess, resulting in respiratory muscular weakness and hypoventilation, which may progress to apnea.
Encourage increased fluid intake if appropriate.	Increased hydration enhances magnesium excretion, but fluid intake must be cautious in event of renal/cardiac failure.
Monitor urinary output and 24-hour fluid balance.	Renal failure is the primary contributing factor in hypermagnesemia; and if present, fluid excess can easily occur.
Promote bedrest, assist with personal care activities as needed.	Flaccid paralysis, lethargy, and decreased mentation reduce activity tolerance/ability.
Recommend avoidance of magnesium-containing antacids if used, e.g., Maalox, Mylanta, Gelusil, Riopan.	Limits oral intake to help prevent recurrence.
Collaborative	
Assist with identification/treatment of underlying cause.	Refer to list of predisposing/contributing factors.
Monitor laboratory studies as indicated: serum magnesium and calcium levels.	Evaluates therapy needs/effectiveness.
Administer IV fluids and thiazide diuretics as indicated.	Promotes renal clearance of magnesium (if renal function is normal).
Administer 10% calcium chloride or gluconate IV.	Antagonizes action/reverses symptoms of magnesium toxicity to improve neuromuscular transmission.
Assist with dialysis as needed.	In the presence of renal disease/failure, dialysis may be needed to lower serum levels.

Acid-Base Imbalances

METABOLIC ACIDOSIS (PRIMARY BASE BICARBONATE DEFICIT)

Reflects an excess of acid (hydrogen) and a deficit of base (bicarbonate) resulting from acid overproduction, loss of intestinal bicarbonate, inadequate conservation of bicarbonate, and excretion of acid, or anaerobic metabolism. Compensatory mechanisms to correct this imbalance include an increase in respirations to blow off excess CO_2, an increase in ammonia formation, and acid excretion (H^+) by the kidneys, with retention of bicarbonate and sodium.

PREDISPOSING/CONTRIBUTING FACTORS

Excess accumulation of ketones (acetoacetic acids and other acids) as may occur in diabetes, ketoacidosis, starvation, alcohol intoxication, high-fat diets/lipid administration.

Loss of bicarbonate from the body as may occur in renal acidosis, lactic acidosis from incomplete carbohydrate metabolism, hyperalimentation, vomiting/diarrhea, small bowel/pancreatic fistulas, and ileostomy.

Systemic infections/sepsis, liver failure.

Poisoning, e.g., salicylate intoxication (after initial stage), paraldehyde intoxication, and drug therapy, e.g., Diamox, NH_4Cl.

Use of IV sodium chloride in presence of preexisting kidney dysfunction.

Use of carbonic anyhdrase inhibitors or anion-exchange resins, e.g., cholestyramine (Questran).

PATIENT ASSESSMENT DATA BASE

ACTIVITY/REST

May report: Lethargy, fatigue; muscle weakness.

CIRCULATION

May exhibit: Hypotension, wide pulse pressure.
Pulse may be weak, irregular (dysrhythmias).

ELIMINATION

May report: Diarrhea.

FOOD/FLUID

May report: Anorexia, nausea/vomiting.

NEUROSENSORY

May report: Headache, drowsiness, decreased mental function.

May exhibit: Changes in sensorium, e.g., stupor, confusion, lethargy, depression, delirium, coma.

RESPIRATION

May report: Dyspnea on exertion.

May exhibit: Hyperventilation, Kussmaul respirations (deep, rapid breathing).

TEACHING/LEARNING

Refer to predisposing/contributing factors.

Discharge Plan Considerations: May require change in therapies for underlying disease process/condition.

DIAGNOSTIC STUDIES

Arterial pH: decreased, <7.35.

HCO₃: decreased, <22 mEq/l.

PCO₂: <35–40 mmHg.

Base excess: decreased, <−2.

Serum potassium: increased.

Serum chloride: increased.

Serum glucose: may be decreased or increased dependent on etiology.

Urine pH: decreased, <6.0.

ECG: cardiac dysrhythmias (bradycardia) and pattern changes associated with hyperkalemia, e.g., tall T wave, prolonged P–R interval, wide QRS.

ACTIONS/INTERVENTIONS	RATIONALE
Independent	
Monitor blood pressure.	Arteriolar dilation/decreased cardiac contractility occurs resulting in systemic shock, e.g., hypotension and tissue hypoxia.
Assess level of consciousness and note progressive changes in neuromuscular status, e.g., strength, tone, movement.	Decreased mental function, confusion, seizures, weakness, flaccid paralysis can occur due to hypoxia, hyperkalemia, and decreased pH of CNS fluid.
Provide seizure/coma precautions, e.g., bed in low position, use of side rails, frequent observation.	Protects patient from injury due to decreased mentation/convulsions.
Monitor heart rate/rhythm.	Acidemia may be manifested by changes in ECG configuration and presence of tachy- or bradydysrhythmias as well as increased ventricular irritability (signs of hyperkalemia). Life-threatening cardiovascular collapse may also occur due to vasodilation and decreased cardiac contractility.
Observe for altered respiratory excursion, rate, and depth.	Deep, rapid respirations (Kussmaul) may be noted as a compensatory mechanism to eliminate excess acid. However, as potassium shifts out of cell in an attempt to correct acidosis, respirations may become depressed. Transient respiratory depression may be the result of overcorrection of metabolic acidosis with sodium bicarbonate.
Assess skin temperature, color, capillary refill.	Evaluates circulatory status, tissue perfusion, effects of hypotension.
Auscultate bowel sounds; measure abdominal girth as indicated.	In the presence of coexisting hyperkalemia, gastrointestinal distress (e.g., distention, diarrhea and colic) may occur.
Monitor intake/output and daily weight.	Marked dehydration may be present due to vomiting, diarrhea. Therapy needs are based on underlying cause and fluid balance.
Test/monitor urine pH.	Kidneys attempt to compensate for acidosis by excreting excess hydrogen in the form of weak acids and ammonia. Maximum urine acidity is pH of 4.0.

ACTIONS/INTERVENTIONS	RATIONALE
Collaborative	
Assist with identification/treatment of underlying cause.	Refer to listing of predisposing/contributing factors.
Monitor/graph serial ABGs.	Evaluates therapy needs/effectiveness. Blood bicarbonate and pH should slowly increase toward normal levels.
Monitor serum electrolytes, e.g., potassium.	As acidosis is corrected, serum potassium deficit may occur as potassium shifts back into the cells.
Replace fluids, as indicated depending on underlying etiology, e.g., D5W/saline solutions.	Choice of solution varies with cause of acidosis, e.g., DKA. Dehydration may be present due to gastric/urinary losses. Note: Lactate-containing solutions may be contraindicated in the presence of lactic acidosis.
Administer medications as indicated, e.g.:	
Sodium bicarbonate/lactate or saline IV;	Corrects bicarbonate deficit. Used cautiously to correct severe acidosis (pH < 7.2) because sodium bicarbonate can cause rebound metabolic alkalosis.
Potassium chloride (KCl);	May be required as potassium reenters the cell, causing a serum deficit.
Phosphate;	May be administered to enhance acid excretion in presence of chronic acidosis with hypophosphatemia.
Calcium.	May be given to improve neuromuscular conduction/function.
Modify diet as indicated, e.g., low-protein, high-carbohydrate diet in presence of renal failure or ADA diet for diabetic.	Restriction of protein may be necessary to decrease production of acid waste products, whereas addition of complex carbohydrates will correct acid production from the metabolism of fats in the diabetic.
Administer exchange resins and/or assist with dialysis as indicated.	May be desired to reduce acidosis by decreasing excess potassium and acid waste products if pH < 7.1 and other therapies are ineffective, or CHF develops. (Refer to CP: Renal Dialysis, p. 567.)

METABOLIC ALKALOSIS (PRIMARY BASE BICARBONATE EXCESS)

A deficit of hydrogen ions and an excess of bicarbonate occurs because of excessive intake of sodium bicarbonate, gastric/intestinal loss of acid, renal excretion of hydrogen and chloride, or prolonged hypercalcemia. Compensatory mechanisms include slow, shallow respirations to increase CO_2 level and an increase of bicarbonate excretion and hydrogen reabsorption by the kidneys.

PREDISPOSING/CONTRIBUTING FACTORS

Prolonged vomiting, gastric lavage; diarrhea (if it has a high chloride content).
Use of potent diuretics (e.g., Thiazides, Lasix, ethacrynic acid) with acid loss (hydrogen and potassium).
Excessive use of salt, laxatives, antacids/baking soda, licorice.
Excessive/overzealous correction of metabolic acidosis with sodium bicarbonate ($NaHCO_3$).
Administration of potassium-free IV solutions, citrated blood.
Primary and secondary hyperaldosteronism.
Adrenocortical hormone disease, e.g., Cushing's syndrome or corticosteroid therapy.
Prolonged hypercalcemia (nonparathyroid), hypokalemia.

PATIENT ASSESSMENT DATA BASE

CIRCULATION

May exhibit: Tachycardia, irregularities/dysrhythmias.

FOOD/FLUID

May report: Nausea/vomiting, diarrhea.

NEUROSENSORY

May report: Dizziness.

May exhibit: Hypertonicity of muscles, tetany, tremors, convulsions.
Confusion, irritability, restlessness, belligerence, apathy, coma.

RESPIRATION

May exhibit: Hypoventilation (increases PCO_2 and conserves carbonic acid).

TEACHING/LEARNING

Refer to predisposing/contributing factors.

Discharge Plan   May require change in therapy for underlying disease process/condition.
Considerations:

DIAGNOSTIC STUDIES

Arterial pH: increased, >7.45.

HCO_3: increased, >26 mEq/l.

PCO_2: slightly increased, >38 mmHg.

Base excess: > +2.

Serum chloride: decreased, <98 mEq/l (if alkalosis is hypochloremia) disproportionately to serum sodium decreases.

Serum potassium: decreased.

Serum calcium: usually decreased.

Urine pH: increased, >7.0

Urine chloride: <10 mEq/l suggests chloride responsive alkalosis, whereas levels >20 mEq/l suggest chloride resistance.

ECG: may show hypokalemic changes including peaked P waves, flat T waves, depressed S–T segment, low T wave merging to P wave, and elevated U waves.

ACTIONS/INTERVENTIONS	RATIONALE
Independent	
Monitor respiratory rate, rhythm, and depth.	Hypoventilation is a compensatory mechanism to conserve carbonic acid and represents definite risks to the individual, e.g., hypoxemia and respiratory failure.
Assess level of consciousness and neuromuscular status, e.g., strength, tone, movement; note presence of Chvostek/Trousseau signs.	The central nervous system may be hyperirritable (increased pH of CNS fluid), resulting in tingling, numbness, dizziness, restlessness, or apathy and confusion. Hypocalcemia may contribute to tetany (although occurrence is rare).
Monitor heart rate/rhythm.	Atrial/ventricular ectopics and tachydysrhythmias may develop.

ACTIONS/INTERVENTIONS	RATIONALE

Independent

Record amount and source of output. Monitor intake and daily weight.

Helpful in identifying source of ion loss; e.g., potassium and HCl are lost in vomiting and GI suctioning.

Restrict oral intake and reduce noxious environmental stimuli; use intermittent/low suction during NG suctioning; irrigate gastric tube with isotonic solutions, rather than water.

Limits gastric losses of hydrochloric acid, potassium, and calcium.

Provide seizure/safety precautions as indicated, e.g., padded side rails, airway protection, bed in low position, frequent observation.

Changes in mentation and CNS/neuromuscular hyperirritability may result in patient harm, especially if tetany/convulsions occur.

Encourage intake of foods and fluids high in potassium and possibly calcium (dependent on blood level), e.g., canned grapefruit and apple juices, bananas, cauliflower, dried peaches, figs, and wheat germ.

Useful in replacing potassium losses when oral intake permitted.

Review medication regimen for use of diuretics (Thiazide, Lasix, ethacrynic acid); and cathartics.

Discontinuation of these drugs may prevent recurrence of imbalance.

Instruct patient to avoid use of excessive amounts of sodium bicarbonate.

Ulcer patients often take baking soda and Milk of Magnesia in addition to prescribed alkaline substances.

Collaborative

Assist with identification/treatment of underlying disorder.

Refer to listing of predisposing/contributing factors.

Monitor laboratory studies as indicated, e.g., ABGs/pH, serum electrolytes (especially potassium), and BUN.

Evaluates therapy needs/effectiveness and monitors renal function.

Administer medications as indicated, e.g.:

Sodium chloride (NaCl) PO/Ringer's solution IV unless contraindicated;

Correcting sodium, water, and chloride defects may be all that is needed to permit kidneys to excrete bicarbonate and correct alkalosis but must be used with caution in patients with CHF or renal insufficiency.

Potassium chloride (KCl);

Hypokalemia is frequently present. Chloride is needed so kidney can absorb sodium with chloride, enhancing excretion of bicarbonate.

Ammonium chloride or arginine hydrochloride;

Increases amount of circulating hydrogen ions. Monitor administration closely to prevent too rapid a decrease in pH, hemolysis of red blood cells. Note: May cause rebound metabolic acidosis and is usually contraindicated in patients with renal/hepatic failure.

Acetazolamide (Diamox);

A carbonic anhydrase inhibitor that increases renal excretion of bicarbonate.

Spironolactone (Aldactone).

Effective in treating chloride resistant alkalosis, e.g., Cushing's.

Avoid/limit use of sedatives or hypnotics.

If respirations are depressed may cause hypoxia/respiratory failure.

Encourage fluids IV/PO.

Replaces extracellular fluid losses.

Administer supplemental oxygen as indicated.

Respiratory compensation for metabolic alkalosis is hypoventilation, which may cause decreased PaO_2 levels/hypoxia.

Assist with dialysis as needed.

Useful when renal dysfunction prevents clearance of bicarbonate.

935

RESPIRATORY ACIDOSIS (PRIMARY CARBONIC ACID EXCESS)

Represents an elevation of P_{CO_2} with resultant excess of carbonic acid (H_2CO_3) due to primary defects in lung function or changes in normal respiratory pattern. Compensatory mechanisms include an increased respiratory rate; Hb (hemoglobin) buffering carbonic acid, forming bicarbonate ions and deoxygenated hemoglobin; and an increased renal formation of ammonia acid excretions, with reabsorption of bicarbonate.

PREDISPOSING/CONTRIBUTING FACTORS

Hypoventilation with retention of CO_2, as in COPD, pneumonia, asthma, airway obstructions, smoke inhalation, acute pulmonary edema, hemo/pneumothorax, atelectasis, mechanical ventilators, or pickwickian syndrome; excessive CO_2 intake, e.g., use of rebreathing mask, CVA therapy.

Decreased function of respiratory center, such as with head trauma, oversedation, barbiturate poisoning, general anesthesia, metabolic alkalosis.

Neuromuscular disorders, such as Guillain–Barré and myasthenia gravis, botulism, spinal cord injuries, or with potassium imbalances.

PATIENT ASSESSMENT DATA BASE

ACTIVITY/REST

May report:	Fatigue.
May exhibit:	Generalized weakness, ataxia, loss of coordination.

CIRCULATORY

May exhibit:	Tachycardia, dysrhythmias.
	Diaphoresis, pallor, and cyanosis (late stage of hypoxia).

FOOD/FLUID

May report:	Nausea/vomiting.

NEUROSENSORY

May report:	Headache, dizziness, visual disturbances.
May exhibit:	Confusion, apprehension, agitation, restlessness, somnolence, coma.
	Tremors, decreased reflexes.

RESPIRATORY

May report:	Dyspnea with exertion.
May exhibit:	Increased respiratory effort with nasal flaring/yawning.
	Decreased respiratory rate.
	Crackles, wheezes, stridor.

TEACHING/LEARNING

Refer to predisposing/contributing factors.

Discharge Plan Considerations:	May require assistance with changes in therapies for underlying disease process/condition.

DIAGNOSTIC STUDIES

Arterial pH: decreased, <7.35.

HCO_3: normal or increased, >26 mEq/l.

PCO_2: increased, >45 mmHg.
PO_2: normal or decreased.
Urine pH: decreased, 6.0.
Serum potassium: normal or increased.
Serum calcium: increased.
Serum chloride: decreased.

ACTIONS/INTERVENTIONS	RATIONALE
Independent	
Monitor respiratory rate, depth and effort.	Corresponding hypoxemia leads to respiratory distress/failure.
Auscultate breath sounds.	Identifies area(s) of decreased ventilation/airway obstruction and therapy needs/effectiveness.
Assess for decreased level of consciousness.	Signals severe acidotic state, which requires immediate attention. Sensorium clears slowly because it takes longer for hydrogen ions to clear from cerebrospinal fluid.
Monitor heart rate/rhythm.	Tachycardia develops in an attempt to increase oxygen delivery to the tissues. Dysrhythmias may occur due to hypoxia (myocardial ischemia) and electrolyte imbalances.
Note skin color, temperature, moisture.	Diaphoresis, pallor, cool/clammy skin are associated with hypoxemia.
Encourage/assist with turning, coughing, and deep breathing. Place in semi-Fowler's position. Suction as necessary. Provide airway adjunct as indicated.	These measures improve ventilation and prevent airway obstruction or decreased alveolar diffusion/perfusion.
Collaborative	
Assist with identification/treatment of underlying cause.	Refer to listing of predisposing/contributing factors.
Monitor/graph serial ABGs; serum electrolyte levels.	Evaluates therapy needs/effectiveness.
Administer oxygen as indicated by mask, cannula, or mechanical ventilation. Increase respiratory rate or tidal volume of ventilator.	Prevents/corrects hypoxemia and respiratory failure. Note: Must be used with caution in presence of emphysema/COPD because respiratory depression/failure may result.
Administer medications as indicated, e.g.:	
Naloxone hydrochloride (Narcan);	May be useful in arousing patient and stimulating respiratory function in presence of drug sedation.
Sodium bicarbonate ($NaHCO_3$);	Given in emergent situations if pH is less than 7.25 and hyperkalemia coexists to correct acidosis. Note: Rebound alkalosis or tetany may occur.
IV solutions of Ringer's lactate or 0.6 M solution of sodium lactate;	May be useful in nonemergent situations to help control acidosis, until underlying respiratory problem can be corrected.
Potassium chloride (KCl).	Acidosis shifts potassium out of cells and hydrogen into cells. Correction of acidosis may then cause serum hypokalemia as potassium reenters the cell. Either imbalance can impair neuromuscular/respiratory function.
Limit use of hypnotic sedatives or tranquilizers.	In the presence of hypoventilation, respiratory depression can occur with the use of sedatives, and CO_2 narcosis may develop.

937

ACTIONS/INTERVENTIONS	RATIONALE
Collaborative	
Maintain hydration (IV/PO)/provide humidification.	Assists in thinning/mobilization of secretions.
Provide aggressive chest physiotherapy, including postural drainage and suctioning as indicated.	Aids in clearing secretions which may improve ventilation, allowing excess CO_2 to be eliminated.
Assist with ventilatory aids, e.g., IPPB in conjunction with bronchodilators.	Increases lung expansion and opens airways to improve ventilation preventing respiratory failure.

RESPIRATORY ALKALOSIS (PRIMARY CARBONIC ACID DEFICIT)

There is a decrease in PCO_2 with a deficit of carbonic acid (H_2CO_3) due to a marked increase in the rate of respirations. Compensatory mechanisms include decreased respiratory rate (if the body is able to respond to the drop in PCO_2) to retain CO_2, increased renal excretion of bicarbonate, and retention of hydrogen.

PREDISPOSING/CONTRIBUTING FACTORS

Hyperventilation caused by nervousness, anxiety, intentional overbreathing, hysteria/extreme emotions; fever; sepsis (usually gram-negative organism), meningitis; severe pain; brain trauma/lesions; multiple pulmonary emboli; or mechanical ventilators.

Restrictive problems, such as asthma, pulmonary fibrosis, pregnancy (abdominal distention with elevation of diaphragm).

Oxygen lack, such as high altitude sickness, severe anemia, hypoxemia.

Congestive heart failure, alcoholic intoxication, cirrhosis, thyrotoxicosis.

Paraldehyde, epinephrine, or early salicylate intoxication.

Rapid correction of metabolic acidosis, e.g., peritoneal dialysis.

PATIENT ASSESSMENT DATA BASE

CIRCULATION

May exhibit:	Hypotension.
	Pulse irregular if dysrhythmias present.

FOOD/FLUID

May report:	Nausea/vomiting.

NEUROSENSORY

May report:	Headache.
	Numbness/tingling of face and hands, circumoral paresthesia.
	Syncope, vertigo.
May exhibit:	Confusion, restlessness, anxiety, obtundation, coma.
	Muscle weakness, hyperreflexia, positive Chvostek's sign, tetany, seizures.

PAIN/COMFORT

May report:	Muscle cramps.

RESPIRATION

May exhibit:	Tachypnea, rapid shallow breathing, dyspnea.

938

TEACHING/LEARNING

Refer to predisposing/contributing factors.

Discharge Plan Considerations: May require change in treatment/therapy of underlying disease process/condition.

DIAGNOSTIC STUDIES

Arterial pH: >7.45.
HCO₃: normal or decreased, <25 mEq/l.
Pco₂: decreased, <38 mmHg.
Serum potassium: decreased.
Serum chloride: increased.
Serum calcium: decreased.
Urine pH: increased, >7.0.

ACTIONS/INTERVENTIONS	RATIONALE
Independent	
Monitor respiratory rate, depth, and effort; ascertain cause for hyperventilation if possible, e.g., anxiety, pain, improper ventilator settings.	Identifies alterations from usual breathing pattern and influences choice of intervention.
Assess level of consciousness and note neuromuscular status, e.g., strength, tone, reflexes and sensation.	Decreased mentation, and tetany or convulsions may occur.
Demonstrate appropriate breathing patterns and review/assist with ordered treatments, e.g., rebreathing mask/bag.	Decreasing the rate of respirations will elevate Pco₂ level.
Provide support by a calm manner and voice.	May help reassure and calm the agitated patient, thereby aiding in reduction of respiratory rate.
Provide safety/seizure precautions, e.g., bed in low position, padded side rails, frequent observation.	Changes in mentation/CNS and neuromuscular hyperirritability may result in patient harm, especially if tetany/convulsions occur.
Collaborative	
Assist with identification/treatment of underlying cause.	Refer to listing of predisposing/contributing factors.
Monitor/graph serial ABGs.	Identifies therapy needs/effectiveness.
Monitor serum potassium. Replace as indicated.	Hypokalemia may occur as potassium is lost (urine) or shifted into the cell in exchange for hydrogen in an attempt to correct alkalosis.
Provide sedation, as indicated.	May be required to reduce psychogenic cause.
Administer CO₂, or use rebreathing mask as indicated. Reduce respiratory rate/tidal volume, or add additional dead space (tubing) to mechanical ventilator.	Increasing CO₂ retention may correct carbonic acid deficit.

BIBLIOGRAPHY

Books/General References

Assessment. Nurse's Reference Library. Nursing84 Books. Springhouse Corp, Springhouse, PA, 1984.

Beland, I and Passos, J: Clinical Nursing Pathophysiological and Psychosocial Approaches, ed 4. Macmillan, New York, 1981.

Benenson, A: Control of Communicable Diseases in Man, ed 14. JD Lucas, Springfield, 1985.

Berkow, R, et al (eds): The Merck Manual of Diagnosis and Therapy, ed 14. Merck, Sharp and Dohme, Rahway, 1982.

Beyers, M and Dudas, S: The Clinical Practice of Medical-Surgical Nursing, ed 2. Little, Brown & Co, Boston, 1984.

Brunner, L and Suddarth, D: The Lippincott Manual of Nursing Practice, ed 4. JB Lippincott, Philadelphia, 1986.

Davidson, S, et al: Nursing Care Evaluation: Concurrent and Retrospective Review Criteria. CV Mosby, St Louis, 1977.

Definitions. Nurse's Reference Library, Nursing84 Books. Springhouse Corp, Springhouse, PA, 1983.

Deglin, J and Vallerand, A: Nurse's Med Deck. FA Davis, Philadelphia, 1986.

Doenges, M and Moorhouse, M: Nurse's Pocket Guide: Nursing Diagnoses With Interventions, ed 2. FA Davis, Philadelphia, 1988.

Fishbach, F: A Manual of Laboratory Diagnostic Tests, ed 2. JB Lippincott, Philadelphia, 1984.

Griffith, HW: Complete Guide to Prescription and Non-Prescription Drugs, ed 2. H P Books Inc, Tucson, 1985.

Holloway, N: Medical Surgical Care Plans. Springhouse Corp, Springhouse, PA, 1988.

Howe, J, et al: The Handbook of Nursing. John Wiley & Sons, New York, 1984.

Jarvis, L: Community Health Nursing: Keeping the Public Healthy. FA Davis, Philadelphia, 1981.

Johanson, B, et al: Standards for Critical Care, ed 2. CV Mosby, St Louis, 1985.

Kenner, CV, Guzzetta, CE, and Dosey, BM: Critical Care Nursing: Body-Mind-Spirit, ed 2. Little, Brown & Co, Boston, 1985.

Kniesl, C and Ames, S: Adult Health Nursing. Addison-Wesley, Reading, Mass, 1986.

Lewis, S and Collier, I: Medical-Surgical Nursing: Assessment and Management of Clinical Problems, ed 2. McGraw-Hill, New York, 1987.

Liu, P: Blue Book of Diagnostic Tests. Saunders Blue Book Series. WB Saunders, Philadelphia, 1986.

Luckmann, J and Sorensen, K: Medical-Surgical Nursing: A Psychophysiologic Approach, ed 3. WB Saunders, Philadelphia, 1987.

Mathewson, M: Pharmacotherapeutics: A Nursing Approach. FA Davis, Philadelphia, 1986.

Moorhouse, M, Geissler, A, and Doenges, M: Critical Care Plans: Guidelines for Patient Care. FA Davis, Philadelphia, 1987.

Neal, M, Cohen, P, and Reighley, J: Nursing Care Planning Guides. Sets 1–5. Nurseco, Inc, Pacific Palisades, 1981.

Nursing86 Drug Handbook. Nursing86 Books. Springhouse Corp, Springhouse, PA, 1985.

Orland, M and Saltman, R: Manual of Medical Therapeutics, ed 25. Little, Brown & Co, Boston, 1986.

Patient Teaching. Nurses Reference Library. Nursing87 Books. Springhouse Corp, Springhouse, PA, 1986.

Phipps, WJ, Long, BC, and Woods, NF: Medical-Surgical Nursing Concepts and Clinical Practice, ed 3. CV Mosby, St Louis, 1987.

Pittiglio, D and Sacher, R: Clinical Hematology and Fundamentals of Hemostasis. FA Davis, Philadelphia, 1987.

Signs and Symptoms. Clinical Pocket Manual Series. Nursing86 Books. Springhouse Corp, Springhouse, PA, 1985.

Swearingen, P: Manual of Nursing Therapeutics. Addison-Wesley, Menlo Park, 1986.

Thomas, C (ed): Taber's Cyclopedic Medical Dictionary, ed 15. FA Davis, Philadelphia, 1985.

Thompson, J, et al: Clinical Nursing. CV Mosby, St Louis, 1986.

Ulrich, S, Canale, S, and Wendell, S: Nursing Care Planning Guides: A Nursing Diagnosis Approach. WB Saunders, Philadelphia, 1986.

Weber, J: Nurses' Handbook of Health Assessment. JB Lippincott, Philadelphia, 1988.

Wilkins, R and Levinsky, N (eds): Medicine: Essentials of Clinical Practice. Little, Brown & Co, Boston, 1983.

Chapter 1: Articles

DeCrosta, T: Megatrends in nursing. Nursing Life 5(3):18, May/June 1985

Higgerson, N, and Slyck, A: Variable billing for services: New fiscal direction for nursing. J Nurs Admin p 20, June 1982.

McHugh, MK: Has nursing outgrown the nursing process? Nursing87 17(8):50, August 1987.

Reinert, R, and Grant, D: A classification system to meet today's needs. J Nurs Admin p 21, January 1981.

Lombard, N and Light, N: On-line nursing care plans by nursing diagnosis. Computers in Healthcare p 22, November 1983.

Chapter 2: Books

Carnevali, D, et al: Diagnostic Reasoning in Nursing. JB Lippincott, Philadelphia, 1984.
Hurley, M (ed): Classification of Nursing Diagnoses: Proceedings of the Sixth Conference. CV Mosby, St Louis, 1986.
Kelly, MA: Nursing Diagnosis Source Book. Appleton-Century-Crofts, Norwalk, CT, 1985.
Kim, MJ, McFarland, GK, and McLane, AM (eds): Classification of Nursing Diagnoses: Proceedings of the Fifth National Conference. CV Mosby, St Louis, 1984.
McLane, AM (ed): Classification of Nursing Diagnoses: Proceedings of the Seventh Conference. CV Mosby, St Louis, 1987.
Tofias, L: A Workbook About Nursing Diagnosis. Dept of Educational Services, Mississauga Hospital, Mississauga, Ontario.

Chapter 2: Articles

American Nurses' Association: Nursing: A social policy statement. Pub Code: NP-63 35M 12/80, Kansas City, 1980.
American Nurses' Association: Standards of nursing practice. Pub Code: NO-41 10M 1:77, Kansas City, 1973.
Baer, C (ed): Nursing diagnosis. Top Clin Nurs 5(4), January 1984.
Bockrath, M: Your patient needs two diagnoses-medical and nursing. Nursing Life p 29, March/April 1982.
Carpenito, LJ: Actual, potential or possible. AJN 85(4):458, April 1985.
Fadden, TC, et al: Nursing diagnosis: A matter of form. AJN 84(4):470, April 1984.
Guzzetta, CE, et al: Nursing diagnosis: Framework, process and problems. Heart Lung, May 1983.
Humbrecht, B, et al: From assessment to´intervention. Nursing82 12(4):34, April 1982.
Kim, MJ: Without collaboration, what's left? AJN 85(3):281, March 1985.
Rooney, V: Question of habit. Nursing Mirror (19 Suppl):ii, vi, 1982.
Shoemaker, J: How nursing diagnosis helps focus your care. RN p 42, August 1979.
Tartaglia, MJ: Nursing diagnosis: Keystone of your careplan. Nursing85 15(3):34, March 1985.

Chapter 3: Books

Gordon, M: Manual of Nursing Diagnosis. McGraw-Hill, New York, 1982.

Chapter 3: Articles

Kieffer, JS: Nursing diagnosis can make a critical difference. Nursing Life 5(4):18, January 1984.
Neel, CJ: Nursing diagnoses work for you . . . every day. Nursing86 86(5):56, May 1986.

Chapter 4: Books

Andreoli, KG, et al: Comprehensive Cardiac Care, ed 6. CV Mosby, St Louis, 1987.
Gulanick, M, Klopp, A, and Galanes, S (eds): Comprehensive Nursing Care Plan Guides. Michael Reese Hospital and Medical Center, Chicago, 1984.
Kim, MJ, McFarland, GK, and McLane, AM: Pocket Guide to Nursing Diagnoses, ed 2. CV Mosby, St Louis, 1987.
Kochar, MS and Woods, KD: Hypertension Control: For Nurses and Other Health Professionals, ed 2. Springer, New York, 1985.
Underhill, SL, et al: Cardiac Nursing. JB Lippincott, Philadelphia, 1982.

Chapter 4: Articles

Ames, R: Hypertension: The demographics of management and control. Health Education, p 11, August/September 1985.
Baum, P: Heed the early warning signs of peripheral vascular disease. Nursing85 15(3):50, March 1985.
Beare, PG: Calcium entry blockers: Action, use and nursing implications. AAOHN 35(16):261, 1987.
Bently, L: Radionuclide imaging techniques in the diagnosis and treatment of coronary heart disease. Focus on Critical Care 14(6):27, December 1987.
Bower, B: Do Type A men have a survival edge? Science News 133(4):53, January 1988.
Burden, L and Atwell, K: The treacherous waters of unstable angina. Nursing83 (12):50, December 1983.
Burge, S, et al: Perceptions of postoperative incisional pain. AJN 86(11):1263, November 1986.
Dennison, R: Cardiopulmonary assessment: How to do it better in 15 easy steps. Nursing86 16(4):34, April 1986.
Cavallo, G: Valvular heart disease. J Cardiovasc Nurs 1(3), 1987.
Challerjee, K: Acute management of unstable angina. Emergency Medicine, p 270, August 15, 1983.
Conti, R and Christie, L: Sorting out chest pain. Emergency Medicine, p 155, February 15, 1984.
Forshee, T: Track down the what, where, when, and how of chest pain. Nursing86 16(5):34, May 1986.
Heggie, J: Pulling your patient through congestive heart failure. RN 43(6):31, September 1980.
Johnson, J: Valvular heart disease in the elderly. J Cardiovasc Nurs 1(2):72, 1987.
Kerr, JA: Adherence and self-care: Patients treated for hypertension. Heart Lung p 24, June 1985.
Kirkpatrick, MK: Self care guide for hypertension risk reduction. AAOHN 35(6):254, 1987.
McCauley, K: Probing the ins and outs of congestive heart failure. Nursing82 12(11):60, November 1982.
Meehan, PA: Hemodynamic assessment using the automated physiologic profile. Crit Care Nurse p 29, January/February 1986.
Meola, D and Walker, V: Responding quickly to tachydysrhythmias. Nursing87 17(11):34, November 1987.
Miracle, V: Anatomy of a murmur. Nursing86 16(7):26, July 1986.
Moreno, C: Concepts of stress management in cardiac rehabilitation. Focus on Critical Care 14(5):13, October 1987.
Murray, M: Chest pain, dyspnea, confusion: When should you sound the alarm? RN p 66, January 1983.
Norsen, L, Telfair, N, and Wagner, A: Detecting dysrhythmias. Nursing86 16(11):34, November 1986.

Pattilo, M and Knox, T: Postmyocardial infarction syndrome: A case study. Focus on Crit Care 14(5):76, October 1987.

Peterson, F and Bastarache, M: Assessing peripheral vascular disease. AJN 83(11):1549, November 1983.

Powers, MJ and Jalowiec, A: Hypertension, psychosocial factors: Profile of the well-controlled, well-adjusted hypertension patient. Nursing Research p 106, March/April 1987.

Pulliam, B: Encouraging compliance with anti-hypertensive treatment. Nursing Life p 31, May/June 1986.

Ryan, A: Stopping CHF while there's still time. RN p 28, August 1986.

Ryan, P: Strategies for motivating life-style change. J Cardiovasc Nurs 1(4):54, 1987.

Scherer, P: ACLS Guidelines: What nurses are saying about the drug changes. AJN 86(12):1352, December 1986.

Schneider, A: Unreported chest pain in a coronary care unit. Focus on Crit Care 14(5):21, October 1987.

Stanley, M: Helping an elderly patient live with CHF. RN p 35, September 1986.

Stuart, EM: Nonpharmacologic treatment of hypertension: A multiple risk-factor approach. J Cardiovasc Nurs 1(4):1, 1987.

Sumner, S and Grau, P: An update on BCLS standards: The latest in cardiopulmonary resuscitation. Nursing86 16(11):48, November 1986.

Taylor, D: Clinical insights: Congestive heart failure, physiology, signs and symptoms. Nursing83 13(19):44, September 1983.

Taylor, D: Thrombophlebitis: Physiology, signs, and symptoms. Nursing83 13(7):52, July 1983.

Urban, N: Integrating hemodynamic parameters with clinical decision-making. Crit Care Nurse p 48, March/April 1986.

Wagner, DW: Hypertension at its worst. Emergency Medicine p 84, April 15, 1985.

Wilkinson, WE: Hypertension: prevention and control program for hospital employees. AAOHN 35(6):259

Chapter 5: Books

Bates, B: A Guide to Physical Examination. JB Lippincott, Philadelphia, 1983.

Carpenito, LJ: Nursing Diagnosis: Application to Clinical Practice. JB Lippincott, Philadelphia, 1983.

Farer, LS: All About TB: Clinical Notes on Respiratory Disease. American Lung Association, New York, 1978.

Giovani, LE and Hayes, JE: Drugs and Nursing Implications. Appleton-Century-Crofts, Norwalk, CT, 1982.

Guyton, AC: Textbook of Medical Physiology. WB Saunders, Philadelphia, 1981.

Robbins, SR: Pathologic Basis of Disease. WB Saunders, Philadelphia, 1978.

Tilkian, SM, Conover, MB, and Tilkian, AG: Clinical Implications of Laboratory Tests. CV Mosby, St Louis, 1983.

Top, FH and Wehrle, PF: Communicable and Infectious Diseases. CV Mosby, St Louis, 1978.

Chapter 5: Articles

Banaszak, E, et al: Home ventilator care. Resp Care 26(12):1262, December 1981.

Baum, P: Taking the PVD patient's history. Nursing86 16(5):30, May 1986.

Biggs, C: The cancer that can cost a patient his voice. RN p 44, April 1987.

Bradley, R: Adult respiratory distress syndrome. Focus on Critical Care 14(5):48, October 1987.

Brandstetter, R: The adult respiratory distress syndrome. Heart Lung 15(3):155, March 1986.

Burkhart, C: After pneumonectomy. AJN 83(11):1562, November 1983.

Carroll, P: Caring for ventilator patients. Nursing86 16(2):43, February 1986.

Coleman, D: Pneumonia, where nursing care really counts. RN p 22, February 1986.

Coleman, D: RN Master Care Plan: The patient with pneumonia. RN p 28, February 1986.

D'Agostino, J: You can breathe new life into your COPD patients. Nursing83 13(9):72, September 1983.

Dennison, R: Cardiopulmonary assessment: How to do it better in 15 easy steps. Nursing86 16(4):34, April 1986.

Feinstein, D: What to teach the patient who's had a total laryngectomy. RN p 53, April 1987.

Fischer, D and Prentice, W: Feasibility of home care for certain respiratory-dependent restrictive or obstructive lung disease patients. Chest 82(6):739, December 1982.

Forshee, T: Track down the what, where, and how of chest pain. Nursing86 16(5):34, May 1986.

Gerdes L: Recognizing the multisystemic effects of embolism. Nursing87 17(12):34, December 1987.

Greifzu, S, Crebase, C, and Winnick, B: Lung Cancer: By the time it's detected, it may be too late. RN p 52, March 1987.

Irwin, M and Openbrier, D: A delicate balance: Strategies for feeding Ventilated COPD patients. AJN 85(3):274, March 1985.

Karnes, N: Don't let ARDS catch you off guard. Nursing87 17(5):34, May 1987.

McHugh, J: Perfecting the 3 steps of chest physiotherapy. Nursing87 17(11):54, November 1987.

McConnell, E: APTT and PT: Two common—but important—coagulation studies. Nursing86 16(5):47, May 1986.

McNaul, F, et al: Lung Cancer: For 6 Continuing Education Credits. AJN 87(11):1427, November 1987.

Nett, L, Morganroth, M, and Petty, T: Weaning from the ventilator: For CE credit. AJN 87(9):1173, September 1987.

Openbrier, D, Hoffman, L, and Wesmiller, S: Home oxygen therapy: Evaluation and prescription. AJN 88(2):192, February 1988.

Patry-Lahey, R: Helping a laryngectomy patient go home. Nursing85 15(3):63, March 1985.

Quinn, A: Thora-Drain III, closed chest drainage made simpler and safer. Nursing86 16(9):46, September 1986.

Taylor, D: Clinical Applications: Assessing breath sounds. Nursing85 15(3):60, March 1985.

Weiss, R: TB troubles, Tuberculosis is on the rise again. Science News 133(6):92, February 1988.

Chapter 6: Books

Adams, R and Victor, M: Principles of Neurology. McGraw-Hill, New York, 1985.

Albequerque, EX and Edelfrawi, AT (eds): Myasthenia Gravis. Chapman and Hall, New York, 1983.

Asbury, A, et al: Diseases of the Nervous System, Vol II. WB Saunders, Philadelphia, 1986.

Burrell, L and Burrell, Z: Critical Care, ed 4. CV Mosby, St Louis, 1982.

Dau, PC: Plasmapheresis and the immunobiology of Myasthenia Gravis. Houghton Mifflin, Boston, 1987.

Heston, L and White, J: Dementia: A Practical Guide to Alzheimer's Disease and Related Illnesses. WH Freeman & Co, New York, 1983.

Hickey, J: The Clinical Practice of Neurological and Neurosurgical Nursing. JB Lippincott, Philadelphia, 1986.

Hudak, C: Critical Care Nursing, ed 3. JB Lippincott, Philadelphia, 1982.

Kimura, J: Electrodiagnosis in Diseases of Nerve and Muscle: Principles and Practice. FA Davis, Philadelphia, 1983.

Lisak, RP and Barchi, RL: Myasthenia Gravis. WB Saunders, Philadelphia, 1982.

Reisberg, B: Alzheimer's Disease: The Standard Reference. The Free Press, New York, 1983.

Sacks, O: The Man Who Mistook His Wife for a Hat and Other Clinical Tales. Summit Books, New York, 1985.

Spencer, R, et al: Clinical Pharmacology and Nursing Management. JB Lippincott, Philadelphia, 1986.

Stephens, G: Pathophysiology for Health Practitioners. Macmillan, New York, 1980.

Swearingen, P (ed): Photo-atlas of Nursing Procedures. Addison-Wesley, Menlo Park, 1984.

Szobar, A: Crises in Myasthenia Gravis. Hafner, New York, 1970.

Chapter 6: Articles

Anderson, F: Sexual problems of patients with neuromuscular diseases. Medical Aspects of Human Sexuality 18(11):82, November 1984.

Beam IM: Alzheimer's disease: Helping families survive. AJN 85(2):229, February 1984.

Baum, P: Carotid endarterectomy: One strike against stroke. Nursing83 13(3):50, March 1983.

Boylan, A and Brown, P: Neurological observations. Nursing Times 3(9):36, July 1985.

Callanan, M: Epilepsy: Putting the patient back in control. RN p 48, February 1988.

Craven, R and Curry, T: When the diagnosis is Raynauds. AJN 81(5):1007, May 1981.

Jones, HR: Diseases of the peripheral motor-sensory unit. Clinical Symposia 37(2):12.

Chance, P: Life after head injury. Psychology Today p 62, October 1986.

Ferguson, J: Helping an MS patient live a better life. RN p 22, December 1987.

Friedman, D: Taking the scare out of caring for seizure patients. Nursing88 18(2):52, February 1988.

Gary, R, Jermier, B, and Hickey, A: Stroke: How to contain the damage. RN p 36, May 1986.

Hackett, C: Limbering up your neurovascular assessment technique. Nursing83 13(3):40, March 1983.

Hinkle, J: Treating traumatic coma. AJN 86(5):551, May 1986.

Kassirer, M and Osterberg, D: Pain in Multiple Sclerosis. AJN 87(7):968, July 1987.

Kunkel, R, et al: Pitfalls in headache management. Patient Care p 71, March 30, 1987.

Mauss-Clum, N: Bringing the unconscious patient safely back. Nursing82 12(8):34, August 1982.

Mikati, MA and Browne, TR: Tonic-clonic seizure. Hospital Medicine p 19, March 1987.

Nursing Grand Rounds: Small hopes: Care of the patient with head trauma. Nursing86 16(5):52, May 1986.

Nursing Grand Rounds: A man alone . . . and afraid: Caring for the patient with Guillain-Barré syndrome. Nursing87 17(12):44, December 1987.

Pajik, M: Alzheimer's disease: Inpatient care. AJN 84(2):215, February 1984.

Reisberg, B: Alzheimer's disease: Stages of cognitive decline. AJN 84(2):225, February 1984.

Santilli, N and Sierzant, T: Advances in the treatment of epilepsy. J Neurosurg Nurs 19(3):141, March 1987.

Saper, J: Approaches to chronic headache. Hospital Practice p 21, May 30, 1987.

Scherer, P: Assessment: The logic of coma. AJN 86(5):542, May 1986.

Shapira, J, Schleslinger, R and Cummings, J: Distinguishing dementias. AJN 86(6):698, June 1986.

Sullivan, J: Using Neuman's Model in the acute phase of spinal cord injury. Focus on Critical Care 13(5):34, October 1986.

Webster, M: Trends and controversies in head trauma. Nursing Life 4(6):46, November/December 1984.

Whitney, L: Assessing your patient for increased ICP. Nursing87 17(6):34, June 1987.

Chapter 7: Articles

Carver, J: Cataract care made plain. AJN 87(5):626, May 1987.

Lent-Wunderlich, E and Ott, M: Helping your patient through eye surgery. RN p 43, June 1986.

Tooke, MC, Elders, J, and Johnson, DE: Corneal transplantation. AJN 86(6):685, June 1986.

Tumulty, G and Resler, M: Eye Trauma. AJN 84(6):740, June 1984.

Chapter 8: Books

Broadwell, DC and Johnson, DE: Principles of Ostomy Care. CV Mosby, St Louis, 1982.

Do More With Your Life Than Just Cope With It: Managing Your Ostomy. Hollister Inc, 1985.

Ebbitt, J: Spinning: Thought Patterns of Compulsive Eaters. Parkside, Parkridge, IL, 1987.

Givens, BA and Simmons, SJ: Gastroenterology in Clinical Nursing, ed 2. CV Mosby, St Louis, 1975.

Chapter 8: Articles

Arnet, G and Basehore, L: Dentofacial reconstruction. AJN 84(12):1488, December 1984.

Barisonek, K, Newman, E, and Logio, T: "My Stomach Hurts." Nursing84 14(11):34, November 1984.

Black, J and Arnold, J: Facial fractures. AJN 82(7):1086, July 1982.

Brozenec, S: Caring for the postoperative patient with an abdominal drain. Nursing85 15(4):54, April 1985.

Cargile, N: Buying time when you face a bowel obstruction. RN p 40, August 1985.

Decker, S: The life-threatening consequences of a GI bleed. RN p 18, October 1985.

Deters, G: Managing complications after abdominal surgery. RN p 27, March 1987.

Donovan S: When your patient faces jaw reconstruction. RN p 43, January 1987.

Feickert, D: Gastric surgery: Your crucial pre- and postop role. RN p 24, January 1987.

Hedrick, J: Effects of ET nursing intervention on adjustment following ostomy surgery. J Enterostom Ther 14(6):229, December 1987.

Kearns, P: Exercises to ease pain after abdominal surgery. RN p 45, July 1986.
McConnell, E: Meeting the challenge of intestinal obstruction. Nursing87 17(7):34, July 1987.
Miller, B and Gavant, M: Biliary catheter care. AJN 85(10):1115, October 1985.
Neufeldt, J: Helping the IBD patient cope with the unpredictable. Nursing87 17(8):47, August 1987.
Peternel, E: A high-tech approach to a GI problem. RN p 44, June 1985.
Quinless, F: Severe liver dysfunction: Client problems and nursing actions. Focus on Critical Care 12(1):24, February 1985.
Smith, B: CE: The ostomy: How is it managed? AJN 85(11):1246, November 1985.
Watt, R: CE: The ostomy: Why is it created? AJN 85(11):1242, November 1985.

Chapter 9: Books

Gulan, M, Klopp, A, and Galanes, S (eds): Nursing Care Plans: Nursing Diagnosis and Intervention. CV Mosby, St Louis, 1986.
Hodgkin's Disease and the Non-Hodgkin's Lymphomas, Research Report. National Cancer Institute. US Dept of Health and Human Services, 1987.
Jones, D, Dunbar, C, and Jirovec, M: Medical-Surgical Nursing: A Conceptual Approach, ed 2. McGraw-Hill, New York, 1982.
Kee, L: Laboratory and Diagnostic Tests with Nursing Implications, ed 2. Appleton & Lange, Norwalk, CT, 1987.
Lamb, J: Laboratory Tests for Clinical Nursing. Robert J Brady Co, Bowie, MD, 1984.
Leukemia Research Report. National Cancer Institute. US Dept of Health and Human Services, 1987.
Patrick, M, et al: Medical Surgical Nursing: Pathophysiological Concepts. JB Lippincott, Philadelphia, 1986.
Price, S and Wilson, L: Pathophysiology: Clinical Concepts of Disease Processes, ed 3. McGraw-Hill, New York, 1986.
Reich, PR: Hematology: Physiopathologic Basis for Clinical Practice, ed 2. Little, Brown & Co, Boston, 1984.
Taylor, CM and Cress, SS: Nursing87 Nursing Diagnosis Cards. Springhouse Corp, Springhouse, PA, 1987.

Chapter 9: Articles

Carter, Y: Nursing management of Sickle Cell anemia. RN p 47, October 1975.
Conley, CL: Anemia: Accurate diagnosis and appropriate therapy. Hospital Practice 19(9):57, September 1984.
Consalvo, K and Gallagher, M: Winning the battle against Hodgkin's disease. RN p 20, December 1986.
Gibbons, D: Transfusion therapy in Sickle Cell disease. Nurs Clin of North Am 18(1):201, March 1983.
Godwin, M and Baysinger, M: Understanding anti-sickling agents and the sickling process. Nurs Clin North Am 18(1):207, March 1983.
Hagan, SJ: Bring help and hope to the patient with Hodgkin's disease. Nursing83 13(8):58, August 1983.
Hays, K and Rafferty, D: Care of the patient with malignant lymphoma. Nurs Clin North Am 17(4):677, December 1982.
Luksenberg, H and Lessin, L: Anemia: From classification to cause. Diagnosis p 80, September 1982.
Rozzell, M, Hijazi M, and Pack, B: The painful episode. Nurs Clin North Am 18(1):185, March 1983.
Terry, BA: Hodgkin's disease and Non-Hodgkin's Lymphomas. Nurs Clin North Am 20(1):207, March 1985.
Walters, I, et al: Complications of Sickle Cell disease. Nurs Clin North Am 18(1):139, March 1983.
Williams, I, Earles, A, and Pack, B: Psychological considerations in Sickle Cell disease. Nurs Clin North Am 18(1):215, March 1983.

Chapter 10: Books

Broadwell, DC and Johnson, DE: Principles of Ostomy Care. CV Mosby, St Louis, 1982.
Do More With Your Life Than Just Cope With It: Managing Your Ostomy. Hollister Inc, 1985.
Fluid Removal Management. Cobe Laboratories Inc, 1976.
Smith, DB and Johnson, DE (eds): Ostomy Care and the Cancer Patient. Grune & Stratton Inc, Orlando, 1986.
Standards of Clinical Practice, Section III: Peritoneal Dialysis. American Association of Nephrology Nurses and Technicians, Parkridge IL, 1977.

Chapter 10: Articles

Andriani, R and Carson, C: Urolithiasis. Clinical Symposia 38(3):14, March 1986.
Frank, A, Murray, S: A no-guess guide for urinary color assessment. RN p 46, June 1988.
Hahn, D: The many signs of renal failure. Nursing87 17(6):34, August 1987.
Malti, J and Wellons, D: CAPD: A dialysis breakthrough with its own burdens. RN p 46, January 1988.
Ruge, C: Shock (wave) treatment for kidney stones. AJN 86(4):400, April 1986.
Reilly, N and Torosian, L: The new wave in lithotripsy: Implications for nursing. RN p 44, March 1988.
Solomon, J: Does renal failure mean sexual failure? RN p 41, August 1986.
Strangio, L: Believe it or not . . . peritoneal dialysis made easy. Nursing88 18(1):43, January 1988.
Stark, J: A quick guide to urinary tract assessment. Nursing88 18(7):56, July 1988.
Stark, J and Hunt, V: Helping your patient with chronic renal failure. Nursing83 13(9):56, September 1983.
Weigel, JW: Urinary incontinence. J Enterost Ther 15(1):24, January/February 1988.

Chapter 11: Books

Byrne, J, et al: Laboratory Tests: Implications for Nursing Care. Addison-Wesley, Menlo Park, 1986.
Muir, BL: Pathophysiology, an Introduction to the Mechanisms of Disease. John Wiley & Sons, New York, 1980.
Sodeman, W and Sodeman T: Sodemans' Pathologic Physiology, Mechanisms of Disease, ed 7. WB Saunders, Philadelphia, 1985.
Stephens, G: Pathophysiology for Health Practitioners. Macmillan, New York, 1980.
Taylor, CM and Cress, SS: Nursing87: Nursing Diagnosis Cards. Springhouse Corp, Springhouse, PA, 1987.

Chapter 11: Articles

Bagdade, JD: Endocrine emergencies. Med Clin North Am 70(15):1117, 1986.

Bille, DA: Tailoring your diabetic patient's care plan to fit his life-style. Nursing86 16(2):54, February 1986.

Brunicardi, C, et al: Current status of adrenalectomy for Cushing's disease. Surgery 98(6):1127, June 1985.

Callahan, M and Bradley, DJ: Why you should teach your diabetic patients to chart. Nursing88 18(3):48, March 1988.

Christman, C and Bennett, J: Diabetes-new names, new test, new diet. Nursing87 17(1):34, January 1987.

Gavin, J: Diabetes and exercise. AJN 88(2):178, February 1988.

Grace, T: Hyperosmolar nonketotic diabetic coma. AFP 32(2):119, 1985.

Haire-Joshu, D, et al: Controlling the insulin balance. AJN 86(11):1239, November 1986.

Hermus, A, et al: Responsivity of adrenocortiocotropin to corticotropin-releasing hormone and lack of suppressibility by dexamethasone are related phenomena in Cushing's disease. J Clin Endocrinol Metab 62(4):634, April 1986.

Hernandez, CM: Surgery and diabetes, minimizing the risks. AJN 87(6):788, June 1987.

Hughes, B: Diabetes management: The time is right for tight glucose control. Nursing87 17(5):63, May 1987.

Leske, J: Hyperglycemic hyperosmolar nonketotic coma: A nursing care plan. Critical Care Nurse 5(5):49, May 1985.

Nath, C, Murray, S, and Ponte, C: Lessons in living with type II diabetes mellitus. Nursing88 18(8):45, August 1988.

Miller, VG: Diabetes: Let's stop testing urine. AJN 86(1):54, January 1986.

O'Neil, J: Action Stat! Thyroid crisis. Nursing87 17(11):33, November 1987.

Ramsey, PW: Hyperglycemia at dawn. AJN 87(11):1424, November 1987.

Robertson, C: When the patient is also a diabetic. RN p 33, July 1987.

Saruta, T, et al: Multiple factors contribute to the pathogenesis of hypertension in Cushing's syndrome. J Clin Endocrinol Metab 62(2):275, February 1986.

Sypniewski, E, et al: Hyperosmolar, hyperglycemic, nonketotic coma in a patient receiving home total parenteral nutrient therapy. Clin Pharm 87(6):72, June 1987.

Thurkauf, G: How do you manage DKA with continuous IV insulin? AJN 88(5):727, May 1988.

Chapter 12: Books

Breast Cancer: Understanding Treatment Options. US Dept of Health and Human Services, 1986.

Hagan, RM: Human Sexuality–A Nursing Perspective, ed 2. Appleton-Century-Crofts, Norwalk, CT, 1985.

The Breast Cancer Digest: A Guide to Medical Care, Emotional Support, Educational Programs and Resources, ed 2. US Dept of Health and Human Services, 1984.

Chapter 12: Articles

Anderson, B: When is a hysterectomy really needed? Patient Care p 62, January 15, 1987.

Bernhard, LS and Dan, AJ: Redefining sexuality from women's own experiences. Nurs Clin North Am 21(1), 1986.

Faulkner, A: Mastectomy; reclaiming a body image. Community Outlook p 11, May 1985.

Hassey, K, Bloom, L, and Burgess, S: Radiation: Alternative to mastectomy. AJN 83(11):1567, November 1983.

Hutcheson, HA: TAIF: New option for breast reconstruction. Nursing86 86(2):52, February 1986.

Hysterectomy. Women's Health and Fitness News. Weight Watchers 2(12):3, August 1988.

Greiner, L and Weiler, C: Early-stage breast cancer: What do women know about treatment choices? AJN 83(11):1570, November 1983.

Levinger, GE: Working through recovery after mastectomy. AJN 80(6):118, June 1980.

New treatments shrink enlarged prostates without surgery. Men's Health 4(7):7, July 1988.

PDQ Information for Patients with Breast Cancer. The Cancer Information Service of Colorado. Courtesy of Penrose Cancer Hospital, Colorado Springs, CO, and AMC Cancer Research Center, Denver, CO.

Schain, WS: Breast cancer and psychosexual sequelae: Implications for remediation. Semin Oncol Nurs 1(3):200, August 1985.

Townsend, C: Management of Breast Cancer, Surgery and Adjuvant Therapy. Reprinted material courtesy of Amilu Rothhammer, M.D.

Chapter 13: Books

Adams, R and Victor, M: Principles of Neurology. McGraw-Hill, New York, 1985.

Asbury, A, et al: Diseases of the Nervous System, Vol II. WB Saunders, Philadelphia, 1986.

Brashear, R and Raney, B: Handbook of Orthopedic Surgery, ed 10. CV Mosby, St Louis, 1986.

Hilt, N and Cogburn, S: Manual of Orthopedics. CV Mosby, St Louis, 1980.

Larson, C and Gould, SB: Manual of Orthopedics, ed 9. CV Mosby, St Louis, 1978.

Orthopedic Nursing Practice: Practice and Outcome Criteria for Selected Diagnoses. ANA, Kansas City, 1986.

Sculco, TP: Orthopedic Care of the Geriatric Patient. CV Mosby, St Louis, 1985.

The AML Modular Head Total Hip System. DePuy, Warsaw, IN, 1987.

Chapter 13: Articles

Barker-Stotts, KA: Traumatic amputation. Nursing88 18(5):51, May 1988.

Bourne, B and Kutcher, J: Amputation: Helping a patient face loss of a limb. RN p 38, February 1985.

Cochran, S: Action stat! Open fracture. Nursing87 17(5):33, May 1987.

Gamron, R: Taking the pressure out of compartment syndrome. AJN 88(8):1076, August 1988.

Hackett, C: Limbering up your neurovascular assessment technique. Nursing83 13(3):40, March 1983.

Jones, A, et al: Side effects following metrizamide myelography and lumbar laminectomy. J Neurosurg Nurs 19(2):94, 1987.

Miller, B: Osteoarthritis in the primary health care setting. Orthopedic Nursing 6(5):42, September/October 1987.

Morris, L, et al: Nursing the patient in traction. RN p 26, January 1988.
Morris, L, et al: Special care for skeletal traction. RN p 24, February 1988.
Nurse's Drug Alert: Methotrexate therapy and arthritic joint degeneration. AJN 88(3):333, March 1988.
Reich, N and Otten, P: What to wear: A challenge for disabled elders. AJN 87(2):207, February 1987.

Chapter 14: Books

Artz, CP, Moncrief, JA, and Pruitt, BA: Burns: A Team Approach. WB Saunders, Philadelphia, 1979.
Baxter, CR: Crystalloid Resuscitation of Burn Shock. Little, Brown & Co, Boston, 1979.
Feller, I and Archembeault, C: Nursing the Burned Patient. The Institute for Burn Medicine, Ann Arbor, 1973.
Fletcher, BJ: Critical Care Nursing. JB Lippincott, Philadelphia, 1983.
Holloway, MN. Nursing the Critically Ill Adult, ed 2. Addison-Wesley, Menlo Park, 1984.

Chapter 14: Articles

Baxter, CR, et al: Fluid and electrolyte therapy of burn care. Heart Lung 2(5):707, 1973.
Bayley, E: The three degrees of burn care. Nursing87 17(3):34, March 1987.
Freeman, JW: Nursing care of the patient with a burn injury. Crit Care Nurse 4(6):52, November/December 1984.
Hurt, R: More than skin deep, guidelines for caring for the burn patient. Crit Care Update 7:24, October 1980.
Robertson, K, Cross, P, and Terry, J: CE: Burn care: The crucial first days. AJN 85(1):29, January 1985.
Tobes, SA and Bowden, ML: Teaching coping strategies for pain management. Bulletin and Clinical Review of Burn Injuries 2(33), 1985.

Chapter 15: Books

Altman, D: AIDS in the Mind of America. Anchor Press/Doubleday, New York, 1986.
Chinn, PL: Ethical Issues in Nursing. Aspen, Rockville, MD, 1986.
Hilt, NE and Cogburn, SB: Manual of Orthopedics. CV Mosby, St Louis, 1980.
Larson, C and Gould, M: Orthopedic Nursing, ed 9. CV Mosby, St Louis, 1987.

Chapter 15: Articles

Aspects of the rheumatic patient. Scand J of Rheumatology 16(4):229; 16(6):395; and Suppl 65, 1987.
AIDS prevention for heterosexuals. Men's Health 4(7):1, July 1988.
Bennell, J: CE: AIDS. What we know about AIDS. AJN 86(9):1015, September 1986.
Brennan, L: The battle against AIDS: A report from the nursing front. Nursing88 18(4):60, April 1988.
Coleman, D: How to care for an AIDS patient. RN p 16, July 1986.
Dhundale, K and Hubbard, P: Home Care for the AIDS patient: Safety first. Nursing86 16(9):34, September 1986.
Diagnostic tests for AIDS. The Medical Letter on Drugs and Therapeutics 771(30):73, July 29, 1988.
Hamilton, D and Mallory, M: For AIDS patients, little things can mean a alot. Nursing88 18(5):61, May 1988.
Haulley, DG: Arthritis and related rheumatic diseases. Nurs Clin North Am 19(4), December 1984.
Henning, LM and Burrnus, SK: Keeping up on arthritis medications. RN p 32, February 1986.
Kloser, P: AIDS NEWS: Special report from the fourth international AIDS conference: Stockholm, June 12–16. Medical Aspects of Human Sexuality p 16, August 1988.
Oerlemans-Bunn, M: On being gay, single, and bereaved. AJN 88(4):472, April 1988.
Saunders, J and Buckingham, S: Suicidal AIDS patients: When depression turns deadly. Nursing88 18(7):59, July 1988.

Chapter 16: Articles

Bond, G, et al: Septicemia from an unexpected source . . . transducer heads. RN p 48, July 1982.
Fox, B and Stegall, B: Take precautions now—patients receiving total parenteral nutrition (TPN) run the risk of sepsis. Nursing85 15(5):48, May 1985.
Hall, KV: Detecting septic shock before it's too late. RN p 29, September 1981.
Hart, LH and Dennis, SL: Two hyperthermias prevalent in the ICU: Fever and heatstroke. Focus on Critical Care 15(4):49, August 1988.
Pritchard, V: Preventing and treating geriatric infections. RN p 36, March 1988.

Chapter 17: Books

A Cancer Source Book for Nurses. American Cancer Society, 1981.
Bouchard-Kurtz, R and Speese-Owens, N: Nursing Care of the Cancer Patient. CV Mosby, St Louis, 1981.
Adams, CG and Macione, A: A Handbook of Psychiatric Mental Health Nursing. John Wiley & Sons, New York, 1983.
Alpers, D, et al: Manual of Nutritional Therapeutics. Little, Brown & Co, Boston, 1983.
Burkhalter, P: Nursing Care of the Alcoholic and the Drug Abuser. Gardner Press, New York, 1984.
Chernecky, CC and Ramsey, PW: Critical Nursing Care of the Client with Cancer. Appleton-Century-Crofts, Norwalk, CT, 1984.
Chemotherapy and You: A Guide to Self-Help During Treatment. US Dept of Health and Human Services, Bethesda, 1981.
Cohen, S, et al: Frequently Prescribed and Abused Drugs. Haworth, New York, 1982.
Eating Hints: Recipes and Tips for Better Nutrition During Cancer Treatment. US Dept of Health and Human Services, National Institutes of Health, Bethesda, 1982.
Doenges, M, Townsend, M, and Moorhouse, M: Psychiatric Care Plans: Guidelines for Client Care. FA Davis, Philadelphia, 1989.
Goldberg, R and Tull, RM: The Psycho-Social Dimensions of Cancer. The Free Press, New York, 1977.

Grant, JB: Handbook of Total Parenteral Nutrition. WB Saunders, Philadelphia, 1980.

Janosik, E and Davies, J: Psychiatric Mental Health Nursing. Jones & Bartlett, Boston, 1986.

Johnson, BS: Psychiatric-Mental Health Nursing: Giving Emotional Care. Prentice-Hall. JB Lippincott, Philadelphia, 1986.

Kastenbaum, RJ: Death, Society and Human Experience. CV Mosby, St Louis, 1981.

LeFever, KJ: Laboratory and Diagnostic Tests with Nursing Implications, ed 2. Appleton & Lange, Norwalk, VA, 1987.

Lehy, IM, St Germain, JM, and Varricehio, CG: The Nurse and Radiotherapy: A Manual for Daily Use. CV Mosby, St Louis, 1979.

Lynn, G, et al: The Nurse's Role During the Living/Dying Interval; A Self-Instructional Unit. Community Oncology Nursing Committee of Dayton, Ohio, and Kettering Medical Center, 1985.

Marino, LB: Cancer Nursing. CV Mosby, St Louis, 1981.

McNally, JC, et al: Guidelines for Cancer Nursing Practice. Grune & Stratton, Orlando, 1985.

Neal, M, et al: Nursing Care Planning Guides for Psychiatric and Mental Health Care, ed 2. Nurseco, Inc, Pacific Palisades, 1985.

Nursing Care Guidelines for the Patient With Cancer. Southern Colorado Cancer Program, Colorado Springs, Colorado, 1982 (unpublished, used with permission).

Nutrition: For Patients Receiving Chemotherapy and Radiation Treatment. American Cancer Society, 1987.

Piepmeyer, J, et al: Tube Feeding At Home. A Manual of Instruction for Tube-Feeding Care. Division of Nutrition, Dept of Medicine, University of Cincinnati College of Medicine.

Rombeau, J and Caldwell, M (eds): Clinical Nutrition, Vol. 1. Enteral and Tube Feeding. WB Saunders, Philadelphia, 1984.

Rubin, P: Clinical Oncology for Medical Students and Physicians, ed 6. American Cancer Society, 1983.

Smith, D, Milkman, H, and Sunderwirth, S: Addictive Disease: Concept and Controversy. In: The Addictions: Multidisciplinary Perspectives and Treatments. Health. Lexington, MA, 1984.

Silverberg, E and Hubera, J: Cancer Statistics, 1987. American Cancer Society, 1987.

Chapter 17: Articles

Archer, D and Smith, A: Sorrow has many faces. Nursing88 18(5):61, May 1988.

Barash, D: Defusing the violent patient before he explodes. RN p 34, March 1984.

Barta, M: Correcting electrolyte imbalances. RN p 30, February 1987.

Bennett, HL: Why patients don't follow instructions. RN p 45, March 1986.

Beers, L: "I want to live until I die." Nursing88 18(10):70, October 1988.

Beteemps, E: Management of the withdrawal syndrome of barbiturates and other central nervous system depressants. J of Psychosocial Nursing and Mental Health Services 19(19):31, September 1981.

Burden, N: Regional anesthesia: What patients and nurses need to know. RN p 56, May 1988.

Calloway, C: When the problem involves magnesium, calcium, or phosphate. RN p 30, May 1987.

Cassell, BL: Treating pressure sores stage by stage. RN p 37, January 1986.

Campbell, E, Williams, M, and Mlynarczyk, S: After the fall—confusion. AJN 86(2):151, February 1986.

Crossley, M: Watch out for nutritional complications of cancer. RN p 22, March 1985.

DeLapp, T: Helping the elderly live longer and better. Nursing83 13(11):61, November 1983.

Detzer, E and Huston, L: When schizophrenia complicates med/surg care. RN p 51, January 1986.

Faulk, D: What tomorrow holds for cancer nursing. RN p 37, August 1987.

Forlaw, L and Bayer, L: Symposia on nutrition. Nurs Clin of North Am 18(1):3, March 1983.

Fox, B and Stegall, B: Take precautions now (TPN). Nursing85 15(5):48, May 1985.

Goodman, L: Would your assessment spot a hidden alcoholic? RN p 56, August 1986.

Gray-Vickrey, M: Color them special—A sensible guide to caring for elderly patients. Nursing87 17(5):59, May 1987.

Green, C: How to recognize hostility and what to do about it. AJN 86(11):1230, November 1986.

Guiness, R: How to use the new small-bore feeding tubes. Nursing86 16(4):51, April 1986.

Henderson, M: Assessing the elderly: Part II. Altered presentations. AJN 85(10):1103, October 1985.

Herth, KA: Laughter, a nursing RX. AJN 84(8):991, August 1984.

Hudson, M: Safeguard your elderly patient's health through accurate physical assessment. Nursing83 13(11):58, November 1983.

Hughes, C: Giving cancer drugs IV: Some guidelines. AJN 86(1):34, January 1986.

Kearns, PC: Exercises to ease pain after abdominal surgery. RN p 45, July 1986.

Keithley, J and O'Donnell, J: Look out for these drug-nutrient interactions. Nursing86 16(2):42, February 1986.

Kline, P and Chernecky, C: Heading off depression in the chronically ill. RN p 44, October 1987.

Lindsey, AM, Piper, BF, and Stotts, NA: Clinical reviews: The phenomena of cancer cachexia. Oncology Nursing Forum 8(2):38, Spring, 1982.

McGee, L: Feeding gastrostomy: Part III. Nursing care. J Enterost Ther 14(5):201, October 1987.

Moore, MC: Do you still believe these myths about tube feeding? RN p 51, May 1987.

Mortensen, M and McMillin, C: Discharge score sheet for surgical outpatients. AJN 86(12):1347, December 1986.

Mulhern, R: When there's no treatment left but the truth. RN p 26, March 1986.

Olsen, E, McEarue, J, and Greenbavor, DM: Recognition, general considerations, and techniques in the management of drug intoxication. Heart Lung 12(2):110, March 1983.

Ostchega, Y and Jacob, J: Providing "safe conduct": Helping your patient cope with cancer. Nursing84 14(4):42, April 1984.

Orne, R: Nurses' views of near-death experiences. AJN 86(4):419, April 1986.

Papowitz, L: Life, death, life. AJN 86(4):416, April 1986.

Pettom, S: Your role in radiation therapy. RN p 32, February 1985.

Powell, AF and Minick, MP: Alcohol withdrawal syndrome. AJN 88(3):312, March 1988.

Quiring, J, Futrell, M, and Heidebrecht, D: Helping the patient and family adjust to LTC living. Nursing86 16(10):60, October 1986.

Santo-Novak, D: Seven keys to assessing the elderly. Nursing88 18(8):60, August 1988.

Sarsany, S: Violent Behavior. RN p 64, September 1988.

Schwartz, M: Potassium Imbalances: for CE Credit. AJN 87(10):1292, October 1987.

Seaman, DJ: Shortcuts to a more complete PAR transfer summary. Nursing83 13(9):47, September 1983.

Smith, SA: Theories and intervention of nutritional deficit in neoplastic disease. Oncology Nursing Forum 9(2):43, Spring 1982.

Speciale, J and Kaalaas, J: Infuse-A-Port, new path for IV chemotherapy. Nursing85 15(10):40, October 1985.

Strassman, R: Adverse reactions to psychedelic drugs: A review of the literature. J Nerv Ment Dis 17(10):577, October 1984.

Thompson, L: When caring is the only cure: Managing the chronically ill patient. Nursing87 17(1):58, January 1987.

Toto, KH: When the patient has hypokalemia. RN p 38, March 1987.

Toto, KH: When the patient has hyperkalemia. RN p 34, April 1987.

Troutman, J: Step-by-step guide to trouble-free IV chemotherapy. RN p 32, September 1985.

Ufema, J: How to talk to dying patients. Nursing87 17(8):43, August 1987.

Ward, GA, Bailey, LR, and Gates, JW: Advanced cancer pain management in a community setting. Oncology Nursing Forum 9(1):32, Winter 1981.

Welch, DA: Waiting, worry and the cancer experience. Oncology Nursing Forum 8(2):14, Spring 1981.

Wilhelm, L: Helping your patient "settle in" with TPN. Nursing85 15(4):60, April 1985.

INDEX OF NURSING DIAGNOSES

APPENDIX

Abbreviations

A-a DO$_2$ ratio: Alveolar to arterial oxygen gradient
ABG: arterial blood gas
a.c.: before meals
ACE: angiotension converting enzyme
ACh RAb: acetylcholine receptor antibody
ACT: activated clotting time
ACTH: adrenocorticotropic hormone
AD: Alzheimer's disease; autonomic dysreflexia
ADA: American Diabetes Association
ADH: antidiuretic hormone
ADLs: activities of daily living
ADRA: Alzheimer's Disease and Related Disorders Association
AED: antiepileptic drug
AF: atrial fibrillation
AIDS: acquired immunodeficiency syndrome
ALS: amyotrophic lateral sclerosis
ALT: alanine aminotransferase (equivalent SGPT)
ANA: nuclear antibody
AntiDNA: deoxyribonuclease
AP: anterior-posterior
APTT: activated partial thromboplastic time
AR: aortic valve regurgitation
ARC: AIDS-related complex
ARDS: adult respiratory distress syndrome
ARF: acute renal failure
AS: aortic valve stenosis
ASA: acetylsalicylic acid
ASI: addiction severity index
ASHD: arteriosclerotic heart disease
ASL: antistreptolysin
ASO: antistreptolysin-O titer
AST: aspartate aminotransferase (equivalent SGOT)
ATN: acute tubular necrosis
AV: aortic valve; atrioventricular; arteriovenous
AVF: augmented unipolar foot lead of electrocardiogram

BAERs: brainstem auditory evoked responses
BBB: bundle branch block
BEAM: brain electrical activity map
BEE: basal energy expenditure
BFP: biologically false positive
b.i.d.: twice a day
BKA: below-knee amputation
BM: bowel movement
BMR: basal metabolic rate
B & O: belladonna and opium
BP: blood pressure

BPM: beats per minute
BSP: bromsulphalein
BUN: blood urea nitrogen

C: centigrade
Ca^{2+}: calcium
CABG: coronary artery bypass graft
CAD: coronary artery disease
CAPD: continuous ambulatory peritoneal dialysis
CAVH: continuous arteriovenous hemofiltration
CBC: complete blood count
cc: cubic centimeters
CCPD: continuous cycling peritoneal dialysis
CEA: carcinogenic embryonic antigen
CHF: congestive heart failure
CHI: creatinine height index
Cl$^-$: chloride
cm: centimeter
CMV: cytomegalovirus
CNS: central nervous system
CO: carbon monoxide
CO$_2$: carbon dioxide
COHbg: carboxyhemoglobin
COPD: chronic obstructive pulmonary disease
CPB: cardiopulmonary bypass (machine)
CPK: creatinine phosphokinase
CPP: cerebral perfusion pressure
CPR: cardiopulmonary resuscitation
CPT: chest physiotherapy
Cr: creatinine
CRF: chronic renal failure
CRP: c-reactive protein
C&S: culture and sensitivities
CSF: cerebrospinal fluid
CT: computerized axial tomography
CTZ: chemoreceptor trigger zone
cu: cubic
CVA: cerebrovascular accident; costovertebral angle
CVP: central venous pressure

DI: diabetes insipidus
DIC: disseminated intravascular coagulation
DIPs: distal interphalangeal joints
DKA: diabetic ketoacidosis
dl: decaliter
DM: diabetes mellitus
DOB: date of birth
DOM: dimethoxymethylamphetamine, STP (used as street drug)

DRG: diagnosis-related group
DSA: digital subtraction angiography
DST: dexamethasone suppression test
DT: delirium tremens
DTIC: dicarbazine (synthetic chemotherapeutic agent)
DTRS: deep tendon reflexes
DUI: driving under the influence
D5W: dextrose 5% water
DVT: deep vein thrombosis

EACA: epsilon aminocaproic acid
ECF: extracellular fluid
ECG: electrocardiogram
ECT: electroconvulsive therapy
EEG: electroencephalogram
ELISA: enzyme-linked immunosorbent assay
ESR: erythrocyte sedimentation rate
ESWL: extracorporeal shock-wave lithotripsy
ET: endotracheal tube

F: Fahrenheit
FAS: fetal alcohol syndrome
FBS: fasting blood sugar
FEV_1: forced expiratory volume in 1 second
FFP: fresh frozen plasma
FIO_2: fraction of inspired oxygen
FRC: functional reserve capacity
FVC: forced vital capacity

GF: glomerular filtration
GFR: glomerular filtration rate
GH: growth hormone
GI: gastrointestinal
Gly-Hb: glycosylated hemoglobin
gm: gram
GU: genitourinary

H: hydrogen
HAA: hepatitis associated antigen
HAV: hepatitis A virus
Hb: hemoglobin
HBIg: hepatitis B immunoglobulin
HBsAg: hepatitis B surface antigen
HCG: human chorionic gonadotropin
HCl: hydrochloric acid
HCO_2: carbonate
HCO_3: bicarbonate
Hct: hematocrit
Hg: mercury
H&H: hemoglobin and hematocrit
HHNC: hyperglycemic, hyperosmotic nonketotic
    coma
HIV: human immunodeficiency virus
HOB: head of bed
HNP: herniated nucleus pulposus
H_2O: water
HR: heart rate
HS: hour of sleep
HSV: herpes simplex virus

IABP: intraaortic balloon pump
ICF: intracellular fluid

ICP: intracranial pressure
ICU: intensive care unit
ID: iron deficiency (anemia)
I&D: incision and drainage
I:E: inspiratory/expiratory ratio
Ig: immune globulin
IHSS: idiopathic hypertrophic subaortic stenosis
IICP: increased intracranial pressure
IM: intramuscular
IMV: intermittent mandatory ventilation
I&O: intake and output
IOL: intraocular lens
IOP: intraocular pressure
IP: identified patient
IPPB: intermittent positive pressure breathing
IV: intravenous
IVP: intravenous pyelogram

JVD: jugular vein distention

K^+: potassium
kg: kilogram
KS: Karposi's sarcoma
KUB: kidneys, ureters, bladder

l: liter
LAP: leucine aminopeptidase
LDH: lactate dehydrogenase
LE cell: neutrophil
LOC: level of consciousness
LP: lumbar puncture
LR: lactated Ringer's
LSD: D-lysergic acid (used as street drug)
LTC: long-term care
LUQ: left upper quadrant
LV: left ventricle
LVEDP: left ventricular end-diastolic pressure
LVF: left ventricular failure

MAO: monoamine oxidase inhibitors
MAP: mean arterial pressure
MAT: multiple atrial tachycardia
MCL_1: Modified chest lead (V_1)
MCL_6: Modified chest lead (V_6)
MCT: medium chain triglycerides
MCV: mean corpuscular volume
MDA: methylenedioxymethamphetamine
MDF: myocardial depressant factor
mEq: milliequivalent
Mg^{2+}: magnesium
mg: milligram
MG: myasthenia gravis
MI: myocardial infarction
min: minute
ml: milliliter
mm: millimeter
mOsm: milliosmol
MR: mitral regurgitation
MRI: magnetic resonance imaging
MS: mitral valve stenosis
MSG: monosodium glutamate
MSH: melanocyte-stimulating hormone

MTM: Modified-Thayer-Martin (culture media for gonococcus)
MUGA: radioactive heart scan
MV: mitral valve
MVP: mitral valve prolapse

Na: sodium
NaHCO$_3$: sodium bicarbonate
NG: nasogastric
NIDDM: non-insulin-dependent diabetes mellitus
NMR: nuclear magnetic resonance
NPO: nothing by mouth
NS: normal saline
NSAID: nonsteroid antiinflammatory drugs
NSR: normal sinus rhythm
NSU: nonspecific urethritis
NTG: nitroglycerin
n/v: nausea/vomiting

O$_2$: oxygen
OR: operating room
Osm: osmolality
OTC: over-the-counter
OT: occupational therapy

PA: posterior-anterior
PAC: premature atrial contraction
PaCO$_2$: arterial carbon dioxide pressure
PAO$_2$: alveolar oxygen pressure
PaO$_2$: arterial oxygen pressure
PAP: pulmonary artery pressure
PAT: paroxysmal atrial tachycardia
PAWP: pulmonary artery wedge pressure
pc/hs: after meals and at bedtime
PCA: patient-controlled analgesia
PCO$_2$: partial pressure of carbon dioxide
PCP: pneumocystis carinii pneumonia; phencyclidine (used as street drug)
PCWP: pulmonary capillary wedge pressure
PE: pulmonary embolus; physical examination
PEEP: positive end-expiratory pressure
PET: positron emission tomography
PG: phostidylglycerol
pH: acid base
PI: phosphotidylinositol
PIPs: proximal interphalangeal joints
PJC: premature junctional contraction
PMI: point of maximal impulse
PO: per os (by mouth)
PO$_2$: partial pressure of oxygen
PO$_4$: phosphate
PPD: purified protein derivative
p.r.n.: as necessary
PT: prothrombin time; physical therapy
PTCA: percutaneous transluminal coronary angioplasty
PTH: parathyroid hormone
PTT: partial thromboplastin time
PTU: propylthiouracil
PUL: percutaneous ultrasonic lithotripsy
PVC: premature ventricular contractions
PWP: pulmonary wedge pressure

q.i.d.: four times a day
QP/QS: shunt measurement pulmonary vs systemic flow
QS/QT: shunt measure-quantity shunted/quantity total (respiratory)
QRS: electrocardiogram measure of electrical activity of ventricle

R: electrocardiogram wave representing ventricular innervation
RA: rheumatoid arthritis
Rad: right axis deviation; radiation dosage
RAI: radioactive iodine
RAP: right atrial pressure
RBC: red blood cell
RCVA: right cerebral vasculor accident
REM: rapid eye movement
RIA: radioimmunoassay
RL: renal electrolytes
ROM: range of motion
RPR: rapid plasma reagin (serologic test)
RUQ: right upper quadrant
RV: right ventricle
RVF: right ventricular failure

S$_1$, S$_2$, S$_3$, S$_4$: heart sounds
SB: sinus bradycardia
SC: subcutaneous
SCI: spinal cord injury
sec: second
SGOT: serum glutamic-oxaloacetic transaminase
SGPT: serum glutamic pyruvic transaminase
SIADH: syndrome of inappropriate antidiuretic hormone
SIMV: synchronized intermittent mandatory ventilation
SLE: systemic lupus erythematosus
SMA: serum chemistry profile
SO: significant other(s)
SPF: sun protective factor
SR: sinus rhythm
ST: sinus tachycardia, electrocardiographic wave representing ventricular repolarization
STD: sexually transmitted disease
STP: (serendipity, tranquility, peace) dimethoxymethyl-amphetamine
ST/T: segment/interval measure on ECG
SVO$_2$: systemic venous oxygen
SVR: systemic vascular resistance

T$_3$: triiodothyronine
T$_4$: thyroxine
TB: tuberculosis
TBSA: total body surface area
TCDB: turn, cough, deep breath
TENS: transcutaneous electrical nerve stimulator
THC: total hydrocarbons; tetrahydrocannabinol (used as a street drug)
TIA: transient ischemic attacks
TIBC: total iron binding capacity
t.i.d.: three times a day
TKO: to keep open
TLC: total lung capacity

959

TMJ: temporomandibular joint
TPN: total parenteral nutrition
TRF: thyrotropin-releasing factor
TRH: thyrotropin-releasing hormone
TSH: thyroid-stimulating hormone
TUR: transurethral resection
TVC: true vomiting center
T-tube: T-shaped drainage tube generally for the common bile duct

UA: urinalysis
UC: ulcerative colitis
UO: urinary output
URI: upper respiratory infection
UTI: urinary tract infection

V, V$_1$, V$_5$, V$_6$: electrocardiogram chest leads
V̇$_E$: minute ventilation
VC: vital capacity
VCU: voiding cystourethrogram.
VF: ventricular fibrillation
VMA: vanillylmandelic acid
VNA: visiting nurse association
V/Q: ventilation/perfusion
VS: vital signs
V$_T$: tidal volume
VT: ventricular tachycardia

WBC: white blood cell
WNL: within normal limits

Classification of NANDA Nursing Diagnoses by Gordon's Functional Health Patterns*

Health Perception-Health Management Pattern
  Health maintenance, altered
  Noncompliance (specify)
  Infection, potential for
  Injury, potential for
  Injury, potential for: trauma
  Injury, potential for: poisoning
  Injury, potential for: suffocating
Nutritional-Metabolic Pattern
  Nutrition, altered: potential for more than body requirements
  Nutrition, altered: more than body requirements
  Nutrition, altered: less than body requirements
  Swallowing, impaired
  Tissue integrity, impaired: oral mucous membrane
  Fluid volume deficit: potential
  Fluid volume deficit: actual (1)
  Fluid volume deficit: actual (2)
  Fluid volume excess
  Skin integrity, impaired: potential
  Skin integrity, impaired: actual
  Tissue integrity, impaired
  Body temperature, altered: potential
  Thermoregulation, ineffective
  Hyperthermia
  Hypothermia
Elimination Pattern
  Bowel elimination, altered: constipation
  Bowel elimination, altered: diarrhea
  Bowel elimination, altered: incontinence
  Urinary elimination, altered patterns
  Incontinence, functional
  Incontinence, reflex
  Incontinence, stress
  Incontinence, urge
  Incontinence, total
  Urinary retention
Activity-Exercise Pattern
  Activity intolerance: potential
  Activity intolerance
  Mobility, impaired physical
  Self-care deficit: bathing/hygiene
  Self-care deficit: dressing/grooming
  Self-care deficit: feeding
  Self-care deficit: toileting
  Diversional activity, deficit
  Home maintenance management, impaired
  Airway clearance, ineffective
  Breathing pattern, ineffective

Gas exchange, impaired
  Cardiac output, altered: decreased
  Tissue perfusion, altered: renal, cerebral, cardiopulmonary, gastrointestinal, peripheral
  Growth and development, altered
Sleep-Rest Pattern
  Sleep pattern disturbance
Cognitive-Perceptual Pattern
  Comfort, altered: pain
  Comfort, altered: chronic pain
  Sensory/perceptual alterations: visual, auditory, kinesthetic, gustatory, tactile, olfactory
  Unilateral neglect
  Knowledge deficit (specify)
  Thought processes, altered
Self-Perception-Self-Concept Pattern
  Fear
  Anxiety
  Hopelessness
  Powerlessness
  Self-concept, disturbance in: body image
  Self-concept, disturbance in: personal identity
  Self-concept, disturbance in: self-esteem
Role-Relationship Pattern
  Grieving, anticipatory
  Grieving, dysfunctional
  Role performance, altered
  Social isolation
  Social interaction, impaired
  Family processes, altered
  Parenting, altered: potential
  Parenting, altered: actual
  Communication, impaired verbal
  Violence, potential for: self-directed or directed at others
Sexuality-Reproductive Pattern
  Sexual dysfunction
  Sexuality, altered patterns
  Rape trauma syndrome
  Rape trauma syndrome: compound reaction
  Rape trauma syndrome: silent reaction
Coping-Stress Tolerance Pattern
  Coping, ineffective individual
  Adjustment, impaired
  Post-trauma response
  Coping, family: potential for growth
  Coping, ineffective family: compromised
  Coping, ineffective family: disabled
Value-Belief Pattern
  Spiritual distress (distress of the human spirit)

---

*Based on Gordon, M.: Nursing Diagnosis: Process and Applications. McGraw-Hill, New York, 1986, with permission.

Taxonomy 1R

Conceptual base for identifying and classifying nursing diagnoses. (Approved by NANDA General Assembly 1986.)

1. **EXCHANGING:** A human response pattern involving mutual giving and receiving.
  1.1. Alterations in Nutrition
    1.1.1. (Cellular)*
    1.1.2. (Systemic)*
      1.1.2.1. More than body requirements
      1.1.2.2. Less than body requirements
      1.1.2.3. Potential for more than body requirements
  1.2 (Alterations in Physical Regulation)*
    1.2.1. (Immune)*
      1.2.1.1. Potential for Infection
    1.2.2. Alteration in Body Temperature
      1.2.2.1. Potential
      1.2.2.2. Hypothermia
      1.2.2.3. Hyperthermia
      1.2.2.4. Inffective Thermoregulation
    1.2.3. (——)*
      1.2.3.1. Dysreflexia
  1.3. Alterations in Elimination
    1.3.1. Bowel
      1.3.1.1. Constipation
        1.3.1.1.1. Perceived Constipation
        1.3.1.1.2. Colonic Constipation
      1.3.1.2. Diarrhea
      1.3.1.3. Bowel Incontinence
    1.3.2. Altered Patterns of Urinary Elimination
      1.3.2.1. Incontinence
        1.3.2.1.1. Stress
        1.3.2.1.2. Reflex
        1.3.2.1.3. Urge
        1.3.2.1.4. Functional
        1.3.2.1.5. Total
      1.3.2.2. Retention [Acute/Chronic]
    1.3.3. (Skin)*
  1.4. (Alterations in Circulation)*
    1.4.1. (Vascular)*
      1.4.1.1. Tissue Perfusion
        1.4.1.1.1. Renal
        1.4.1.1.2. Cerebral
        1.4.1.1.3. Cardiopulmonary
        1.4.1.1.4. Gastrointenstinal
        1.4.1.1.5. Peripheral
      1.4.1.2. Fluid Volume
        1.4.1.2.1. Excess
        1.4.1.2.2.1. Deficit (1) and (2)
        1.4.1.2.2.2. Potential
    1.4.2. (Cardiac)*
      1.4.2.1. Decreased Cardiac Output
  1.5. (Alterations in Oxygenation)*
    1.5.1. (Respiration)*
      1.5.1.1. Impaired Gas Exchange
      1.5.1.2. Ineffective Airway Clearance
      1.5.1.3. Ineffective Breathing Pattern

1.6 (Alterations in Physical Integrity)*
  1.6.1. Potential for Injury
    1.6.1.1. Potential for Suffocating
    1.6.1.2. Potential for Poisoning
    1.6.1.3. Potential for Trauma
    1.6.1.4. Potential for Aspiration
    1.6.1.5. Potential for Disuse Syndrome
  1.6.2. Impairment
    1.6.2.1. Tissue Integrity
      1.6.2.1.1. Oral Mucous Membrane
      1.6.2.1.2.1. Skin Integrity
      1.6.2.1.2.2. Potential
2. **COMMUNICATING:** A human response pattern involving sending messages.
  2.1. Alterations in Communication
    2.1.1. Verbal
      2.1.2.1. Impaired
    2.1.2. (Nonverbal)*
3. **RELATING:** A human response pattern involving establishing bonds.
  3.1. (Alterations in Socialization)*
    3.1.1. Impaired Social Interaction
    3.1.2. Social Isolation
  3.2. (Alterations in Role)*
    3.2.1. Altered Role Performance
      3.2.1.1.1. Altered Parenting
      3.2.1.1.2. Potential
    3.2.1.2. Sexual
      3.2.1.2.1. Dysfunction
    3.2.1.3. (Work)*
    3.2.2. Family Processes
      3.2.2.1. Parental Role Conflict
  3.3. Altered Sexuality Patterns
4. **VALUING:** A human response pattern involving the assigning of relative worth.
  4.1. Alterations in Spiritual State
    4.1.1. Distress
5. **CHOOSING:** A human response pattern involving the selection of alternatives.
  5.1. Alterations in Coping
    5.1.1. Individual
      5.1.1.1. Ineffective
        5.1.1.1.1. Impaired Adjustment
        5.1.1.1.2. Defensive Coping
        5.1.1.1.3. Ineffective Denial
    5.1.2. Family
      5.1.2.1. Ineffective
        5.1.2.1.1. Disabled
        5.1.2.1.2. Compromised
      5.1.2.2. Potential for Growth
    5.1.3. (Community)*
  5.2. (Alterations in Participation)*
    5.2.1. (Individual)*
      5.2.1.1. Noncompliance
    5.2.2. (Family)*
    5.2.3. (Community)*
      5.3.1.1. Decisional Conflict (specify)
  5.4. Health Seeking Behaviors (specify)

6. **MOVING:** A human response pattern involving activity.
   6.1. (Alterations in Activity)*
      6.1.1. Physical Mobility
         6.1.1.1. Impaired
         6.1.1.2. Activity Intolerance
            6.1.1.2.1. Fatigue
         6.1.1.3. Potential Activity Intolerance
      6.1.2. (Social Mobility)*
   6.2. (Alterations in Rest)*
      6.2.1. Sleep Pattern Disturbance
   6.3. (Alterations in Recreation)*
      6.3.1. Diversional Activity
         6.3.1.1. Deficit
   6.4. (Alterations in Activities of Daily Living)*
      6.4.1. Home Maintenance Management
         6.4.1.1. Impaired
      6.4.2. Health Maintenance
   6.5. Alterations in Self-Care
      6.5.1. Feeding
         6.5.1.1. Impaired Swallowing
         6.5.1.2. Ineffective Breast Feeding
      6.5.2. Bathing/Hygiene
      6.5.3. Dressing/Grooming
      6.5.4. Toileting
   6.6. Altered Growth and Development
7. **PERCEIVING:** A human response pattern involving the reception of information.
   7.1. Alterations in Self-Concept
      7.1.1. Disturbance in Body Image
      7.1.2. Disturbance in Self-Esteem
         7.1.2.1. Chronic Low Self-Esteem
         7.1.2.2. Situational Low Self-Esteem
      7.1.3. Disturbance in Personal Identity
   7.2. Sensory/Perceptual Alteration
      7.2.1. Visual

         7.2.1.1. Unilateral Neglect
      7.2.2. Auditory
      7.2.3. Kinesthetic
      7.2.4. Gustatory
      7.2.5. Tactile
      7.2.6. Olfactory
   7.3. (Alterations in Meaningfulness)*
      7.3.1. Hopelessness
      7.3.2. Powerlessness
8. **KNOWING:** A human response pattern involving the meaning associated with information.
   8.1. Alterations in Knowledge
      8.1.1. Deficit
   8.2. (Alterations in Learning)*
   8.3. Alterations in Thought Processes
      8.3.1. (Confusion)*
9. **FEELING:** A human response pattern involving the subjective awareness of information.
   9.1. Alterations in Comfort
      9.1.1. Pain
         9.1.1.1. Chronic
         9.1.1.2. Acute
      9.1.2. (Discomfort)*
   9.2. (Alterations in Emotional Integrity)*
      9.2.1. Grieving
         9.2.1.1. Dysfunctional
         9.2.1.2. Anticipatory
      9.2.2. Potential for Violence: self-directed or directed at others
      9.2.3. Post-Trauma Response
         9.2.3.1. Rape Trauma Syndrome
            9.2.3.1.1. Compound Reaction
            9.2.3.1.2. Silent Reaction
      9.3.1. Anxiety
      9.3.2. Fear

---

*Recommended by The Taxonomy Committee but not yet approved by NANDA.

Diagnosis Qualifiers _____

A common set of definitions for frequently used qualifiers.

Category 1

Actual: Existing at the present moment; existing in reality.
Potential: Can, but has not yet, come into being; possible.

Category 2

Ineffective: Not producing the desired effect; not capable of performing satisfactorily.
Decreased: Smaller; lessened; diminished; lesser in size, amount, or degree.
Increased: Greater in size, amount, or degree; larger, enlarged.
Impaired: Made worse, weakened; damaged, reduced; deteriorated.
Depleted: Emptied wholly or partially; exhausted of.
Deficient: Inadequate in amount, quality, or degree; defective; not sufficient; incomplete.
Excessive: Characterized by an amount or quantity that is greater than is necessary, desirable, or usable.
Dysfunctional: Abnormal; impaired or incompletely functioning.
Disturbed: Agitated; interrupted, interfered with.
Acute: Severe but of short duration.
Chronic: Lasting a long time; recurring; habitual; constant.
Intermittent: Stopping and starting again at intervals; periodic; cyclic.

DIAGNOSTIC DIVISIONS

ACTIVITY/REST
Activity intolerance
Activity intolerance, potential
Disuse syndrome, potential for
Diversional activity deficit
Fatigue
Sleep pattern disturbance

CIRCULATION
Cardiac output, altered: decreased
Dysreflexia
Tissue perfusion, altered: (specify)

EGO INTEGRITY
Adjustment, impaired
Anxiety [specify]
Coping, defensive
Coping, ineffective individual
Decisional conflict (specify)
Denial, ineffective
Fear
Grieving, anticipatory
Grieving, dysfunctional
Hopelessness
Post-trauma response
Powerlessness
Rape trauma syndrome
Self-concept, disturbance in: body image; personal identity; role performance; self-esteem
  Self-esteem, chronic low
  *Self-esteem, disturbance in
  Self-esteem, situational low
Spiritual distress (distress of the human spirit)

ELIMINATION
Bowel elimination, altered: constipation
  Constipation, colonic
  Constipation, perceived
Bowel elimination, altered: diarrhea
Bowel elimination, altered: incontinence
Incontinence, functional
Incontinence, reflex
Incontinence, stress
Incontinence, total
Incontinence, urge
Urinary elimination: altered patterns
Urinary retention [acute/chronic]

FOOD/FLUID
Breastfeeding, ineffective
Fluid volume, altered: excess
Fluid volume deficit, actual 1 [regulatory failure]
Fluid volume deficit, actual 2 [active loss]
Fluid volume deficit, potential
Nutrition, altered: less than body requirements
Nutrition, altered: more than body requirements
Nutrition, altered: potential for more than body requirements

Oral mucous membranes, altered
Swallowing, impaired

HYGIENE
Self-care deficit: feeding; bathing/hygiene; dressing/grooming; toileting

NEUROSENSORY
Neglect, unilateral
Sensory-perceptual alteration: visual; auditory; kinesthetic; gustatory; tactile; olfactory
Thought processes, altered

PAIN/COMFORT
Comfort, altered: pain, acute
Comfort, altered: pain, chronic

RESPIRATION
Airway clearance, ineffective
Aspiration, potential for
Breathing pattern, ineffective
Gas exchange, impaired

SAFETY
Body temperature, potential altered
Health maintenance, altered
Home maintenance management, impaired
Hyperthermia
*Hypothermia
Infection, potential for
Injury, potential for: poisoning; suffocation; trauma
Mobility, impaired physical
Skin integrity, impaired: actual
Skin integrity, impaired: potential
Thermoregulation, ineffective
Tissue integrity, impaired
Violence, potential for: directed at self/others

SEXUALITY (Component of Social Interaction)
Sexual dysfunction
Sexuality patterns, altered

SOCIAL INTERACTION
Communication, impaired: verbal
Coping, family: potential for growth
Coping, ineffective family: compromised
Coping, ineffective family: disabling
Family process, altered
Parental role conflict
Parenting, altered: actual or potential
Self-concept, disturbance in: role performance
Social interaction, impaired
Social isolation

TEACHING/LEARNING
Growth and development, altered
Health seeking behaviors (specify)
Knowledge deficit [learning need] (specify)
Noncompliance [compliance, altered] (specify)

---

*Revised.